CLINICAL SONOGRAPHY

A PRACTICAL GUIDE

FOURTH EDITION

ROGER C. SANDERS, MA, BM, BCH (OXEN), MRCP, FRCR, FACR
Clinical Professor of Radiology
University of New Mexico
Albuquerque, New Mexico

THOMAS C. WINTER, III, MD, MA
Professor of Radiology
Director of Ultrasound
University of Wisconsin
Madison, Wisconsin

WITH

Sarah M. Baker, RDMS, RVT, RI(R)
Teresa Bieker, MBA-H, RDMS, RDCS, RVT
Carolyn Taylor Coffin, MPH, RDMS, RDCS, RVT
Joyce Cordier, BS, RDCS, RDMS
Barbara Del Prince, BS, RDMS, RVT
Jag Dhanju, RDMS, RT(R)
Gretchen M. Dimling, BS, RDMS
Julia A. Drose, BA, RDMS, RDCS, RVT
Roger Gent, DMU, AMS, Honorary Fellow ASUM
Beverly E. Hashimoto, MD, FACR
Christine Labinski, RDMS
Michael E. Ledwidge, BS, RDMS, RVT, CNMT
Lyndal Macpherson, AMS, BAppSc Grad Dip U/S
Mary McGrath-Ling, BS, RDMS
Nancy Smith Miner, RT(R), RDMS
Carol Mitchell, PhD, RDMS, RDCS, RVT, RT(R)
Susan Murphy, RDMS
Lisa A. Parsons, BS, RDMS, RDCS
Cynthia L. Rapp, BS, RDMS
Gail Sandager-Hadley, RN, RVT, FSVU
Mimi Maggio Sayler, RDMS, RDCS
Heather Schierloh, MS, RDMS, RVT, RT(R)
Rebecca Schilling, RDMS, RCVT
Marilyn J. Siegel, MD
Deroshia B. Stanley, RN
Tim Walker, RDMS, RDCS, RVT
Barbara Vanderwerff, RDMS, RDCS, RVT

Lippincott Williams & Wilkins
a Wolters Kluwer business
Philadelphia • Baltimore • New York • London
Buenos Aires • Hong Kong • Sydney • Tokyo

Acquisitions Editor: Peter Sabatini
Managing Editor: Kevin C. Dietz
Marketing Manager: Mary Martin and Allison M. Noplock
Production Editor: Kevin P. Johnson
Designer: Holly McLaughlin
Compositor: Maryland Composition Co., Inc.
Printer: Courier Kendallville

351 West Camden Street
Baltimore, MD 21201

530 Walnut Street
Philadelphia, PA 19106

The publisher is not responsible (as a matter of product liability, negligence, or otherwise) for any injury resulting from any material contained herein. This publication contains information relating to general principles of medical care that should not be construed as specific instructions for individual patients. Manufacturers' product information and package inserts should be reviewed for current information, including contraindications, dosages, and precautions.

Printed in the United States of America

Library of Congress Cataloging-in-Publication Data

Clinical sonography: a practical guide/[edited by] Roger C. Sanders, Thomas C. Winter III ;
with Teresa Bieker. . . [et al.].— 4th ed.
p. ; cm.
Includes bibliographical references and index.
ISBN 0-7817-4869-0
1. Diagnosis, Ultrasonic. I. Sanders, Roger C., 1936- . II. Winter, Thomas C.
(Thomas Charles), 1958- . II. Title.
[DNLM: 1. Ultrasonography—methods. WN 208 C6405 2007]
RC78.7.U4C585 2007
616.07'543—dc22

2005035265

The publishers have made every effort to trace the copyright holders for borrowed material. If they have inadvertently overlooked any, they will be pleased to make the necessary arrangements at the first opportunity.

To purchase additional copies of this book, call our customer service department at **(800) 638-3030** or fax orders to **(301) 223-2320.** International customers should call **(301) 223-2300.**

Visit Lippincott Williams & Wilkins on the Internet: http://www.LWW.com. Lippincott Williams & Wilkins customer service representatives are available from 8:30 am to 6:00 pm, EST.

10 9 8 7 6 5 4 3 2 1

CLINICA
SONOG Y

A PRACTICAL GU

FOURTH EDITION

To my wife Barri, possessor of a literary style and critical mind far superior to mine, who has been of great help in the preparation of this book.

—Roger C. Sanders

To Susan, Rhys, Carys, and Aeddan, for all the love and joy you bring to my life.

—Thomas C. Winter

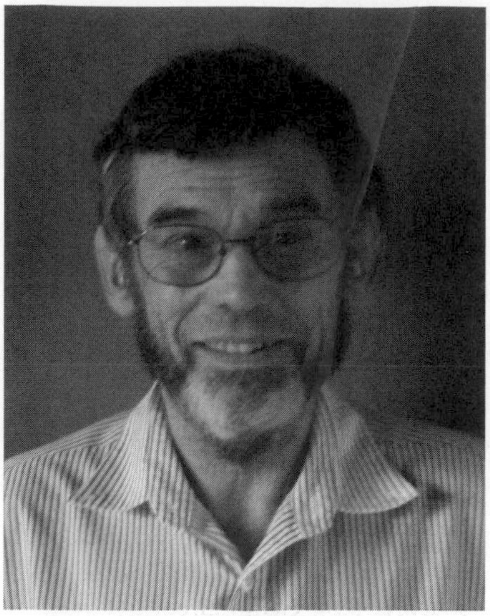

Roger C. Sanders

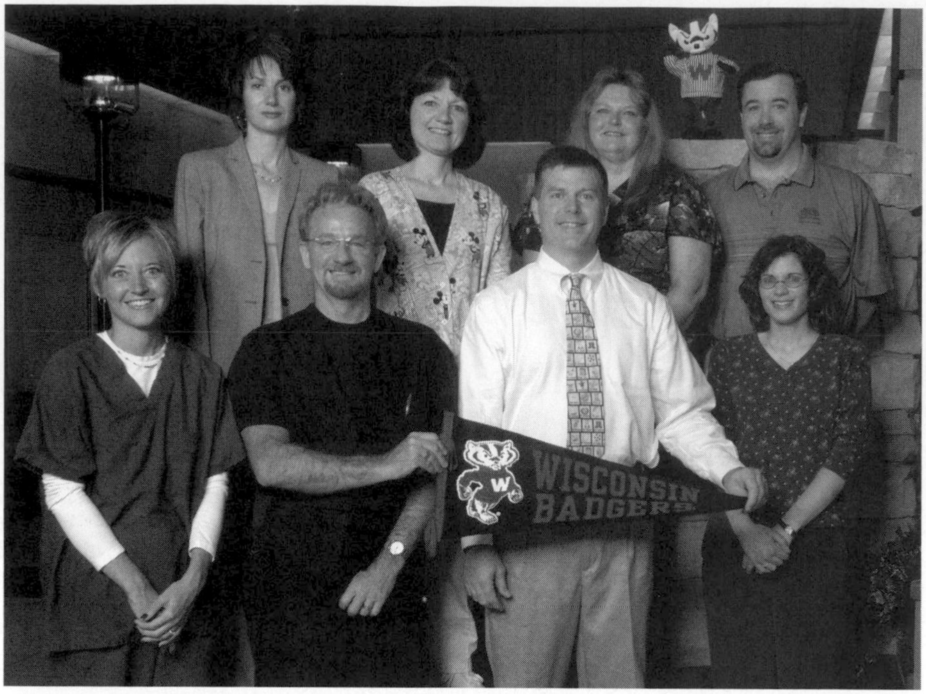

Front row, left to right: Sara Baker, Tim Walker, Thomas C. Winter, Heather Schierloh; back row, left to right: Carol Mitchell, Christine Labinski, Barbara Vanderwerff, Mike Ledwidge.

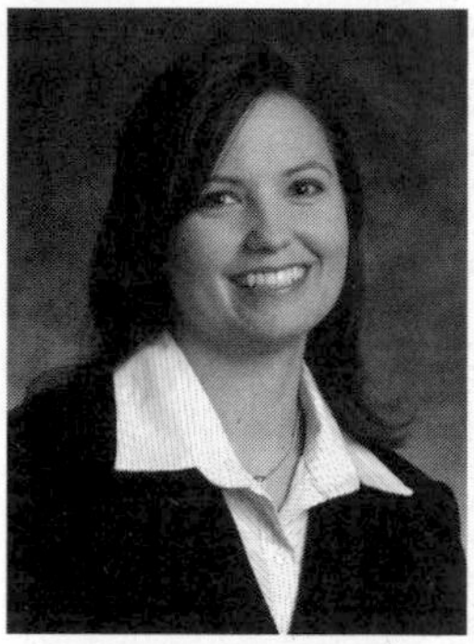

Teresa Bieker

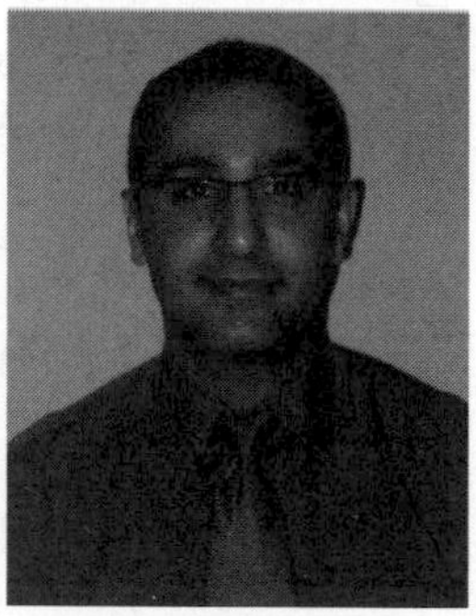

Jag Dhanju

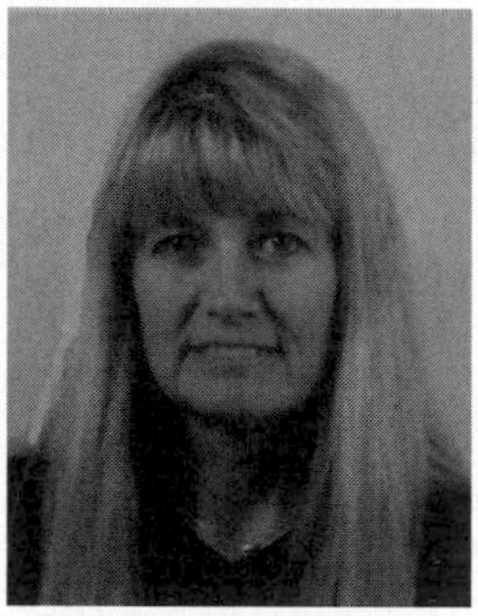

Julia Drose

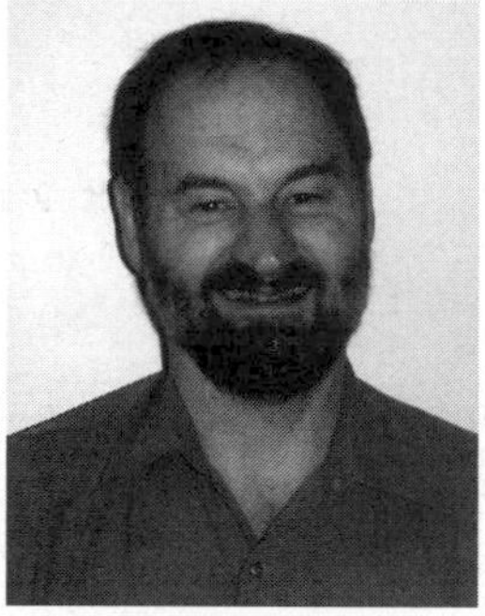

Roger Gent

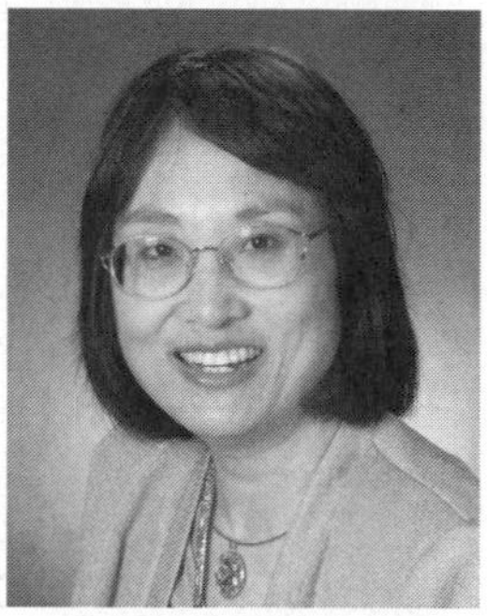

Beverly Hashimoto

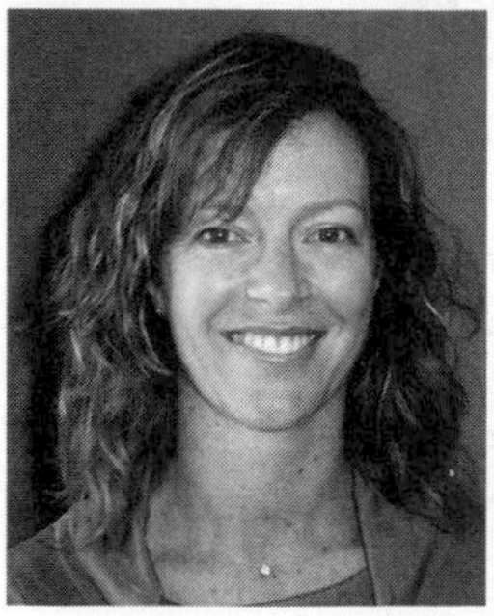

Lyndal Macpherson

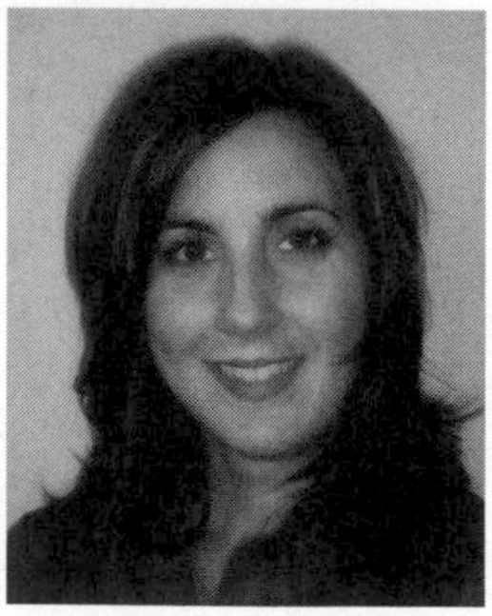

Lisa Parsons

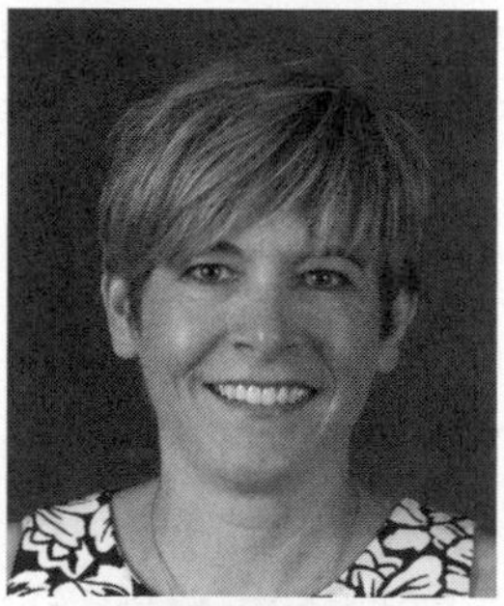

Cynthia L. Rapp

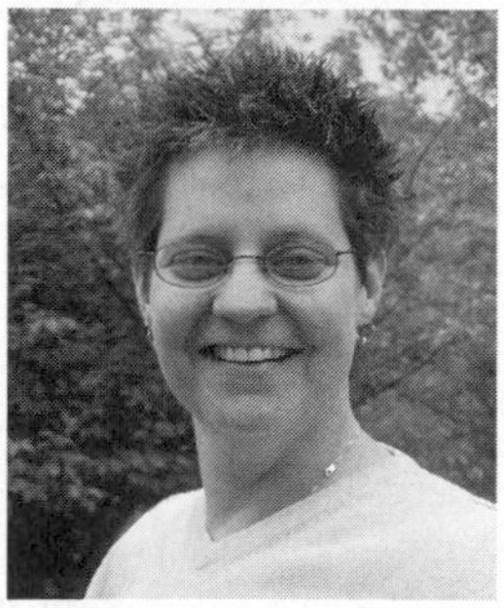

Rebecca Schilling

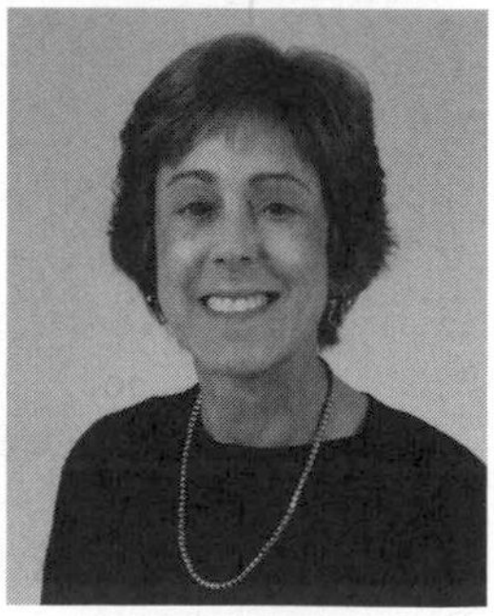

Marilyn Siegel

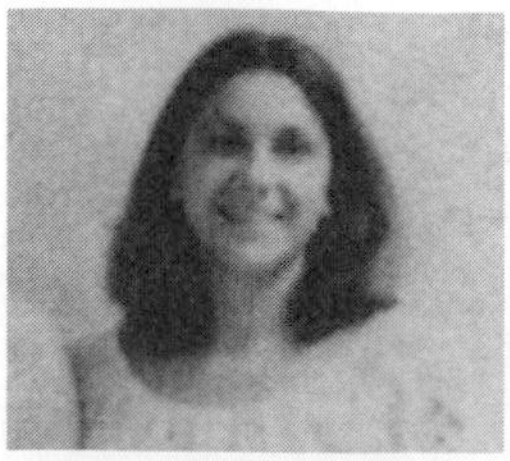

Nancy Smith Miner

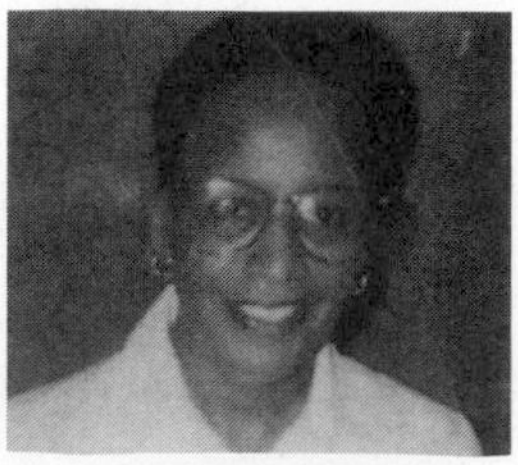

Deroshia Stanley

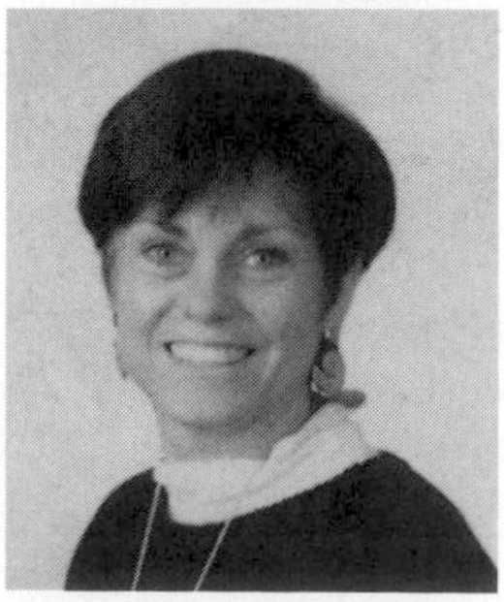

Gail Sandager-Hadley

Contributors

Sara M. Baker, RDMS, RVT, RI(R)
Ultrasonographer
Department of Radiology/Ultrasound
University of Wisconsin Hospital and Clinics
Madison, Wisconsin

Teresa Bieker, MBA-H, RDMS, RDCS, RVT
Lead Diagnostic Medical Sonographer
Division of Ultrasound
University of Colorado Hospital
Denver, Colorado

Carolyn Taylor Coffin, MPH, RDMS, RDCS, RVT
Diagnostic Medical Sonography Program
Division of Health and Public Services
Doña Ana Branch Community College
Las Cruces, New Mexico

Joyce Cordier, BS, RDCS, RDMS
Pediatric Cardiac Sonographer
Children's Hospital
Columbus, Ohio

Barbara Del Prince, BS, RDMS, RVT
Senior Market Manager
Siemens Medical Solutions
Ultrasound Division
Mountainview, California

Jag Dhanju, RDMS, RT(R)
Director of Imaging
Canadian Centre for Musculoskeletal Ultrasonography
North York, Ontario, Canada

Gretchen M. Dimling, BS, RDMS
Freelance Sonographer
Baltimore, Maryland

Julia A. Drose, BA, RDMS, RDCS, RVT
Associate Professor of Radiology
University of Colorado Health Sciences Center
Chief Sonographer
Department of Ultrasound
University of Colorado Hospital
Denver, Colorado

Roger Gent, DMU, AMS, Honorary Fellow ASUM
Pediatric Ultrasound Department
Women's and Children's Hospital
Adelaide, South Australia

Beverly E. Hashimoto, MD, FACR
Virginia Mason Medical Center
Seattle, Washington

Christine Labinski, RDMS
Ultrasonographer
Department of Radiology/Ultrasound
University of Wisconsin Hospital and Clinics
Madison, Wisconsin

Michael E. Ledwidge, BS, RDMS, RVT, CNMT
Ultrasonographer
Department of Radiology/Ultrasound
University of Wisconsin Hospital and Clinics
Madison, Wisconsin

Lyndal Macpherson, AMS, BAppSc Grad Dip U/S
Clinical Sales Specialist
Ultrasound
Siemens Medical Solutions
Mountainview, California

Mary McGrath-Ling, BS, RDMS
Rockville, Maryland

Nancy Smith Miner, RT(R), RDMS
Adjunct Faculty in Diagnostic Ultrasound
New Hampshire Technical Institute
Concord, New Hampshire

Carol Mitchell, PhD, RDMS, RDCS, RVT, RT(R)
Associate Researcher
Department of Cardiology
University of Wisconsin
Program Director
Department of Radiology
School of Diagnostic Medical Sonography
University of Wisconsin Hospital and Clinics
Madison, Wisconsin

Susan Murphy, RDMS

Lisa A. Parsons, BS, RDMS, RDCS
Ultrasonographer
Department of Maternal-Fetal Medicine
Evergreen Hospital Medical Center
Kirkland, Washington

Cynthia L. Rapp, BS, RDMS
Sonographer Practitioner
Radiology Imaging Associates
Greenwood Village, Colorado

Gail Sandager-Hadley, RN, RVT, FSVU
Technical Director
Vascular Ultrasound Core Laboratory
Massachusetts General Hospital
Boston, Massachusetts

Roger C. Sanders, MA, BM, Bch (Oxen), MRCP, FRCR, FACR
Clinical Professor of Radiology
University of New Mexico
Albuquerque, New Mexico

Mimi Maggio Sayler, RDMS, RDCS
Troy, Idaho

Heather Schierloh, MS, RDMS, RVt, RT(R)
Medical Imaging Specialist IV
Prenatal Diagnosis Center
Meriter Hospital
Ultrasonographer
Department of Radiology/Ultrasound
University of Wisconsin Hospital and Clinics
Madison, Wisconsin

Rebecca Schilling, RDMS, RCVT
Vascular Sonography Director
University of Maryland at Baltimore County
Baltimore, Maryland

Marilyn J. Siegel, MD
Professor of Radiology and Pediatrics
Mallinckrodt Institute of Radiology
Washington University Medical School
Radiologist
Mallinckrodt Institute of Radiology
Barnes-Jewish Hospital
St. Louis, Missouri

Deroshia B. Stanley, RN
Russell H. Morgan Department of Radiology and Radiological Science
Johns Hopkins Medical Institutions
Baltimore, Maryland

Tim Walker, RDMS, RDCS, RVT
Ultrasonographer
Department of Radiology/Ultrasound
University of Wisconsin Hospital and Clinics
Madison, Wisconsin

Tom Winter, MD, MA
Professor of Radiology
Director of Ultrasound
University of Wisconsin
Madison, Wisconsin

Barb Vanderwerff, RDMS, RVT, RDCS
Lead Sonographer
Department of Radiology/Ultrasound
University of Wisconsin Hospital and Clinics
Madison, Wisconsin

Preface

The attributes of a sonographer are increasingly being defined, as befits a growing profession. Criteria for accreditation of ultrasound laboratories have been established (see Chapter 62); guidelines for virtually all sonographic examinations have been laid out (see Appendices 32–43); and the Society of Diagnostic Medical Sonographers (SDMS) has approved a Code of Ethics, which we have included as Appendix 44. As welcome as these guidelines are, they fail to convey that "extra something" that is the intangible essence of the quality sonographer. Managed care may be requesting speed at the expense of competence—indeed, a good sonographer has both speed and competence—but a high-quality sonographer can accomplish an efficient examination without sacrificing intellectual curiosity. What separates a top-flight sonographer from the average? The real diagnosis is one that may require creative scanning that goes beyond a hastily filled-out requisition. True sonographers, given a patient complaining of right upper quadrant pain, do not stop at an empty gallbladder and normal duct crossing the portal vein. They keep looking until they find the mass in the bowel or the lobar pneumonia. They pursue pathology aggressively. They are detectives on the trail of a diagnosis.

This has always been our approach. The tools available, of course, continue to change. Life is a little easier with color and three-dimensional imaging, for instance, although not much. For the most part, these new tools are just adjuncts which make the diagnosis faster and more definitive. Three-dimensional imaging may bring out that cleft lip that was difficult to see. There are a few places where color makes a diagnosis we could not have made before. Although color prints are still expensive, quality grayscale imaging prices have decreased, and a big change in this edition is the inclusion of many ultrasound images in addition to the diagrams we have largely used in previous editions.

In the Western world, other imaging modalities such as computed tomography (CT) and magnetic resonance imaging (MRI) have become the preferred method for some areas of study—such as the liver, adrenals, and pancreas—but in other parts of the world, ultrasound remains the primary imaging technique. There are occasions when ultrasound still gives the answer after those other modalities fail. Because of this, and because incidental pathology is uncovered in these anatomical regions during other ultrasonic examinations, these chapters remain in the text.

A number of new areas have come to be important over the last few years. Most of these areas are included in the book, notably orthopaedic imaging (see Chapters 38, 52, and 53). Repetitive stress injury has regrettably become commonplace among sonographers as work pace and pressure increase, so we have inserted a chapter on ergonomics (Chapter 56). Litigation and accreditation issues are an increasing worry for sonologists and sonographers, and we have added separate chapters on malpractice (Chapter 61) and accreditation (Chapter 62). Much enhanced chapters on ultrasound-guided procedures (Chapter 54) and artifacts (Chapter 57) are a feature of this edition. Many other chapters have been substantially revised as a new crop of sonographers have become involved with the book.

I now only perform obstetrical and gynecological ultrasound, so I am lucky Tom Winter has joined as co-editor. Tom is Professor of Radiology at the University of Wisconsin. He has authored many original papers in several different ultrasonic areas and shares my interest in promoting sonographers as clinicians and in discovering and describing the quirks of hands-on sonography. As Harris Finberg has pointed out (Finberg, 2004), the current generation of radiologist/sonologists has few replacements as budding radiologists succumb to the lure of easy money from CT and MRI. Fortunately Tom has not.

Nancy Smith Miner is an obvious absence from this new edition, which is too bad because she is a great sonographer and magnificent editor. Her insights and felicitous phraseology have lit up all the previous editions. She is sorely missed.

New to this edition is the utilization of an Online Student Resource Center. The Appendices mentioned throughout the book are now located on the following site: http://connection.lww.com/go/sanders. The student can access the Resource Center anytime and print the appropriate Appendices as needed.

There are various other areas we could have included, such as endoluminal, transesophageal, gastrointestinal endoscopic, and ophthalmic ultrasound. We did not include them because these procedures are performed almost exclusively by physicians rather than sonographers. The focus of this book continues to be on the sonographer, although we know this text is read by those physicians who are involved in hands-on scanning. This book is dedicated to all those who go beyond the merely adequate.

Roger C. Sanders

REFERENCES

Finberg HJ. Whither (wither?) the ultrasound specialist? *J Ultrasound Med* 2004;23:1543–1547.

Contents

Color Plate pages appear between pages 18 and 19.

Appendices

Available online at http://connection.lww.com/go/sanders

Basic Physics

ROGER C. SANDERS
MIKE LEDWIDGE

1

SONOGRAM ABBREVIATIONS

Bl	Bladder
D	Diaphragm
Gbl	Gallbladder
K	Kidney
L	Liver
P	Pancreas
Th	Thyroid
Ut	Uterus

KEY WORDS

Acoustic Impedance. Density of tissue times the speed of sound in tissue. The speed of sound waves in body tissue is relatively constant at approximately 1,540 meters per second.

Amplitude. Strength or height of the wave, measured in decibels.

Attenuation. Progressive weakening of the sound beam as it travels through body tissue, caused by scatter, absorption, and reflection.

Beam. Directed acoustic field produced by a transducer.

Crystal. Substance within the transducer that converts electrical impulses into sound waves and vice versa.

Cycle. Per-second frequency at which the crystal vibrates. The number of cycles per second determines frequency.

Decibel (dB). A unit used to express the intensity of amplitude of sound waves; does not specify voltage.

Focal Zone. The depth of the sound beam where resolution is highest.

Focusing. Helps to increase the intensity and narrow the width of the beam at a chosen depth.

Fraunhofer Zone (Far Field). Area where transmitted beam begins to diverge.

Frequency. Number of times the wave is repeated per second as measured in hertz. Usable frequencies, except in the eye where higher frequencies can be used, lie between 2.5 and 13 million per second.

Fresnel Zone (Near Field). Area close to the transducer where the beam form is uneven.

Hertz (Hz). Standard unit of frequency; equal to one cycle per second.

Interface. Occurs whenever two tissues of different acoustic impedance are in contact.

Megahertz (MHz). 1,000,000 Hz.

Piezoelectric Effect. Effect caused by crystals (such as zirconate and titanate) changing shape when in an electrical field or when mechanically stressed, so that an electrical impulse can generate a sound wave or vice versa.

Power (Acoustic). Quantity of energy generated by the transducer, expressed in watts.

Pulse Repetition Rate. The number of times per second that a transmit-receive cycle occurs.

Resolution. Ability to distinguish between two adjacent structures (interfaces).

Specular Reflector. Reflection from a smooth surface at right angles to the sound beam.

Transducer (Probe). A device capable of converting energy from one form to another (see Piezoelectric Effect). In ultrasonography, the term is used to refer to the crystal and the surrounding housing.

Velocity. Speed of the wave, depending on tissue density. The speed of sound in soft tissues is between 1,500 and 1,600 meters per second. Velocity is standardized at 1,540 meters per second on all current systems.

Wavelength. Distance a wave travels in a single cycle. As frequency becomes higher, wavelengths become smaller.

Physics for Successful Scanning

In order to obtain the best image possible, basic fundamentals of ultrasound wave physics must be understood and applied.

AUDIBLE SOUND WAVES

Audible sound waves lie between 20 and 20,000 Hz. Ultrasound uses sound waves with a far greater frequency (i.e., between 1 and 30 MHz).

SOUND WAVE PROPAGATION

Sound waves do not exist in a vacuum, and propagation in gases is poor because the molecules are widely separated. The closer the molecules are, the faster the sound wave moves through a medium, so bone and metals conduct sound exceedingly well (Fig. 1-1).

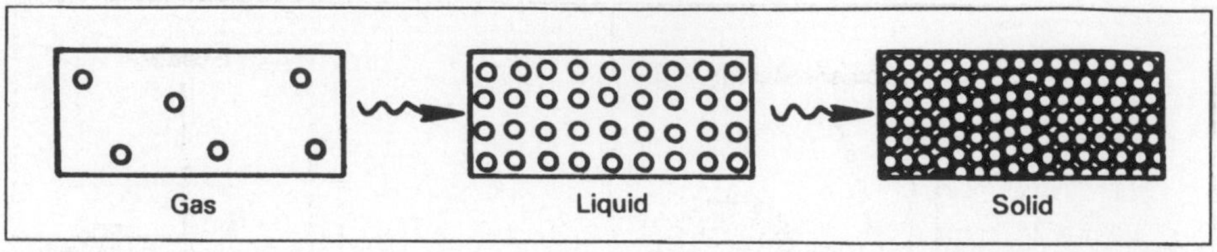

Figure 1-1. ■ *Sound propagation is worse in gas because molecules are widely separated. It is better in liquids and best in solids.*

Effect on Image

Air-filled lungs and bowel containing air conduct sound so poorly that they cannot be imaged with ultrasound instruments. Structures behind them cannot be seen. A neighboring soft-tissue or fluid-filled organ must be used as a window through which to image a structure that is obscured by air (Fig. 1-2). An acoustic gel must fill the space between the transducer and the patient, otherwise sound will not be transmitted across the air-filled gap. Bone conducts sound at a much faster speed than soft tissue. Because ultrasound instruments cannot accommodate the difference in speed between soft tissue and bone, current systems do not image bone or structures covered by bone.

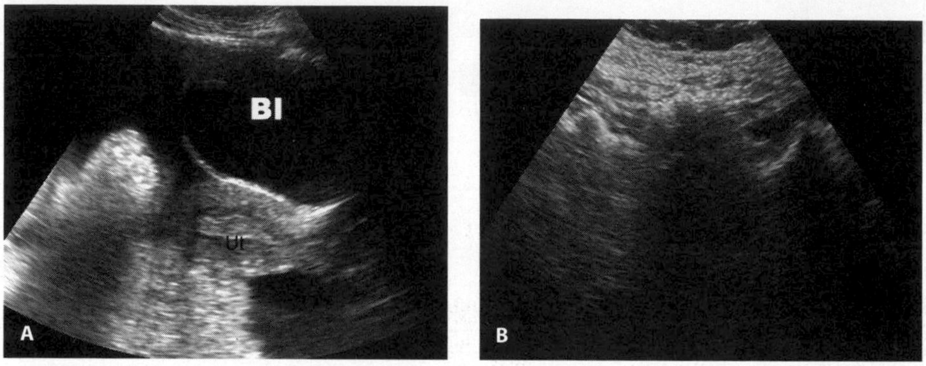

Figure 1-2. ■ *Sound propagation: effects on image.* ***A.*** *A distended urinary bladder* (Bl) *serves as a window for the uterus(Ut).* ***B.*** *With an empty urinary bladder, the uterus cannot be seen.*

THE PULSE-ECHO PRINCIPLE

Because the crystal in the transducer is electrically pulsed, it changes shape and vibrates, thus producing the sound beam that propagates through tissues. The crystal emits sound for a brief moment and then waits for the returning echo reflected from the structures in the plane of the sound beam (Fig. 1-3). When the echo is received, the crystal again vibrates, generating an electrical voltage comparable to the strength of the returning echo.

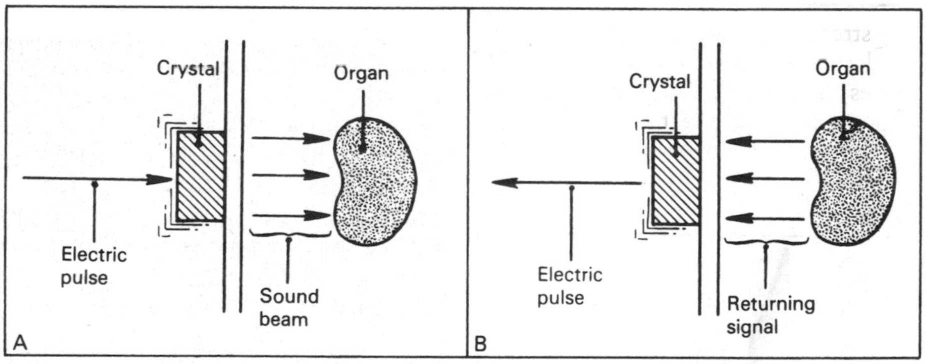

Figure 1-3. ■ *The pulse-echo principle.* ***A.*** *The electrical pulse strikes the crystal and produces a sound beam, which propagates through the tissues.* ***B.*** *Echoes arising from structures are reflected back to the crystal, which in turn vibrates, generating an electrical impulse comparable to the strength of the returning echo.*

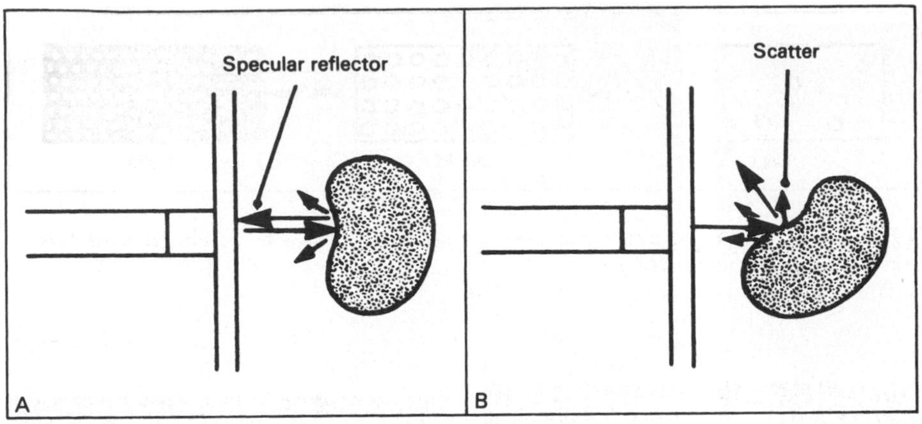

Figure 1-4. ■ *Angle of sound beams. A. When the sound beam is perpendicular to the organ interface, specular echoes are produced. B. When the sound beam is not perpendicular to the organ interface, scatter is seen.*

Effect on image

Grayscale imaging shows echoes in varying levels of grayness, depending on the strength of the interface. Some livers are homogeneously echogenic when fat is deposited. On the other hand, in acute hepatitis, overall echogenicity is lowered so that the portal vein's borders stand out more brightly.

BEAM ANGLE TO INTERFACE

The strength of the returning echo is related to the angle at which the beam strikes the acoustic interface. The more nearly perpendicular the beam is, the stronger the returning echo will be; smooth interfaces at right angles to the beam are known as *specular reflectors* (Fig. 1-4A). Echoes reflected at other angles are known as *scatter* (Fig. 1-4B).

Effect on Image

To demonstrate the borders of a body structure, the transducer must be placed so that the beam strikes the borders at a more-or-less right angle. It is worthwhile attempting to image a structure from different angles to produce the best representation. Some smaller echoes returning from structures that are not at right angles to the beam help to define the borders and contents of an organ or lesion (Fig. 1-5).

TISSUE ACOUSTIC IMPEDANCE

The returning echo's strength also depends on the differences in acoustic impedance between the various tissues in the body. Acoustic impedance relates to tissue density: the greater the difference in density between two structures is, the stronger the returning interface echoes defining the boundaries between those two structures on the ultrasound image will be.

Effect on Image

Structures of differing acoustic impedance (such as the gallbladder and the liver) are much easier to distinguish from one another than structures of similar acoustic texture (e.g., kidney and liver) (Fig. 1-6).

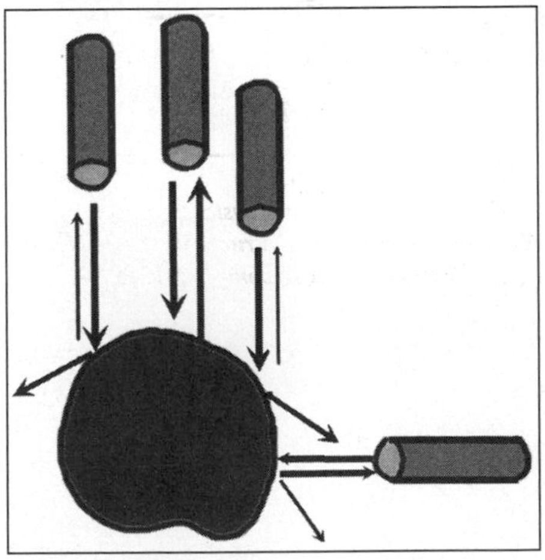

Figure 1-5. ■ *When visualizing a structure, it is important to scan at several different angles to find the best possible interface* (thick arrows). *Only a few echoes return from the interfaces at an oblique angle to the beam—specular reflections* (thin arrows). *Most of the echoes are scattered.*

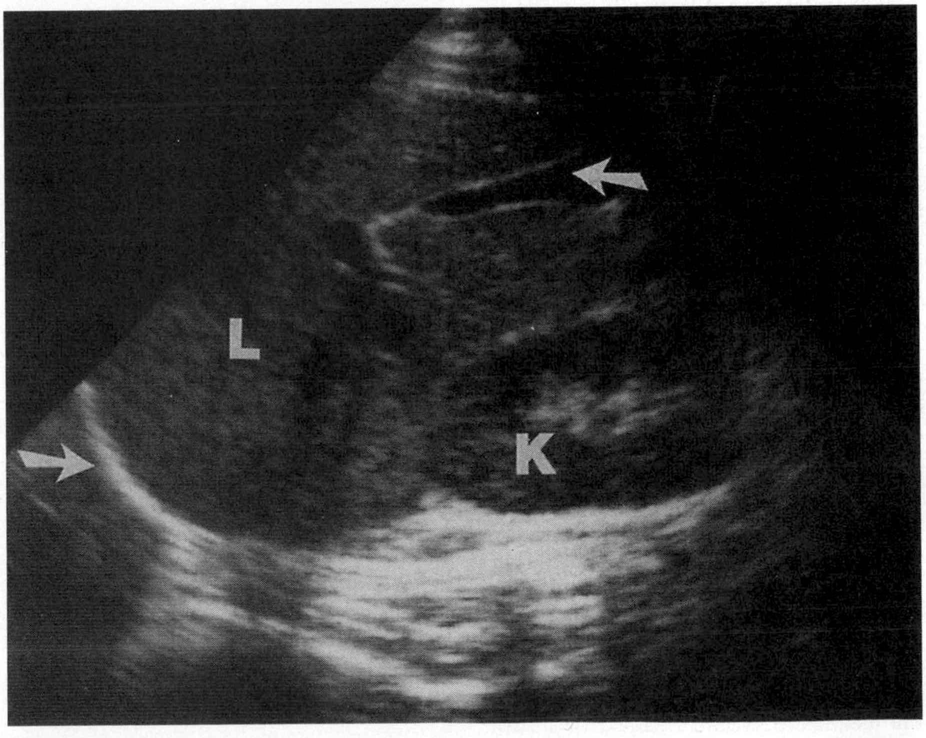

Figure 1-6. ■ *Tissue acoustic impedance. The bright interfaces at the gallbladder* (right arrow) *and the diaphragm* (left arrow) *are due to large differences in acoustic impedance (density) compared with the liver* (L). *The kidney* (K), *which is similar in texture to the liver, is not as easy to see.*

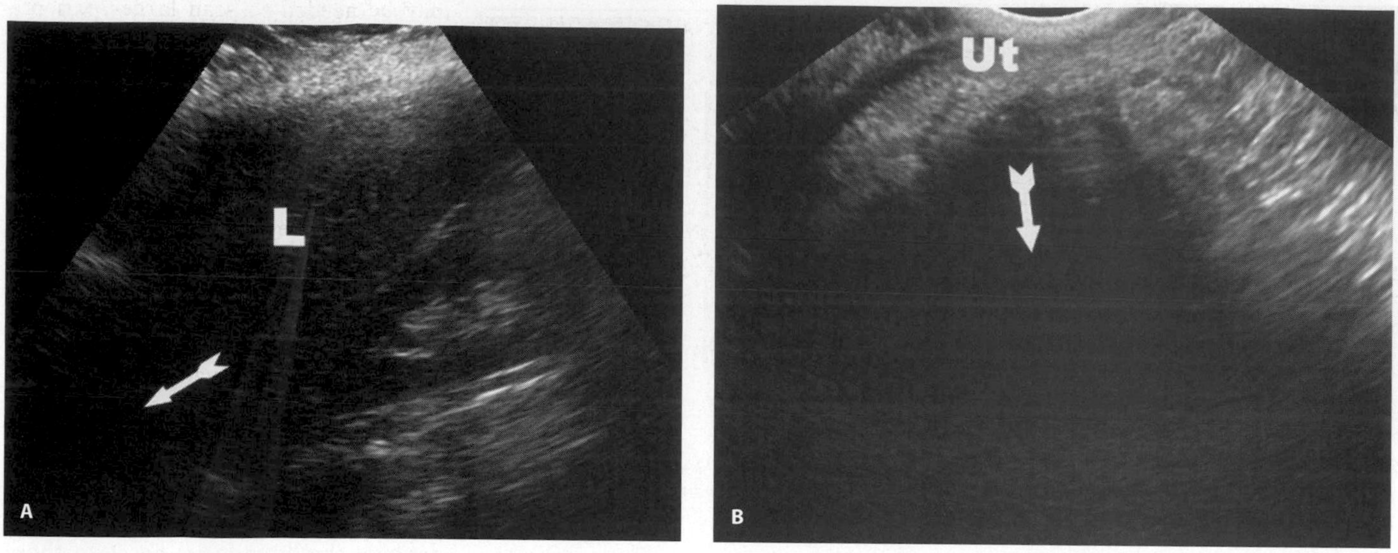

Figure 1-7. ■ *Absorption and scatter. A. In this longitudinal scan of a fatty liver* (L), *the diaphragm is not seen* (arrow). *B. Posterior borders of a large fibroid uterus* (Ut) *are not well delineated* (arrow).

ABSORPTION AND SCATTER

Because much of the sound beam is absorbed or scattered as it travels through the body, it undergoes progressive weakening (attenuation).

Effect on Image

Increased absorption and scatter prevent one from seeing the distal portions of a structure. In obese patients, the diaphragm is often not visible beyond the partially fat-filled liver (Fig. 1-7A). Fibroids may absorb so much sound that their posterior border may be difficult to define although no sizable mass is present (Fig. 1-7B).

TRANSDUCER FREQUENCY

Transducers come in many different frequencies—typically 2.5, 3.5, 5, 7, and 10 MHz. Increasing the frequency improves resolution but decreases penetration. Decreasing the frequency increases penetration but diminishes resolution.

Effect on Image

Transducers are chosen according to the structure being examined and the size of the patient (Fig. 1-8). The highest possible frequency should be used because it will result in superior resolution. Pediatric patients can be examined at 5 to 7.5 MHz. Lower frequencies (e.g., 2.5 MHz) permit greater penetration and

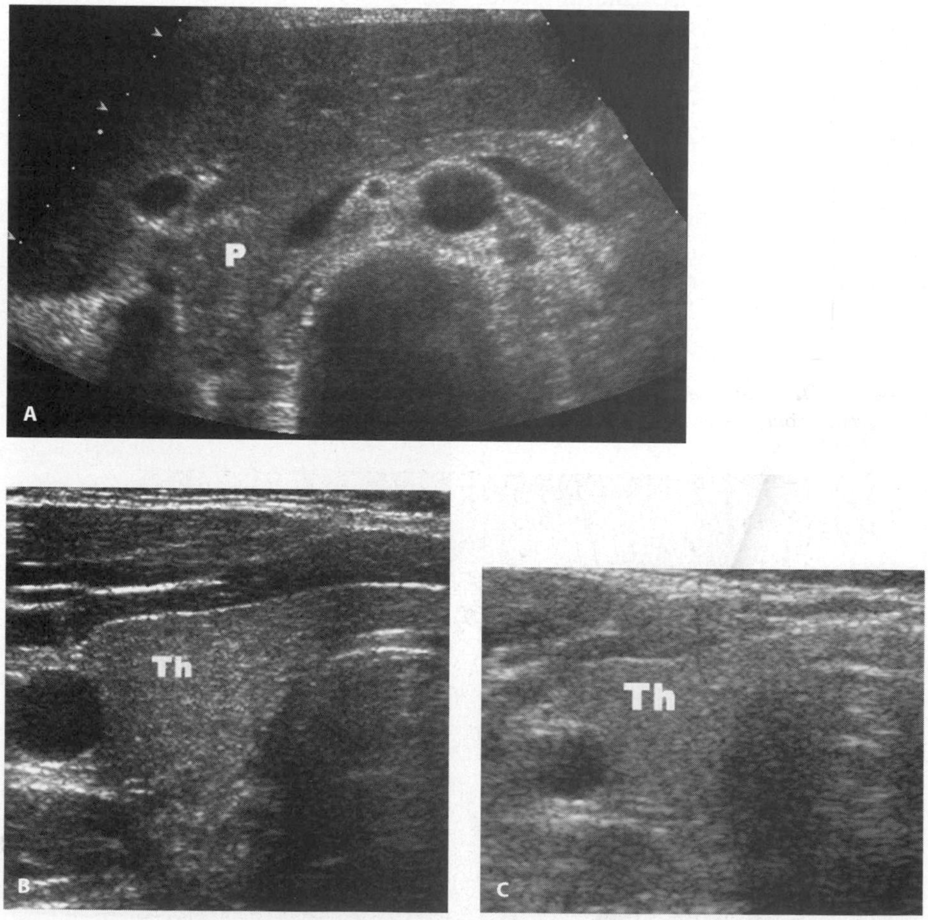

Figure 1-8. ■ *Transducer focal zones. A. A superficial pancreas* (P) *is seen well using a 6-MHz short-focus transducer. B. A thyroid* (Th) *scan using a 10-MHz short-focus transducer. Note image detail. C. A less-detailed thyroid* (Th) *scan with a 5-MHz short-focus transducer; this frequency is inappropriately low for such a superficial structure.*

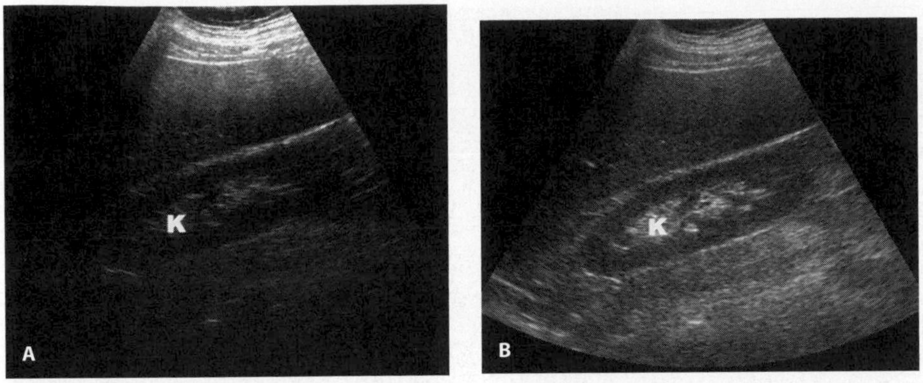

Figure 1-9. ■ *Low-frequency transducers. A. A longitudinal scan using a 5-MHz transducer does not penetrate to the posterior aspect of the kidney* (K). *B. A 3-MHz transducer penetrates adequately in this obese patient.*

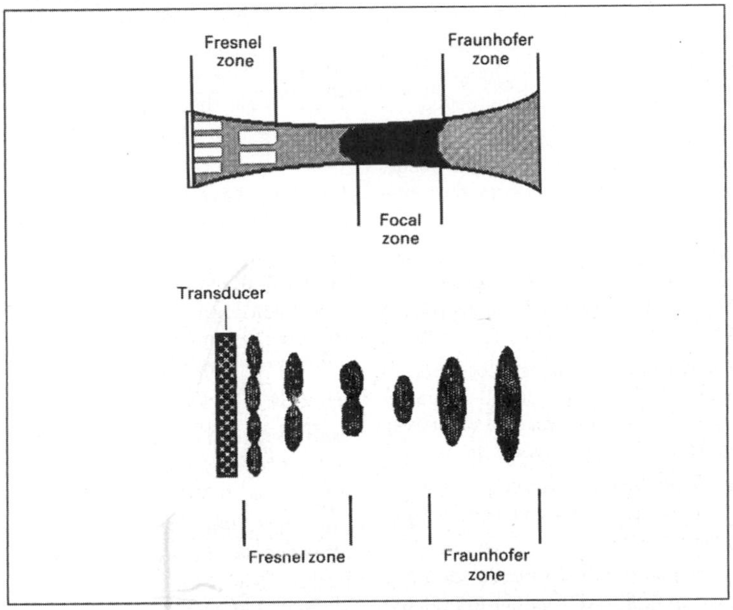

Figure 1-10. ■ *Diagram of the waveforms in a sound beam. Unequal waveforms in the near field (Fresnel zone). Widening of focal beam (Fraunhofer zone) beyond the focal zone.*

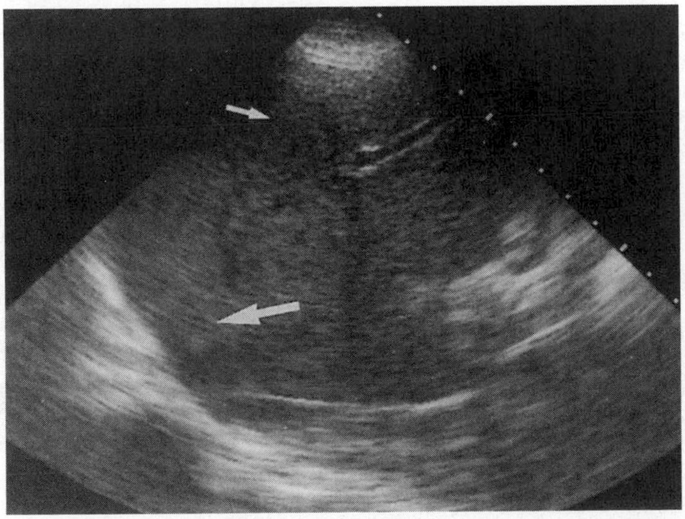

Figure 1-11. ■ *Longitudinal view of liver. Information is lost in the first 4 cm of the liver* (small arrow). *Pinpoint structures are distorted in the far field* (large arrow).

may be needed to scan larger patients (Fig. 1-9).

BEAM PROFILE

The sound beam varies in shape and resolution. Close to the skin, it suffers from the effect of turbulence, and resolution here is poor. Beyond the focal zone, the beam widens (Fig. 1-10).

Effect on Image

Information that appears to be present in the near field may actually be an artifact. Structures beyond the focal zone are distorted and difficult to see. A structure as small as a pinhead may appear to be half a centimeter wide (Fig. 1-11).

TRANSDUCER FOCAL ZONE

Sound beams can be focused in a similar fashion to light. Most systems use electronic focusing, which permits the transducer to be focused at one or more variable depths. The sonographer can alter the focus level electronically.

Effect on Image

To achieve high resolution, select a transducer with the proper focal zone or use electronic focusing set at the right depth for the study. For example, imaging the thyroid with a 3.5-MHz transducer using a focal zone set at 10 cm would provide poor-quality images (Fig. 1-8B,C).

SELECTED READING

Hykes D, Hedrick WR, Starchman D, eds. *Ultrasound Physics and Instrumentation,* 4th ed. Philadelphia: Mosby; 2005.

Kremkau FW, ed. *Diagnostic Ultrasound: Physical Principles and Exercises,* 5th ed. Philadelphia: WB Saunders; 2002.

Zagzebski J. *Essentials of Ultrasound Physics.* St. Louis: CV Mosby; 1996.

2 Instrumentation

BARBARA DEL PRINCE
ROGER C. SANDERS

KEY WORDS

A-Mode (Amplitude Modulation). A one-dimensional image displaying the amplitude strength of the returning echo signals along the vertical axis and the time (and, therefore, the distance from the transducer) along the horizontal axis (see Fig. 2-1).

Annular Array. A type of phased array transducer utilizing several concentric ring-shaped elements. Not commonly used in modern equipment.

Axial. Depth axis. Resolution along the axis of the ultrasound beam. Represents the smallest spacing required between two reflectors to be resolved as independent reflectors.

B-Mode (Brightness Modulation). A method of displaying the intensity (amplitude) of an echo by varying the brightness of a dot to correspond to echo strength (see Fig. 2-2). Real-time scanners are based on B-mode.

Backing Material. See *Damping Material* (see also Fig. 2-7).

Beam Steering. The ability to steer the beam of a linear transducer to the left or right in two-dimensional (2D) (grayscale) imaging.

Cine Loop. The system memory stores the most recent sequence of image frames before the freeze button is pressed. The operator can then review the sequence of images frame by frame or in real time.

Cathode Ray Tube (CRT). The term used to describe the monitor on which the image is displayed.

Curved Linear Transducer (Curved Array). Linear array transducers with a curved scan head. Focusing is electronically controlled. Useful in abdominal and obstetric/gynecologic imaging (see Fig. 2-22F).

Damping Material. Material attached to the back of the transducer crystal to decrease ring time (continued vibration of the crystal after the internal responses; see Fig. 2-7).

Dynamic Clip. Term used to describe the capture and storage of a cine loop of images. Allows review a real-time clip after the examination is ended.

Dynamic Focusing. The ability to select focal zones at different depths throughout the image. As the number of focal zones increases, the frame rate decreases.

Dynamic Range. The range of signals that a system's components can process. Relates echo amplitude to the assigned grayscale value. Unit of measure is decibels (dB).

Electronic Focusing. Each element, or group of elements, within a transducer is pulsed separately to focus the beam at a particular area of interest. Used in array technology of all types.

Endocavity Transducer. High-frequency transducer that is designed to be used for endorectal as well as endovaginal imaging.

Endorectal Transducer. High-frequency transducer that is placed into the rectum to evaluate the prostate and rectal wall. Some probes have both longitudinal and transverse transducers mounted on the same probe head (biplane transducers).

Endovaginal Transducer. A high-frequency probe, which is introduced into the vagina for evaluating the pelvic organs.

Focusing. The act of narrowing the ultrasound beam to a small width (slice thickness). Image detail increases within the narrowed region.

Footprint. Term used to describe the portion of the transducer that is in contact with the patient.

Frame Rate (Image Rate). Rate at which the image is refreshed in a real-time system display. Frame rate varies with system settings such as focal zones, depth of the image display, preprocessing settings, and image width.

Freeze Frame. Control that stops a moving real-time image for photography or prolonged evaluation.

Linear Array. A transducer with many small electronically coordinated elements oriented side by side, producing a rectangular image. Useful in small parts, intraoperative, and vascular imaging. The long bar shape interferes with imaging between the ribs, making abdominal imaging difficult.

Matching Layer. Minimizes the difference in acoustic impedance between the transducer crystal and skin (see Fig. 2-7).

Mechanically Steered Transducer. The physical movement of the element or mirror that causes the sound beam to sweep through the tissue, providing a real-time image.

Monitor. Term used for the TV display.

Multi-D Array Transducers. Utilize multiple rows of transducer elements fired in sequence to improve imaging slice thickness.

MultiHertz. The ability to cycle between two or more sending frequencies within a given transducer.

Oscilloscope. The TV display screen. Not used in modern equipment. May be found on dedicated A-mode machines.

Phased Array. Electronically steered system in which many small elements are electronically coordinated to produce a focused wavefront. Used in curved linear, linear, sector, and phased-array transducers.

Real-Time (Dynamic) Imaging. Type of imaging in which many frames are run together to create a cinematic view of the tissue.

Ring-Time. Length of time that a transducer crystal vibrates after it has been activated.

Scan Converter. A device that gathers all of the signals and organizes them on the basis of their location to give a 2D display.

Sector Scanner. Transducer with a small head that produces a pie-shaped image. May be a mechanical, or phased array (see Figs. 2-16 and 2-22D,E).

Transrectal Transducer. See *Endorectal Transducer.*

Transvaginal Transducer. See *Endovaginal.*

Vector Array. Small footprint transducer that utilizes the entire transducer face to form the image. Produces a trapezoid image with a larger field of view than the traditional sector (see Fig. 2-22C).

Virtual Format Imaging. Allows a linear transducer to be displayed as a trapezoidal image format. Increases the field of view of a linear transducer for easier measurements and display of larger regions of interest.

Types Of Ultrasound Display

AMPLITUDE MODULATION OR MODE

In amplitude modulation or mode (A-mode), the most basic form of diagnostic ultrasound, a single beam of ultrasound is analyzed. The distance between the transducer and the structure determines where an echo is seen along the time axis. The time elapsed from the transmission to the return of the signal is converted to distance. An echo (sound wave) is assumed to travel at a constant speed of 1,540 m/sec in soft tissue; thus, the time it takes for the echo to return to the transducer represents a distance. Isolated use of the A-mode is almost obsolete, however, it may be helpful to differentiate a cystic lesion from a solid lesion on some equipment. A cystic lesion will appear as a flat line with a prominent back wall echo (Fig. 2-1). A-mode imaging may also be used in ophthalmic applications for measuring ocular dimensions.

BRIGHTNESS MODE

An A-mode signal can be converted to dots, which vary in brightness depending on the strength of the returning echo (amplitude). A stronger (high-amplitude) echo will display a brighter dot than a weaker (low-amplitude) echo (Fig. 2-2). The depth of the reflector is displayed by the dot's location. Multiple brightness mode (B-mode) images may be displayed together to form a 2D B-scan.

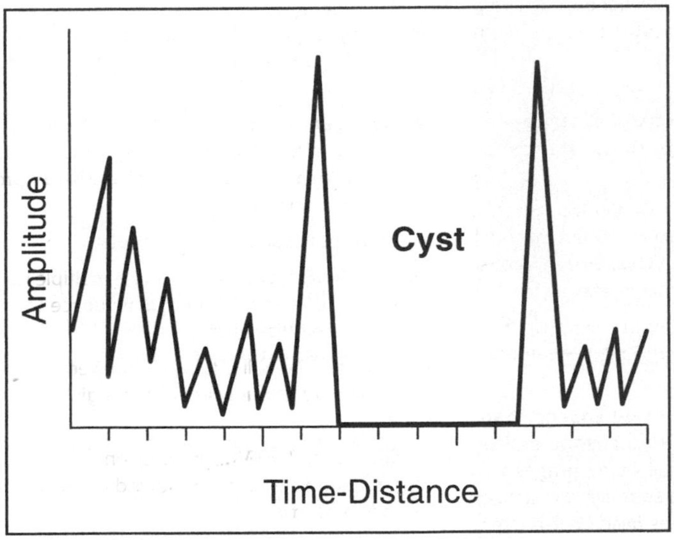

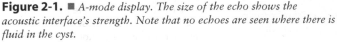

Figure 2-1. ■ *A-mode display. The size of the echo shows the acoustic interface's strength. Note that no echoes are seen where there is fluid in the cyst.*

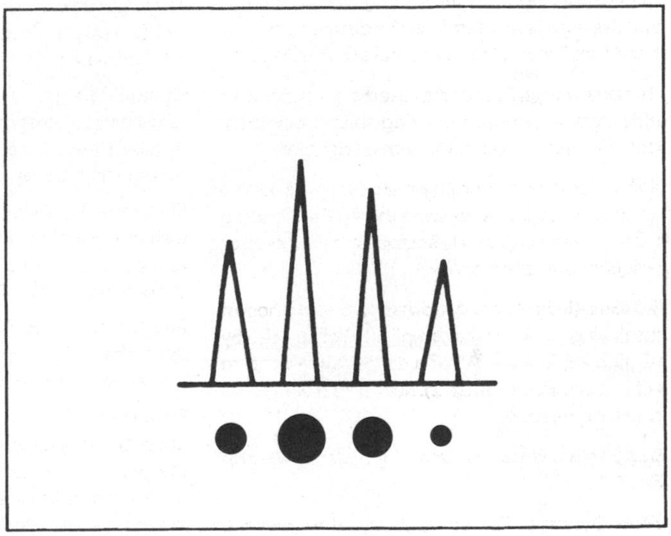

Figure 2-2. ■ *B-mode. The amplitude of an echo is displayed as the brightness of a dot comparable to the echo strength on the A-mode display.*

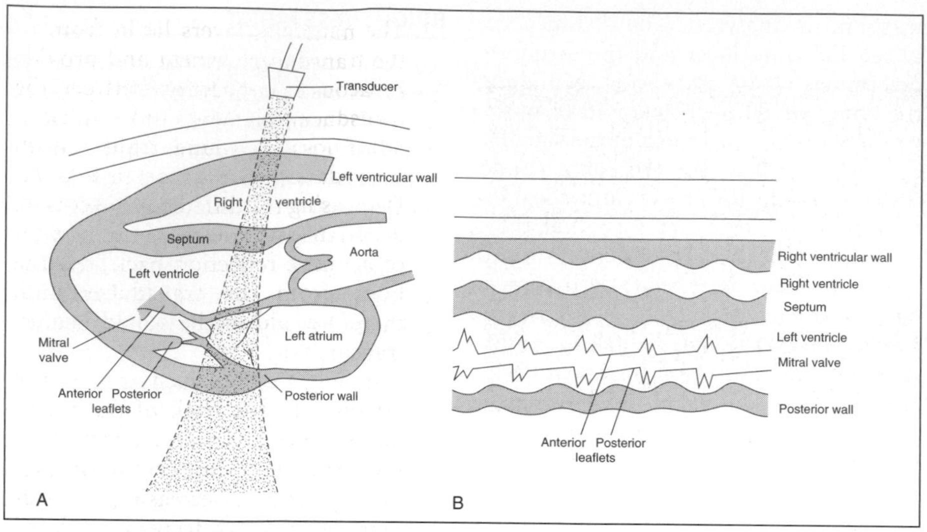

Figure 2-3. ■ *M-mode. A. Diagram demonstrating the sound beam angled through specific heart structures. B. The M-mode readout of those structures within the sound beam.*

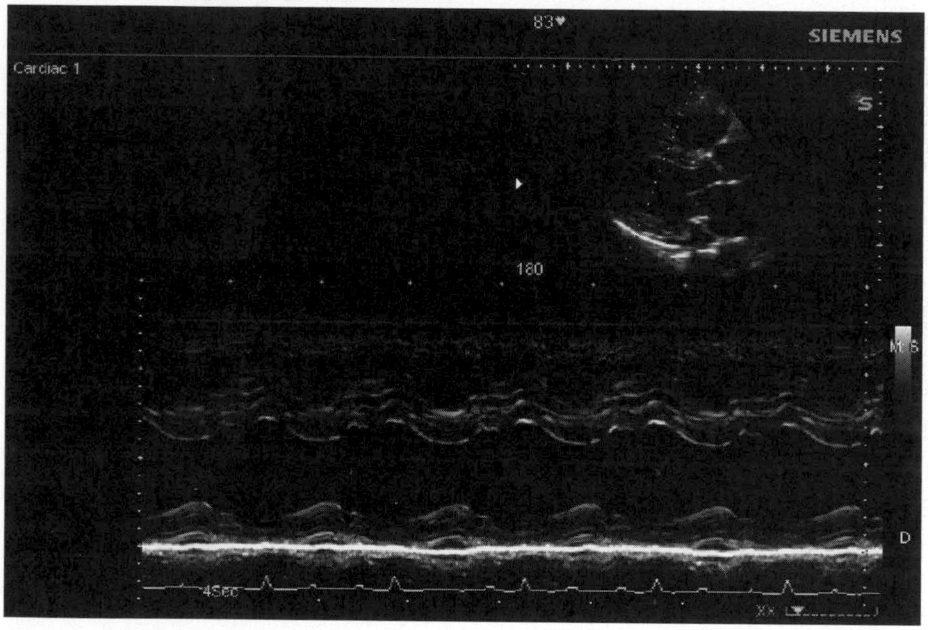

Figure 2-4. ■ *M-mode display of the adult heart demonstrating motion of the intraventricular septum and ventricular wall.*

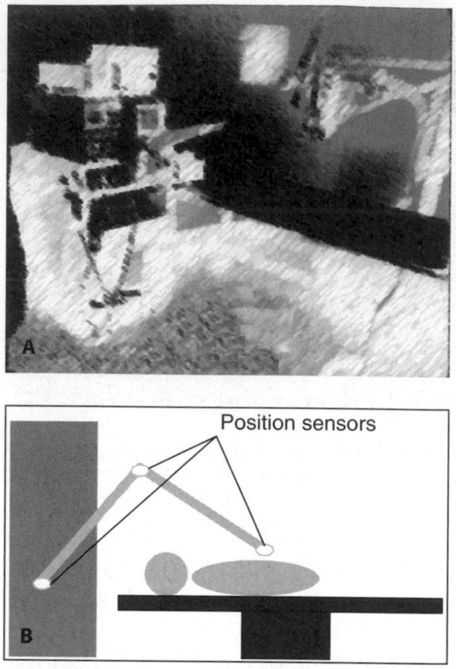

Figure 2-5. ■ *A. An articulated arm B-scan machine from the 1970s. B. Articulated arm scanners contained position sensors throughout the arm to track the orientation transducer throughout the scan.*

M-MODE (Motion Mode)

In motion mode (M-mode), a series of B-mode dots is displayed on a moving time base graphing the motion of mobile structures. M-mode imaging formed the basis of echocardiography prior to real-time (Figs. 2-3 and 2-4). M-mode is currently used in conjunction with real-time imaging in adult, pediatric, and fetal echocardiography.

B-SCAN (STATIC SCAN)

The B-scan uses a series of B-mode images to "build" a 2D view of the tissue. The transducer is attached to an articulated arm, which provides the ultrasound system with information on transducer position and orientation (Figs. 2-5 and 2-6). Although a large field-of-view image is produced, this type of imaging is not used in modern equipment because of the numerous drawbacks. These disadvantages are as follows:

1. Scanning motion and planes are limited because of the articulated arm.
2. Examinations are lengthy and require a great deal of patient cooperation.
3. A high level of operator skill is required.
4. Movement cannot be displayed.
5. Equipment is large and unwieldy. A portable examination cannot be performed.

REAL-TIME, B-MODE

Real-time systems provide a cinematic view of the area being evaluated by displaying a rapid series of images sequentially (see Fig. 2-22A–E). The following features are advantages of real-time scanning:

1. Scanning planes that best demonstrate the area of interest can be found easily.
2. A rapid examination can be performed because there is constant visual feedback on the display screen.
3. Extended structures such as vessels can be followed, allowing them to be traced to their origin.

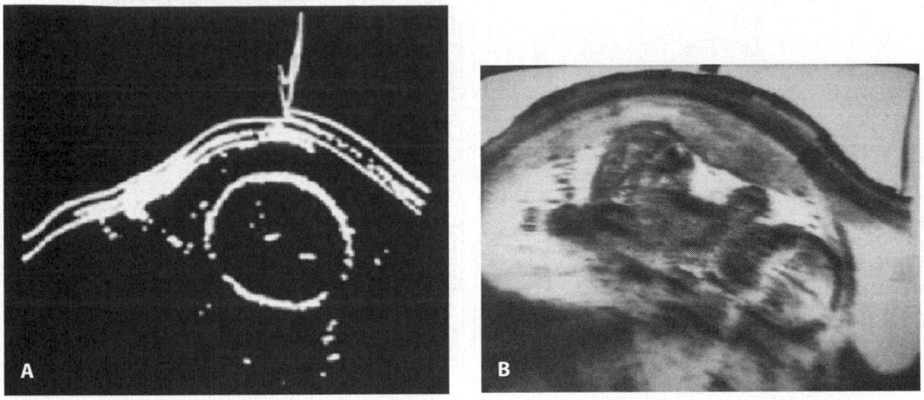

Figure 2-6. ■ *A. Bistable image from an articulated arm B-scanner. B. Early grayscale image from an articulated arm B-scanner.*

4. Movement observation may aid in organ identification (e.g., mass vs. bowel).
5. Infants, children, and uncooperative patients can be examined easily.
6. Critically ill patients and those with acute conditions can be studied portably.
7. Pulsed and color-flow Doppler can be performed coincident with the real-time examination.

Real-Time Imaging

All modern imaging systems use a real-time approach. Real-time B-mode ultrasound systems use a transducer, which contains a crystal that can convert ultrasound impulses into electrical impulses. These signals are integrated by a computer, known as a *scan converter*, into a 2D image. A description of the components of the basic system follows.

SCAN CONVERTER

The scan converter is the portion of the imaging system in which the image data are stored and converted for display on the cathode ray tube. Analog scan converters are the oldest form of imaging and are not used in modern equipment. An electron gun is used to fire electrons on a grid, which stores the charges and then displays the information on the cathode ray tube. Digital scan converters, now found in all new systems, use computer memory to digitize the image and transfer it to the display monitor.

Preprocessing and postprocessing of the image information occurs in the scan converter. The brightness level for an electronic signal derived from an ultrasound echo can be varied, depending on whether strong or weak signals need to be emphasized.

TRANSDUCERS

The transducer-assembly consists of five main components: the transducer crystal, the matching layers, damping material, the transducer case, and the electric cable (Fig. 2-7).

1. The transducer crystal is composed of a piezoelectric material, most commonly lead zirconate titanate. The transducer crystal converts the electrical voltage into acoustic energy upon transmission, and acoustic energy to electrical energy upon reception.
2. The matching layers lie in front of the transducer element and provide an acoustic connection between the transducer element and the skin. Some loss of sound transmission (impedance) occurs at this layer. Decreasing the difference in acoustic impedance will decrease the amount of acoustic reflection back into the body from the transducer and, therefore, aid in the sound beam's transmission.
3. Damping material such as rubber is attached to the back of the transducer element to decrease secondary reverberations of the crystal with returning signals. Decreasing the ring-time results in an increase in depth (axial) resolution.
4. The transducer case provides a housing for the crystal, a damping material layer, and insulation from interference by electrical noise.
5. The electronic cable contains the bundle of electrical wires used to excite the transducer elements and receive the returned electrical impulses. There must be an individual wire for excitation and for reception of each individual transducer element.

There are several types of transducer elements:

1. Mechanical Transducers. The transducer crystal is physically moved to provide steering for the beam. Most

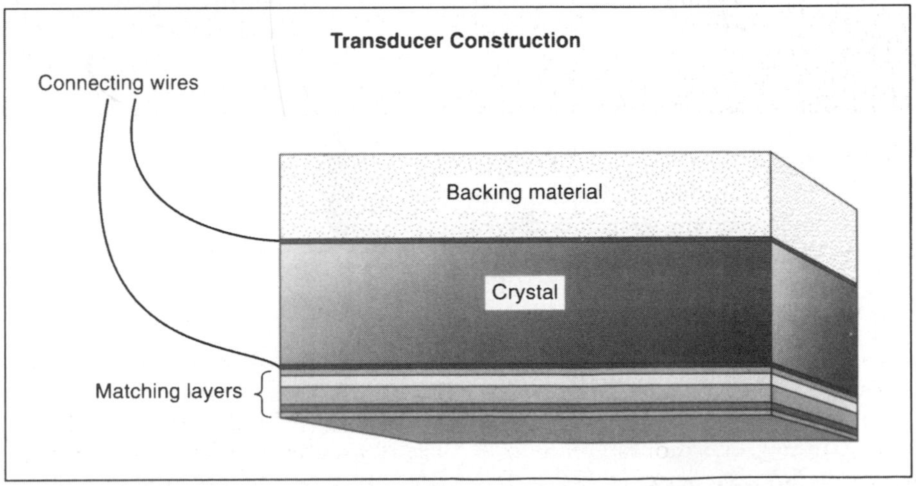

Figure 2-7. ■ *Diagram showing transducer construction. Matching layers of material decrease the size of the main bang acoustic interface that occurs between the crystal and the skin. Backing material acts as a damping tool to stop secondary reverberations of the crystal. The crystal is constructed of piezoelectric material, which can convert electrical impulses into sound waves and vice versa.*

of these probes provide a sector image with a fixed focus. Although mechanical steering is less commonly used in modem equipment than phased-array transducers, mechanical transducers are often used in 3D or 4D applications.

a. Rotary Type (Wheel). In mechanically steered systems using a rotary type transducer, one or more transducer elements are arranged in a wheel-like housing that moves the beam through an arc-shaped sector (Fig. 2-8). The small size of the transducer face allows intercostal access for scanning organs such as the liver and heart.

b. Oscillating Transducer (Wobbler). The drive motor and transducer element are housed in a small container in mechanically steered systems using an oscillating transducer. The motor drives the transducer element back and forth, producing a sector image (Fig. 2-9).

c. Transducer with Oscillating Mirror. In this type of mechanically steered system, the transducer element is stationary, but the beam is moved by oscillating a mirror that reflects the sound (Fig. 2-10).

2. Electronically Steered Systems. In this type of transducer, multiple piezoelectric elements are used. A separate electrical supply is provided for each element. Steering and focusing occur by sequentially exciting individual elements across the face of the transducer. Focusing is controlled electronically by the operator. The images are displayed in a sector, vector, linear, or curved linear format.

a. Linear Sequenced Arrays. Multiple transducer elements are mounted on a straight or curved bar. Groups of elements are electronically pulsed at once to act as a single larger element. Pulsing occurs sequentially down the length of the transducer face, moving the sound beam from end to end (Fig. 2-11).

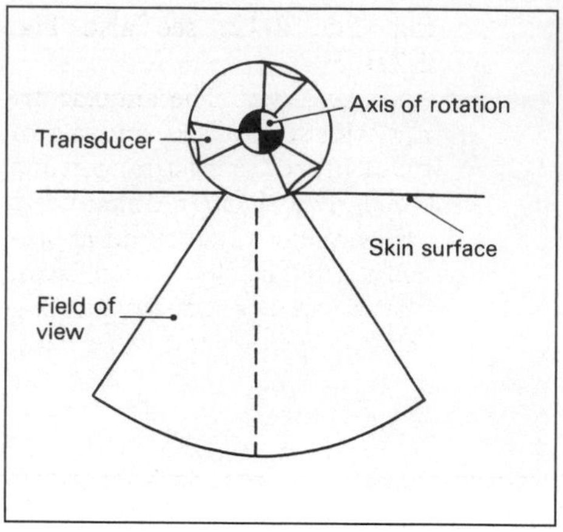

Figure 2-8. ■ *Mechanical rotary sector scanner.*

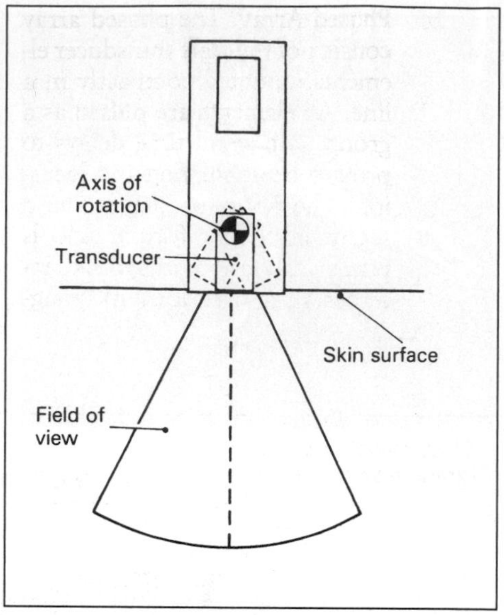

Figure 2-9. ■ *Oscillating transducer (wobbler).*

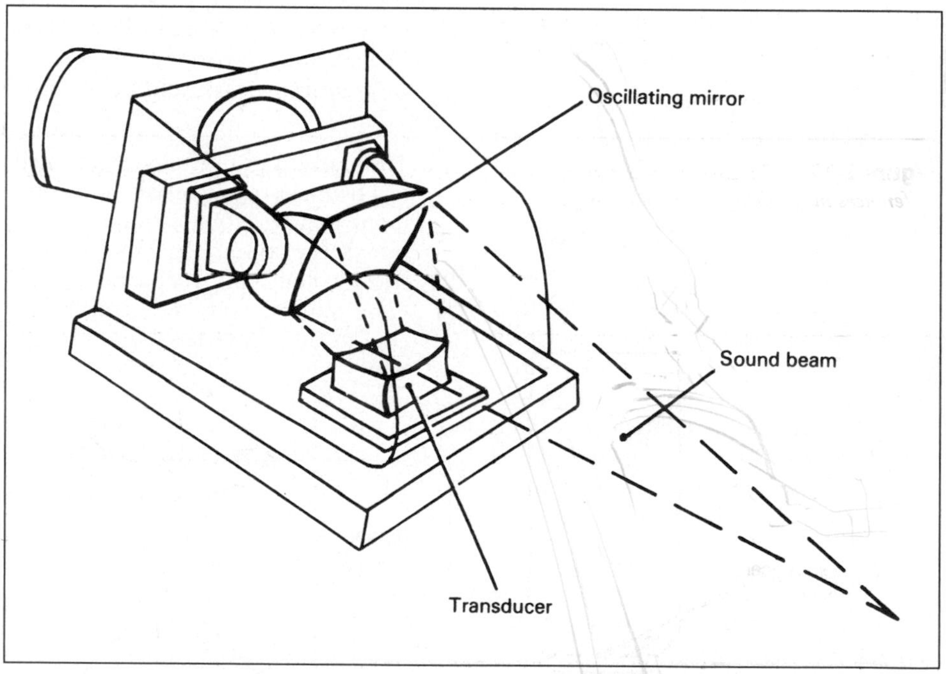

Figure 2-10. ■ *Stationary transducer with oscillating mirror.*

b. Phased Array. The phased array consists of multiple transducer elements mounted compactly in a line. All elements are pulsed as a group with small time delays to provide beam steering and focusing. The resulting image is in a sector or vector format and is particularly useful in cardiac, intercostal, and endocavity imaging (Fig. 2-12; see also Fig. 2-22E,F).

c. Annular Array. The annular array system employs crystals of the same frequency arranged in a circle. The circular transducers are electronically focused at several depths (Fig. 2-13). The beam may be reflected off an oscillating acoustic mirror into a water bath.

Multi-D Array (1.5D Array, 2D Array) Transducers

This type of transducer utilizes multiple rows of elements to form a matrix of crystals (Fig. 2-14). Through the use of multiple pulses, these crystals may be pulsed in sequence to create a very thin slice thickness, which yields increased resolution.

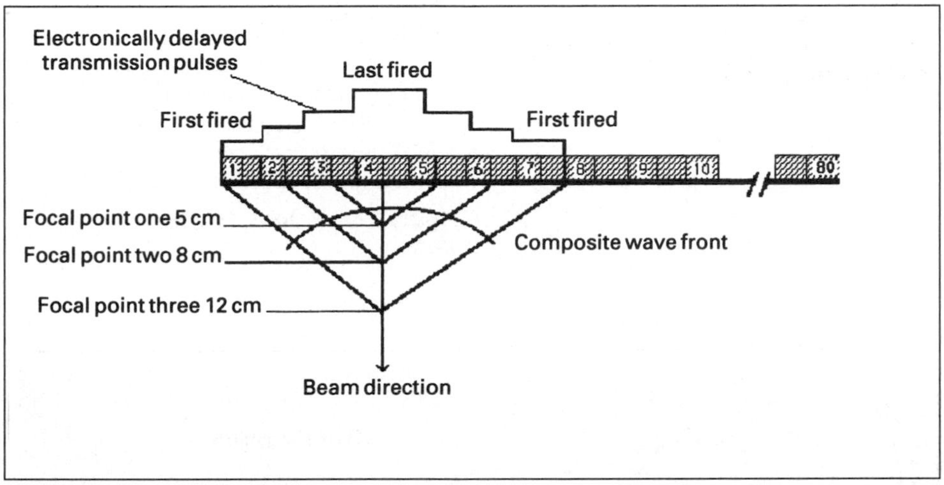

Figure 2-11. ■ *Linear sequenced array. Multiple transducer elements are pulsed in groups. Time differences in the delay of the returning signal allow focusing at different depths.*

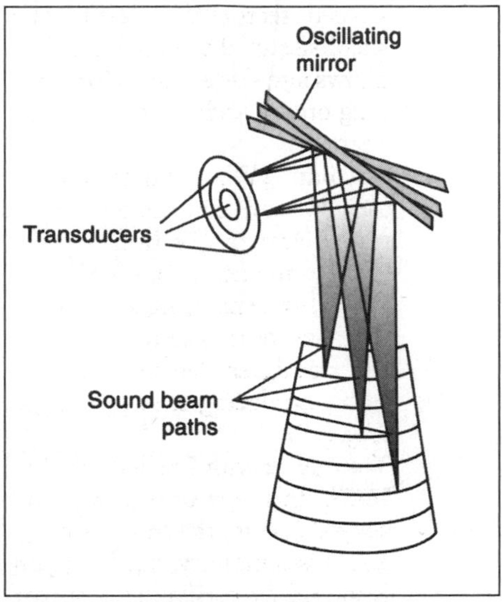

Figure 2-13. ■ *Annular array transducer.*

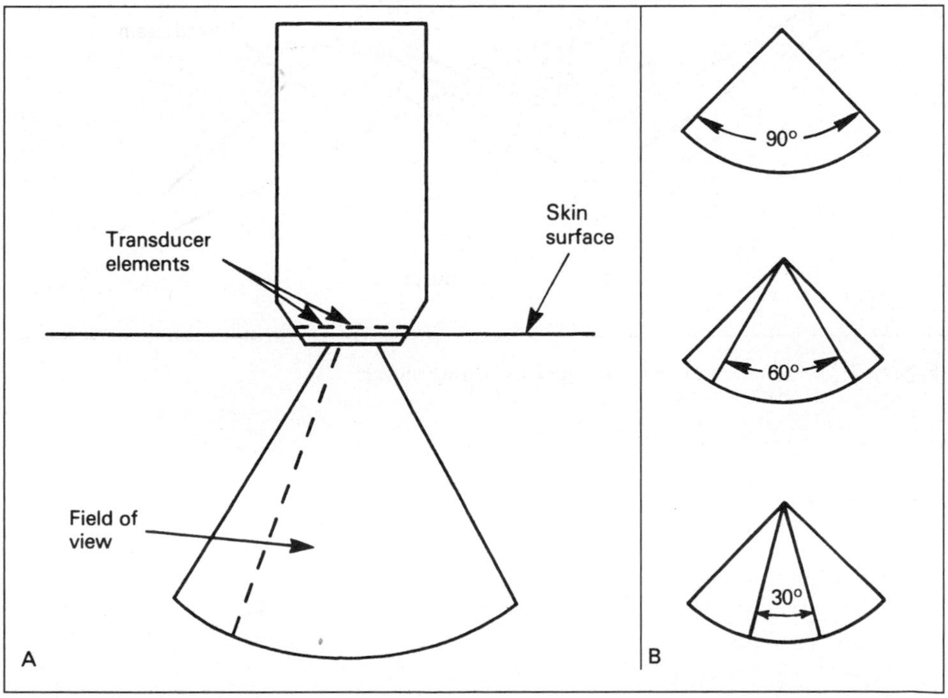

Figure 2-12. ■ *Wedged-shaped field. A. Phased (steered) array. B. Different size fields of view. Smaller fields provide better resolution.*

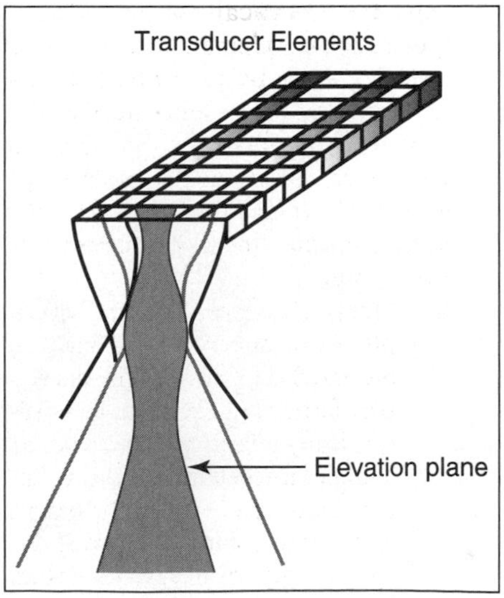

Figure 2-14. ■ *Multiple rows of transducer crystals allow for a more uniform elevation plane and improved resolution.*

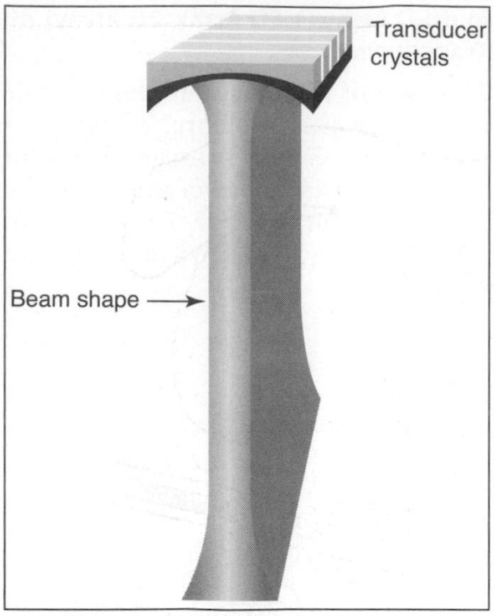

Figure 2-15. ■ *Hanafy lens transducer. The plano-concave design of the transducer crystals provides a uniform slice thickness.*

Hanafy Lens Technology

Hanafy lens technology is another technique used to create a very thin slice thickness that is uniform throughout the field of view. With this technology, the transducer crystals are cut in a plano-concave fashion (Fig. 2-15). This cutting method creates crystals, which are thin in the center and thicker at the edges. The thinner center will ring at a higher frequency (focusing in the near field), and the thicker edges will ring at a lower frequency (focusing in the far field) automatically creating a uniform slice thickness throughout the field of view.

Specialized Ultrasound Transducers And Systems

SPECIAL TRANSDUCERS

Special transducers (Fig. 2-16) have been produced to help view specific areas:

1. Small parts (7.5- to 15-MHz) transducer
2. Rectal transducers in longitudinal (linear) and transverse (radial) configurations (biplane) (Figs. 2-17 and 2-18)
3. Biopsy transducer
4. Doppler probes

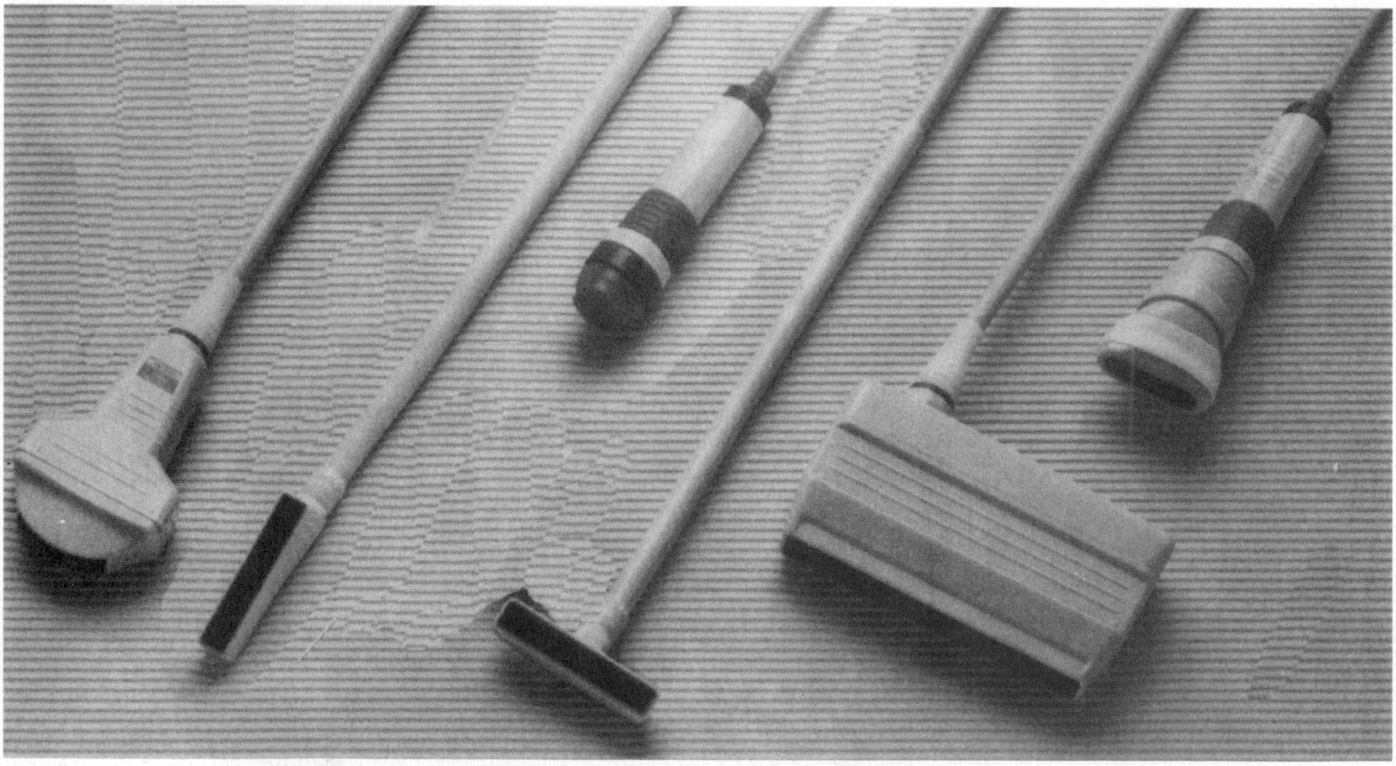

Figure 2-16. ■ *A variety of transducers are available for specific purposes. The transducers shown on this image (from left to right) are a curved linear array, a sagittal transrectal probe, a mechanical wobbler, a transverse intraoperative linear array, an obstetrical linear array, and a small footprint cardiac transducer for use between ribs.*

ENDOCAVITY ULTRASOUND SYSTEMS

The transducer, which can be a linear, phased array (or mechanical sector scanner) is placed on the end of a rod. This rod is inserted into the rectum or vagina (see Figs. 2-17 and 2-18).

TRANSESOPHAGEAL TRANSDUCERS

A transesophageal transducer may be introduced into the esophagus to visualize the heart. This transducer provides a higher-resolution image than transthoracic echocardiography (Fig. 2-19).

INTRALUMINAL AND INTRACARDIAC TRANSDUCERS

Smaller transducers on the end of catheters can be introduced into vessels, the biliary duct, or the ureter (transluminal transducers). These transducers allow close visualization of the anatomy that is being examined. These transducers are not commonly used and may be found more frequently in research applications.

An intracardiac catheter has been developed more recently. A 10F catheter, which may be introduced into the right heart (Fig. 2-20), provides very high-resolution imaging and may be used for interventional and electrophysiology applications.

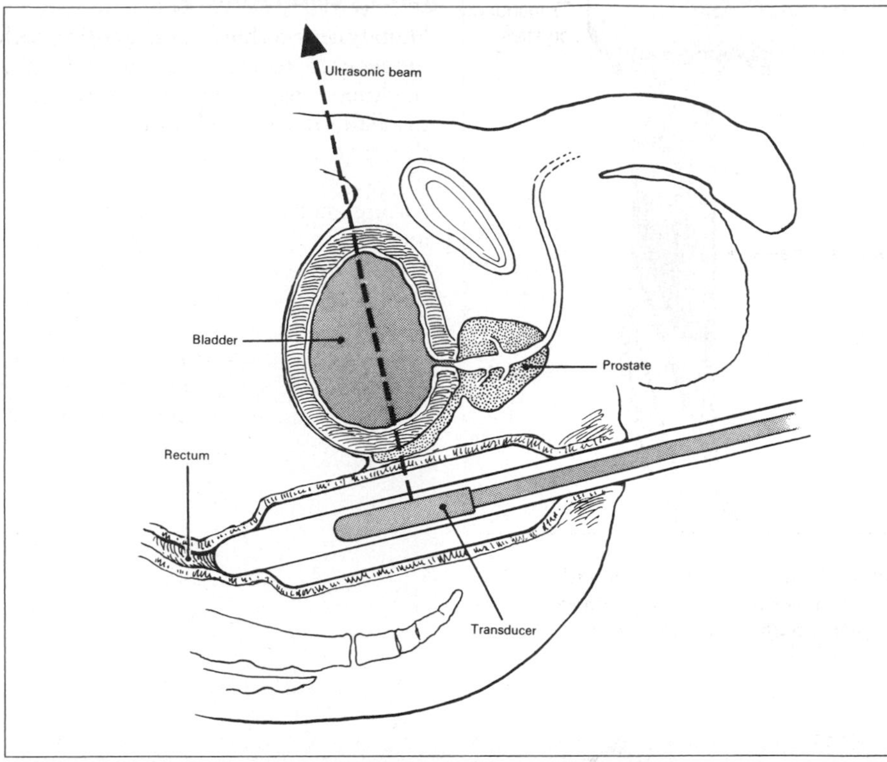

Figure 2-17. ■ *Rectal scanner. An ultrasound probe in a balloon filled with water is placed in the rectum adjacent to the prostate. The probe is moved or rotated to create an image of the prostate and bladder.*

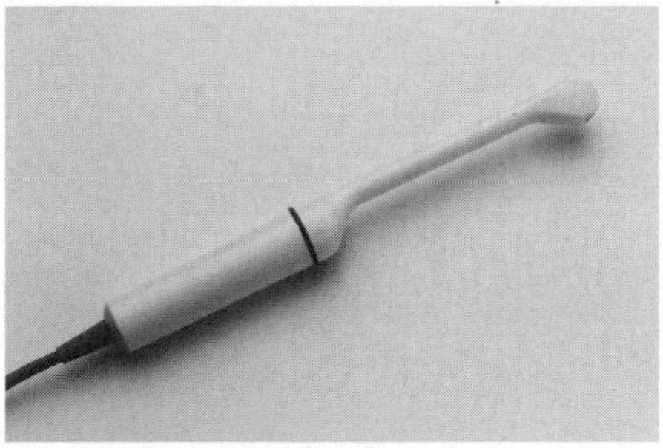

Figure 2-18. ■ *Photo of a endovaginal transducer.*

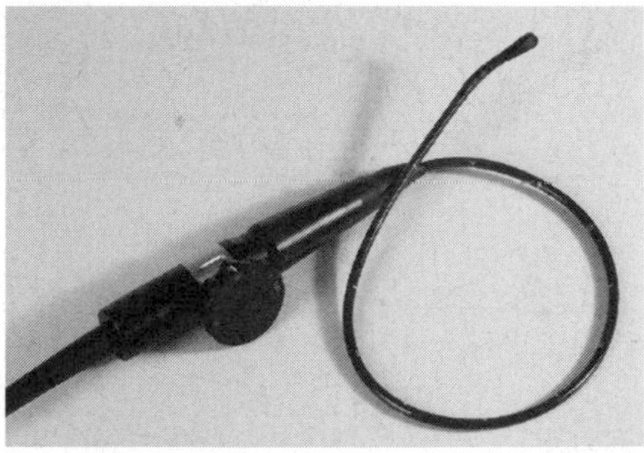

Figure 2-19. ■ *Photo of a transesophageal echocardiography transducer.*

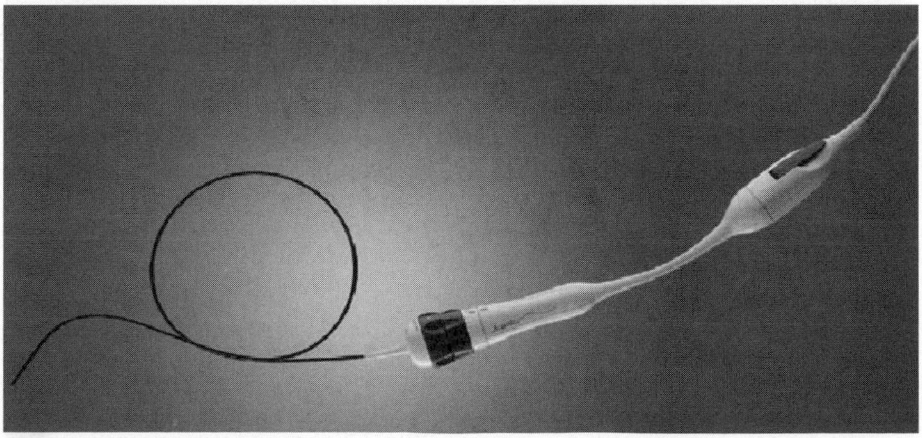

Figure 2-20. ■ *Photo of the AcuNav Intracardiac ultrasound catheter.*

OPERATIVE SYSTEMS

Standard ultrasound systems are modified so they can be used in a sterile fashion in the operating room. Special high-frequency ultrasound probes are used for this purpose (Fig. 2-21). Intraoperative transducers are designed with a size and shape to allow easy handling and positioning during intraoperative procedures.

Transducer Formats

There are a variety of transducer formats available in modern equipment, each suited to particular scanning applications.

- Linear Array. The linear format provides a rectangular image (Fig. 2-22A). This transducer is most useful in "small parts" and vascular imaging. Some linear-array transducers provide additional formats, increasing the variety of applications they may be used for:
    - Beam Steering. The ability to steer the grayscale image (Fig. 2-22B).
    - Virtual Format. The ability to display a trapezoidal image shape from a linear transducer, providing a wider field of view for imaging and measurements (Fig. 2-22C).
- Vector. A vector format provides a trapezoidal image (Fig. 2-22D). This small footprint transducer is often used in abdominal, gynecologic, and obstetric applications.
- Sector. The sector image is pie-shaped and is commonly used in cardiac, abdominal, gynecologic, obstetric, and transcranial imaging (Fig. 2-22E).
- Curved Array. A curved array transducer will provide a large field of view with a convex near field (Fig. 2-22F). This transducer is most commonly used in obstetrics; however, other applications include abdominal and gynecologic imaging.

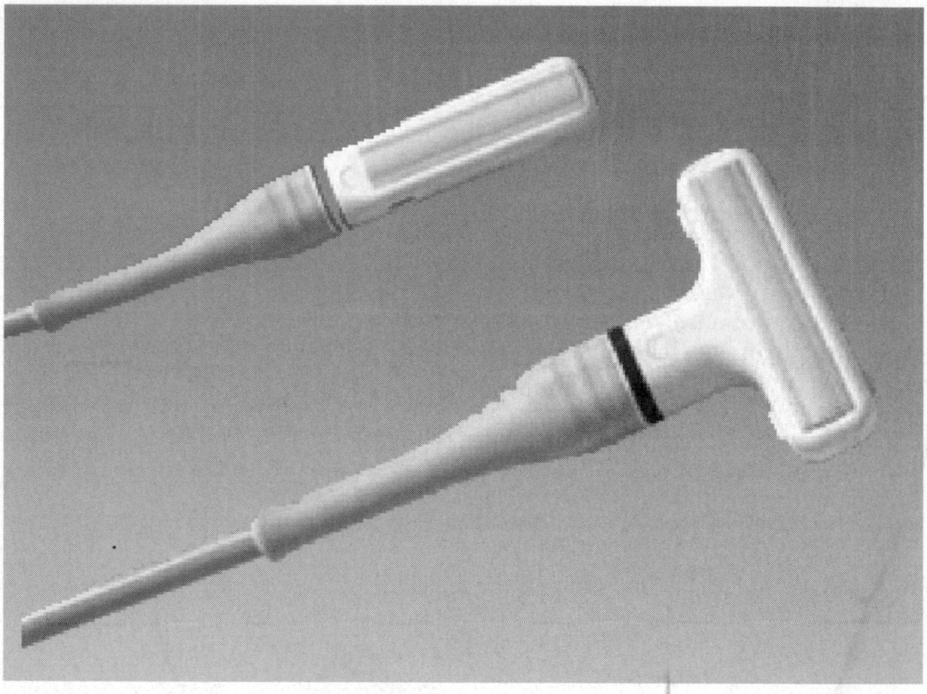

Figure 2-21. ■ *Intraoperative transducers are designed to allow easy access to anatomy. The transducers in this photograph are designed for abdominal, vascular, and gynecological applications.*

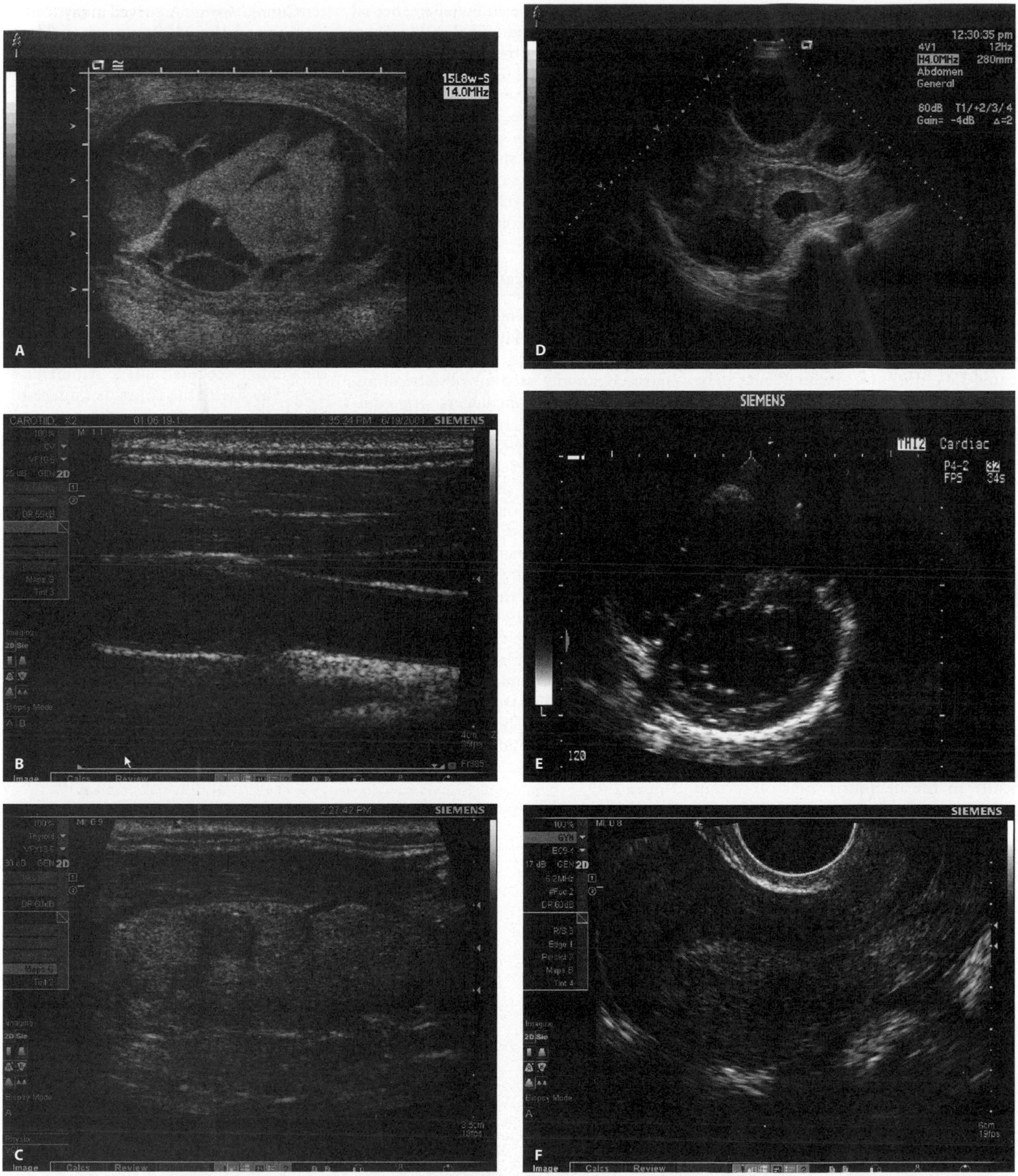

Figure 2-22. ■ *A. Note the square image in this linear array view of a complex mass. B. View of the carotid artery using beam steering. Note that the image is obliqued to the left to show plaque in the vessel. C. Trapezoid image of the thyroid. D. Vector format image of liver masses. E. Sector format image of the heart. F. Curved array image of the uterus.*

New Techniques For Improving The Image

3D IMAGING SYSTEMS

3D imaging capabilities have been increasing in popularity over recent years. The technologies used to acquire 3D images vary widely. Position-sensing techniques use specialized transducers or magnetic sensors attached to transducers to relate the transducer's position to the ultrasound system. This method allows for a very accurate display of the acoustic echoes. These systems are usually dedicated 3D ultrasound machines but can be "add-on" systems used in conjunction with standard ultrasound systems to display 3D images. Freehand 3D imaging is the least expensive and most commonly used technology. With freehand imaging, the ultrasound system assumes the transducer is moved at a particular speed and direction. This information is used in conjunction with specific algorithms to create a 3D image.

3D images may be displayed in two different ways: surface rendering or multiplanar rendering (MPR). In surface rendering, the ultrasound information is used to create a 3D display of an object's surface (Fig. 2-23). This technique is commonly used in obstetrics to display the face of a fetus. It may be helpful clinically in the demonstration of certain pathologies such as cleft lip/palate, neural tube defects, and abdominal wall defects.

MPR displays the ultrasound information in three orthogonal (perpendicular) planes from one sweep (Fig. 2-24). For example, by sweeping the transducer through the region of the kidney, the MPR display will show images in the sagittal, transverse, and coronal planes. The user can then cycle through different image frames to display the desired anatomy.

4D IMAGING SYSTEMS

4D imaging systems use specialized transducers to display the real-time motion of a 3D image. These systems are most commonly used for obstetrical applications. The transducers are commonly mechanical transducers, which are held in place while the ultrasound system controls the acquisition of the images by "rocking" the transducer crystals and displaying the 4D images.

The 4D image display usually comprises four components. The MPR display longitudinal, transverse, and coronal components of the volume-rendered display (Fig. 2-24). As in 3D imaging, the MPR display represents three imaging planes (Color Plate 2-1), which are orthogonal (perpendicular) to one another. These planes are known as the X-, Y-, and Z-axis. The acquisition plane (the direction in which the transducer is held) determines the orientation of the remaining two planes. It is important to understand the MPR planes and their orientation to one another when manipulating 4D images.

The amount of information within the MPR and volume-rendered images is determined at acquisition. The region of interest (ROI) is a tool that allows the user to determine the amount of data to be displayed in the 4D image (Color Plates 2-1 and 2-2). The ROI and volume rate are inversely proportional; therefore, it is imperative to choose an ROI that will allow you to demonstrate the anatomy while maximizing volume rate.

The volume of interest determines the amount of information displayed in the volume-rendered image (Color Plate 2-3). The size of the volume of interest is also used to maximize the volume rate of the 4D image. The 4D volume rendering is determined through manipulation of the MPR quadrants. All quadrants may be rotated around their X-, Y-, and Z-axis. The user may then synchronize the volume image to the desired quadrant. In Color Plate 2-5, the volume image was synchronized to the coronal image in the bottom left corner to display the endometrium. The small view plane (solid line in the upper left quadrant) determines the amount of information displayed in the volume-rendered image. In this example, a very thin view plane allows the user to display the endometrium clearly without obstruction by the anterior myometrium. Positioning the view

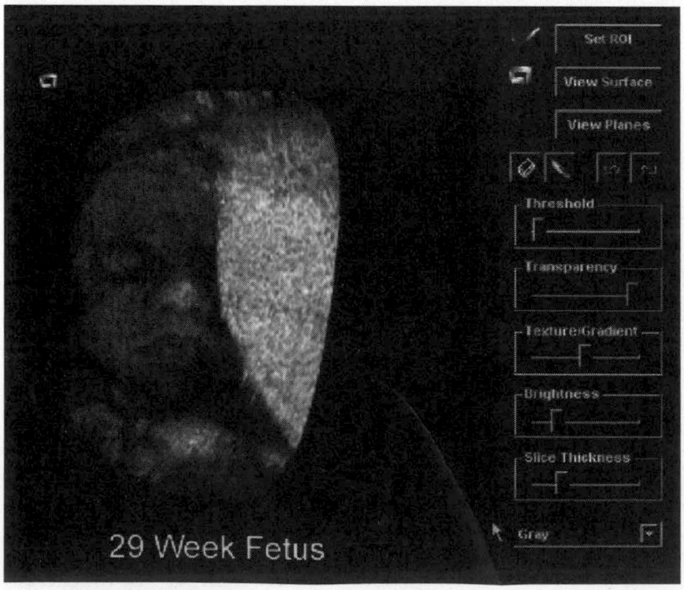

Figure 2-23. ■ *3D surface-rendered image of the fetal face.*

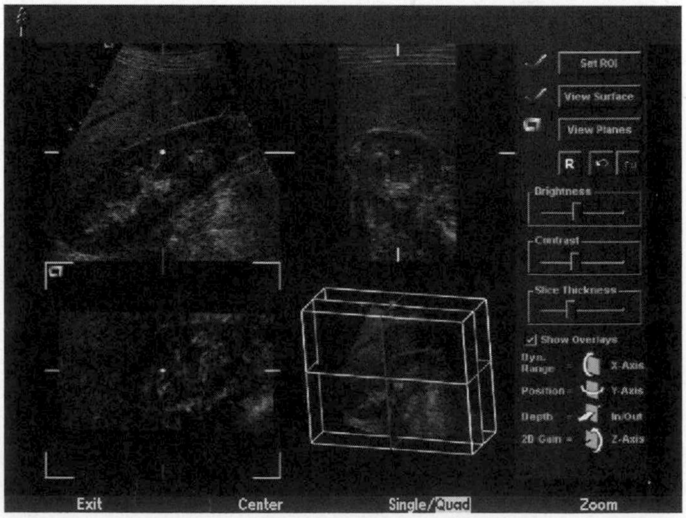

Figure 2-24. ■ *3D MPR image of an adult kidney. The longitudinal plane is demonstrated in the upper left quadrant; transverse in the upper right; coronal lower left; reference cube lower right.*

plane will help to remove unwanted information from the volume-rendered display.

Various types of rendering methods also affect the presentation of the volume-rendered display. The most common types of rendering methods are opacity, maximum intensity projection (IP), minimum IP, and mean IP. The opacity mode (Color Plates 2-3 and 2-5) blends volume data to demonstrate an object's surface anatomy. This technique is commonly used to show surface anatomy such as a fetal face or extremity. Opacity mode may be useful in diagnosing obstetrical anomalies such as cleft lip. Maximum IP (Color Plates 2-3 and 2-6) is used to highlight the maximum intensity signals in a volume-rendered image. This technique is used to emphasize hyperechoic structures such as fetal skeletal anatomy. Minimum IP is used to demonstrate the minimum values in the volume-rendered display. This method is used to emphasize hypoechoic structures such as hypoechoic lesions or large vascular structures. Mean IP (Color Plates 2-3 and 2-7) (also known as *x-Ray Mode*) is used to show the mean value of the pixels in the volume-rendered display. This method is used to enhance contrast resolution.

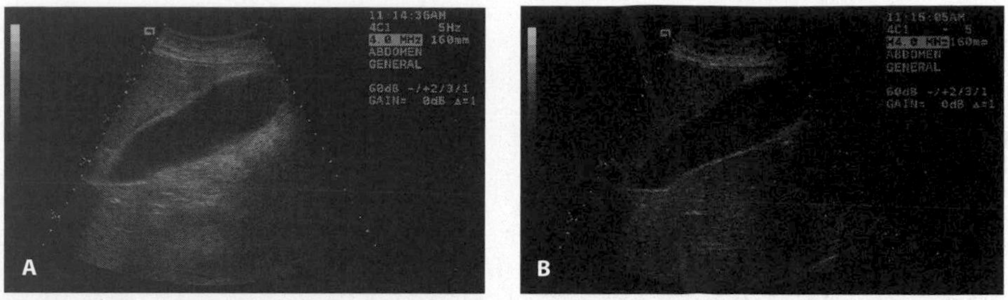

Figure 2-25. ■ *A. Standard image of the gallbladder on a technically difficult patient. B. Harmonic image of the same patient using tissue harmonic imaging. The overlying noise is removed, leaving a clean image demonstrating gallbladder sludge.*

HARMONIC IMAGING

Images are obtained from returning signals, which are a multiple of the transmitted (fundamental) frequency. The harmonic signal is created from the compression and relaxation of tissues during sound propagation.

Native Tissue Harmonic Imaging, Phase Inversion

With traditional ultrasound techniques, the ultrasound system transmits a pulse of a specific frequency and receives a pulse of the same frequency. This frequency is known as the *fundamental frequency*. As this fundamental frequency travels through tissues, the tissues compress and expand with the variations in acoustic pressure. This compression and expansion results in the generation of additional ultrasound frequencies, known as *harmonics*.

The harmonic frequencies are multiples of the transmitted fundamental frequency. (For example, if the transmitted signal is 2 MHz, the second harmonic frequency will equal 4 MHz.) The body's tissues generate these harmonic frequencies and therefore are only subjected to aberrations by the body wall once resulting in a cleaner signal. The challenge for the ultrasound system is to separate the clean harmonic signals from the fundamental signals (Fig. 2-25A,B). Tissue harmonic imaging removes noise from images, especially in patients that are difficult to image.

The simplest separation method is to lengthen the transmitted pulse. This technique will result in a clear separation of the fundamental and harmonic signals; a filter may then be applied to remove the fundamental signals. Although this type of separation is easy to implement, using a lengthened transmit pulse will result in a narrow bandwidth harmonic signal and degradation of image resolution.

Phase inversion techniques utilize multiple pulses on transmit. These transmit pulses vary in phase, which is maintained on transmit and receive. The harmonic signals generated by the tissue have a different shape and phase than that of the transmitted pulse (Fig. 2-26). By summing the received pulses, the ultrasound system cancels the fundamental frequencies (destructive interference) and adds the harmonic signals (construc-

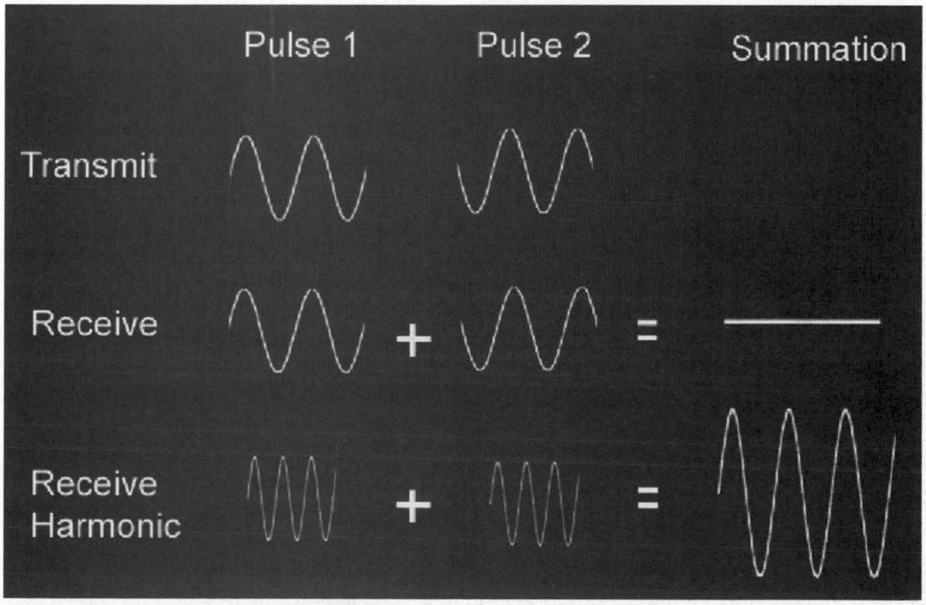

Figure 2-26. ■ *Phase inversion cancellation provides cancellation of fundamental signals while maintaining harmonic signal resolution.*

tive interference). The final result is clear separation of the harmonic signal.

IMAGE COMPOUNDING

Multiple ultrasound frames are averaged together to produce an image with increased contrast resolution.

SieClear Multiview Spatial Compounding, SonoCT

Image compounding averages multiple ultrasound frames to produce an image with increased contrast resolution. Image compounding may use image frames of varying frequency (transmit or frequency compounding) or by utilizing image frames from varying angles (spatial compounding).

Frequency Compounding

Frequency compounding uses multiple transmit pulses to obtain images of the same area with different frequencies. By varying the frequency, the system obtains varying speckle patterns, which are reduced when added together (Fig. 2-27). Frequency compounding will provide an increase in contrast resolution and may also provide an increase in penetration as compared to a similar noncompounded frequency. Compounding may occur by sending multiple fundamental frequencies or by sending a combination of fundamental and harmonic frequencies.

Spatial Compounding

Spatial compounding techniques interrogate the same area of interest from various locations. By averaging these ultrasound frames, the speckle pattern is reduced and will provide an image with increased contrast resolution. Spatial compounding may occur by varying the transmitted beam's location, varying the transducer position, or by varying the location of the receive beam.

Varying the transmitted beam's location occurs electronically by pulsing crystals in sequences that steer the ultrasound beam in a particular direction. This type of compounding will result in a decrease in frame rate, as multiple pulses are needed. Caution must be used with transmit techniques, as they may also result in a decrease in the appearance of acoustic markers such as posterior acoustic enhancement and shadowing. This is caused by obtaining image frames from oblique angles versus perpendicular to anatomy or pathology (Fig. 2-28).

Spatial compounding may also be achieved by using a single transmit pulse and varying the crystals that "listen" on receive. This technique typically maintains higher frame rates, as less transmit pulses are used (Fig. 2-29).

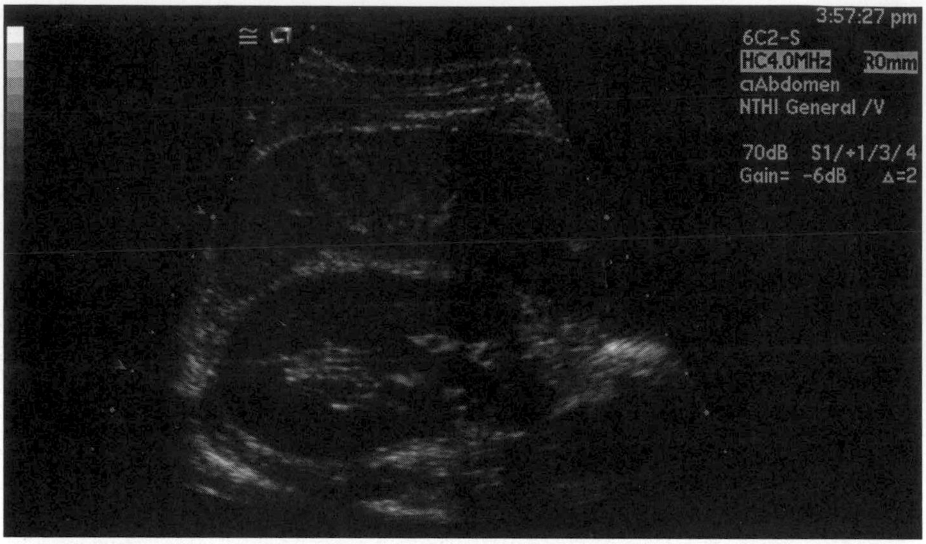

Figure 2-27. ■ *Compounding occurs by using two pulses of varying frequency. In this case, pulse 1 is fundamental and pulse 2 is harmonic. Varying frequency will result in increased contrast resolution.*

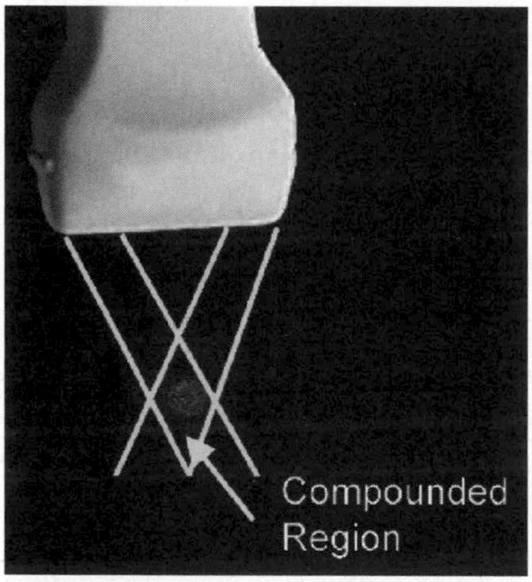

Figure 2-28. ■ *Spatial compound technique utilizing varying transmit angles. The area of compounding occurs in the region where transmit beams overlap.*

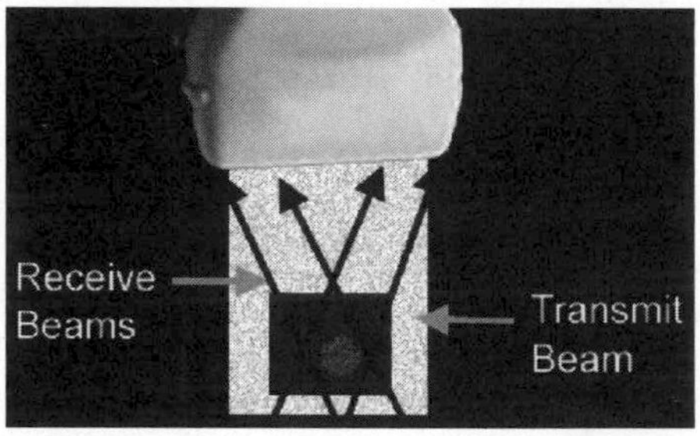

Figure 2-29. ■ *Spatial compound technique using varying receive angles. The area of compounding occurs in the region where receive beams overlap.*

SELECTED READING

Hykes D, Hedrick WR, Starchman D, eds. *Ultrasound Physics and Instrumentation,* 4th ed. Philadelphia: Mosby; 2005.

Kremkau FW. *Diagnostic Ultrasound: Principles and Instruments,* 6th ed. Philadelphia: WB Saunders; 2002.

Zagebski J. *Essentials of Ultrasound Physics.* St. Louis: CV Mosby; 1996.

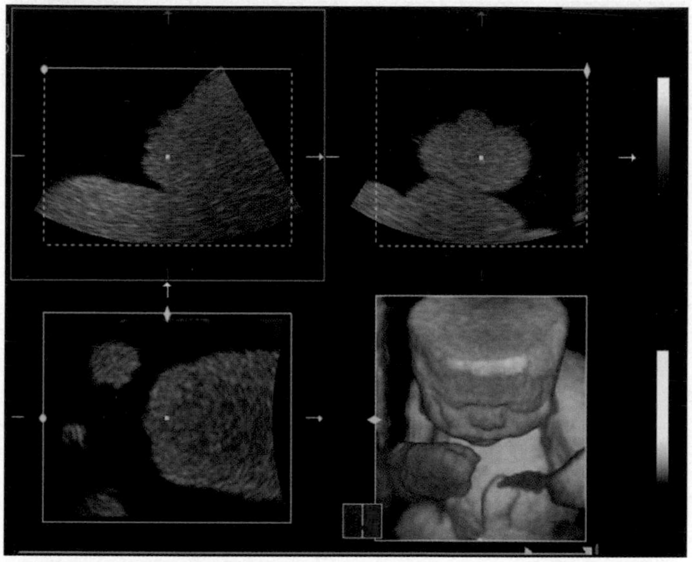

Color Plate 2-1. ■ *Four-dimensional views of a phantom. The longitudinal plane (acquisition plane) is demonstrated in the upper left quadrant, coronal in the upper right, transverse in the lower left. The volume rendered image is lower right.*

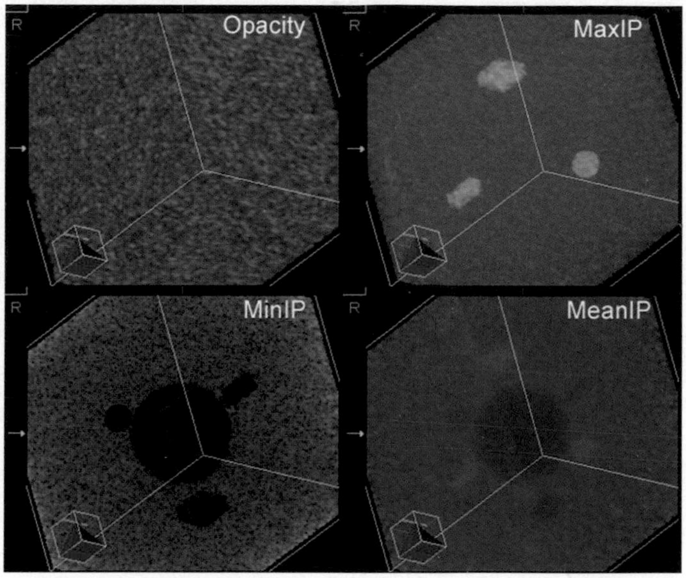

Color Plate 2-3. ■ *Comparison of opacity, max IP, min IP, and mean IP rendering modes using a contrast target phantom.*

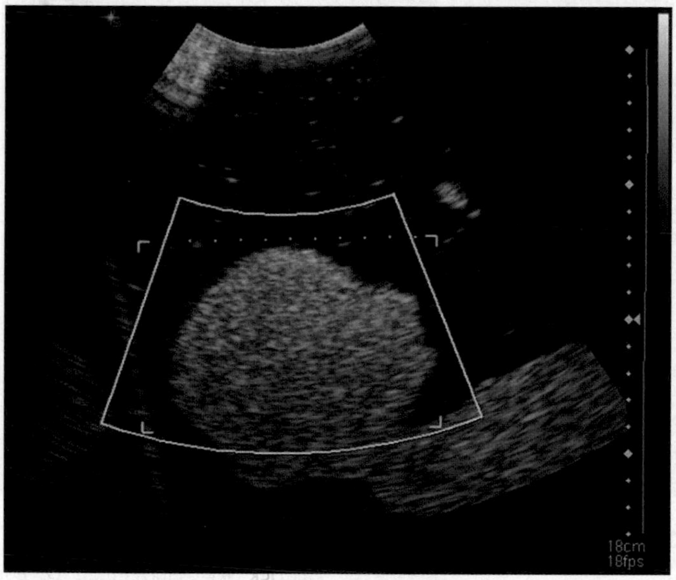

Color Plate 2-2. ■ *During acquisition setup, the region of interest (ROI) is used to determine the amount of information in the multiplanar rendering (MPR) and volume images. In this example, the ROI is outlined by the solid line. The volume of interest (VOI) is represented by the dotted rectangle.*

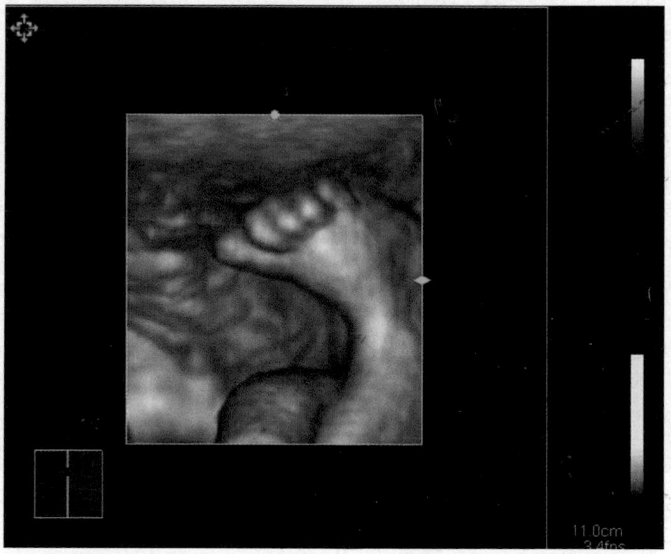

Color Plate 2-4. ■ *The opacity rendering mode is used to demonstrate surface anatomy, as seen in this image of a second trimester fetal foot.*

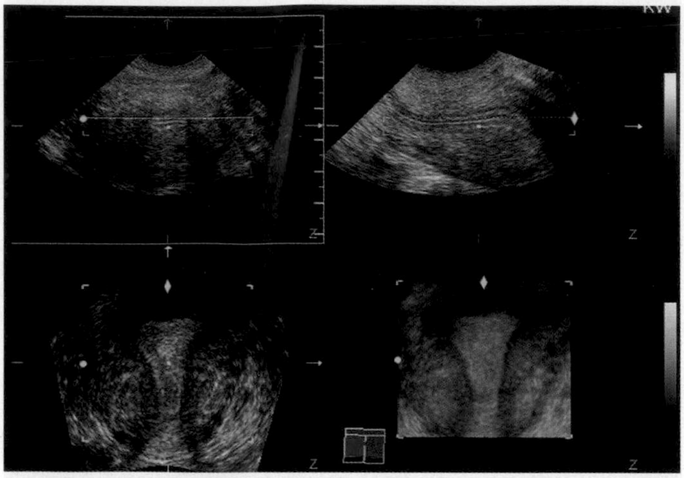

Color Plate 2-5. ■ *Four-dimensional views of the uterus. Transverse plane (acquisition plane) is demonstrated in the upper left quadrant, sagittal in the upper right, coronal in the lower left. The volume rendered image is the lower right image.*

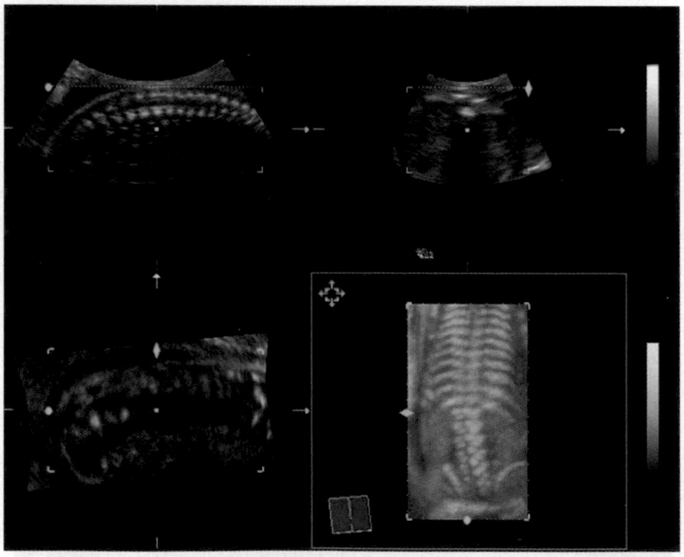

Color Plate 2-6. ■ *The max IP mode is used to highlight the fetal skeletal anatomy.*

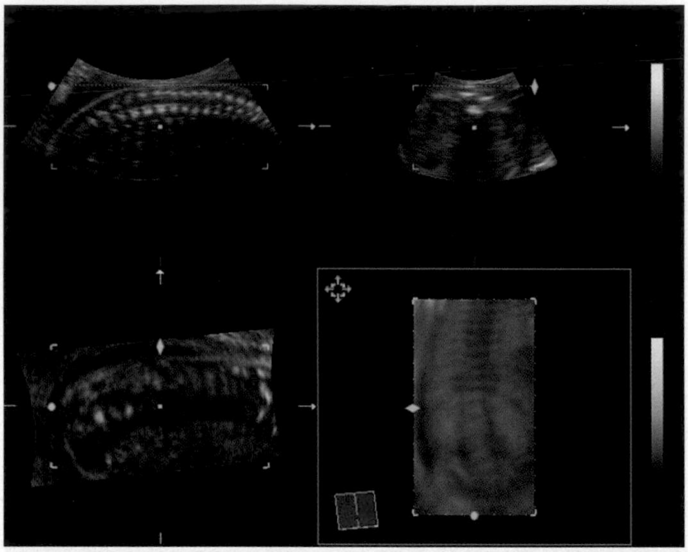

Color Plate 2-7. ■ *The mean IP is used to demonstrate the average pixel intensity to emphasize contrast resolution. In this image, one is able to see easily the fetal skeletal anatomy, as well as the soft tissue such as the fetal kidneys.*

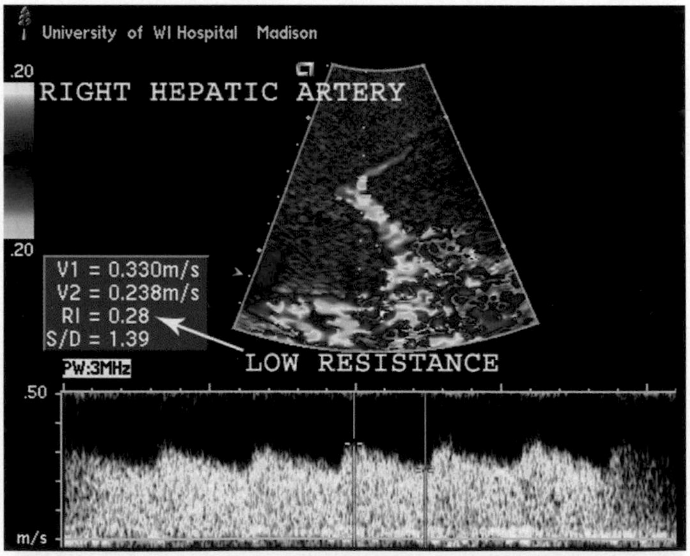

Color Plate 4-1. ■ *Pulsed Doppler sonogram from a low-resistance system (resistance index [RI] = 28%).*

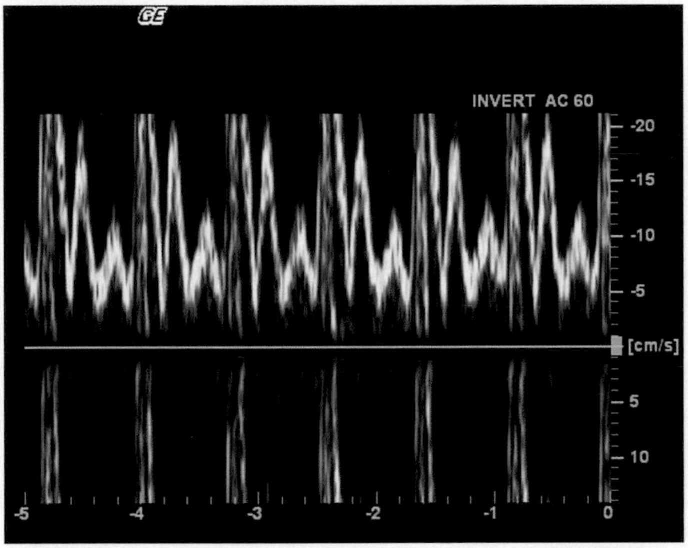

Color Plate 4-2. ■ *Pulsed Doppler aliasing. The velocity is too high to be displayed above the baseline; those velocities that exceed the set scale are therefore projected below the baseline (aliasing).*

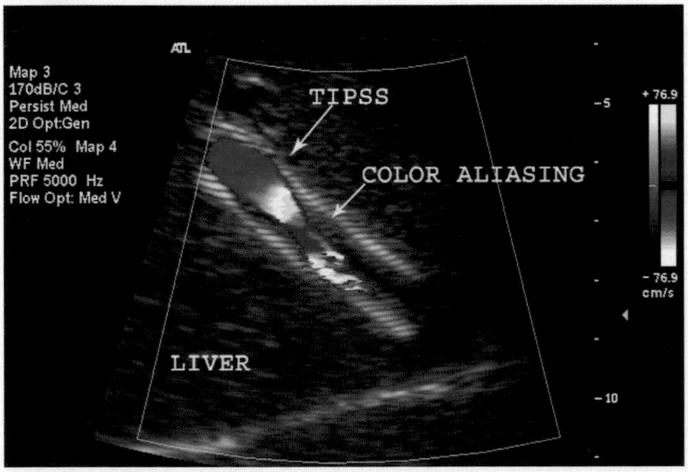

Color Plate 4-3. ■ *Color Doppler aliasing shows what happens with too low a pulse repetition frequency* (PRF)*—the color appears to change direction ("wrap around"). Note how flow going away from the transducer is initially blue and then increases to white before wrapping around to yellow and various shades of red.*

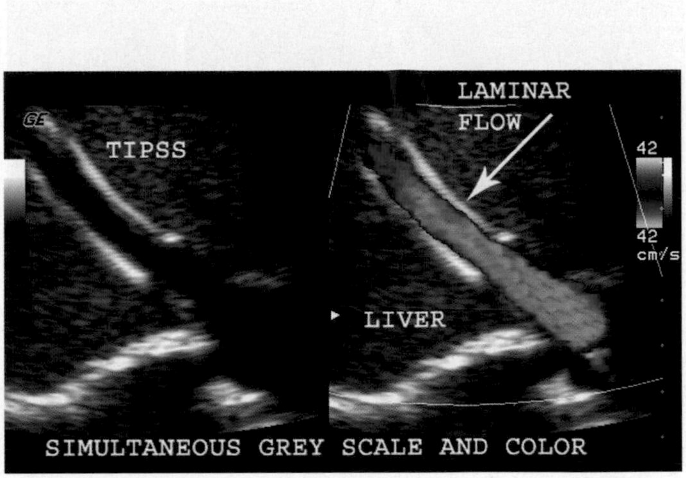

Color Plate 4-4. ■ *Color Doppler with correct setting of pulse repetition frequency* (PRF) *to remove aliasing. Note how flow going away from the transducer is represented.*

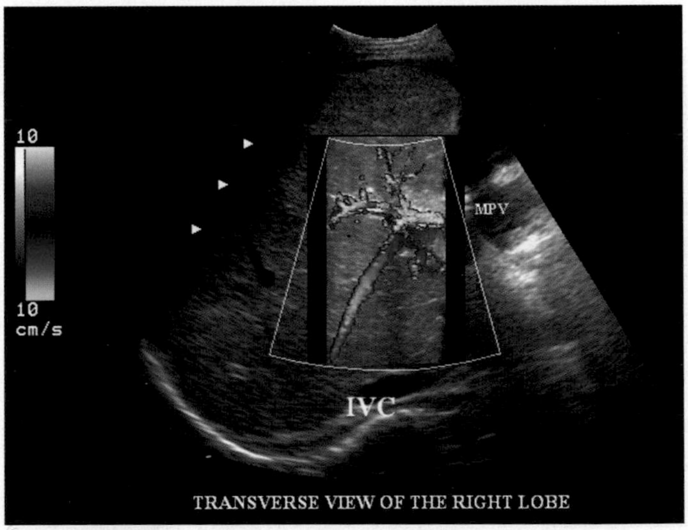

Color Plate 8-1. ■ *Budd-Chiari syndrome. Failure to visualize the hepatic veins should prompt one to consider hepatic vein thrombus. In this color Doppler image, the main portal vein* (MPV) *and its branches are well seen, but on this and other views, both grayscale and color, none of the hepatic vein branches could be seen flowing into the inferior vena cava* (IVC). *(Images courtesy of Phil Thompson.)*

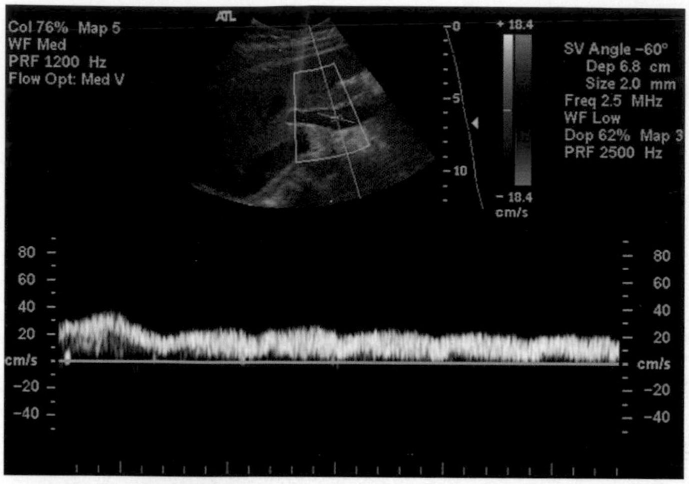

Color Plate 10-1. ■ *Pulsed Doppler waveform of the main portal vein* (MPV) *showing normal monophasic flow.*

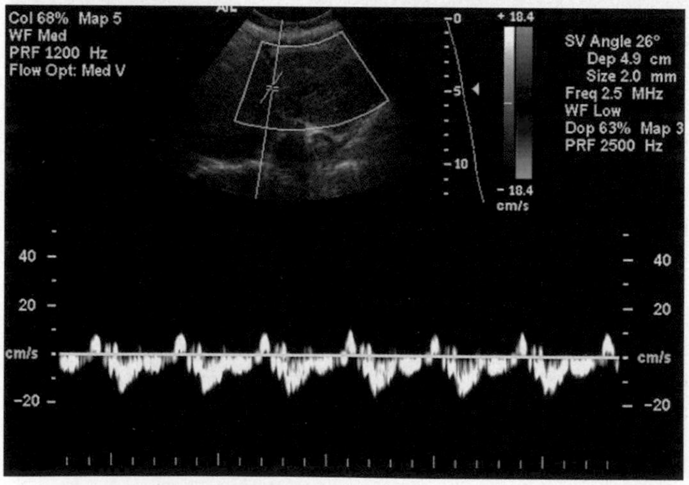

Color Plate 10-2. ■ *Pulsed Doppler waveform of the middle hepatic vein* (MHV) *showing normal pulsatile flow.*

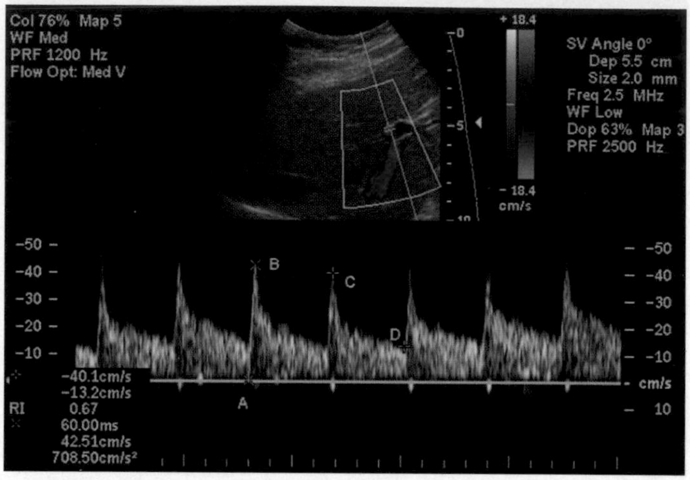

Color Plate 10-3. ■ *Pulsed Doppler waveform of the proper hepatic artery showing normal low resistance, pulsatile flow. Points A and B show the appropriate points to measure acceleration time. Point C corresponds with peak systolic velocity, and point D corresponds with end-diastole, both of which are used to calculate resistive index.*

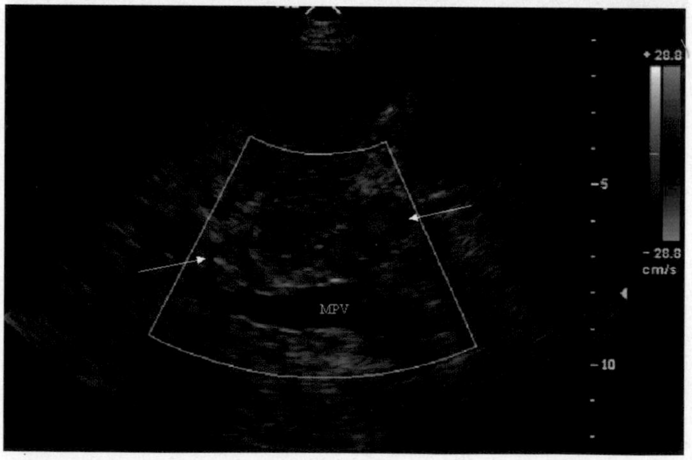

Color Plate 10-4. ■ *Cavernous transformation. Numerous collateral vessels are seen surrounding a thrombosed portal vein within the porta hepatis.*

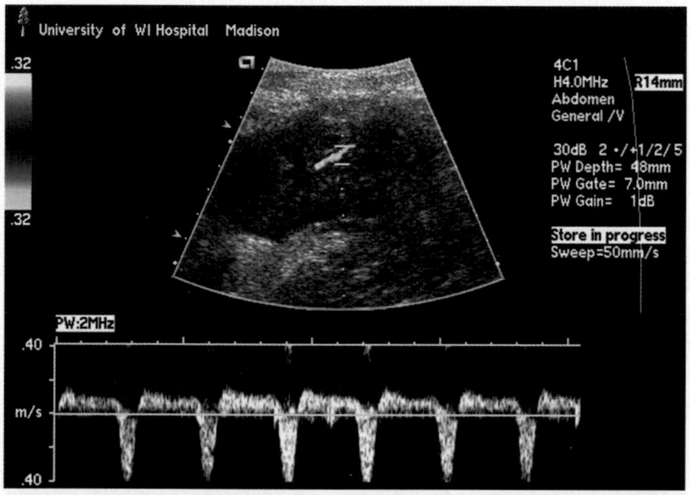

Color Plate 22-11. ■ *Reversed diastolic flow in a patient with venous thrombosis of his pancreatic transplant.*

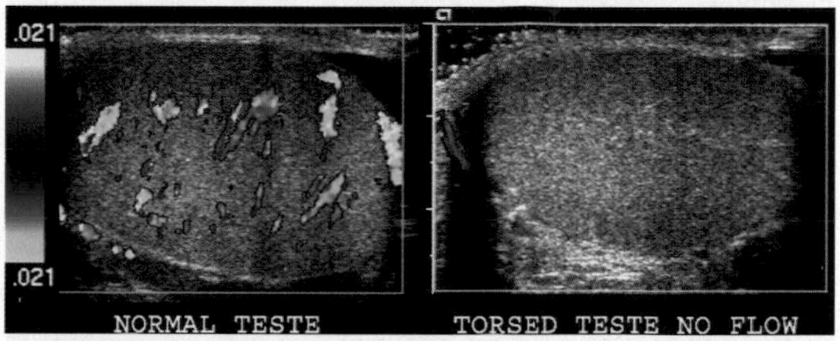

Color Plate 25-2. ■ *Left testicular torsion. The right testis shows a normal vascular flow pattern; there is a complete absence of color flow in the left testicle. Remember that when comparing the flow between the two testicles, do not change any technical parameters from side to side. This ensures an accurate assessment of flow in these paired organs.*

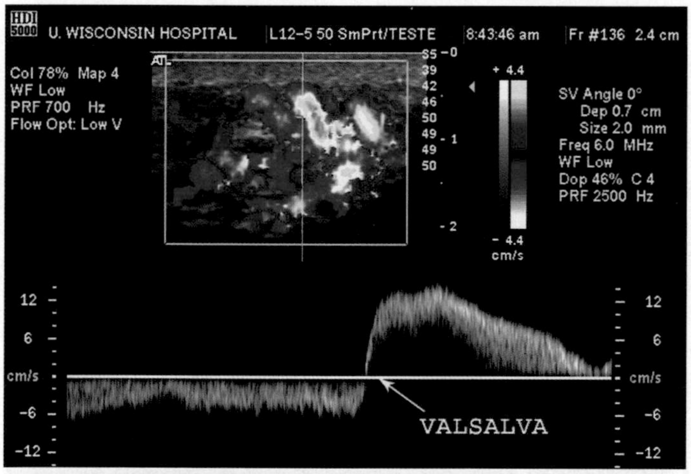

Color Plate 25-1. ■ *Doppler interrogation of the veins shows the venous flow reversing as intra-abdominal pressure increases when the Valsalva maneuver is performed.*

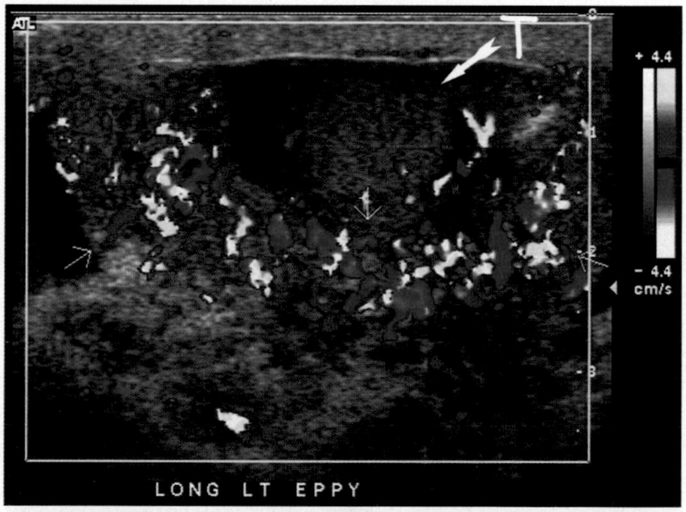

Color Plate 25-3. ■ *Epididymitis. The left testicle* (large arrow) *has normal blood flow within it. Contrast this to the surrounding epididymis* (multiple small arrows), *which is markedly hyperemic, demonstrating greatly increased color flow. A normal epididymis should only have a small amount of flow, less than the corresponding testicle.*

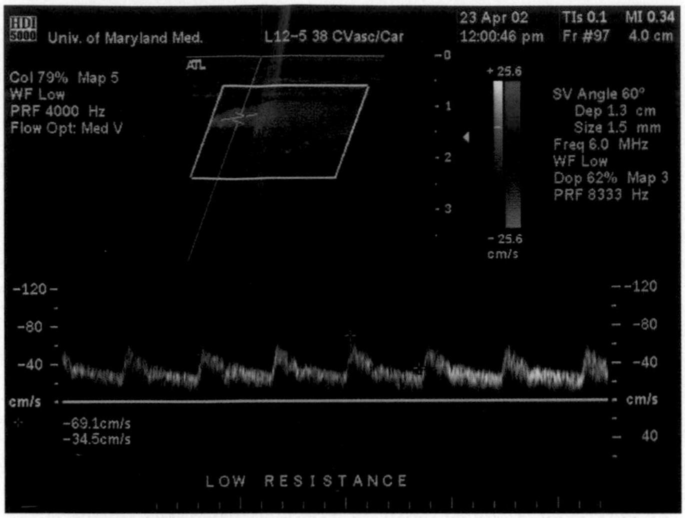

Color Plate 48-1. ■ *Low-resistance flow.*

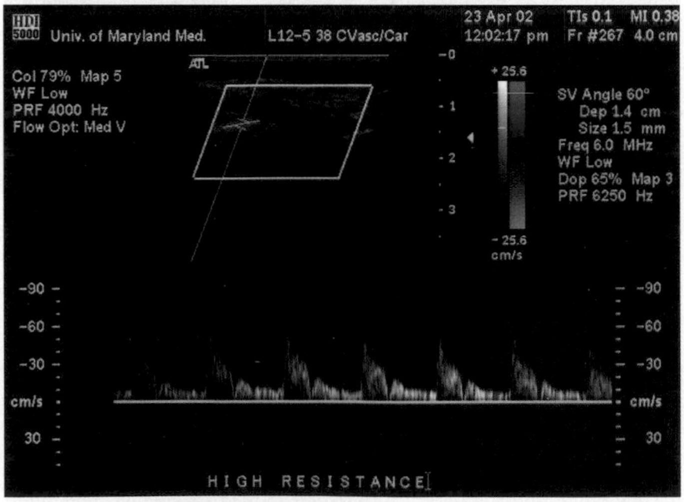

Color Plate 48-2. ■ *High-resistance flow.*

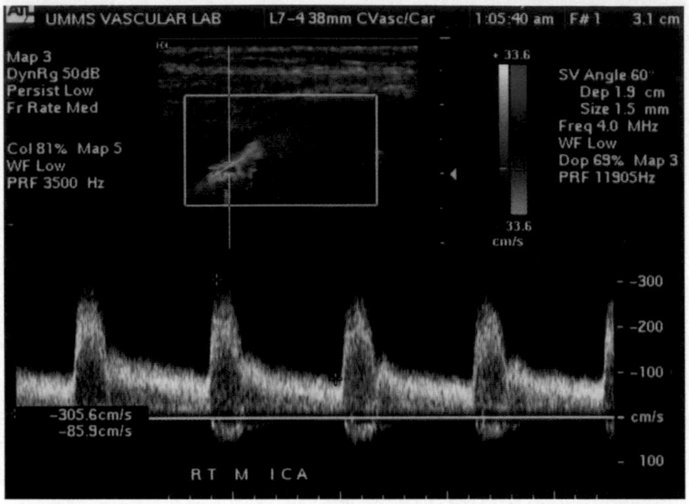

Color Plate 48-3. ■ *Fifty to seventy percent stenosis.*

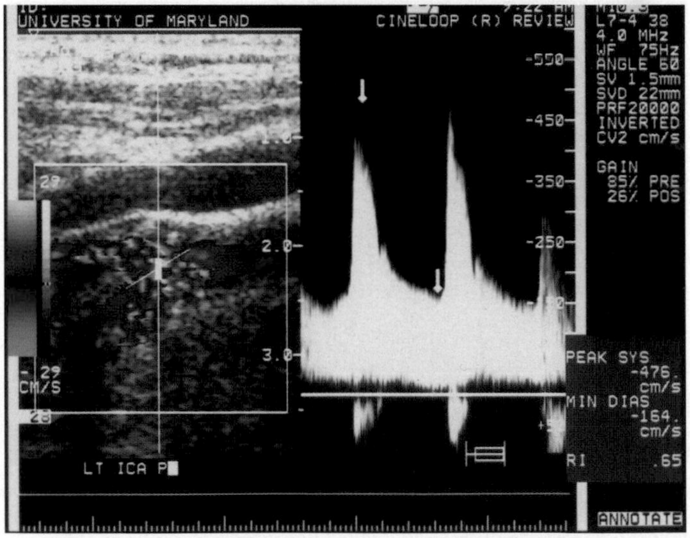

Color Plate 48-4. ■ *Eighty to ninety-nine percent stenosis.*

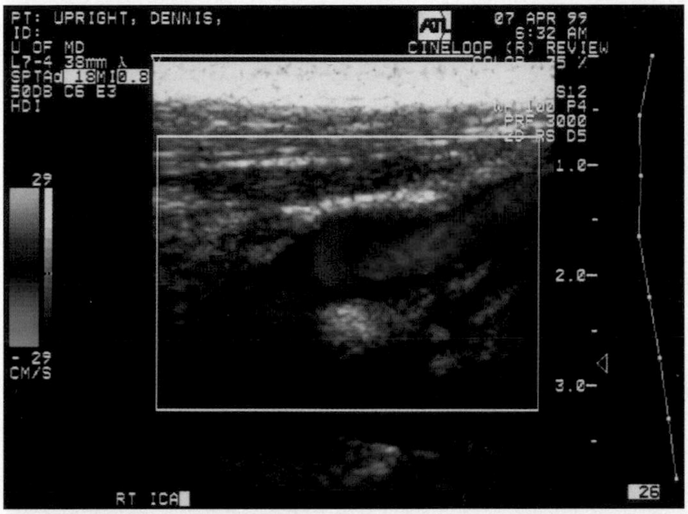

Color Plate 48-5. ■ *Occluded ICA.*

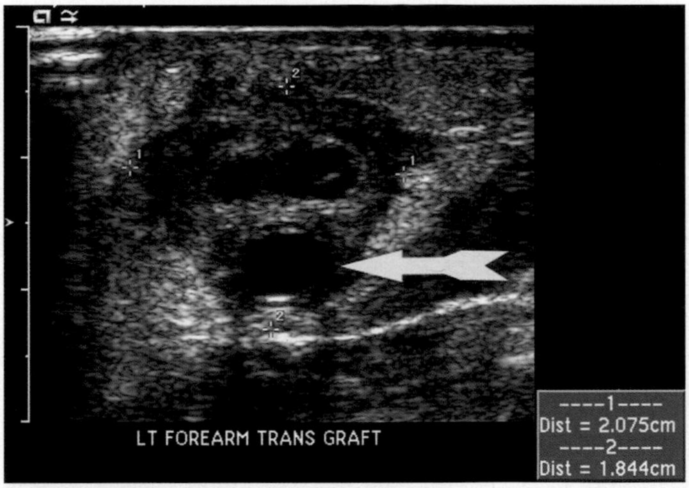

Color Plate 50-2. ■ *Transverse view of dialysis graft. The thick smooth walls of the shunt can be seen* (arrow). *The hematoma lies anterior to the shunt.*

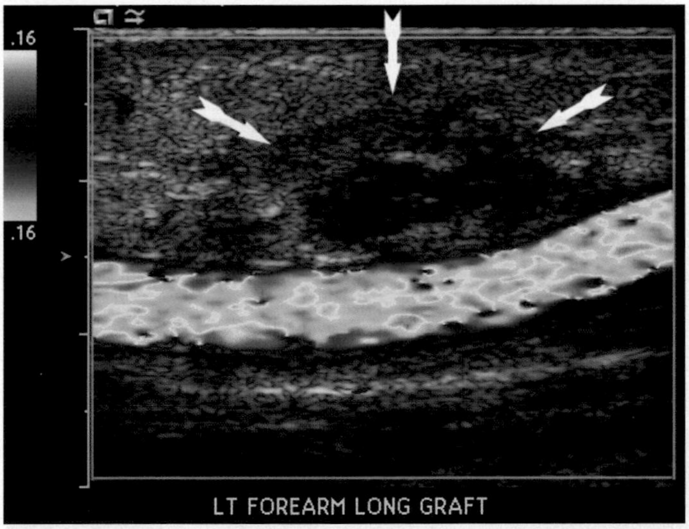

Color Plate 50-1. ■ *Sagittal view of dialysis graft. Pulsatile swelling around the graft was clinically suspected to be a pseudoaneurysm. Sonography showed that the mass was a hematoma* (arrows).

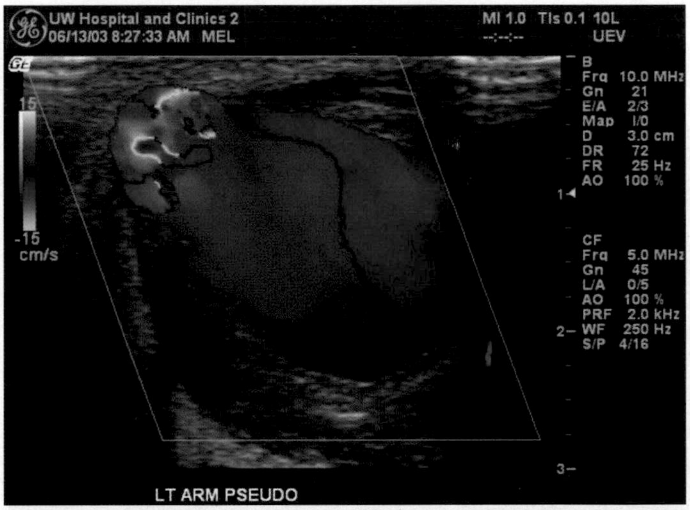

Color Plate 50-3. ■ *Large pseudoaneurysm of the area after surgical trauma. Notice that blood is flowing to and from the aneurysm, which is surrounded by a wall of clot.*

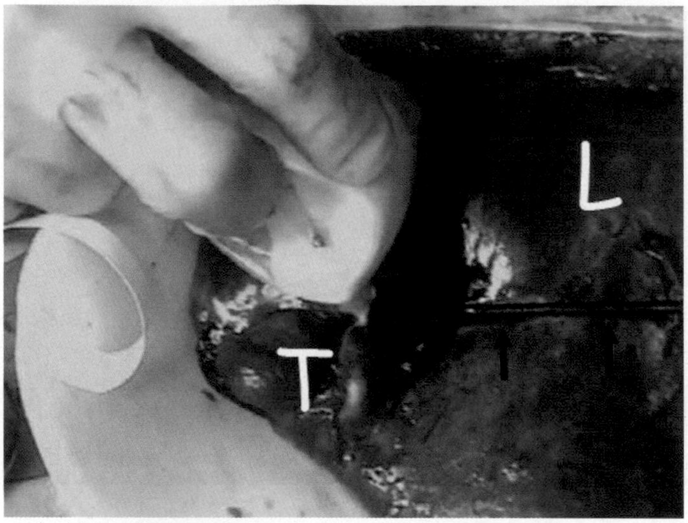

Color Plate 54-1. ■ *Intraoperative liver ultrasound. A sterilely draped, broad bandwidth (8–4 MHz), dedicated intraoperative ultrasound probe (under radiologist's fingers) is placed directly over a liver tumor* (T) *that is being ablated with an experimental microwave system* (black arrows). *Normal liver* (L).

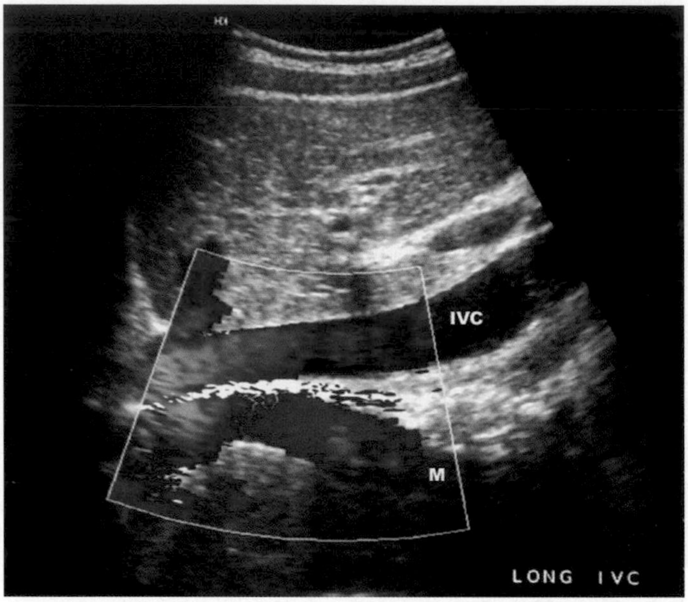

Color Plate 57-2. ■ *Longitudinal view of the right upper quadrant, showing a mirror image of the inferior vena cava* (M), *which fills with color signals just as the "true" inferior vena cava* (IVC) *does. The IVC and flow within it are mirrored in lung during deep inspiration. The mirror image shows red and blue because of the sector scan and curvature of the mirror.*

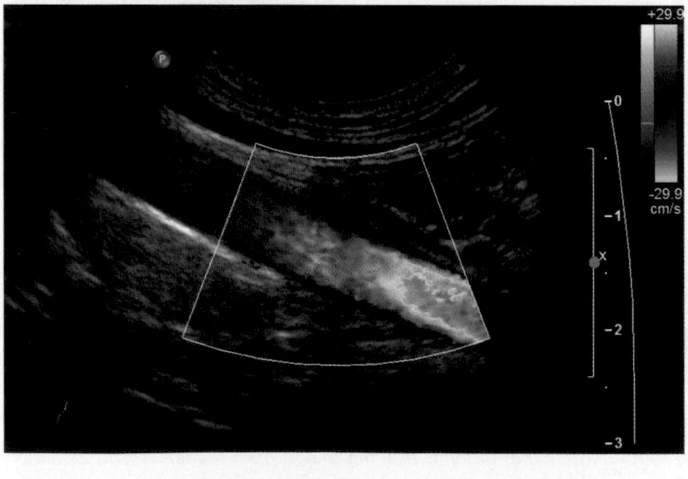

Color Plate 57-1. ■ *Color Doppler image of carotid artery. The abrupt color change from orange to blue represents aliasing, not change of flow direction. There is no black line between the orange and blue.*

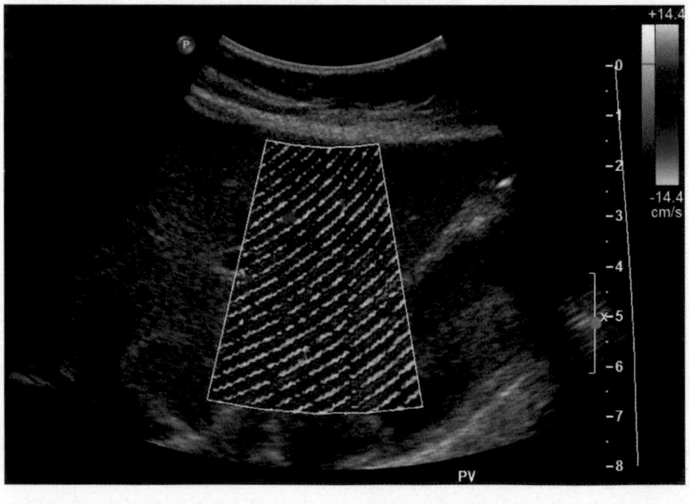

Color Plate 57-3. ■ *Color Doppler artifact resulting from electrical interference. (Image courtesy of Lino Piotto.)*

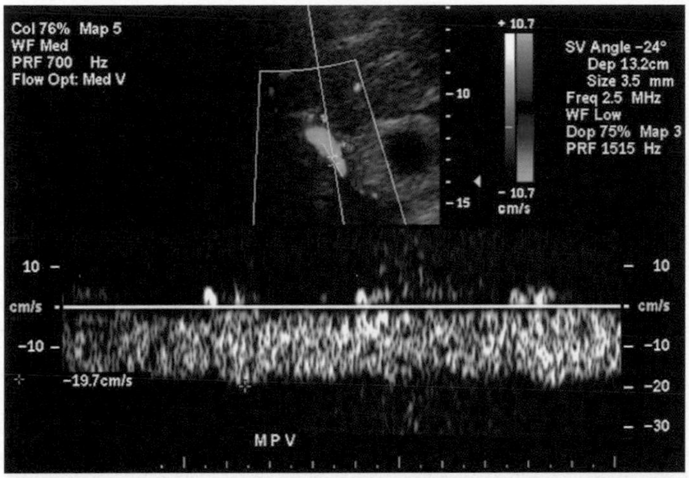

Color Plate 10-5. ■ *Hepatofugal flow within the main portal vein* (MPV) *in a patient with portal hypertension.*

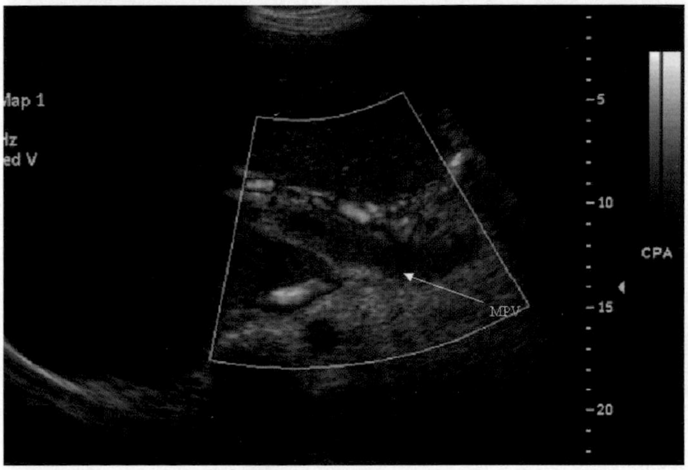

Color Plate 10-6. ■ *Longitudinal image of a thrombosed main portal vein* (MPV). *Clot can be seen with the vessel. Power Doppler depicts the presence of flow within surrounding collateral vessels, but not within the MPV.*

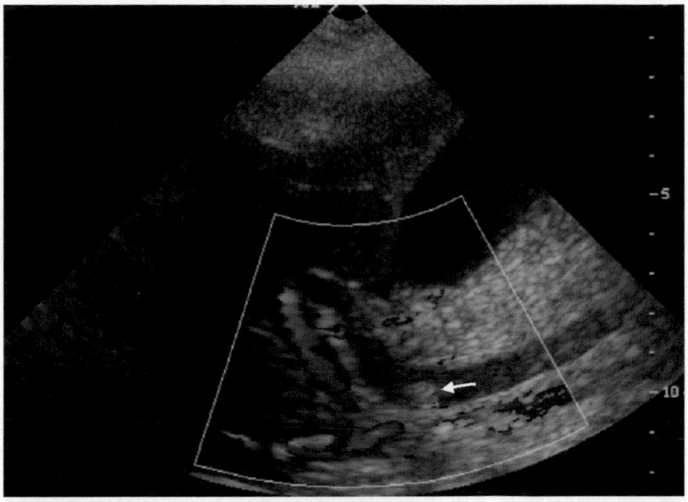

Color Plate 10-7. ■ *Longitudinal image of the common bile duct* (CBD) *containing a stone in the midportion.*

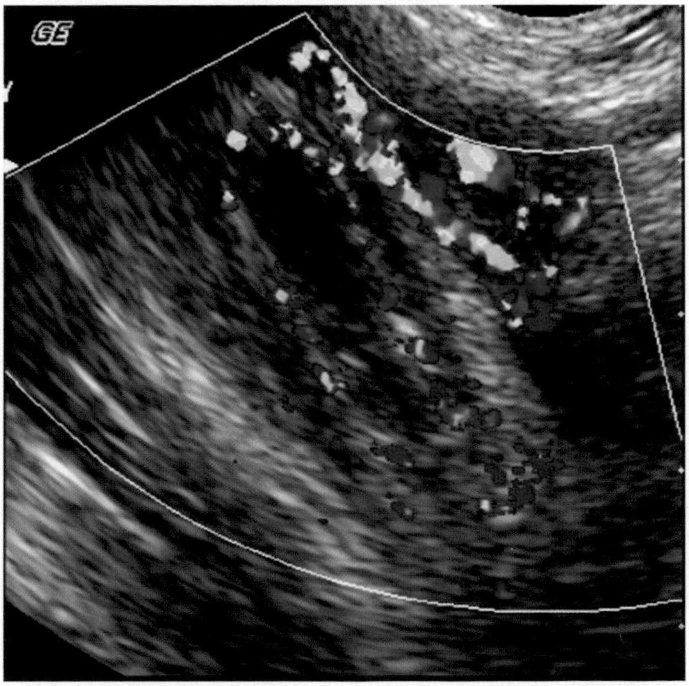

Color Plate 15-1. ■ *Inflamed appendix. Despite graded compression, the appendix is over 6 mm in diameter with thick walls. It is extremely tender. Note the echogenic inflamed omentum* (T) *alongside the appendix giving the appearance of thyroid tissue. Color flow shows increased vascularity along the walls of the appendix.*

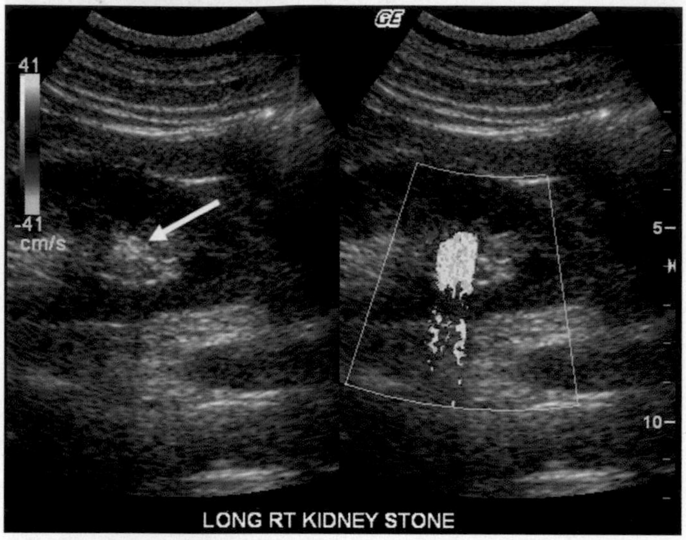

Color Plate 20-1. ■ *A subtle 1-cm stone in the lower pole of the kidney could easily be missed on grayscale imaging* (left, white arrow) *but is dramatically highlighted by twinkle artifact* (right).

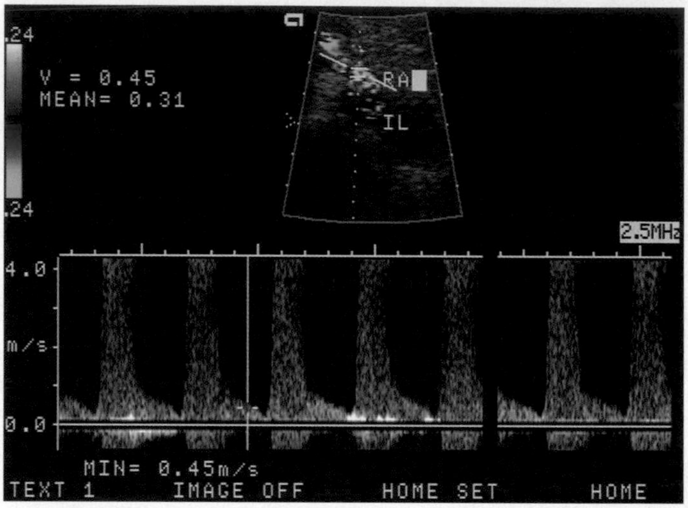

Color Plate 22-1. ■ *Increased velocities greater than 3.0 m/sec, indicating renal artery stenosis.*

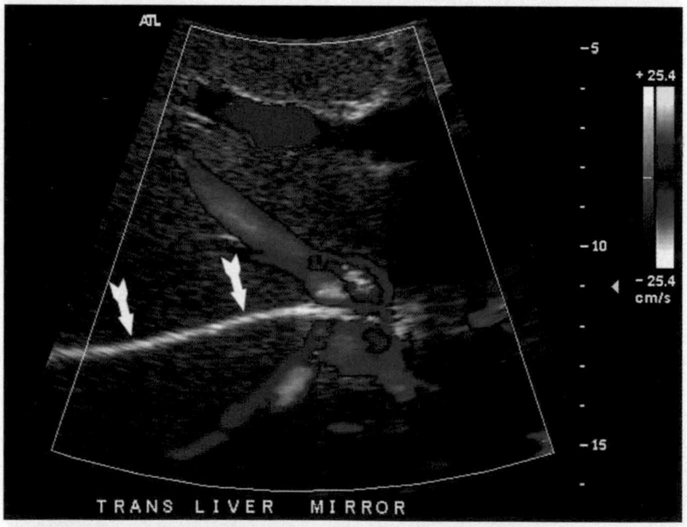

Color Plate 21-1. ■ *Ultrasound showing mirror artifact projecting right hepatic vein above the diaphragm* (arrows), *mimicking blood flow within the lung. Blue is the normal right hepatic vein, whereas red vessel on the other side of the diaphragm is the mirror artifact.*

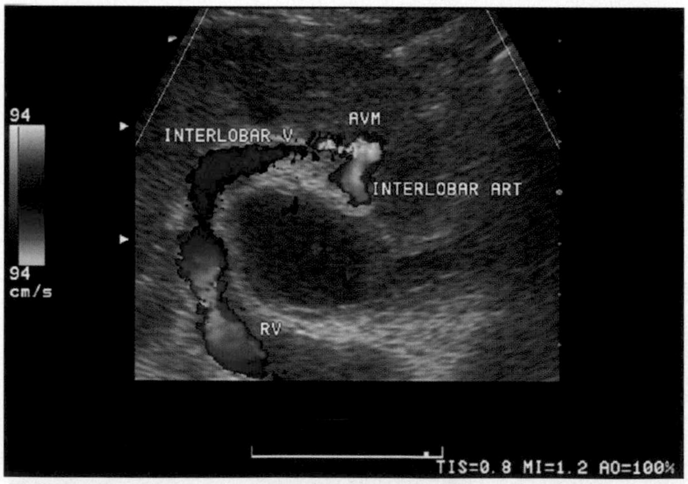

Color Plate 22-2. ■ *Intrarenal arteriovenous fistula* (AVM) *after a renal biopsy.*

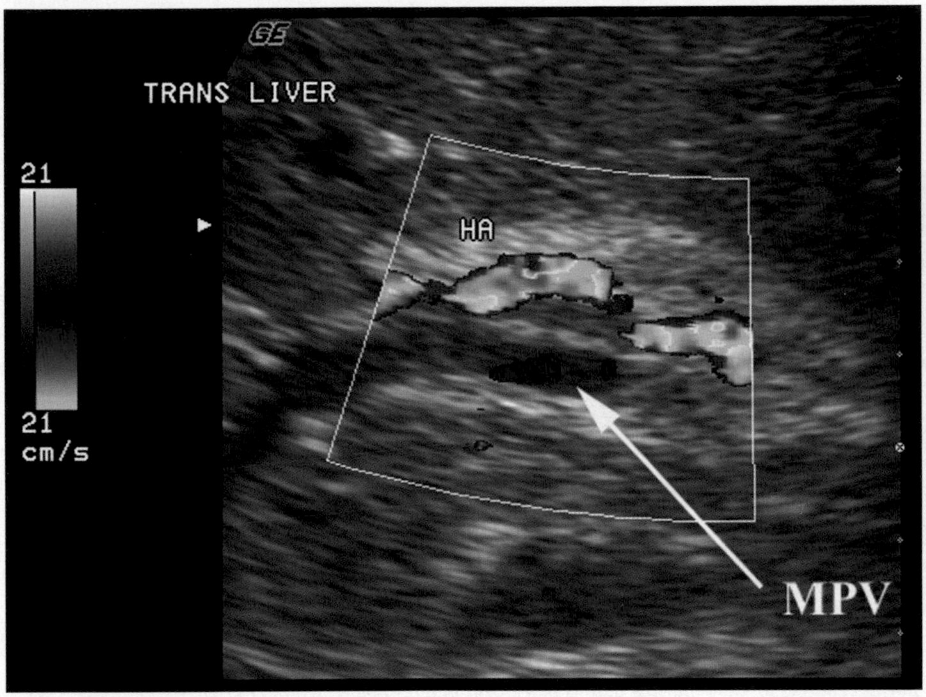

Color Plate 22-3. ■ *A magnified image of the normal proper hepatic artery after liver transplant.*

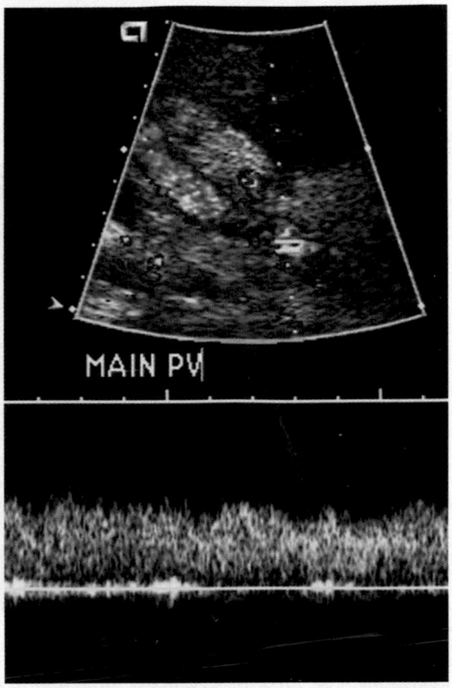

Color Plate 22-5. ■ *Normal Doppler signal from the main portal vein in a liver transplant patient.*

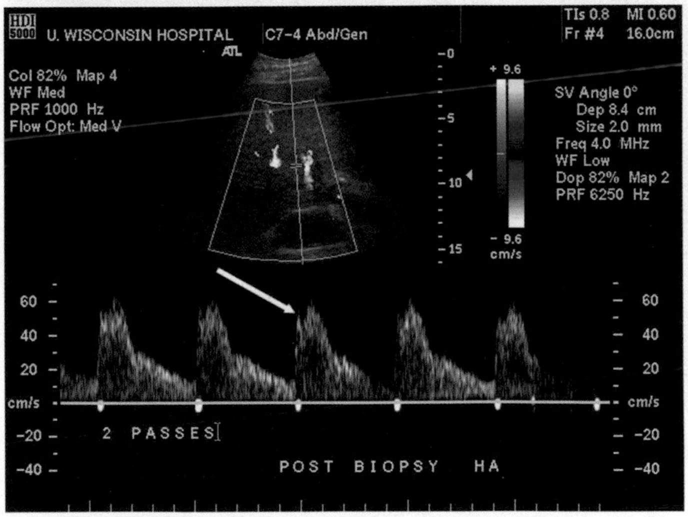

Color Plate 22-4. ■ *Doppler signal of a normal hepatic artery. Note early systolic peak* (ESP, arrow) *and rapid early systolic rise time, both indicators of a widely patent feeding artery.*

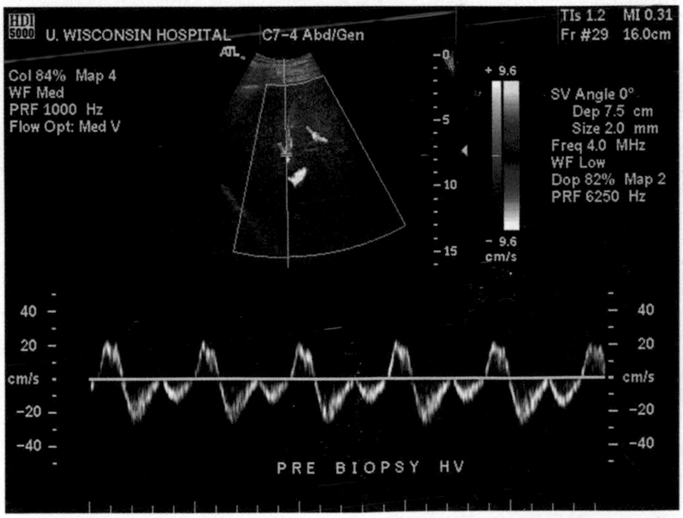

Color Plate 22-6. ■ *Normal hepatic vein signal. Note the direction of flow is predominantly toward the inferior vena cava* (IVC), *although the normal triphasic waveform with atrial kick can be seen.*

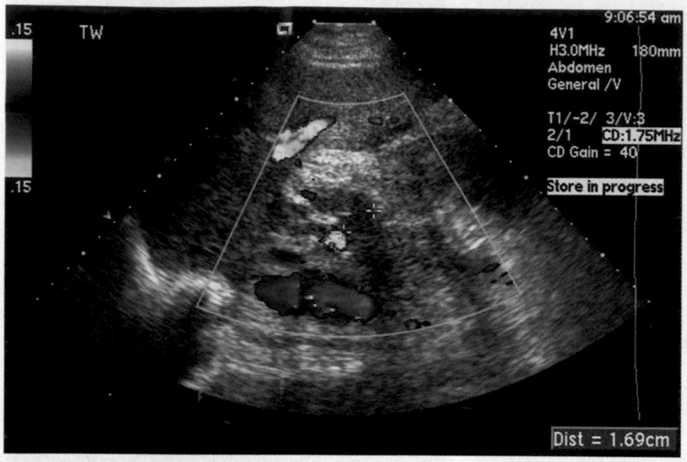

Color Plate 22-7. ■ *Portal vein thrombosis in a patient status after liver transplant showing absence of flow within the portal vein* (cursors).

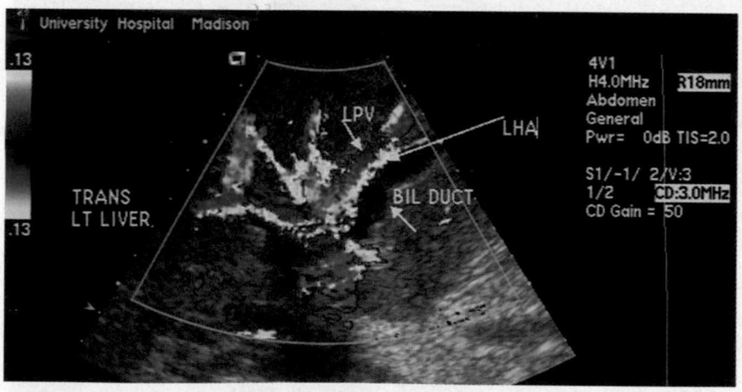

Color Plate 22-8. ■ *Classic biloma. Color Doppler shows dilated bile duct adjacent to left portal vein (LPV) and artery (LHA).*

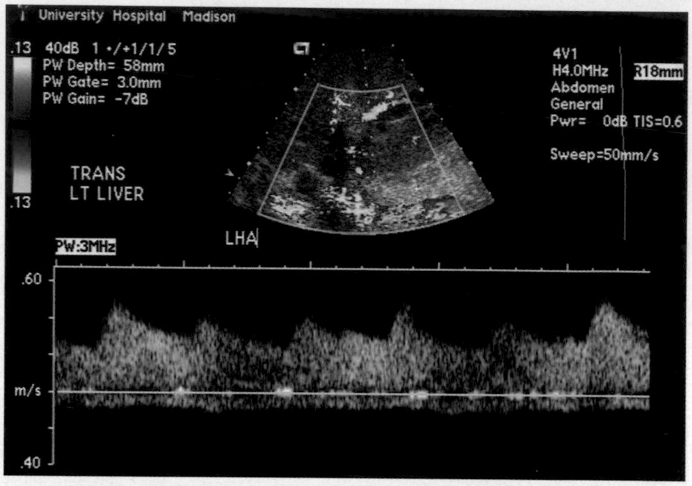

Color Plate 22-9. ■ *Classic biloma. Pulsed Doppler depicts classic tardus parvus waveform in left hepatic artery (LHA).*

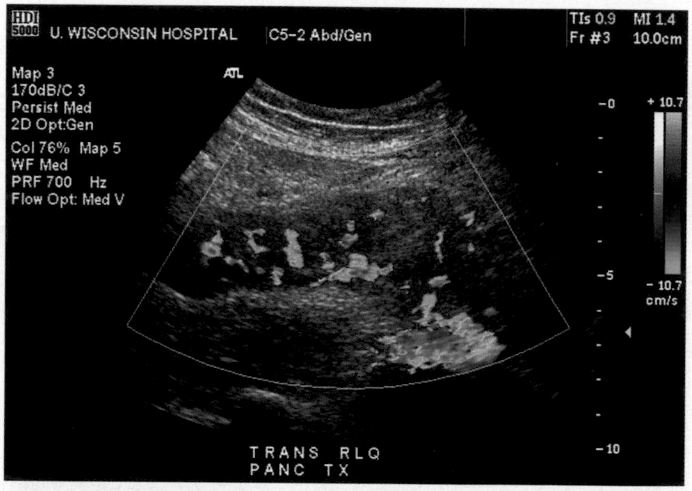

Color Plate 22-10. ■ *Normal flow within a pancreas transplant.*

Knobology

MIMI MAGGIO SAYLER
BARBARA DEL PRINCE

3

KEY WORDS

Acoustic Power/Transmit Power. A control that varies the amount of energy the transducer transmits to the patient; power should be used at the lowest level consistent with satisfactory image quality.

Alternate Color. A control that switches between various forms of color (e.g., color Doppler and color Doppler energy).

Annotation Keys. Allow labeling of the image. May consist of preprogrammed keys or a keyboard for typing.

B-Color. Colorizes the grayscale to enhance contrast resolution.

Body Markers. Provide a drawing of the specific area being examined (e.g., abdomen, pelvis, breast) to aid in labeling of the image.

Calipers. Measurement tool.

Caps Lock. Allows either lower- or uppercase characters to be typed.

Caret. Arrow denoting the location of the transmit zone or focal zone.

Cine Loop/Playback. The system memory stores the most recent sequence of image frames before the freeze button is pressed. The operator can then review the sequence of images.

Color Doppler. Activates the system's color Doppler mode.

Delta. A control that varies the contrast resolution in an image without sacrificing detail resolution.

Depth. Varies the depth to which the echoes are displayed. The maximum depth varies depending on the transducer used.

Dual Image. Allows the display screen to be split in order to show two views of an image or to compare the anatomy of the abnormal side with that of the normal side.

Dynamic Range/Log Compression. The range of intensity from the largest to the smallest echo that a system can display.

Edge. A two-dimensional edge enhancement function. Enhances contrast or detail resolution by adding more or less smoothing to the image pixels.

Ellipse. Measurement tool used in circumference measurements.

Freeze. All display data (real-time image frames) start and stop with this control. An image cannot be printed or measured until it is frozen.

Gain. Regulates the degree of echo amplification (the brightness of the image).

M-Mode. Activates the motion mode (M-mode) used in cardiac imaging to trace movements of the cardiac tissue.

MultiHertz. Allows the user to choose between different sending frequencies of the transducers.

Needle Guide (Biopsy Guide). Activates graphics on the display screen corresponding to the intended path of the needle during invasive procedures.

Persistence. Control that allows the accumulation of echo information over a longer period. Subtle texture differences can be enhanced using this control.

Postprocessing. This control may be adjusted in real time or while the image is frozen. The postprocessing alters image aesthetics by placing more or less emphasis on specific echo levels.

Preprocessing. Control that adjusts edge enhancement of image pixels. This control must be used before freezing an image.

Print. This control activates the camera to document the image on the screen.

Pulsed-Wave Doppler. Activates the spectral Doppler mode.

Exam/Recall Application/Recall Set/Program Select. Pre-established parameters that are specific for the different studies performed. Preprocessing, persistence, and postprocessing are among the preset parameters.

Slide Pots. Time gain compensation (TGC) controls can be adjusted in short segments with the use of slide pots.

Space-Time. Allows the user to enhance the image for increased frame rate or increased resolution.

Tissue Equalization Technology. Adjusts the overall gain, lateral gain and the depth gain compensation (DGC) curve to display an image of uniform brightness.

Time Gain Compensation (TGC), Time Compensation Gain (TCG), Depth Gain Compensation (DGC). These controls compensate for the loss (attenuation) of the sound beam as it passes through tissue.

Trace. Measurement tool that allows the user to trace the outline of an area that is being measured. Often used to obtain circumference measurements.

Trackball/Joystick. Controls the movements of the annotation cursor, calipers, focal zone carets, and cine loop.

Transducer Choice. Permits the activation of the different transducer ports.

Transmit Zone/Focal Zone. The transmit zone enhances the resolution of an area in the image by electronic focusing. The frame rate is lowered when multiple foci are used on an image.

Triplex. Allows the simultaneous use of grayscale imaging and spectral, as well as color Doppler.

Use of Knobs

The basics of knobology are interchangeable between different types of real-time systems. Controls specific to Doppler technology are described in Chapter 4 (Doppler and Color Flow Principles). Learning to use the knobs effortlessly is an important part of the art of ultrasonic scanning.

GAIN

The system gain controls the degree of echo amplification, or brightness of the image. The gain control is usually measured in decibels, an arbitrary measurement of sound amplitude (Fig. 3-1). Care must be taken with the use of gain. Too much overall gain can fill artifactual echoes into fluid-filled structures, whereas too little gain can negate real echo information.

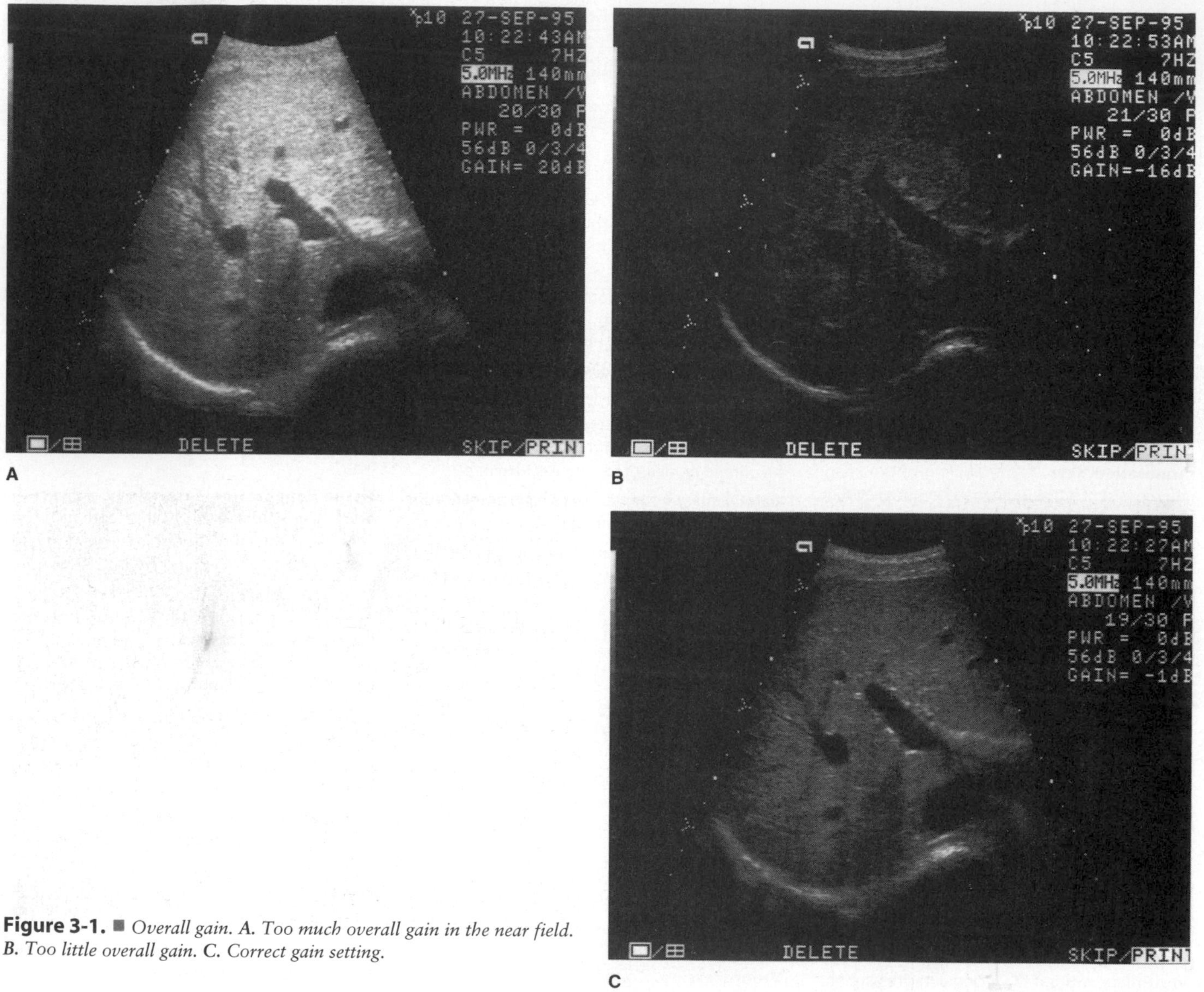

Figure 3-1. ■ *Overall gain. A. Too much overall gain in the near field. B. Too little overall gain. C. Correct gain setting.*

DEPTH GAIN COMPENSATION

The depth gain compensation (DGC) attempts to compensate for the acoustic loss by absorption, scatter, and reflection and to show structures of the same acoustic strength with the same brightness, no matter what the depth is. Individual controls for small segments of the display, known as *slide pots*, are available from most manufacturers. The DGC and gain controls should be used together to provide a uniform image (Fig. 3-2).

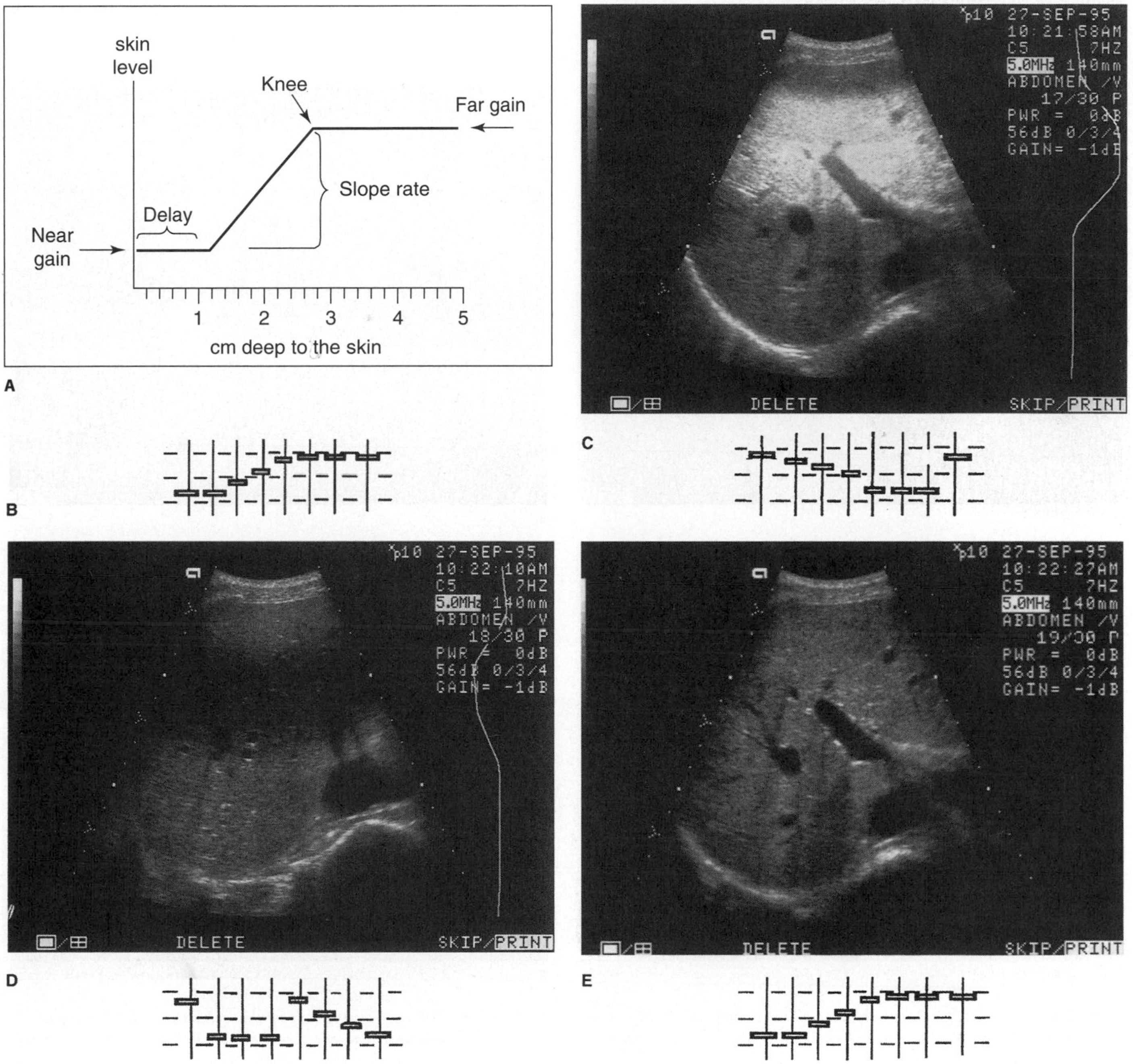

Figure 3-2. ■ *A. Diagram showing the components of the time gain compensation curve. B. Slide pots are used in modern systems rather than separate controls. The slide pots are often prearranged to compensate for tissue attenuation and are all set at the same level. C. DGC curve: Too much emphasis on midfield echoes. D. DGC curve: Too little emphasis on midfield echoes. E. Correct DGC setting.*

DYNAMIC RANGE (LOG COMPRESSION)

The dynamic range (log compression) is the range of intensities from the largest to the smallest echo that a system can display. Changing the log compression does not affect the number of gray shades in the image; instead, it varies the display of the gray shades. For example, a signal will appear more sonolucent at a lower log compression than the same amplitude signal at a high-log compression setting. The log compression may be used to remove reverberation artifacts from cystic structures or to enhance the display of low-level echoes such as gallbladder sludge or soft plaque (Fig. 3-3).

PREPROCESSING (EDGE ENHANCEMENT)

The preprocessing control alters the edges of the image pixels to accentuate the transition between areas of different echogenicities. Altering the preprocessing may aid in performing measurements by making borders sharper (Fig. 3-4).

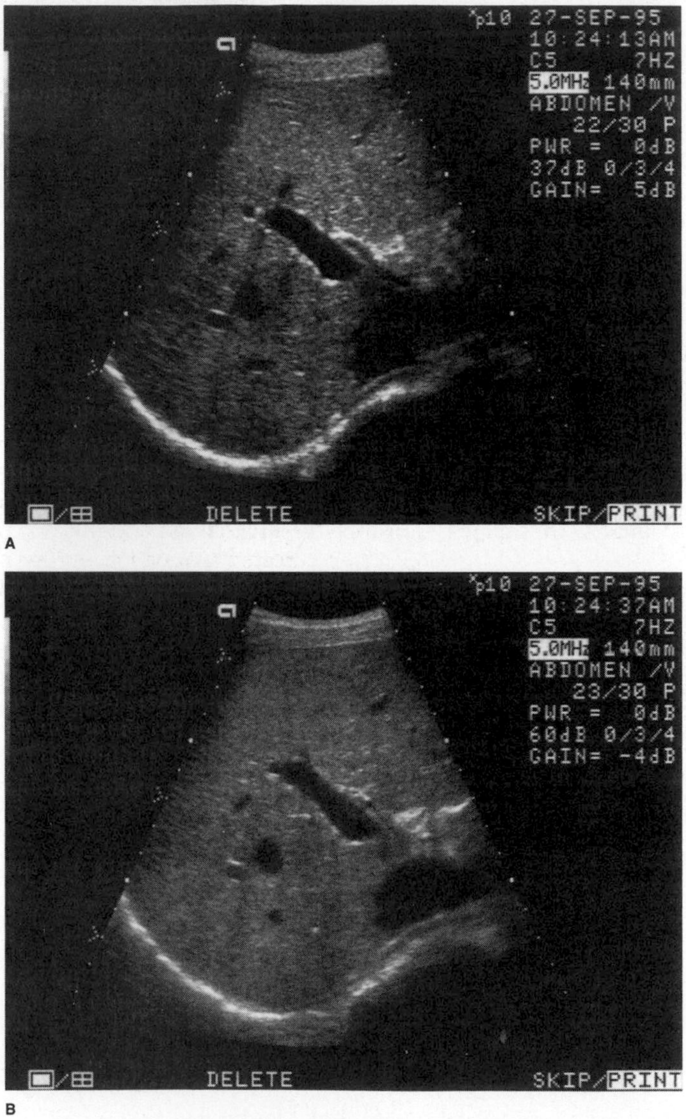

Figure 3-3. ■ *Dynamic range. **A.** Low dynamic range of 37 dB creates an image with more contrast (more black and white). **B.** High dynamic range of 60 dB creates a softer image appearance.*

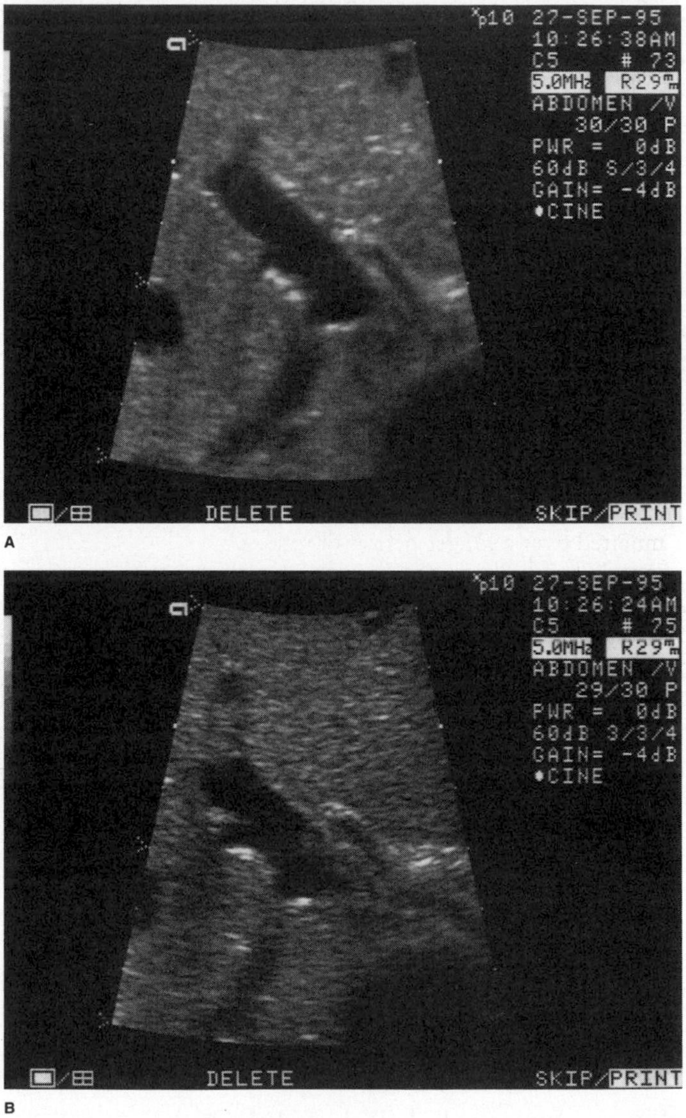

Figure 3-4. ■ *Preprocessing (edge enhancement). **A.** The setting of S creates a soft appearance to the pixel borders. **B.** The high preprocessing setting of 3 creates a crisp appearance to the pixel borders.*

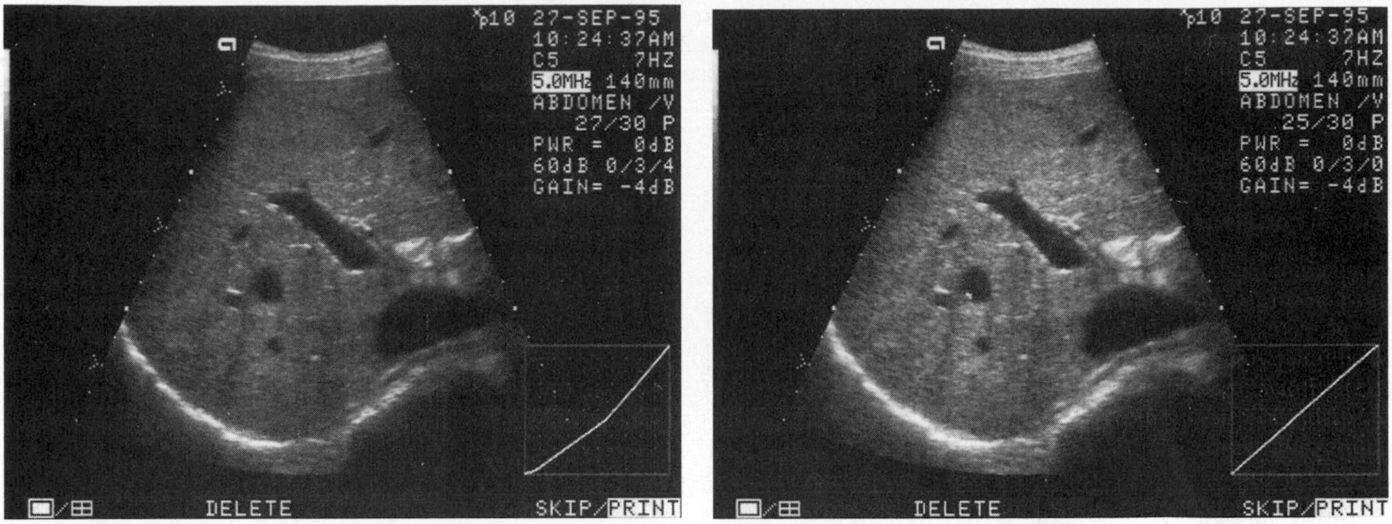

A B

Figure 3-5. ■ *Postprocessing. A. This postprocessing setting de-emphasizes midlevel echoes, as seen in the graph in the lower right-hand corner, providing a soft image. **B.** This postprocessing setting provides equal emphasis of all echoes resulting in a more contrasty appearance.*

PERSISTENCE

Persistence is a frame-averaging function that allows echo information to be accumulated over a longer period of time. By increasing the persistence, subtle tissue texture differences will be enhanced. Decreasing the persistence allows the user to evaluate moving structures more easily.

POSTPROCESSING

Postprocessing alters image aesthetics by placing more or less emphasis on specific echo intensities. Changing the postprocessing map may aid the user in evaluating pathology (e.g., emphasizing bones in obstetric patients) or in evaluating technically difficult patients. Postprocessing may be changed after the image is frozen (Fig. 3-5).

ZOOM

The zoom function allows image magnification by increasing the pixel size, although this change results in image degradation.

WRITE ZOOM (RES)

With write zoom, a box is placed on the screen, and the area seen within the box can be expanded to fill the screen. The number of scan lines remains the same, and the lines are reallocated so that the image is a true magnification of the area under examination.

TRANSDUCER SELECTION

The transducer selection feature allows the user to activate the transducer of choice.

CALIPERS

Caliper markers are available to measure distances. The ellipsoid measurement is an added feature in most units. A dotted line can be created around the outline of a structure to calculate either the circumference or the area.

SELECTED READING

Hykes D, Hedrick WR, Starchman D, eds. *Ultrasound Physics and Instrumentation*, 4th ed. Philadelphia: Mosby; 2005.

Kremkau FW. *Diagnostic Ultrasound: Principles and Instruments*, 6th ed. Philadelphia: WB Saunders; 2002.

Zagebski J. *Essentials of Ultrasound Physics*. St. Louis: CV Mosby; 1996.

4 Doppler and Color Flow Principles

MIKE LEDWIDGE
TOM WINTER
BARBARA DEL PRINCE

KEY WORDS

Aliasing. A technical artifact that leads to ambiguity in the measurement of high-frequency Doppler shifts. It occurs when the sampling frequency (pulse repetition frequency [PRF]) is not at least twice that of the Doppler shift being assessed. Typically occurs with deep abdominal arteries that contain high-velocity flow. The waveform wraps around so that peak signals appear at the bottom of the display. The problem is corrected by increasing the PRF, reducing the transmitted frequency, or adjusting the baseline.

Autocalculations. Machine-specific algorithms that attempt to calculate Doppler parameters automatically.

B-flow. Grayscale-coded imaging of blood flow. Advantages include absence of aliasing, lack of blooming outside of vessel walls, and good resolution of blood flow. Cine clips are useful to show dynamic blood flow because still images may look like thrombus.

Diastole. The second part of the spectral waveform and the second part of the cardiac cycle, when lower velocities are seen. At this time, the heart muscles are relaxing, and the ventricular chambers fill with blood.

Duplex Imaging. The simultaneous display of the grayscale image and the Doppler waveform.

Frame Rate. The number of times per second (Hz) that the image is refreshed.

Frequency Shift. The amount of change in the returning frequency when compared to the transmitted frequency, occurring when the sound wave hits a moving target such as blood in an artery.

Hepatofugal. Flow away from the liver in the portal venous system. Seen when pressure within the portal system is increased to the point that flow cannot enter the liver through the portal vein and instead goes to the heart via collaterals. Hepatofugal flow is also normally seen in the opposite portal vein in the setting of a patent transjugular intrahepatic portosystemic shunt (TIPS); for example, in the left portal vein when there is a patent transjugular intrahepatic portosystemic shunt starting in the right portal vein.

Hepatopetal. Portal vein flow toward the liver (the normal condition).

Intima. The inner lining of an artery. The adventitia and media are the other components of the arterial wall.

Laminar. Normal pattern of blood flow in a vessel; the flow in the center of the vessel is faster than at the walls.

Linear Steering. Some units offer this feature with linear-array transducers. The angle of the sound beam can be obliqued independently in all three different modes (B-scan image, Doppler, and color); for example, the grayscale image can be obliqued to the left while the Doppler image is steered to the right.

Power Doppler. Another type of Doppler flow imaging in which the integrated power of the Doppler signal is displayed, rather than the mean frequency shift used in conventional color Doppler.

Parvus and Tardus Flow Changes. Flow patterns seen distal to arterial obstruction or narrowing. There is a slowly ascending systolic flow signal with overall decreased signal amplitude, and increased end-diastolic flow (low resistive index).

Pulse Repetition Frequency (PRF). Also known as *flow velocity range* or *scale*. This control sets the number of pulses of ultrasound transmitted per second for a given viewing depth. The deeper the depth is, the lower the PRF will be, as more time must be allowed for a returning signal. With a shallow depth, a higher velocity range and higher PRF can be used. Many systems program the PRF for a selected structure or depth. PRF can be adjusted with the velocity range control knob. Use of a PRF that is too low for a specified velocity gives rise to aliasing.

Resistance. As arterial flow enters an organ such as the kidney, the density of the tissue creates pressure against the flow. When the pressure is abnormally increased, as in organ rejection or arterial stenosis, a high-resistance flow pattern develops. High-resistance flow patterns can be normal in some locations (e.g., femoral artery). A high-resistance pattern has high systolic peak and low diastolic flow levels. Low-resistance flow has low systolic levels and more prominent flow in diastole.

Sample Volume (Gate). The sample site from which the signal is obtained with pulsed Doppler. The size and position of the box (gate) outlining the site being sampled can be varied.

Spectral Analysis/Waveform. Evaluation of the entire frequency display characteristics.

Spectral Broadening. Echo fill-in of the spectral window proportional to the severity of the vessel stenosis. It may also result from poor technique, with too much gain, or if the sample volume is too large.

Spectral Window. The area that is being sampled by the Doppler system.

Systole. The first half of the spectral waveform and of the cardiac cycle; high velocities are seen. This signal reflects the contraction of the heart muscle as it propels blood to the body.

Triplexing. Grayscale, color Doppler, and spectral waveform all being acquired simultaneously. The image quality is somewhat degraded because the machine must process much data simultaneously to obtain an image.

Velocity. Speed of blood flow in a vessel.

Velocity Display Mode. This function allows the operator to adjust the displayed colors to correspond to the desired flow velocity range to be measured.

Doppler

Doppler physics as it relates to diagnostic ultrasonography concerns the behavior of high-frequency sound waves as they are reflected off moving fluid (usually blood) (Fig. 4-1).

THE DOPPLER EFFECT

When a high-frequency sound beam meets a moving structure, such as blood flow in a vessel, the reflected sound returns at a different frequency. The speed (velocity) of the moving structure can be calculated from this frequency shift (Fig. 4-2). The returning frequency will be increased if flow is toward the sound source (transducer) and will be decreased if flow is away from the sound source. The frequency of the returning wave can be converted to an audible signal. The Doppler effect is responsible for the variation in the pitch of the sound wave from an ambulance siren as it moves toward and away from you. The siren pitch becomes higher as the ambulance approaches and lowers as the vehicle departs.

Clinical Correlation

The Doppler effect is helpful in localizing blood vessels and determining optimal sites for velocity measurements. Veins typically have a low-pitched hum, whereas arteries have an alternating pattern with a high-pitched systolic component and a low-pitched diastolic component.

CONTINUOUS WAVE DOPPLER

The sound beam is continuously emitted from one transducer and is received by a second. Both transducers are encased in one housing. Because this is a simple system, it is inexpensive, but it can only be used when superficial vessels are examined. Many current high-end ultrasound systems do not have continuous wave (CW) probes. CW does not allow the operator to generate an image, thereby limiting its usefulness in many situations.

Clinical Correlation

Vascular surgeons use CW Doppler to check for the presence or absence of flow in superficial arteries. CW Doppler is also sometimes used to monitor umbilical artery flow. Because the cord lies in the amniotic fluid, no other confusing vessels are within the ultrasonic beam.

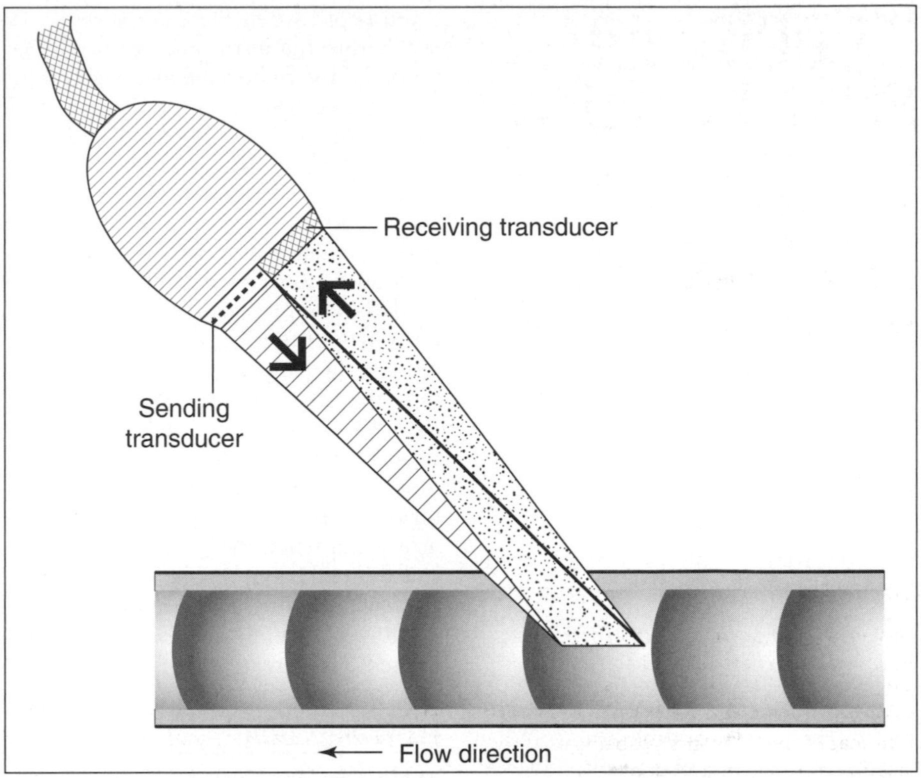

Figure 4-1. ■ *Diagram of a pulsed Doppler transducer demonstrating the direction of the transmitted sound beam toward the flow of blood and the receiving sound beam back to the transducer.*

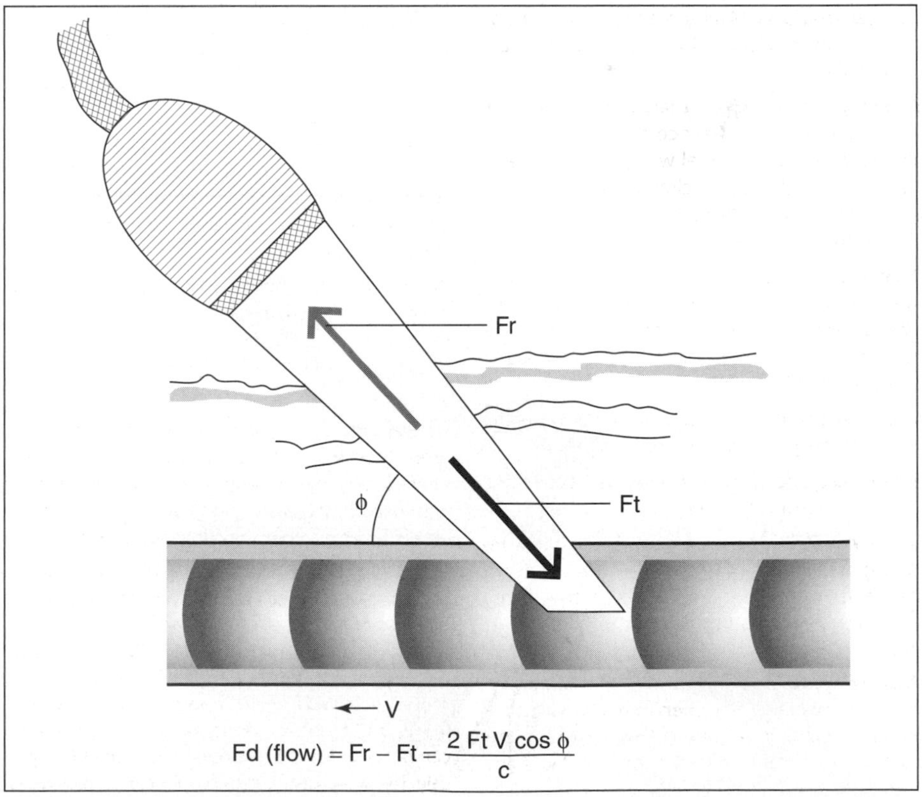

Figure 4-2. ■ *Diagram showing the components of the Doppler equation. Fr, return frequency; Ft, sending frequency; ϕ, angle of insonation of the vessel; V, blood flow velocity; c, speed of sound in tissue (~1,540 m/sec).*

PULSED DOPPLER

A Doppler sound beam is sent and received (pulsed) over a short period of time (Fig. 4-3). Because the time that the Doppler signal takes to reach the target can be converted to distance (similar to estimating distance to a lightning strike by counting the number of seconds between seeing the lightning and hearing the thunder and then using the known speed of sound in air to convert to distance), the depth of the site sampled is known.

The pulsed sound beam is "gated." Only those signals from a vessel at a known depth are displayed and analyzed (Fig 4-3). The size of the gate controls the volume of waveform data that are retrieved. A larger gate is not necessarily better, as it diminishes the sensitivity of the signal detection and averages blood flow of different velocities. To obtain the highest velocity in a stenotic vessel, move a smaller gate through the vessel and listen for the highest audible sound. When a large clot is present in a vein, however, using a large sample volume may help detect some area of flow within the vein.

Clinical Correlation

Pulsed Doppler is used to detect the presence of blood flow in a select vessel at a given depth when there are several vessels within the ultrasonic beam. For example, if the right renal artery shows no flow, an occlusion can be diagnosed although the portal vein and inferior vena cava lie close to the right renal artery because the gate does not include those vessels. Clots can appear echo-free, so a real-time image may erroneously appear to show a normal vessel even if it is occluded. Doppler will detect no flow. Flow from other vessels outside the region of the gate is not analyzed because only the gated area is examined. Pulsed Doppler can be used to differentiate between the hepatic artery and the common bile duct, as these structures lie anterior to the portal vein (the hepatic artery can reach the size of a pathologically dilated common bile duct). Doppler confirmation of flow within arteries and no flow within bile ducts is helpful when dilated ducts create confusion.

FLOW DIRECTION

The direction of blood flow can be discovered by assessing whether the frequency of the returning signal is above or below the baseline in a suspect vessel. Flow toward the transducer is traditionally displayed above the baseline, and flow away from the transducer is shown below the baseline (Fig. 4-4). Flow direction can also be established by comparing the flow pattern in a vessel in which the flow direction is known with the flow pattern in a neighboring vascular structure in which the flow might be in either direction. Note of caution—the spectral display can be reversed by adjusting the setting on the machine (user-preference). Be sure it is set correctly before suggesting pathologic reversed flow.

Clinical Correlation

Flow in the portal vein is sometimes reversed when pressure in the liver increases in portal hypertension; flow away from the liver is known as *hepatofugal* and indicates that the portal pressure is so high that flow has been reversed. A memory aid that some sonographers find useful to remember this often-confusing terminology is "fugitives flee." Flow toward the liver is known as *hepatopetal*. Flow direction analysis allows the diagnosis of the abnormal hepatofugal flow.

FLOW PATTERN

The pattern of flow can be assessed with Doppler ultrasound. Typically, a vein shows a continuous rhythmic flow in diastole and systole and emits a lower-pitched signal than arterial flow. Arterial flow has an alternating high-pitched systolic peak and a much lower diastolic level (Fig. 4-4).

Clinical Correlation

Veins may be confused with arteries on real time. For example, if the patient has portal hypertension, it may be difficult to

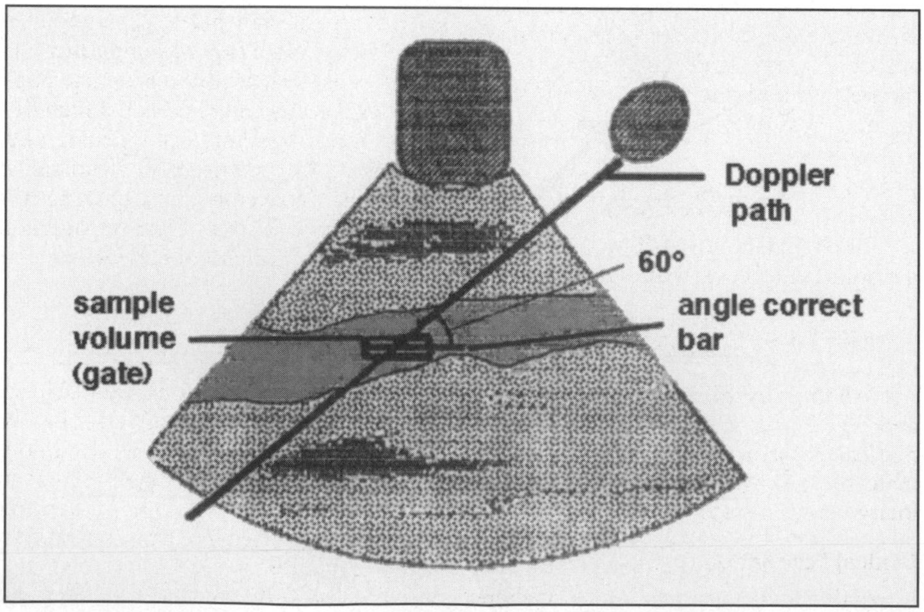

Figure 4-3. ■ *Real-time image displaying the gate (sample volume) and the angle correct bar within the blood vessel. Note the 60-degree angle of the beam to vessel flow. Only timed signals from the area within the gate are displayed and analyzed in the Doppler signal.*

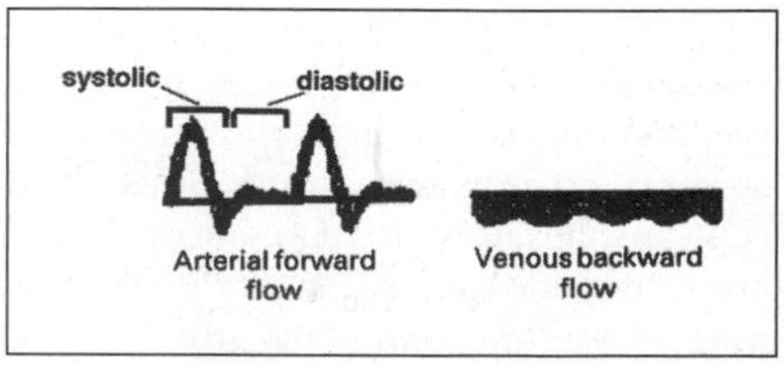

Figure 4-4. ■ *Arterial waveform demonstrating flow above the baseline; venous flow is displayed below the baseline (flow in the other direction). Note the phases of systole and diastole in arterial pulse.*

decide whether the hepatic artery is patent because many venous collaterals are seen alongside the portal vein. The hepatic artery and venous collaterals are, however, easily distinguished using pulsed Doppler.

FLOW VELOCITY

The velocity of blood flow can be deduced from the arterial waveform. If the peak systolic flow frequency and the angle at which the beam intersects the vessel are known, a simple formula allows the calculation of velocity (Fig. 4-2). The velocity calculation formula is only accurate if the angle of the Doppler beam to the interrogated vessel is less than 60 degrees (Fig. 4-3). At a 70-degree angle, the velocity error is 25%, and it is proportionately larger as the angle is increased up to 90 degrees.

Clinical Correlation

Velocity is an important factor in calculating the severity of carotid stenosis. Generally, the more severe the stenosis is, the greater the velocity through the narrowed vessel will be. As the vessel becomes critically occluded, however, flow velocity will diminish.

LOW- VERSUS HIGH-RESISTANCE FLOW

Doppler flow analysis allows the detection of two types of arterial flow: a high-resistance (Fig. 4-5 and Color Plate 22-11) and a low-resistance (Fig. 4-6 and Color Plate 4-1) pattern. The high-resistance pattern has a high systolic peak and a low diastolic flow. Low-resistance arterial systems demonstrate a biphasic systolic peak and a relatively high level of flow in diastole (Fig. 4-6). Resistance is commonly calculated using a simple formula:

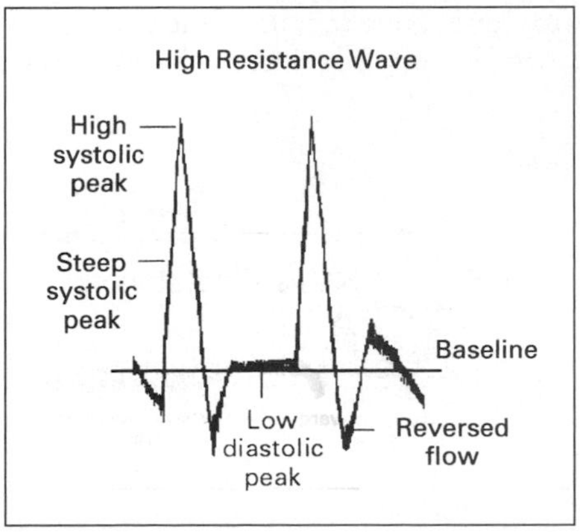

Figure 4-5. ■ *Diagram of an arterial spectral waveform in a high-resistance bed. Note the low diastolic flow. See Color Plate 22-11, a pulsed Doppler sonogram from a high-resistance system.*

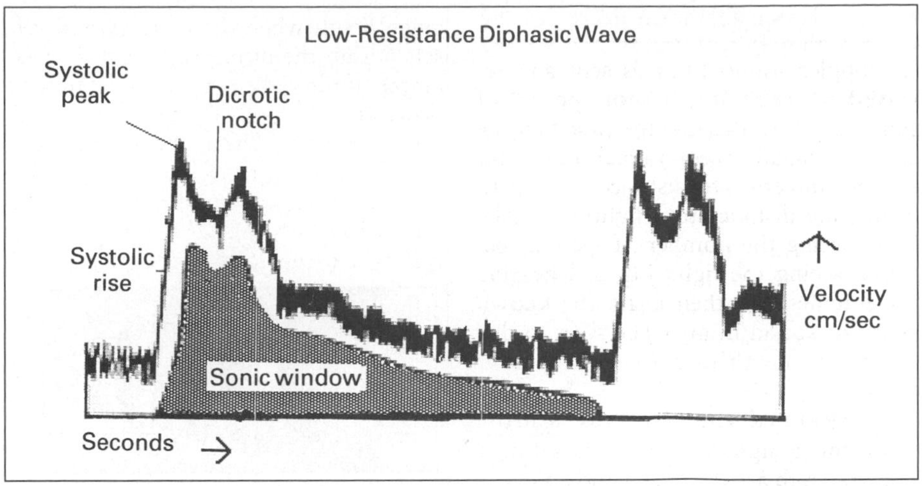

Figure 4-6. ■ *Diagram of an arterial spectral waveform in a low-resistance bed. Note the relatively high diastolic flow. See Color Plate 4-1.*

Resistive index (RI)

$$= \frac{\text{(Systolic velocity − Diastolic velocity)}}{\text{(Systolic velocity)}}$$

An alternative technique, known as the *pulsatility index* (PI), evaluates the diastolic flow in a different fashion. A cursor is run along the superior aspect of the systolic and diastolic flow envelope, and the mean is calculated by the system.

$$\text{PI} = \frac{\text{(Systolic velocity − Mean Flow)}}{\text{(Systolic velocity)}}$$

In obstetrics, the A/B or systolic-to-diastolic ratio is commonly used:

$$\text{S/D} = \text{A/B} = \frac{\text{(peak systolic velocity)}}{\text{(end diastolic velocity)}}$$

All three of these parameters (RI, PI, and S/D ratio) are just different mathematical constructs that attempt to estimate the relative difference in flow velocity between systole and diastole.

Clinical Correlation

If a high-resistance pattern is seen where there is normally a low-resistance appearance, such as in the common carotid or renal artery, vessel narrowing is present. For example, a completely occluded internal carotid artery may create a high-resistance waveform in the common carotid artery. Increased resistance is also a feature of a number of renal diseases such as rejection and hydronephrosis. Quantifying the severity of the resistance may help in clinical management.

A high-resistance pattern is usually seen in the vessel supplying the ovaries in the proliferative phase of the cycle. If a low-resistance pattern ($RI < 0.4$) is seen within an ovarian mass, carcinoma is more likely. Note that although this observation is statistically true in large populations, because there is such a high degree of overlap between normal and abnormal, RI measurement is typically of little use in reliably distinguishing between benign and malignant ovarian masses in any individual patient.

FLOW PATTERN WITHIN A VESSEL (LAMINAR FLOW)

In a normal vessel, the velocity of blood is highest in the center of a vessel and is lowest closer to the wall. This condition is termed *laminar flow*. When there is a wall irregularity or if the artery is angled, the flow is distorted and may be greatest when it is closest to the vessel wall. Stenosis markedly increases the flow velocity through an area of narrowing, whereas vessel dilatation decreases the speed of flow (Fig. 4-7).

Clinical Correlation

To accurately measure the flow velocity in a tortuous carotid artery, place the sample volume (the area that is gated) at the center of the highest flow. Listening to the audible signal is very useful in determining the site for optimal measurement. A high-grade stenosis will have a shrill, chirping sound.

FLOW DISTORTION

Normal laminar flow at and immediately beyond an area of wall irregularity or stenosis is disturbed, resulting in abnormal spectral waveforms. Flow distortion (nonlaminar) is characterized by high velocities in both systole and diastole. The presence of many echoes within the sonic window is termed *spectral broadening* and may indicate considerable flow disturbance. Eddies occur because the high-velocity jet suddenly hits flow in an undisturbed vessel (Fig. 4-8). Grayscale visualization of soft echo-free plaques as the source of a wall irregularity may be limited.

Clinical Correlation

Flow disturbance in an artery such as the carotid may indicate pathologic atheromatous changes (see the section under Pitfalls later in this chapter).

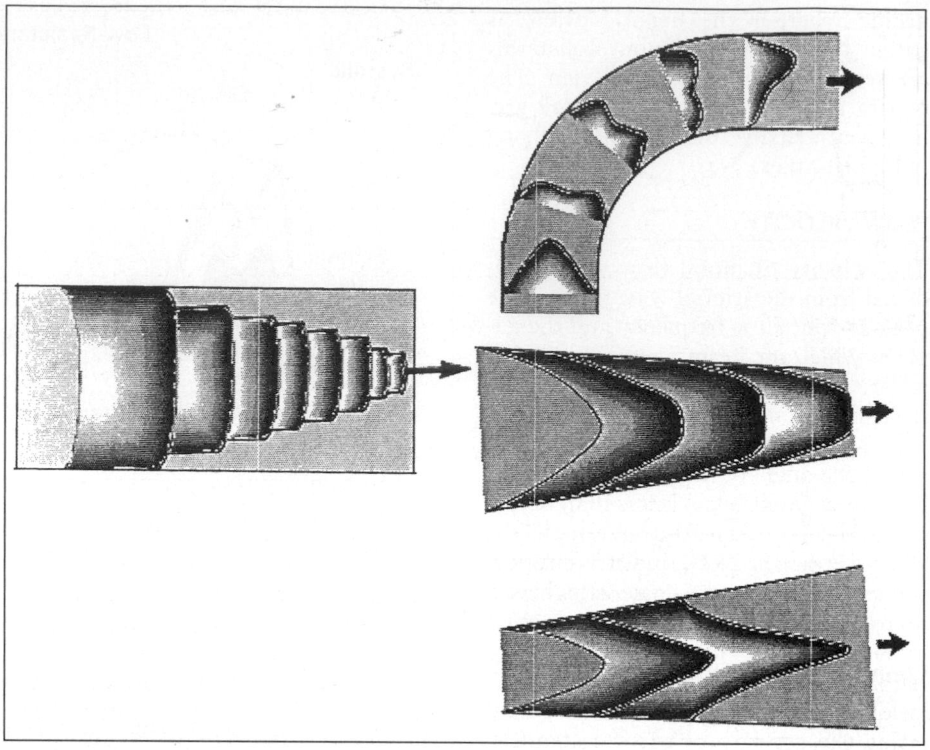

Figure 4-7. ■ *Due to the narrowing of the vessel lumen, the tortuosity, or the vessel's diameter, the blood flow pattern will vary.*

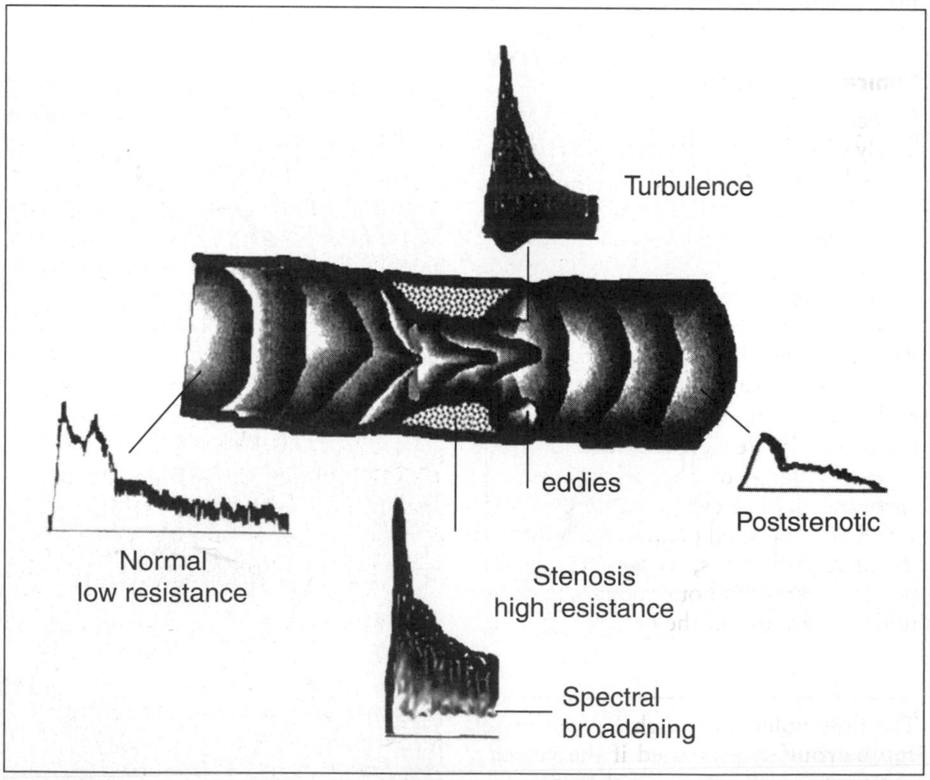

Figure 4-8. ■ *Diagram showing typical flow pattern before, at, just beyond, and distal to an arterial stenosis. Note that at the level of the stenosis, there is high systolic and diastolic flow with much spectral broadening. Just beyond the stenosis, there is considerable turbulence with a continued relatively high systolic level. Beyond the stenosis in the poststenotic region, there is a slow ascent to the systolic pulse with a low-amplitude flow.*

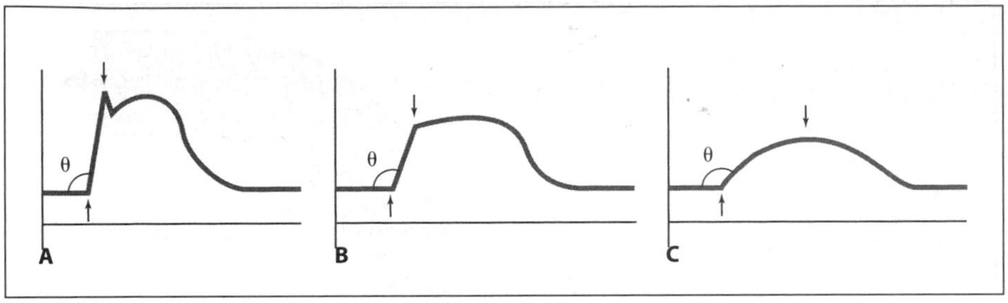

Figure 4-9. ■ *Flow alterations distal to an area of stenosis. A. Normal steep slope to systole* (between arrows). *B. Moderate stenosis with less steep angle* (between arrows). *C. Slow upswing and smooth peak with severe stenosis* (between arrows), *the classic* tardus et parvus *waveform.*

FLOW CHANGES BEYOND A NARROWED AREA (POSTSTENOTIC CHANGES)

Poststenotic changes in arterial flow may be seen in the next few centimeters beyond a narrowed area. When there is severe stenosis, the systolic peak in the poststenotic area will be lower (more rounded) with lower velocities throughout diastole (Figs. 4-8 and 4-9). The acceleration slope of the systolic peaks (peak systole) will be diminished. This pattern is known as the *tardus et parvus* abnormality. In less severe obstruction, the spectral waveform may resume the normal high- or low-resistance flow appropriate for that artery.

Clinical Correlation

Detecting a poststenotic pattern is particularly valuable in evaluating the renal arteries because the usual site of stenosis, adjacent to the aorta, is rarely seen owing to the presence of bowel gas. Poststenotic changes may also be seen in the common carotid artery when the stenosis involves the origin of the common carotid. A dampened signal may be displayed (Fig. 4-9). Keep in mind that this dampened signal may be the result of an overall systemic problem (e.g., low cardiac output). The waveform of the other common carotid should be evaluated for comparison. Large calcified plaques may obscure the area of stenosis, so one may be dependent on poststenotic changes to determine the severity of the narrowing.

FLOW VOLUME

The flow volume through a given vessel can be roughly estimated if the velocity of flow (using the formula shown in Fig. 4-2) and the vessel diameter are known.

Clinical Correlation

The calculation of flow volume is important in situations in which a low level of flow is associated with inadequate function (e.g., penile arterial flow).

ALIASING

If there is a marked frequency shift with a high measured velocity, the signal may return after the next pulse has started (Fig. 4-10 and Color Plate 4-2). This condition is called *aliasing*. To compensate for aliasing, increase the velocity range (PRF). Most machines will allow the operator to freeze the real-time image, and a wider measurable range of velocities can then be obtained on the spectral waveform. Lower the velocity range (PRF) to display slower velocities accurately. Lowering the baseline may also prevent aliasing.

Clinical Correlation

If aliasing is present, the peak signal will be inaccurately measured as lower than it really is, and the severity of the stenosis will be incorrectly measured.

COLOR-FLOW IMAGING

Color flow assigns different hues to the red blood cells in a vessel depending on their velocities and the direction of the blood flow relative to the transducer. This allocation is based on the Doppler principle; therefore, some of the same guidelines will apply to both techniques. This color assignment to the flow velocities is performed very rapidly, so a real-time image is generated.

Clinical Correlation

The site of maximum flow can be visualized quickly so that the pulsed Doppler gate can be inserted where the flow is highest. This technique prevents a tedious hunt with conventional Doppler.

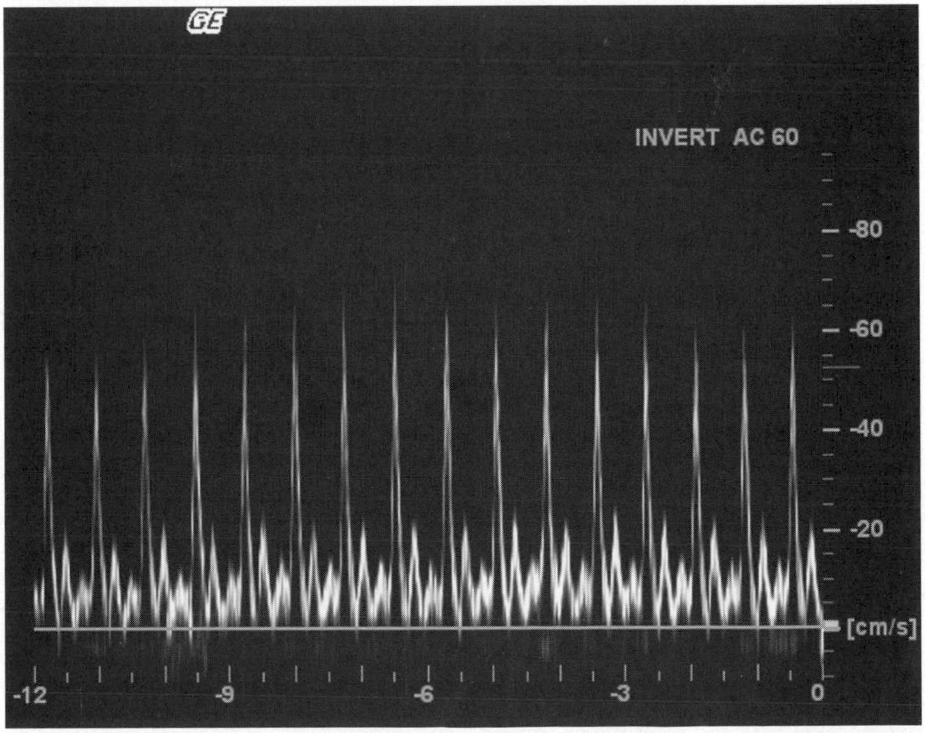

Figure 4-10. ■ *Pulsed Doppler aliasing. In Color Plate 4-2, the velocity is too high to be displayed above the baseline; those velocities that exceed the set scale are therefore projected below the baseline (aliasing). This figure shows the corrected image, with adjustments in PRF and baseline, which allows one to display the entire spectrum appropriately.*

Aliasing (see the section under Pitfalls) is readily visible, as there will be a color change with higher velocities.

COLOR-FLOW DISPLAY AND DIRECTION WITHIN A VESSEL

In most systems, flow toward the transducer is allocated red, and flow away from the transducer is allocated blue. The flow velocity is displayed with faster velocities in brighter colors and slower velocities in darker colors (Color Plates 4-3 and 4-4). The fastest velocity may be displayed in yellow or white. Turbulent flow will demonstrate a mixture of colors. Usually, the operator is given several choices of color scale in the menu for the velocity display mode. As with pulsed Doppler, optimal images are only obtained at an oblique angle. If a vessel runs a straight course, flow at 90 degrees to the color box will not be displayed. The angle of the color box region of interest (ROI) can be adjusted to the left or right when linear steering is available; otherwise, the probe can be manually angled to provide the angle needed to receive the returning signals. Keep in mind that if the vessel still does not fill in with color, you may need to widen the dynamic range, allowing lower velocities to be displayed. It should then be fairly straightforward to determine the degree of luminal stenosis. Scanning the vessel in the transverse plane allows for the most accurate calculation of lumen diameter stenosis.

Clinical Correlation

Soft plaque may be missed on grayscale, but a flow void will be seen using color flow. Sometimes, soft plaques may show no changes on grayscale. Once correct color allocation has been made, normal vessels will fill with color.

Knobology: Doppler and Color Flow

RANGE GATE CURSOR (SAMPLE VOLUME)

The Doppler sample volume is displayed on the B-scan image (Fig. 4-3). This cursor, which may be presented as a box or two parallel bars, indicates the depth and area from which the Doppler signal is obtained. The size of the box can vary, depending on the volume of blood to be evaluated.

REGION OF INTEREST

This box is used to restrict the color display of a blood flow image and to eliminate an unnecessary display of color (Color Plate 4-3). A narrower box generally improves the frame rate.

INVERSION AND DIRECTION OF FLOW AND ITS RELATION TO BASELINE (DOPPLER)

When blood flow is moving toward the transducer, sound waves of high frequency are reflected, and positive signals are seen above the baseline (Fig. 4-4). Blood cells that are moving away from the transducer appear as negative signals below the baseline (Fig. 4-4). Both veins and arteries can show flow in either direction because interpreting flow direction depends on the angle of the vessel to the transducer.

COLOR INVERSION

The display color can be inverted. With the invert on, flow coming toward the probe is blue, and flow away from the probe is red. This should be noted so that it is clear to a person who is interpreting the images at a later time.

COLOR-FLOW BASELINE

Blood flow toward the transducer will be shown within the measurable range of colors (usually red) above the color bar baseline. Blood flow away from the probe will be displayed in the range of colors below the baseline, usually blue (Color Plates 4-3 and 4-4). If the range of velocities is too high, reversed colors will appear within the color image. This situation can be corrected by lowering the baseline, so the color display will remain above the baseline, and the highest velocities will be displayed in white or yellow.

VELOCITY SCALE/VELOCITY RANGE/PRF (DOPPLER)

The range of velocities that can be seen in the spectral display is determined by the PRF value. A superficial structure (e.g., carotid) requires a high PRF; therefore, the velocity range should be increased. For deep structures such as the inferior vena cava, a low PRF is used.

PRF (COLOR FLOW)

The range of velocities used in color flow is lower compared to the spectral waveform because the average Doppler shift frequency is displayed, rather than the peak velocity. With lower PRF values, there will be a shift to a different color, representing a slightly higher velocity flow (i.e., white or yellow).

SWEEP SPEED (DOPPLER ONLY)

The rate at which the spectral information is displayed can be adjusted using the sweep speed controls. A slow speed (e.g., 25 mm/sec), a moderate speed (e.g., 50 mm/sec), or a fast speed (e.g., 100 mm/sec) can be selected. A slow sweep speed is easier to measure, and a fast sweep speed allows more cardiac cycles to be displayed in one image.

WALL FILTER (DOPPLER)

Blood flow signals that are not wanted can be eliminated by using the wall filter. For example, pulsatile signals from the vascular wall and artifact from respiration can be filtered out by increasing the filter setting. If the filter is set too high, however, the true flow signal itself may also be deleted if the true flow is slow. A lower wall filter setting will display more information in the Doppler signal. This setting is helpful when evaluating venous flow, a slow flow state.

FILTER (COLOR FLOW)

A phenomenon called *color flash*, caused by cardiac or peristaltic motion or by transducer movement, produces a flash of spurious color in an area where there is no real flow. The area of interest can be concealed by the flash artifact. Flash may be unavoidable, but check the color filter to determine whether this condition can be corrected by increasing the filter level.

GAIN (DOPPLER AND COLOR FLOW)

The gain controls alter the spectral waveform and the color-flow image. Inadequate gain results in an image in which the vessel is incompletely filled with color or in which no conventional Doppler signal can be obtained in areas of slow flow. When too much color gain is used, the color display image and the neighboring tissue will be saturated with color noise, and pixels of color will appear throughout the image. Correct this problem by lowering the color gain so there is no artifactual flow outside the vessel; a range of colors will then be seen within the vessel. Too much Doppler gain will fill in the "sonic window" with noise and will create artifactual spectral broadening. In the absence of color flow, make sure the color gain is not set too low. On some current systems, there is an "infinite" gain control, which may need to be adjusted a large amount to increase or decrease sensitivity.

ANGLE CORRECT BAR (FLOW VECTOR)

An angle correct bar is situated within the range gate cursor (Fig. 4-3). This bar should be aligned with the direction of blood flow. The angle created by the insonating ultrasound beam and this bar must be known if the flow velocity is to be deduced from the frequency of the returning Doppler signal. The angle should be less than 60 degrees. A quantitative calculation of velocity is especially important when evaluating the carotid because velocity changes are correlated with the degree of stenosis and are used in patient management. Changing the angle (linear steering) helps one achieve the optimum angle in color flow and pulse Doppler mode. At the same time, an optimal B-scan image can be obtained.

DYNAMIC RANGE (COLOR FLOW)

A wide range of velocities can be displayed by changing the dynamic range. The artery will fill with more color, and more velocities will be displayed. Remember that some individuals have lower velocities (lower cardiac output) in their arteries.

POWER DOPPLER

Movement is visualized, and flow in all directions can be visualized. This technique is more sensitive for subtle flow than conventional color-flow Doppler on lower-quality machines, while on current high-end machines, the sensitivity of color Doppler and power Doppler is essentially the same. Power Doppler is particularly useful in seeing low flow or small subtle vessels (e.g., in an ovarian mass). Clutter and flash (movement) artifacts are accentuated with this technique.

AUDIO VOLUME

The Doppler sound will be heard from the built-in speakers. Usually, there are independent speakers for both forward and reverse flow. The control varies the volume of the Doppler sound.

CURSOR MOVEMENT CONTROL

The cursor (range gate cursor and ROI) movement can be manipulated by means of a trackball or a joystick.

MEASUREMENTS

The standard measurement unit used in displaying the spectral waveform is velocity (m/sec or cm/sec). When dealing with a high-grade stenosis, obtain maximum velocities at and just beyond the area of lumen narrowing.

Pitfalls

INCORRECT ANGLE

A waveform that appears to indicate a distal obstruction is displayed in a vessel; however, no plaque is seen in the vessel.

Correction Technique. Check the position of the ultrasound beam relative to the direction of flow. If the angle is greater than 60 degrees, then the velocity is not being accurately calculated, and an abnormal waveform is created (Fig. 4-3). This abnormal waveform may mimic a high-resistance waveform (see the section under Angle Correct Bar).

LITTLE OR NO DOPPLER SIGNAL IN AN ARTERY

The spectral waveform shows apparent low systolic flow and minimal diastolic flow.

Explanation A

There may be a severe obstruction proximal to this area and in an area too difficult to evaluate with the ultrasound beam (e.g., origin of the common carotid artery).

Explanation B

This patient may have diminished cardiac output. In order to document this condition, scan the corresponding vessel on the other side and document the symmetry of the waveform abnormality.

Explanation C

The sample volume (gate) may not be placed where maximum flow is present.

Correction Technique. Do not depend solely on the visualization of the vessel. Color flow highlights the higher velocities in the artery and helps in gate placement, but a keen ear is more sensitive. A higher velocity may be evident as the sound beam is angled slightly off the center of the stream.

Explanation D

The sample volume is too large for the small amount of flow.

Correction Technique. A larger sample size may be needed when scanning to locate the site of flow, but to obtain a more precise flow measurement within an artery, decrease the gate size.

Explanation E

The wall filter's level is set too high.

Correction Technique. The wall filter should be set at the lowest setting that does not introduce artifacts, especially when scanning a vein (a low-flow state). Adjust the Doppler gain and volume as you lower the filter.

Explanation F

Try the following maneuvers before giving up.

1. Change to another acoustic window or different incident angle.
2. Open up the gate setting.
3. Lower the velocity range.
4. Use a lower-frequency transducer. The patient may be too obese for a higher-frequency transducer.

A HIGH-RESISTANCE WAVEFORM IN A LOW-RESISTANCE BED

Explanation

There may be soft plaque distal to this area. If the B-scan gain is too low, soft plaque may be missed. Use color flow to outline the true patent lumen.

ALIASING

A tight stenosis causes such high velocities at the site of flow and immediately distal to the narrowed area that flow is seen above the baseline and at the lower edge of the spectral display. When color is used, there may be peaks of color from the other end of the spectrum. A chirping sound may be heard as you angle through the stenotic area.

Explanation

The velocity is so high that the signal wraps around itself, and peak velocities are displayed below the baseline (Fig. 4-10 and Color Plate 4-2). This problem arises because the selected PRF is too low to accurately pick up the high velocities that are occurring.

Correction Techniques.

1. Place the baseline at its lowest site to allow the systolic peaks to be displayed.
2. Increase the PRF (velocity range).
3. Some units allow the B-scan image to be frozen while the Doppler signal is obtained. This will also widen the measurable velocity range.
4. Increase the Doppler angle, but do not exceed 60 degrees.
5. Decrease the insonating frequency. Most units offer a choice of several Doppler frequencies for each transducer. Otherwise, change to a lower-frequency transducer.
6. Change to CW (not widely available on most current machines).

INADEQUATE VENOUS SIGNAL

Venous flow is difficult to detect even when the vessel is clearly demonstrated.

Explanation A

There may be little venous flow at rest.

Correction Technique. Respiration affects venous flow. With inspiration and the descent of the diaphragm, pressure increases in the abdomen. Ask the patient to perform a Valsalva maneuver. (A Valsalva maneuver is performed by taking a deep breath, holding it, and tensing the abdomen.) As the breath is released, venous flow increases, and the venous signal will become more pronounced.

Explanation B

The vein may be compressed by patient position, for example, extension of the leg.

Correction Technique. Ask the patient to flex the leg slightly and re-evaluate. Use color flow in these instances to accentuate subtle flow.

Explanation C

The B-scan gain may be too low to demonstrate the clot within the vein.

Correction Technique. Increase the gain and apply gentle compression to see if the vein collapses.

AUDIBLE SIGNAL BUT VESSEL NOT SEEN

A venous signal can be heard, but a patent vessel cannot be visualized. The vein may be subtotally occluded or the presence of adjacent collaterals may cause the audible signal.

Correction Technique. Color flow will demonstrate the smaller collateral vessels as well as a small amount of residual flow in an almost-occluded vessel.

SPECTRAL BROADENING

Apparent spectral broadening may be caused by too much gain or by scanning too close to the vessel wall, picking up lower velocities.

Correction Technique. Make sure the supposed spectral broadening reflects true pathology, and is not just noise, by comparing it to an area known to be normal.

A FLICKERING IMAGE

Sometimes, it is difficult to evaluate color flow when obtaining a pulsed Doppler signal because the image flickers.

Explanation

A large amount of data is being processed to generate the image for each frame of information when obtaining the Doppler signal or color flow. Therefore, the frame rate is lowered, and a flicker may occur.

Correction Technique. To reduce this flicker, evaluate one mode at a time (e.g., use color flow only) or reduce the width of the color flow box.

COLOR MISREGISTRATION ARTIFACT (COLOR FLASH)

If the transducer is rapidly moved, a flash of color related to transducer movement and not to vascular flow may develop.

Correction Technique. Use the filter to reduce noise and move the transducer slowly, using caution not to remove real vascular flow from the image.

TISSUE VIBRATION OR TRANSMITTED PULSATION

In the region of a highly pulsatile structure such as an artery, neighboring structures may move, causing some color artifact in the surrounding tissues.

Correction Technique. Scan from a different axis, if possible.

ACTIVE PERISTALSIS

Active peristalsis may induce a color-flow artifact.

UNDUE COLOR GAIN

The outline of vessels may be misregistered owing to excessive gain, so the flow appears to fill in some of the surrounding tissues ("color bleed").

Correction Technique. Decrease gain so the color image corresponds to the vessel outline.

SELECTED READING

Gent R. *Applied Physics and Technology of Diagnostic Ultrasound.* Prospect, South Australia: Milner Publishing; 1997.

Kremkau FW. *Doppler Ultrasound Principles and Instrumentation,* 6th ed. Philadelphia: WB Saunders; 2002.

MacSweeney JE, Cosgrove DO, Arenson J. Colour Doppler energy (power) mode ultrasound. *Clin Radiol* 1996;51:387–390.

Polak JF, ed. *Peripheral Vascular Sonography: A Practical Guide,* 2nd ed. Philadelphia: Lippincott Williams & Wilkins; 2004.

Wachsberg RH. B-flow, a non-Doppler technology for flow mapping: early experience in the abdomen. *Ultrasound Quarterly* 2003;19(3):114–122.

Zagzebski J. *Essentials of Ultrasound Physics.* St. Louis: CV Mosby; 1996.

5

Basic Principles

NANCY SMITH MINER

SONOGRAM ABBREVIATIONS

Ao	Aorta
Du	Duodenum
F	Fibroid
GBL	Gallbladder
IVC	Inferior vena cava
K	Kidney
L	Liver
P	Pancreas
SMA	Superior mesenteric artery
Sp	Spleen
Spa	Splenic artery
Spv	Splenic vein
St	Stomach
Ut	Uterus

KEY WORDS

Acoustic Enhancement. Because sound traveling through a fluid-filled structure is barely attenuated, the structures distal to a cystic lesion appear to have more echoes than neighboring areas. Also referred to as *through transmission* (information to follow; see and Fig. 5-1).

Anechoic. Without internal echoes. Not necessarily cystic unless there is distal echo enhancement (good through transmission).

Complex. A structure that has both fluid-filled (echo-free) and solid (echogenic) areas.

Contralateral. On the other side of the body.

Cyst. Spherical, fluid-filled structure with well-defined walls that contains few or no internal echoes and exhibits good acoustic enhancement.

Cystic. In ultrasonography, the word *cystic* does not necessarily refer to a cyst. The term is used (inaccurately) by some to describe any fluid-filled structure (e.g., urine-filled bladder or bile-filled gallbladder; see Fig. 5-1).

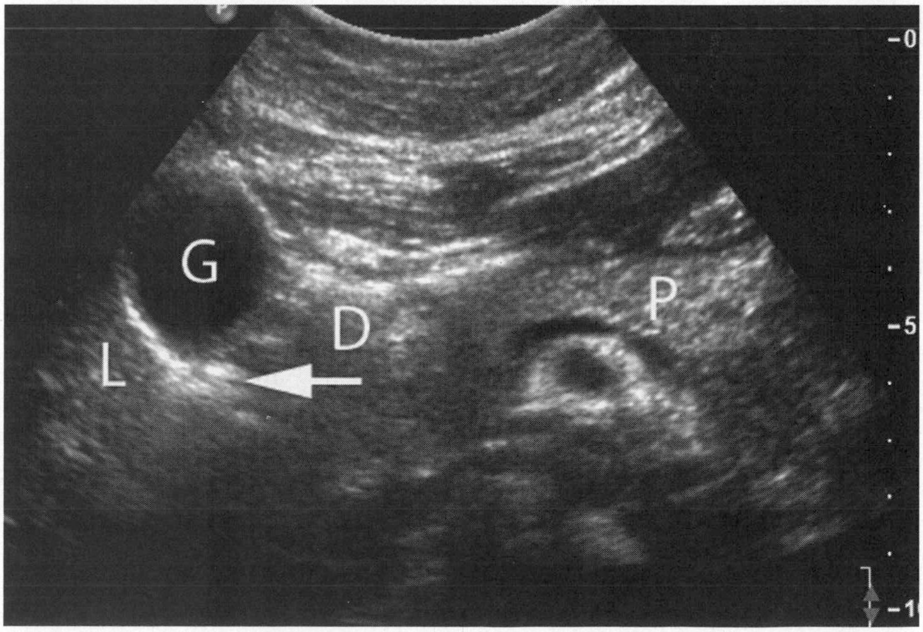

Figure 5-1. ■ *Transverse section of the upper abdomen showing the usual echogenicity of the organs in a young adult. Note that the pancreas* (P) *contains more echoes than the liver* (L). *The gallbladder* (G), *a "cystic" (fluid-filled) structure, shows acoustic enhancement behind it* (arrow), *in the region of the duodenum* (D). *The spleen is slightly more echogenic than the liver.*

Distal. The extremity (limb) end of a body structure.

Echo-free. See *Anechoic.*

Echogenic. Describes a structure that produces echoes. Usually a relative term. For example, Figure 5-1 shows the normal texture of the liver and pancreas; the pancreas is slightly more echogenic. A change in the normal echogenicity signifies a pathologic condition.

Echogram. Term used by some to describe an ultrasonic examination, especially in cardiac work; an echocardiogram is frequently referred to as an "echo."

Echolucent. Without internal echoes; not necessarily cystic.

Echopenic. A few echoes within a structure; less echogenic. The normal kidney is echopenic relative to the liver (see Fig. 5-1).

Echo-poor. See *Echopenic.*

Echo-rich. See *Echogenic.*

Fluid-Fluid Level. Interface between two fluids with different acoustic characteristics. This interface has a horizontal level that varies with patient position.

Footprint. Descriptive term for the amount of transducer face in contact with the patient (i.e., a small-head transducer has a small footprint).

Gain. The strength of the echoes throughout the image can be varied by changing the power output from the system.

Homogeneous. Of uniform composition. The normal texture of several parenchymal organs is homogeneous (e.g., liver, thyroid, and pancreas).

Hyperechoic. See *Echogenic.*

Hypoechoic. See *Echopenic.*

Interface. Strong echoes that delineate the boundary of organs and that are caused by the difference between the acoustic impedance of two adjacent structures. An interface is usually more pronounced when the transducer is perpendicular to it (Fig. 5-2).

Ipsilateral. On the same side of the body.

Isoechoic. Of the same echogenicity as a neighboring area, but not necessarily of the same texture.

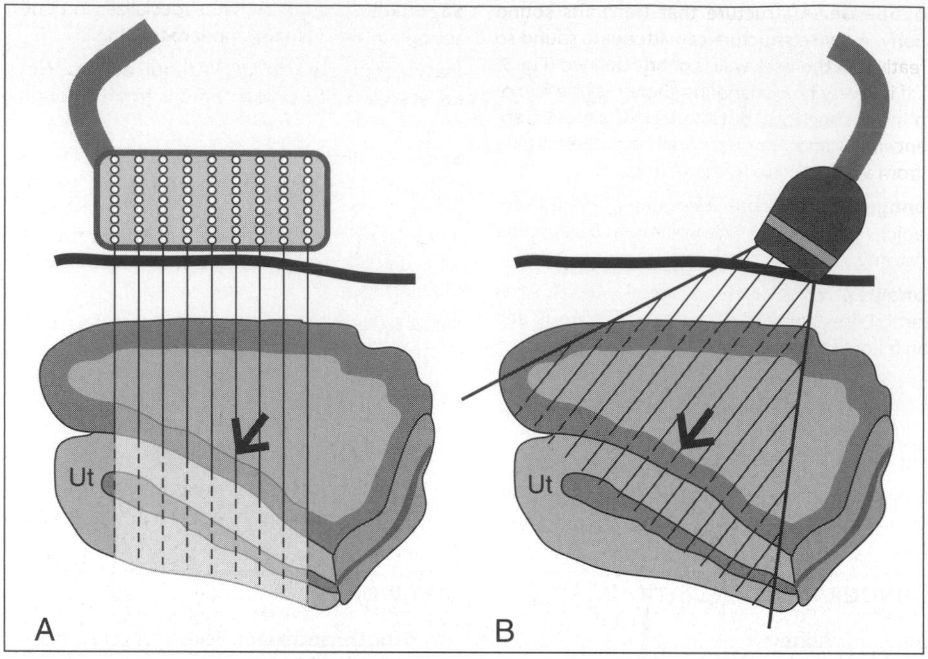

Figure 5-2. ■ *Interface. A. The "interface" between the bladder* (black arrow) *and the uterus* (Ut) *is poorly defined because the linear array beam is not perpendicular to the uterine wall. B. The sector beam was angled perpendicular to the interface* (black arrow) *and is now well seen. The use of a small-headed scanner can bring out interfaces that are oblique to the linear array beam.*

Noise. Artifactual echoes resulting from too much gain rather than from true anatomic structures.

Proximal. The trunk end of a limb or organ.

Reverberation. An artifact that results from a strong echo returning from a large acoustic interface to the transducer. This echo returns to the tissues again, causing additional echoes parallel to the first.

Ring Down. Extreme form of reverberation artifact that occurs when a long series of echoes caused by a very strong acoustic interface and consequent reverberations are seen.

Scan. Verb: to perform an ultrasound scan. Noun: a sonographic examination.

Shadowing. Failure of the sound beam to pass through an object. This blockage is caused by reflection or absorption of the sound and may be partial or complete. For example, air bubbles in the duodenum allow poor transmission of the sound beam because most of the sound is reflected. A calcified gallstone does not allow any sound to pass through, and shadowing is pronounced (Fig. 5-3). These degrees of acoustic shadowing may help in diagnosis.

Solid (Homogeneous). A mass or organ that contains uniform low-level echoes because the cellular tissues are acoustically very similar.

Sonodense. A structure that transmits sound poorly. A dense structure can attenuate sound so greatly that the back wall is poorly defined (Fig. 5-4). If it is very homogeneous, there may be few or no internal echoes, but the lack of acoustic enhancement and poor back wall help differentiate it from a cystic, echo-free structure.

Sonogenic. Handsome ultrasound image (photogenic), such as a good example of vascular anatomy.

Sonographer. A health professional who has learned how to perform quality sonography and can tailor the examination to individual patients.

Sonologist. A physician who specializes in ultrasonography and has appropriate training.

Sonolucent (Anechoic). Without echoes. Not necessarily cystic unless there is good through transmission.

Specular Reflector. Structure that creates a strong echo because it interfaces at right angles to the sound beam and has significantly different acoustic impedance from a neighboring structure (e.g., diaphragm/liver or posterior bladder wall/bladder).

Static Scan. Not real time. B-scans produced with a fixed-arm system. Obsolete technique.

Texture. The echo pattern within an organ; could be homogeneous or irregular.

Through Transmission. The amount of sound passing through a structure (see Fig. 5-1). Same as acoustic enhancement (mentioned previously).

Transonicity. Term used to indicate the amount of sound passing through a mass or cyst, usually qualified as good or poor. Same as acoustic enhancement.

Trendelenburg. A position in which a recumbent patient is tilted so that the feet are higher than the head.

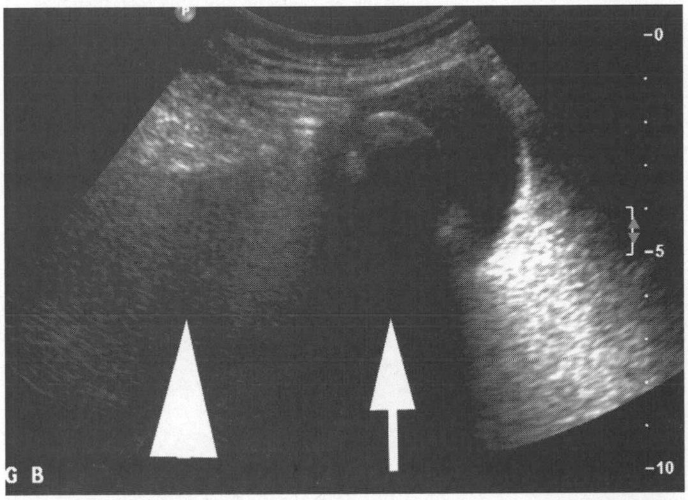

Figure 5-3. ■ *The acoustic shadowing from the stones in the gallbladder* (GB) *is "sharp"* (small arrow), *whereas the shadowing from the bowel gas is "soft"* (large arrow).

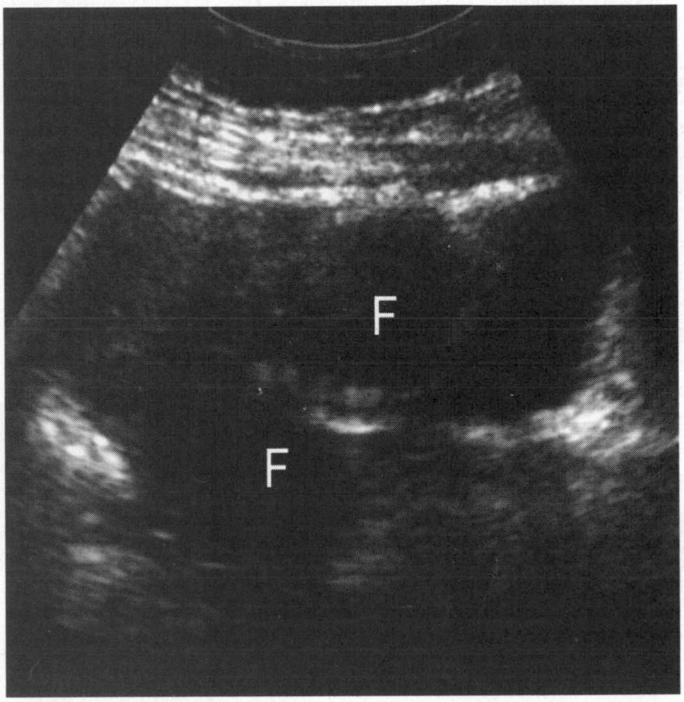

Figure 5-4. ■ *The fibroid* (F) *at the posterior aspect of the uterus is a solid homogenous mass with some internal echoes. Its density attenuates sound, so the internal echogenicity diminishes near the back wall, and there is poor through transmission.*

Terms Relating to Orientation

ANATOMIC TERMS

See Figures 5-5, 5-6, and 5-7.

Anterior or Ventral. Structure lying toward the front of the patient.

Distal. Away from the origin.

Inferior or Caudal. Terms denoting a structure closer to the patient's feet.

Lateral. Structure lying away from the midline.

Medial or Mesial. Structure lying toward the midline.

Posterior or Dorsal. Structure lying toward the back of the patient.

Prone. The patient lies on his or her stomach.

Proximal. Nearer to the center of the body.

Quadrant. The abdomen is divided into four quarters, each known as a *quadrant*.

Superior, Cranial, or Cephalad. Interchangeable terms denoting a structure closer to the patient's head.

Supine. The patient lies on his or her back.

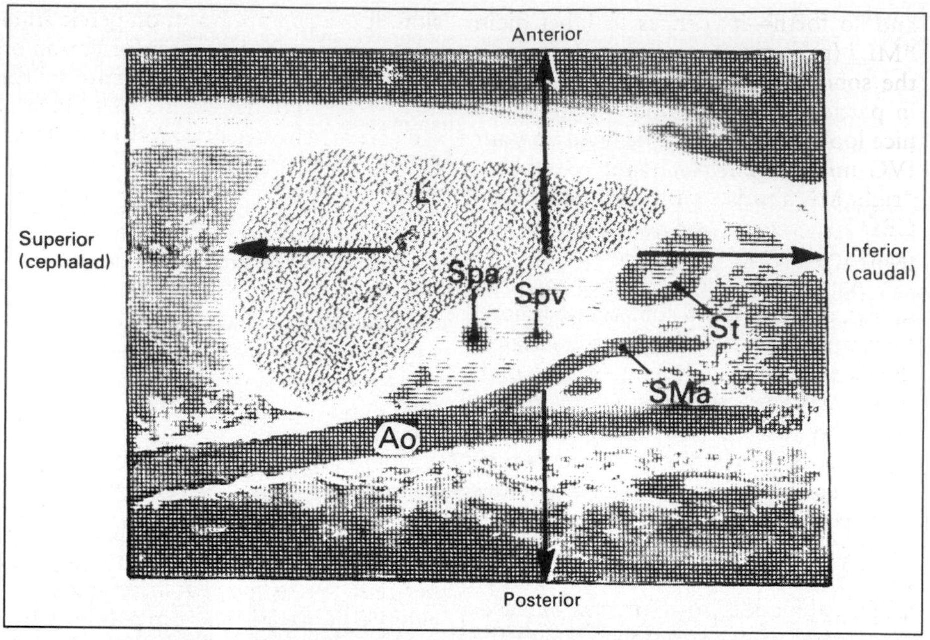

Figure 5-6. ■ *A longitudinal scan to the left of the midline showing normal structures and orientation.*

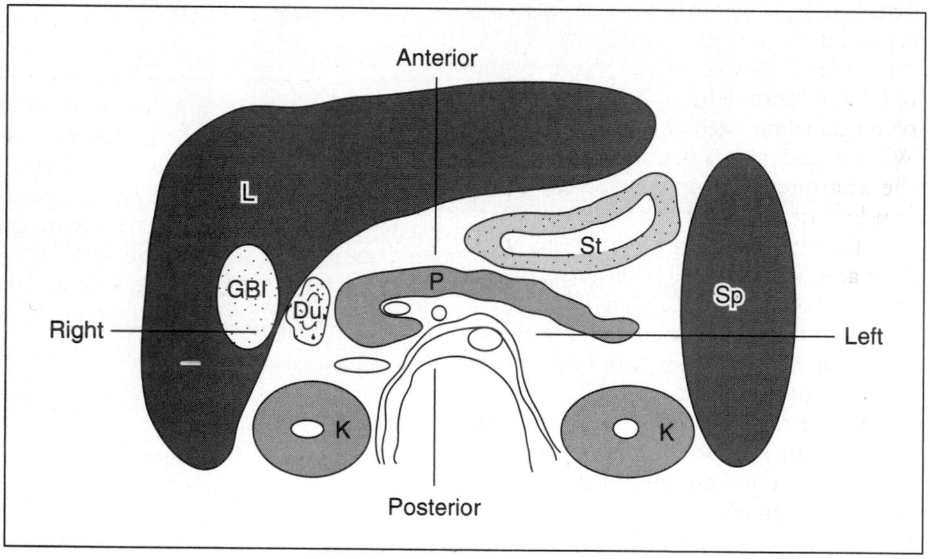

Figure 5-7. ■ *Transverse scan. The sonographic right and left are the opposite of the viewer's right and left.*

Terms Relating to Labeling

The American Institute of Ultrasound in Medicine has established standards for labeling studies so that a sonogram done in Columbus, Ohio, can be interpreted with no misunderstanding in Baltimore, Maryland.

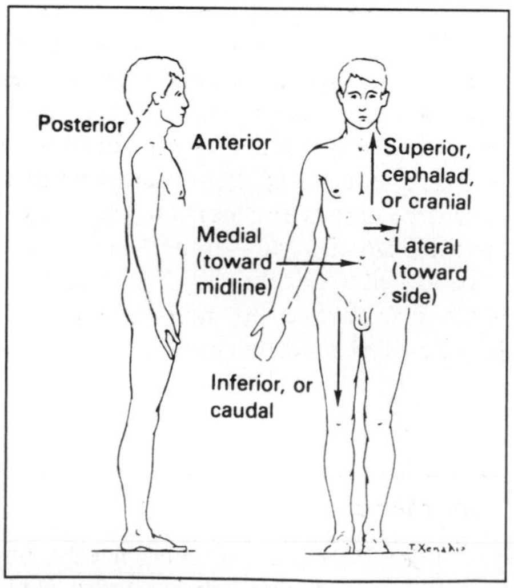

Figure 5-5. ■ *Standard labeling nomenclature used to show where structures lie in relation to each other.*

These standards are occasionally revised and are available on request from The American Institute of Ultrasound in Medicine.

One of the great features of real-time ultrasound is that structures can be visualized in their long axis, which may be oblique and may not fall neatly into a sagittal or transverse plane. The basic principle of examining everything in at least two planes is a sound one, however, so suggestions for labeling an abdomen and a pelvis in longitudinal and transverse planes are discussed here.

LONGITUDINAL (SAGITTAL) SCANS

In the abdomen, the aorta and the inferior vena cava (IVC) may not follow an exact longitudinal plane but should be imaged in their long axes if possible. Because these images also include other anatomy of interest—left lobe of liver, superior mesenteric artery, pancreas, and so forth—it suffices to label them "ML" (midline) unless you wish to draw the sonologist's attention to something in particular. For instance, if you get a nice look at the pancreatic head on your IVC image, you may want to label it "right ML, head of panc" or "ML, distal CBD" (common bile duct) if that appears in the head of the pancreas.

As you scan left, "left sag" will do unless, again, there is something of note. "Right sag" will suffice for the longitudinals on the right, although some sonologists may wish to know which images were obtained more coronally, so as you scan through the patient's ribs and come in through his or her side, "rt sag obl" is more precise. It is not generally necessary to label each organ; however, smaller organs or subtle structures such as the CBD, gallbladder, or pancreas are usually named (i.e., a section through the CBD will be labeled *CBD*).

TRANSVERSE SCANS

Transversely, whether you are angling cephalad or not, on inspiration or not, "trans left," "trans right," "trans right obl," and "trans left obl" will cover most of the labeling needed in the abdomen. When a patient has pathology distorting the anatomy, or normal variants that you had to trace to the source to figure out, throw all those rules out the window and label copiously on-screen even at the risk of insulting your sonologist. Always remember that someone may review that sonogram a month later, when you are not on hand to explain.

In the normal pelvis, the following labels do nicely, provided that you are certain that these are indeed the ovaries you are imaging:

ML

long. uterus

long. (or sag) right (or left) ovary

trans right (or left) ovary

trans C (cervix)

trans uterus or, perhaps, trans uterine fundus

Because patients often neglect to say things like, "Oh yes, they removed my right ovary when they did my appendectomy 10 years ago," it is unwise to blithely label any lump of tissue in the adnexa "ovary." If unsure, stick to "right sag," "right trans," and "right adnexa."

It may be helpful to label all "endovag" images as such to avoid confusion. It is also important, on pelvic studies, to include the patient information on each image. Make sure the date of the last menstrual period or last normal menstrual period is recorded, even if that date is "10 years ago." An otherwise unremarkable scan of a plump endometrial cavity takes on new meaning when it is made clear that the patient is postmenopausal or at an inappropriate stage of her cycle.

DECUBITUS

These are scans taken with the patient lying on either side; following the traditional radiology standard, the label is for the side down (closest to the x-ray film) (Fig. 5-8). For example, an image of the left kidney taken with the patient on his or her right side is labeled "right lateral decubitus." Frankly, this terminology is confusing, and is better labeled simply "left side up." The exception is the gallbladder, which is routinely examined with the right side up: "decub" will suffice, no matter what the plane, in this case.

CORONAL

The term *coronal* implies a specific plane. The image is taken from the patient's side, whether he or she is decubitus or supine, if you are scanning the abdomen (see Fig. 5-8). In the neonatal head, *coronal* refers to images taken through the fontanelle, from side to side (see Chapter 36).

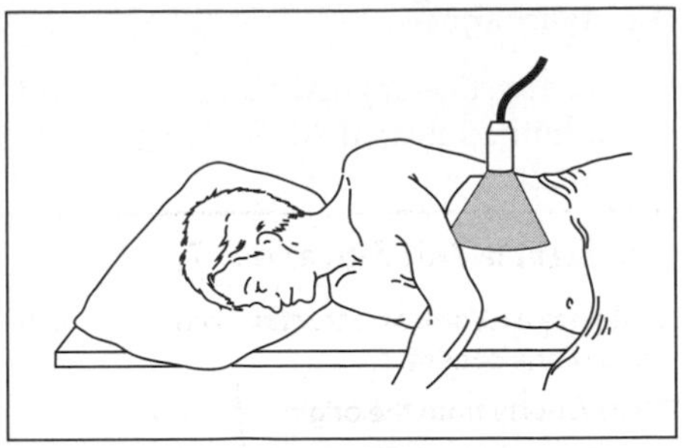

Figure 5-8. ■ *Left coronal, right decubitus, or left-side-up view.*

Scanning Techniques and Choices

GENERAL PRINCIPLES

Regardless of the type of exam or transducer being employed, the following guidelines help ensure meaningful images.

1. The beam should be as perpendicular as possible to the structure being imaged. (Note: This is always true unless you are using Doppler—see Chapter 4.)
2. Scan through the best acoustic window possible—this may be the liver, a mass, or the distended bladder. If no window is available, consider creating one by having the patient drink water to fill the bladder or filling the stomach with water.
3. Get in the habit of demonstrating the long axis. Ultrasound is flexible in scanning planes, unlike computed tomography, and any plane can be used as long as bone or gas does not interfere. The longest axis of the kidney, the aorta, or a tumor can be shown on real-time; then turn 90 degrees and demonstrate the short axis.
4. Never carelessly photograph an image that is suspicious for pathology when you think it is a scanning artifact, such as a pseudotumor caused by a rib shadow or the suggestion of gallstones created by artifact.

TRANSDUCERS

Selecting the proper transducer is critical to the success of a scan. The wrong transducer shape or frequency can give you a passable scan in which the anatomy is demonstrated, but the pathology never shows up. Keep the following factors in mind, and don't be lazy about changing transducers from patient to patient or in the middle of a study.

FREQUENCY

Use the highest frequency that will let you penetrate your object. Note, however, that you will defeat your purpose if the frequency is so high that your gain and time gain compensation settings are at their upper limits. In addition to the absence of flexibility in changing controls, you've now put noise in your image that hides subtle changes.

SHAPE-SECTOR OR SMALL FOOTPRINT SCANNER

Advantages

- Useful for areas of small access: between ribs, through a urinary bladder, through a fontanelle.
- Good for angling up under or for wedging in between tight spots.

Disadvantages

- The wedge-shaped image gives you a limited near field of view (see Fig. 2-22C).

CURVED LINEAR ARRAY

Advantages

- Much bigger field of view, good for large structures and overviews.
- Near field is wider than sector (see Fig. 2-22F).
- Useful for second- and third-trimester obstetric patients, anywhere in abdomen that it will fit.

Disadvantages

- Larger transducer face than sector, may not fit in acoustic window.
- May acquire artifacts along sides of image due to poor contact.
- Near field is still more limited than linear array, but not by much, so it is the most popular transducer design.

LINEAR ARRAY

Advantages

- "Block" shape of image allows for large field of view in superficial areas; excellent for small parts, renal transplants, subfacial hematomas, and other superficial imaging (see Fig. 2-22A).
- Possible to hook up two images to form one very large field of view in cases when it is important not to extrapolate measurements (e.g., when measuring renal transplants or large masses undergoing radiation therapy, or when demonstrating hepatomegaly or polyhydramnios).

Disadvantages

- Can only be used where there is a large window, such as in the midline or in a pregnant uterus. Cannot get between ribs.
- Even where there are no ribs, the flat surface of the transducer makes it difficult to angle around pockets of gas or through small windows.

ENDOVAGINAL

Advantages

- No full bladder needed.
- Better resolution because decreased distance allows higher frequency.
- Good way to assess cervix without distortion caused by full bladder.
- Can see anatomy and fetal heart motion sooner than transabdominally (see Chapter 39).
- Using the transducer as a palpating tool allows recognition of the source of pain.

Disadvantages

- Limited field of view (difficult to visualize a fibroid or large ovarian mass).
- More invasive; sometimes, the patient may object. Note: The sonographer's gender has to be considered here. Medicolegally, it is wise to have a woman in the room during insertion and probably during the use of an endovaginal transducer.

There are many specialized transducers, including endorectal and intraoperative, that are described in other chapters. Most transducers, however, even small parts, generally fall into one of these categories. Transesophageal and endoluminal transducers are not commonly used by sonographers or general sonologists so far and will not be considered further.

COLOR

The use of color is constantly being refined; currently, it is predominantly used to demonstrate fluid motion, and therefore flow, if the velocity is great enough. The color is coded to show the direction of the flow.

Helpful

- Good as an adjunct to duplex Doppler scanning; maps out the vessels.
- Clarifies confusing Doppler values, such as those due to reversal of flow, etc.
- Establishes vascularity of an organ, as when questioning a torsed testicle.
- Establishes direction of flow at a glance, such as in the portal vein.

Not Helpful

- In instances of slow flow; if a tumor doesn't "light up" with color, it may still be a vascular tumor with low-velocity flow. A venous lake may contain blood, but the blood moves so slowly that it does not light up with color (see Chapter 42).
- In precisely assessing flow. Color gives an image of the actual flow in the lumen, but spectral analysis, which quantifies flow, is obtained from the traditional pulsed Doppler.

CINE LOOP

Most machines offer this option to "rewind" the real-time images for several frames, a boon to those with a slow finger on the freeze button.

Helpful

- In catching a moving target, such as a four-chamber view of a fetal heart. Check back to make sure your frozen image is indeed the longest femur length, etc.
- When patients can't hold their breath, and the desired part flashes in and out of view.
- In fighting the "Was That a Real Lesion?" Syndrome. By all means, go back and look at it again.

Not Helpful

- When rerunning the cineloop causes you to violate one of the basic principles of scanning. If you can't duplicate a "lesion," maybe it was artifact in the first place. Beware of creating pathology where it doesn't exist.
- When students of scanning become too dependent on it. That stripped-down unit in Labor and Delivery probably won't offer it at 3:00 AM.

CONTRAST MEDIA

So far, contrast media are not commonly available except in echocardiography, but they can be helpful in showing subtle intraluminal or intraparenchymal masses, enhancing color flow, and showing fallopian tube spill.

Patient Preparation

GALLBLADDER AND PANCREAS SCANS

Patients scheduled for upper abdominal scans should ingest nothing that will make the gallbladder contract for at least 8 hours preceding the sonogram. Water is acceptable, but often the patient is scheduled for an upper gastrointestinal series on the same day. This situation can be a problem if good visualization of the pancreas is required, as water in the stomach is frequently crucial to the ultrasound exam. In those cases requiring the ingestion of water, the gastrointestinal series should be scheduled for the following day.

PELVIC SCANS

The bladder should be distended to provide an acoustic window to the pelvic structures in patients undergoing a transabdominal pelvic scan. Outpatients should be instructed to drink enough fluid—at least 16 ounces—to make their bladder slightly uncomfortable at the time of the exam. Because an endovaginal examination is now routinely used as a follow-up except in young girls, we now recommend not emptying the bladder 2 hours before an exam rather than drinking water when a transvaginal exam is likely to be performed. Inpatients instructed to ingest nothing by mouth require alternative arrangements: an indwelling Foley catheter can be clamped ahead of time, an IV flow rate can be increased, or permission can be obtained to insert a catheter so that the bladder can be filled in the ultrasound lab.

The endovaginal transducer has made bladder filling unnecessary in many situations. Remember that the bladder can be too full. An overdistended bladder can distort or displace pathology enough to hide it altogether. For rectal and endovaginal scanning, the bladder should be empty or only slightly filled for use as a landmark. Some prefer that patients undergoing a rectal scan should be prepped with an enema, although it generally makes little difference.

OBSTETRIC SCANS

For early transabdominal obstetric scans, the bladder should be distended enough to visualize the lower uterine segments. After 20 weeks, the bladder should be empty to properly evaluate the cervix and its relationship to the placenta.

Patient–Sonographer Interaction

Talking to your patients will not only relieve anxiety, but will also reassure them that you are interested in helping to diagnose their problem. Because sonography requires so much time and patient contact, a sonographer is in an excellent position to elicit pertinent information from the patient.

The information provided with outpatients is usually limited, so questions such as "What kind of trouble are you having?" or "Is this the first time you've been in the hospital?" can trigger a flood of information that can be relayed to the physician. With inpatients, it should be standard procedure to read the synopsis of a patient's chart. Even with inpatients, however, conversation can yield information that helps focus a study: consider the case of a patient sent for a sonogram to rule out gallstones who casually mentions that pesky renal stone he passed 5 years ago.

Patients often ask the sonographer what the study shows. It is important to understand how much information the sonologist and the patient's clinician are willing to let the sonographer reveal. One way to answer questions without being too evasive is to explain that although sonographers are well versed in anatomy, diagnosing pathology from the images is up to the doctors. Questions about bioeffects should never be evaded; the sonographer has a responsibility to keep up to date and answer the patient. At this time, no side effects from the levels of ultrasound used for diagnostic imaging have been documented, but power levels have been increasing.

Sonographer–Sonologist Interaction

The sonographer and the sonologist should work together as a team. Once the sonographer performs a preliminary scan, both should discuss the findings, and the sonologist should rescan any confusing or unusual areas. Additional views can be made before the patient is removed from the table. The sonologist can benefit from watching the sonographer rescan a difficult area for which a specific scanning technique has been devised. If the sonologist is not available, it can be helpful to videotape confusing areas that are clarified by some dynamic process, for example, peristalsis in a very suspicious-looking "mass," or an alarming arrhythmia in a fetus when Doppler or M-mode is not available.

The physician should be informed about any problems encountered during scanning that may pertain to pathology—for instance, you may turn in a nice, homogeneous image of a liver, but to get that pretty picture, you had to change to a much lower-frequency transducer than you thought you'd need. This issue might bring fatty liver into question.

Perhaps one of the most significant contributions a sonographer can make to the diagnosis is to determine the source of a localized area of tenderness or of a palpable mass. The sonographer is in a unique position to see what lies directly beneath the patient's most tender spot. A good example is the patient with right upper-quadrant pain in whom no gallstones are found. The presence of acute pain at the site of the gallbladder makes acute cholecystitis likely. The borders of a palpable mass can be defined on film by placing arrows where the edges are felt.

The value of this type of information is diminished if the films are read later in the day by a physician. Physician-to-patient contact may be essential to confirm such an important pathologic finding. A combined approach, using the expertise of both a sonographer and a sonologist, ensures that the best possible examination is made. As it becomes increasingly more common for the physician to see neither the patient nor the sonographer, it becomes increasingly important for the sonographer to leave an impression in writing for the sonologist.

SELECTED READING

American Institute of Ultrasound in Medicine. Safety statement. Approved March 1995. Current versions are available to the public upon request or at http//www.airum.org.

Barnett SB. Ultrasound safety in obstetrics: what are the concerns? *Ultrasound Quart* 1995;13:228–239.

Barnett SB, Ter Haar GR, Ziskin MC, et al. International recommendations and guidelines for the safe use of diagnostic ultrasound in medicine. *Ultrasound Med Biol* 2000;26:355–366.

Benacerraf BR. Filling of the bladder for pelvic sonograms: an ancient form of torture. *J Ultrasound Med* 2003;22:239–241.

Sonographic Abdominal Anatomy

JULIA A. DROSE

6

SONOGRAM ABBREVIATIONS

Ao	Aorta
Azv	Azygous vein (ascending lumbar vein)
Ca	Celiac artery
CBD	Common bile duct
CHa	Common hepatic artery
CHD	Common hepatic duct
Cla	Common iliac artery
Cr	Crus of the diaphragm
Du	Duodenum
GBl	Gallbladder
Gda	Gastroduodenal artery
Hea	Hepatic artery
Hev	Hepatic vein
IMa	Inferior mesenteric artery
IMv	Inferior mesenteric vein
IVC	Inferior vena cava
K	Kidney
L	Liver
LGa	Left gastric artery
LGv	Left gastric vein
LHev	Left hepatic vein
LPv	Left portal vein
LRa	Left renal artery
LRv	Left renal vein
MHev	Middle hepatic vein
P	Pancreas
PHa	Proper hepatic artery
Ps	Psoas muscles
Pv	Portal vein
QL	Quadratus lumborum
RA	Rectus abdominis
RGv	Right gastric vein
RHev	Right hepatic vein
RPv	Right portal vein
RRa	Right renal artery
RRv	Right renal vein
S	Spine
SGv	Splenogastric vein
SMA	Superior mesenteric artery
SMV	Superior mesenteric vein
Spa	Splenic artery
Spv	Splenic vein
St	Stomach

Because the bony landmarks visible with other imaging modalities are not available and gas may limit the ultrasound field of view, recognizing normal anatomic landmarks is crucial for proper orientation. Vascular structures are the most important in defining location, but normal muscular structure and organ position must also be known.

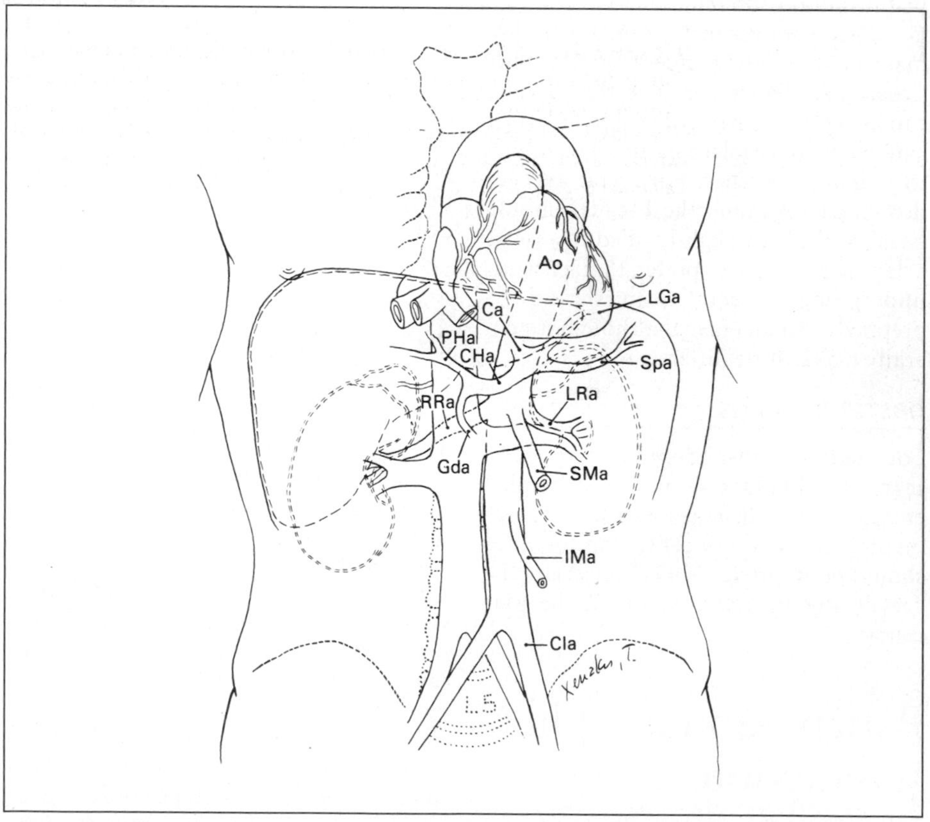

Figure 6-1. ■ *Commonly visualized vessels arising from the aorta are the celiac artery, splenic artery, left gastric artery, common hepatic artery, proper hepatic artery, gastroduodenal artery, right and left renal arteries, superior mesenteric artery, inferior mesenteric artery, and—below the aortic bifurcation at the level of the fourth lumbar vertebra—the right and left common iliac arteries. Only the portion of the aorta below the diaphragm is visualized on an abdominal study.*

KEY ANATOMICAL STRUCTURES

ARTERIES

Aorta (Abdominal). Main trunk of the arterial system (see Figs. 6-1 and 6-5). Lies anterior to the spine and bifurcates into the right and left common iliac arteries at the level of the umbilicus.

Celiac Artery (Axis, Trunk). Arises just below the liver from the anterior aorta and is usually only 2 to 3 cm in length (see Figs. 6-1, 6-2, and 6-5). It almost immediately divides into the splenic artery, left gastric artery, and common hepatic artery.

Common Femoral Arteries. Seen in the inguinal region, the common femoral arteries arise from the iliac arteries and extend into the upper thigh (see Fig. 50-1). A branch—the profunda femoris—originates just below the inguinal ligament.

Common Iliac Arteries. Originate from the aorta at the level of the umbilicus and extend toward the groin (Fig. 6-1). Less than 15 mm in diameter at their origin is normal.

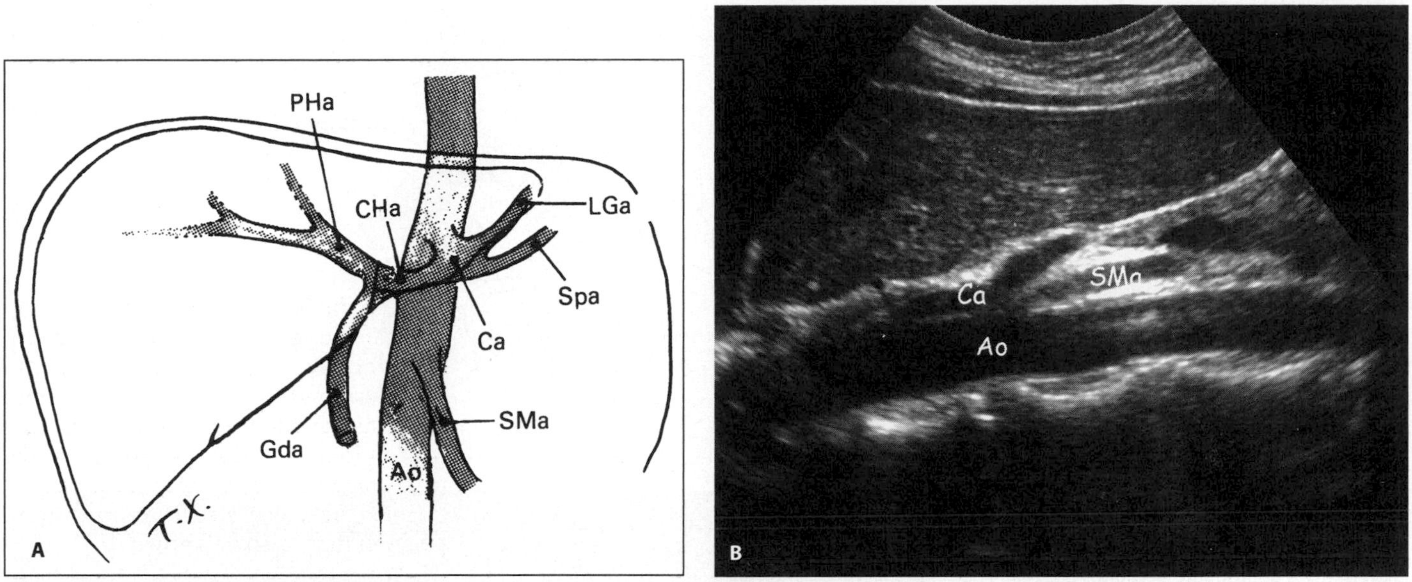

Figure 6-2. ■ *A. The vessel arising from the aorta, closest to the diaphragm is the celiac artery. This vessel is a 1- to 2-cm trunk that bifurcates into the splenic and common hepatic arteries. The common hepatic artery then bifurcates into the proper hepatic artery and gastroduodenal artery. The superior mesenteric artery (SMA) arises from the anterior surface of the aorta at a level just inferior to the celiac artery. The less-frequently visualized left gastric artery originates from the celiac artery. **B.** Longitudinal ultrasound of the aorta showing the celiac artery arising anteriorly, with the SMA arising below it.*

Gastroduodenal Artery. Originates from the common hepatic trunk and supplies the stomach and duodenum (Figs. 6-1, 6-2, and 6-3). It is a landmark delineating the anterolateral aspect of the head of the pancreas.

Hepatic Artery (Common). Originates from the celiac trunk and courses toward the liver. It branches into the proper hepatic artery and the gastroduodenal artery (Figs. 6-1 and 6-2). Supplies the stomach, pancreas, duodenum, liver, gallbladder, and greater omentum.

Hepatic Artery (Proper). A branch of the common hepatic artery that supplies the liver and gallbladder (Figs. 6-1 and 6-2). It runs medial to the common bile duct and anterior to the portal vein into the liver within the porta hepatis.

Inferior Mesenteric Artery. Originates from the abdominal aorta close to the umbilicus (Fig. 6-1). Supplies the left portion of the transverse colon, the descending and sigmoid colon, and part of the rectum. It is not usually visualized by ultrasound except at its origin.

Left Gastric Artery. Arises from the superior margin of the celiac axis and can be seen by ultrasound for only 1 or 2 cm (Figs. 6-1 and 6-2); supplies the stomach.

Renal Arteries, Right and Left. Originate from the abdominal aorta just below the level of the SMA. They supply the kidneys, adrenals, as well as the ureters, and are often best seen when the patient is in the appropriate decubitus position. The left renal artery arises from the posterolateral wall of the aorta and enters the left renal hilum. The right arises from the posterolateral wall of the aorta, runs posterior to the inferior vena cava (IVC), and enters the right renal hilum (Fig. 6-1).

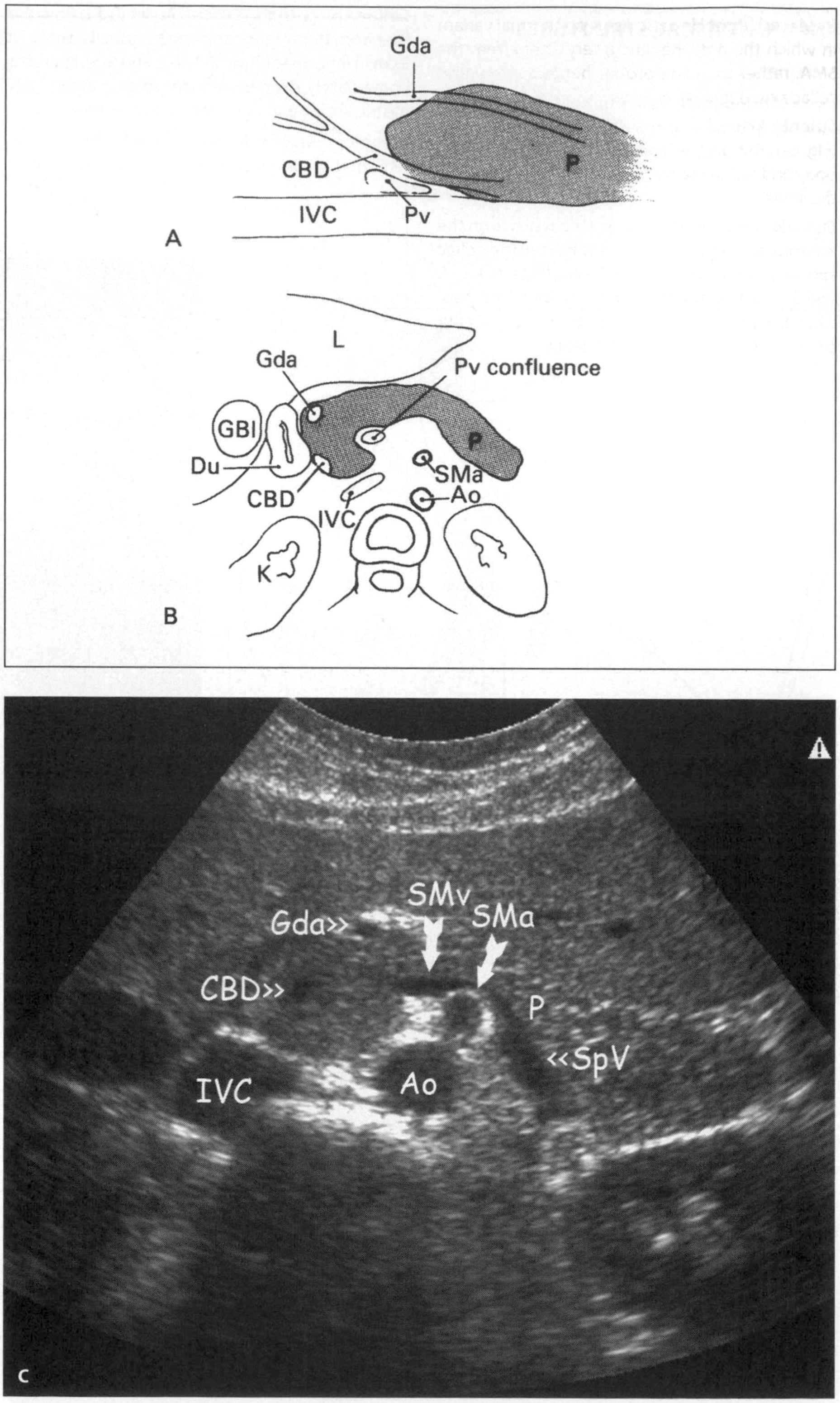

Figure 6-3. ■ *The gastroduodenal artery outlines the anterolateral margin of the head of the pancreas, whereas the common bile duct marks the posterolateral margin. A. Longitudinal diagram. B. Transverse diagram. C. Transverse ultrasound image.*

Replaced Right Hepatic Artery. A normal variant in which the right hepatic artery arises from the SMA, rather than the proper hepatic artery and celiac axis. (Fig. 6-4).

Splenic Artery. Originates from the celiac trunk (Fig. 6-1, 6-2, and 6-5) and courses superior to the body and tail of the pancreas. It primarily supplies the spleen.

Superior Mesenteric Artery. Originates from the anterior abdominal aorta, just below the celiac axis and runs parallel to the aorta (Figs. 6-1, 6-4, and 6-5). It lies posterior to the body of the pancreas. Supplies the small bowel, cecum, ascending colon, and part of the transverse colon.

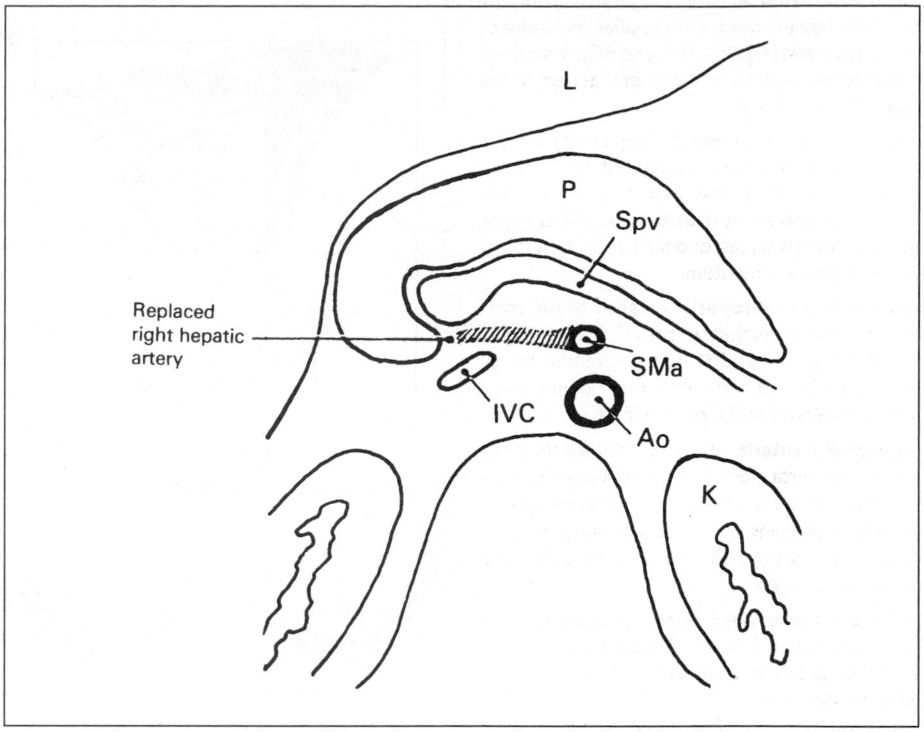

Figure 6-4. ■ *At the level of the splenic vein and pancreas, a normal variant can sometimes be visualized. The replaced right hepatic artery originates from the superior mesenteric artery to supply the liver.*

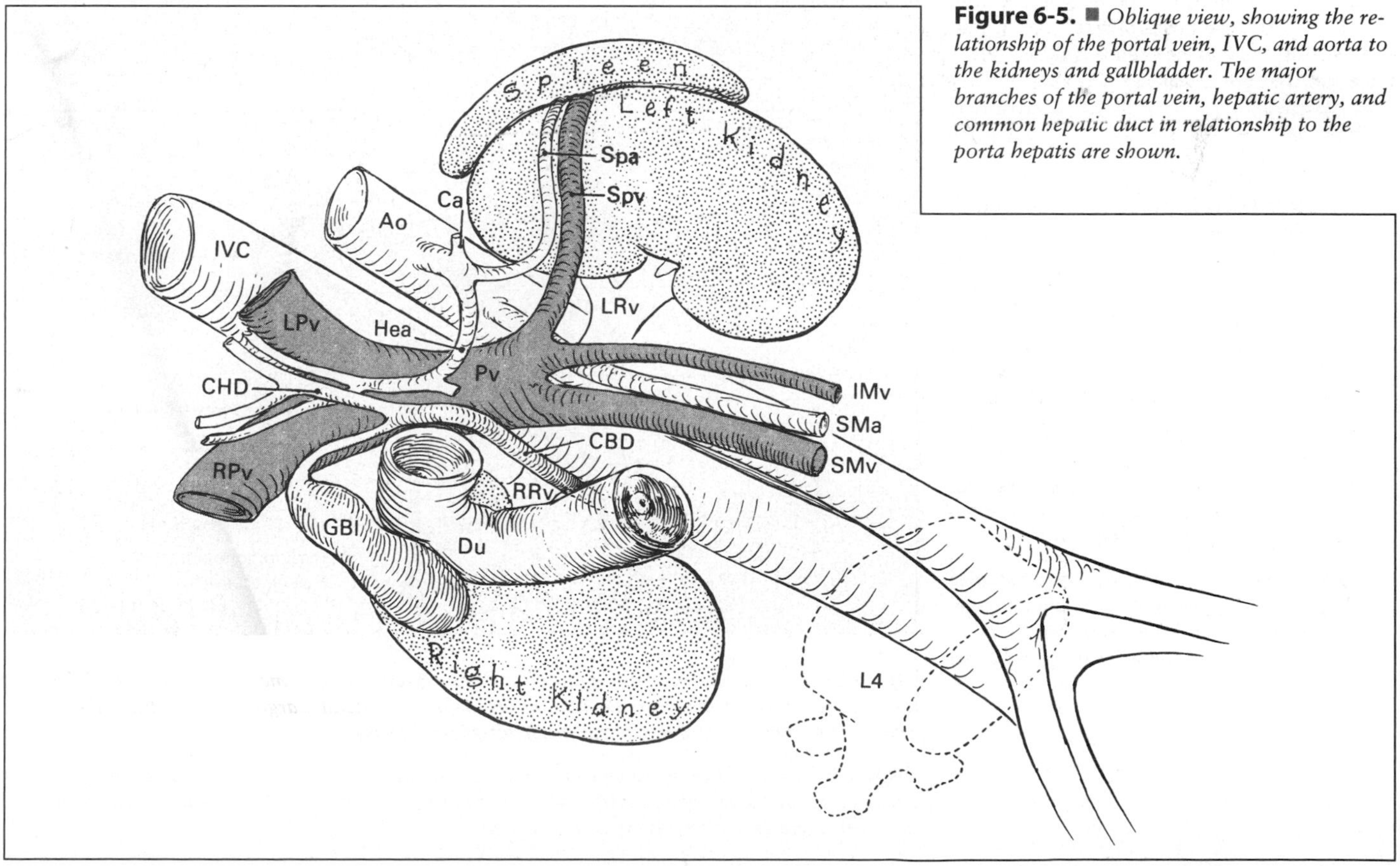

Figure 6-5. ■ *Oblique view, showing the relationship of the portal vein, IVC, and aorta to the kidneys and gallbladder. The major branches of the portal vein, hepatic artery, and common hepatic duct in relationship to the porta hepatis are shown.*

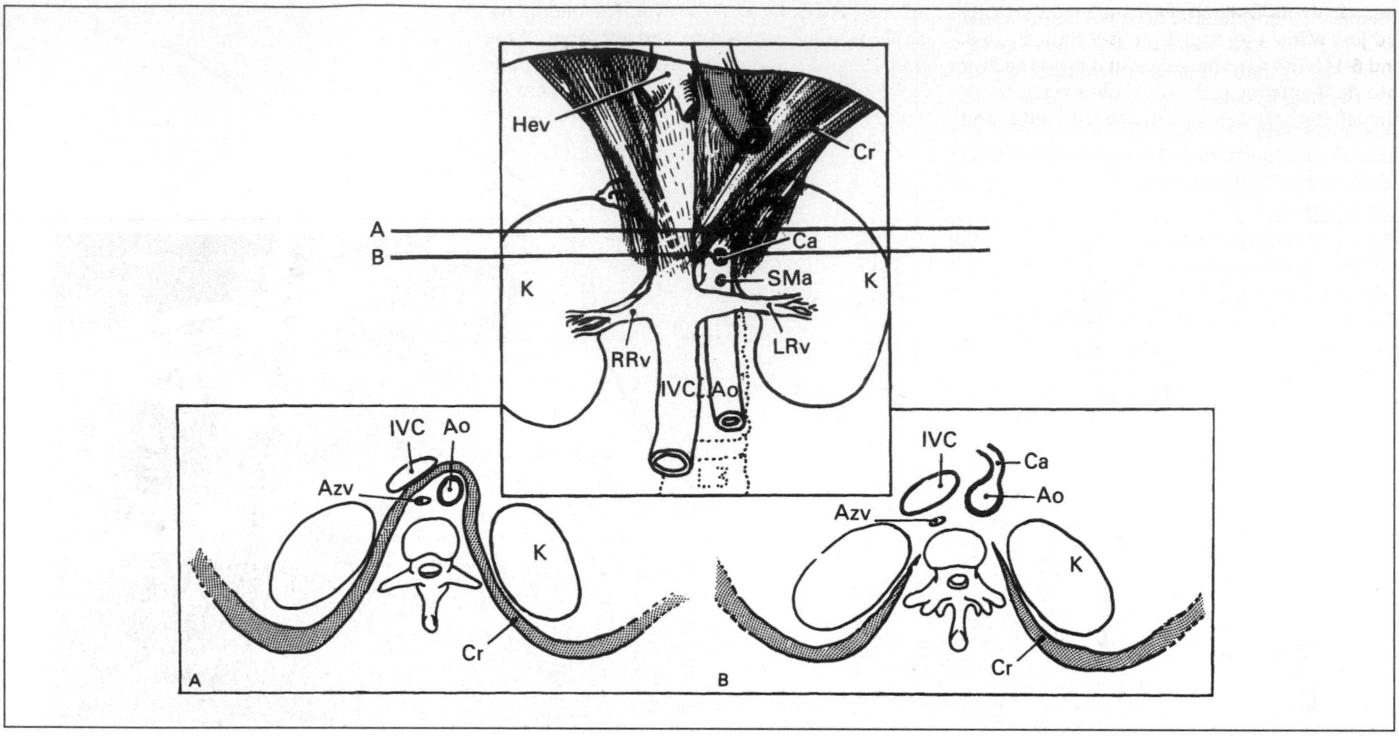

Figure 6-6. ■ *The crus of the diaphragm can be visualized anterior to the aorta above the level of the celiac artery. Below that level, it extends along the lateral aspects of the vertebral column only.* ***A.*** *A transverse section at a higher level shows the crus posterior to the IVC and anterior to the aorta. The infrequently visualized azygos vein is seen posterior to the crus.* ***B.*** *At a lower level, transversely, the crus is seen only at the lateral vertebral margins extending posteriorly.*

VEINS

Azygous Vein. Lies posterior to the IVC and is not usually seen unless enlarged secondary to congestive heart failure or portal hypertension (see Fig. 6-7).

Collaterals. Accessory vessels that develop when portal vein pressure is increased (e.g., portal hypertension) (Fig. 6-6). Collaterals can be seen in the region of the pancreas, around the esophagogastric junction (anterior to the upper portion of the aorta), in the porta hepatis, and in the splenic hilum (Fig. 6-7).

Confluence. The junction of the superior mesenteric vein and splenic vein, which forms the main portal vein (see Figs. 6-5 and 6-9).

Femoral Veins. Lie medial to the femoral arteries in the groin and upper thigh. They are normally larger than the arteries. These veins normally compress easily and do not pulsate (see Figs. 50-2 and 50-3).

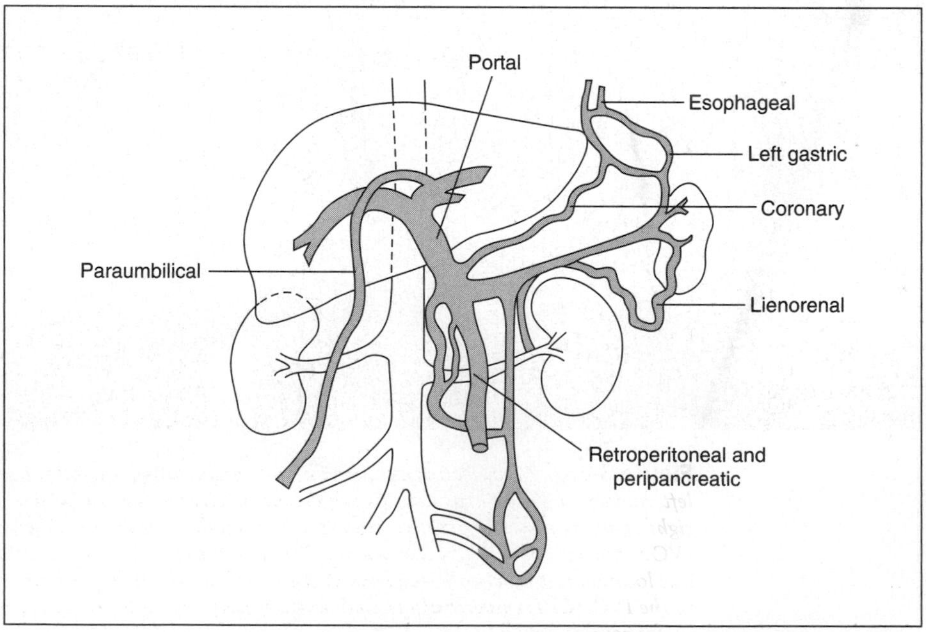

Figure 6-7. ■ *Diagram showing some of the collateral routes established when portal hypertension exists. The paraesophageal, left gastric, coronary, paraumbilical, lienorenal, retroperitoneal, and peripancreatic collaterals are demonstrated.*

Hepatic Veins. Drain the liver and empty into the IVC just below the diaphragm (see Figs. 6-8, 6-9, and 6-14). The right hepatic vein divides the liver into right anterior and right posterior segments. The left hepatic vein divides the left medial and left lateral segments of the liver. The middle hepatic vein divides the right and left lobes of the liver. (See Chapter 8 for a discussion of hepatic anatomy and the Couinaud-Bismuth system for describing parts of the liver.)

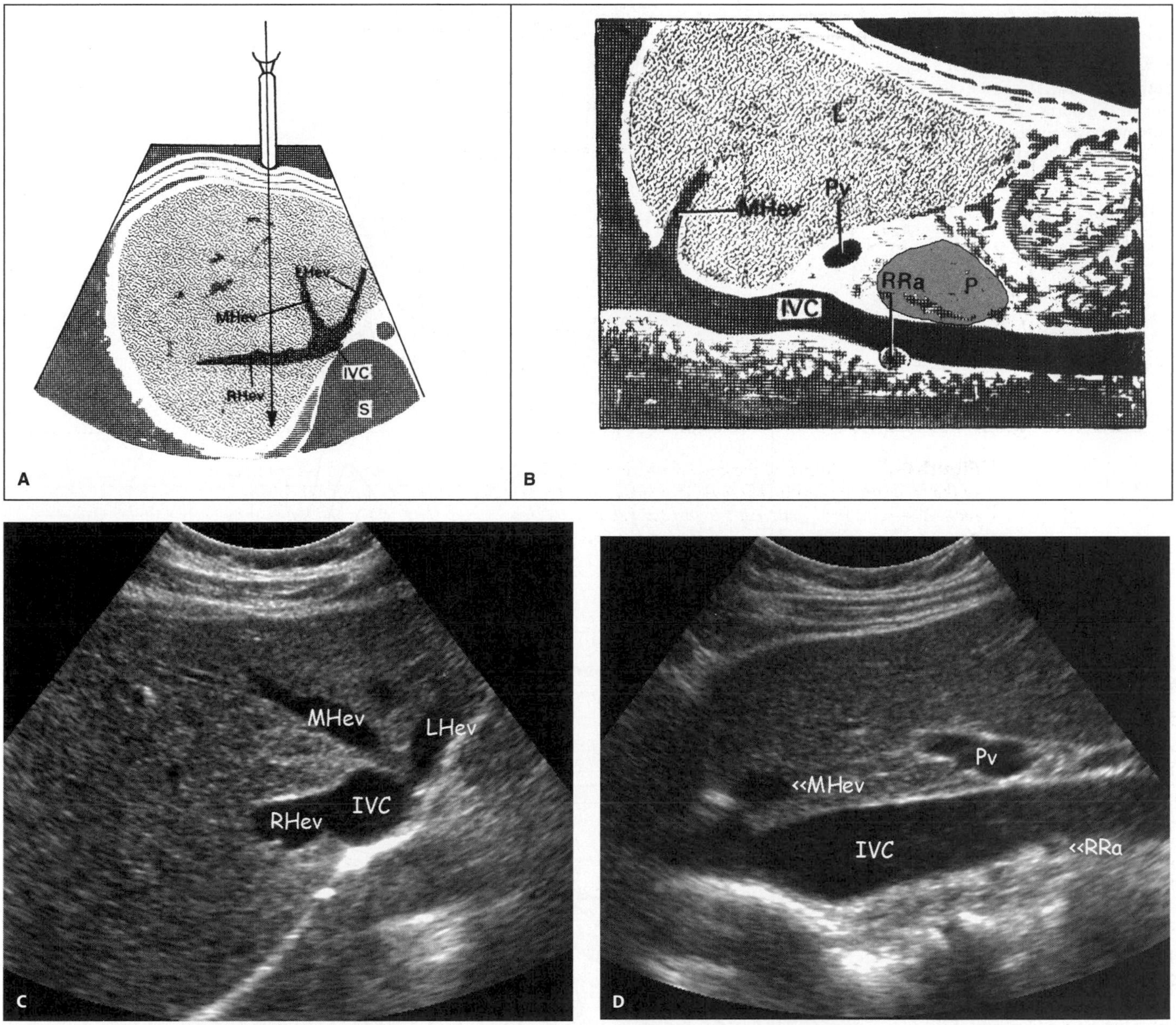

Figure 6-8. ■ *Hepatic veins. **A.** Transverse diagram, using a slightly cephalad angulation. The left, middle, and right hepatic veins can be imaged as they empty into the IVC just beneath the right diaphragm. **B.** Longitudinal diagram. The middle hepatic vein is shown as it empties into the IVC at the level of the right diaphragm. The main branch of the portal vein is seen in its extrahepatic location just superior to the head of the pancreas. The right renal artery is visualized posterior to the IVC. (C) Transverse ultrasound image corresponding to (A). (D) Longitudinal ultrasound image corresponding to (B).*

Inferior Mesenteric Vein. Courses to the left of the superior mesenteric vein to join the splenic vein (Fig. 6-9). It is usually too small to visualize by ultrasound. Drains the left third and upper portion of the colon.

Inferior Vena Cava. Returns blood from the lower half of the body and enters the right atrium of the heart (Figs. 6-5, 6-6, and 6-8B). It is formed by the union of the iliac veins. A marked change in caliber can be appreciated with respiration (Fig. 6-10).

Left Renal Vein. Drains the left kidney. Runs anterior to the aorta and posterior to the superior mesenteric artery to enter the lateral wall of the IVC. (see Figs. 6-5, 6-6, and 6-12). The left renal vein is much longer than the right renal vein.

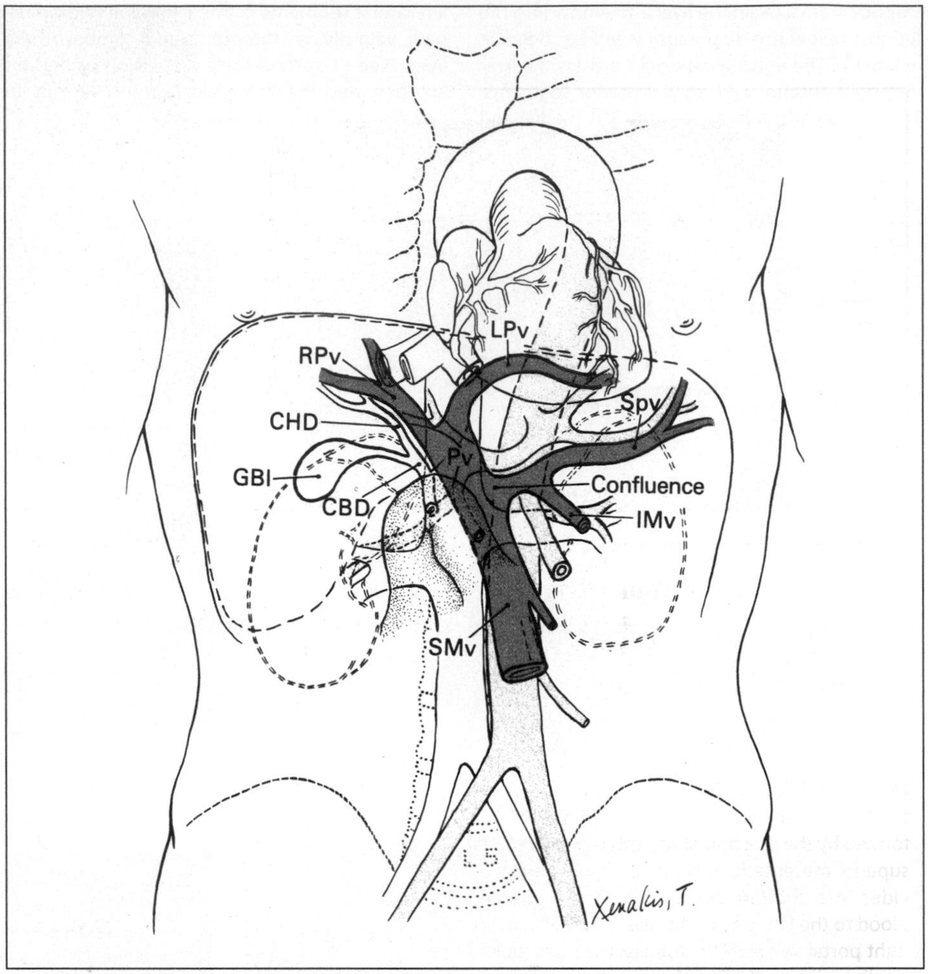

Figure 6-9. ■ *The splenic vein and superior mesenteric vein join (at the confluence) to form the main portal vein. The portal vein then branches into the liver, forming the left portal vein and the right portal vein.*

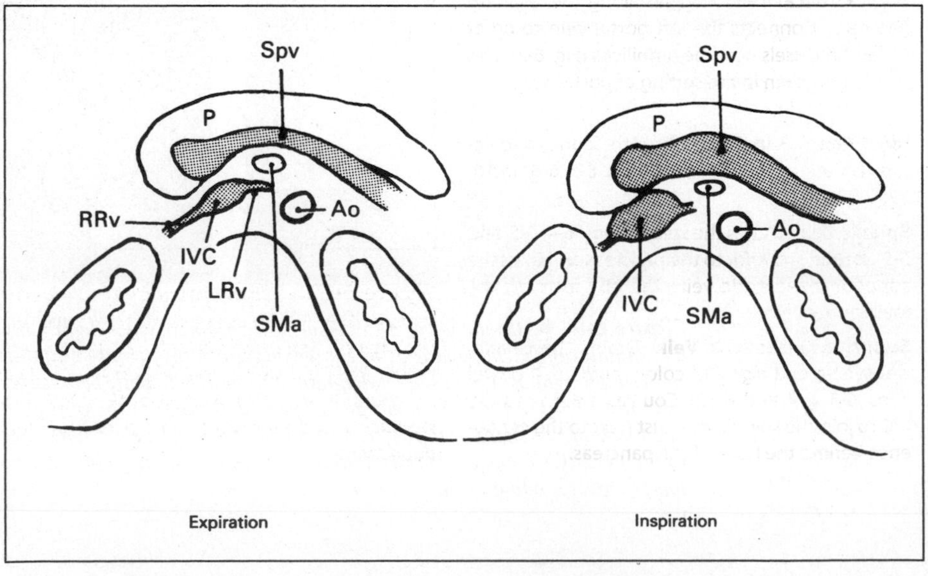

Figure 6-10. ■ *Venous structures should dilate at the end of deep inspiration or Valsalva maneuver. This maneuver can help confirm the venous nature of the vessels and enlarge the vessels to make it easier to image.*

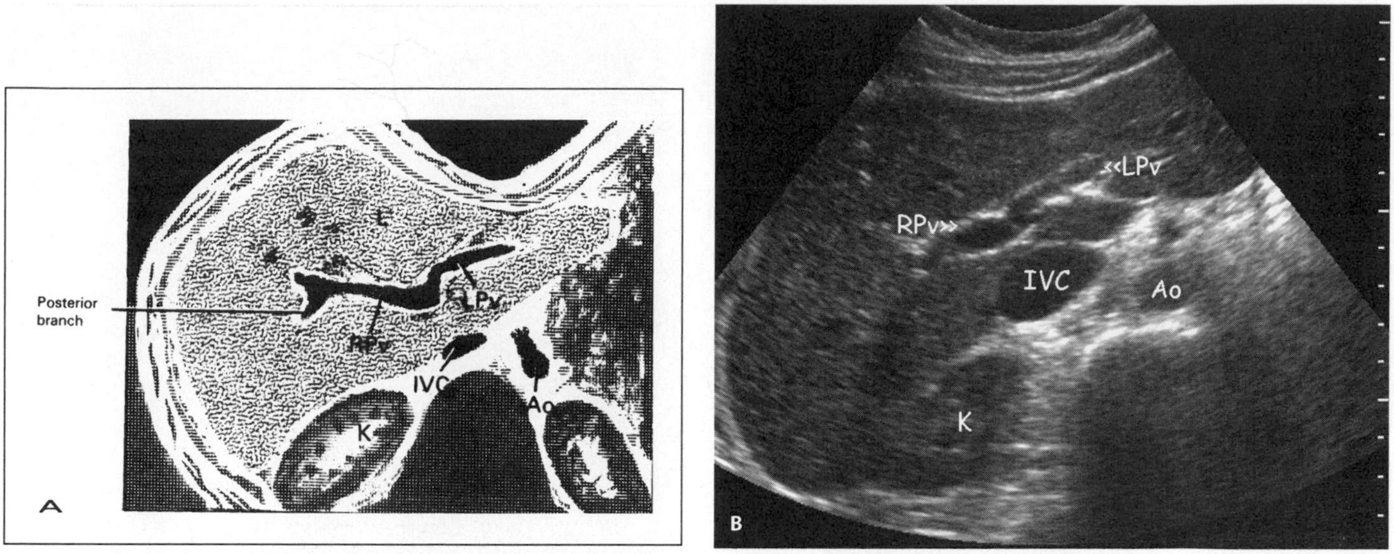

Figure 6-11. ■ *Transverse view within the liver. The portal vein branches into the left and right portal veins. The right vein again bifurcates the posterior branch supplying the posterior right lobe of the liver. A. Diagram. B. Ultrasound image.*

Main Portal Vein. Drains blood from the digestive tract and empties into the liver (Fig. 6-9). It is formed by the junction of the splenic vein and the superior mesenteric vein. The main portal vein divides into the left portal vein, which supplies blood to the left lobe of the liver (Fig. 6-9) and the right portal vein, which supplies the right lobe of the liver (Fig. 6-11). Portal veins characteristically run in triads with the hepatic arteries and bile ducts and branch away from the porta hepatis. They can be identified by their echogenic walls that occur due to acoustic reflection arising from the fibrous tissue that surrounds these triads.

Paraumbilical Vein. Courses along the falciform ligament. Connects the left portal vein to other collateral vessels near the umbilicus (Fig. 6-7). This vein is only seen in the setting of portal hypertension.

Right Renal Vein. Drains the right kidney and enters the lateral wall of the IVC (Figs. 6-5, 6-6, and 6-12).

Splenic Vein. Drains the spleen (Figs. 6-4, 6-5, and 6-9). It runs posterior to the pancreas and joins the superior mesenteric vein, thereby forming the main portal vein.

Superior Mesenteric Vein. Drains the cecum, transverse and sigmoid colon, and small bowel (Figs. 6-5, 6-9, and 6-12). Courses anterior to the IVC to join the splenic vein just next to the confluence behind the head of the pancreas.

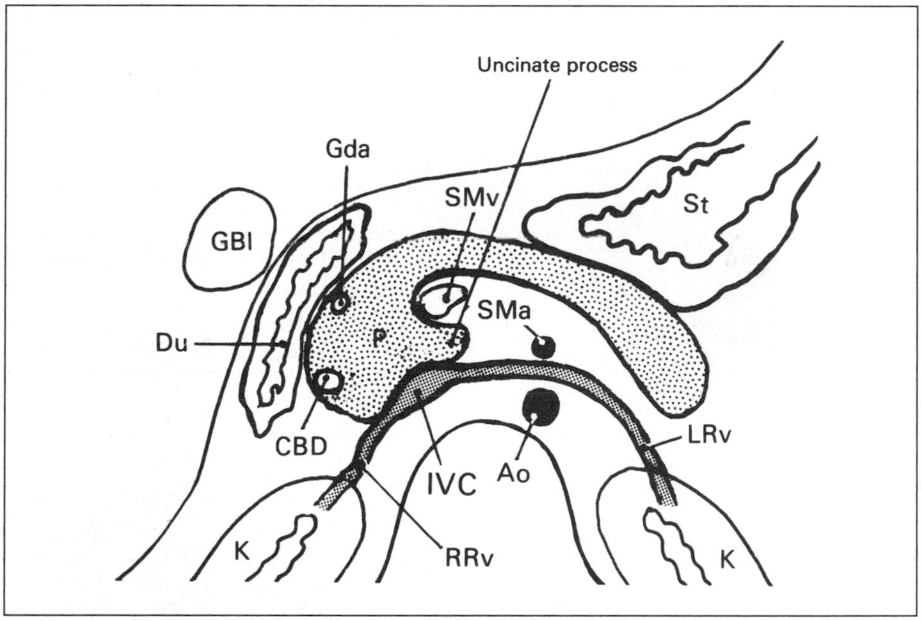

Figure 6-12. ■ *Many vascular structures can be visualized on a transverse section in the midabdomen. The IVC gives rise to the right and left renal veins; the latter passes between the aorta and the superior mesenteric artery. The superior mesenteric vein lies anterior to the IVC. The pancreas can be imaged anterior to these vessels. The gastroduodenal artery and the common bile duct assist in outlining the lateral margin of the head of the pancreas. When empty, the antrum walls of the stomach and the duodenum are seen as echo-free linear structures. The gallbladder is lateral to the duodenum.*

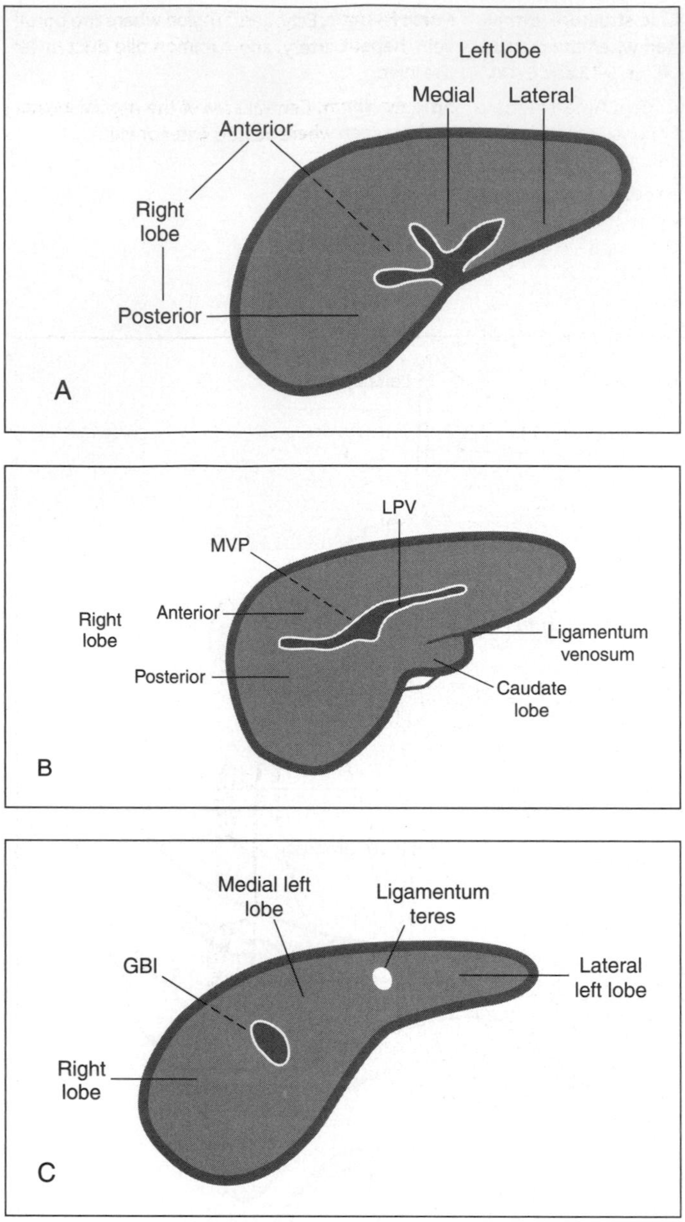

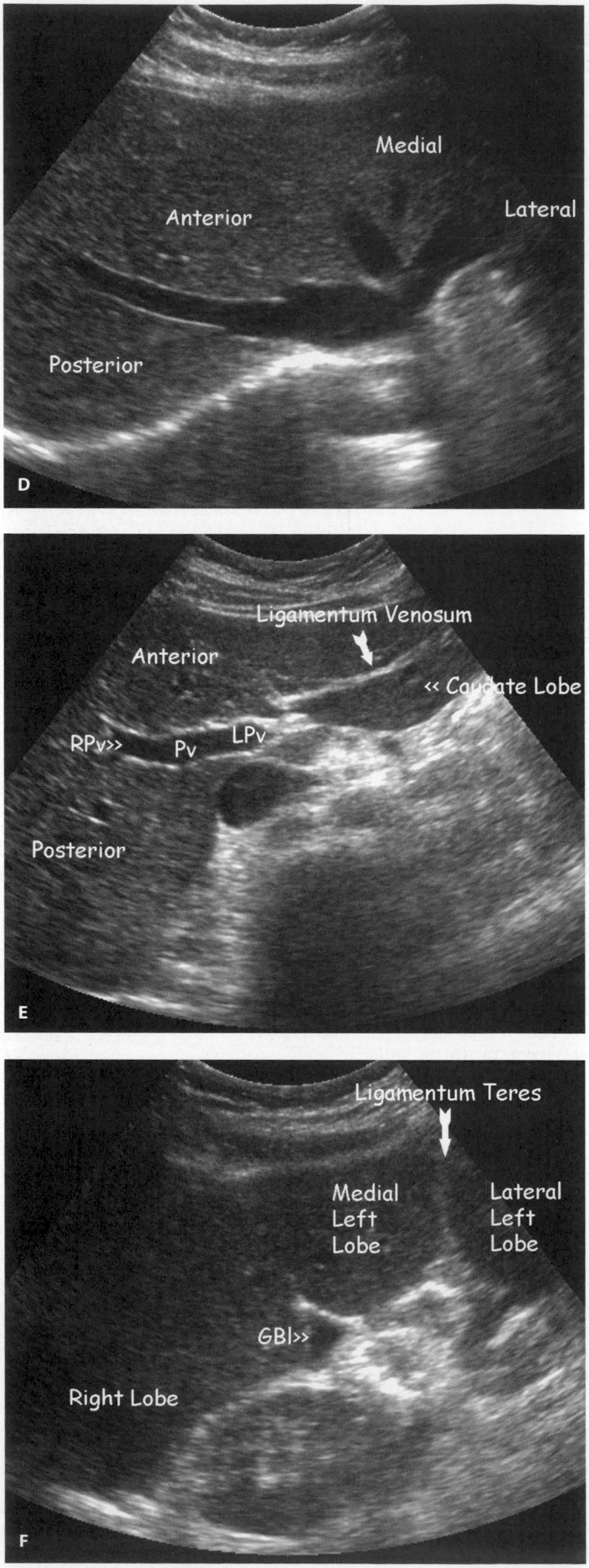

Figure 6-13. ■ *Series of transverse views of the liver to show vascular supply at different levels. Level A (diagram) and D (ultrasound image) are taken close to the diaphragm and show the hepatic veins. Level B (diagram) and E (ultrasound image) are taken in midliver and show the left and right portal veins. Level C (diagram) and F (ultrasound image) are taken at the level of the gallbladder.*

OTHER STRUCTURES

Crus of the Diaphragm. A tubular muscular structure seen anterior to the aorta and posterior to the IVC above the level of the celiac axis and superior mesenteric artery (Fig. 6-6). The right crus of the diaphragm arises from the lateral aspect of the first three lumbar vertebral bodies. The left crus arises from the first two lumbar vertebral bodies. Sonographically, the crus is seen as a thin hypoechoic band.

Ligamentum Teres. Echogenic structure within the left lobe of the liver, formed when the ductus venosus atrophies after birth. (Figs. 6-13 and 6-14).

Ligamentum Venosum. Echogenic line anterior to the caudate lobe and posterior to the left lobe of the liver (Figs. 6-13 and 6-14).

Main Lobar Fissure. Runs between the right and left lobes of the liver. Can be visualized between the gallbladder and the right portal vein (Fig. 6-14).

Porta Hepatis. Echogenic region where the portal vein, hepatic artery, and common bile duct enter the liver.

Splenic Hilum. Central area of the medial aspect of the spleen where vessels enter or exit.

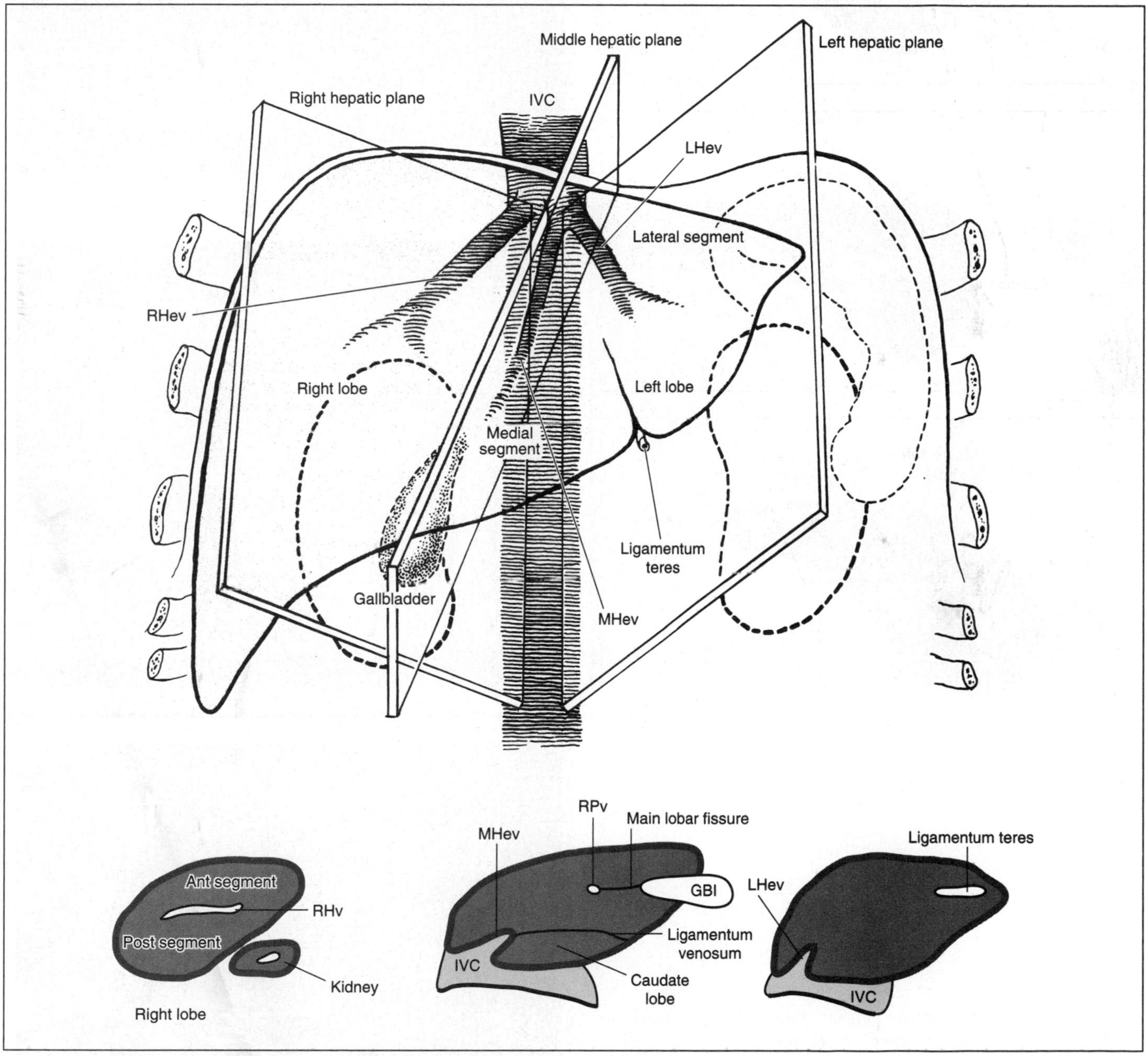

Figure 6-14. ■ *Diagram of the upper abdomen showing the liver, spleen, gallbladder, and kidneys. The hepatic veins represent the divisions between the lobes and segments of the liver. The middle hepatic vein divides the right and left lobes of the liver. The left hepatic vein separates the medial and lateral segments of the left lobe; the right hepatic vein separates the anterior and posterior segments of the right lobe of the liver. The gallbladder represents the inferior end of the separation between right and left lobes of the liver; the ligamentum teres represents the inferior end of the separation between the medial and lateral segments of the left lobe.*

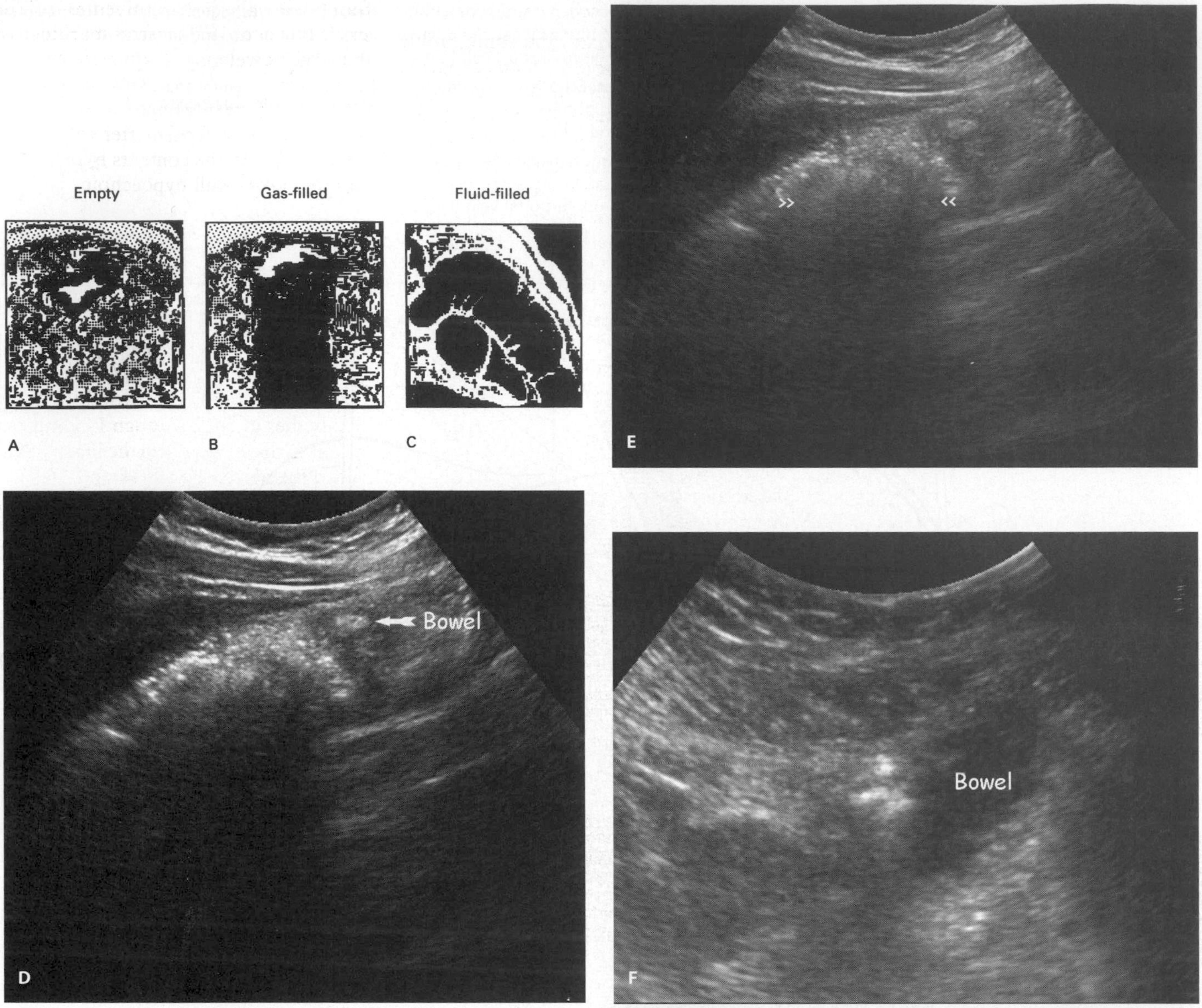

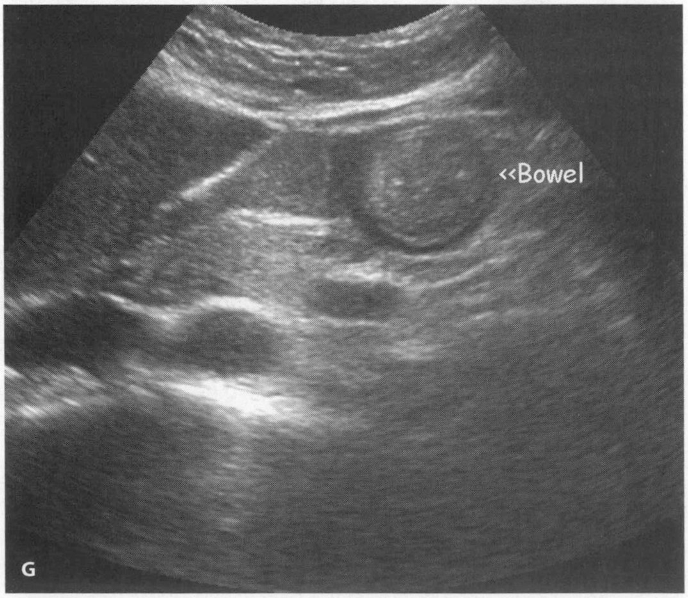

Figure 6-15. ■ *Bowel can have different sonographic appearances depending on its contents. A (diagram) and D (ultrasound image): When empty, there is a hypoechoic wall around an echogenic center. B (diagram) and E (ultrasound image): When gas-filled, there is acoustic shadowing. C (diagram) and F (ultrasound image): When fluid-filled, one may be able to make out the haustral markings of the colon or valvulae conniventes of the small bowel in the wall of the fluid-filled bowel. G (ultrasound image): bowel filled with echogenic fecal matter surrounded by hypoechoic bowel wall.*

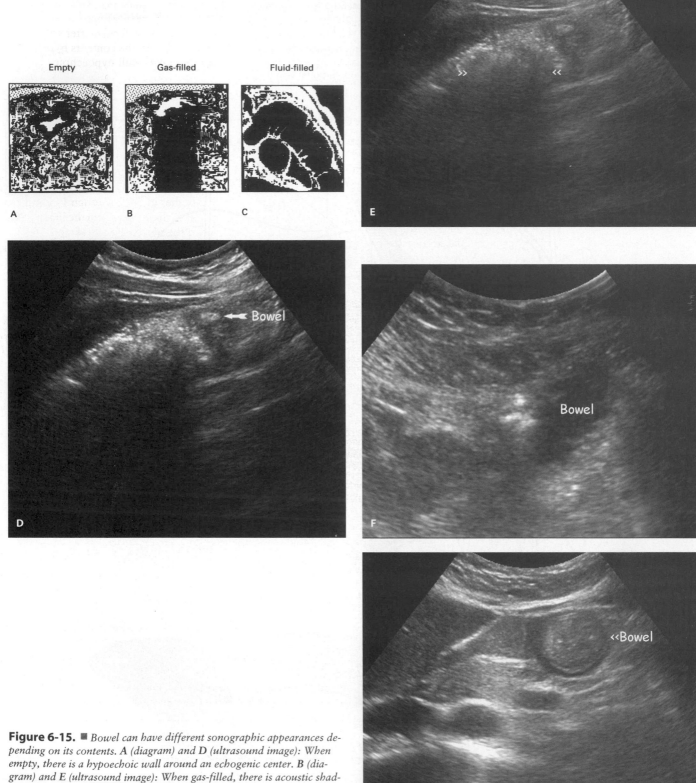

BOWEL

Sonographic visualization of the gastrointestinal tract can be challenging due to the intraluminal air usually present. The bowel wall is composed of five layers. These appear alternately echogenic (first, third, and fifth layers) and hypoechoic (second and fourth layers) by ultrasound. Bowel can have different sonographic appearances depending on its contents (Fig. 6-15). In general, small bowel is more difficult to visualize than large bowel. Peristalsis, air movement, or movement of intraluminal contents may be appreciated by ultrasound in normal bowel.

Empty Bowel

When bowel is empty, the sonographic appearance can range from an echogenic center surrounded by a thin sonolucent ring, to visualization of all five layers, depending on patient size and transducer frequency. Normal bowel wall thickness is less than 3 mm, but incompletely distended bowel or the gastric antrum may be thicker than this.

Gas-Filled Bowel

When bowel is gas-filled, distal acoustic shadowing will occur. This shadowing usually has a mottled sonographic appearance.

Fluid-Filled Bowel

Fluid-filled bowel often presents as dilated tubular structures coursing through the abdomen. When bowel contains fluid, the valvulae conniventes of the small bowel or the haustral markings of the large bowel may be appreciated.

Intraluminal Contents

Bowel filled with fecal matter will appear distended, with the contents hyperechoic and the bowel wall hypoechoic.

MUSCLES

The larger muscle groups within the abdomen may also serve as useful anatomical landmarks.

Psoas Muscles

The psoas muscles arise from the vertebral bodies of T-12 through L-5 and run lateral to the spine to join the iliacus muscles in the pelvis (Figs. 6-16 and 6-17).

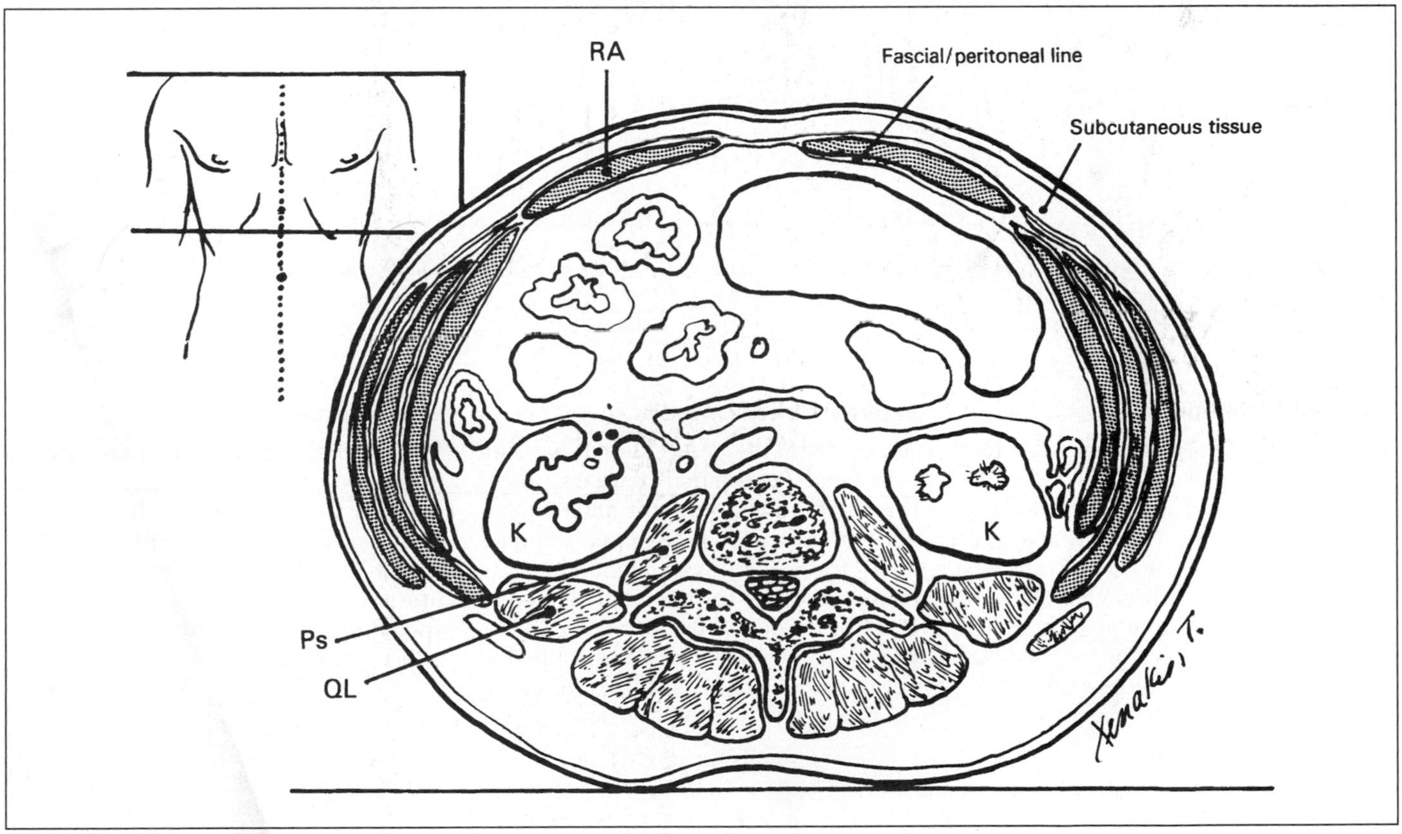

Figure 6-16. ■ *The rectus abdominis muscles lie on either side of the midline, anteriorly deep to the subcutaneous tissues. The psoas and quadratus lumborum muscles are shown in transverse section.*

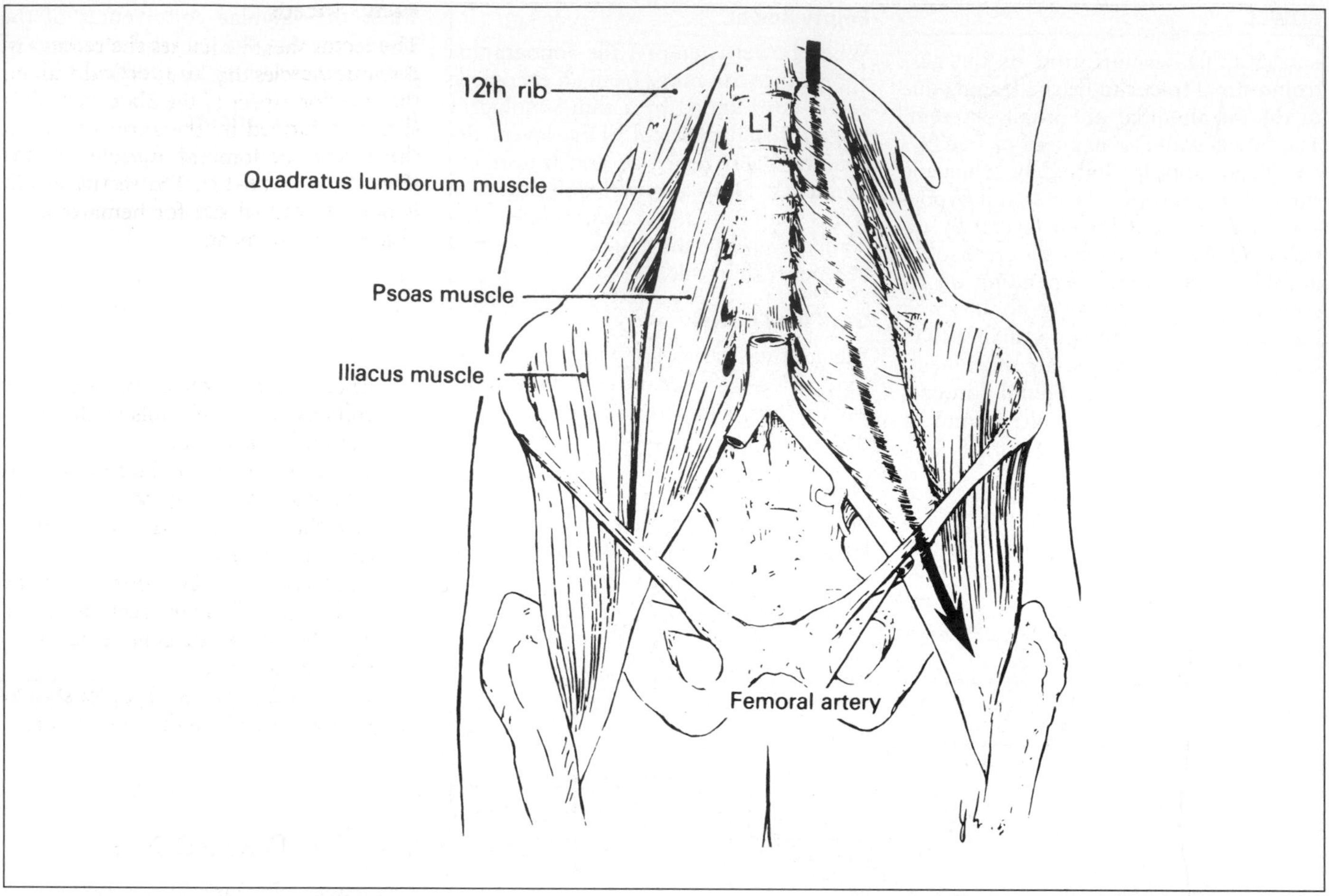

Figure 6-17. ■ *Diagram showing the normal location of the psoas, iliacus, and quadratus lumborum muscles.*

Quadratus Lumborum

The quadratus lumborum muscles form the posterior wall of the abdomen behind the kidneys. They arise from the inferior border of the 12th ribs and insert into the apices of the transverse processes of the first through fourth lumbar vertebra, the iliolumbar ligament, and the posterior third of the iliac crest (Figs. 6-16 and 6-17). They can be mistaken for pathology behind the kidneys.

External Oblique Muscles

Along with the internal oblique and transverse abdominal muscles, these three flat muscles form the anterolateral abdominal wall. The external obliques arise from the lower eight ribs and course medially to insert into the outer anterior portion of the iliac crest, the inguinal ligament, the pubic tubercle and crest, and the edge of the anterior rectus sheath muscle.

Internal Oblique Muscles

The internal oblique muscles lie deep to the external oblique muscles. They arise from the anterior two thirds of the iliac crest and lateral two thirds of the inguinal ligament and insert into the inferior borders of the 10th to 12th ribs, the aponeurosis of the rectus sheath, and the pubic symphysis.

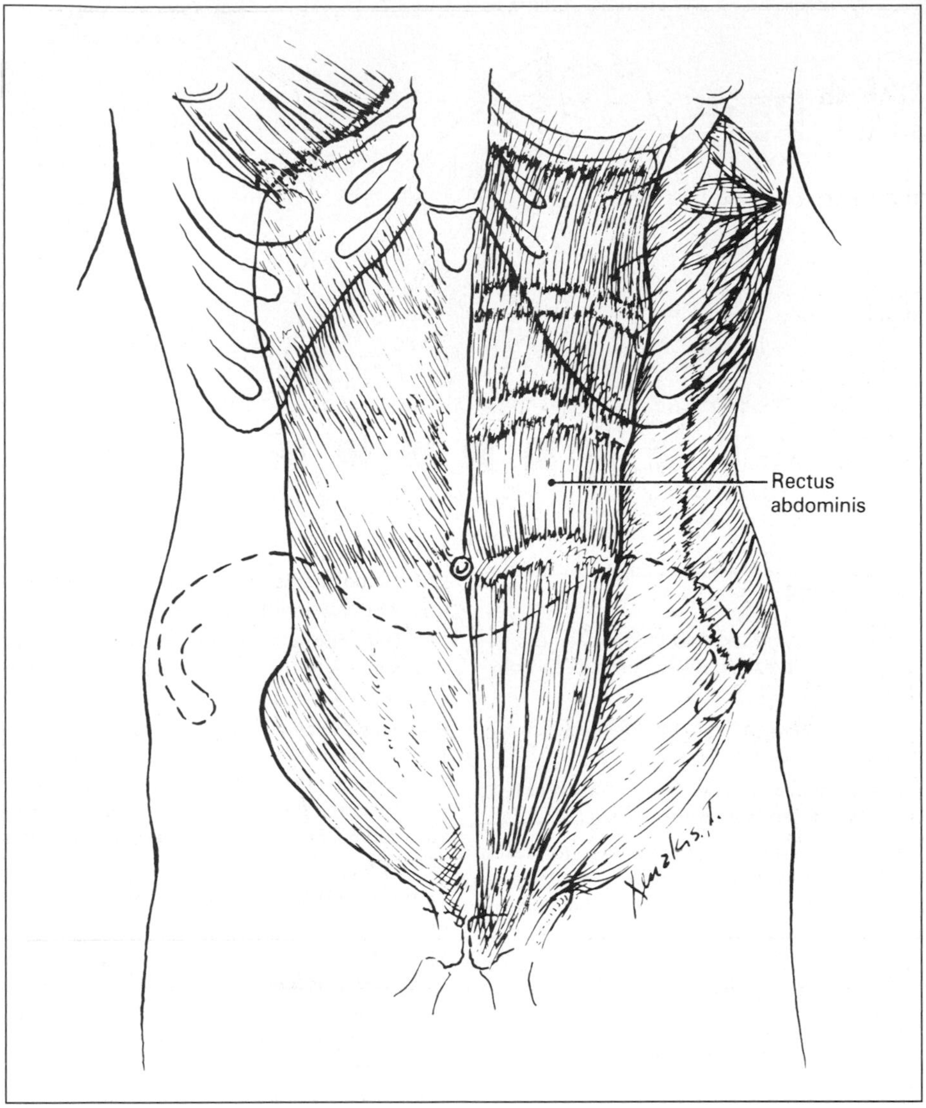

Figure 6-18. ■ *Diagram showing the location of the rectus abdominal muscles.*

Rectus Sheath

The rectus sheath encloses the rectus abdominis muscles that run vertically along the anterior aspect of the abdomen. This sheath is formed by the aponeuroses to the lateral abdominal muscle groups (Figs. 6-16 and 6-18). The rectus sheath is not an unusual site for hematoma or abscess development.

Pitfalls

1. Excessive transducer pressure can collapse the vessel walls so that they cannot be visualized.
2. Veins can sometimes be too small to visualize. Deep inspiration will allow them to expand and be more easily identified.
3. Catheters may be confused with pathology. They are seen as linear parallel echoes or echogenic areas with shadowing.
4. Color and/or pulsed Doppler should be used to confirm that a structure is a blood vessel.

SELECTED READING

Hagen-Ansert SL. *Textbook of Diagnostic Ultrasonography*, vol.1, 5th ed. St. Louis: Mosby, Inc; 2001.

Kawamura DM. *Diagnostic Medical Sonography, A Guide to Clinical Practice: Abdomen and Superficial Structures*, 2nd ed. Philadelphia: Lippincott; 1997.

Netter FH. *Digestive System: Upper Digestive Tract*. Part I, vol. 3. CIBA (The Collection of Medical Illustrations). New York: CIBA Pharmaceuticals; 1987.

Rumack DM, Wilson SR, Charboneau JW. *Diagnostic Ultrasound*, vol. 1, 3rd ed. St. Louis: Mosby, Inc; 2004.

Epigastric Pain (Upper Abdominal Pain)

Pancreatitis?

JULIA A. DROSE

7

SONOGRAM ABBREVIATIONS

AO	Aorta
CA	Celiac axis
CBD	Common bile duct
CD	Common duct
CHD	Common hepatic duct
DU	Duodenum
GB	Gallbladder
GDA	Gastroduodenal artery
HA	Hepatic artery
IVC	Inferior vena cava
K	Kidney
L	Liver
LRV	Left renal vein
P	Pancreas
PD	Pancreatic duct
PV	Portal vein
RRV	Right renal vein
SMA	Superior mesenteric artery
SMV	Superior mesenteric vein
SP	Spleen
SA	Splenic artery
SV	Splenic vein
ST	Stomach

KEY WORDS

Amylase. Enzyme secreted by the pancreas, responsible for breaking down complex carbohydrates.

Grey-Turner's Sign. Bruising of flanks secondary to retroperitoneal bleeding.

Hyperlipidemia. Elevated concentration of lipid in the blood. Can cause pancreatitis.

Ileus. Dilated bowel secondary to decreased motility. Causes include acute pancreatitis, peritonitis, bowel ischemia, myocardial infarction, infection, and certain medications.

Leukocytosis. Increase in number of white blood cells in bloodstream. Can be due to infection.

Lipase. Digestive enzyme secreted by the pancreas that breaks down fats. Usually elevated along with amylase in acute pancreatitis.

Pancreatic Ascites. Fluid that results from a ruptured pancreatic pseudocyst.

Pancreatic Pseudocyst. Accumulation of pancreatic fluid in a cyst-like loculus, but without an epithelial lining. May occur within or outside the pancreas.

Pancreatitis. Acute or chronic inflammation of the pancreas.

> **Acute.** Edematous, enlarged pancreas. Most commonly caused by alcohol or biliary disease.
>
> **Chronic.** Histological changes within the pancreas secondary to repeated episodes of acute pancreatitis. Results in gland atrophy as well as stone and cyst formation.
>
> **Hemorrhagic.** Bleeding within the pancreas, associated with acute pancreatitis.
>
> **Phlegmonous.** Inflammatory process that spreads to the soft tissues surrounding the pancreas.

Pancreas Divisum. Congenital variant in which the dorsal and ventral pancreatic ducts fail to fuse. This condition may result in inadequate enzyme drainage, predisposing the individual to pancreatitis. More recent thinking casts doubt upon this possible association.

Peptic Ulcer Disease (PUD). Ulceration in the wall of the stomach or duodenum.

Serum Amylase. Laboratory test that is elevated in the setting of acute pancreatitis. Also elevated with mumps, ischemic bowel disease, pelvic inflammatory disease, acute cholecystitis, renal failure, and PUD.

Total Parenteral Nutrition. Liquid form of nutrition administered through a central line.

Uncinate Process. Portion of the head of the pancreas that lies posterior to the superior mesenteric vein.

RELEVANT LABORATORY VALUES

Lipase: 0 to 160 U/L

Serum amylase: 23 to 85 U/L

White blood cell count: 5,000 to 10,000 U/L

Specific values may vary between laboratories

The Clinical Problem

Epigastric pain, whether acute or chronic, is frequently caused by peptic ulcer disease (PUD) or pancreatitis. Acute cholecystitis and hepatic disorders such as an abscess may also be characterized by epigastric pain. Sonography is not the imaging modality of choice to evaluate uncomplicated PUD. Computed tomography may also be more beneficial when evaluating the pancreas for pancreatitis; however, there are several primary and secondary sonographic characteristics of pancreatitis that may be useful in confirming the diagnosis.

Pancreatitis is defined as inflammation of the pancreas. It may be classified as acute or chronic, with symptoms ranging from mild to severe. The most common cause of pancreatitis in the United States is biliary tract disease, followed by ethyl alcohol abuse. Other less common causes include PUD, trauma, pregnancy, drug use, and infectious agents. Pancreatic carcinoma, hypercalcemia, hyperlipoproteinemias, and invasive procedures involving the pancreas or biliary system may also result in pancreatitis.

Congenital pancreatitis or idiopathic fibrosing pancreatitis has also been reported. When pancreatitis is diagnosed in children or young adults, it is frequently due to a hereditary cause such as pancreas divisum, cystic fibrosis, von Hippel-Lindau syndrome, Cushing syndrome, or autosomal dominant polycystic kidney disease.

ACUTE PANCREATITIS

Acute pancreatitis is the result of damage to the acinar cells within the pancreas. This tissue destruction causes pancreatic enzymes to be released into the surrounding tissue, resulting in inflammation of the gland.

Elevated serum amylase and lipase, as well as leukocytosis, may be present in patients with acute pancreatitis.

Clinical symptoms of acute pancreatitis include epigastric pain, abdominal distension secondary to an ileus, hypoxia, fever, and malaise. Nausea and vomiting may also occur. Acute pancreatitis usually occurs suddenly and lasts for a short period of time before resolving. It is more common in men than women.

Individuals affected with acute pancreatitis can develop serious complications, including pseudocysts, phlegmon, peritonitis, hemorrhage, or obstruction of the bowel or bile ducts. In severe cases, heart, lung, or kidney failure (or death) can occur.

Treatment for acute pancreatitis depends on its severity. Acute pancreatitis often resolves on its own. Treatment may not be necessary in these cases or may only consist of intravenous (IV) fluid administration to prevent dehydration. If it does not resolve, total parenteral nutrition may be required for 3 to 6 weeks to allow the pancreas to heal.

If gallstones cause the pancreatitis, cholecystectomy is indicated.

If infection develops, antibiotics are usually prescribed. In the setting of extensive infection or hemorrhage, surgery may be necessary. Surgery or percutaneous draining may also be necessary to treat pseudocysts.

CHRONIC PANCREATITIS

Chronic pancreatitis results from recurrent bouts of acute pancreatitis. In this setting, the continuous destruction and fibrosis of pancreatic parenchyma can result in glandular failure. Chronic pancreatitis is more common in men than in women, and up to 70% of cases occur secondary to alcoholism.

An increase in serum amylase and lipase may also be present with chronic pancreatitis, although they may remain within normal limits.

Patients with chronic pancreatitis may be asymptomatic in the early stages, but they eventually develop progressive epigastric pain, nausea, vomiting, and jaundice secondary to common bile duct (CBD) obstruction. The pain may worsen after eating, spreading to the back. Epigastric pain associated with chronic pancreatitis often becomes chronic and disabling. As the condition progresses, however, pain may resolve secondary to complete cessation of enzyme production by the pancreas.

Complications associated with chronic pancreatitis include diabetes, pancreatic pseudocyst, or portal or splenic vein thrombosis.

Treatment for chronic pancreatitis usually includes pain control via medication or surgery, dietary changes, and pancreatic enzyme replacement medication.

As with acute pancreatitis, percutaneous procedures or surgery may be necessary to treat complications such as hemorrhage or pseudocyst.

Anatomy

The pancreas is a nonencapsulated, retroperitoneal structure that lies between the duodenal loop and the splenic hilum. The normal length of the pancreas ranges from 12.5 to 15 cm. In an anterior to posterior (AP) dimension, the head of the pancreas normally measures 2 to 3.5 cm. Normal AP dimensions for the body and tail of the pancreas are 2 to 3 cm and 1 to 2 cm, respectively.

The pancreas can be divided into the head, uncinate process, body, and tail. The pancreatic head sits within the C-loop of the duodenum. The body is located beneath the antrum of the stomach, with the tail extending into the splenic hilum. The uncinate process is the portion of pancreatic tissue that extends posterior and medial from the head.

Understanding the relationship between surrounding vessels and the pancreas can be a very useful means of identifying pancreatic anatomy (Fig. 7-1).

In cross section, the pancreas' head lies anterior to the inferior vena cava (IVC) and to the right of the confluence of the splenic vein and superior mesen-

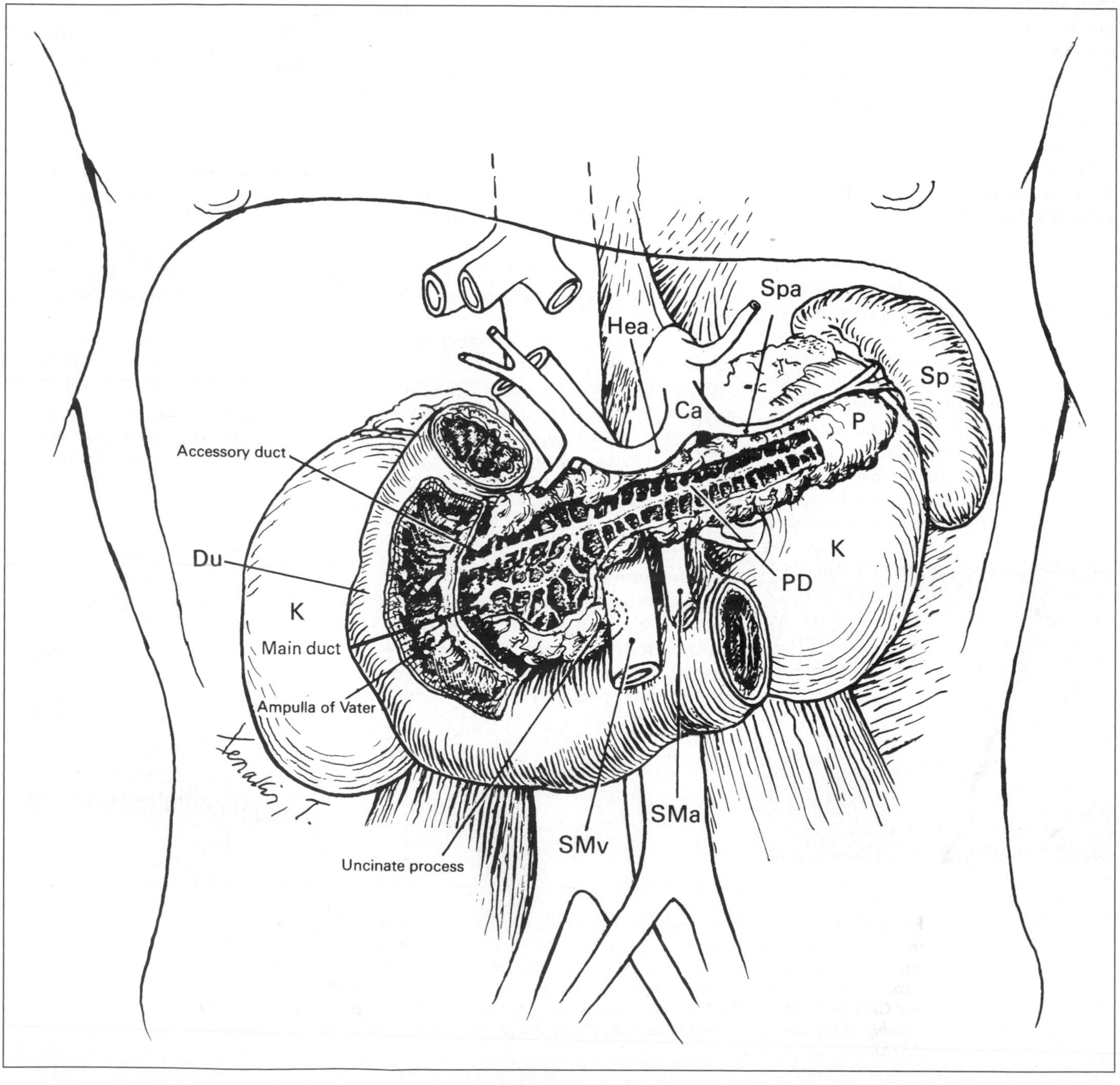

Figure 7-1. ■ *Diagram showing the relationship of the pancreas to surrounding vessels and organs. Note that the main pancreatic duct (duct of Wirsung) runs through the center of the pancreas to the ampulla of Vater. The splenic artery lies superior to the pancreas.*

teric vein (SMV). The uncinate process can be seen wrapping around the SMV. The splenic vein forms the posterior, medial border of the pancreas' body and tail (Fig. 7-2).

The aorta is posterior to the body of the pancreas. The celiac axis, which originates from the aorta, gives rise to the splenic artery, common hepatic artery, and the left gastric artery. The splenic artery runs along the superior border of the pancreatic body and tail. The common hepatic artery courses along the superior aspect of the body and head, giving rise to the gastroduodenal artery and the proper hepatic artery. The gastroduodenal artery is seen lateral and anterior to the pancreatic head.

The superior mesenteric artery (SMA), which also arises from the aorta, is located posterior to the body of the pancreas (Fig. 7-3).

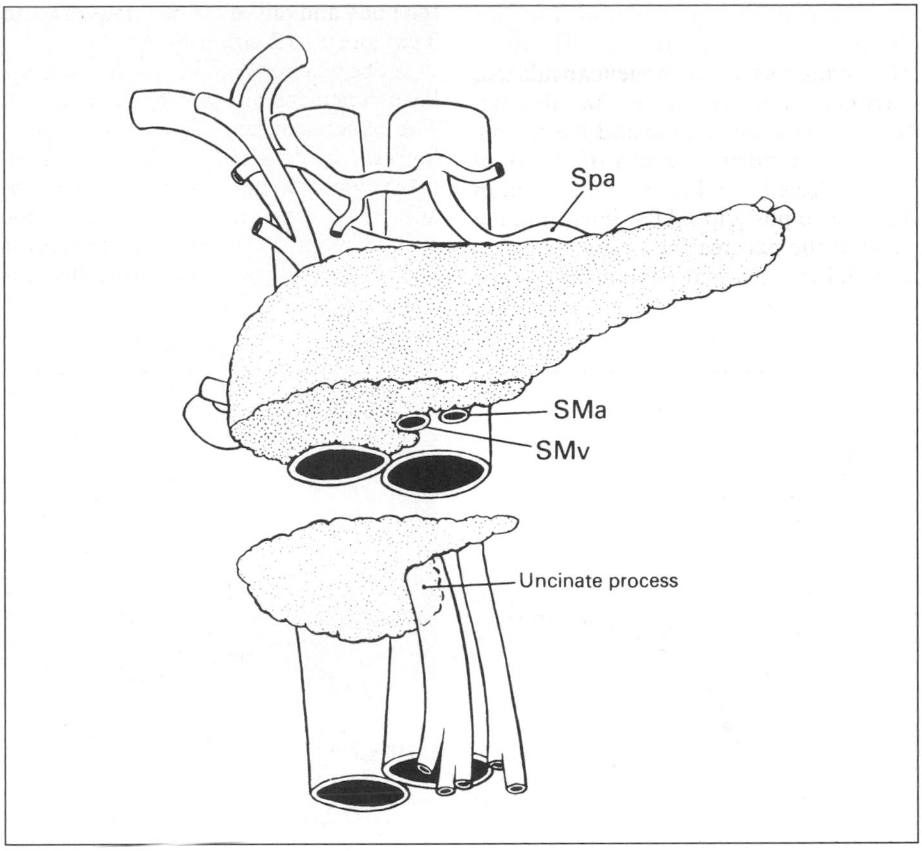

Figure 7-2. ■ *Diagram showing the relationship of the vessels to the pancreas. The exploded view through the uncinate process shows the relationship of the superior mesenteric artery* (SMA) *and the vein to the uncinate process.*

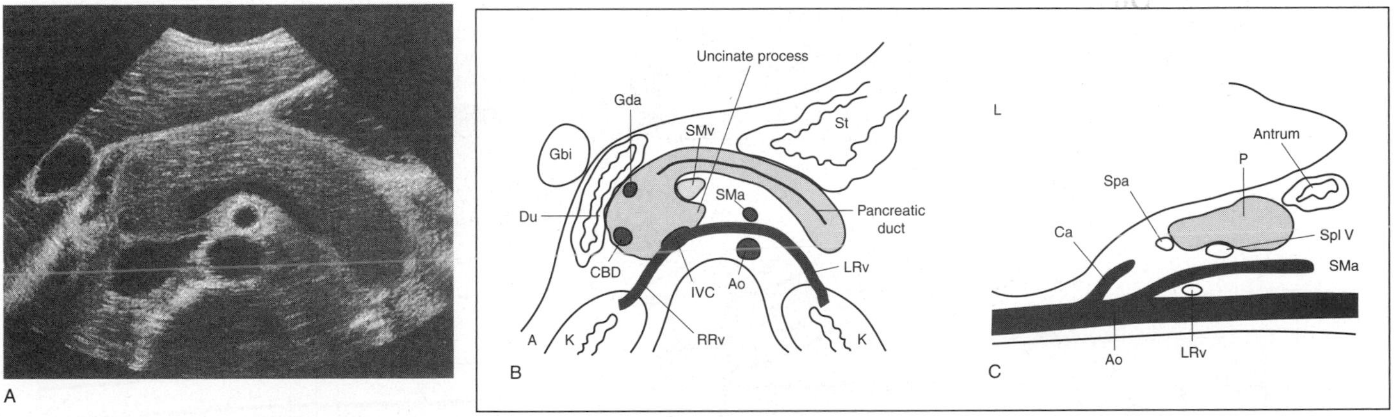

Figure 7-3. ■ *A. Transverse image of the pancreas showing the common bile duct and the gastroduodenal artery. **B.** Transverse diagram. The uncinate process lies between the superior mesenteric vein* (SMV) *and the inferior vena cava* (IVC). *The gallbladder, duodenum, and pancreas form a constant threesome. The SMV lies medial to the head of the pancreas. The gastroduodenal artery and CBD lie in the lateral aspect of the head of the pancreas. **C.** Sagittal diagram showing the relationship of the pancreas to the splenic vein, splenic artery, and the superior mesenteric artery* (SMA).

Two ducts are responsible for drainage within the pancreas. The main pancreatic duct is the primary pancreatic duct in the body and tail of the pancreas. It bifurcates into the duct of Wirsung and the duct of Santorini in the head of the pancreas. The duct of Wirsung joins the CBD at the ampulla of Vater and enters the duodenum. A normal duct of Wirsung measures approximately 2 mm or less in AP dimension and may be visualized by ultrasound (Fig. 7-4). The accessory pancreatic duct is the duct of Santorini. This duct is responsible for draining the upper aspect of the head of the pancreas. It enters the duodenum approximately 2 cm above the ampulla of Vater, at the minor papilla. The duct of Santorini is normally small and difficult to visualize by ultrasound.

The CBD is also a useful landmark that can normally be seen entering the posterior aspect of the pancreatic head (Fig. 7-5).

RELATIONSHIP TO OTHER ORGANS

The pancreas' relationship to other organs remains constant. The gallbladder lies to the right of the duodenum, which in turn lies to the right of the head of the pancreas (Fig. 7-3). The tail of the pancreas lies anterior to the left kidney and posterior to the left colic flexure and transverse colon. The tail extends toward the splenic hilum. The antrum of the stomach lies anterior and somewhat inferior to the pancreas.

Although the pancreas usually has an oblique axis with the head inferior to the tail, the axis is variable, and the gland is often horizontal.

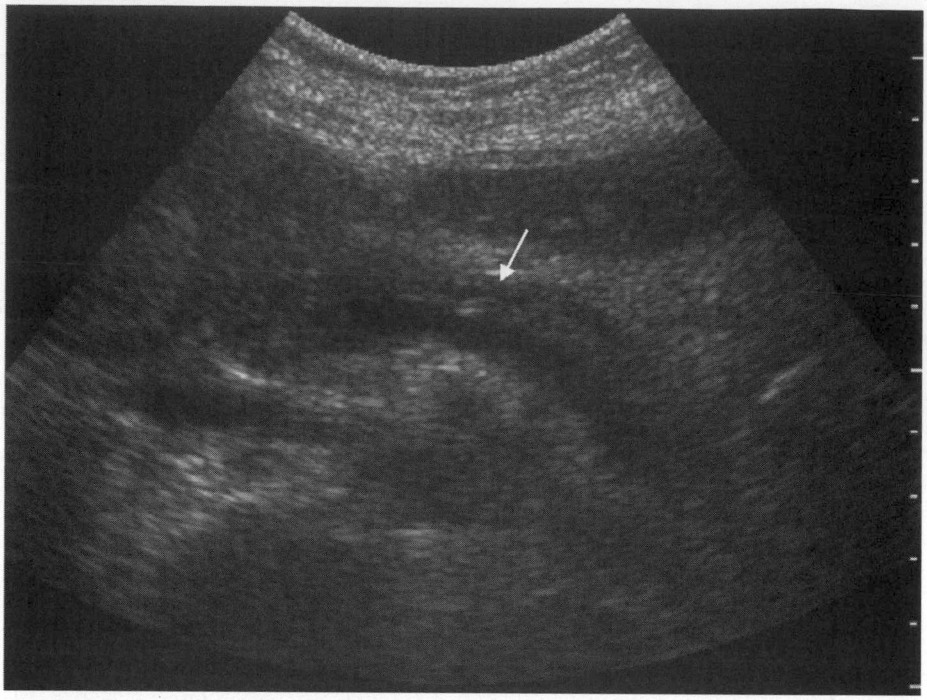

Figure 7-4. ■ *Transverse image of a normal pancreas showing the small caliber of a normal pancreatic duct* (arrow).

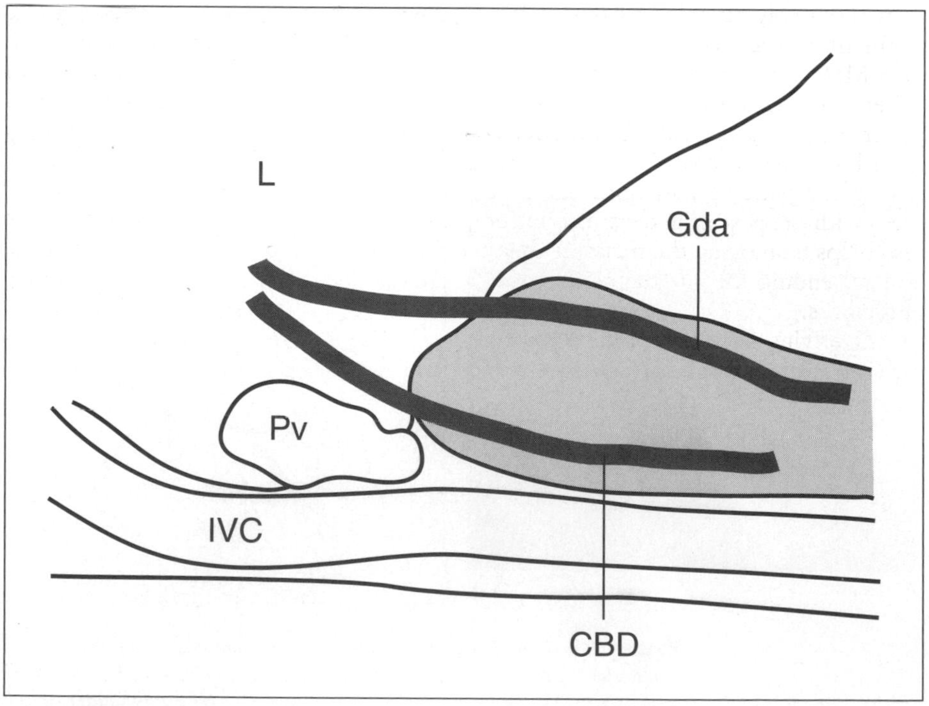

Figure 7-5. ■ *Longitudinal diagram of head of the pancreas showing the normal location of the gastroduodenal artery* (Gda) *and common bile duct* (CBD).

TEXTURE

The normal pancreas is slightly more echogenic than the liver and surrounding retroperitoneum. In older individuals, the pancreas may increase in echogenicity secondary to fatty infiltration and fibrous tissue formation. This condition often makes it difficult to distinguish the pancreas sonographically from surrounding retroperitoneal fat. The size of the pancreas may also decrease with age. In children, the normal pancreas is often less echogenic than the liver.

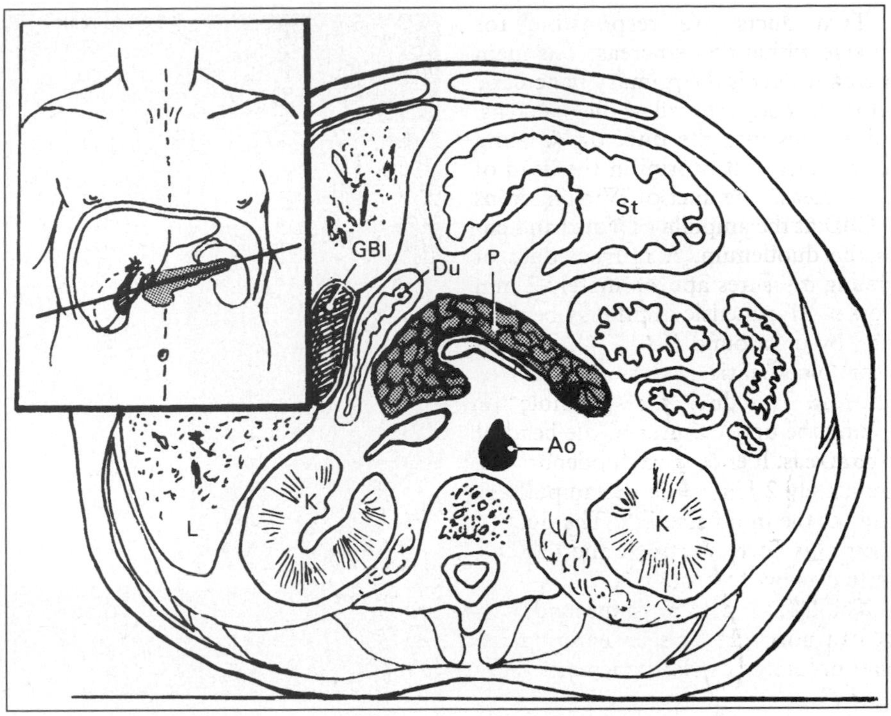

Figure 7-6. ■ *Diagram showing the appropriate transducer angulation for evaluating the pancreas.*

Technique

Individuals undergoing ultrasound to evaluate the pancreas should be given nothing by mouth for 8 to12 hours before the examination to minimize overlying bowel gas.

Sonographically, the pancreas is usually best visualized in a transverse plane. With the patient supine, the transducer is placed in a subxiphoid position with the transducer slightly obliqued from the patient's left shoulder to the right hip (Fig. 7-6). It may also be useful to angle slightly caudal using the left lobe of the liver as an acoustic window. A 4- or 5-MHz sector or curved linear transducer is usually sufficient to visualize the pancreas. The previously described vascular landmarks are very helpful in identifying the pancreas. Imaging the pancreas with the patient in deep inspiration also helps by moving the pancreas down and distending the surrounding venous landmarks.

Overlying bowel gas often impedes the ability to visualize the pancreas with ultrasound. Several maneuvers may be necessary to alleviate the problem.

Changing the patient's position from supine to right posterior oblique, left posterior oblique, or even erect may displace the overlying gas into another part of the gastrointestinal tract. An additional benefit of the erect position is that the liver moves down over the pancreas, allowing an improved acoustic window.

If the pancreas is still not readily visualized, having the patient ingest degassed water to fill the stomach, which will then act as an acoustic window, may be beneficial. Instruct the patient to drink at least 12 ounces of water through a straw to prevent ingesting air, preferably in a left lateral decubitus or erect position. Allow sufficient time to dissipate remaining air bubbles (2 to 5 minutes). The patient can then be scanned in the erect position, which allows the body and tail of the pancreas to be visualized as the antrum of the stomach fills. As the water moves into the duodenum, the

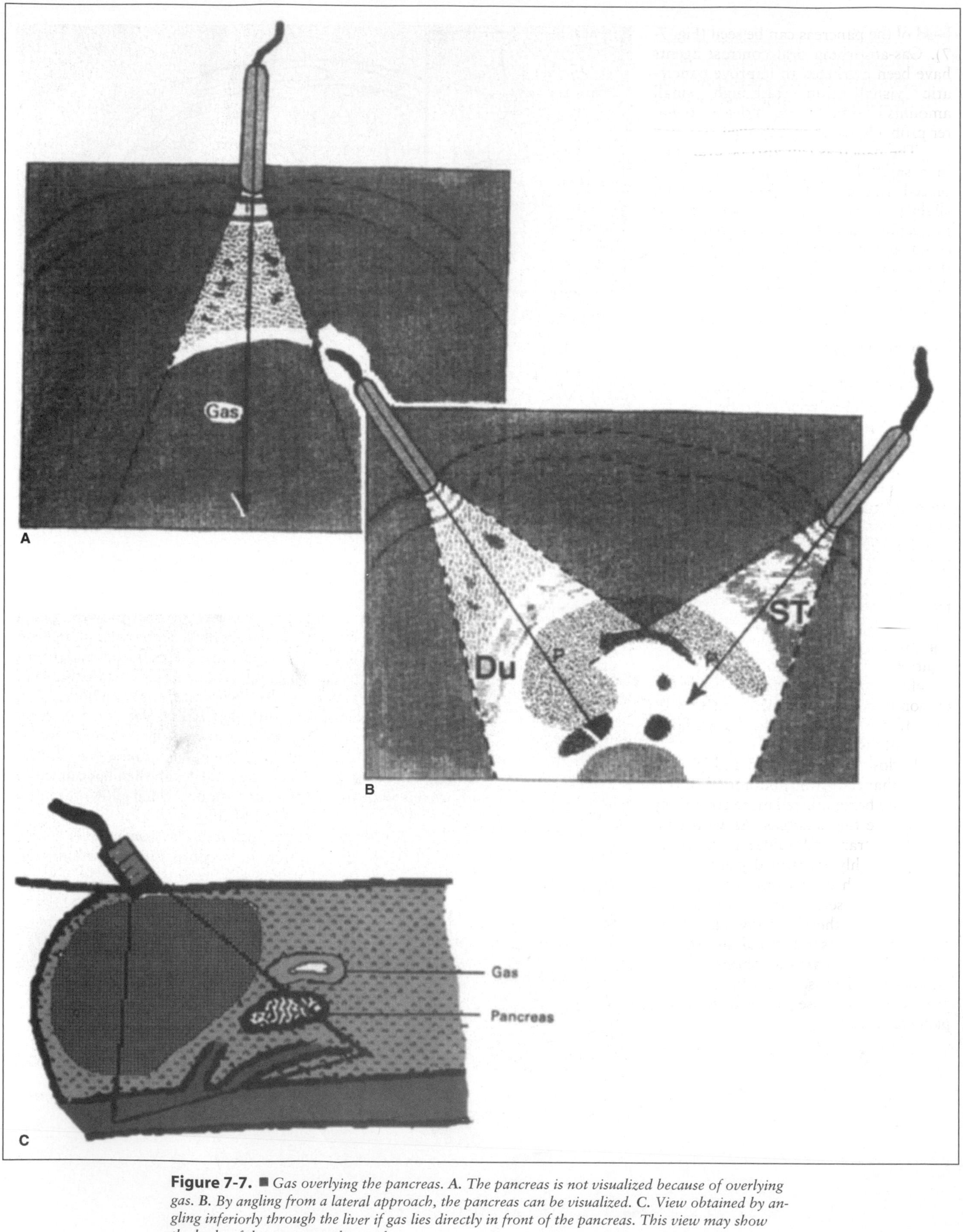

Figure 7-7. ■ *Gas overlying the pancreas. A. The pancreas is not visualized because of overlying gas. B. By angling from a lateral approach, the pancreas can be visualized. C. View obtained by angling inferiorly through the liver if gas lies directly in front of the pancreas. This view may show the body of the pancreas adequately.*

head of the pancreas can be seen (Fig. 7-7). Gas-absorbing oral contrast agents have been marketed to improve pancreatic visualization, although small amounts of simethicone in degassed water probably work equally well.

The pancreas can also be evaluated in a sagittal plane. The transducer is placed longitudinally below the xiphoid, slightly to the right of midline. In this projection, the head of the pancreas is located anterior to the IVC and inferior to the portal vein (Fig. 7-8). As the transducer is moved to the left of midline, the body of the pancreas should be seen anterior to the aorta and SMA (Fig. 7-9). Deep inspiration is also useful in the sagittal plane.

Finally, placing the patient in the right lateral decubitus or prone position and using the left kidney or spleen as an acoustic window to visualize the tail of the pancreas can be attempted.

A newer advance in ultrasound imaging, which may aid in both visualizing the pancreas and identifying smaller focal lesions, is compound imaging. This concept utilizes beam-steering technology to maneuver the ultrasound beam off axis. This method is carried out internally by machines equipped with this feature and results in multiple off-axis transmit angles. The benefit of this technique is that visualization of borders and interfaces may be improved by reducing inherent artifacts, such as bowel gas.

Endoscopic ultrasound and IV contrast-enhanced transabdominal ultrasound are being utilized more commonly to evaluate the pancreas. As with conventional transabdominal ultrasound, these are highly operator-dependent procedures. With endoscopic ultrasound, the probe is inserted into the duodenum and stomach, thereby allowing factors that impede transabdominal ultrasound, such as bowel gas and obesity, to be eliminated. Endoscopic ultrasound is most commonly used to evaluate small pancreatic lesions.

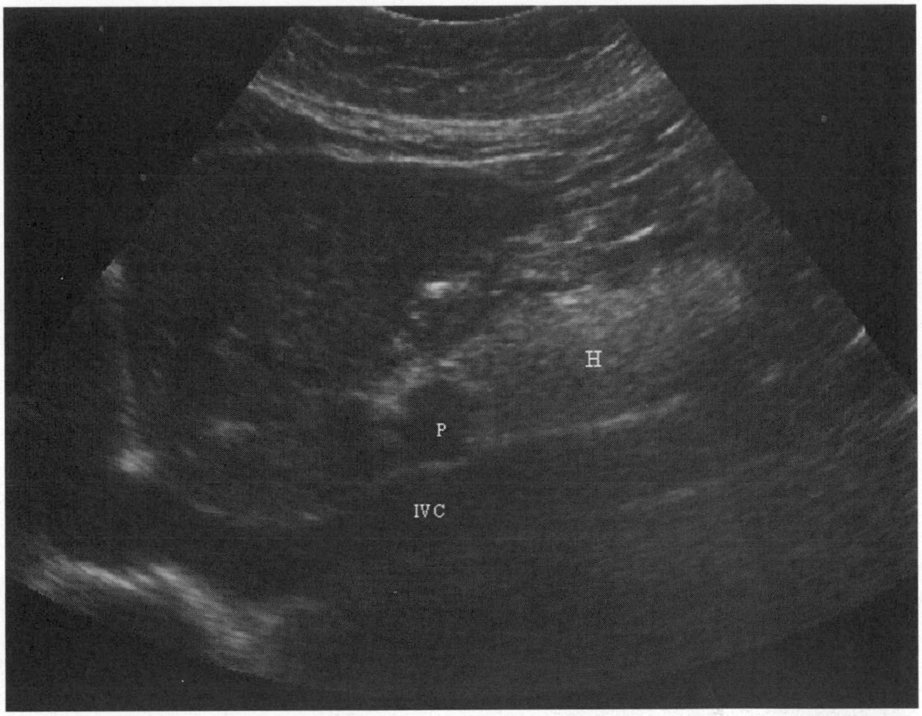

Figure 7-8. ■ *Sagittal image of the head of the pancreas* (H), *anterior to the inferior vena cava* (IVC), *and inferior to the portal vein* (P).

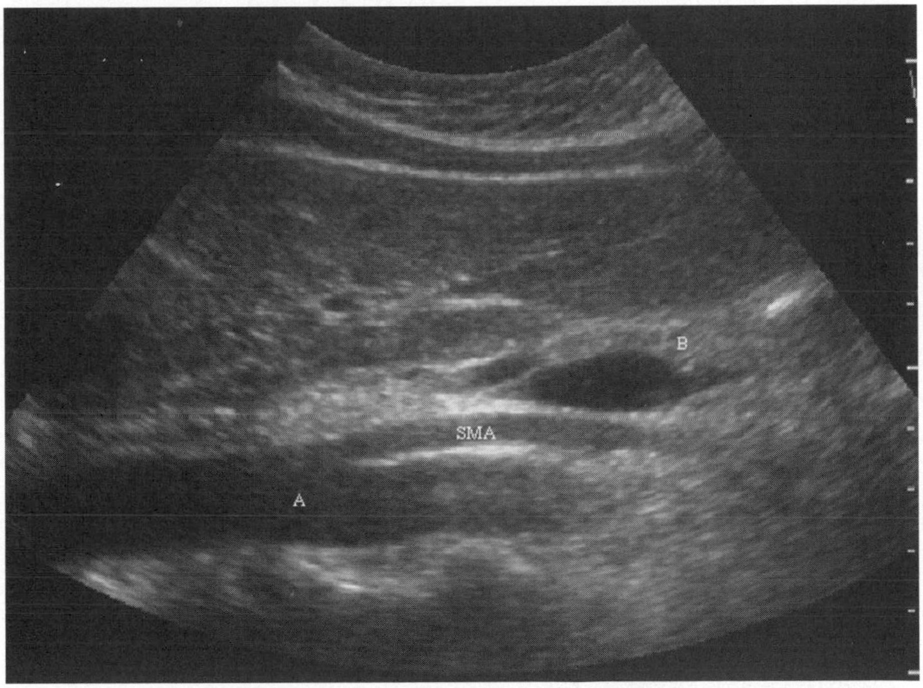

Figure 7-9. ■ *Sagittal image of the body of the pancreas* (B) *anterior to the aorta* (A) *and superior mesenteric artery* (SMA).

Contrast-enhanced (or dynamic) sonography has been reported to be useful in identifying and characterizing pancreatic lesions. Although currently used mainly in a research setting, this type of imaging involves IV injection of a contrast agent while observing the pancreas. Both grayscale imaging utilizing tissue harmonics and complex pulse-shaping technologies, as well as color or power Doppler, can be used to localize focal areas with increased contrast enhancement or increased blood flow associated with malignant lesions.

Pathology

ACUTE PANCREATITIS

Acute pancreatitis has a variety of sonographic appearances. In many cases, the pancreas may appear normal. As it becomes edematous, it can enlarge and appear hypoechoic (Fig. 7-10). Edema may cause focal or diffuse enlargement, with the gland's borders becoming irregular. When focal enlargement occurs, it is usually within the head of the pancreas. The pancreatic duct may also enlarge, allowing it to be more easily visualized. Additionally, 40% to 60% of patients with acute pancreatitis will have gallstones.

Several complications of acute pancreatitis may also be visualized by ultrasound.

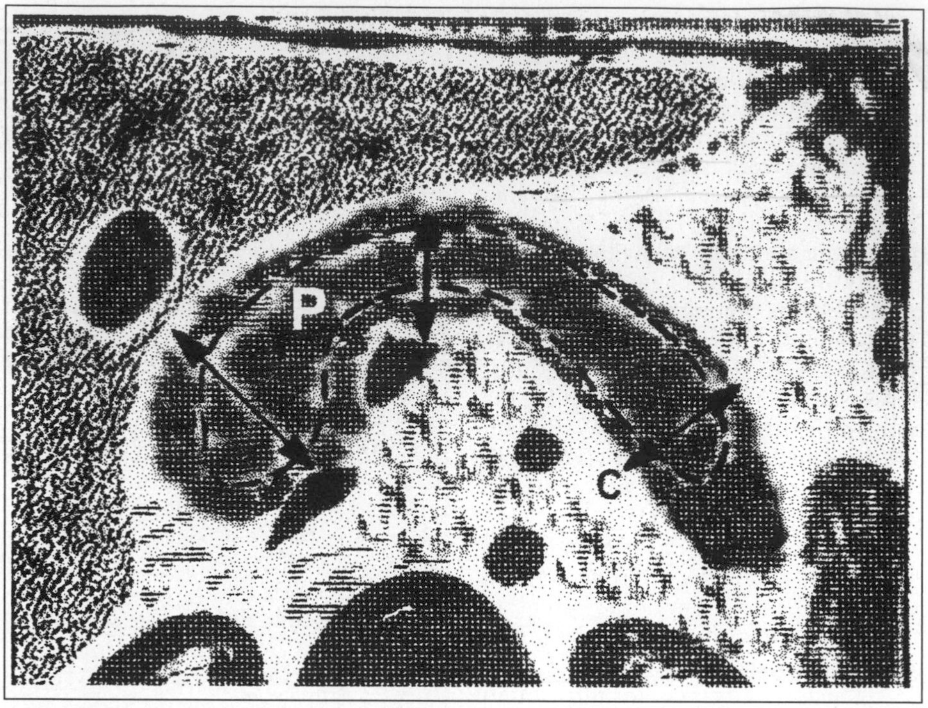

Figure 7-10. ■ *In acute pancreatitis, the pancreas swells and becomes more sonolucent than usual. The dotted lines show the normal size of the pancreas; the arrows show the increase that occurs with pancreatitis.*

HEMORRHAGIC PANCREATITIS

If a patient develops hemorrhagic pancreatitis, focal areas of fat necrosis or extravasated blood may be visualized within the pancreas. Over time, these focal masses may appear cystic with solid components or septations. Eventually, the hemorrhage may appear entirely cystic. Blood vessel necrosis can result in discoloration of the flanks, which is referred to as *Grey-Turner's sign*. Patients who develop hemorrhagic pancreatitis have a high mortality rate.

PHLEGMONOUS PANCREATITIS

Phlegmonous pancreatitis refers to diffuse spreading of inflammation throughout the pancreas, which often results in abscess. Extension outside the gland occurs in 20% of patients with acute pancreatitis. Sonographically, the pancreas with phlegmonous pancreatitis will appear as a hypoechoic ill-defined mass. Phlegmon may be seen extending into the lesser sac or left anterior pararenal space.

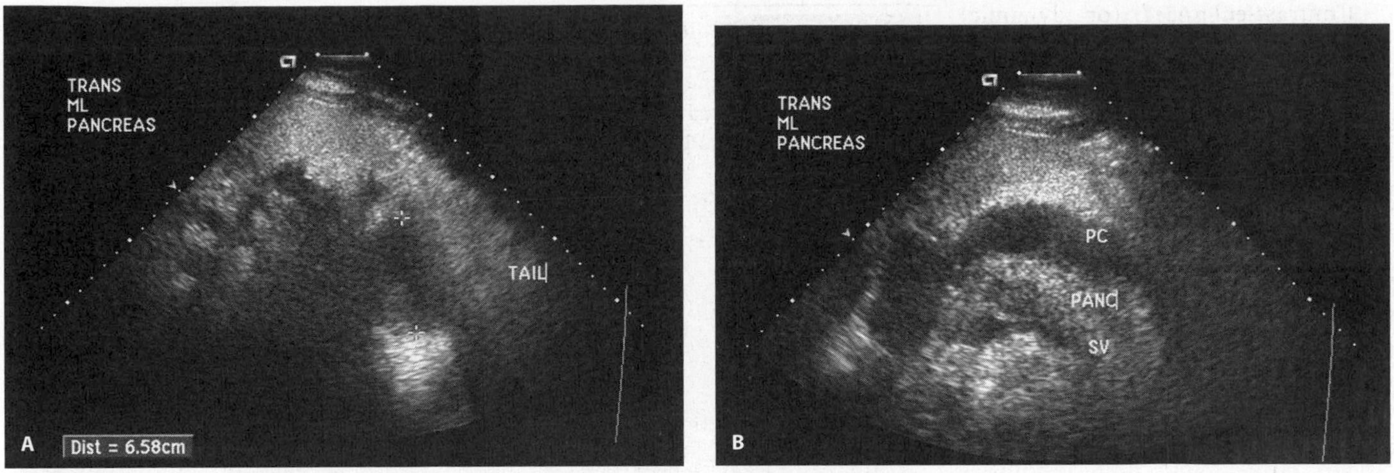

Figure 7-11. ■ *Peripancreatic fluid collections in a patient with acute pancreatitis. **A.** 6.6-cm complex fluid collection posterior to the tail of the pancreas. **B.** Fluid collection* (PC) *anterior to the pancreas.*

PSEUDOCYST

Pseudocysts occur in 10% to 20% of cases of acute pancreatitis. A pseudocyst is defined as a fluid collection with a well-defined nonepithelialized wall, occurring in response to extravasated enzymes that escape from the pancreas and break down tissue. Pseudocysts may develop in a variety of locations; the most common location is within the pancreas or in the lesser sac (Fig. 7-11A,B). Other locations include the anterior pararenal space, mesentery, mediastinum, and the pelvis. Pseudocysts can also dissect into adjoining organs such as the liver or spleen. Sonographically, pseudocysts commonly appear as well-defined cystic structures with increased acoustic enhancement (Fig. 7-12). They may be hypoechoic or may contain internal echoes or septations when hemorrhage or infection is present. Because pseudocysts often take on the contour of the space they occupy, their shape is variable. They may be singular or multiple. Over time, the walls of a pseudocyst become thicker, and calcifications may develop. Pseudocyst rupture occurs in approximately 5% of cases. This rupture, in turn, leads to peritonitis and carries a mortality rate of 50%.

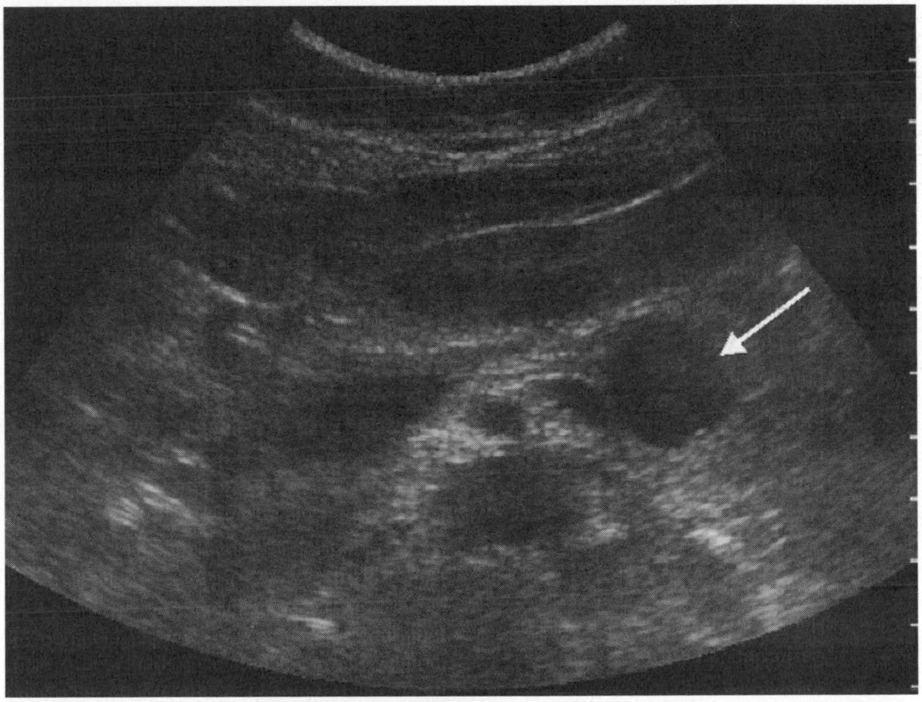

Figure 7-12. ■ *Transverse image of the pancreas with a well-circumscribed pseudocyst* (arrow) *in the tail.*

CHRONIC PANCREATITIS

Chronic pancreatitis occurs when recurrent episodes of acute pancreatitis cause continuing destruction of the pancreatic parenchyma.

The classic sonographic appearance of chronic pancreatitis is a small gland that is hyperechoic secondary to fibrotic and fatty changes (Fig. 7-13). The pancreas' contour can be irregular or nodular, and it is not uncommon for calcifications to occur within the parenchyma or more commonly within the pancreatic duct (Fig. 7-14A,B). As with acute pancreatitis, the pancreatic duct may be enlarged. Focal hypoechoic lesions or pseudocysts may also occur.

Biliary obstruction or portosplenic vein thrombosis may also arise as a complication of chronic pancreatitis.

PANCREATIC CARCINOMA

Many of the sonographic characteristics of pancreatic carcinoma can mimic those of pancreatitis. The clinical symptoms of pancreatic carcinoma, including increased amylase and epigastric pain, are also similar to pancreatitis. Additionally, patients with a history of chronic pancreatitis are at a slightly increased risk of developing pancreatic carcinoma.

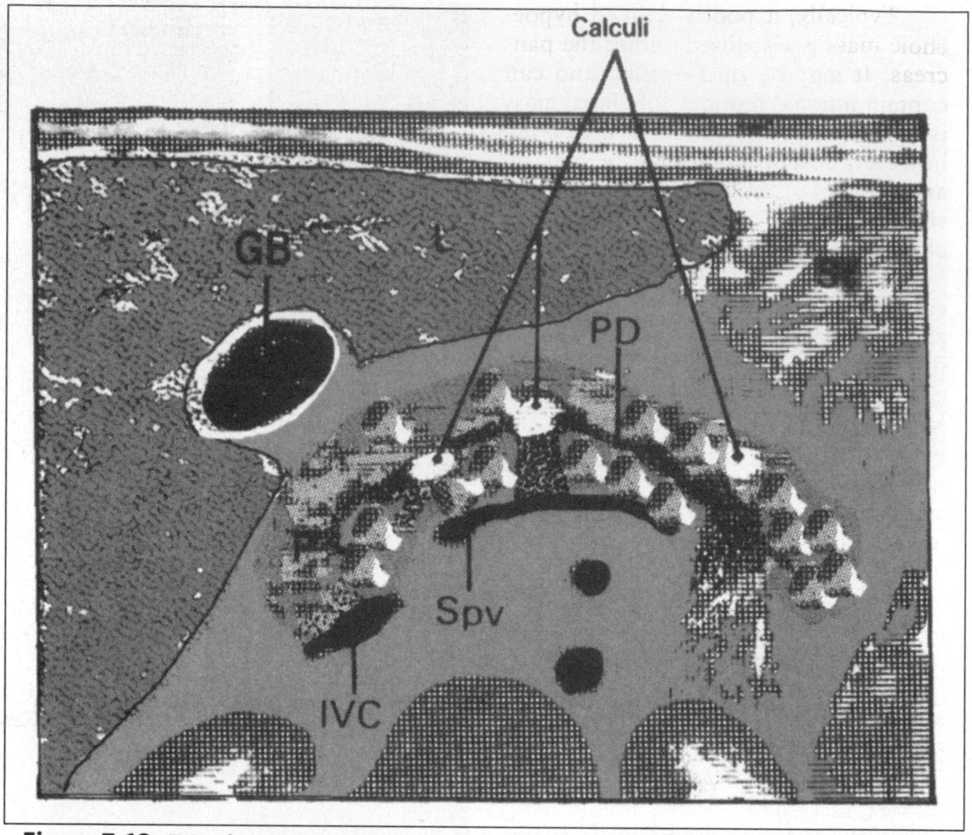

Figure 7-13. ■ *In chronic pancreatitis, calculi develop within the pancreas (some with acoustic shadowing), and the pancreatic duct enlarges. The outline of the pancreas is more irregular, and its overall echogenicity is increased.*

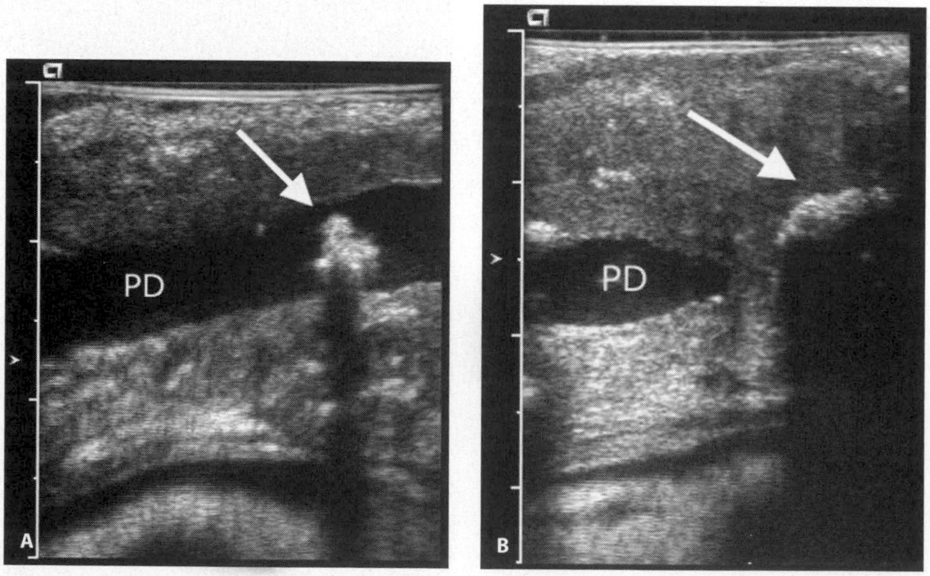

Figure 7-14. ■ *Intraoperative ultrasound nicely demonstrating calcifications* (arrows) *within the pancreatic ductal system. A. Main pancreatic duct. B. Side branch.*

Typically, a poorly defined hypoechoic mass is visualized within the pancreas. It may be thick-walled and can contain internal septa. A lobulated mass is more likely to represent a carcinoma; however, keep in mind that the appearance of some carcinomas may be very similar to pseudocyst (Fig. 7-15) or chronic pancreatitis.

Approximately 80% of pancreatic carcinomas occur in the head of the pancreas and may cause gland enlargement (Fig. 7-16). Pancreatic carcinoma can cause dilatation of both the pancreatic duct and the biliary system. *Courvoisier gallbladder* refers to a palpable gallbladder that results from ductal obstruction secondary to a pancreatic head mass.

As a carcinoma enlarges, displacement of the surrounding vascular structures can be seen. Metastatic spread to the liver and paraortic lymph nodes is not uncommon.

The most common primary neoplasm of the pancreas is adenocarcinoma. Cystadenocarcinomas, islet cell tumors, metastatic disease, and a variety of rare tumors may also occur.

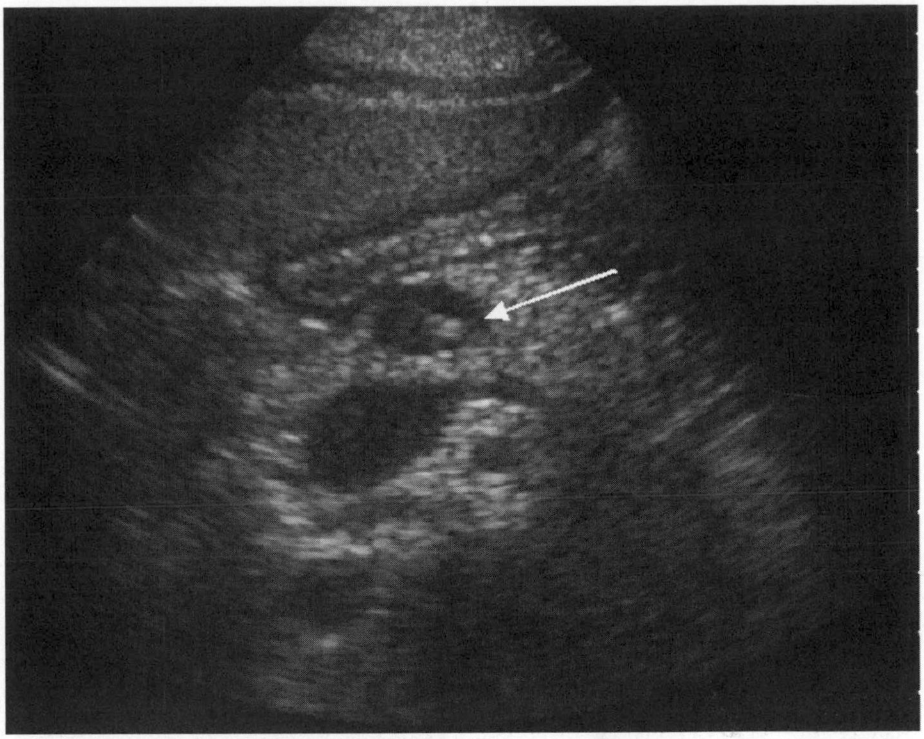

Figure 7-15. ■ *Transverse image of the pancreas with an adenocarcinoma in the body of the pancreas that has a sonographic appearance similar to a pseudocyst* (arrow).

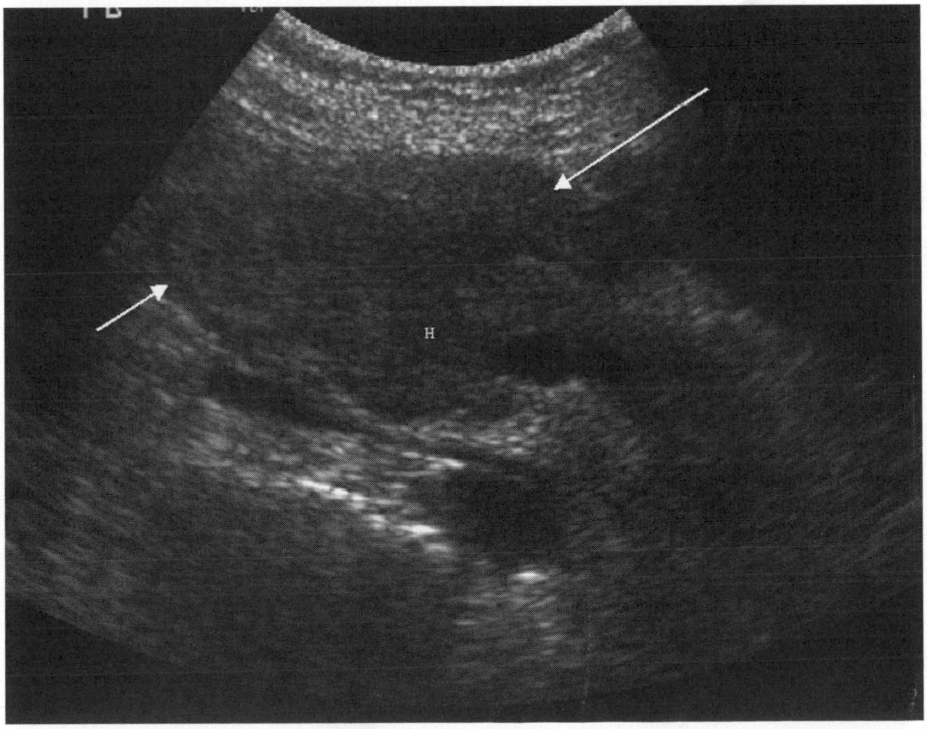

Figure 7-16. ■ *Transverse image of the pancreas with a large carcinoma* (arrows) *enlarging the head* (H) *of the pancreas.*

Pitfalls

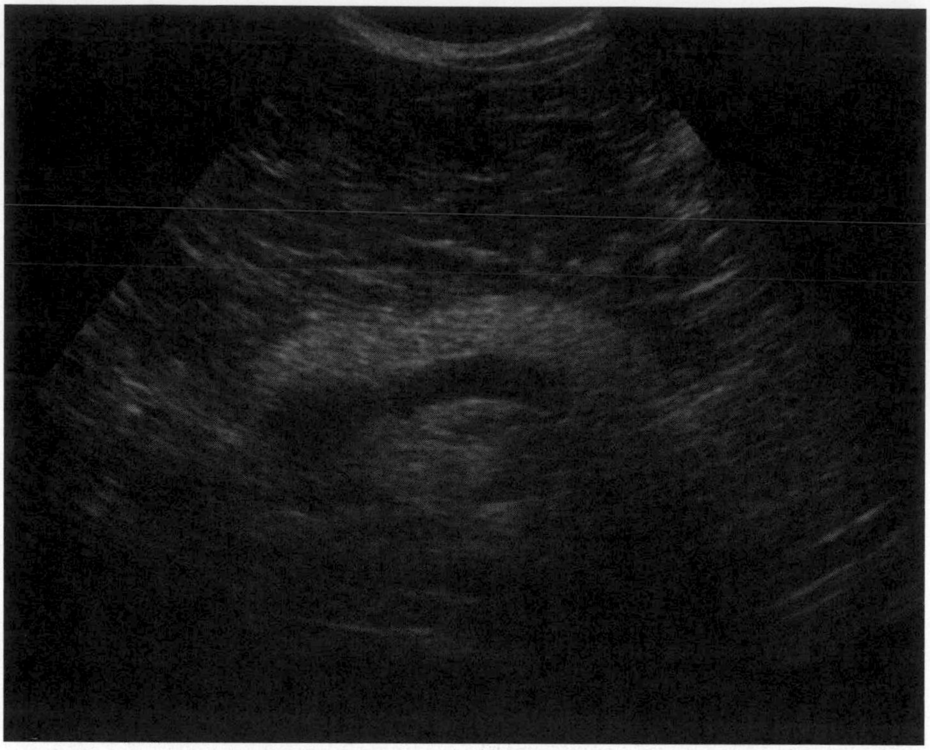

Figure 7-17. ■ *Transverse image of the pancreas in a 70-year-old patient, showing increased echogenicity secondary to fatty replacement.*

1. Posterior wall of the stomach versus the pancreatic duct. The posterior stomach wall can be mistaken for the pancreatic duct. Following the stomach wall around the entire outline of the stomach differentiates it from the pancreatic duct. The stomach will not extend the entire length of the pancreas, as will the duct.
2. Fatty changes versus chronic pancreatitis. The pancreas becomes more echogenic with age secondary to fatty infiltration. Do not confuse normal aging changes (where the border of the pancreas remains smooth) with chronic pancreatitis (which causes heterogeneity of the parenchyma and a nodular contour of the gland) (Fig. 7-17).
3. Bowel versus pseudocyst. Cystic structures near the pancreas are not always pseudocysts. Make sure that the cystic structure is not a fluid-filled stomach or colon. Identification of peristalsis or passage of a nasogastric tube will aid in differentiation.
4. Splenic artery versus pancreatic duct. The splenic artery may be confused with the pancreatic duct and occasionally runs through the center of the pancreas. Pulsed or color Doppler can be used to distinguish the two.
5. Gallbladder versus pseudocyst. Confusion between gallbladder and a pseudocyst may occur, but the gallbladder will contract with fat administration, whereas a pseudocyst will not. Pseudocysts may develop in the gallbladder fossa in patients who have undergone cholecystectomy.
6. Duodenum versus head of pancreas. The duodenum may be mistaken for a mass in the head of the pancreas when the gut contents have a similar echogenicity to the pancreas. Having the patient ingest water and watching for peristalsis should differentiate duodenum from pancreatic head.
7. Pancreatic calcification versus gut. Calcifications in the pancreatic head and body may resemble air in the gut. Be sure to use landmarks and recognize borders between the pancreatic head and duodenum.
8. Caudate lobe versus pancreatic mass. The caudate lobe of the liver may extend medially and may mimic a pancreatic neoplasm. Careful sonographic analysis will show that the caudate lobe connects to the liver and is separate from the pancreas.
9. Uncinate process versus pancreatic mass. The uncinate process posterior to the SMV may be relatively large as a normal variant. It should not be mistaken for a pancreatic mass. If a mass is present, the uncinate should not have a normal-appearing contour.
10. Horseshoe kidney versus pancreas. The isthmus of a horseshoe kidney can resemble the body of the pancreas. A horseshoe kidney's connecting tissue will be directly anterior to the aorta and the IVC. The pancreas is separated from the aorta by a fat-filled space containing the mesenteric vessels.

Where Else To Look

1. If a mass is found, the head of the pancreas, the CBD, intrahepatic ducts, gallbladder, and pancreatic duct should be evaluated for obstruction.
2. A mass in the pancreas may be a carcinoma. Look for liver metastases, para-aortic or porta hepatis nodes, and vascular invasion.
3. If pancreatitis is found, look for associated findings such as:
   - Abnormal liver texture due to cirrhosis, hepatitis, or fatty liver.
   - Splenomegaly.
   - Portal hypertension: dilated splenic, portal, superior mesenteric, or coronary veins, as well as evidence of collateral vessels in the porta hepatis or splenic hilum. Pulsed or color Doppler should be used to determine the direction of flow in the portal vein.
   - Ascites, which may be secondary to liver disease or pancreatic ascites from a ruptured pseudocyst.
   - Gallstones.
4. If the pancreatic duct is dilated (Fig. 7-18), make sure that there is not an obstructing mass in the head of the pancreas or at the level of the ampulla of Vater. Scanning in the transverse plane with the patient in a sitting position often allows the best visualization of the distal CBD for a potential obstructing stone.

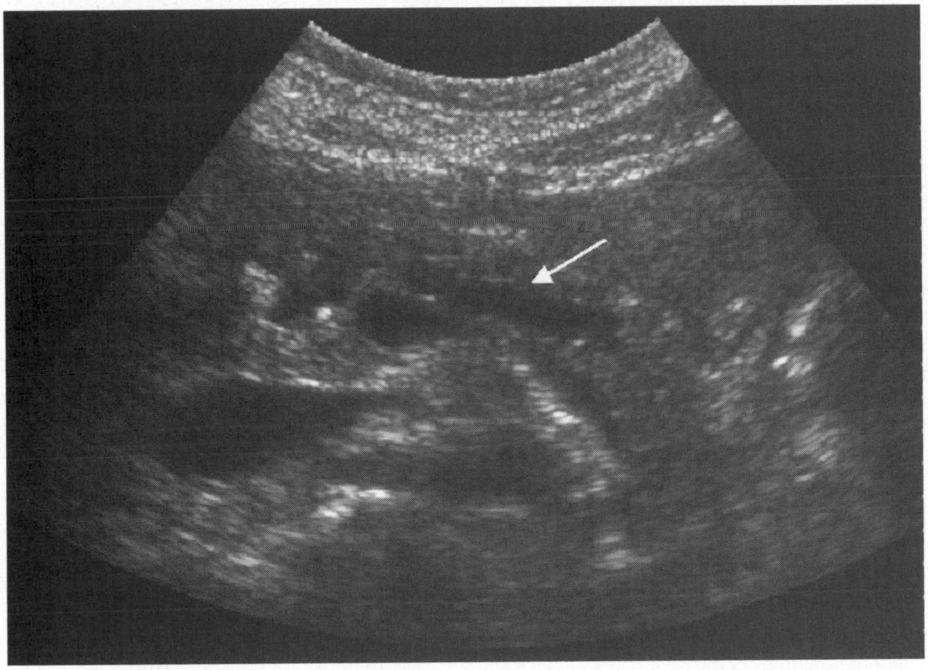

Figure 7-18. ■ *Transverse image of the pancreas with a dilated pancreatic duct* (arrow).

SELECTED READING

Atri M, Finnegan PW. The pancreas. In: Rumack CM, Wilson SR, Charboneau JW, eds. *Diagnostic Ultrasound*, vol 1, 2nd ed. St. Louis, MO: Mosby; 1998:225–277.

Baun J. Pancreas. In: Kawamura DW, ed. *Diagnostic Medical Sonography, A Guide to Clinical Practice. Abdomen and Superficial Structures*, 2nd ed. Philadelphia, PA: Lippincott; 1997:241–261.

Brand B, Pfaff T, Binmoeller KF, et al. Endoscopic ultrasound for differential diagnosis of focal pancreatic lesions, confirmed by surgery. *Scand J Gastroenterol* 2000;35(11):1221–1228.

Hagan-Ansert SL. The pancreas. In: Hagan-Ansert SL, ed. *Textbook of Diagnostic Ultrasonography*, 5th ed. St. Louis, MO: Mosby; 2001:194–224.

John TG, Greig JD, Carter DC, Garden OJ. Carcinoma of the pancreatic head and periampullary region: tumor staging with laparoscopy and laparoscopic ultrasonography. *Ann Surg* 1995;221:156–164.

Marks WM, Filly RA, Callen PW. Ultrasonic evaluation of normal pancreatic echogenicity and its relationship to fat deposition. *Radiology* 1980;137:475–479.

Oshikawa O, Tanaka S, Ioka T, et al. Dynamic sonography of pancreatic tumors: comparison with dynamic CT. *AJR Am J Roentgenol* 2002;178(5):1133–1137.

Ozawa Y, Numata K, Tanaka K, et al. Contrast-enhanced sonography of small pancreatic mass lesions. *J Ultrasound Med* 2002; 21(9):983–991.

Rickes S, Unkrodt K, Neye H, et al. Differentiation of pancreatic tumours by conventional ultrasound, unenhanced and echo-enhanced power Doppler sonography. *Scand J Gasteroenterol* 2002;37(11):1313–1320.

Robertson JK, Gill KA. Pancreas. In: Gill KA, ed. *Abdominal ultrasound. A practitioner's guide*. Philadelphia, PA: W.B. Saunders Company; 2001:149–168.

Shawker TH, Garra BS, Hill MC, et al. The spectrum of sonographic findings in pancreatic carcinoma. *J Ultrasound Med* 1986; 5:169–177.

Right Upper Quadrant Mass

Possible Metastases to Liver

8

LISA PARSONS
TOM WINTER

SONOGRAM ABBREVIATIONS

Ao	Aorta
Bl	Bladder
Ca	Celiac artery
CD	Common duct
D	Diaphragm
GBl	Gallbladder
Hea	Hepatic artery
Hev	Hepatic vein
Ip	Iliopsoas muscle
IMv	Inferior mesenteric vein
IVC	Inferior vena cava
K	Kidney
L	Liver
LHev	Left hepatic vein
MHev	Middle hepatic vein
Pv	Portal vein
RHev	Right hepatic vein
RPv	Right portal vein
RUQ	Right upper quadrant
S	Spine
SMA	Superior mesenteric artery
Sp	Spleen
Spa	Splenic artery
St	Stomach

KEY WORDS

Adenopathy. Abnormally enlarged lymph nodes.

Alpha-Fetoprotein. Biochemical marker that, when elevated, may indicate hepatocellular cancer in the liver.

Ameboma. Abscess caused by amebic infection. Common in Mexico and southern United States.

Budd-Chiari Syndrome. Thrombosis of the hepatic veins. Associated with ascites and liver failure.

Carcinoembryonic Antigen (CEA). CEA is a colorectal tumor marker. Abnormal values are specific neither for colon cancer nor for malignancy. CEA determination may have prognostic value for patients with colon cancer and may be used to monitor treatment, but it fails to detect recurrent disease in more than 50% of patients. CEA usually returns to normal within 1 to 2 months of surgery.

Caudate Lobe. Lobe of the liver that lies posterior to the left lobe and anterior to the inferior vena cava.

Cold Defect. Area of decreased radionuclide uptake on nuclear liver-spleen scan.

Couinaud-Bismuth. Nomenclature describing segmental anatomy of the liver.

Courvoisier's Sign. A right upper quadrant mass with painless jaundice implies that there is a cancer in the head of the pancreas that is causing biliary duct obstruction. The palpable mass is due to an enlarged gallbladder.

Echinococcal Cyst. Infected cyst caused by hydatid disease. Frequently calcified. Seen in individuals who are in contact with sheep and dogs.

Hemangioma. Benign vascular tumor of the liver.

Hepatoblastoma. Liver tumor that is common in childhood.

Hepatoma (Hepatocellular Carcinoma). Tumor of the liver that is associated with end-stage cirrhosis. Common in the Far East and Africa, where toxins from certain fungi can precipitate the disease, in patients with viral infections of the liver, and in ethanol-induced cirrhosis.

Hydatid. See *Echinococcal Cyst.*

Ligamentum Teres. Echogenic focus in the left lobe of the liver; remnant of the fetal umbilical vein.

Quadrate Lobe. Obsolete term for the medial segment of the left lobe of the liver.

Riedel's Lobe. Change in shape that occurs when the right lobe of the liver is longer than usual but the left is smaller—a normal variant.

RELEVANT LABORATORY VALUES

AFP (alpha-fetoprotein): 0.0 to 8.5 ng/mL

Serum carcinoembryonic antigen: <2.5 ng/mL in an adult nonsmoker and <5.0 ng/mL in a smoker.

The Clinical Problem

Patients can present with a right upper quadrant (RUQ) mass for a great variety of reasons. Palpable causes include everything from enlarged organs to primary or metastatic tumors. Hepatomegaly can result from infection, leukemia, bone marrow transplant, anemia, congestive heart failure, or portal hypertension. These are often accompanied by splenomegaly. An important underlying cause of hepatomegaly is a malignancy.

Liver tumors or metastases may be suspected because biochemical tumor markers (carcinoembryonic antigen and alpha-fetoprotein) or liver function test results are elevated. Alternatively, a patient may be referred because a previous computed tomography (CT) scan or other imaging technique demonstrated a concern.

CT is usually the first modality used in the United States when metastases are suspected because it produces a more comprehensive survey of the liver and is not as operator-dependent as ultrasound. The kinds of problems referred to ultrasound from CT are generally lesions that are difficult to characterize as cystic or solid, or to determine the possibility of performing ultrasound-guided liver biopsy (the preferred method to biopsy a liver lesion). A CT scan performed without contrast can yield ambiguous results that ultrasound can resolve. Some tumors can be seen with ultrasound but not with CT. Contrast-enhanced ultrasound can be used to delineate isoechoic liver lesions and to help characterize focal lesions. Current contrast research is focused on identifying liver masses by their vascular pattern during arterial and venous phases (Fig. 8-1).

Primary liver tumors may also be suspected in cirrhotic patients experiencing a rapid downhill course if liver function tests rapidly worsen. Delineating the precise site of a primary liver tumor is important because it influences surgical resectability. When both right and left lobes are involved, tumor resection is much more difficult. The margins between the individual segments of each lobe can be defined with ultrasound, both preoperatively and intraoperatively. In some cases, inoperable lesions may be candidates for radiofrequency ablation (heating) or cryoablation (freezing). These ultrasound-guided procedures use thermal mechanisms to kill tumor cells and may increase life expectancy for some patients or convert inoperable patients to operable.

Anatomy

LIVER POSITION

The major structure in the RUQ is the liver. This more-or-less triangular organ hugs the right diaphragm. The gallbladder hangs from its inferior aspect, and the right kidney lies to the right posteriorly (see Fig. 6-14). The porta hepatis (a fibrous structure containing the hepatic artery, the portal vein, lymph nodes, and the common bile duct) enters the liver from its inferior aspect close to the midline. Adjacent to the porta hepatis are the duodenum, gallbladder, and head of the pancreas. The inferior vena cava (IVC) runs through the posterior aspect of the liver to the right of the midline. The aorta lies just to the left of the midline behind the left lobe of the liver.

LOBES OF THE LIVER

The liver is divided into three lobes: right, left, and caudate (see Fig. 6-14). A fissure known as the *ligamentum teres*, in which lies a remnant of the fetal umbilical vein, appears to be a logical separation between the right and left lobes, but in reality, it separates the left lobe into two segments. The medial segment of the left lobe (the one closest to the right lobe) was formerly known as the *quadrate lobe*. This is now an obsolete term.

The division between the right and left lobes is visible sonographically only where certain anatomic landmarks appear (see Fig. 6-14):

1. Main lobar fissure. This shows up on ultrasound as an echogenic line superior to the gallbladder, which seems to connect the right portal vein to the gallbladder fossa.
2. Middle hepatic vein. More superiorly, the middle hepatic vein runs between the right and left lobes.

The left lobe is divided into medial and lateral segments superiorly by the left hepatic vein and more inferiorly by the ligamentum teres. Between those two points, the segment of the left portal vein that turns sharply anterior marks the division between the medial and lateral segments of the left lobe. The right lobe is divided into anterior/posterior segments by the right hepatic vein. The caudate lobe, which has its own blood supply, is posterior to and separated from the left lobe by the ligamentum venosum (a remnant of the fetal sinus venosus), which appears as an echogenic interface posterior to the left lobe.

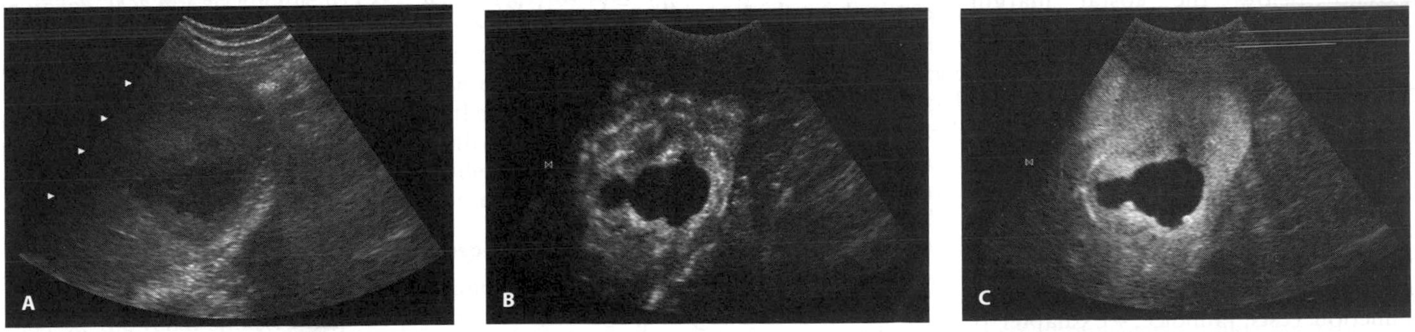

Figure 8-1. ■ *Hepatoma (A), imaged after a 1.3-mL bolus of contrast (B), and again 90 seconds later (C). (Courtesy of Phil Thompson.)*

Right Upper Quadrant Pain

MIKE LEDWIDGE
TOM WINTER

9

SONOGRAM ABBREVIATIONS

Ao	Aorta
CBD	Common bile duct
GB, Gbl	Gallbladder
IVC	Inferior vena cava
K	Kidney
L	Liver
Pv	Portal vein
S	Spine

KEY WORDS

Acute Abdomen. Sudden onset of abdominal pain. Causes include appendicitis, perforated peptic ulcer, strangulated hernia, acute cholecystitis, pancreatitis, and renal colic.

Adenomyomatosis. A chronic gallbladder condition causing right upper quadrant (RUQ) pain with several sonographic manifestations—the most common are multiple, small polypoid masses arising from the gallbladder wall.

AIDS. Acquired immunodeficiency syndrome (see Chapter 11).

Amebiasis. Infection with amebic parasite, common in Mexico, the southern United States, and warm climates.

Ameboma of the Liver. Abscess caused by amebiasis.

Cholangitis. Inflammation of a bile duct.

Cholecystitis. Inflammation of the gallbladder.

Acute. Usually caused by gallbladder outlet obstruction.

Chronic. Inflammation persisting over a longer period.

Choledochojejunostomy. Surgical procedure in which the bile duct is anastomosed to jejunum; food and air may reflux into the bile ducts.

Choledocholithiasis. Gallstone in a bile duct.

Cholelithiasis. Gallstones in the gallbladder.

Cholesterosis (Cholesterolosis). Variant of adenomyomatosis in which cholesterol polyps arise from the gallbladder wall.

Hartmann's Pouch. Portion of the gallbladder that lies nearest the cystic duct where stones often collect.

Junctional Fold. Septum usually arising from the posterior midaspect of the gallbladder, a normal variant.

Murphy's Sign. Tenderness when an inflamed gallbladder is palpated clinically, usually on deep inspiration.

Phrygian Cap. Variant gallbladder shape in which the gallbladder's fundus is separated from the body of the gallbladder by a junctional fold.

Pyogenic. Producing pus.

Rokitansky-Aschoff Sinuses (RAS). Multiple pouches in the wall of the gallbladder, which often fill with cholesterol crystals.

Sphincterotomy. Procedure in which the sphincter of Oddi is widened surgically. Gas will reflux into the bile ducts.

Wall Echo Shadow (WES), Wall Echo Shadow Complex (WESC), or Double Arc Shadow Sign. Sonographic pattern seen when the gallbladder is filled with stones. The WES consists of two curved, parallel bright lines separated by a thin, anechoic space, accompanied by posterior acoustic shadowing.

RELEVANT LABORATORY VALUES*

Alkaline phosphatase: 40 to 135 U/L

ALT (SGPT): 5 to 60 U/L

AST (SGOT): 5 to 42 U/L

Bilirubin

Direct: 0.0 to 0.3 mg/dL
Total: 0.1 to 1.6 mg/dL

GGT: 1 to 50 U/L

White blood cell count: 3,800 to 10,500/uL

*See Chapter 10 for definitions. Numbers listed for each measurement are the range of normal values.

The Clinical Problem

RUQ pain, either chronic or acute, may be caused by disease in the gallbladder, liver, porta hepatis, pancreas, right kidney, adrenal gland, lung, or diaphragmatic pleura. Differential diagnosis is sometimes difficult and often requires the use of many modalities, including the patient's history and physical examination, laboratory tests, computed tomography (CT) scans, nuclear medicine, magnetic resonance imaging, and ultrasound. Important physical signs and symptoms include the presence or absence of jaundice, acute pain, fever, and vomiting.

Ruling out gallstones is perhaps the most common indication for an RUQ scan. Although stones in the gallbladder and ducts certainly can cause pain, they are often asymptomatic. Because choledocholithiasis may be indicated by increases in liver function tests before any pain is experienced, this condition will be discussed in Chapter 10. The clinician asks for concrete evidence from the sonographer before referring the patient to a surgeon: Does the gallbladder have stones? A thickened wall? Fluid around it? Is it locally tender? Is it enlarged? Is there biliary tree dilatation? Is there any evidence of a gallbladder tumor?

When RUQ pain is acute, rapid and accurate diagnosis on an emergency basis may be crucial. Many of the internal disasters that precipitate an acute abdomen, such as renal colic with secondary hydronephrosis, and pancreatitis, are readily detectable with ultrasound. Others, however, such as perforated ulcer, are not. Due to the proximity of the gallbladder and pancreas to the right hemidiaphragm, patients with cholecystitis and pancreatitis sometimes experience referred pain in the right shoulder area. Pain may also be referred into the RUQ from inflammation of the diaphragmatic pleura. Thus, the sonographic finding of an unsuspected pleural effusion may shift the focus of the work-up to the chest. Pyelonephritis and renal stones (see Chapter 20), as well as liver tumor or abscess, may present as RUQ pain.

Sometimes, RUQ pain is the result of chronic disease, as when oncology patients have viscous bile from prolonged stasis and develop acute acalculous cholecystitis or gallstones, or when AIDS patients develop cholangitis. RUQ abnormalities may be incidental findings in these patients because the pain may not be marked, or because the signs and symptoms wind up buried in a very complex clinical picture. These patients require a careful search for any problem that can be treated to alleviate pain.

Anatomy

GALLBLADDER

The gallbladder is situated on the inferior aspect of the liver, medial and anterior to the kidney, and lateral and anterior to the inferior vena cava. The main lobar fissure is a sonographic landmark leading to the gallbladder fossa, seen as an echogenic line (Fig. 9-1) that runs from the right portal vein to the gall-

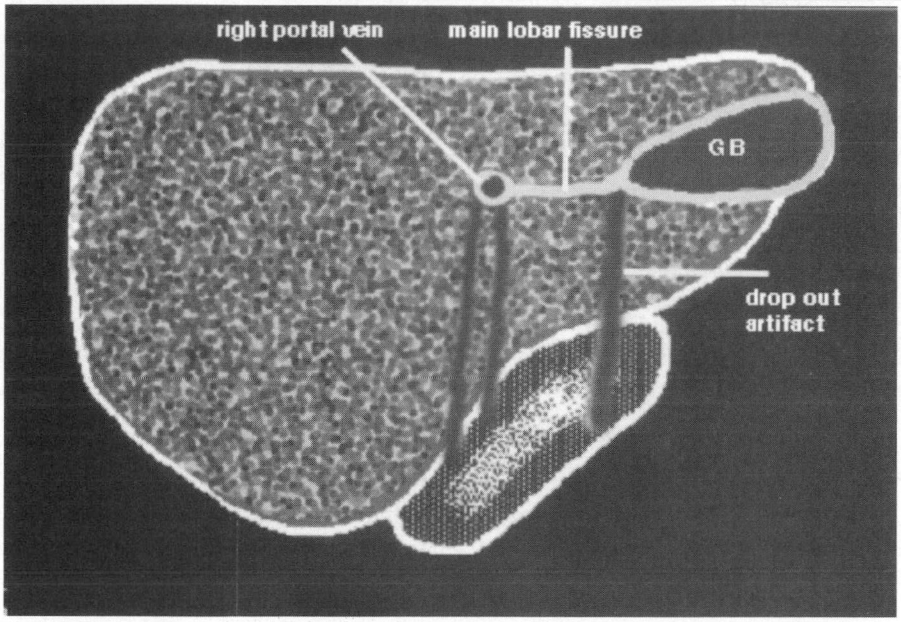

Figure 9-1. ■ *Diagram showing the main lobar fissure between the right portal vein and the gallbladder. Note the refractive acoustic shadowing from the gallbladder wall and the portal vein wall. There is no echo source for these areas as there would be if a gallstone were present.*

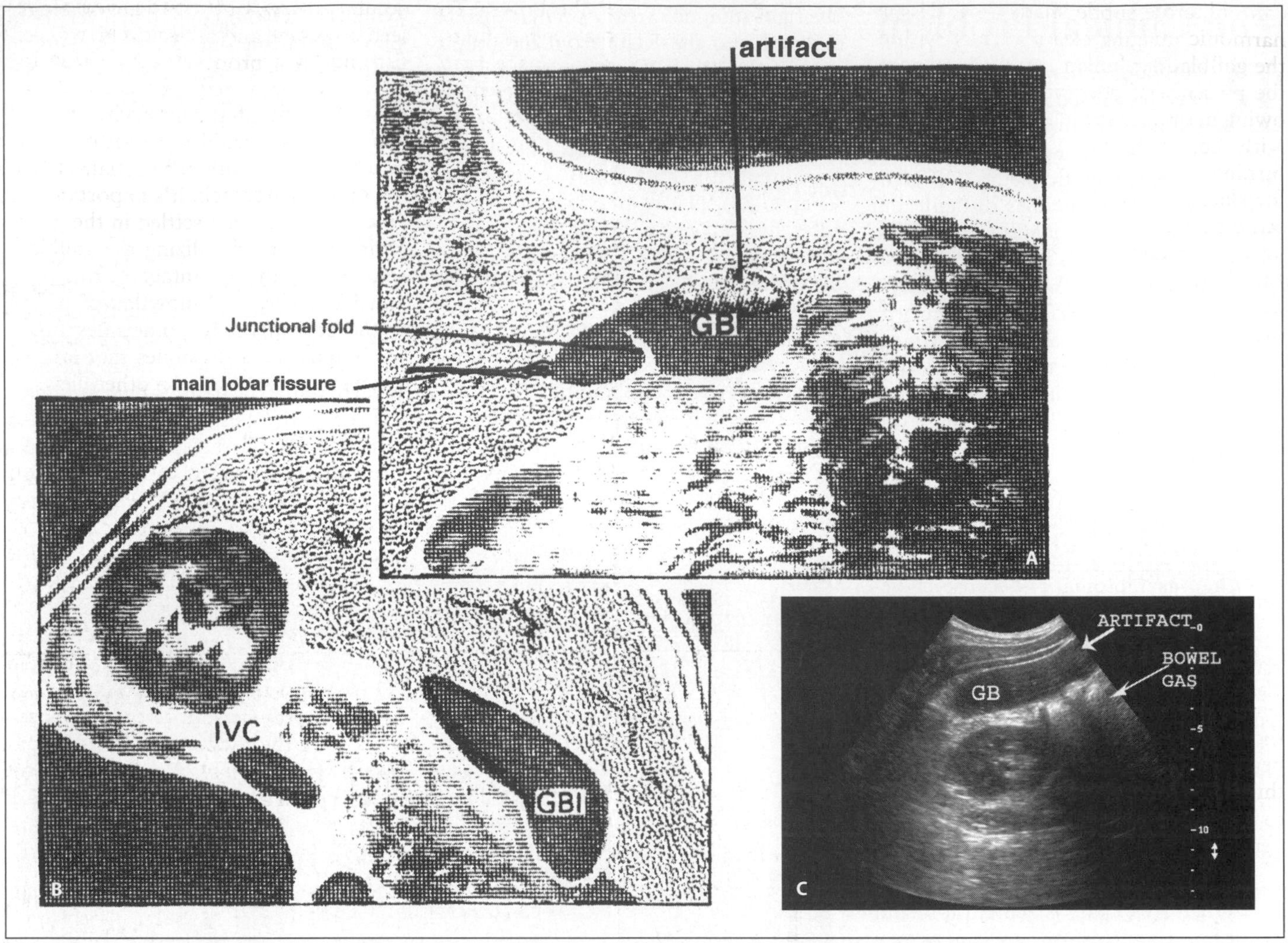

Figure 9-2. ■ *Reverberation artifacts. A. Reverberations are a common problem in the anterior aspect of the gallbladder (artifact). The gallbladder is easily located by following the main lobar fissure from the right portal vein to the gallbladder fossa. The fold at the neck of the gallbladder could cause confusion if caught in a plane that demonstrated only a portion of it. B. Increasing the gallbladder's distance from the transducer by turning the patient in a decubitus position moves the gallbladder wall into the focal zone of the transducer and decreases reverberations. The decubitus position allows the fundus to fall and the kink to straighten out. C. In this grayscale image showing reverberation artifact filling gallbladder lumen with false echoes, note the nearby bowel forming a "dirty" shadow.*

bladder. The gallbladder is pear-shaped and varies in size. It may contain a kink (the junctional fold) close to the neck (Fig. 9-2). It is divided into the fundus (the distal tip area), the body, and the neck (Hartmann's pouch is that portion of the gallbladder between the junctional fold and the neck). The gallbladder has an echogenic wall that should not be more than 3 mm thick in a fasting patient. See Chapter 10, Abnormal Liver Function Tests: Jaundice, for anatomy of the biliary tree.

Technique

PATIENT PREPARATION

Gallbladder studies should be performed after an overnight fast of 8 to 12 hours. Water (and oral contrast for CT, which has only a weak contracting effect on the gallbladder) is permitted, but be sure the patient is not scheduled for other exams for which he or she should be without fluids, such as an upper gastrointestinal series.

Even if the gallbladder is not present, abdominal sonograms benefit from the patient's fasting; there is less air in the stomach, and it makes a better window if there is a need to fill it with water.

TRANSDUCER

The two most important points to remember in scanning gallbladders are to use a transducer with a high frequency and to set the focal zone at the back wall where stones collect. The frequency must be adequate to penetrate the entire organ, but you may need to change the transducer from the one used to demonstrate the right lobe of the liver, or you can obliterate subtle shadowing. Tissue harmonic imaging clears artifact within the gallbladder lumen and may enhance the presence of posterior acoustic shadowing in smaller stones. If using a system with spatial compounding, consider turning off compounding while looking for shadows, as compounding may obscure subtle shadows. A high-frequency linear transducer can be used when the gallbladder is located close to the abdominal wall to aid in accurate wall measurements and to enhance shadowing in very small stones.

PATIENT POSITION

Supine Position

The gallbladder is first examined with the patient in a supine position using a sector or curvilinear scanner (a linear probe may be used to show Rokitansky-Aschoff sinuses and to obtain more accurate gallbladder wall measurements). Try to obtain long-axis views by varying the obliquity of the transducer until the maximum length of the gallbladder is seen. Scan through the short axis of the gallbladder, beginning at the neck and sweeping through the fundus. It is often necessary to angle caudally through the body to demonstrate the entire fundus well, as it can be tucked up under the bowel. To view the gallbladder, it may be helpful to scan through an intercostal space with the right arm raised above the head (if possible), or to scan from a subcostal approach with breathhold on inspiration.

Decubitus Position

It is mandatory to obtain additional gallbladder views in the left lateral decubitus (right side up), oblique, prone, or upright position because stones may be missed if only supine views are obtained (Fig. 9-2). They might be small and therefore undetectable along the back wall. Changing position can pile stones together and can create enough volume to produce shadowing. The decubitus position allows the liver to act as an acoustic window for visualizing the gallbladder. Stones and gravel will fall into the most dependent portion—usually the fundus—whereas polyps or adherent stones will stay put. Sludge will only gradually level off in the bottom. Think of sludge movement as similar to that of molasses or honey—it may take some time to shift noticeably after a change in position.

Prone Position

If the most dependent part of the gallbladder becomes obscured by bowel on a decubitus view, or if there are no stones seen on supine and decubitus views, persist and try a prone view. Position the transducer on the patient's side and scan coronally through the liver when the patient is in a decubitus position, then watch while the patient rolls flat (or flatter) onto the stomach. It's important not to let the patient get settled in the prone position before visualizing the gallbladder, because the advantage of this position is in seeing the "snowflakes" falling as the patient turns. Sometimes prone positioning picks up stones that layered and were undetectable on other views.

Upright Position

The upright position is awkward for both patient and sonographer, but in patients with a small, high liver and large anteroposterior diameter, it may be the best alternate view. Don't just sit the patient up on the stretcher, as the bowel may push up in front of the gallbladder (Fig. 9-3). Have the patient stand and brace against the stretcher. Don't waste all this effort—be sure to scan the pancreas while the patient is upright. In patients with this build, it's often the best way to get an acoustic window, and so it is worth the trouble.

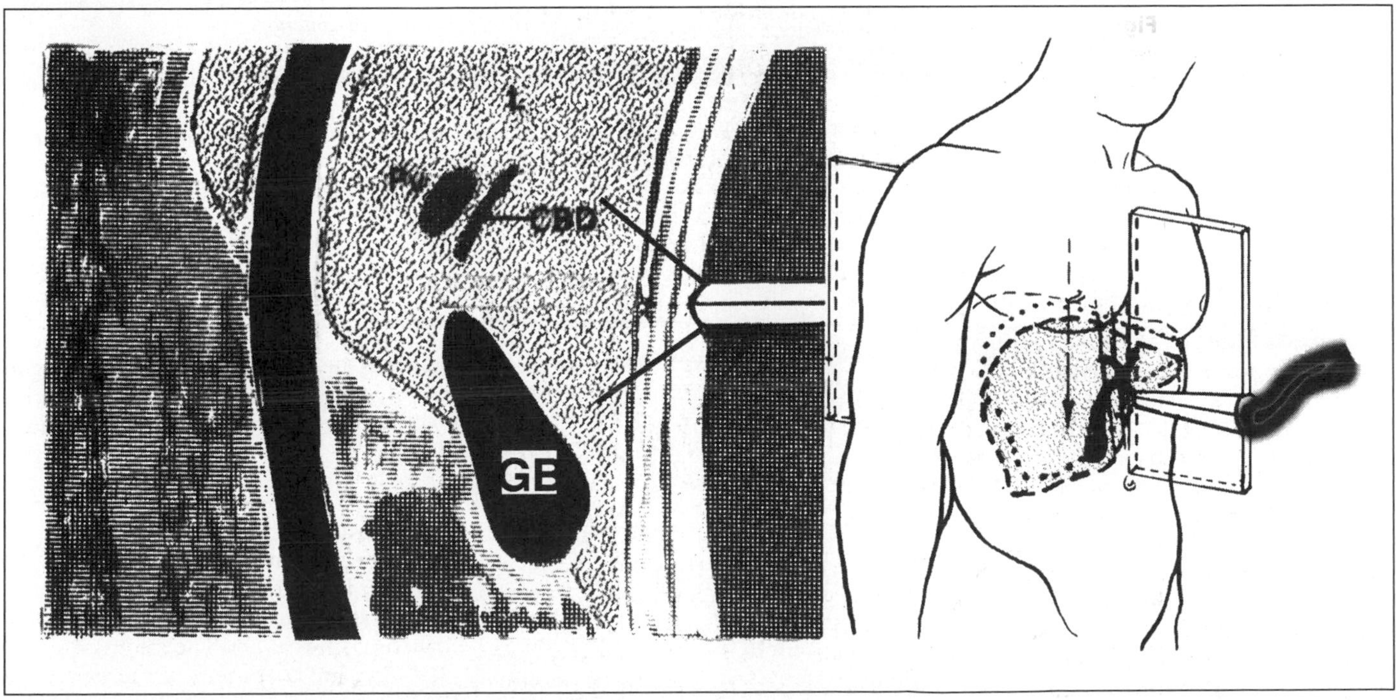

Figure 9-3. ■ *Gravity and redistribution of abdominal organs may allow better access to the liver, gallbladder, and pancreas when the patient is upright.*

LOCAL TENDERNESS

A positive ultrasonic Murphy's sign is an excellent indicator that RUQ pain is indeed localized to the gallbladder. Press the transducer subcostally over the gallbladder and ask the patient if that hurts (the answer is irrelevant if you are scanning between ribs). Because this is a somewhat subjective assessment, double-check a positive result by pressing in the epigastric region and right lower quadrant. If these areas also hurt, this is not a valid Murphy's sign, although the gallbladder may still be the source of the pain. Another approach is to scan continuously from just left of midline to the right midaxillary line once or twice for practice, then do it again and ask the patient to lift his or her finger (assuming that he or she is holding his or her breath in inspiration and should not speak) when the probe is over the point of maximum tenderness and see if that correlates with the gallbladder.

If uncertain, turn the patient into a decubitus position and let the gallbladder move into the midline. Press on the gallbladder in the new location and see whether it still hurts. If it doesn't hurt here, where the transducer may have even better access, think again and check the right kidney for stones, or the liver for abscess. Ask the patient to put one finger on the point of maximum pain, and take a look there with the probe.

Pathology

GALLSTONES

Gallstones are seen with acute and chronic cholecystitis but may be found in symptom-free patients as well. They may have several different sonographic appearances. The larger the stone is, the less likely it will cause problems in the future. Smaller stones are mobile and may move into the cystic duct or common duct and cause obstruction.

Gallstone with Shadowing

A stone surrounded by bile appears as a dense specular reflector within fluid. The density of the stone will absorb and reflect sound, so that a column of acoustic shadowing is seen posterior to the gallstone (Fig. 9-4).

Shadowing from a stone is "clean" with sharp borders and few internal echoes, whereas shadowing from air is less well defined with more echoes, that is, soft or "dirty" (Fig. 9-2C).

Color Doppler may be employed in an attempt to show the "twinkle" artifact as a sign of a gallstone (see Fig. 9-15), similar to use of this artifact in detecting renal calculi (see Chapter 20).

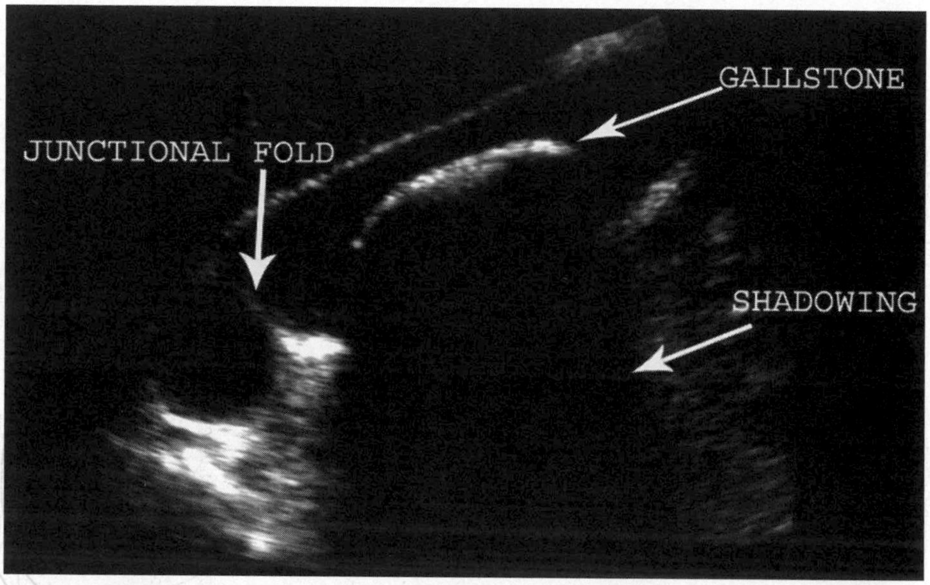

Figure 9-4. ■ *Solitary gallstone casting a "clean" shadow. Note that the echo source is within the gallbladder. Also note the incidental junctional fold.*

Gallstones without Shadowing

Figure 9-5 shows gallstones without shadowing. Very small stones may not be associated with acoustic shadowing using standard transducers, although improvements in technology now often allow us to show shadowing, even from small stones. If an echogenic focus (a possible stone) can be shown to move when the patient is repositioned—for example, in the left lateral decubitus or prone position—the lesion is a stone; if the focus does not move, the echoes probably represent a polyp or a septum (although stones can be adherent and immobile).

Gravel

If many tiny stones are present, they will layer out in the most dependent portion of the gallbladder. It is sometimes difficult to discern each separate stone; an irregular pattern of bright echoes is displayed along the gallbladder's posterior wall. Shadowing may or may not be seen. Gravel will layer out immediately along the dependent wall of a gallbladder in the decubitus position.

Gallbladder Filled with Stones

Sometimes when the gallbladder contains many stones, no echo-free bile can be seen around them. The stones appear as a group of dense echoes with acoustic shadowing located near the liver edge but within the liver on all views. Because this condition looks suspiciously like a gas-filled duodenum, it can represent a

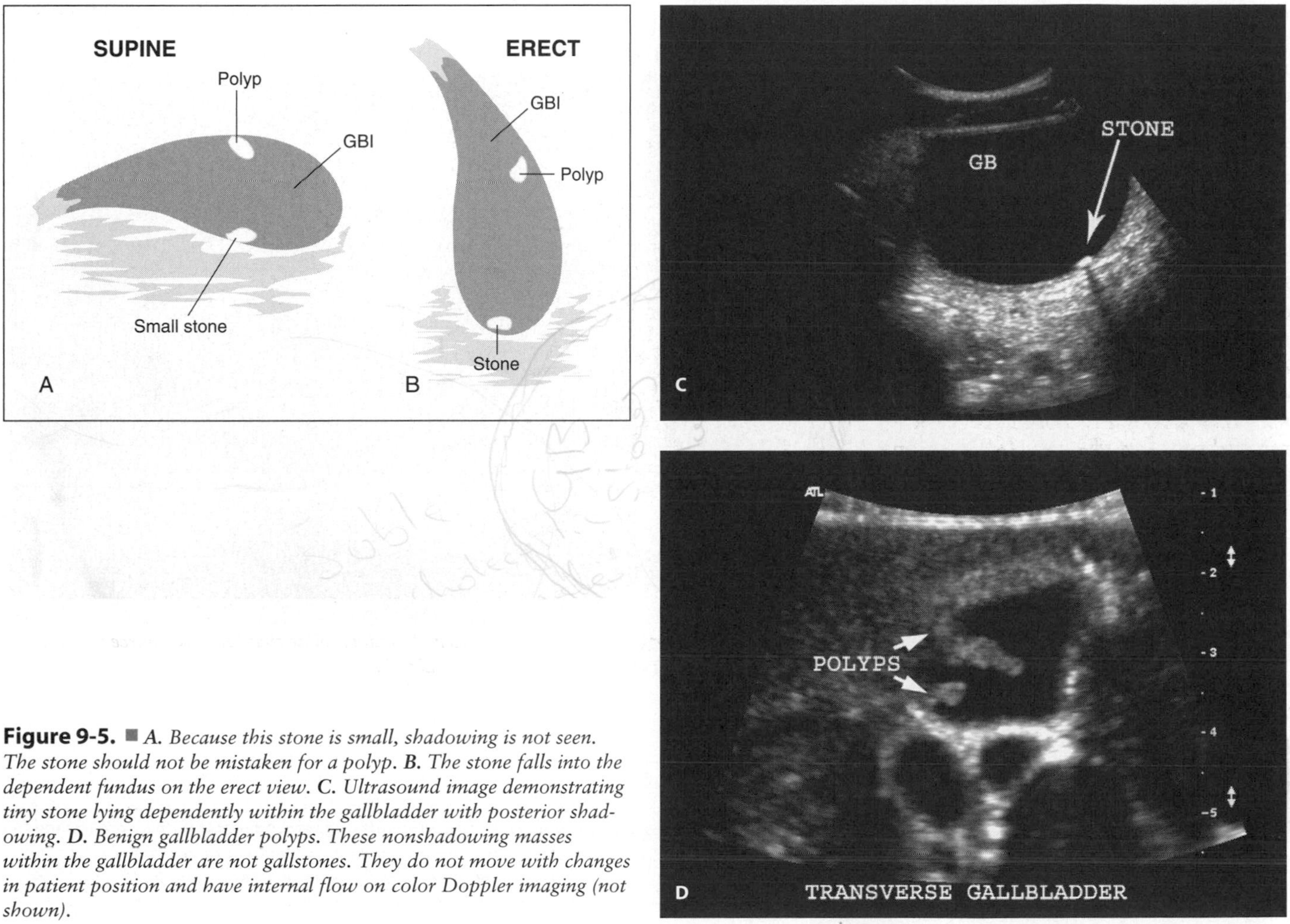

Figure 9-5. ■ *A. Because this stone is small, shadowing is not seen. The stone should not be mistaken for a polyp.* ***B.*** *The stone falls into the dependent fundus on the erect view.* ***C.*** *Ultrasound image demonstrating tiny stone lying dependently within the gallbladder with posterior shadowing.* ***D.*** *Benign gallbladder polyps. These nonshadowing masses within the gallbladder are not gallstones. They do not move with changes in patient position and have internal flow on color Doppler imaging (not shown).*

diagnostic problem (Fig. 9-6), and special techniques are required:

1. Make sure another candidate for gallbladder is not visible somewhere else in the RUQ.
2. Trace the main lobar fissure to the gallbladder fossa to prove that this is the gallbladder, as opposed to the duodenum.
3. Change the patient's position. This step may cause stones to settle in the dependent portion of the gallbladder and a thin layer of bile to appear across the top (Fig. 9-6).
4. Have the patient drink water; peristalsis will be seen in the true duodenum.
5. Evaluate the acoustic shadow. Air causes shadowing that has a less well-defined pattern than dense stones (Fig. 9-2). The borders of a shadowed area caused by stones are generally sharper and more clearly outlined than those caused by gas.
6. Look for the WES (Fig. 9-6C). Echoes are seen both from the wall of the gallbladder and from the layer of stones. By contrast, air in the duodenum will be right against the mucosa.
7. Make sure the patient has not had a prior cholecystectomy—some patients forget their medical history (check for surgical scars on the patient's abdomen).

Stones as a Fluid Level

Occasionally, stones float and will be seen as a fluid level within the gallbladder, particularly when the gallbladder contains radiographic contrast material. The stones appear singly or as an irregular echogenic line floating in the bile; when the patient's position is changed, the floating line re-forms.

Adherent Stones

Small adherent stones may appear as echoes in the gallbladder with or without shadowing. If the echoes do not change position with alternate views, the possibilities include adherent stones, gallbladder polyps, or a tumor. Color Doppler, at a high sensitivity setting, may show flow in small intraluminal tumors. Watch out for artifactual color resonance ("twinkle" artifact) mimicking flow. Pulsed Doppler may be used to show actual flow versus artifact (see Fig. 9-15).

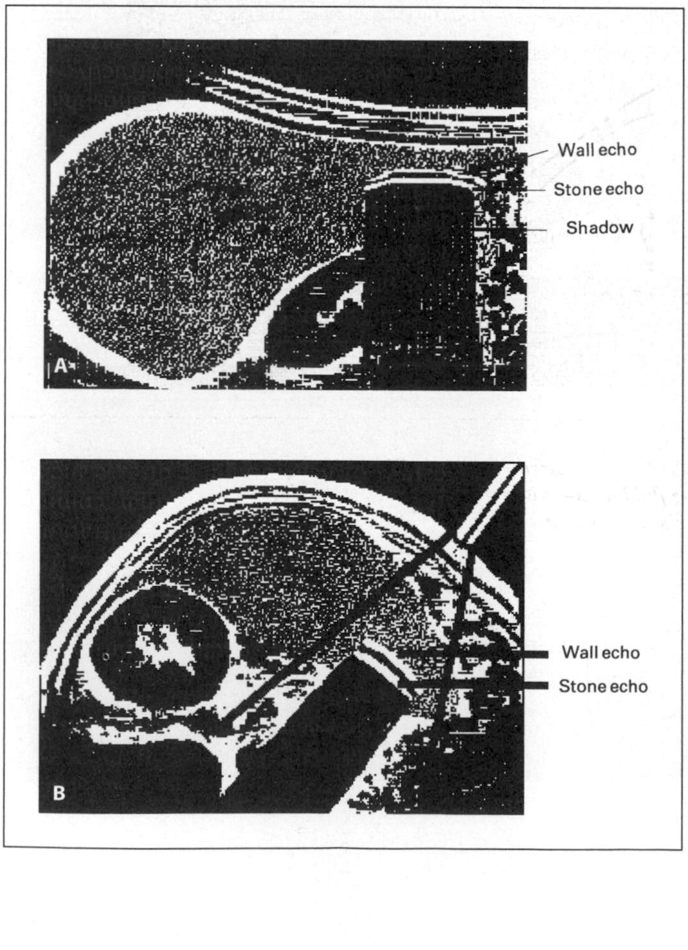

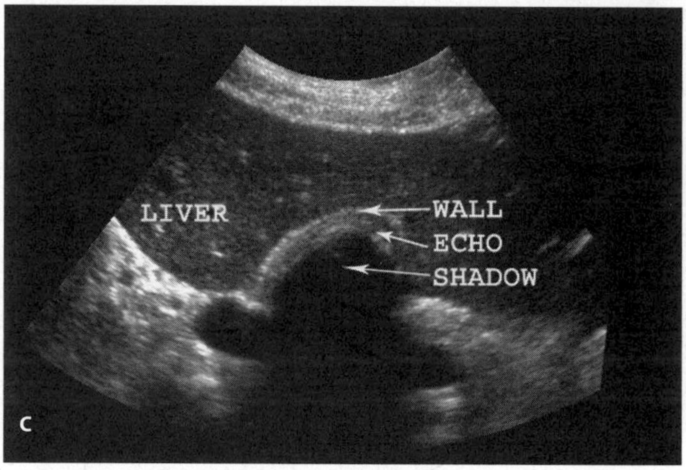

Figure 9-6. ■ *Acoustic shadowing. A. Clear, well-defined shadowing is evidence that this is a gallbladder full of stones and not gas shadowing from adjacent structures (the wall echo shadow; there is an echo from the gallbladder wall and from the layer of stones). The shadowing arises within the liver contour. B. If a gallbladder full of stones is examined on a decubitus view, a thin layer of bile may appear, supporting the diagnosis of gallstones. C. Grayscale image showing the wall echo shadow arising from within the liver.*

Viscid Bile (Sludge)

Viscid bile usually causes low-level echoes in the dependent portion of the gallbladder akin to those seen with numerous small stones but unaccompanied by shadowing. The fluid level associated with viscid bile is usually not entirely horizontal. If the patient is placed in the erect or decubitus position, the fluid level takes several minutes to reaccumulate (Fig. 9-7), whereas many small stones almost immediately fall into a dependent site. Viscid bile is seen mainly in patients with obstructive jaundice, liver disease, hyperalimentation, or sepsis (think "ICU" patient). A focal area of viscid bile can simulate a polyp or nonshadowing stone. Gallstones with definite shadowing may be mixed in with the sludge.

Acute Cholecystitis

When a patient has acute RUQ pain, acute cholecystitis must be considered. If the patient's most tender area turns out to be exactly where the gallbladder is located, this information should be documented for the clinician, because it indicates acute cholecystitis (sonographic Murphy's sign). Pain may be the only finding suggestive of cholecystitis, because this condition is not always accompanied by gallstones (acute acalculous cholecystitis). Note, however, that absence of a sonographic Murphy's sign does not exclude cholecystitis, particularly in very severe cases of cholecystitis; Murphy's sign may be present in only one third of patients with gangrenous cholecystitis.

Checking to see whether a patient has local tenderness over the gallbladder should be part of a routine gallbladder or RUQ examination. If the gallbladder is palpable, it is usually obstructed. A nuclear medicine hepatobiliary scan may be used to establish whether or not the cystic duct is obstructed. Keep in mind that because the radioisotope cannot enter a flaccid, bile-filled gallbladder, it produces false-positive results in patients on treatment protocols that include par-

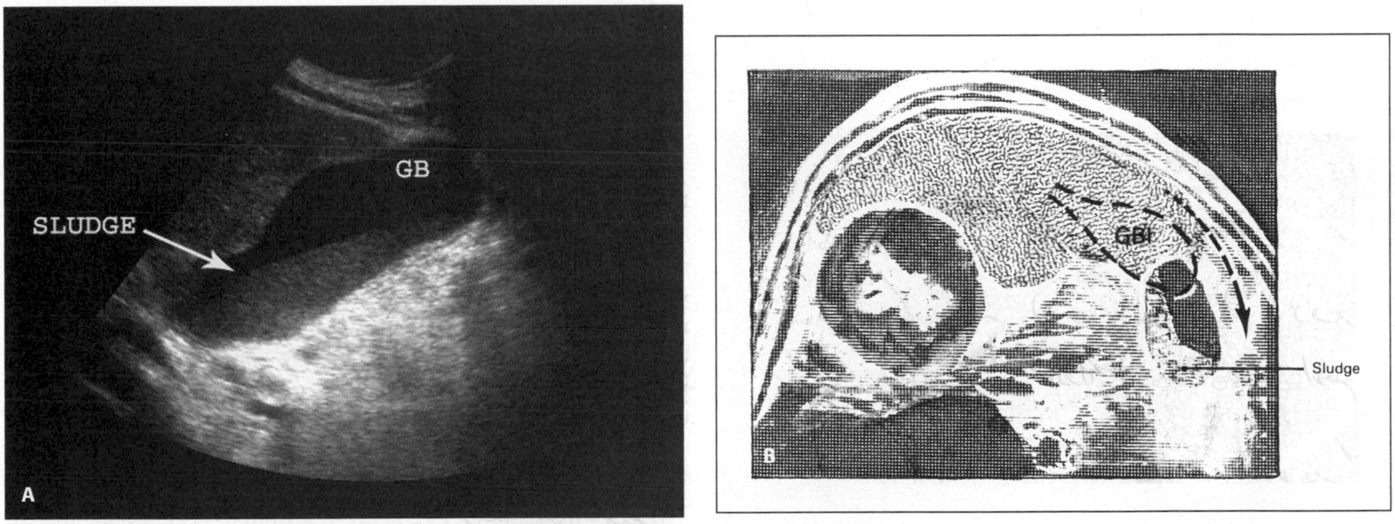

Figure 9-7. ■ *Presence of sludge. A. Irregular echoes in the posterior aspect of the gallbladder—forming a poorly defined, gravity-dependent layering fluid level—suggests the presence of sludge. B. If the patient is placed in a decubitus position, the sludge may not re-form a fluid-fluid level for many minutes.*

enteral nutrition, large doses of narcotics, antibiotics, or long-term fasting (Fig. 9-8).

Sonographic signs of inflammation include the following:

1. Cholelithiasis
2. Focal tenderness over gallbladder (Murphy's sign)
3. Wall thickening (more than 3 mm) and irregularity
4. Fluid in the pericholecystic space
5. Gas in the gallbladder (emphysematous cholecystitis)
6. Tense distention of the gallbladder (hydrops)

Wall Thickening

Wall thickening is not specific for acute cholecystitis. Diffuse wall thickening can be seen in patients with AIDS, sepsis, hepatitis, congestive heart failure, or ascites. Some of the most striking examples of wall thickening are seen in hepatitis rather than cholecystitis. The wall thickening seen in ascites may be uniformly echogenic, whereas in acute cholecystitis there is usually an echopenic rim. Striated wall thickening has been associated with acute gangrenous cholecystitis and AIDS (Fig. 9-8). The "wall" should not be more than 3-mm thick; if the outermost echogenic interface is included, the normal thickness should not exceed 5 mm.

Perigallbladder (Pericholecystic) Fluid Collection

A discrete fluid collection, which represents a small abscess, may be seen around the gallbladder, often near the fundus. This is sometimes the most definitive evidence of acute cholecystitis (Fig. 9-8A,C).

Gas in the Gallbladder

With emphysematous cholecystitis, the gallbladder or gallbladder wall is filled with gas, which reflects sound back and forth in a reverberation pattern. The appearance is therefore different from that of a gallbladder filled with stones, which blocks the sound completely. The gallbladder may be acutely tender.

Adenomyomatosis

Adenomyomatosis is considered a noninflammatory disease of the gallbladder wall with hyperplasia and intramural diverticula (Rokitansky-Aschoff sinuses). It can cause mild recurrent RUQ pain. There are three sonographic appearances:

1. Multiple septa within the gallbladder
2. Multiple polyps in the gallbladder

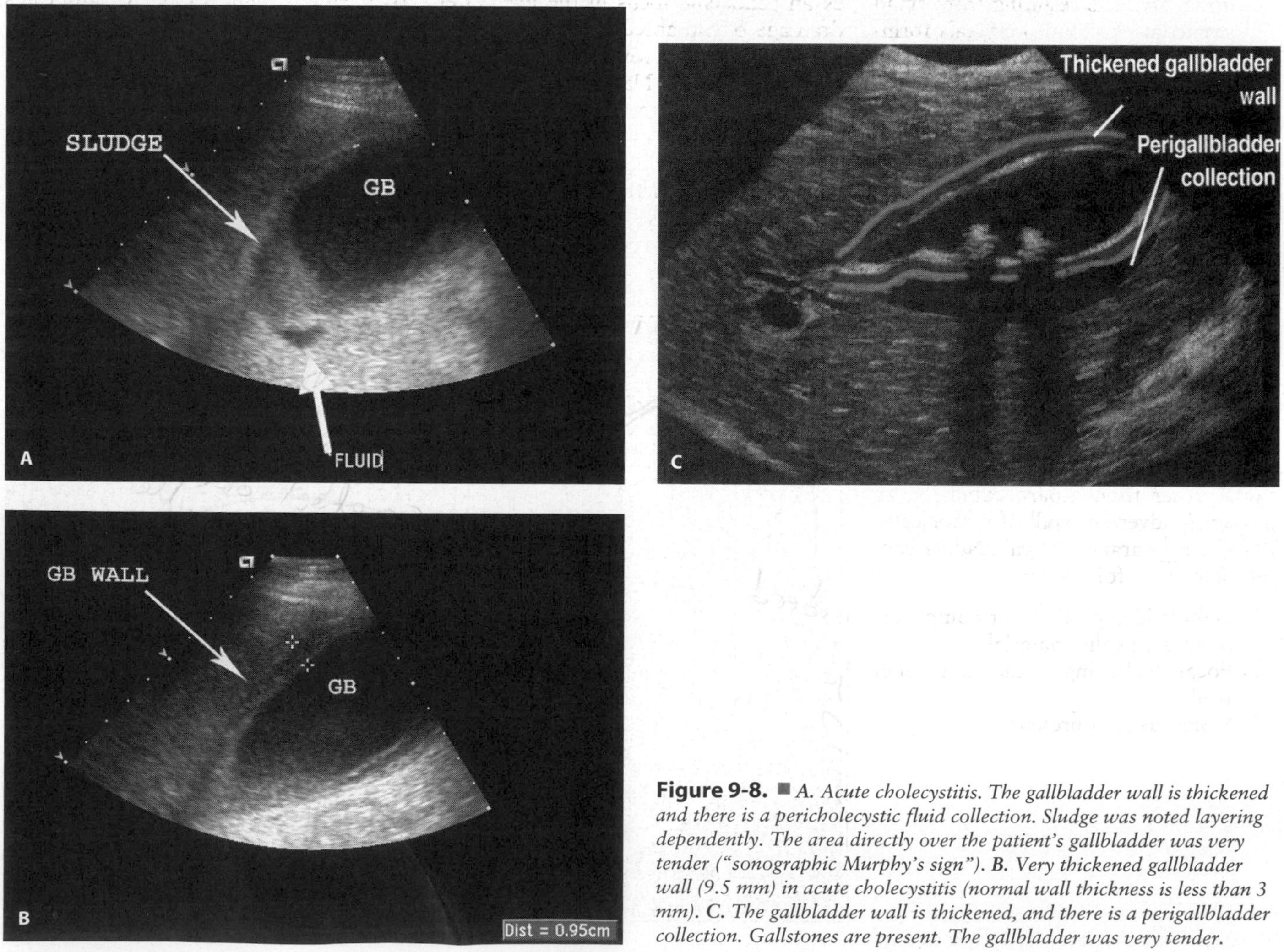

Figure 9-8. ■ *A. Acute cholecystitis. The gallbladder wall is thickened and there is a pericholecystic fluid collection. Sludge was noted layering dependently. The area directly over the patient's gallbladder was very tender ("sonographic Murphy's sign"). B. Very thickened gallbladder wall (9.5 mm) in acute cholecystitis (normal wall thickness is less than 3 mm). C. The gallbladder wall is thickened, and there is a perigallbladder collection. Gallstones are present. The gallbladder was very tender.*

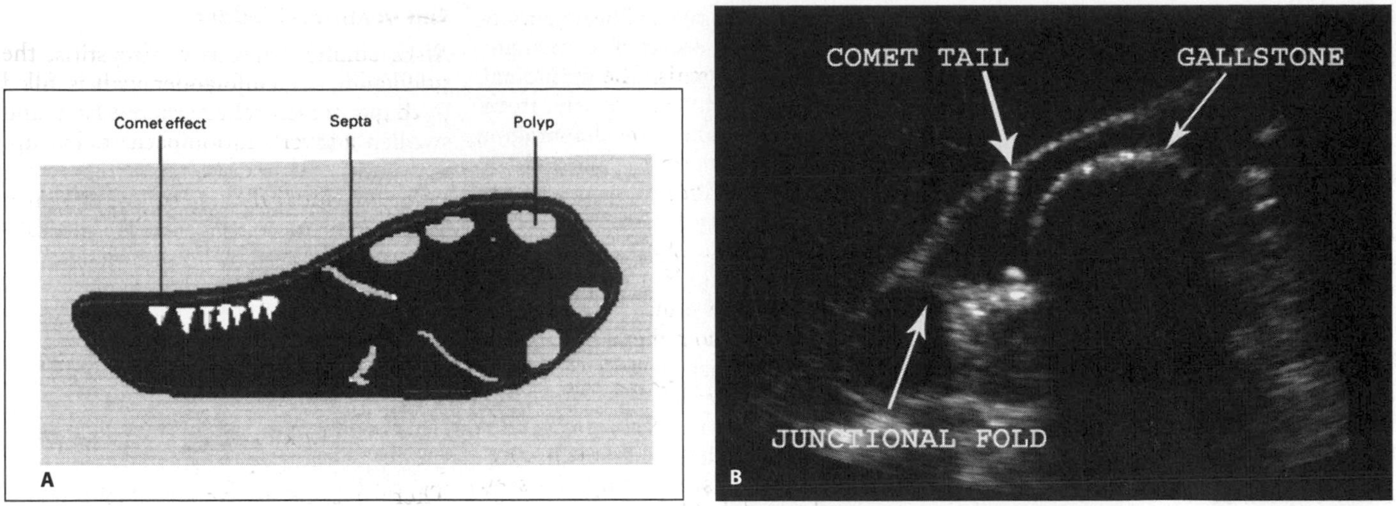

Figure 9-9. ■ *A. Adenomyomatosis. Small stones and/or cholesterol crystals in the gallbladder wall cause the comet effect diagnostic of adenomyomatosis. Septa may be seen. Small polyps are common. B. Comet tail artifact arising from the anterior gallbladder wall, as well as large shadowing gallstone and junctional fold.*

3. Multiple "comet effects"—ring-down artifacts resulting from small stones or cholesterol crystals forming in the intramural diverticula (Fig. 9-9)

Carcinoma of the Gallbladder

On rare occasions, carcinoma of the gallbladder causes pain; more often, it is an unexpected finding on a study performed for other reasons. This is a very important diagnosis to make, as gallbladder cancer has its best prognosis when detected incidentally before invasion into the liver or other structures. Also, knowledge of gallbladder cancer is important for the surgeon because gallbladder cancer should always be removed with a conventional large incision, rather than laparoscopically, to prevent inadvertent spill of tumor cells. Possible appearances of gallbladder cancer include the following:

1. Gallbladder partially or completely filled with solid material
2. Focal thickening of the gallbladder wall
3. Stones usually present

Nongallbladder Causes of RUQ Pain

ABSCESSES

Abscesses in the liver usually have an echopenic center with good through transmission and a thickened wall; sometimes, the collapsed wall shows up as an echogenic focus in the liver after drainage of the abscess. Some pyogenic abscesses exhibit low-level echoes on high-gain settings. Necrotic liver tumors also have fluid-filled centers and may be confused with abscesses, but they generally have thicker walls. Color flow may help depict flow in vessels in the wall of an abscess. The subhepatic and subphrenic spaces are also common sites for abscesses, particularly in the postoperative patient. Multiple small abscesses with echogenic centers are seen in immunosuppressed patients owing to fungal infection (Fig. 9-10). Until intravascular ultrasound contrast agents become widely available, some hepatic abscesses may be very difficult to detect; when in doubt, contrast-enhanced CT should be performed.

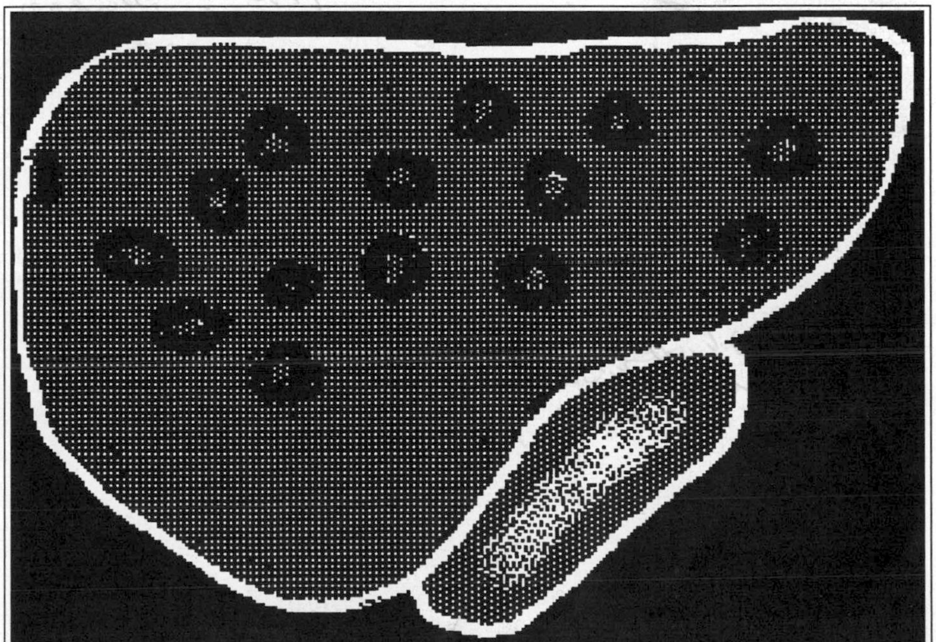

Figure 9-10. ■ *View showing multiple fungal abscesses within the liver. They are echopenic but have an echogenic center.*

ECHINOCOCCAL (HYDATID) CYSTS

Echinococcal cysts, round or oval in shape, are caused by the parasite *Echinococcus granulosus* and can have any one or a combination of the following appearances:

1. Simple cyst with a parallel line (a laminar membrane) inside the wall. Loose, mobile debris may be seen ("falling snowflakes")
2. Cyst containing smaller daughter cysts; these can deflate, and the walls cave in to form the "drooping lily sign" (Fig. 9-11)
3. Homogeneous material filling cyst or surrounding internal contents
4. Calcifications within; calcified walls
5. Collapsed cyst within the "parent" cyst
6. Echogenic, with or without the other signs; poor acoustic enhancement

A second type of parasite, alveolar echinococcus, is seen principally in the Far East. Masses have irregular borders and are echopenic, resembling a neoplasm.

PERIHEPATIC FLUID COLLECTIONS

A collection of fluid on either side of the diaphragm is an important finding and should be easily shown on longitudinal scans through the liver.

A pleural effusion usually appears as an echo-free, wedge-shaped area superior to the diaphragm on a longitudinal view (see Fig. 21-3). Transversely, there is an echo-free rim above the diaphragm. A subdiaphragmatic collection, which may be less well defined, is an area of decreased echogenicity inferior to the diaphragm.

Subphrenic fluid can be differentiated from a pleural effusion (Fig. 9-12) on transverse views. In the latter, the diaphragm will be adjacent to the liver, not separated by fluid. The bare area prevents fluid from lying between the diaphragm and the liver in the midline, whereas a pleural effusion may extend posterior to the heart alongside the spine.

Pyelonephritis

The tenderness may be localized to the kidney. The kidney itself can look normal even when acute inflammation (pyelonephritis) is present. There may be a focal swollen, relatively echopenic area of the kidney that represents an area of acute pyelonephritis. Occasionally, especially in thin patients, color or power Doppler imaging may show an area of absent perfusion to correspond to the focus of infection within the kidney. Renal calculi may be seen with or without hydronephrosis and can be the cause of RUQ pain (see Chapter 20).

Pancreatitis

Although the patient complains of right-sided pain, the tenderness may be caused by pancreatitis. The pancreas may be swollen and more sonolucent than normal if pancreatitis is acute (see Chapter 7), but remember that the most common imaging finding (either CT or ultrasound) in pancreatitis is a normal scan.

Pitfalls

1. Artifact versus stone. Scattered echoes adjacent to the anterior wall of the gallbladder may be due to reverberation, and near the posterior wall of the gallbladder, they may be due to the partial volume effect (see Chapter 57). To diminish these artifacts:
   a. Be sure the electronic focus on the transducer is set at the correct level; this is operator-dependent on most real-time equipment.
   b. Use a transducer with the correct focal zone and frequency. A short focus, high frequency is usually correct. Tissue harmonic imaging is usually of benefit. Turn spatial compounding on and off, and try a linear transducer.
   c. Change the patient's position to obtain a decubitus or erect view,

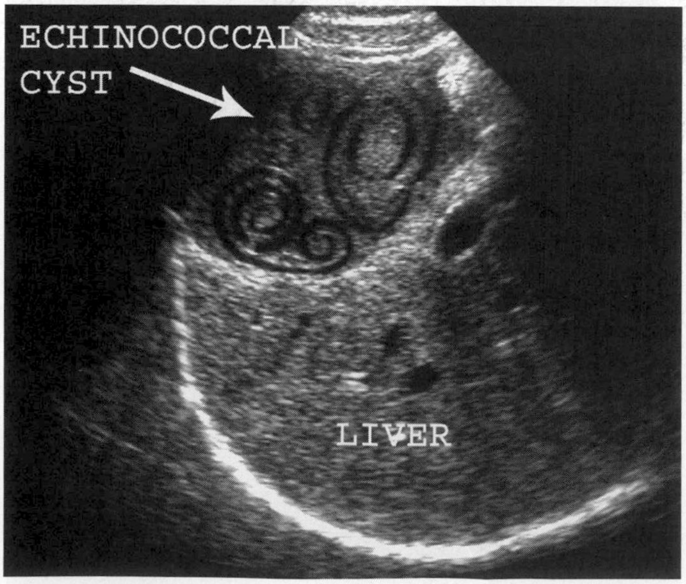

Figure 9-11. ■ *Hydatid cyst. A 13-year-old from the Middle East presents with fever and RUQ pain. Sonogram shows a classic appearance of echinococcal granulosus infection.*

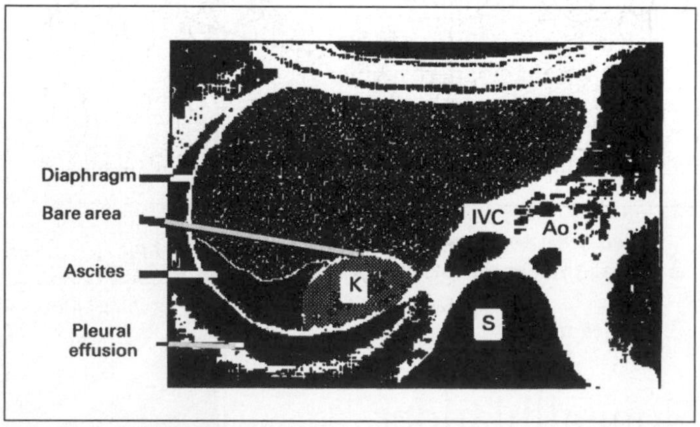

Figure 9-12. ■ *A transverse scan above the xiphoid shows a collection of pleural fluid above the diaphragm. Some ascites is seen below the diaphragm outlining the "bare area."*

thereby increasing the distance between the gallbladder and the transducer. This step will eliminate near-field reverberation artifacts (Fig. 9-2).

d. Lower the overall gain to decrease echogenicity, producing an artifact-free gallbladder. Remember that a good setting for viewing the gallbladder may not be appropriate for imaging other soft-tissue organs.

2. Apparently absent gallbladder. When the gallbladder is small, it can be missed entirely. The main lobar fissure is seen at the right portal vein bifurcation, running directly to the gallbladder fossa, serving as a guide. Also, look for surgical scars on the patient (either several small laparoscopic port sites or one long RUQ incision following the costal margin). Some patients forget that they have had their gallbladder removed! In patients with gangrenous cholecystitis, it can be impossible to image the gallbladder due to air filling the gallbladder lumen or wall. CT is excellent at assessing for gas in the gallbladder lumen or wall.
3. Polyp versus nonshadowing stone. Acoustic shadowing can be enhanced by using a high-frequency transducer, which places the stone in the correct focal zone. Overgaining can obscure shadowing. Changing patient position helps determine whether a polyp or a stone is present by demonstrating a change in the stone's location. A polyp will not move dependently with changes in the patient's position (Fig. 9-5). Beware of "floating" gallstones that move but do not rest on the dependent portion of the gallbladder.
4. Gallbladder wall thickening. Although wall thickening suggests acute cholecystitis; other possible causes include the following:
   a. A recent meal, coffee or candy, which causes subsequent gallbladder contraction
   b. Ascites (Fig. 9-13)
   c. Hypoalbuminemia
   d. Hepatitis and other hepatic dysfunction
   e. Some chemotherapeutic drugs
   f. AIDS
   g. Chronic heart failure
5. Food in the gallbladder. After a choledochojejunostomy or sphincterotomy, where a communication between the gallbladder and the gut is created surgically, it is possible for food or gas to reflux into the gallbladder; there may even be acoustic shadowing owing to gas in the gallbladder or biliary tree. Be sure to try and obtain all relevant patient surgical history.

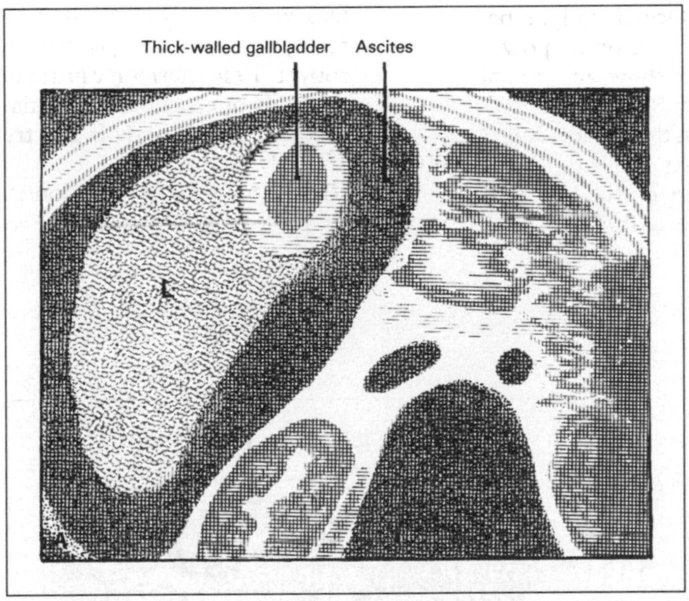

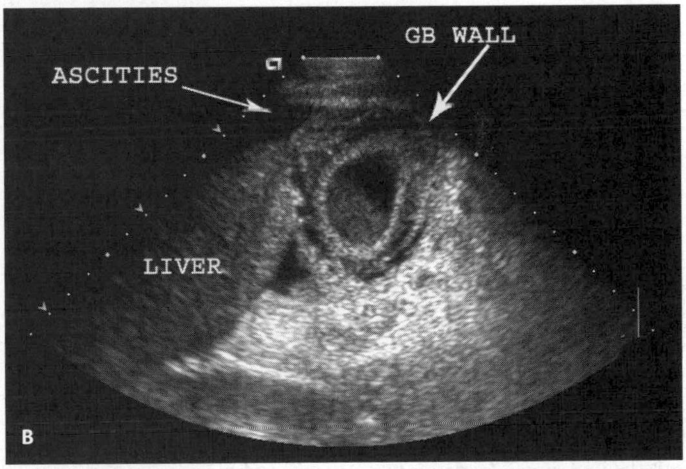

Figure 9-13. ■ *A. Ascites and the liver disease that often produces it can cause a thick gallbladder wall. B. Gallbladder wall thickening noted in a patient with ascites but no gallbladder disease. Incidentally noted is gallbladder sludge due to the patient's chronic illness.*

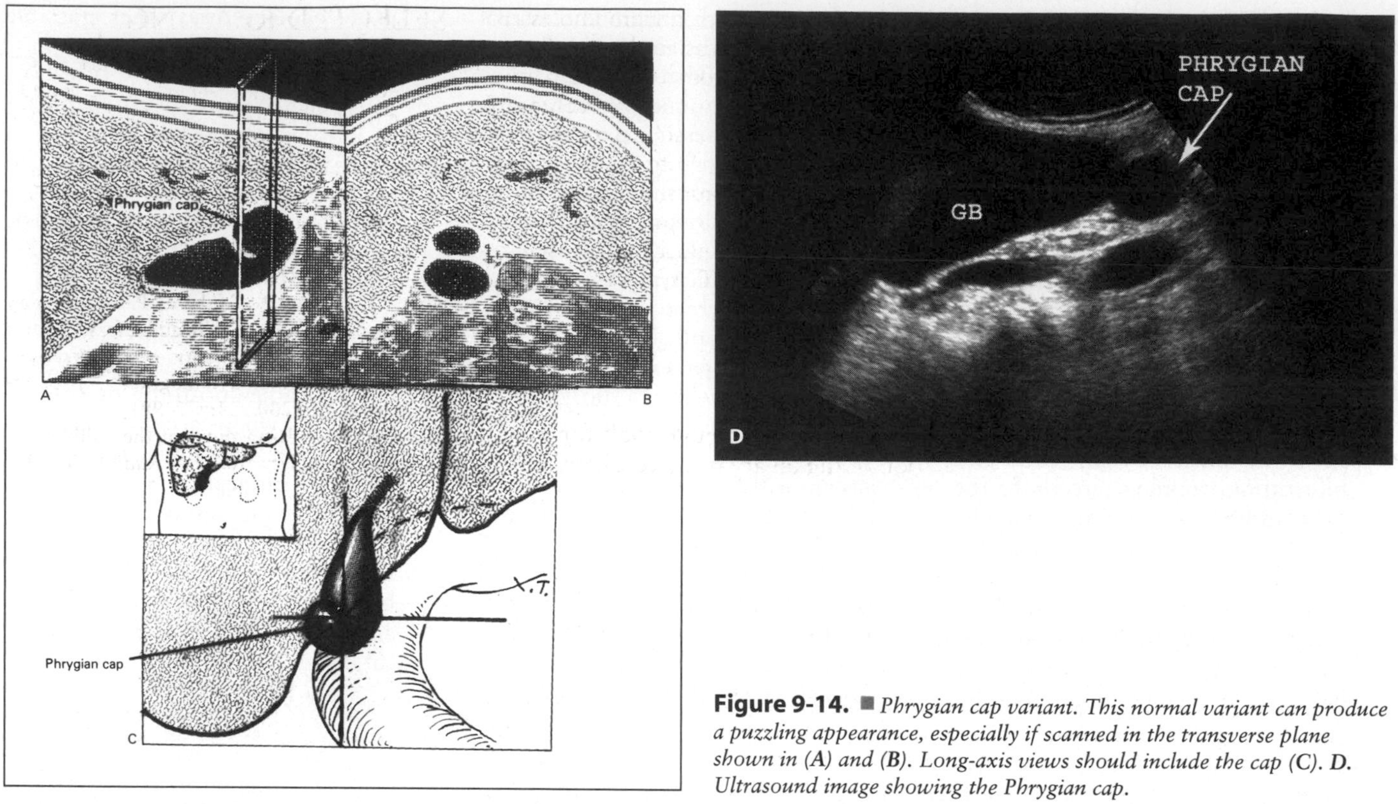

Figure 9-14. ■ *Phrygian cap variant. This normal variant can produce a puzzling appearance, especially if scanned in the transverse plane shown in (**A**) and (**B**). Long-axis views should include the cap (**C**). **D.** Ultrasound image showing the Phrygian cap.*

6. Kink or septum in the gallbladder. Gallbladders often fold over on themselves or contain a septum, usually in the region where the neck and body meet (the junctional fold) (Fig. 9-4). If only a portion of the septum is seen on a single cut, it can resemble a gallstone or polyp in the dependent portion of the gallbladder (Fig. 9-14A). A decubitus or erect view can straighten out a folded gallbladder and reveal that a suspected stone is only a kink.
7. Phrygian cap. Sometimes a septum develops in the fundus of the gallbladder, forming a "Phrygian cap." This is a normal variant (Fig. 9-14).
8. Portal vein collaterals mimicking a perigallbladder collection. A sonolucent space medial to the gallbladder in the region of the porta hepatis can be caused by multiple collaterals from portal vein hypertension. These vessels generally light up on color flow imaging (Fig. 9-15).

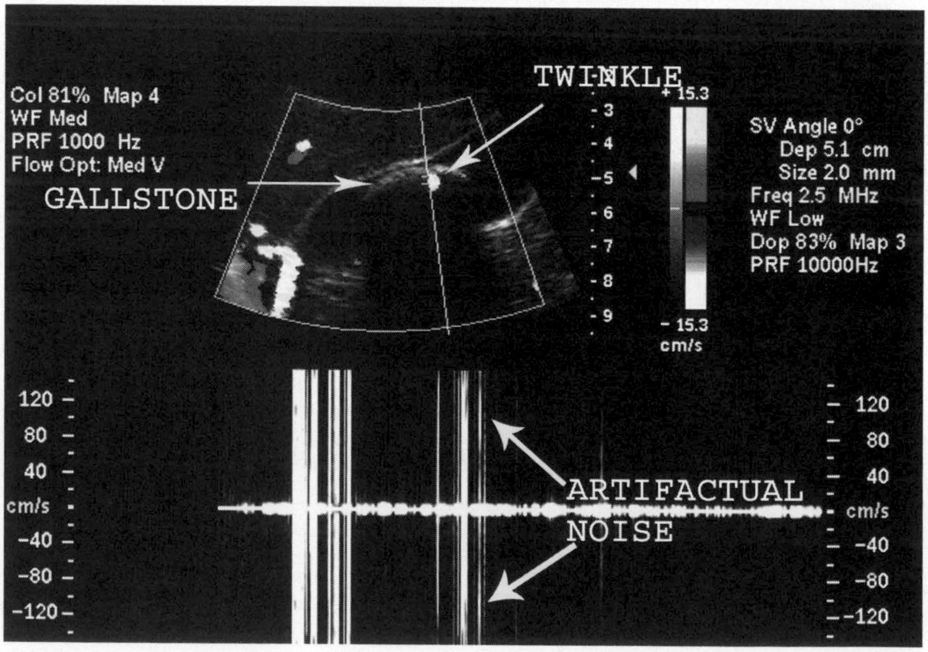

Figure 9-15. ■ *Gallstone demonstrated within gallbladder lumen by the "twinkle" artifact. On color Doppler there is a "twinkle" artifact mimicking flow. Pulsed wave Doppler shows no normal vascular flow, only artifactual noise, which sometimes produces a ringing sound on Doppler.*

9. Refractive shadowing mimicking stones. An apparent shadow at the neck of the gallbladder with no echogenic focus at its source is due to refraction of the beam from the wall (Fig. 9-1).
10. Surgical clips mimicking gallbladder with calculi. Clips at the site of cholecystectomy can shadow and resemble stones. Look at the patient's incisions and check the medical record. Remember that the gallbladder can be removed from appendectomy incisions or laparoscopically. Most surgical clips have a ring-down artifact, similar to the comet tail artifact arising from cholesterol crystals in the gallbladder wall.
11. Adenomyomatosis (cholesterol crystals) mimicking emphysematous cholecystitis. The echo patterns from both of these reflectors may be similar; differentiation between these two entities rests upon clinical correlation, and in worrisome cases, on plain film or CT assessment for air.

Where Else to Look

If gallstones are found, look for dilatation of the biliary tree (see Chapter 10).

SELECTED READING

Bennett GL, Balthazar EJ. Ultrasound and CT evaluation of emergent gallbladder pathology. *Radiol Clin N Am* 2003;41:1203–1216.

Khalili K, Wilson SR. The biliary tree and gallbladder. In: Rumack CM, Wilson SR, Charboneau JW, et al., eds. *Diagnostic Ultrasound*. 3rd ed. St. Louis: Mosby; 1998:171–212.

Khan O, Naipaul R, Maharaj P. Is same-day sonography of the gallbladder feasible after intravenous urography or contrast-enhanced computed tomography? *J Ultrasound Med* 2002;21:977–981.

Yarmenitis SD. Ultrasound of the gallbladder and the biliary tree. *Eur Radiol* 2002;12:270–282.

Abnormal Liver Function Tests

Jaundice

JULIA A. DROSE

10

SONOGRAM ABBREVIATIONS

A	Ascites
Ao	Aorta
CA	Celiac axis
CBD	Common bile duct
CHD	Common hepatic duct
Du	Duodenum
GB	Gallbladder
HA	Hepatic artery
HV	Hepatic vein
IMV	Inferior mesenteric vein
IVC	Inferior vena cava
K	Kidney
L	Liver
LHV	Left hepatic vein
LLS	Left lateral segment
LMS	Left medial segment
LPV	Left portal vein
MHV	Middle hepatic vein
MPV	Main portal vein
P	Pancreas
PV	Portal vein
RAS	Right anterior segment
RPS	Right posterior segment
RPV	Right portal vein
S	Spine
SMA	Superior mesenteric artery
SMV	Superior mesenteric vein
SA	Splenic artery
SV	Splenic vein

KEY WORDS

Alkaline Phosphatase. Enzyme that catalyses the cleavage of inorganic phosphate. Elevated with biliary obstruction.

ALT. Alanine aminotransferase. Enzyme involved in protein metabolism. Increased in alcoholic hepatitis, jaundice, and cirrhosis. Formerly called *serum glutamic-pyruvic transaminase* (SGPT).

Ampulla of Vater. The point at which the common bile duct and pancreatic ducts enter the duodenum.

AST. Aspartate aminotransferase. Enzyme involved in synthesis of amino acids. Elevated in acute hepatitis and cirrhosis. Formerly called *serum glutamic oxaloacetic transaminase* (SGOT)

Biliary Atresia. Progressive obliteration of the extrahepatic and proximal intrahepatic bile ducts, as well as the gallbladder. Usually diagnosed within the first 2 weeks of life.

Bilirubin. Yellowish pigment in bile formed by red blood cell breakdown. Increases with hepatic disorders in which metabolism is impaired, such as cirrhosis or hepatitis. Also increases with obstructive disease such as gallstones. Bilirubin is classified as direct or indirect. Direct (conjugated) bilirubin is excreted in urine, whereas indirect (unconjugated) is not. Most laboratories report total and direct bilirubin. Indirect is calculated by subtracting the direct value from the total.

Cavernous Transformation of the Portal Vein. The extrahepatic portal vein becomes thrombosed and is replaced by numerous collateral veins in the porta hepatis.

Cholangiocarcinoma. A malignant neoplasm arising from the bile ducts.

Choledochal Cyst. Congenital dilatation of the common bile duct. Usually found in children but may not be diagnosed until adulthood.

Choledocholithiasis. Stones in the biliary tree.

Cirrhosis. Progressive hepatocellular disease. Common causes include excessive alcohol or drug use and viral infection, although there are many other etiologies. May result in fibrosis, jaundice, portal hypertension, and liver failure.

Collaterals. Also called *varices*. Dilated veins that occur with portal hypertension. Seen principally in the region of the porta hepatis, pancreas, and splenic hilum.

Common Bile Duct. Portion of the biliary duct formed by the confluence of the common hepatic duct and the cystic duct.

Common Hepatic Duct. Portion of the biliary duct formed by the confluence of the right and left hepatic ducts.

Coronary Vein. Vein that arises from the splenic vein in the midline and courses superior and to the left. Becomes dilated in the setting of portal hypertension.

Courvoisier Gallbladder. Enlarged, palpable gallbladder. Results from distal obstruction of the common bile duct (CBD) secondary to a pancreatic head mass.

Cystic Duct. Drains the gallbladder. Joins the common hepatic duct to form the CBD.

Fatty Infiltration. Infiltration of hepatocytes by lipids. Eventually results in fat cells being surrounded by fibrous material. Common causes include hepatitis, diabetes, metabolic disorders, and pregnancy. May be focal or diffuse.

GGT. Gamma glutamyl transferase. Biliary enzyme that increases with obstructive jaundice and liver disease.

Glisson's Capsule. Fibrous membrane that surrounds the liver, as well as the portal triads within the liver.

Glycogen Storage Disease. Disease process in which large quantities of glycogen are abnormally deposited within the liver, resulting in fatty infiltration and tumors.

Hemolytic Anemia. Anemia resulting from destruction of red blood cells. Either congenital or acquired from a variety of causes including various infections.

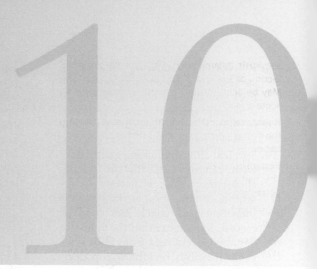

Hepatitis. Inflammation of the liver due to viral infection or less commonly, autoimmune disease. May be acute or may become chronic after an acute episode.

Hepatocellular Disease. Diffuse disease affecting the liver parenchyma such as cirrhosis, fatty infiltration, or hepatitis.

Hepatofugal. Portal vein flow away from the liver. This pattern can be seen in patients with severe portal hypertension.

Hepatopetal. Normal portal vein flow, toward the liver.

Jaundice (Icterus). Yellow pigmentation of the skin due to excessive bilirubin accumulation. Usually secondary to liver or biliary disease.

Klatskin Tumor. A type of cholangiocarcinoma, an adenocarcinoma of the common hepatic duct bifurcation.

LDH. Lactic dehydrogenase. Enzyme that catalyses the formation and removal of lactate. Elevated with liver disease.

Porta Hepatis. Transverse fissure on the visceral surface of the liver in which the CBD, proper hepatic artery, and main portal vein (MPV) run alongside each other as they leave or enter the liver.

Portal Hypertension. Increased portal venous pressure usually secondary to liver disease (most commonly cirrhosis); leads to dilatation of the portal vein with splenic and superior mesenteric vein enlargement, splenomegaly, and formation of collaterals. Can also be caused by portal or splenic vein thrombosis.

Portal Triad. Portal vein, hepatic artery, biliary duct.

Primary Biliary Cirrhosis. Autoimmune disease resulting in irreversible destruction of the liver and bile ducts.

Regenerating Nodule. Regenerating areas of hepatocytes surrounded by fibrotic septa.

Sphincter of Oddi. Annular sheath of muscle contracting around the ampulla of Vater.

Varices. Dilated veins.

RELEVANT LABORATORY VALUES*

*Reference ranges for individual laboratories may vary slightly.

Alkaline phosphatase		40 to 135 U/L
ALT (SGPT)		5 to 60 U/L
AST (SGOT)		5 to 42 U/L
Bilirubin		
	Direct	0.0 to 0.3 mg/dL
	Total	0.1 to 1.6 mg/dL
GGT		1 to 50 U/L
LDH		115 to 255 U/L

INCREASED LABORATORY VALUES DIFFERENTIAL

↑ALK	Fatty infiltration Alcoholic hepatitis Primary biliary cirrhosis Liver tumor (benign or malignant) Drug-induced liver disease Cholecystitis Cholelithiasis Primary biliary cirrhosis
↑ALT	Liver disease
↑AST	Liver disease
↑Bilirubin (total)	Hepatitis Cirrhosis Liver tumor Biliary tract obstruction Cholangitis
↑Bilirubin (direct)	Hepatitis Cirrhosis Metastatic liver disease Fatty infiltration Biliary tract obstruction
↑Bilirubin (indirect)	Cirrhosis Hepatitis
↑GGT	Chronic alcoholic hepatitis Liver neoplasm or metastases Cholestasis Pancreatic carcinoma
↑LDH	Liver disease

THE CLINICAL PROBLEM

There are three basic mechanisms by which jaundice occurs: red blood cell destruction, hepatocellular disease, or obstruction of the intrahepatic or extrahepatic bile ducts.

RED BLOOD CELL DESTRUCTION

Destruction of red blood cells in hemolytic anemias results in jaundice. In this setting, red cells are destroyed so rapidly that an elevated bilirubin results. Hemolytic anemias are caused by infection, certain medications, autoimmune disorders, and inherited conditions. The spleen and the liver, the principal sites of red blood cell removal, may become enlarged.

HEPATOCELLULAR DISEASE

Hepatocellular disease causes impaired hepatic cell function and cell death, which leads to a buildup of bilirubin and elevates the serum enzymes AST, ALT, and GGT. Alcoholic liver disease is the most common form; it progresses from alcoholic hepatitis to fatty infiltration of the liver to cirrhosis. Other common causes of hepatocellular disease include hepatitis, metabolic disorders, and malaria.

OBSTRUCTION OF INTRAHEPATIC OR EXTRAHEPATIC BILE DUCTS

Bile ducts dilate proximal to the site of obstruction. Unlike hemolytic anemia or hepatocellular disease, obstruction of the biliary system is treated surgically.

When bile excretion is blocked, urine and serum bilirubin, serum cholesterol, and serum alkaline phosphatase are elevated. Severe nonobstructive liver disease can also elevate these enzymes.

Common causes of bile duct obstruction include gallstones and choledocholithiasis, pancreatic tumors, or tumors in the bile ducts, such as Klatskin tumors. Primary sclerosing cholangitis and biliary strictures will also result in obstruction. In the infant and small child, two other important obstructive processes occur. Biliary atresia is the most common type of biliary obstructive disease in this age group. It is a progressive obliteration of the extrahepatic bile ducts and often the gallbladder. The proximal aspects of the intrahepatic bile ducts may also be involved. Symptoms usually present between 2 and 6 weeks after birth. Treatment includes surgically created drainage of bile into the intestine if the obstruction is extrahepatic. With intrahepatic obstruction, liver transplant is the only treatment option.

A choledochal cyst is a segmental dilatation of either the intra- or extrahepatic bile ducts. This is a congenital anomaly that can result in biliary dilation proximal to the cyst formation. Usually diagnosed in childhood, this condition may also be discovered later in life, and is treated surgically.

Ultrasound is often able to ascertain the cause of jaundice, allowing the clinician to determine the appropriate treatment method.

Anatomy

Diagnosis of biliary obstruction requires a thorough knowledge of the normal anatomy of the liver and biliary system, as well as vascular structures within the liver (Fig. 10-1).

LIVER ANATOMY

Liver anatomy may be described anatomically, based on external markings, or segmentally based on internal lobar divisions. From an anatomic standpoint, the liver can be divided into right, left, and caudate lobes. The right lobe is separated from the left lobe by the main lobar fissure. The right lobe is divided into anterior and posterior segments by the right intersegmental fissure. The left lobe is divided into medial and lateral segments by the left intersegmental fissure. The caudate lobe is bordered posteriorly by the inferior vena cava (IVC), anteriorly and superiorly by the left medial lobe of the liver, and inferiorly by the MPV.

Segmentally, the middle hepatic vein divides the liver into left and right lobes. The left hepatic vein divides the left lobe into medial and lateral segments, and the right hepatic vein divides the right lobe into anterior and posterior segments.

BILIARY TREE

Normally, only a small segment of the biliary tree is seen by ultrasound within the liver—the common hepatic duct, which is formed by the confluence of the left and right hepatic ducts. As the duct crosses the portal vein and exits the liver, it is still considered the common hepatic duct until it merges with the cystic duct. At this point, it becomes the CBD. The cystic duct's precise location is often difficult to visualize by ultrasound, however. Sonographically, the common hepatic duct lies within the porta hepatis, anterior to the right hepatic artery (RHA) and undivided right portal vein (Fig. 10-2). After joining the cystic duct, the CBD normally descends anterior and lateral to the MPV. The proper hepatic artery can be seen anterior and medial to the MPV (Fig. 10-3).

The normal diameter for the common hepatic duct and CBD varies within the literature. Additionally, recent reports have expressed concern that increased bile duct size associated with increased age and increased bile duct size after cholecystectomy, both historically thought to be normal findings, may not be. Although the bile ducts may enlarge slightly with age or status post cholecystectomy, any measurement above 6 to 7 mm in young patients and 8.5 mm in the elderly should be considered abnormal and followed accordingly.

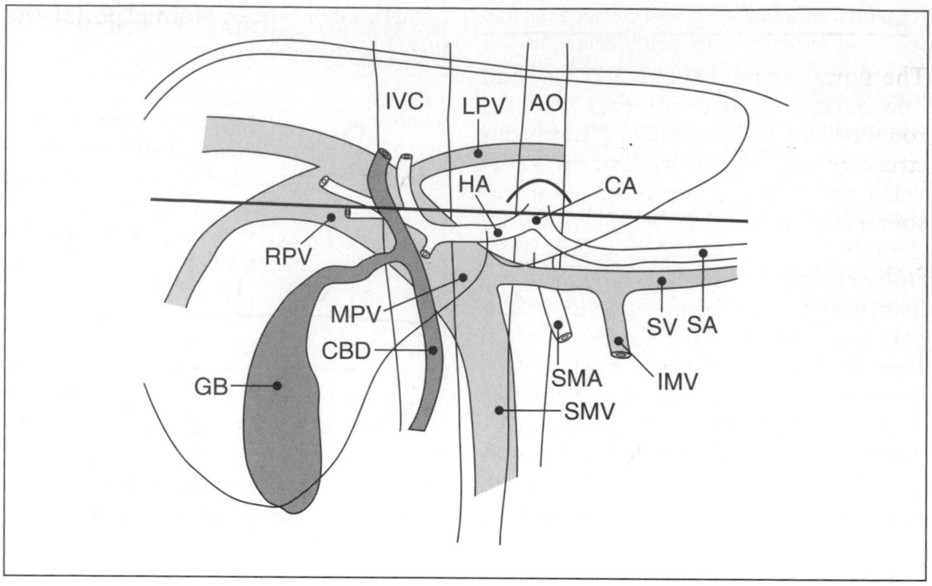

Figure 10-1. ■ *Diagram of the relationships between the biliary system and vascularity within the liver.*

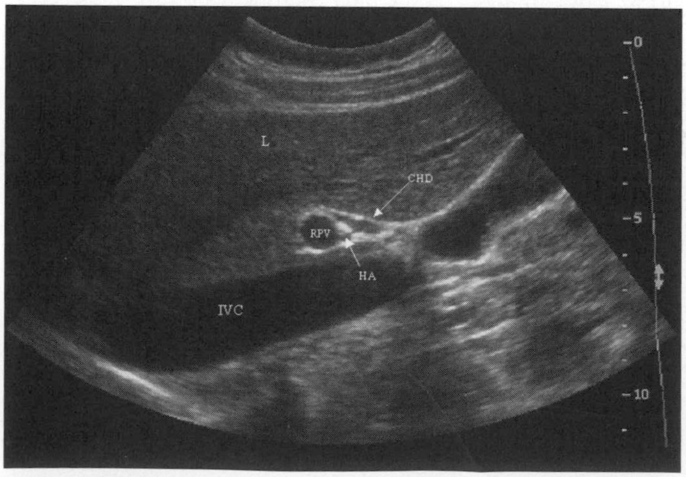

Figure 10-2. ■ *Longitudinal image of the liver, showing the relationship of the common hepatic duct to the right hepatic artery and undivided right portal vein.*

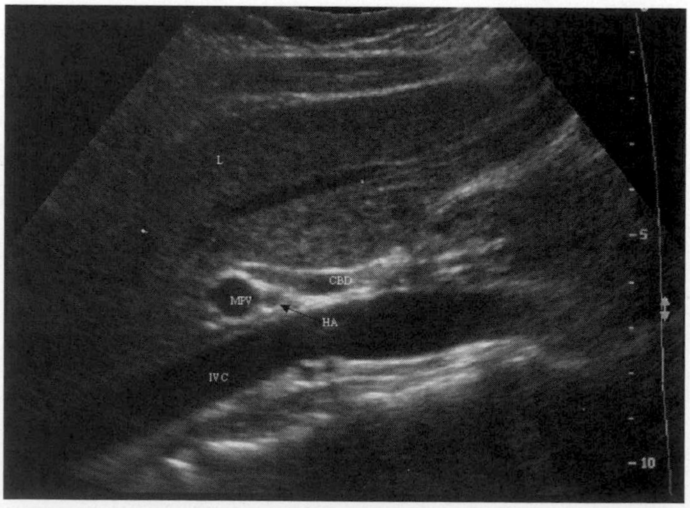

Figure 10-3. ■ *Longitudinal image of the liver showing the relationship of the common bile duct to the main portal vein and the proper hepatic artery.*

PORTAL VEINS

The portal veins, hepatic arteries, and bile ducts run in triads that are surrounded by Glisson capsule. This fibrous structure results in the walls of the portal veins appearing hyperechoic on ultrasound (Fig. 10-4). The MPV arises from the confluence of the splenic and superior mesenteric veins. As it enters the liver, it branches into the undivided right and left portal veins. The right branch then bifurcates within the right lobe of the liver into anterior and posterior segments. The left portal vein courses leftward within the left lobe. Smaller branches may occasionally be visualized. The portal veins run centrally, within the segments of the liver. Normal portal vein flow is hepatopetal.

HEPATIC VEINS

Hepatic veins (Fig. 10-5) are easily differentiated from portal veins because they are not surrounded by an echogenic wall. Hepatic veins course between the lobes and segments of the liver and drain into the IVC (Fig. 10-6).

HEPATIC ARTERIES

The common hepatic artery takes off from the celiac axis and courses over the anterior, superior edge of the pancreas. It gives rise to the gastroduodenal artery, the supraduodenal artery, and the right gastric artery. At this point, it is termed the *proper hepatic artery* and runs cephalad into the porta hepatis. It courses anterior to the MPV and to the left of the CBD. Once the proper hepatic artery enters the liver, it bifurcates into left and right branches. The RHA crosses between the common hepatic duct and the right portal vein. It may double back on itself (Fig. 10-7). Hepatic arteries can be a source of confusion in the region of the porta hepatis because they can be mistaken for a bile duct. Color or pulsed Doppler will easily make the distinction by showing flow if the vessel is hepatic artery. Hepatic artery flow is hepatopetal.

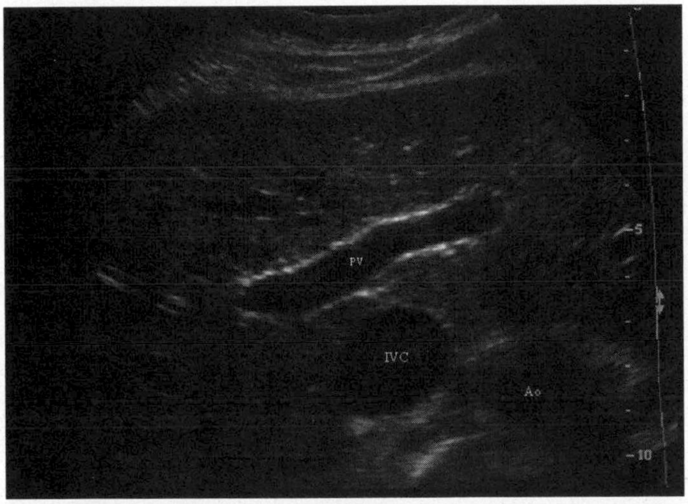

Figure 10-4. ■ *Transverse image of the liver showing the echogenic walls that surround the normal portal veins.*

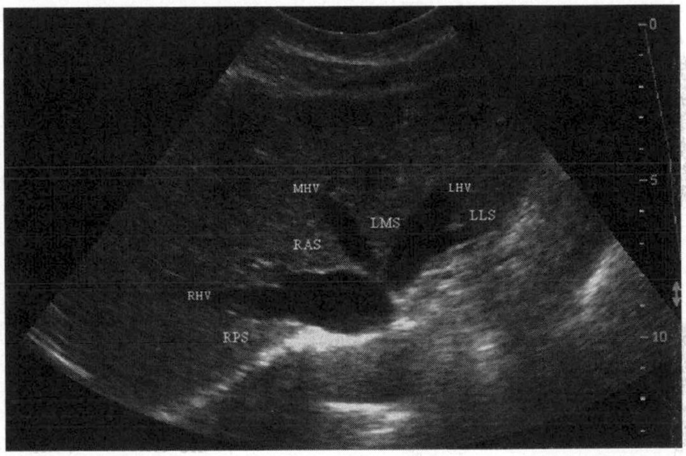

Figure 10-5. ■ *Transverse image of the liver showing the right, middle, and left hepatic veins dividing the segments of the liver and draining into the inferior vena cava. Unlike the portal veins, the walls of the hepatic veins are not echogenic.*

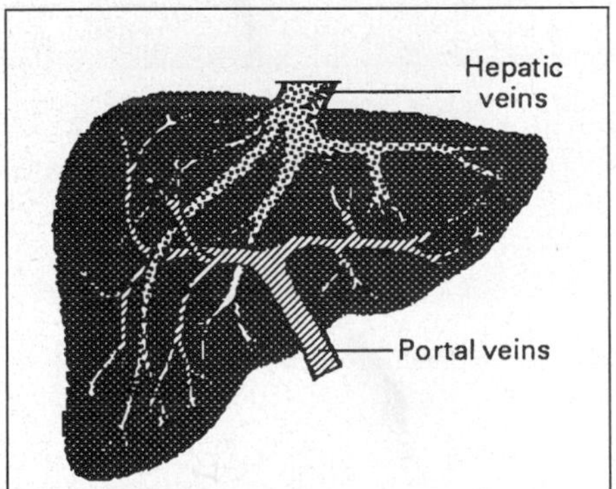

Figure 10-6. ■ *Diagram showing the relationship of the portal and hepatic veins.*

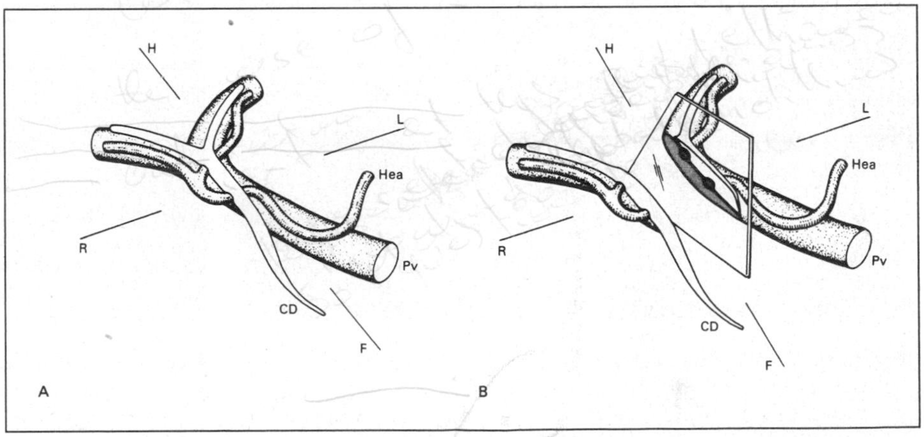

Figure 10-7. ■ *A variant situation in which the hepatic artery bends to the right and then turns back to the left again. (Reprinted with permission from Berland L, Foley D. Porta hepatis sonography: discontinuation of bile ducts from artery with pulsed Doppler anatomic center.* AJR *1982;138:833.)*

Technique

LIVER ANATOMY

The liver should always be evaluated in both transverse and sagittal planes. Sagittal images of the liver should be documented starting at the most lateral aspect of either the right or left lobe and moving continuously through the entire liver to the opposite lateral aspect. Liver length should be measured at the level of the right kidney, from the diaphragm to the most inferior aspect of the liver.

Transverse images are best acquired by placing the transducer in a subxiphoid position and angling cephalad. It may also be necessary to move subcostally or between the ribs to visualize the entire extent of the right lobe.

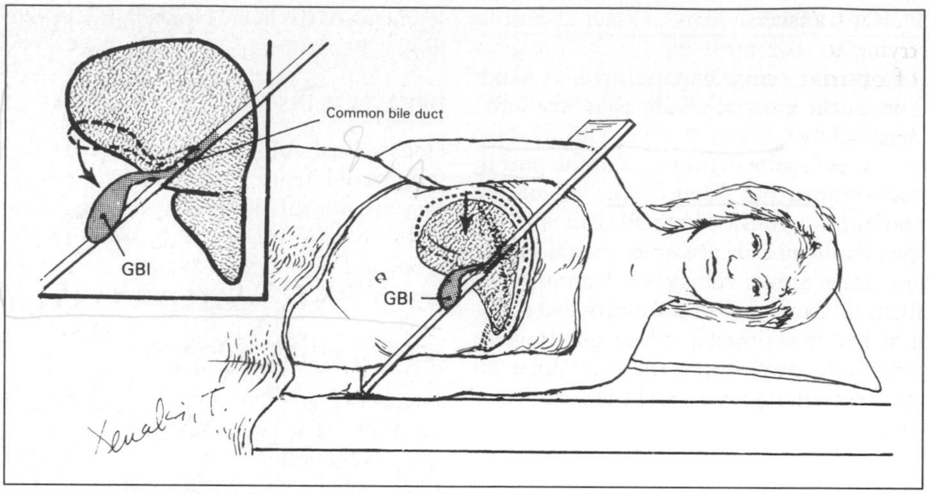

Figure 10-8. ■ *Positioning the patient in a left posterior oblique position to use the liver as an acoustic window and angling the transducer from the patient's right shoulder to left hip often aids in visualizing the common bile duct.*

COMMON HEPATIC DUCT AND COMMON BILE DUCT

Because the common hepatic duct courses in a plane that is somewhat perpendicular to the right costal margin, a parasagittal plane with the transducer angled from the right shoulder to the left hip is required to visualize more than a small segment of it. Turning the patient up toward his or her left side (into a left posterior oblique position) is helpful in using the liver to provide a better acoustic window (Fig. 10-8). The standardized level to measure the common hepatic duct is at the point it crosses anterior over the right portal vein and RHA (see Fig. 10-17). This same transducer angulation should allow visualization of the proximal CBD anterior to the MPV. If the duct is still not well visualized, the patient can be turned all the way on his or her side into a left lateral decubitus position.

DISTAL CBD

The axis of the CBD changes from oblique to sagittal at the superior margin of the pancreas. The distal CBD is best evaluated in the sagittal plane, angling under the duodenum if necessary, to see the proximal intrapancreatic portion (Fig. 10-9). At this point, the duct curves laterally and eventually disappears into the sphincter of Oddi (Fig. 10-10).

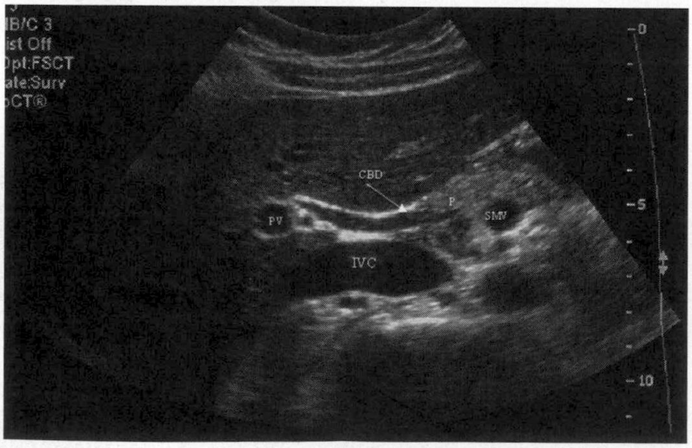

Figure 10-9. ■ *Sagittal image of the distal common bile duct as it enters the head of the pancreas.*

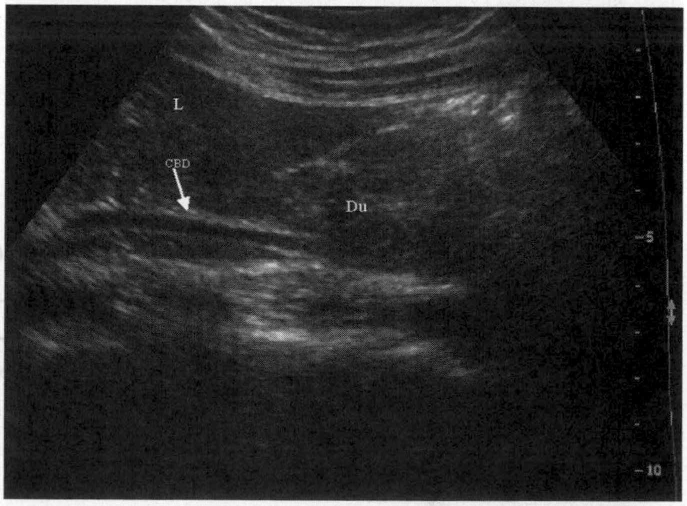

Figure 10-10. ■ *Sagittal image of the distal common bile duct as it enters the duodenum at the sphincter of Oddi.*

A transverse plane is often useful in trying to determine the precise location of obstruction, particularly when it occurs at the most distal aspect of the CBD (Fig. 10-11).

Gas in the antrum and duodenum can obscure the distal CBD. Placing the patient in an erect right posterior oblique position helps displace the air. If bowel gas interference still exists, have the patient drink 16 ounces of degassed water and rest in a right lateral decubitus position for 2 to 3 minutes. Then rescan in the erect right posterior oblique position, transversely.

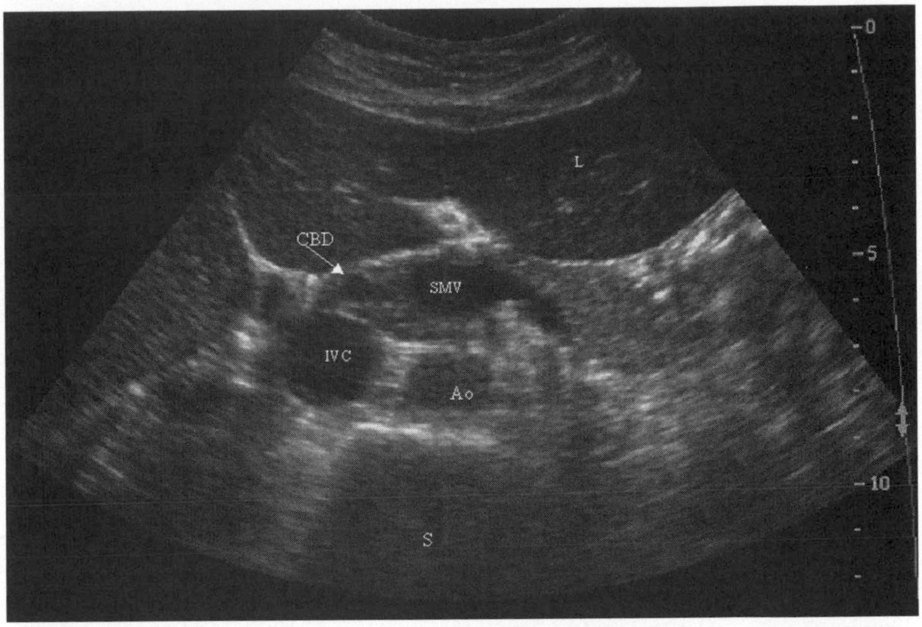

Figure 10-11. ■ *Transverse image of the common bile duct within the head of the pancreas.*

INTRAHEPATIC DUCTS

Although intrahepatic ducts will often only be seen if they are dilated, as the resolution of newer equipment increases, it is becoming easier to visualize nondilated intrahepatic ducts. When dilated, intrahepatic ducts often appear tortuous and will cause posterior acoustic enhancement (Fig. 10-12). Blood vessels within the liver do not cause posterior acoustic enhancement because blood attenuates sound more than bile. Therefore, when a tubular structure with posterior acoustic enhancement is seen, intrahepatic biliary dilation should be suspected. Another sonographic sign of intrahepatic biliary dilation is the "double barrel" sign (Fig. 10-13). This sign is also referred to as "too many tubes" or the "parallel channel" sign. In this setting, the dilated duct can be seen running anterior to its accompanying portal vein. It is important to examine the entire liver parenchyma, because isolated biliary duct obstruction can occur.

DOPPLER IMAGING OF HEPATIC VESSELS

Pulsed Doppler interrogation of the hepatic vessels may provide a variety of information, including normal velocity and direction of blood flow, altered velocity secondary to stenosis or thrombosis, or reversal of blood flow, which occurs with portal hypertension. Absence of blood flow may indicate occlusion. Lower-frequency transducers are often necessary to obtain adequate Doppler information, particularly in the setting of hepatocellular disease. Color Doppler is also useful when evaluating the vessels within the liver, both to identify their location and determine direction of blood flow. It also allows a large area of vessels to be sampled at the same time.

Vessels in the liver are often perpendicular to the angle of insonation, making it difficult to maintain a Doppler angle of less than 60 degrees. Creative positioning is often necessary. Turning

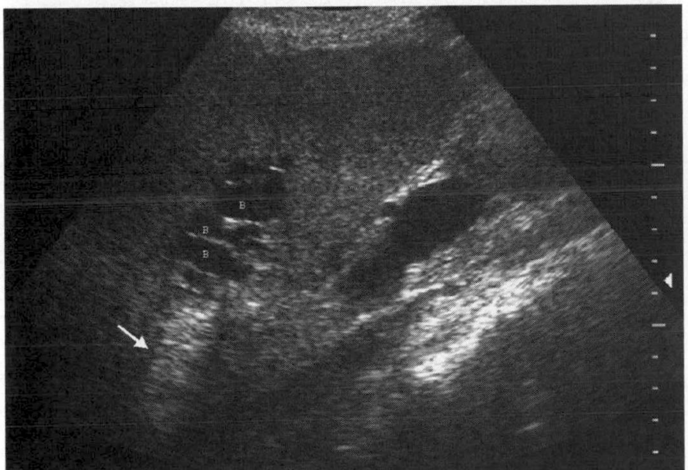

Figure 10-12. ■ *Longitudinal image of the liver showing dilated intrahepatic biliary ducts with increased posterior enhancement.*

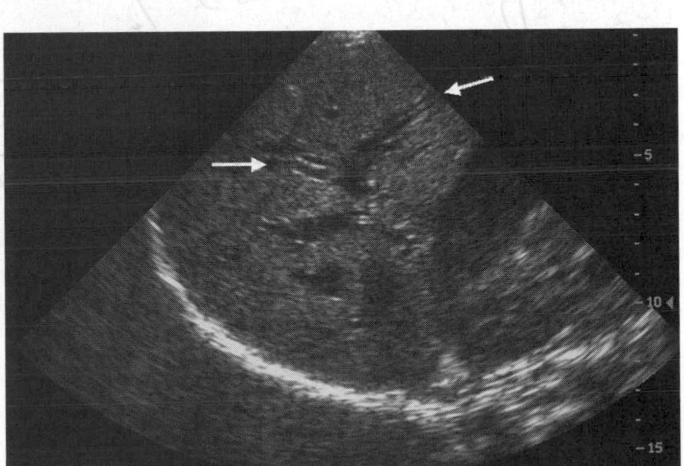

Figure 10-13. ■ *Longitudinal image of the liver showing dilated intrahepatic biliary ducts running parallel with portal veins.*

the patient into a left posterior oblique or left lateral decubitus position and scanning from the right side may be helpful.

The MPV can be imaged sagittally, as it enters the portal hepatis. As it enters the liver, the undivided right and subsequently the anterior and posterior right segmental portal veins can be interrogated. The left portal vein is best evaluated by following its origin from the MPV into the left lobe of the liver. Normal portal vein flow is continuous and monophasic with little pulsatility (Color Plate 10-1). As stated previously, the normal direction of portal vein flow is hepatopetal. If portal vein flow is reversed, portal hypertension should be considered. A Doppler angle as close to 0 degrees as possible should be attempted.

The hepatic veins are best interrogated from a transverse subcostal approach. The normal hepatic vein waveform is pulsatile, secondary to transmitted pulsations from the heart (Color Plate 10-2). Two peaks will be seen, which correspond with the tricuspid valve's movement. A transient flow reversal will also be seen, and it corresponds to atrial contraction. In the setting of severe liver disease, hepatic vein flow may become monophasic. This condition is termed "portalized" flow because the waveform takes on portal vein characteristics, and it is thought to occur secondary to compression of the hepatic vein by the surrounding liver parenchyma.

Hepatic arterial flow is normally low-resistance, pulsatile flow. Both resistive indices and acceleration time can be measured by pulsed Doppler when evaluating hepatic arteries for liver disease (Color Plate 10-3).

Pathology

DIFFUSE LIVER DISEASE

Diffuse parenchymal liver disease has a number of sonographic features, however, most are nonspecific. The sonographic appearance of some conditions, such as fatty infiltration of the liver or alcoholic liver disease, may improve rapidly when the primary cause is removed. The following are the most typical patterns.

Fatty Infiltration

The liver becomes enlarged with fatty infiltration. Echogenicity is increased. Visualization of the right hemidiaphragm and blood vessels within the liver, even with a low-frequency transducer, is difficult due to the increased acoustic attenuation (Fig. 10-14). Comparing liver echogenicity to that of the right renal parenchyma helps to assess the degree of fatty infiltration. Liver parenchyma is normally only slightly more echogenic than the kidney. Because the spleen is usually slightly more echogenic than the normal liver, the diagnosis of fatty infiltration of the liver may be suggested when the echogenicity difference between the liver and right kidney is greater than that between the spleen and left kidney. With severe fatty infiltration, the acoustic impedance can be so great that it is difficult to penetrate more than a few centimeters of liver, completely obscuring any posterior structures.

Early Alcoholic Liver Disease

Subtle changes in the liver's shape may indicate the presence of alcoholic liver disease. The edge of the right lobe becomes rounded. A large left lobe or a prominent caudate lobe may also be seen. Alcoholic liver disease also causes increased echogenicity. Over time, cirrhosis will occur, causing the liver to become very small and dense.

Acute Hepatitis

In acute hepatitis, the portal triads are more prominent than usual. This characteristic is secondary to decreased liver echogenicity caused by diffuse swelling and is often termed the "starry sky" appearance. The liver and spleen can become enlarged, and the gallbladder wall can become markedly thickened. Keep in mind, however, that in many cases of acute hepatitis, the liver will appear normal by ultrasound.

Chronic Hepatitis

Livers with chronic hepatitis are also sonographically normal in many cases. Once cirrhosis develops, the liver may become small, and the echotexture becomes coarse, secondary to fibrosis.

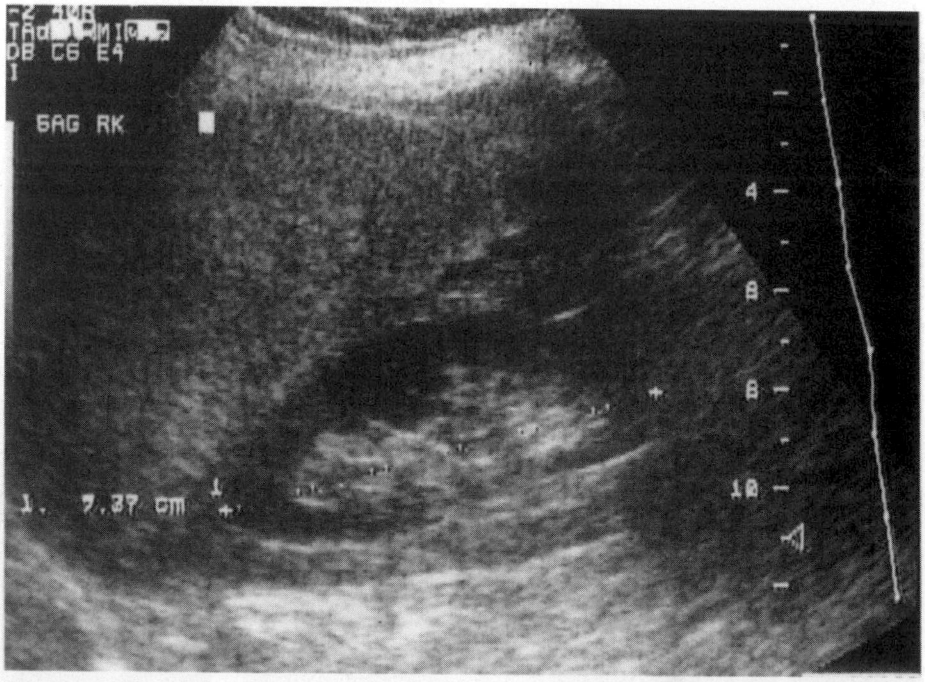

Figure 10-14. ■ *Longitudinal image of a liver with fatty infiltration. The liver is enlarged with an abnormally coarse echo texture. The liver parenchyma is much more echogenic than the right kidney.*

Cirrhosis

In cirrhosis, the liver becomes hyperechoic, decreases in size, and starts to develop a nodular border. In long-standing, end-stage cirrhosis, the liver becomes atrophied and very echogenic (Fig. 10-15). Splenomegaly and ascites may be present. Portal hypertension will occur with advanced cases. Recanalization of the paraumbilical vein may also occur. This condition is diagnosed by visualizing a dilated vein running from the left portal vein back toward the umbilicus. Other collateral vessels may be seen in the porta hepatis and the splenic hilum (Fig. 10-16).

If the cause of the cirrhosis is removed before the liver is too adversely affected, areas of parenchyma may begin regenerating over time. If regeneration occurs, focal, hypoechoic areas within the liver may be visualized.

PORTAL HYPERTENSION

Increased pressure in the portal vein is a consequence of liver fibrosis or of portal vein obstruction secondary to clot or tumor. The most common cause of intrahepatic portal hypertension is cirrhosis. Features of portal hypertension include:

1. Portal vein diameter larger than 1.3-cm diameter. Portal vein size may return to normal if collateral circulation develops.
2. Recanalization of the paraumbilical vein within the ligamentum teres. The ligamentum teres is the remnant of the umbilical vein in the fetus and contains small vessels that dilate when the intrahepatic pressure increases. The ligamentum teres runs from the ascending left portal vein to the anterior surface of the liver. It is best visualized in a sagittal plane.
3. Collateral vessels (varices). These are seen as small tortuous vessels in the porta hepatis, around the gastric fundus, in the pancreatic bed, and in the splenic hilum. Pulsed and color Doppler will help in confirming that these are vessels. The portal vein may become thrombosed and replaced by numerous small collaterals. This occurrence is known as cavernous transformation of the portal vein (Color Plate 10-4).
4. Dilation of the splenic vein, the superior mesenteric vein, and sometimes the coronary vein
5. Ascites
6. Reversal of flow in the portal veins on pulsed or color Doppler. Blood flow in the portal vein and hepatic artery are normally in the same direction, toward the liver (hepatopetal). In severe portal hypertension, flow in the portal veins becomes reversed, away from the liver (hepatofugal) (Color Plate 10-5).
7. Splenomegaly (see Fig. 10-16)

PORTAL AND SPLENIC VEIN THROMBOSIS

Portal vein thrombosis may precipitate a sudden deterioration in the condition of a patient with portal hypertension. Causes of thrombosis within the portal or splenic vein include:

1. Portal hypertension
2. Tumor compression or involvement
3. Pancreatitis causing compression of the splenic vein
4. Trauma
5. Sepsis

Sonographic features can include the following:

1. Nonvisualization of the vessel
2. Clot within the lumen (Color Plate 10-6)
3. Absence of blood flow on pulsed or color Doppler
4. Collaterals, which will develop in the porta hepatis (cavernous transformation of the portal vein)
5. Marked splenomegaly

HEMOLYTIC ANEMIA

In most types of hemolytic anemia, the only sonographic characteristics are enlargement of the liver and spleen. Gallstones may be present. If hemolytic anemia is a result of lymphoma, nodal enlargement may also be seen.

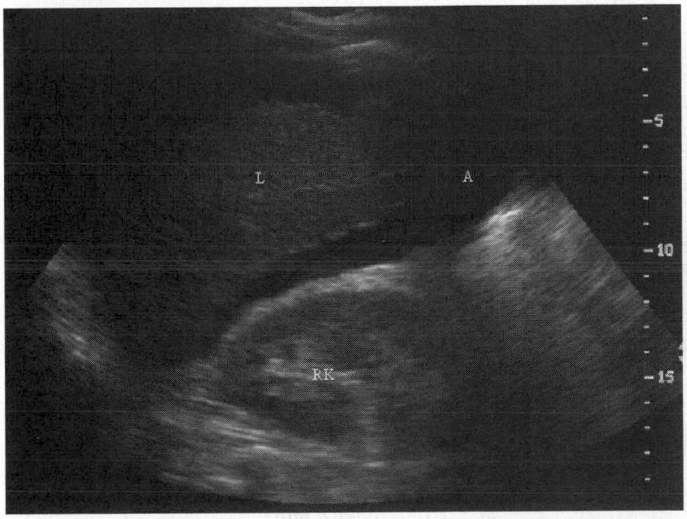

Figure 10-15. ■ *Longitudinal image through the liver in a patient with cirrhosis. The liver is small and echogenic, with a nodular surface. Ascites is seen surrounding the liver.*

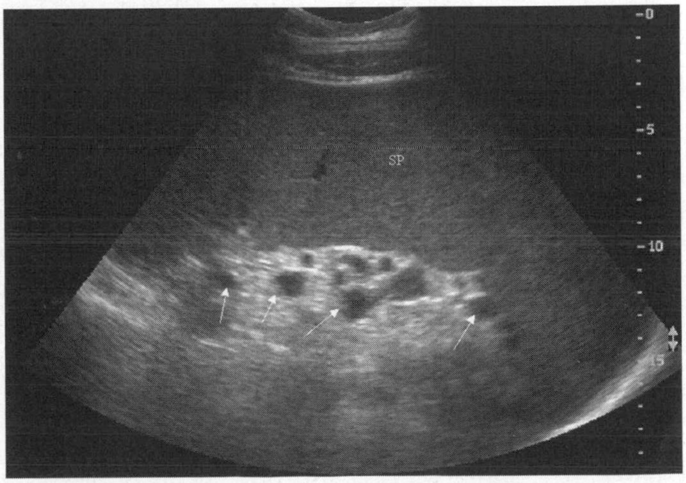

Figure 10-16. ■ *Transverse image through an enlarged spleen in a patient with cirrhosis. Numerous collateral vessels are present in the splenic hilum.*

INFILTRATIVE DISORDERS

Most infiltrative disorders such as glycogen storage disease cause a diffuse increase in echogenicity throughout the liver as well as hepatomegaly and splenomegaly. This increase is similar to the sonographic appearance of diffuse fatty infiltration. Glycogen storage disease manifests itself in the neonatal period. Patients may survive to childhood or early adulthood. In this population, focal adenomas or hepatocellular carcinoma may occur.

BILIARY OBSTRUCTION

Bile Duct Measurements

When evaluating for biliary obstruction, both the common hepatic and CBD should be measured.

The diameter of the common hepatic duct is measured intrahepatically, at the level of the undivided right portal vein (Fig. 10-17). The CBD can be measured at its point of largest dimension (Fig. 10-18). If the cause of the biliary obstruction is mechanical (e.g., a stone or tumor), dilated ducts will be seen proximal to the level of obstruction.

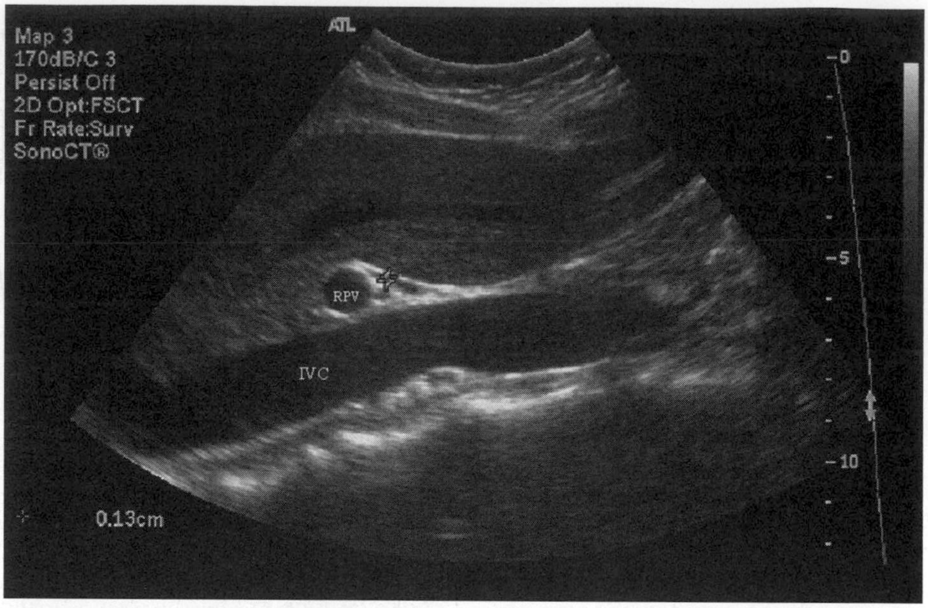

Figure 10-17. ■ *Longitudinal image of the liver showing the appropriate level to measure the common hepatic duct.*

Dilated Intrahepatic Ducts

Intrahepatic ducts run anterior to the portal veins. When they are dilated, two parallel structures representing the portal vein branch and the dilated bile duct may be seen (Fig. 10-13).

Unlike portal veins, bile ducts branch repeatedly, are tortuous, and show acoustic enhancement. Suspicious tubular structures should be traced to their origins, if possible, to ensure that they are part of the biliary system and not hepatic arteries. Color or pulsed Doppler is also useful in determining whether a structure is a vessel or a duct.

Dilated peripheral ducts often splay out from a central point, giving them a starlike appearance.

Unlike blood, which attenuates sound, bile transmits it; so acoustic enhancement posterior to dilated biliary ducts should be appreciated (Fig. 10-12). Unlike hepatic veins, obstructed bile ducts will not dilate with a Valsalva maneuver; they will stay the same. Normal ducts usually decrease in size.

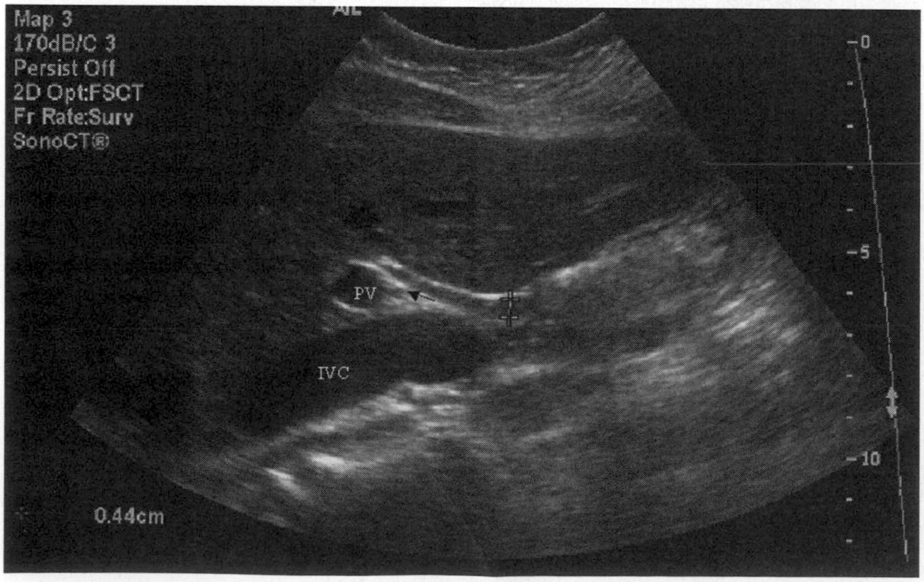

Figure 10-18. ■ *Longitudinal image of the liver showing the appropriate level to measure the CBD.*

CAUSES OF BILIARY DILATATION

Bile Duct Stones

Most stones can be seen if the distal CBD is thoroughly evaluated. An area of acoustic shadowing with an echogenic source represents a stone (Color Plate 10-7). Most biliary duct stones lie in the distal-most portion of the CBD. As shown in Figure 10-11, a transverse plane may be useful in identifying biliary duct dilation at the level of the pancreatic head, as well as following the distal course of the duct to the duodenum to identify the stone's presence.

Mirizzi Syndrome

This is an uncommon condition in which the obstructing stone lies in the cystic duct. This situation results in compression of the common hepatic duct. Sonographic findings include intrahepatic biliary dilatation, a large stone in the cystic duct or neck of the gallbladder, and a normal-caliper CBD. In some cases, the stone may penetrate the common hepatic duct or gut, causing a cholecystobiliary or cholecystenteric fistula.

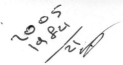

Bile Duct Carcinoma

Rarely, a tumor may be seen within a bile duct (cholangiocarcinoma). Most cholangiocarcinomas originate within the CBD or common hepatic duct (Fig. 10-19). In approximately 25% of cases, cholangiocarcinoma occurs at the junction of the right and left intrahepatic ducts, referred to as a Klatskin tumor. In the setting of cholangiocarcinoma, the bile ducts will be dilated proximal to the tumor. A specific mass may not be visualized, but isolated intrahepatic biliary dilation should raise the possibility of cholangiocarcinoma.

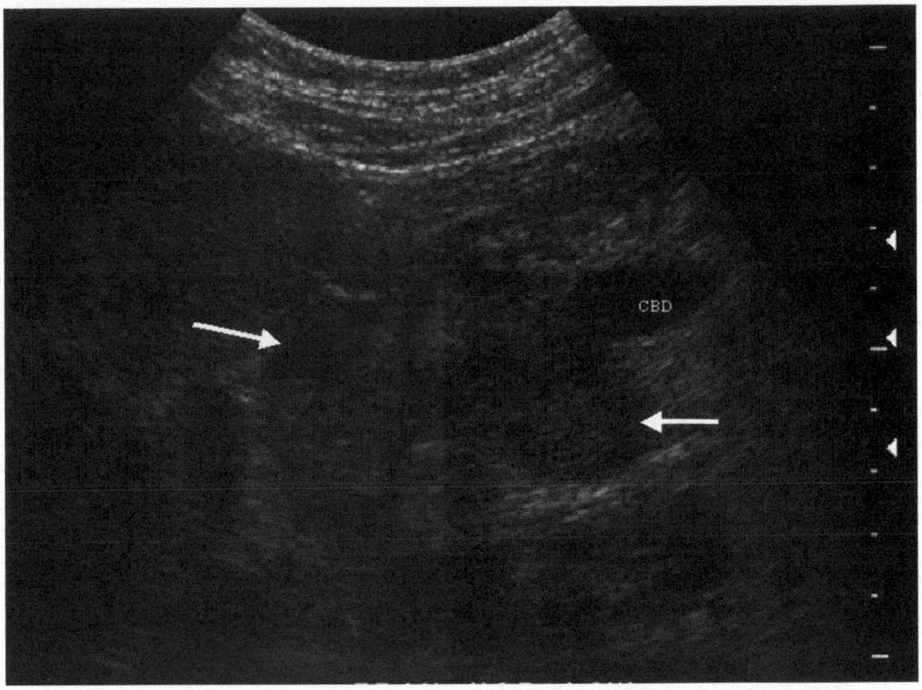

Figure 10-19. ■ *Longitudinal image of the common bile duct infiltrated with cholangiocarcinoma* (arrows), *causing dilation of the duct.*

Biliary Parasites

Biliary parasites are rare. The most common parasite is *Ascaris lumbricoides*. Sonographically, patients may present with a worm or worms visualized within the extrahepatic bile duct. *Clonorchis sinensis*, a liver fluke that affects Far East populations, may also be seen sonographically. Characteristic sonographic findings include intrahepatic ductal dilation, with echogenic thickening of the bile duct walls. Finally, *Fasciola hepatica* is a liver fluke that has been reported to occur in humans infected by drinking or eating contaminated water or plants. These parasites usually appear sonographically as echogenic foci within the gallbladder or dilated extrahepatic ducts. In all cases of parasites, motion of the worm or fluke may be observed, which can confirm the diagnosis.

AIDS Cholangitis

Intrahepatic bile duct changes often occur in patients with AIDS cholangitis. The ducts may not appear dilated, but irregular wall thickening may be observed (Fig. 10-20). This appearance is identical to that of primary sclerosing cholangitis.

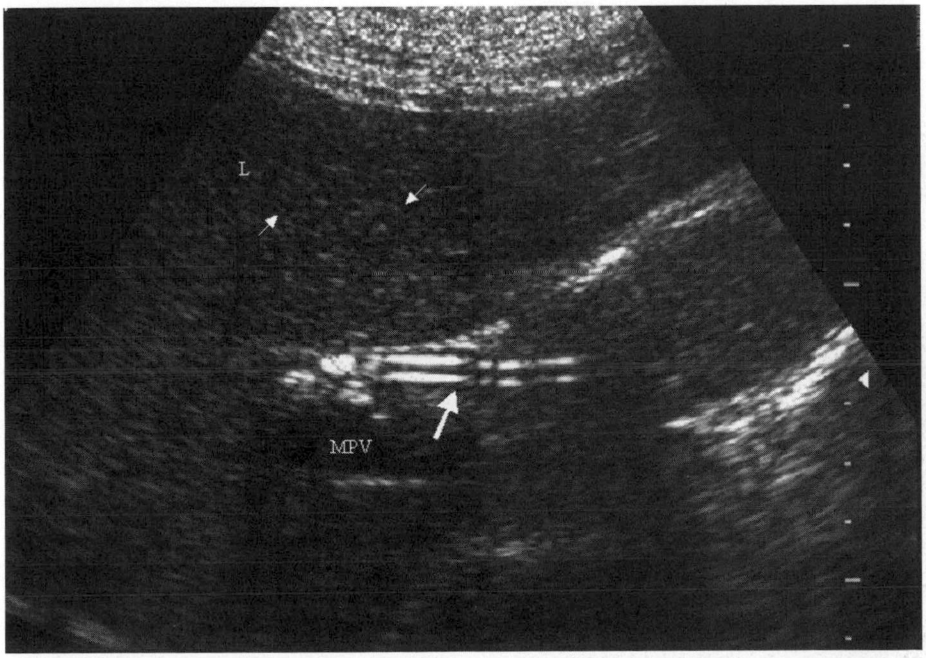

Figure 10-20. ■ *Longitudinal image of the liver in a patient with AIDS cholangitis.* Arrows *show the thickened walls of the intrahepatic biliary ducts. A stent is seen within the common bile duct.*

Caroli Disease

Caroli disease is a congenital abnormality that results in saccular areas being formed within the intrahepatic bile ducts. Identifying communication between the sac-like structures and the bile ducts can differentiate this entity from polycystic liver disease. Intrahepatic biliary dilation, stones, or abscess may also be present.

There is also a childhood form of Caroli disease in which intrahepatic biliary dilation may not be as prevalent, but hepatic fibrosis may be present. Ultimately, portal hypertension and liver failure will occur. This form of Caroli disease has been associated with choledochal cyst and infantile polycystic kidney disease.

Choledochal Cyst

Todani has categorized choledochal cysts into five types. The most common form is a fusiform dilation of the CBD (Fig. 10-21). Less commonly, a diverticulum protruding from the wall of the CBD or a herniation of the CBD into the duodenum may be seen. Sonographically, an extrahepatic cystic structure will be seen, often with the CBD entering it. Bile duct dilation may or may not be present elsewhere.

Courvoisier Gallbladder

In patients who present with jaundice and a palpable right upper quadrant mass, Courvoisier gallbladder should be considered. With this entity, the gallbladder and distal CBD are markedly enlarged secondary to a pancreatic head mass.

Hepatic Duct Calculi

Stones may develop in the gallbladder and then reflux into the biliary tree, causing focal dilatation of a segment of the biliary tree. These patients present with pain rather than jaundice. Liver function tests may be normal because the bulk of the biliary tree is unaffected.

Biliary Atresia

Biliary atresia is a rare disease of newborns, usually diagnosed by 2 to 3 weeks of age. It is the progressive sclerosis of the extrahepatic and proximal intrahepatic bile ducts. Secondary to decreased or absent bile flow, the gallbladder is very small or absent in most cases. Neonates typically present with jaundice. Sonographically, the gallbladder and extrahepatic ducts will not be visualized. The intrahepatic ducts may be dilated. Additionally, cystic areas may be present within the liver.

Metastatic Tumor

Focal liver metastasis can block peripheral intrahepatic bile ducts, causing bile duct dilatation. Depending on the location of the metastatic lesions, biliary dilation may or may not be appreciated.

Pitfalls

1. Pseudo bile duct obstruction
   a. Hepatic artery. The proper hepatic artery runs anterior to the MPV in close proximity to the CBD. The artery occasionally reaches a size of greater than 6 mm and can be mistaken for a dilated CBD. Color or pulsed Doppler should be used to confirm the absence of blood flow when in doubt. Additionally, the hepatic artery can run anterior to the common duct as a normal variant. This condition may also cause confusion. Finally, patients with cirrhosis and portal hypertension can have abnormally large intrahepatic arteries, which look like dilated intrahepatic ducts; these will readily show flow with color or pulsed Doppler.
   b. Neck of gallbladder (Hartmann's pouch). The neck of the gallbladder sometimes lies anterior to the CBD and can fold in such a manner that on some views it may appear to be separate from the body. It can be mistaken for a dilated common hepatic or proximal CBD if not traced into the body of the gallbladder.
2. Gas in the biliary tree versus stones. If communication occurs between the biliary tree and the gastrointestinal tract (e.g., after a sphincterotomy), gas can reflux into the biliary tree and cause pockets of acoustic shadowing. This shadowing should not be mistaken for biliary stones. A posterior comet-tail artifact is usually seen, which contains echoes, as opposed to the clean, echo-free shadowing resulting from a stone (Fig. 10-22). Additionally, gas usually rises to the most anterior loca-

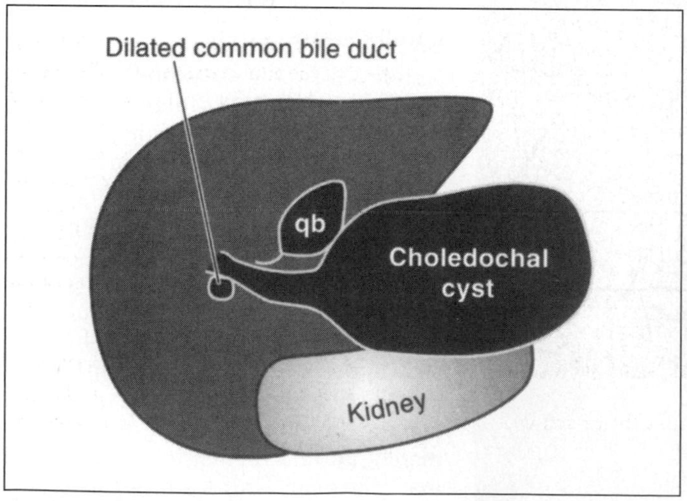

Figure 10-21. ■ *Diagram of the most common location of a choledochal cyst. A dilated duct is seen entering the cyst, and the gallbladder is seen as a separate structure.*

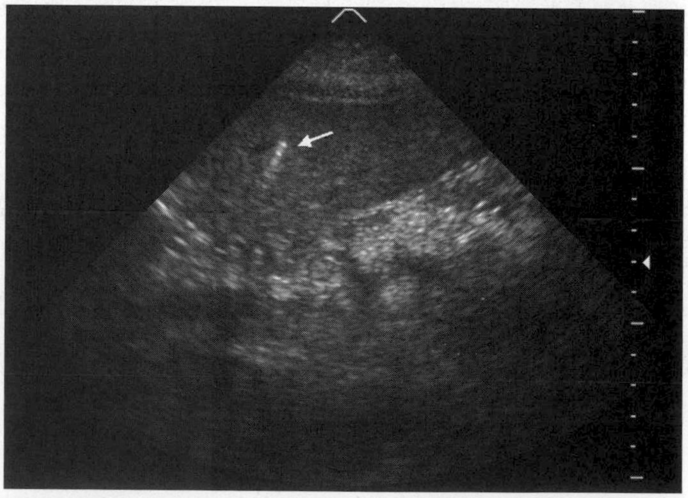

Figure 10-22. ■ *Comet-tail artifact seen posterior to an intrahepatic bile duct containing air.*

tion. Therefore, when the patient is in a supine position, air should be seen in the biliary ducts within the left lobe of the liver. In the gallbladder, air will rise to the most anterior wall (Fig. 10-23). The location of the air should change as the patient changes position.

3. Pseudo diffuse liver disease. A high-frequency transducer used with maximum gain settings in order to penetrate the liver may cause the appearance of coarse echoes in the parenchyma, mimicking diffuse liver disease. With this scenario, it would be more appropriate to use a lower-frequency transducer with gain settings in the midrange. Comparison between the liver and kidney should show the normal liver parenchyma to be slightly more echogenic than the kidney parenchyma. Also, due to lack of penetration if too high a frequency transducer is used, the diaphragm may be poorly seen, making it appear as though there is fatty infiltration.
4. Splenomegaly due to causes other than portal hypertension can result in a dilated portal venous system. No collaterals will be seen in this setting, however.
5. Pseudo absence of blood flow in the portal vein (false-positive portal vein thrombus). If blood flow is not detected in the portal vein, particularly in the absence of other relevant clinical features of portal vein thrombosis, improper technique may be the cause. A pulsed Doppler angle of greater than 60 degrees, or a wall filter that is set too high, can result in slow blood flow not being detected. If blood flow is not detected, all Doppler parameters should be checked and the velocity scale needs to be adjusted to ensure maximum sensitivity.

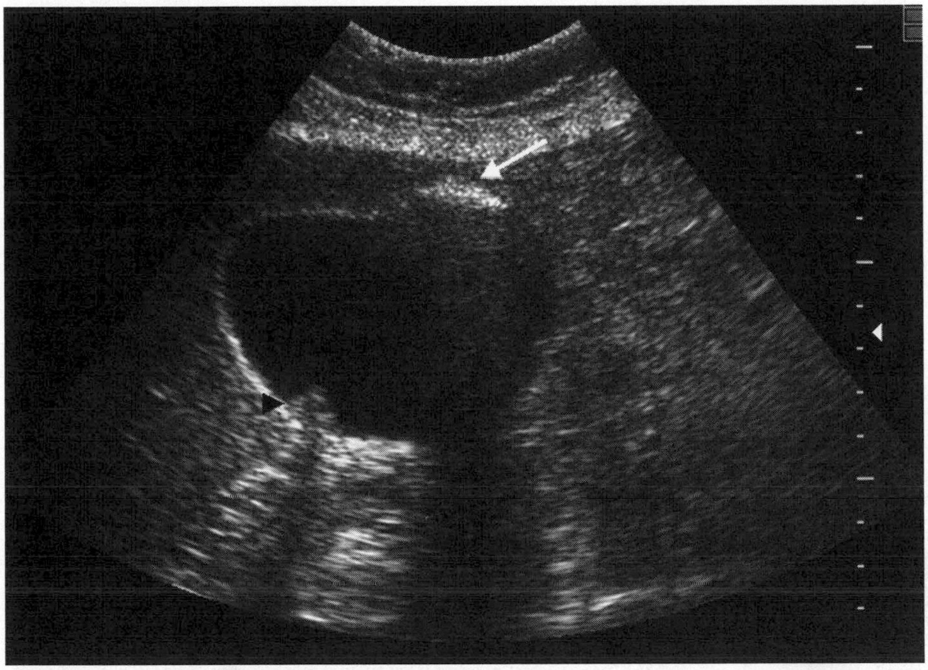

Figure 10-23. ■ *Image of the gallbladder containing air* (white arrow). *A stone* (black arrowhead) *is also noted in the dependent aspect of the gallbladder.*

Where Else to Look

1. Obstructed bile ducts. If obstructed bile ducts are identified, it is important to trace the duct to the point of obstruction. Often, the obstruction is in the region of the pancreas. Mass lesions such as carcinoma of the pancreas, pseudocyst, or focal pancreatitis are often responsible. If a stone is seen within an obstructed bile duct, the gallbladder should also be evaluated for coexisting stones. Rarely, obstructed ducts are due to extrinsic pressure from nodes in the region of the porta hepatis, so this area should also be evaluated.
2. Hepatocellular disease. Diffuse textural changes within the liver are usually caused by alcoholic liver disease. When these changes are found, look for other sequelae of liver disease: a pancreatic pseudocyst, calcification, or pancreatitis; portal hypertension with splenomegaly, enlarged superior mesenteric and splenic veins, visible collaterals, and ascites.
3. Hemolytic jaundice. If the jaundice appears to result from hemolytic anemia with an enlarged liver and spleen, look for enlarged periaortic lymph nodes, because there may be underlying leukemia or lymphoma.

SELECTED READING

Bachar GN, Cohen M, Belenky A, et al. Effect of aging on the adult extrahepatic bile duct: a sonographic study. *J Ultrasound Med* 2003;22(9):879–882.

Bressler EL, Rubin JM, McCracken S. Sonographic parallel channel sign: a reappraisal. *Radiology* 1987;164:343–346.

Feldstein VA, LaBerge JM. Hepatic vein flow reversal at duplex sonography: a sign of transjugular intrahepatic portosystemic shunt dysfunction. *AJR AM J Roentgenol* 1994; 162:839–841.

Gill KA. Gallbladder and biliary tree. In: Gill KA, ed. *Abdominal Ultrasound: A Practitioner's Guide*. Philadelphia: WB Saunders; 2001:123–147.

Grant E, Schiller V, Millener P, et al. Color Doppler imaging of the hepatic vasculature. *AJR Am J Roentgenol* 1992;159:943–950.

Hernanz-Schulman M, Ambrosino MM, Freeman PC, et al. Common bile duct in children: sonographic dimensions. *Radiology* 1995;195:193–195.

Horrow MM, Horrow JC, Niakosari A, et al. Is age associated with size of adult extrahepatic bile duct?: sonographic study. *Radiology* 2002;221:411–414.

Joseph AEA, Saverymuttu SH. Ultrasound in the assessment of diffuse parenchymal liver disease. *Clin Radiol* 1991;44:219–221. Editorial.

Kawamura DM, Carr-Hoeffer C. Liver. In: Kawamur DM, ed. *Abdomen and Superficial Structures. Diagnostic Medical Sonography: A Guide to Clinical Practice*. 2nd ed. Philadelphia: Lippincott; 1997:115–189.

Ladenheim JA, Luba DG, Yao F, et al. Limitations of liver surface US in the diagnosis of cirrhosis. *Radiology* 1992;185: 21–24.

Laing FC. The gallbladder and bile ducts. In: Rumack CM, Wilson SR, Charboneau JW, eds. *Diagnostic Ultrasound*, vol 1, 2nd ed. St. Louis: Mosby; 175–223.

Laing FC, Jeffrey RB, Wing VW, et al. Biliary dilatation: defining the level and cause by real-time US. *Radiology* 1986;160:39–42.

Lin DY, Sheen IS, Chiu CT, et al. Ultrasonographic changes of early liver cirrhosis in chronic hepatitis B: a longitudinal study. *J Clin Ultrasound* 1993;21:303–308.

Mageed AW, Ross B, Johnson AG. The preoperatively normal bile duct does not dilate after cholecystectomy: results of a five-year study. *Gut* 1999;45:741–743.

Matsui O, Kadoya M, Takahashi S, et al. Focal sparing of segment IV in fatty livers shown by sonography and CT: correlation with aberrant gastric venous drainage. *AJR Am J Roentgenol* 1995;164:1137–1140.

Perret RS, Sloop GD, Borne JA. Common bile duct measurements in an elderly population. *J Ultrasound Med* 2000;19(11):727–730.

Quinn RJ, Meredith C, Slade L. The effect of the Valsalva maneuver on the diameter of the common hepatic duct in extrahepatic biliary obstruction. *J Ultrasound Med* 1992; 11:143–145.

Ralls PW. Color Doppler sonography of the hepatic artery and portal venous system. *AJR Am J Roentgenol* 1990;155:517–525.

Ralls PW, Mayekawa DS, Lee KP et al. The use of color Doppler sonography to distinguish dilated intrahepatic ducts from vascular structures. *AJR Am J Roentgenol* 1989; 9152:291–292.

Wachsberg RH, Needleman L, Wilson DJ. Portal vein pulsatility in normal and cirrhotic adults without cardiac disease. *J Clin Ultrasound* 1995;23:3–15.

Zwiebel WJ, Mountford RA, Halliwell MJ, et al. Splanchnic blood flow in patients with cirrhosis and portal hypertension: investigation with duplex Doppler US. *Radiology* 1995;194:807–812.

11 Fever of Unknown Origin

HEATHER SCHIERLOH
TOM WINTER

SONOGRAPHIC ABBREVIATIONS

Ao	Aorta
Bl	Bladder
Bwl	Bowel
GB	Gallbladder
HEM	Hematoma
Ip	Iliopsoas muscle
IVC	Inferior vena cava
K	Kidney
L	Liver
LHA	Left hepatic artery
LHV	Left hepatic vein
LPV	Left portal vein
MPV	Main portal vein
MHV	Middle hepatic vein
P	Pancreas
PHA	Proper hepatic artery
RAt	Right atrium
RHA	Right hepatic artery
RHV	Right hepatic vein
RPV	Right portal vein
RK	Right kidney
Sp	Spine
Spl	Spleen
St	Stomach
Ut	Uterus

KEY WORDS

Abscess. Localized collection of pus caused by pyogenic bacterium.

AIDS. Acquired immunodeficiency syndrome. An immune system disorder caused by the human immunodeficiency virus (HIV) resulting in increased susceptibility to opportunistic infections throughout the body.

Anemia. Too few red blood cells. Causes include decreased blood cell formation, blood cell destruction, and bleeding.

Candidiasis. A fungal infection with the Candida organism (*Candida albicans* is the most common type) that affects the skin, mucous membranes, lungs, and blood system. Occurs in patients who are immune-compromised or patients who have taken multiple antibiotics.

Cholangitis. Infection of the biliary tree.

Cholecystitis. Infection of the gallbladder.

Cystitis. Inflammation of the bladder commonly associated with urinary tract infections (UTIs).

Cytomegalovirus (CMV). A form of the herpes virus that can become pathogenic with immune-compromised patients including those with AIDS, organ transplants, extensive burns, and underdeveloped immune systems.

Erythrocyte Sedimentation Rate (ESR). This laboratory test determines how far red blood cells settle to the bottom of a specially marked test tube within 1 hour. ESR can be used to screen for a variety of pathogens.

Fever. See *Pyrexia*.

Gallbladder Fossa. The area located on the inferior aspect of the liver where the gallbladder is situated.

Gossypiboma. A sterile collection of fluid surrounding a sterile surgical sponge inadvertently left in the body postoperatively.

Gutters. See *Paracolic Gutters*.

Hematocrit. The percentage of erythrocytes in a given volume of blood after centrifugation.

Hematoma. A clot or collection of blood confined to an organ or space within the body.

Hemolysis. Breakdown of red blood cells with release of hemoglobin into the surrounding plasma.

Hemorrhage. An internal or external discharge of blood resulting from damage to the vascular system at the arterial, venous, or capillary levels.

Hypernephroma. Older term for renal cell carcinoma.

Immunosuppressed. A term used to describe the circumstance in which the immune system is not operating on a normal level. Affected patients include those who are being treated with drugs or suffering from an illness that decreases the body's response to infection. Examples of causes include AIDS, steroids, and anticancer drugs.

Leukocyte. A white blood cell (WBC) that acts as a phagocyte to defend the body against infection and aids in the repair of damaged tissues.

Leukocytosis. An increase in the number of leukocytes (WBC).

Lymphadenopathy. Abnormally enlarged lymph nodes that are an indication that a disease process is present within the lymph system.

Murphy's Sign (sonographic). Localized tenderness over the gallbladder.

Paracolic Gutters. Areas in the flanks lateral to the colon where ascites and abscesses can form.

Pneumocystis Carinii Pneumonia (PCP). An otherwise rare type of bacterial pneumonia commonly seen in patients infected with the AIDS virus.

Prostatitis. Inflammation or infection of the prostate gland.

Pyelonephritis. Infection of the kidney(s).

Pyogenic. The production of pus caused by a microorganism infecting an organ or body system.

Pyrexia. A rise in body temperature above 98.6°F (37°C).

Sedimentation Rate. See *Erythrocyte Sedimentation Rate* (ESR).

Sepsis. The presence of pathogenic microorganisms or their toxic products that spread from the originally affected organ into the blood circulatory system.

Septicemia. Infection in the blood.

Staging. Demonstration of the areas that are involved in a malignancy. The more areas that are involved, the more severe the staging grade will be.

Subphrenic. Under the diaphragm.

Subpulmonic. The area located inferior to the lung and superior to the diaphragm.

RELEVANT LABORATORY VALUES

Cultures (aerobic and anaerobic): No range applicable, test indicates type of pathogen

Purified protein derivative (PPD): No range applicable, test is positive or negative. Positive indicates the patient has had exposure to tuberculosis.

Erythrocyte sedimentation rate (ESR): Elevated values are associated with a wide range of infectious and inflammatory diseases.

- Men 18 to 50 years 0 to 15 mm/hr
- Men ≥50 years 0 to 20 mm/hr
- Women 18 to 50 years 0 to 20 mm/hr
- Women ≥50 years 0 to 30 mm/hr

Urinalysis: Abnormal values may be associated with kidney or bladder infections.

- Specific gravity 1.005 to 1.030
- pH 5.0 to 7.5
- Urobilinogen 0.1 to 1.0 mg/dL
- WBC 0 to 5/hpf; RBC 0 to 2/hpf
- Epithelial cells (only squamous) 0 to 2/hpf
- Casts 0 to 1 hyaline cast/lpf

WBC: High values are associated with infection.

- 1 month to 2 years—6.0 to 14.0 K/uL
- 2 to 10 years—4.0 to 12.0 K/uL
- 10 to 18 years—4.0 to 10.5 K/uL
- >18 years 3.8 to 10.5 K/uL

The Clinical Problem

Pyrexia, or fever, is defined as an elevation of body temperature above 98.6°F (37°C) oral temperature and is a common symptom associated with numerous types of pathological etiologies. The cause of the fever can usually be narrowed by examining the patient's history, symptoms, and laboratory results; however, in some cases, this information does not provide sufficient data to explain the fever. If the patient's condition continues over several weeks, it is classified as a fever of unknown origin (FUO). Before beginning a study in a patient with FUO, the history and laboratory data in the patient's chart should be checked for evidence suggesting any of the possibilities mentioned (information to follow; see also Key Words). Understanding the patient's history will help the sonographer concentrate on the most appropriate areas.

The differential diagnosis for patients with FUO relies on a classification based on their clinical history and laboratory results. There are four broad categories of disease that are common in most patients with FUO, including infections, malignancies, autoimmune conditions, and miscellaneous symptoms. Factors affecting the diagnosis include the patient's individual symptoms, the duration of the symptoms, the patient's age, and underlying pathologies.

In cases of FUO, radiographs (x-ray "plain" films) and computed tomography (CT) with oral and/or intravenous contrast are usually the first medical imaging tests ordered to detect the underlining cause of the fever. Ultrasound examinations are routinely ordered as follow-up studies to provide additional information on the gallbladder and biliary tract and to better evaluate abdominal and pelvic abscesses that are identified on x-ray and CT. In cases when venous thrombosis is suspected as a potential cause of the fever, lower and/or upper extremity peripheral Doppler examinations may also be ordered. When tumors, abscesses, and ascites are identified, ultrasound-guided invasive procedures (such as paracentesis and biopsy) can be performed to obtain samples that can be analyzed to identify the exact pathogen causing the fever; this type of examination allows appropriate antibiotic therapy to be started.

ABSCESSES

Patients who have recently undergone invasive or surgical procedures are susceptible to abscesses (wound infection) that can spread throughout the chest, abdomen, and pelvis. Symptoms associated with abscess include fever, localized pain, and an elevated WBC count. Infections usually start approximately on the fifth postoperative day and develop into an abscess approximately on the 10th postoperative day. Risk factors include cancer, diabetes, connective tissue disorders, immunosuppression, and existing hematomas.

ORGAN INFLAMMATION

Infection may progress to actual abscess formation or may be limited to organ inflammation. The following conditions may induce fever, yet there may be no localizing clinical signs. Sonographic findings may be present.

1. Hepatitis
2. Pyelonephritis
3. Cholecystitis
4. Cholangitis
5. Pancreatitis
6. Cystitis
7. Prostatitis

TUMORS

Many tumors are associated with fever and leukocytosis and may mimic the characteristics of infections. Common malignant causes include renal cell carcinoma, lymphoma, and hepatoma (Fig. 11-1).

POSTOPERATIVE COLLECTIONS

Patients who have recently undergone surgery may develop a fluid pocket at the incision site. Cesarean section, hysterectomy, liver surgery, and organ transplantation are often followed by collection development that may be a hematoma, urinoma, abscess, lymphocele, biloma, ascites, or seroma. Hematomas also follow anticoagulant therapy. They may be suspected when a drop in the patient's hematocrit level is present. Any of these fluid collections may become superinfected.

GOSSYPIBOMA

This sterile collection due to a retained surgical sponge has a distinctive appearance on ultrasound (Fig. 11-2).

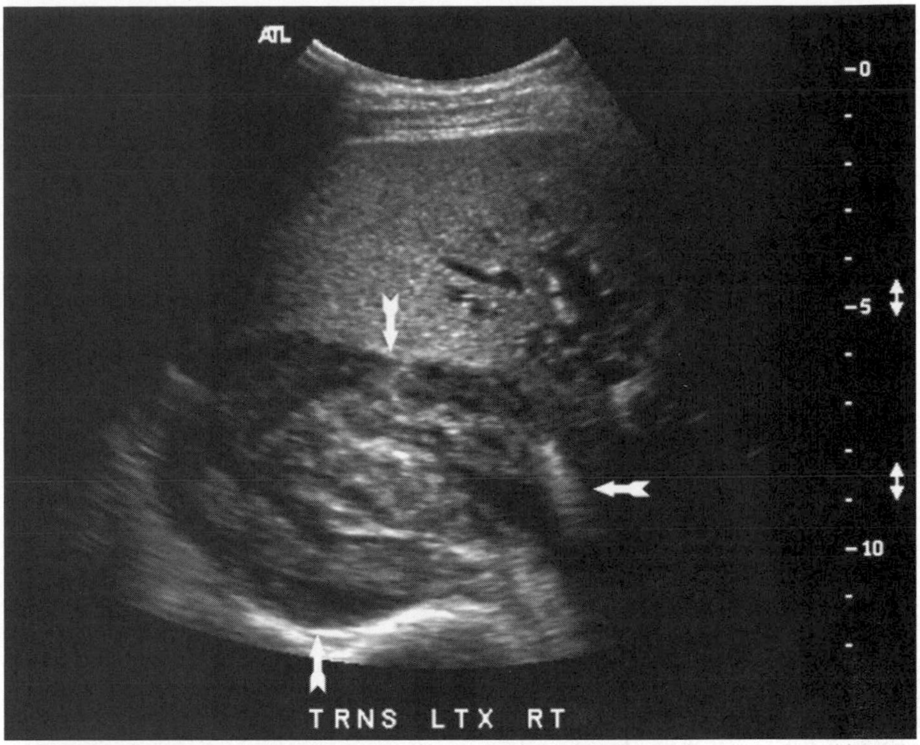

Figure 11-1. ■ *Lymphoma. This liver transplant recipient had a very mild fever and rise in liver function tests 2 years after surgery. Ultrasound shows a large mass* (arrows) *in the posterior segment of the right lobe of the liver that at biopsy proved to be posttransplant lymphoproliferative disorder, a type of lymphoma very common in transplant patients.*

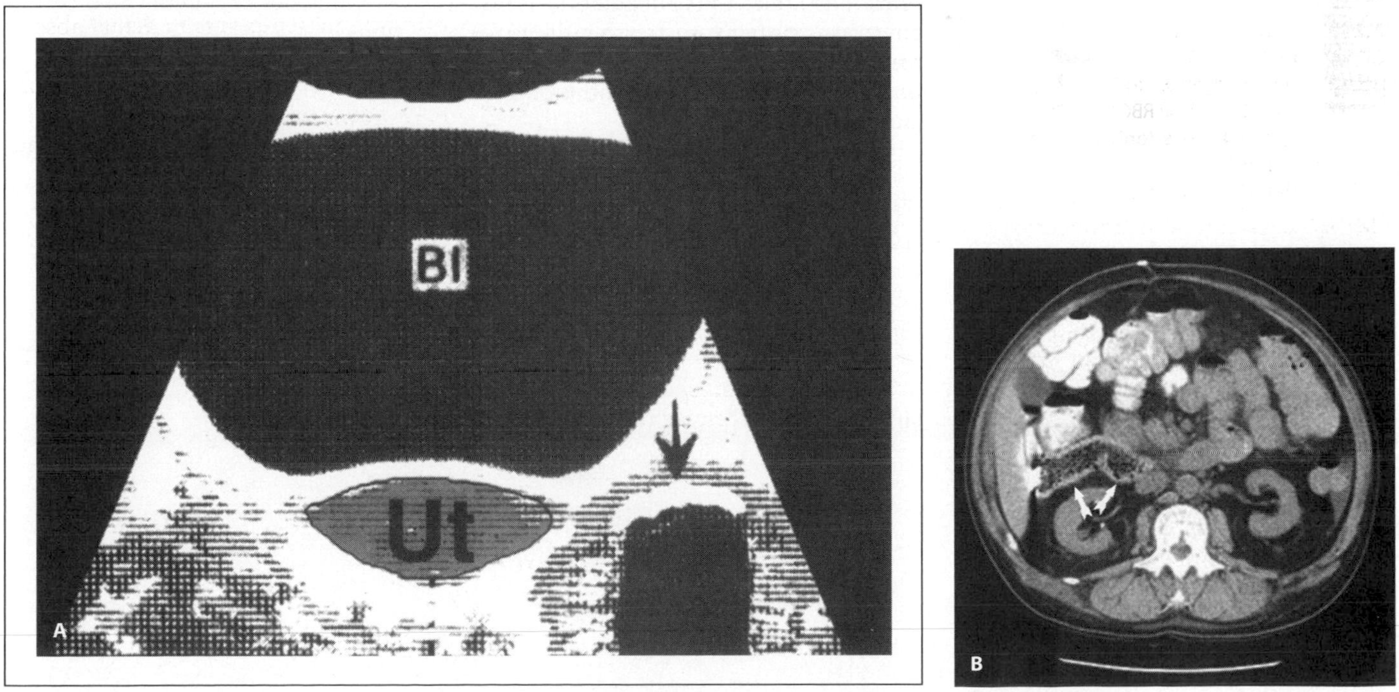

Figure 11-2. ■ *A. Transverse diagram of the female pelvis with a left-sided tubo-ovarian abscess. The abscess contains air, which rises to the top and casts a strong acoustic shadow. Retained sponge (gossypiboma) would be another cause of the same sonographic appearance. B. CT of gossypiboma located in front of the right kidney. Gas bubbles trapped within the cotton surgical sponge will have an echogenic shadowing appearance on ultrasound.*

AIDS

AIDS is a disease transmitted through bodily fluids such as blood and semen. It has many sonographic manifestations and is due to an infection with a virus known as *human immunodeficiency virus* (HIV). A patient with AIDS does not pose a risk of infection to a sonographer unless blood from the infected individual contacts a bleeding surface or mucous membrane on the sonographer. Infections are alleged to have taken place through the conjunctiva of the eye and the mucous membrane of the mouth from blood that splashed from the patient at the time of surgery or biopsy. It is therefore essential to wear a mask and an eye guard if a puncture procedure is being performed on an AIDS patient. Otherwise, contact with AIDS patients is not dangerous and routine universal precautions are adequate.

AIDS almost exclusively affects members of four groups: (1) homosexuals; (2) intravenous drug abusers; (3) hemophiliacs and those who have had multiple blood transfusions; and (4) individuals who have intercourse with an HIV-infected person (this last mode is becoming increasingly common). AIDS is widespread in Haiti and east Africa.

To diagnose AIDS, an HIV test must be performed. This test can be administered only if the patient agrees, because there is a social stigma with a diagnosis of AIDS. It is, therefore, not uncommon for a hospital patient to have undiagnosed AIDS, which is why universal precautions have become the standard in hospital practice (see Chapter 55).

Typical presenting symptoms in patients with AIDS are as follows:

1. Fever
2. Lymphadenopathy
3. Weight loss
4. Diarrhea
5. Right upper quadrant pain
6. Clinical evidence of abdominal masses
7. Gastrointestinal hemorrhage
8. Gastrointestinal obstructions

Many infections are more common in patients with AIDS than in patients with normal immune systems. These include the following:

1. *Pneumocystis carinii*
2. Candidiasis
3. Cytomegalovirus
4. Herpes simplex virus
5. Mycobacterium avium complex

Rare neoplasms are more frequent with AIDS, such as Kaposi's sarcoma and unusual lymphomas (e.g., Burkitt's lymphoma). The success of medical treatment for AIDS in the past decade has markedly decreased the number of infections and unusual tumors seen; however, resistance to treating drugs is rising, and some experts predict a resurgence in the complications of this devastating disease.

Anatomy

See the relevant chapters for each organ.

Technique

ROUTINE VIEWS

All abdominal organs and pathological lesions should be investigated in perpendicular planes. The patient should be instructed to take nothing by mouth for 6 to 8 hours before the ultrasound examination if the gallbladder is suspected of causing the FUO; a normal contracted gallbladder due to a recent meal may be difficult to distinguish from a diseased gallbladder. Scanning the patient in a variety of positions (supine, left posterior oblique, right posterior oblique, etc.) is often useful. If the patient is able to follow breathing instructions, inspiratory and expiratory views should be obtained to ensure that all abdominal organs are seen in their entirety.

1. Start by examining the patient in the supine position. The aorta and the inferior vena cava should be examined from the diaphragm to the bifurcation, looking for enlarged lymph nodes or midline fluid collections.

2. On longitudinal sections, examine the liver, right diaphragm, right kidney, subhepatic space, and gallbladder area (Fig. 11-3). Make sure that the diaphragm moves well and that no pleural effusions are present (if available, cine clips work well when relevant to document diaphragmatic movement). If a psoas problem is being considered (i.e., pain in the psoas area when the leg is moved), obtain longitudinal sections of the psoas by scanning medially to the kidney.
3. Using a transverse approach, start at the xiphoid and sweep down to the umbilicus, watching for nodes around the inferior vena cava and the aorta. Look in the lesser sac area around the pancreas and in the paracolic gutters (Fig. 11-3) for collections. This is also the time to examine the perinephric spaces and to look in the renal pelves for adenopathy.

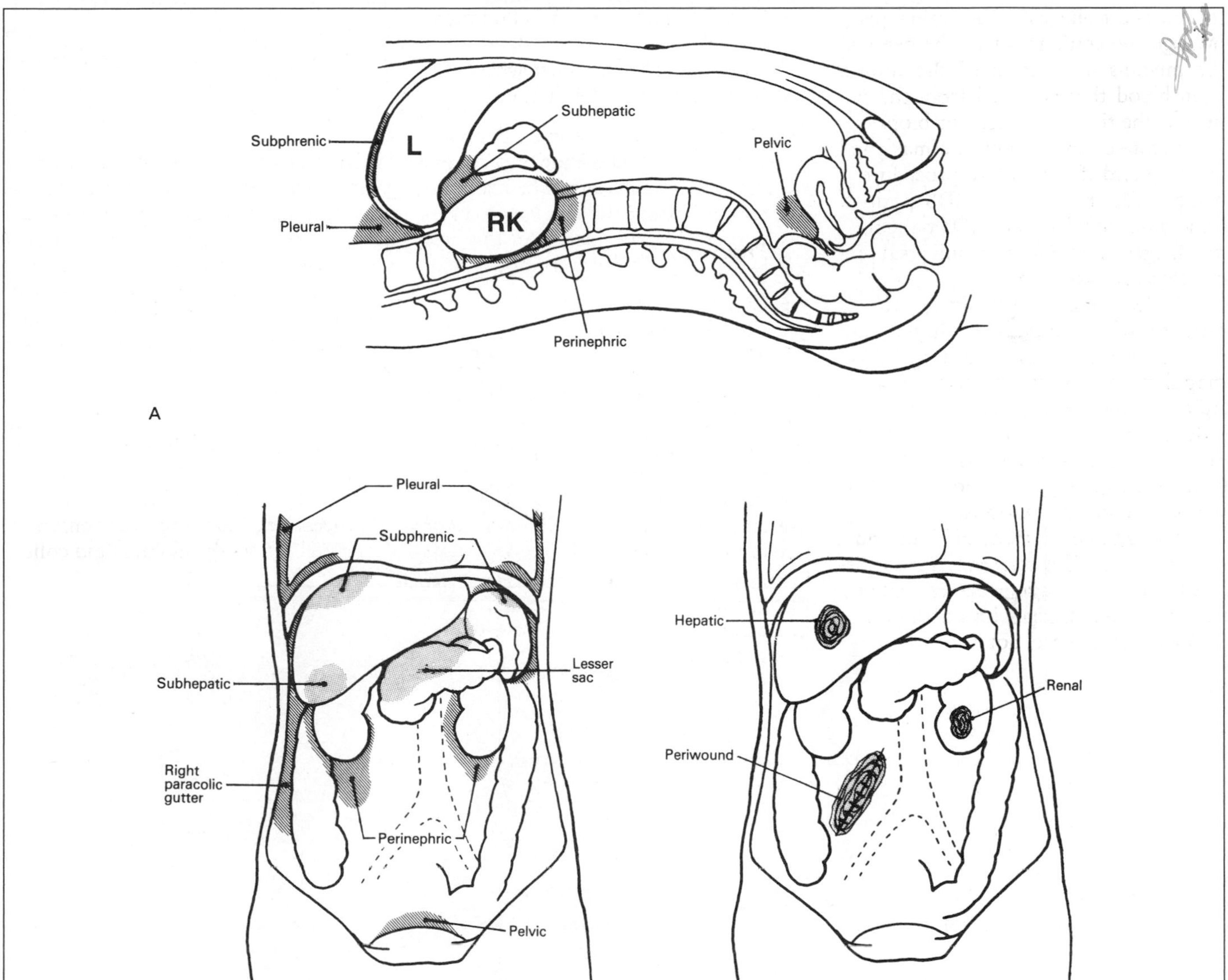

Figure 11-3. ■ *A,B. A number of spaces exist in the abdomen where fluid may collect. Common sites for fluid collection are the pelvic, subphrenic, subhepatic, paracolic gutter, and lesser sac areas. Fluid may collect around the kidneys or in the pleural space. C. Sites where abscesses may form are the spaces already mentioned, as well as within the liver or kidney and around incisions.*

4. With the bladder moderately full, look in the pelvis for ascites, nodes, or a pelvic abscess (Fig. 11-4). Be sure to include the iliopsoas muscles; these may contain an abscess or hematoma or may be surrounded by nodes. If the patient is male, check the prostate and seminal vesicles for enlargement (see Chapter 26). If the patient is female, check the uterus and ovaries (see Chapters 30 and 31). An overdistended bladder may compress and displace pathology into inaccessible sites.
5. Turn the patient left side up and look in the region of the left hemidiaphragm. Vary the inspiration until the diaphragm appears in the costal space (often, deep inspiration is helpful), and rule out collections above and below it. Examine the spleen, the left kidney, and the perinephric area, including the psoas muscles. All of these areas are possible sites for abscesses. The left coronal view is also the best way to evaluate the space between the left kidney and the aorta for nodes (Fig. 11-5).
6. In a postoperative patient, examine the incision area. If the incision is recent, use a sterile approach, as described in Chapter 55. Use sterile gel on the skin. To avoid causing pain, scan only adjacent to the wound,

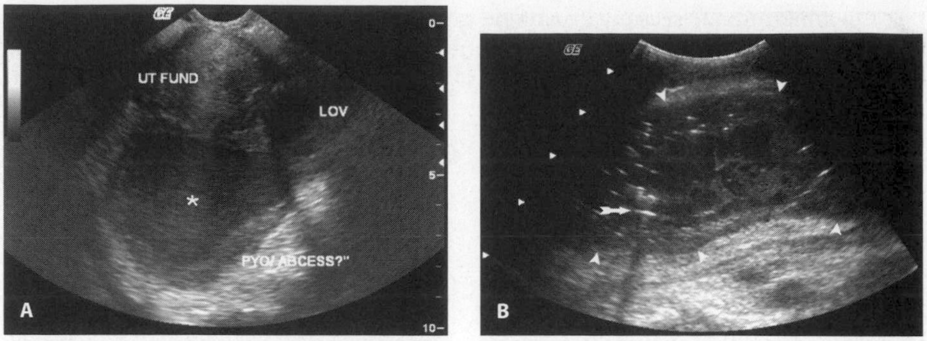

Figure 11-4. ■ *Pelvic abscesses. A. Pelvic inflammatory disease leading to tubo-ovarian abscess* (*). LOV, *left ovary;* UT FUND, *fundus of uterus. B. Parovarian abscess* (arrowheads) *after gynecological surgery. Note small bubbles of gas* (arrow) *within the collection.*

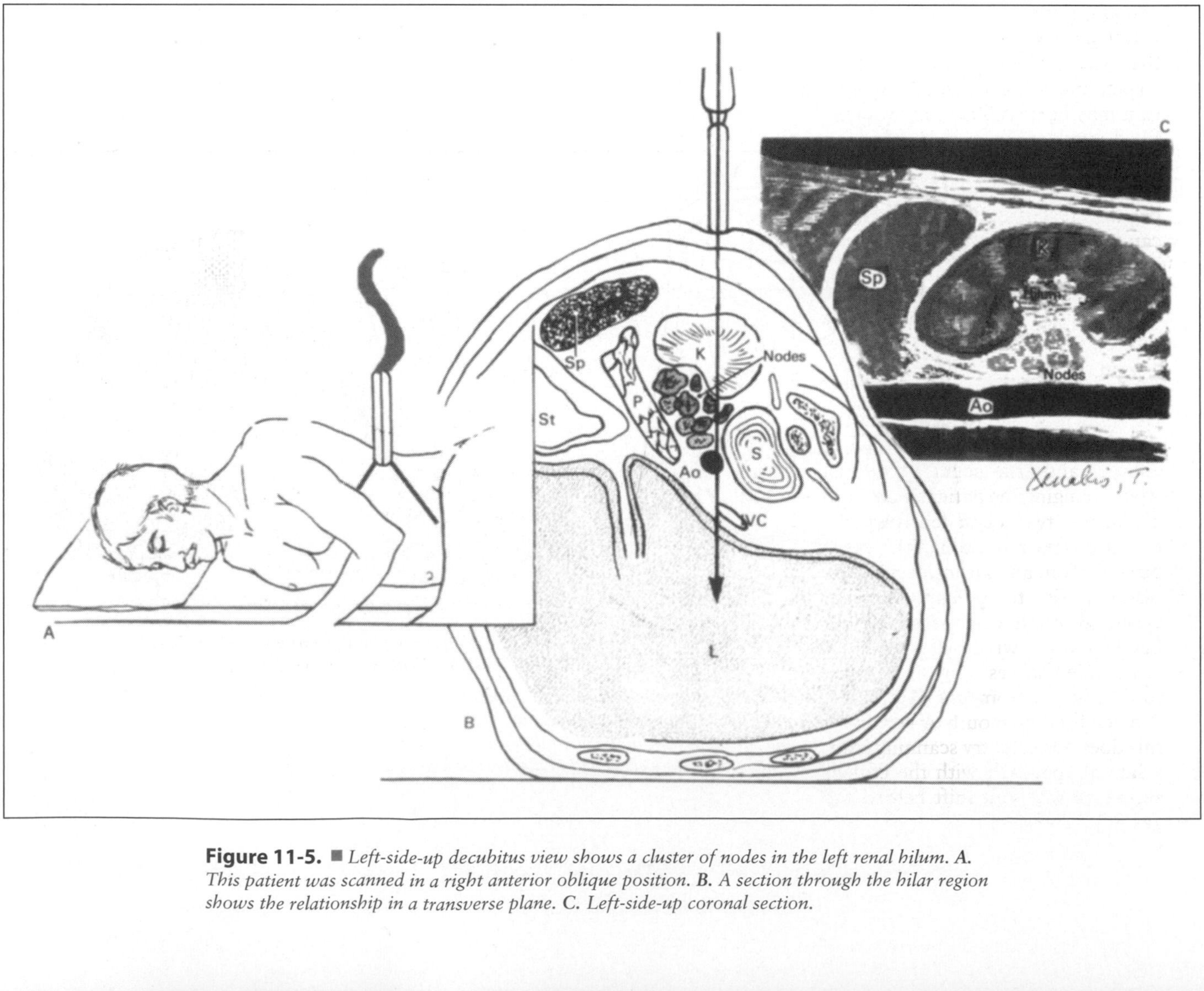

Figure 11-5. ■ *Left-side-up decubitus view shows a cluster of nodes in the left renal hilum. A. This patient was scanned in a right anterior oblique position. B. A section through the hilar region shows the relationship in a transverse plane. C. Left-side-up coronal section.*

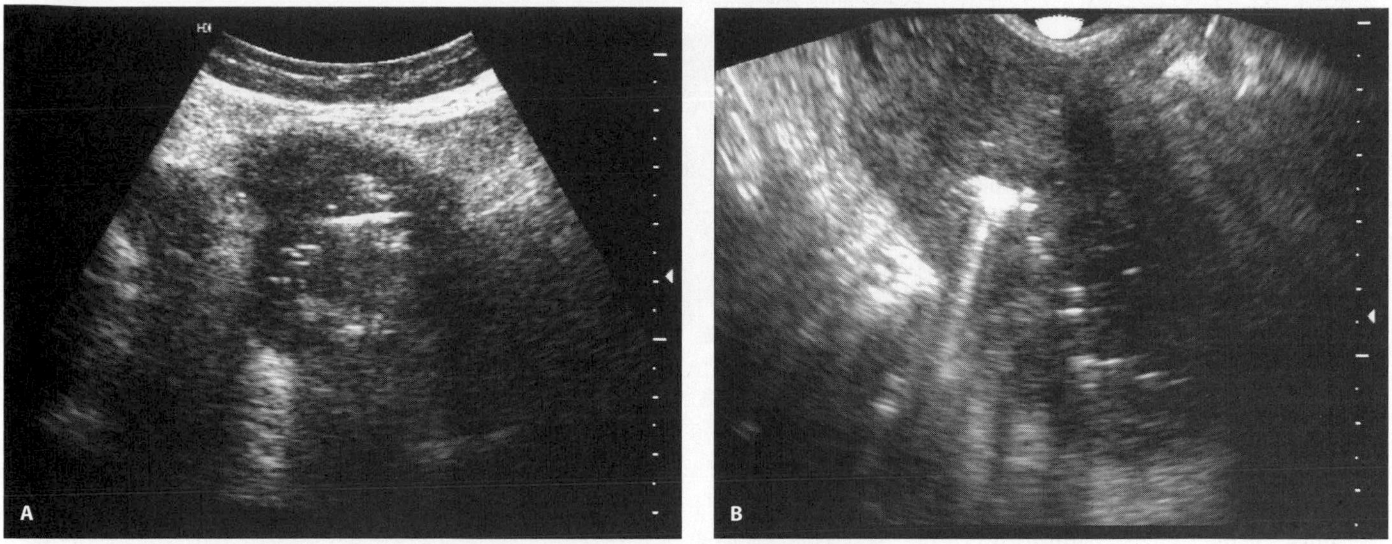

Figure 11-6. ■ *Diverticular abscess. This 65-year-old woman had experienced 6 months of vague left-lower-quadrant pain with low-grade fever. An ultrasound ordered to evaluate the ovaries detected a 5-cm ill-defined mass containing air bubbles adjacent to the sigmoid colon.* ***A.*** *Transabdominal view.* ***B.*** *Transvaginal view. The mass was removed at surgery, and the patient's symptoms completely resolved.*

and angle under it with the beam. A water-path technique may help if the area is extremely sensitive. Depending on how open the wound is, it may be possible to put a water-filled sterile glove over it, allowing the transducer more direct access to the site. There are also sterile membranes, gel-film skin barriers that can be used to cover the wound for scanning (see Chapter 55). Ensure that recent incisions are kept clean, as communal bottles of gel can contain bacteria that may cause infection in the postoperative patient.

7. Examining the contents of a collection may require a higher-frequency transducer to distinguish between artifact and true septa or debris. Also, changing the patient's position can help in two ways: debris will often float and resettle in the dependent portion, and air inside a collection will rise to the top, allowing access through what is perhaps a better acoustic window.
8. A gas-filled abscess may be difficult to distinguish from gut (Fig. 11-6). Provide fluid by mouth or rectum. If this does not help, try scanning from a lateral approach with the patient supine so that you shift behind the gas (Fig. 11-7).

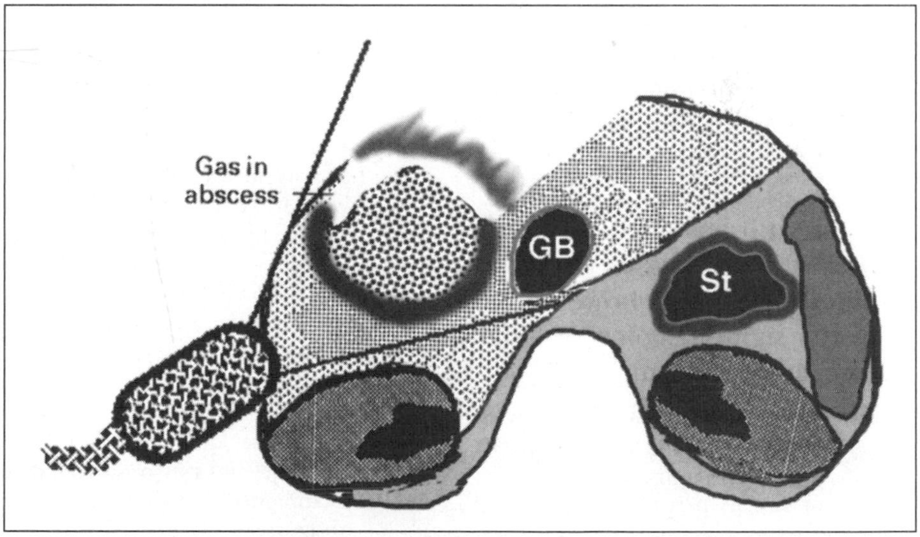

Figure 11-7. ■ *Abscess in the liver with gas rising to the anterior margin. Scan from a posterolateral approach with the patient in a supine position so the beam passes behind the gas.*

9. Sometimes, a subfascial hematoma can follow Cesarean sections (Fig. 11-8). Good near-field visualization is imperative, so use a short focus, high-frequency transducer—linear or curved linear. Set the electronic focus just below the fascial plane. Look for the rectus muscles to determine whether the collection is posterior to them; if this is difficult to discern at the region of the hematoma, start more laterally and trace the posterior surface of the rectus muscles medially. A lower-frequency transducer will be necessary to evaluate the areas posterior to the bladder.

10. The following special techniques may be valuable in difficult circumstances.

    a. Diaphragm obscured. Often, the left diaphragm is difficult to see owing to lung interference. If this is the case, and if the patient is lying in a decubitus position, roll the patient back to the supine position and reach around to scan through the ribs. Use whatever degree of inspiration is needed to bring the diaphragm into view. This can keep the lungs out of the field.

    b. Small liver. If the liver is small and high, and if the edge is obscured by gas, perform intercostal scans from a level superior to the liver edge. Scanning in this manner places the beam more perpendicular to this interface. Turning the patient left side down, or upright, is also helpful in making more liver visible.

    c. Possible pelvic abscess. When trying to find an abscess that could be located between loops of bowel, watch any suspicious area patiently for a few minutes with real time, or return to it occasionally to see if it has changed shape or size. If peristalsis is seen, the question is answered; however, because the sigmoid colon is often inactive, a water enema may be required. Use only enough water to cause flow through or around the questionable mass. Unfortunately for the patient, the bladder must remain distended enough to allow for an adequate acoustic window. When using a water enema technique, it is often just as informative to watch the water being drained back into the bag as it was to watch it go in. This gives you a second chance to observe activity in the questionable area without requiring the patient to go through any extra discomfort.

    d. Possible subacute appendicitis. Ask the patient to point with one finger to the area of maximum pain. Place a linear transducer directly on this spot. An infected appendix is more than 6 mm in transverse diameter, noncompressible, and may be surrounded by inflamed (echogenic) fat or an abscess. See Chapter 15 for a discussion of appendicitis.

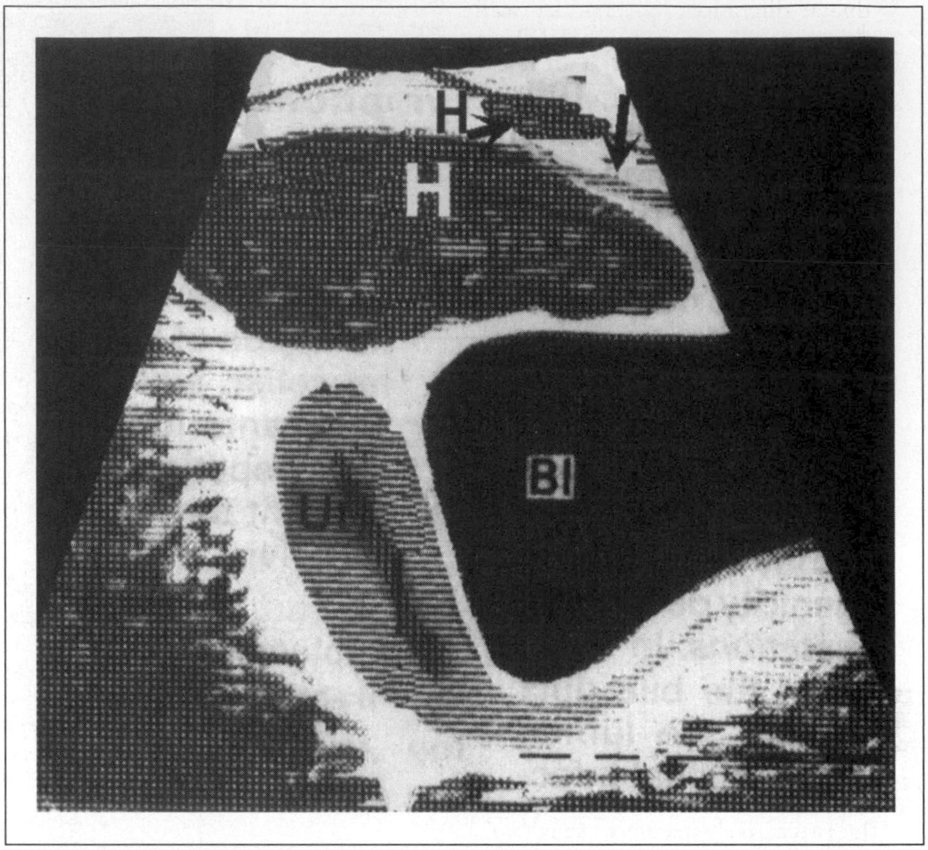

Figure 11-8. ■ *A postoperative pelvis. A hematoma in the abdominal wall is present* (black H). *A subfascial hematoma* (white H), *which is much larger, is also shown. Although the hematoma is echolucent, it does not transmit sound quite as well as a known fluid-filled structure, such as the bladder. The fascia can be seen* (arrow).

Pathology

AIDS: SONOGRAPHIC MANIFESTATIONS

1. Masses. Nodal masses in the usual node sites (i.e., para-aortic and porta hepatis regions) are common. Lymphadenopathy may develop in other sites that are not routine (e.g., within the liver and kidney).
2. Kaposi's sarcoma. Kaposi's sarcoma is normally located in the limbs, but in the presence of AIDS, primary tumors, and metastatic lesions may involve the abdomen, the testes, and the liver. Bulky para-aortic nodes are common.
3. Renal manifestations. Patients with AIDS develop an AIDS-related nephritis. The kidneys become greatly enlarged and densely echogenic (see Fig. 18-8). Renal enlargement may occur before the increased echogenicity develops.
4. Right upper quadrant. In AIDS patients who present to ultrasound for right upper quadrant imaging because of fever, abdominal pain, and elevated alkaline phosphatase, the biliary tree should be scanned carefully for signs of AIDS cholangitis. The initial feature of AIDS cholangitis may be thickening of the bile duct mucosa, followed by stricture formation and resultant intrahepatic

ductal dilatation. Gallbladder wall thickening in patients with AIDS is a common sonographic finding. Acalculous cholecystitis may be diagnosed sonographically by the presence of gallbladder wall edema and a positive sonographic Murphy's sign.

5. Fungal and parasitic infections. Unusual infections (Fig. 11-9), such as cryptococcosis or tuberculosis, are common. Abscesses may develop in any part of the abdomen. These abscesses may contain pus that is densely echogenic and can be confused with a tumor. Multiple abscesses may be present in the liver or spleen that, if fungal, may have an echopenic periphery to an echogenic center (see Chapter 8).
6. Hepatosplenomegaly. The liver and spleen are often massively enlarged, especially in HIV-infected children. Patients with AIDS may well have complications of alcoholism or intravenous drug abuse (e.g., an abnormal pancreas and evidence of portal hypertension).
7. Abdominal malignancies. Cancers such as non-Hodgkin's lymphoma are more common in patients with AIDS than in the general population. Ultrasound is helpful in identifying hepatic lesions in patients with AIDS-related lymphomas, which may appear as large confluent masses or scattered hypoechoic nodular densities throughout the liver. Abdominal lymphadenopathy is also common in the AIDS patient.

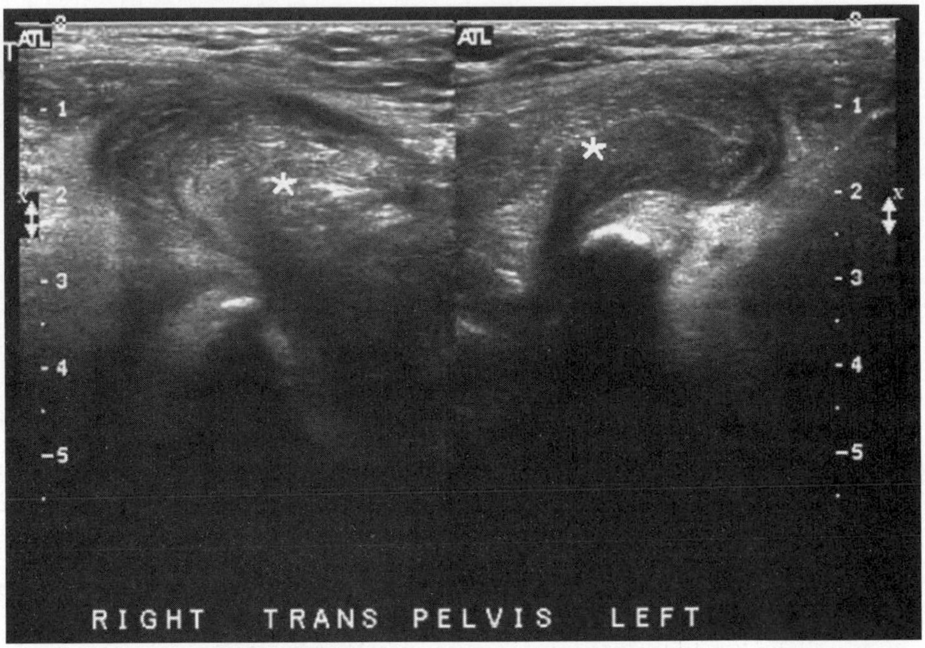

Figure 11-9. ■ *Tuberculous abscesses (*) in the groin in an AIDS patient. Dual image (split-screen) format in transverse orientation over each hip shows a complex mass tracking along the course of each psoas muscle. These proved to be tuberculous ("cold") abscesses. The patient was initially sent up from the surgery clinic for an ultrasound-guided biopsy of palpable bilateral hip masses that the clinicians thought were lymph nodes secondary to lymphoma.*

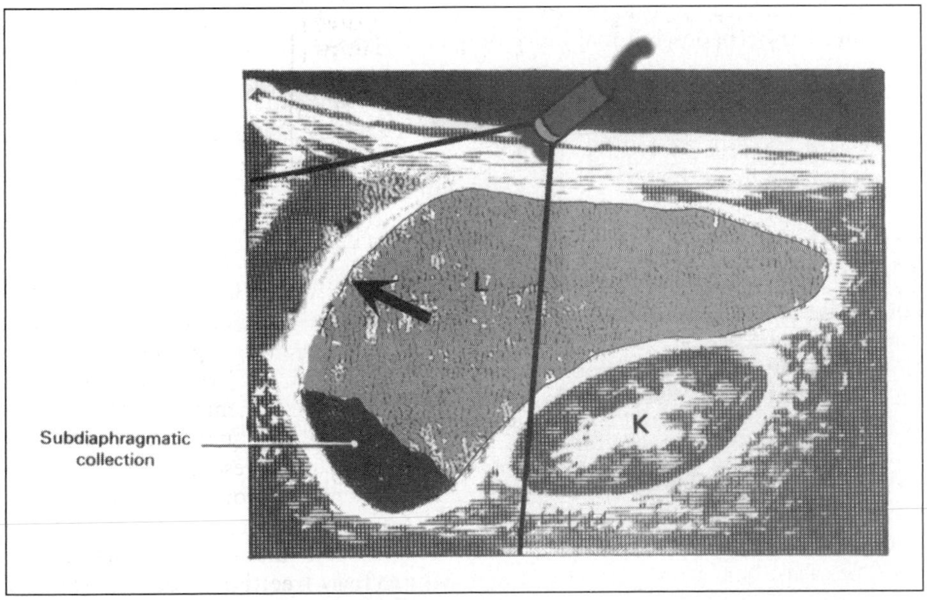

Figure 11-10. ■ *Right longitudinal section. A subphrenic abscess is shown. Subhepatic, perinephric, and subphrenic collections can all elevate and/or immobilize the diaphragm* (arrow).

ABSCESSES

Location

There are a number of potential spaces in the abdomen where fluid can collect and where abscesses commonly form. Abscesses tend to collect in spaces around organs and may displace structures or render them immobile (see Figs. 11-10 and 11-3).

1. Right subphrenic space. Between the diaphragm and the dome of the liver.
2. Subhepatic space (Morison pouch). Between the inferior posterior aspect of the liver and the right kidney.
3. Left subphrenic space. Between the spleen and the left hemidiaphragm.
4. Lesser sac. A large potential space mainly anterior to the pancreas and posterior to the stomach.
5. Pelvis cul-de-sac. Posterior to the uterus and anterior to the rectum.
6. Paracolic gutters. Along the flanks, lateral to the colon.
7. Perinephric space. There are various spaces around the kidneys. These are described in detail in Chapter 18, Renal Failure.

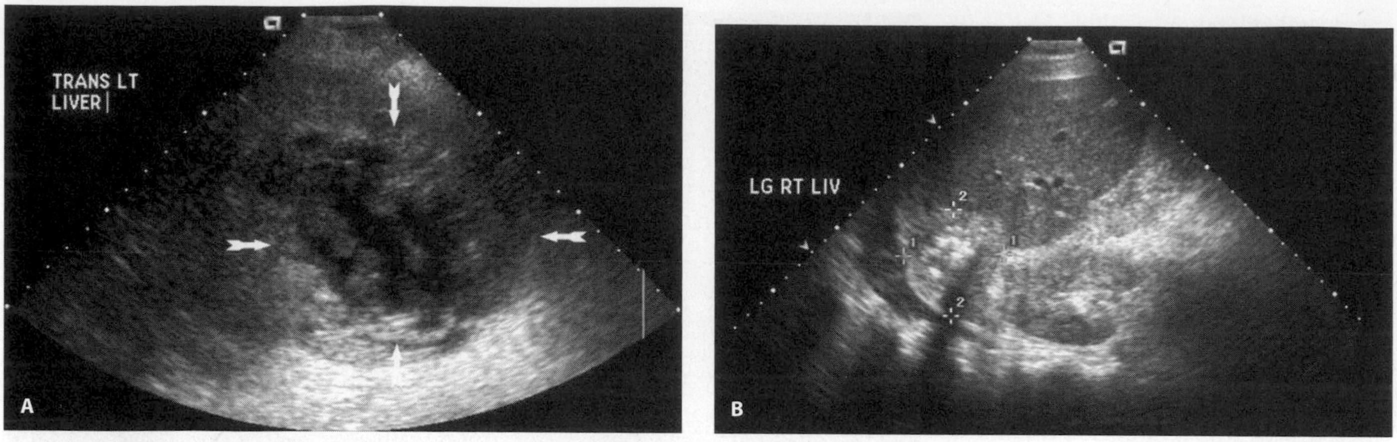

Figure 11-11. ■ *Intrahepatic abscesses in two different patients (both of whom had hepatic artery thrombosis after liver transplant). A. Complex, poorly marginated hypoechoic mass* (arrows) *containing a small amount of fluid. B. More solid and well-demarcated echogenic mass (between cursors) containing gas bubbles.*

8. Intrahepatic (Fig. 11-11)
9. Intranephric
10. Psoas area on either side of the spine medial to the kidney
11. Region of an incision

Remember that infection can originate in a site remote from the region where the abscess eventually settles.

Sonographic Appearance

Abscesses can appear predominantly fluid filled with thick, irregular walls. The amount of through transmission depends on the quantity and composition of the fluid. The contents of an abscess may resemble a dense mass; there are no typical features that consistently set abscesses apart from other entities.

Multiple abscesses may also be found within organs such as the liver (Fig. 11-11) or the kidney. Less frequently, they are found in the spleen and in the prostate. In alcoholics, a pancreatic pseudocyst may become infected, forming a pancreatic abscess. Abscesses in the mesentery may resemble bowel; local tenderness can help identify them. Those surrounded by gut often resemble fluid-filled loops of bowel with irregular shapes (see the section under Technique and Fig. 11-6)

Watch for the following:

1. Local tenderness. This may not be present if the patient is immunosuppressed.
2. Gas. When there is gas inside an abscess, shadowing varies with the amount and location of the gas (Figs. 11-2 and 11-7). Gas is a suspicious finding when it occurs in an unlikely location, such as in the liver or kidney parenchyma, or the abdominal wall. Correlation with a CT scan or an abdominal radiograph is helpful. A radiograph is often the precursor of the sonogram, suggesting, for example, an elevated diaphragm. Scan from a posterior angle in the supine position if there is gas in the abscess so the gas does not obscure the beam as it would if scanning from an anterior approach (Fig. 11-7).
3. Debris. Some collections contain debris, which can appear to be solid and homogeneous but may float or settle in a dependent portion to create a fluid-fluid level. To distinguish from a solid mass, turn the patient and observe the movement of the debris.

Draining an Abscess

Aspirating an abscess under ultrasonic control is considerably helpful in clinical management because it allows identification of the responsible microorganism and may permit curative drainage (Chapter 54). In general, ultrasound-guided interventions in the abdomen and pelvis are cheaper, faster, safer, and more effective than those using CT-guidance. Ultrasound can be used in at least 90% of cases.

INFLAMMATORY CHANGES

Most organs respond to infection in a similar fashion, and without abscess formation. In the involved area, the organ becomes swollen and more sonolucent. Local tenderness is present and should be noted by the sonographer.

DIAPHRAGMATIC MOBILITY

Real time will allow the demonstration of a hemidiaphragm's mobility, which is decreased when inflammation is present or when flanked with fluid. If assessing for paradoxical motion, watch both sides simultaneously. This step is especially easy in an infant; if the patient is on a respirator, take care to observe the motion briefly with the patient breathing on his or her own if possible. Diaphragmatic paralysis may be overlooked if the patient is on the respirator. Because ultrasound is portable, it may be used for this purpose in the intensive care unit. If movement is not easily detected, have the patient sniff. Diaphragmatic motion may be quantified by using M-mode techniques.

GOSSYPIBOMA

A retained sponge has a very distinctive appearance: a dense linear echo in the midgut area with well-defined shadowing seen at the site of tenderness (Fig. 11-2).

HEPATOMAS AND RENAL CELL CARCINOMAS

Hepatomas and hypernephromas are acknowledged causes of fever (see Chapters 8 and 17).

HEMATOMAS

Hematomas, whether occurring postoperatively or due to trauma, can cause fever (Fig. 11-12).

Appearance

Hematoma appearances change rapidly. When fresh, hematomas are usually echo-free. Within a few hours, they generally become echogenic. After a few days, they become partially echopenic, and when older, they may become so echopenic again that a subcapsular hematoma may be mistaken for ascites.

Location

Depending on the type and location of the surgical procedure or trauma, hematomas can form in many different locations. Some common sites for hematoma formation after gynecologic surgery are in the cul-de-sac, in the broad ligament, adjacent to the surgical site, in the anterior abdominal wall, and in the myometrium (Fig. 11-8). Hematomas in coagulopathic patients often occur in the rectus sheath or in the iliopsoas muscles.

Hematomas occurring after Cesarean delivery can be divided into three types (Fig. 11-8): superficial wound hematomas, subfascial hematomas, and bladder-flap hematomas. Patients are usually febrile and have a drop in hemoglobin.

1. The superficial variety is anterior to the rectus muscles (see Chapter 14) and involves the incision.
2. The subfascial type is posterior to the rectus muscles and much more serious, requiring surgical intervention. This space is anterior to the bladder but extends into the retropubic area; 2,500 mL of fluid can collect in this space before a mass may be palpable (Fig. 11-8).
3. A bladder-flap hematoma begins at the incision in the lower uterine segment behind the bladder, but it is covered by a fold of peritoneum that was disrupted during the surgery. Although bleeding is usually confined by the "flap," it can spread along the broad ligaments into the retroperitoneum.

After a renal transplant, hematomas may form in a subcapsular location, in the perinephric area, or in the retroperitoneum.

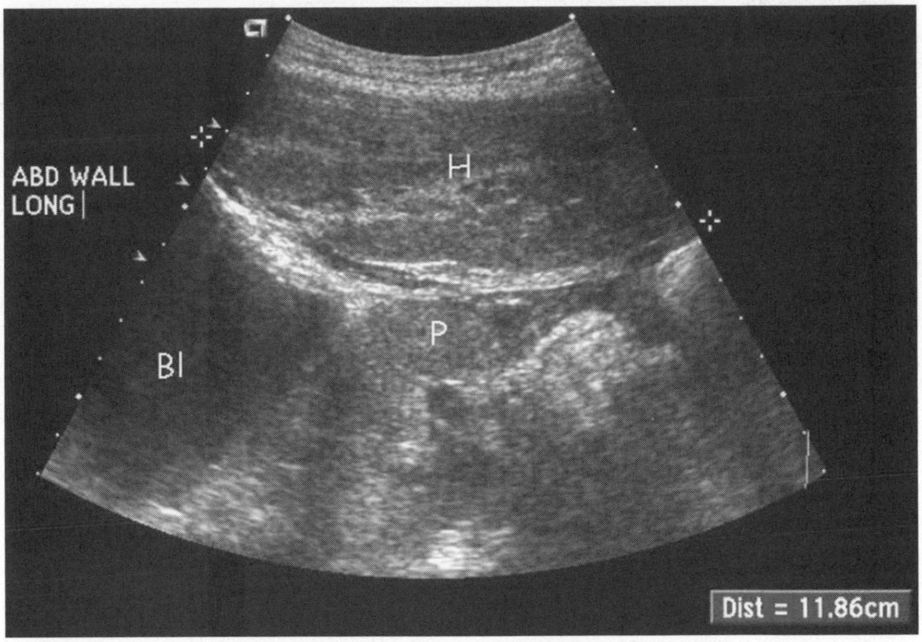

Figure 11-12. ■ *Hematoma (H, between cursors) following biopsy. This pancreatic transplant patient underwent a percutaneous biopsy that inadvertently lacerated the inferior epigastric artery and led to a 12-cm hematoma in the rectus sheath.* P, *pancreas transplant.*

Hematomas generally resolve, but they may also develop into abscesses. Hematomas tend to spread along fascial planes rather than break through tissue planes as abscesses do. If the hematoma is due to trauma, ask the patient's advice on where to start your search.

Pitfalls

1. Bowel versus abscess. Examine the area for several minutes with real time, perform a water enema, or give fluid by mouth. Go back repeatedly to a worrisome area; if it is gut, it often changes. Be careful to duplicate the exact scan plane each time.
2. Gossypiboma versus persistent bowel gas. Depending on location, try a water enema to decide whether you are dealing with a stubborn gas pocket in bowel or a sponge. It may be necessary to rescan on another day to see whether there is no change; CT is also an option because retained sponges have a characteristic CT appearance (Fig. 11-2B).
3. Fat deposits. In obese patients, there may be a deposit of deep subcutaneous fat in the midepigastric region that can resemble an abscess. This fat is symmetrical on both sides of the midline and has well-defined borders.
4. Ascites versus abscess/hematoma. A localized area of ascites may be mistaken for an abscess or echo-free hematoma. Place the patient in the erect, Trendelenburg, or decubitus position: ascites will shift, but an abscess or hematoma will not.
5. Reverberation problems (pseudobladder). "Mirror" reverberations may create an apparent fluid collection deep in the pelvis behind the bladder. The following maneuvers may show the "collection" to be an artifact (Chapter 57).
   a. Scanning through a different part of the bladder or through the psoas muscles may cause the suspicious area to change size or disappear because this will change the distance between the transducer and the bladder border.
   b. Measuring the distance from the skin to the center of the collection may show that the supposed collection lies well behind the patient's back.

Where Else to Look

1. If nodes are present, look for neoplasm or splenic enlargement due to lymphoma.
2. If one abscess is seen, look for more.
3. If a neoplasm is seen, look for metastases.

SELECTED READING

American College of Radiology. ACR Appropriateness Criteria for Imaging Evaluation of Patients with Acute Abdominal Pain and Fever. *Am Coll Radiol* 2001. http://guideline.gov/summary/summary.aspx?ss=15&doc_id=3258&nbr=2484&string=.

Bechtold RE, Dyer RB, Zagoria RJ, et al. The perirenal space: relationship of pathologic processes to normal retroperitoneal anatomy. *Radiographics* 1996;16:841–854.

Keane MAR, Finlayson C, Joseph AEA. A histological basis for the sonographic snowstorm in opportunistic infection of the liver and spleen. *Clin Radiol* 1995;50:220–222.

Gaillot O, Maruejouls C, Abachin E, et al. Nosocomial outbreak of Klebsiella pneumoniae producing SHV-5 extended-spectrum beta-lactamase, originating from a contaminated ultrasonography coupling gel. *J Clin Microbiol* 1998;36:1357–1360.

Molmenti EP, Balfe DM, Kanterman RY, et al. Anatomy of the retroperitoneum: observations of the distribution of pathologic fluid collections. *Radiology* 1996;200:95–103.

Muradali D, Gold WL, Phillips A, et al. Can ultrasound probes and coupling gel be a source of nosocomial infection in patients undergoing sonography: an in vivo and in vitro study. *Am J Roentgenol* Jun 1995; 164(6):1521–1524.

Pantongrag-Brown L, Nelson AM, Brown AE, et al. Gastrointestinal manifestations of acquired immunodeficiency syndrome: radiologic-pathologic correlation. *Radiographics* 1995;15:1155–1178.

Roth AR, Basello GM. Approach to the adult patient with fever of unknown origin. *Am Fam Physician* Dec 2003;1:68(11):2223–2228. Review.

12 Palpable Left Upper Quadrant Mass

TOM WINTER

SONOGRAM ABBREVIATIONS

Ad	Adrenal gland
Ao	Aorta
D	Diaphragm
GBl	Gallbladder
IVC	Inferior vena cava
K	Kidney
L	Liver
P, Pa	Pancreas
PPs	Pancreatic pseudocysts
R	Ribs
Sp	Spleen
St	Stomach

KEY WORDS

Gaucher's Disease. One of the group of "storage" diseases in which fat and proteins are abnormally deposited in the body, typically in the liver, spleen, and bone marrow.

Myeloproliferative Disorder. Term referring to chronic myeloid leukemia, myelofibrosis, and polycythemia vera—a spectrum of hematologic conditions associated with a large spleen. Sometimes one entity will change into another.

Pancreatic Pseudocyst. Fluid collection produced by the pancreas during acute pancreatitis.

Pheochromocytoma. A hormone-producing tumor that generally arises from the adrenal glands.

Portal Hypertension. A rise in the pressure of the venous blood flowing into the liver through the portal venous system, causing an increase in the size of the portal, splenic, and superior mesenteric veins and of the spleen. If portal hypertension is severe, additional vessels known as *collaterals* develop at multiple points within the abdomen (see Fig. 6-7).

Splenomegaly. Enlargement of the spleen.

Subphrenic Abscess. An abscess lying under the left or right diaphragm. Such abscesses commonly follow a surgical procedure in the area, for example, an operation on the stomach.

The Clinical Problem

SPLENOMEGALY

The most frequent left upper quadrant mass is an enlarged spleen. Splenomegaly occurs in a wide variety of disease states.

1. Infectious diseases such as tuberculosis, malaria, infectious mononucleosis ("mono"), and subacute bacterial endocarditis are often accompanied by an enlarged spleen. (The spleen is occasionally the site of an abscess, particularly with subacute bacterial endocarditis or any other bacteremic state.)
2. Myeloproliferative disorders such as myelofibrosis may be characterized by splenomegaly.
3. Splenomegaly occurs when the veins draining the spleen are obstructed, as in portal hypertension or splenic vein thrombosis. Both pancreatic cancer and pancreatitis can cause splenic vein thrombosis.
4. Metastases may occur in the spleen; however, the spleen is not often the site of neoplastic involvement.
5. Lymphoma and leukemia may involve the spleen directly or cause splenomegaly as a secondary phenomenon because blood production is disorganized.
6. Storage disorders such as Gaucher's disease may cause splenomegaly.

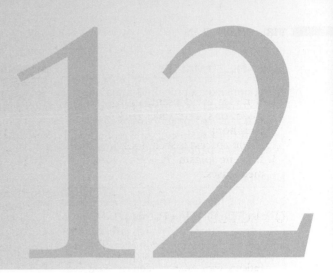

FLUID-FILLED MASSES

A left upper quadrant fluid-filled mass is quite common and may be (1) a renal mass such as hydronephrosis or a large renal cyst, (2) a splenic cyst, (3) an adrenal cyst, or (4) a pancreatic pseudocyst.

NEOPLASMS

Neoplastic masses in the left upper quadrant include (1) retroperitoneal sarcomas; (2) adrenal tumors, which are usually small (e.g., metastases, pheochromocytoma) but occasionally become large; and (3) pancreas and kidney cancers, which can spread into the left upper quadrant and cause a palpable abdominal mass.

The surgical approach is dictated by the origin and nature of the mass. Cysts may be treated conservatively or by cyst puncture rather than by surgery.

ABSCESSES

The left subdiaphragmatic region is a common site for abscess collections, particularly in postoperative patients after removal of the spleen or stomach operations.

Anatomy

SPLEEN

The spleen is the predominant organ in the left upper quadrant. It lies immediately under the left hemidiaphragm and may be difficult to see because of gas in the neighboring lung and ribs. It lies superior to the left kidney and lateral to the adrenal gland and the tail of the pancreas. The left lobe of the liver is often in contact with the spleen.

The splenic texture is more echogenic than the liver or kidney. A group of high-level echoes in the spleen's center at its medial aspect represents the splenic hilum at the entrance of the splenic artery and vein.

ADRENAL GLANDS

See Chapter 16 for information pertaining to the adrenal glands.

Technique

LEFT SIDE VIEW (CORONAL)

The left-side-up position (right lateral decubitus) is the preferred position for investigating the left upper quadrant (Fig. 12-1). Angle the transducer somewhat obliquely so that it passes between the ribs. Place a pillow or a wedge under the patient to improve access to the left kidney (see Chapter 18). To identify your location, find the left kidney; the spleen will be superior to it. There should normally be nothing between the spleen and the left hemidiaphragm. Make sure the scan plane allows visualization above the diaphragm as well.

TRANSVERSE VIEWS

Transverse views are also obtained in the left-side-up position. The best access route is often far posterior. Administering fluids by mouth or through a nasogastric tube helps to define the stomach and its margin. Placing the patient in the supine position and scanning from the lateral aspect helps if lung interference is a problem.

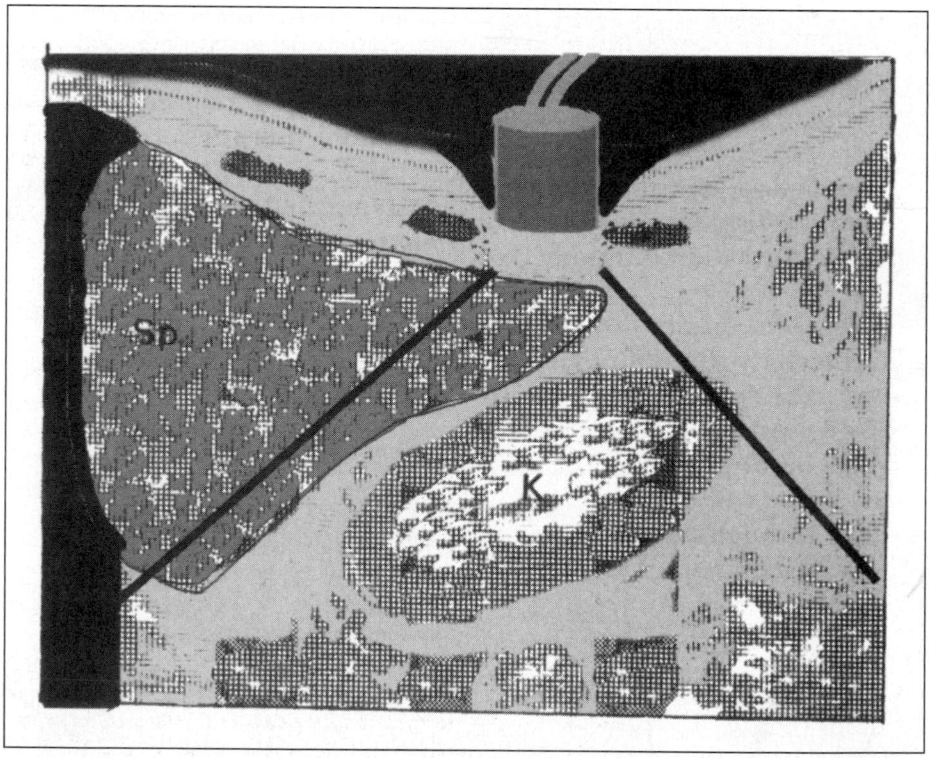

Figure 12-1. ■ *Left-side-up view of the spleen and left kidney. Ribs partially obscure the spleen and kidney.*

Pathology

SPLENOMEGALY

As one gains experience with sonography, it is generally obvious when the spleen is significantly enlarged, but criteria for documenting enlargement are still unsatisfactory. A good rule of thumb is as follows: if the transducer has a 90-degree angle and the superior/inferior border of the spleen cannot fit on an image, the spleen is enlarged. Beware of this method if the patient has a small anteroposterior diameter, because the liver and spleen are often flatter and longer as a normal configuration. Another useful rule of thumb in adults is that 95% of normal people have a spleen with a length smaller than 12 cm.

Splenic echogenicity may be altered when the spleen is enlarged. If it is less echogenic than usual, one should think of lymphoma; if more echogenic, consider myelofibrosis or infection (Fig. 12-2).

FOCAL SPLENIC MASSES

Although unusual, focal lesions may occur in the spleen (Figs. 12-3 through 12-6). Abscesses usually have irregular borders and some internal echoes; they may show shadowing associated with gas. In immunocompromised patients, multiple echopenic abscesses with echogenic centers may be seen in both the liver and the spleen. Metastatic lesions, which are rare, resemble those seen in the liver.

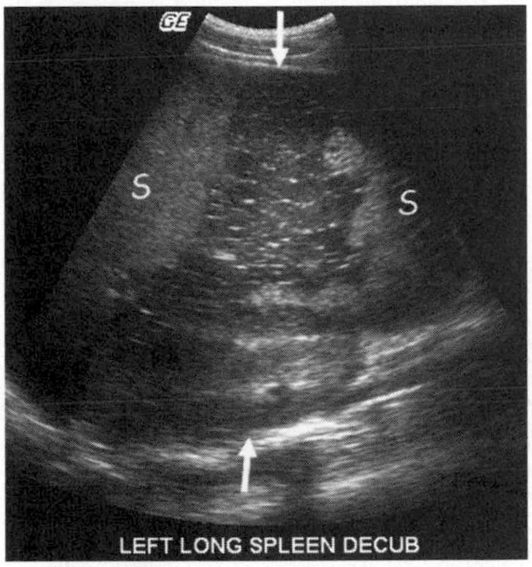

Figure 12-2. ■ *Splenomegaly and splenic infarct. A huge spleen (22 cm long) has a large infarct (heterogeneous region,* arrows*) in this patient with sickle-cell disease.*

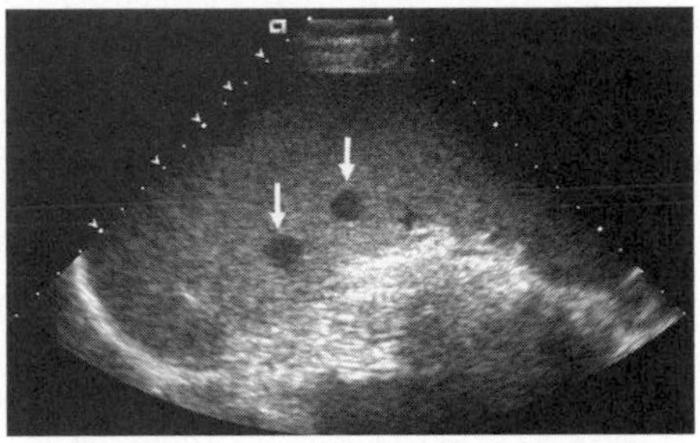

Figure 12-3. ■ *Leukemia. Two small focal deposits* (arrows) *are seen in the spleen.*

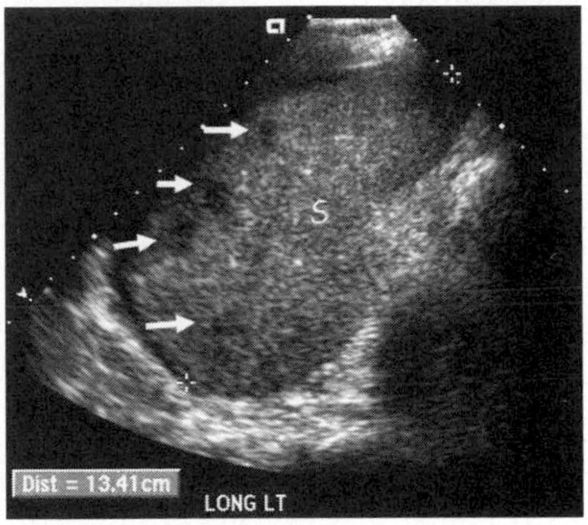

Figure 12-4. ■ *Septic emboli. Multiple infarcts* (arrows) *are seen at the periphery of an enlarged spleen (13.4 cm).*

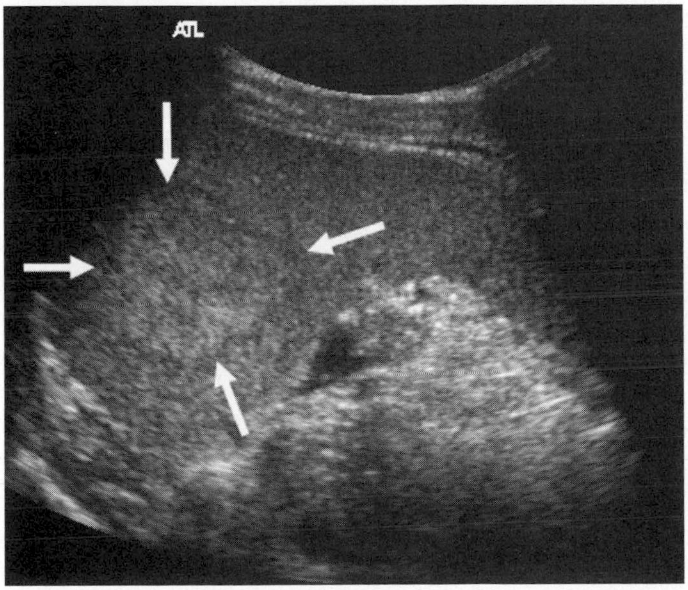

Figure 12-5. ■ *Benign hemangioma. A slightly hyperechoic 3.7-cm solid mass* (arrows) *is seen within the spleen.*

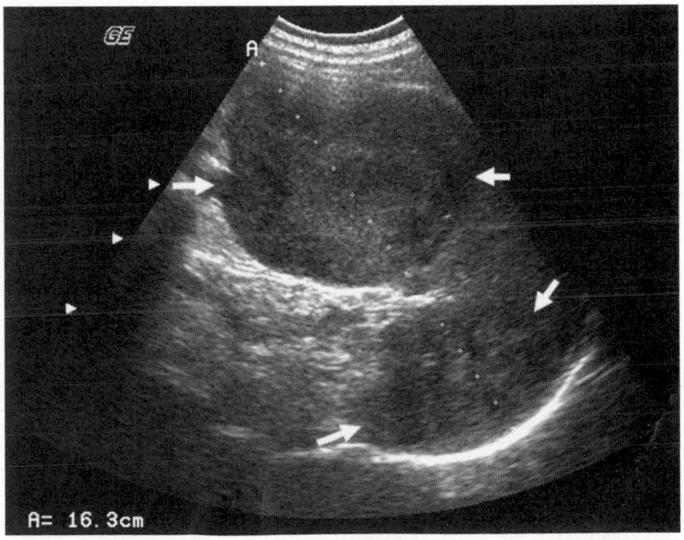

Figure 12-6. ■ *Non-Hodgkin's lymphoma. Two large hypoechoic solid masses are denoted by arrows in this enlarged spleen (16.3 cm).*

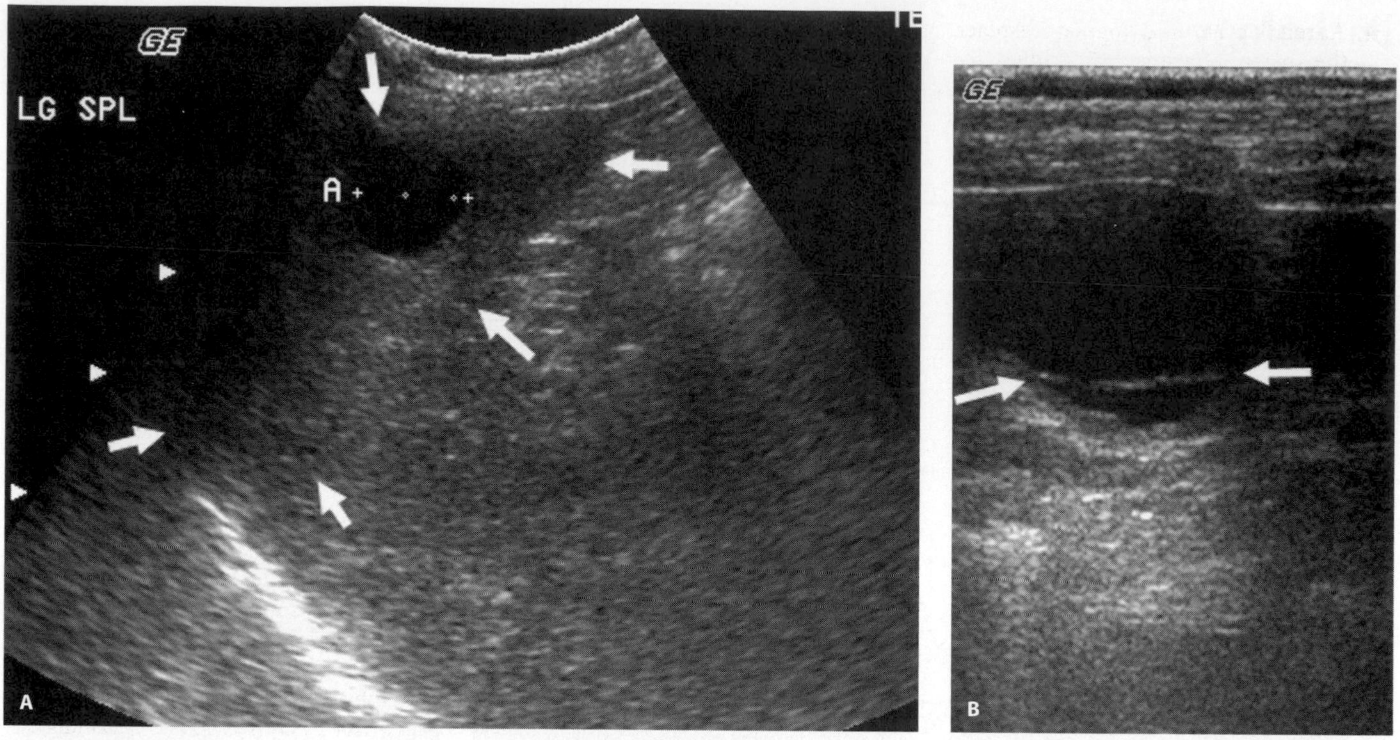

Figure 12-7. ■ *A. Typical benign splenic cyst* (arrows, *splenic outline;* cursors, *cyst). B. A linear transducer was used to obtain better resolution of the cyst, demonstrating a thin septation* (arrows). *This appearance remained stable over 3 years.*

CYSTS

If the left upper quadrant mass is a cyst, make sure you know the organ of origin.

1. Splenic cysts should have a rim of splenic parenchyma around them (Fig. 12-7). Having the patient sit in an upright position may help to show the complete cyst. Splenic cysts may contain many internal echoes and septa. Administer water to the patient in order to distinguish the stomach from a medially located cyst.
2. Renal cysts arise from the kidney, and there is usually a claw-like portion of renal parenchyma surrounding the cyst. The kidney may become very large with hydronephrosis. Differentiation of hydronephrosis from a cyst is simple in most instances (see Chapter 18).
3. Pancreatic pseudocysts often show some connection with the pancreas; they generally displace the spleen superiorly and the kidney inferiorly (Fig. 12-8). A clinical history of pancreatitis is usually easily obtained.

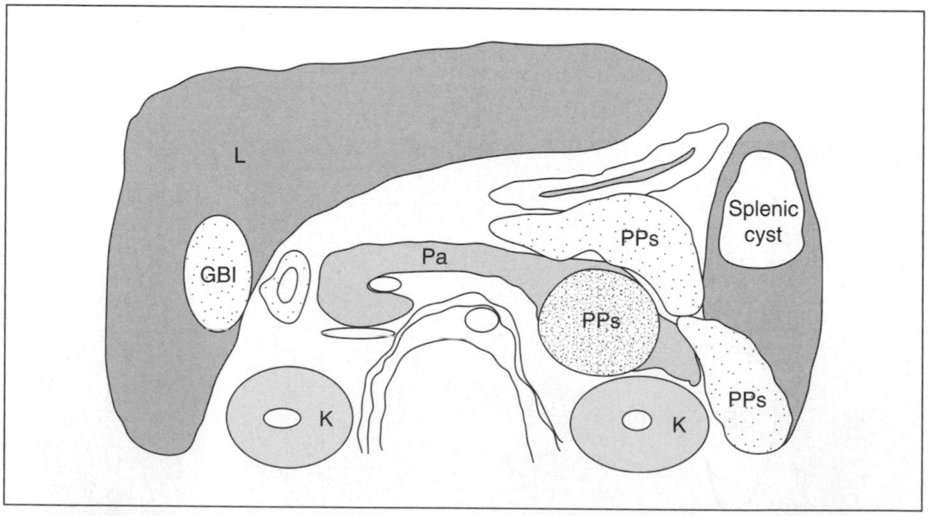

Figure 12-8. ■ *Typical location for pancreatic pseudocysts. Pancreatic pseudocysts are shown in the pancreas, in the lesser sac, and lateral to the left kidney. Pancreatic cysts are usually echo-free but can contain internal echoes. A cyst in the spleen is also shown.*

4. Adrenal cysts and masses displace the spleen anteriorly, the kidney inferiorly, and the pancreas anteriorly (Fig. 12-9). Adrenal cysts may have a calcified border; if so, the rim of the mass lesion will be densely echogenic, and through transmission will not be seen.

SUBPHRENIC ABSCESS

A fluid collection located in the splenic site following splenectomy or between the diaphragm and the spleen may represent a left subphrenic abscess. These abscesses may be difficult to see because this area is so inaccessible unless, as is common, there is a coincident pleural effusion.

An infected hematoma often develops where the spleen used to lie. Bowel may fall into the splenectomy site. Have the patient drink some water to distinguish the two. Look for pleural effusions above the diaphragm.

SOLID MASS

If the mass is solid, displacing the adjacent organs will indicate its origin.

1. Retroperitoneal sarcomas will displace the kidney, spleen, and pancreas anteriorly.
2. Renal neoplasms will lie inferior to the spleen and pancreas.
3. Accessory spleen tissue, a very common incidental finding, appears as a small round solid mass adjacent to the spleen.

Pitfalls

1. Left lobe of the liver versus perisplenic collection. The left lobe of the liver may extend superior to the spleen, especially if a partial hepatectomy has been performed. Trace the suspect "mass" into the normal liver, demonstrating continuity. Follow the left portal vein into the suspect mass. The liver is a little less echogenic than the spleen. There is virtually no interface between the two. Note color Doppler evidence of flow within the liver, a finding not expected in a perisplenic fluid collection.
2. Stomach versus left upper quadrant collection. The stomach may look like a left upper quadrant fluid collection. Give fluid by mouth, and peristalsis and the ingested fluid will be seen.
3. Spleen versus effusion. The spleen may resemble a pleural effusion if the sonographer is not careful to establish where the kidney lies, because in an obese patient, a more or less horizontal diaphragm may not be imaged adequately. If there is any difficulty in determining what represents the diaphragm, have the patient sniff through his or her nose. The diaphragm will move if it is not paralyzed.
4. Splenic hilum. An echogenic area at the site where the splenic vein and splenic artery enter the spleen, the hilum can be mistaken for a neoplasm. Real-time and color Doppler will show vessels in this area.
5. Subphrenic versus subpulmonic collection. It may be difficult to distinguish a subphrenic (below the diaphragm) from a subpulmonic (below the lung but above the diaphragm) collection if the diaphragm is not easily seen. Distinguishing between the spleen and a pleural effusion is the key to recognizing the location of the fluid. The kidney lies just below the spleen and is a useful landmark.

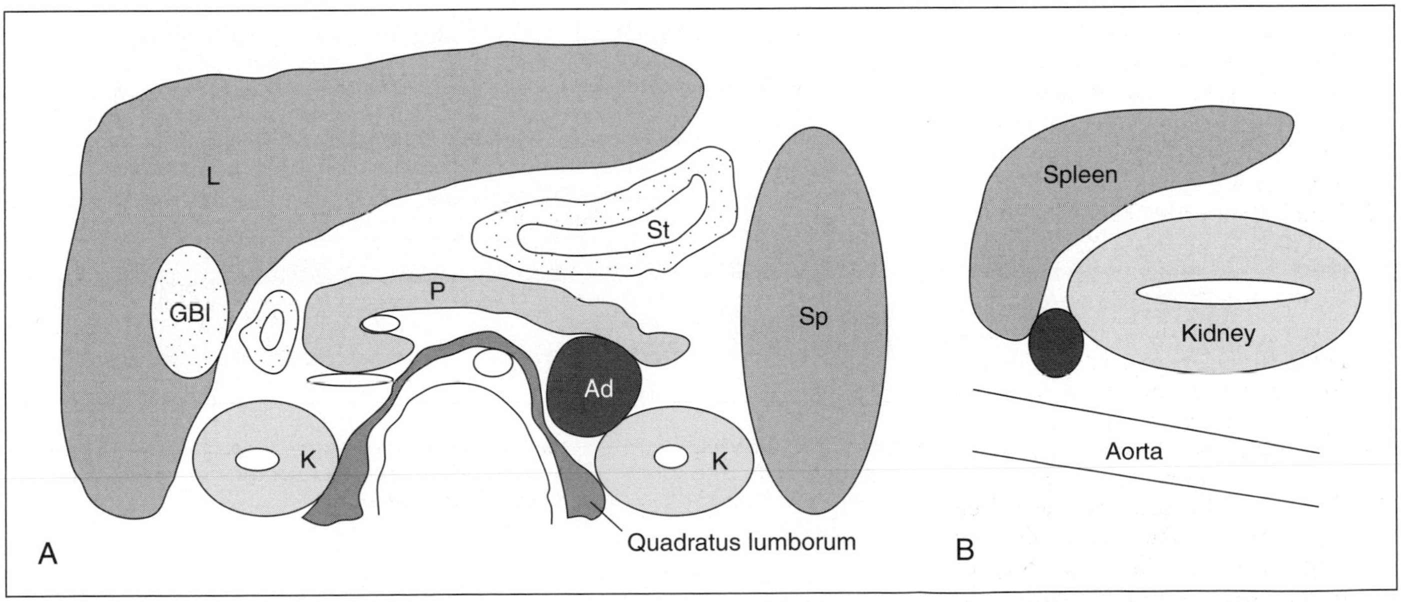

Figure 12-9. ■ *Adrenal mass.* ***A.*** *An adrenal mass* (Ad) *displaces the spleen laterally, the kidney posteriorly, and the pancreas anteriorly.* ***B.*** *On a coronal view, an adrenal mass will displace the kidney inferiorly, the spleen superiorly, and the aorta medially.*

6. Inverted diaphragm. If the left diaphragm is inverted by a left pleural effusion, an apparent left upper quadrant cystic mass may develop. A longitudinal section will show the true site of the diaphragm and reveal that the cystic area—the pleural effusion—is intrathoracic (Fig. 12-10).
7. Accessory spleens. Additional round or ovoid echopenic circular masses may be seen around the spleen, representing accessory spleens. The acoustic texture will be the same as the spleen.
8. Calcified granulomas form echogenic foci, often with acoustic shadowing within the spleen and are relatively common. In the United States, they usually indicate that the patient has been exposed to histoplasmosis (a generally benign and often undetected infection found with high frequency in those who live along the Mississippi and St. Lawrence river valleys).

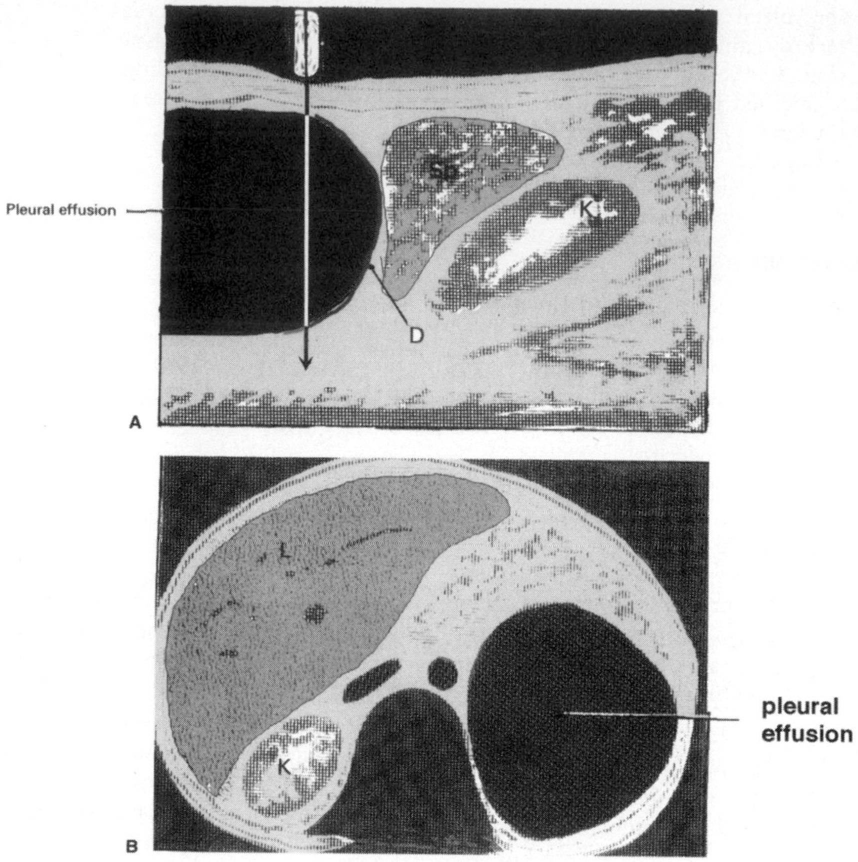

Figure 12-10. ■ *Pleural effusion. **A.** A very large pleural effusion may appear as a left upper quadrant mass. The diaphragm may be inverted, and the spleen and kidney may be displaced inferiorly. **B.** On a transverse view, a large pleural effusion inverting the diaphragm can look like a large cyst.*

Where Else to Look

1. If splenomegaly is present:
   a. Examine the liver for evidence of diffuse liver disease (cirrhosis), portal and splenic vein enlargement, and collaterals with portal hypertension.
   b. Note whether nodes are present in association with splenomegaly and lymphoma.
2. If the mass appears to be a pancreatic pseudocyst, look for the stigmata of alcoholism elsewhere and evidence of pancreatitis in the remainder of the pancreas.
3. If the left upper quadrant mass is hydronephrosis, look for the cause of obstruction in the pelvis along the course of the ureter.

SELECTED READING

Goerg C, Schwerk WB, Goerg K. Splenic lesions: sonographic patterns, follow-up, differential diagnosis. *Eur J Radiol* 1991;13:59–66.

Lamb PM, Lund A, Kanagasabay RR, et al. Spleen size: how well do linear ultrasound measurements correlate with three-dimensional CT volume assessments? *Br J Radiol* 2002;75:573–577.

Megremis SD, Vlachonikolis IG, Tsilimigaki AM. Spleen length in childhood with US: normal values based on age, sex, and somatometric parameters. *Radiology* 2004;231:129–134.

Siniluoto TMJ, Tikkakoski TA, Lahde ST, et al. Ultrasound or CT in splenic diseases? *Acta Radiol* 1994;35:597–605.

Ultrasound of Abdominal Wall Masses

CYNTHIA L. RAPP

13

SONOGRAM ABBREVIATIONS

CFA	Common femoral artery
CFV	Common femoral vein
IEA	Inferior epigastric artery
LA	Linea alba
SP cord	Spermatic cord

KEY WORDS

Aponeurosis. A sheet-like fibrous membrane, resembling a flattened tendon, which serves as a fascia to bind muscles together or as a means of connecting muscle to bone.

Fascia. Dense connective tissue layer.

Hernia. A protrusion of a part or structure through the tissues normally containing it.

Epigastric Hernia. Midline hernia superior to the umbilicus.

Femoral Hernia. Herniation of the abdominal contents though the femoral canal, leading to a bulge below the inguinal ligament.

Hypogastric Hernia. Midline hernia inferior to the umbilicus.

Incarcerated Hernia. The trapping of abdominal contents within the hernia itself, which cannot be reduced or pushed back.

Inguinal Hernia ("Groin Hernia"). The most common (75%) of all abdominal hernias. Subdivided anatomically into direct and indirect, although this distinction is generally not of surgical importance.

Direct. Acquired groin hernia, ~25% of all hernias.

Indirect. Congenital groin hernia, ~50% of all hernias.

Interstitial Hernia. Hernia contents that extend between muscle or fascial layers.

Recurrent Hernia. A hernia that has been previously repaired surgically and now has returned.

Spigelian Hernia. Protrusion of properitoneal or intraperitoneal contents through the semilunar line.

Strangulated Hernia. Injury to the blood circulation to the intestine caused by incarceration that results in dead bowel and a surgical emergency.

Umbilical/Paraumbilical Hernia. Hernia that develops in and around the area of the umbilicus (belly button or naval).

International Normalized Ratio (INR). A laboratory test that measures one aspect of the blood's ability to clot. Commonly used to monitor patients taking warfarin (Coumadin) as a blood thinner, the INR has replaced the older prothrombin time (PT) test that was used to measure how much blood coagulation has been inhibited. Values that are too high predispose the patient to spontaneous hemorrhage.

Linea Alba. The median vertical tendinous line formed of fibers from the aponeuroses of the two rectus abdominis muscles that extends from the xiphoid process to the pubic symphysis.

Peritoneal Membrane. Inner abdominal cavity lining; it fully surrounds the intestines and abdominal organs. It lies between the muscles of the abdominal wall and intestines.

Process Vaginalis. A pouch of peritoneum that is carried into the scrotum by the descent of the testicle and which in the scrotum forms the tunica vaginalis.

Properitoneal. Lying between the parietal peritoneum and the ventral musculature of the body cavity (herniated mass, fat).

Semilunar Line. A curved line on the ventral abdominal wall parallel to the midline and halfway between it and the side of the body that marks the lateral border of the rectus abdominis muscle. Also known as the *linea semilunaris*.

Tunica Vaginalis. The inner covering of the spermatic cord, continuous above the deep inguinal ring with the transversalis fascia.

Valsalva Maneuver. Performed by attempting to forcibly exhale while keeping the mouth and nose closed.

Volvulus. A twisting of the bowel on itself, causing intestinal blockage.

RELEVANT LABORATORY VALUES

INR: 0.9 to1.1 (normal). When the patient is taking a blood thinner such as warfarin (Coumadin), one generally tries to maintain the INR between 2 and 3.5 (depending on the disease being treated). Values greater than 5 dramatically increase the risk of a spontaneous hemorrhage.

Clinical Problem

Abdominal wall masses are a common clinical problem. Hernias are one of the most common causes of abdominal wall masses and may be difficult to diagnose by clinical acumen alone. Sonography is an accurate means of identifying abdominal wall hernias when the clinical diagnosis is uncertain. The clinical diagnosis of hernias is particularly difficult in females, obese, and postoperative patients, and those with recurrent pain or swelling after hernia repair. Even when the physical findings alone establish the diagnosis of hernia, they cannot accurately characterize individual hernia features. Ultrasound can diagnose hernias in cases when the clinical findings are nonspecific. Additionally, it can accurately characterize the individual hernia features that impact treatment. Sonography can determine the hernia's anatomic location, its contents, and complications such as incarceration, bowel obstruction, volvulus, and strangulation. Sonography is the only imaging modality that allows real-time evaluation of the hernia and its contents. Keep in mind that sonographic diagnosis of hernias may be difficult. Therefore, it is essential to be familiar with the sonographic anatomy, the variable appearances, and the common locations of hernias.

Other causes of abdominal wall masses include hematomas, infections, and soft-tissue tumors. Ultrasound and clinical clues permit rapid and accurate assessment of the first two of these possibilities. Although ultrasound is generally not accurate in fully evaluating true soft-tissue tumors, it alerts one to the fact that a tumor is present and may assist in performing a needle biopsy of the mass in the appropriate clinical setting.

Anatomy

Hernia type is determined by site of origin, which is limited to areas where aponeurosis and fascia are not protected by overlying striated muscle. There are two main categories: groin hernias and anterior abdominal wall hernias. Groin hernias include inguinal (both indirect and direct varieties) and femoral types. Anterior abdominal wall hernias include umbilical, linea alba (epigastric and hypogastric), Spigelian, and incisional types. The anatomy differs for each hernia type; however, the scanning principles remain the same.

Hernia contents vary. Not all hernias contain bowel. In fact, the majority of hernias diagnosed by sonography contain only fat and membranes, with only a small percentage containing bowel and/or peritoneal fluid. Preoperative recognition of the hernia contents helps to assess the risk of complications such as strangulation.

Hernias are defined as "a protrusion of a part or structure through the tissues normally containing it." Thus, the fat within a hernia need not be intraperitoneal in origin (Fig. 13-1). Symptomatic, indirect inguinal, femoral, Spigelian, and linea alba hernias may contain only properitoneal fat. Unfortunately, it is not always possible to determine sonographically whether fat is intraperitoneal or properitoneal in origin.

Technique

Because the sonographic contrast between hernia contents and surrounding abdominal wall tissues is minimal, the key to diagnosis in most cases is demonstrating the movement of hernia contents during dynamic maneuvers. During the Valsalva maneuver, hernia contents move distally, and the hernia widens. During the relaxation after Valsalva, hernia contents move back toward the abdomen, and the sac narrows. Compression with the transducer reduces the hernia and pushes contents back toward the abdomen, whereas release of the transducer results in the opposite effect. Most hernias enlarge (and some are present only) in the upright position. Therefore, when a hernia is not demonstrable in the supine position, even after Valsalva maneuvers, it is important to scan the patient in the upright position. Failure to do so will result in some hernias being

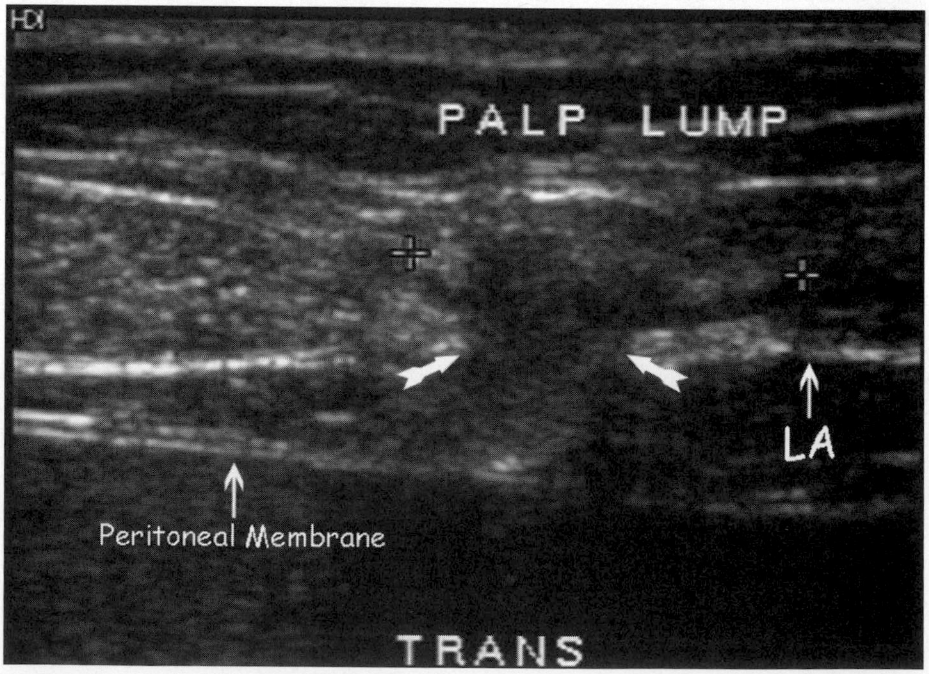

Figure 13-1. ■ *Transverse midline image demonstrates an epigastric (superior to the umbilicus) hernia containing properitoneal fat (between cursors). There is a defect* (arrows) *in the linea alba allowing the fat that normally lies between the peritoneal membrane and linea alba to be herniated.*

missed. Additionally, many hernias are symptomatic only in the upright position. Some hernias that are completely reducible in the supine position are nonreducible in the upright position. Competing diagnostic imaging studies, like computed tomography or magnetic resonance imaging, are not capable of evaluating patients in the upright position or in real time during dynamic maneuvers.

Pathology

INGUINAL HERNIAS

Inguinal hernias are the most common type of abdominal wall hernia, comprising about 75% of all hernias. There are two types of inguinal hernias: direct and indirect. Indirect hernias outnumber direct hernias by about two to one. To diagnose inguinal hernias, locate the internal inguinal ring by identifying the inferior epigastric vessels. While scanning in a transverse plane directly over the rectus muscle, three vessels can be visualized just posteriorly, one artery with two paired veins (Fig. 13-2). These are the inferior epigastric vessels.

Follow the inferior epigastric artery (IEA) to its origin from the external iliac artery. The IEA's origin marks the internal inguinal ring.

Indirect hernias arise in the internal (deep) inguinal ring and extend superficially and inferomedially down the inguinal canal anterior to the spermatic or the round ligament. Congenital indirect inguinal hernias can extend as far inferiorly as the processus vaginalis is patent—into the scrotum in males and the labium majorum in females. They are far more common in males than females; therefore, this type of hernia is more often clinically unsuspected in females. Patients with indirect inguinal hernias generally present with groin pain and/or swelling.

Indirect inguinal hernias may present with a wide or narrow neck (Fig. 13-3). Hernias with a wide neck are typically the sliding type. In hernias with a narrow neck and relatively volu-

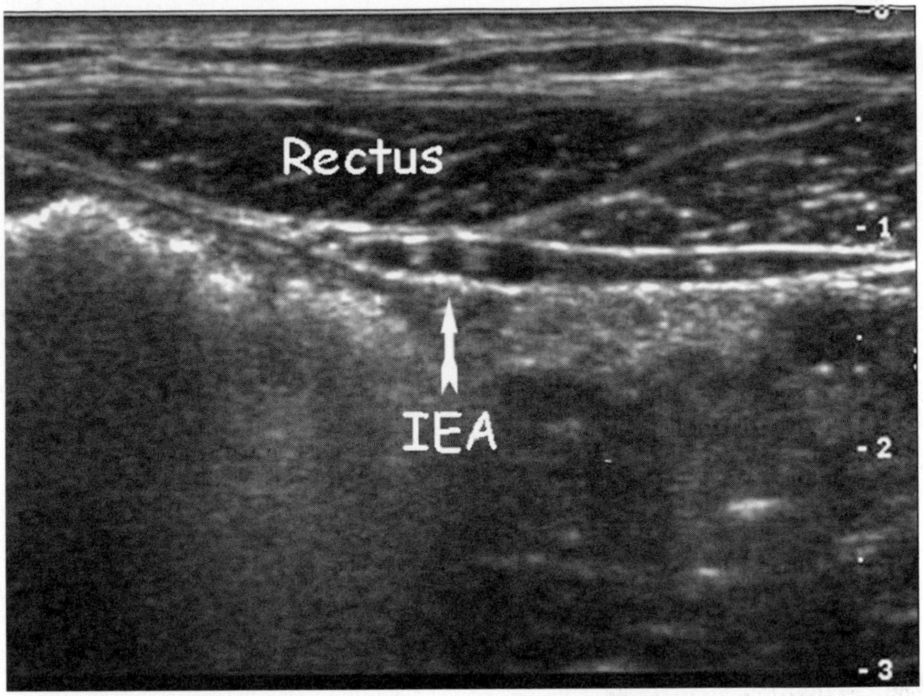

Figure 13-2. ■ *Transverse image scanning over the right rectus muscle showing the central IEA* (arrow) *with the paired epigastric veins on either side.*

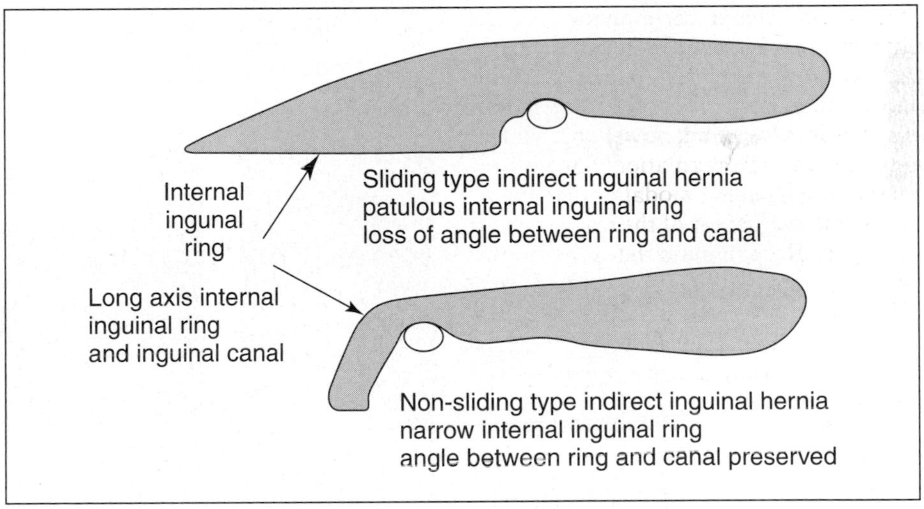

Figure 13-3. ■ *Diagram showing wide- and narrow-necked indirect inguinal hernias.*

minous sacs, strangulation is most likely to occur (Fig. 13-4). Strangulation, the most common and serious complication of a groin hernia, increases mortality and morbidity as well as the need for general anesthesia and hospitalization. In a strangulated hernia, the sac's contents are compressed, usually at the neck of the hernia, resulting in compromised blood supply with intestinal necrosis and obstruction. Incarceration is distinguished from strangulation, in that an incarcerated hernia's contents are also nonreducible, but the vascular supply is intact.

DIRECT INGUINAL HERNIAS

Direct inguinal hernias are the second most common type of hernia. They are acquired and occur as a result of a developed weakness of the transversalis fascia below the conjoined tendon. Direct inguinal hernias can occur from two different mechanisms: a thinning, stretching, and bulging of the transversalis fascia or an actual tear of the fascia.

Direct inguinal hernias (Fig. 13-5) originate in the transversalis fascia/conjoined tendon complex inferior and medial to the internal inguinal ring and the IEAs. Unlike indirect hernias, they do not pass through the inguinal ring and do not pass anterior to the IEA. The position of direct hernias relative to the spermatic cord also differs from that of indirect hernias. Direct hernias lie posterior and medial to the spermatic cord, whereas indirect hernias lie anterior. The direct hernia location posterior to the cord prevents them from extending all the way into the scrotum or labium majorum.

FEMORAL HERNIAS

Femoral hernias are difficult to diagnose clinically because of their deep location within the femoral canal. They are protrusions of the transversalis fascia and may contain either properitoneal fat or intraperitoneal contents.

Femoral hernias are far less common than inguinal hernias and occur mostly in women. Increased intrapelvic pressure and relaxation of ligaments during pregnancy probably contributes to the higher incidence. There is a high risk of incarceration and strangulation in femoral hernias because they tend to be

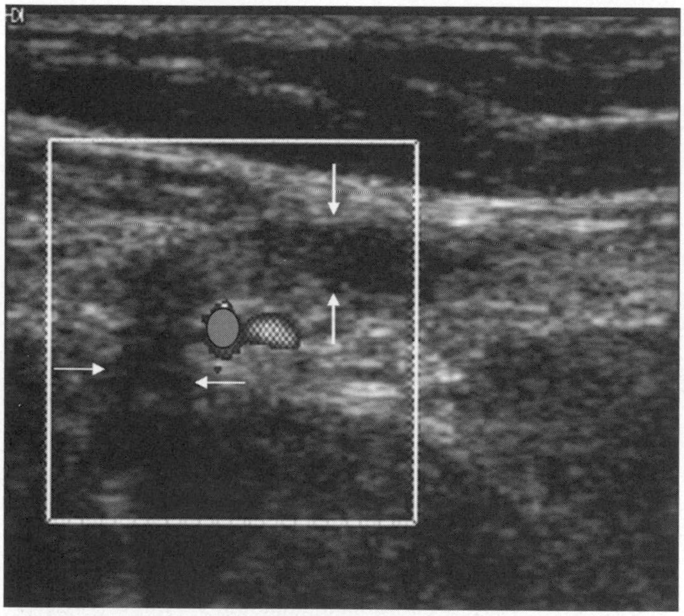

Figure 13-4. ■ *Longitudinal image of a small, narrow-necked, fat-containing indirect inguinal hernia* (arrows). *The keys to diagnosing an indirect inguinal hernia are that (1) it goes up and over (or anterior to) the IEA (oval in image) and (2) it is anterior to the spermatic cord.*

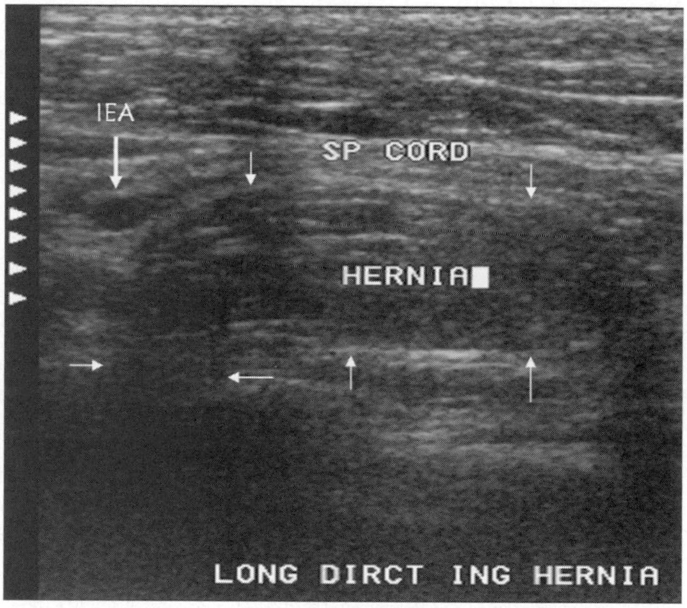

Figure 13-5. ■ *Longitudinal image showing a fat-containing direct inguinal hernia* (arrows). *The keys to diagnosing a direct inguinal hernia are that (1) it is inferior and medial to the internal inguinal ring, (2) it is a defect through the conjoined tendon, (3) it is posterior to the spermatic cord, and (4) it will never pass anterior to the IEA.*

long and have narrow necks. Femoral hernias (Fig. 13-6) protrude through the femoral canal into a potential empty space that is posterior to the inguinal ligament. The most common location is medial to the common femoral vein (CFV), but occasionally they can be found anterior or posterior to the CFV (Fig. 13-7).

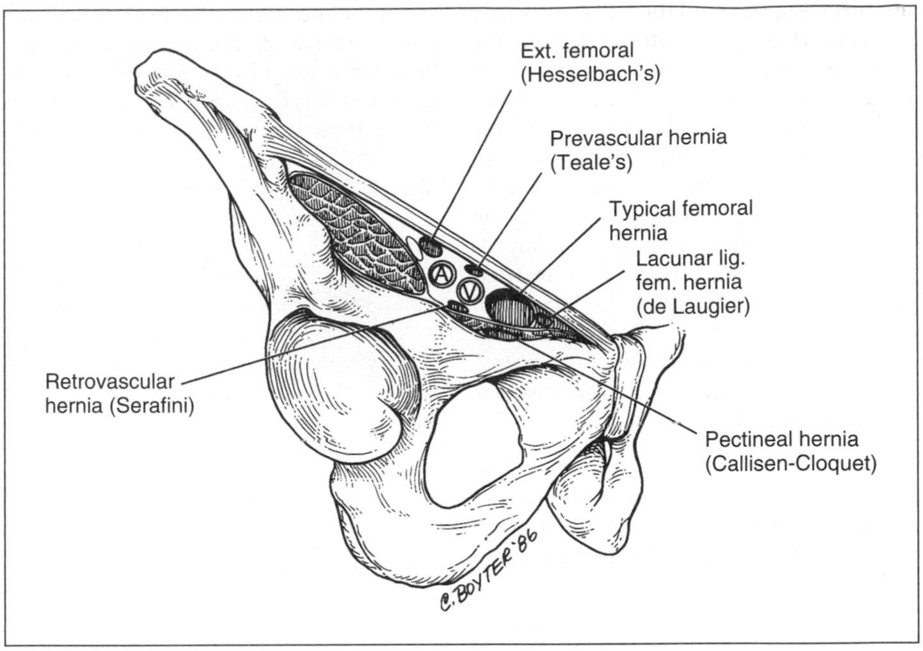

Figure 13-6. ■ *Diagram showing the possible locations of a femoral hernia.*

SPIGELIAN HERNIAS

Spigelian hernias (Fig. 13-8) are protrusions of properitoneal fat or intraperitoneal contents through deeper layers of the linea semilunaris, which lies between the lateral edge of the rectus abdominus muscle and the medial edge of the internal oblique muscle. Spigelian hernias may occur anywhere along the length of the semilunar line. They are most commonly found just above the point where the inferior epigastric vessels pierce the posterior wall of the rectus sheath, where the semilunar line is widest, and where the vessels penetrate the aponeuroses.

Spigelian hernias are rare and have a high frequency of incarceration. Clinical diagnosis of Spigelian hernias is particularly difficult because they are frequently intraparietal (interstitial), extending between muscle or fascial layers of the anterior abdominal wall rather than protruding all the way through the wall.

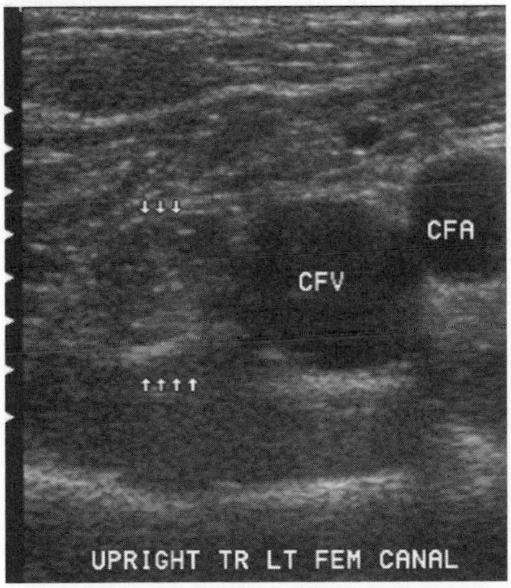

Figure 13-7. ■ *Transverse image of the left femoral canal demonstrating a fat-containing hernia* (arrows) *during a Valsalva maneuver. It is medial to the CFV, a typical location for femoral hernias.*

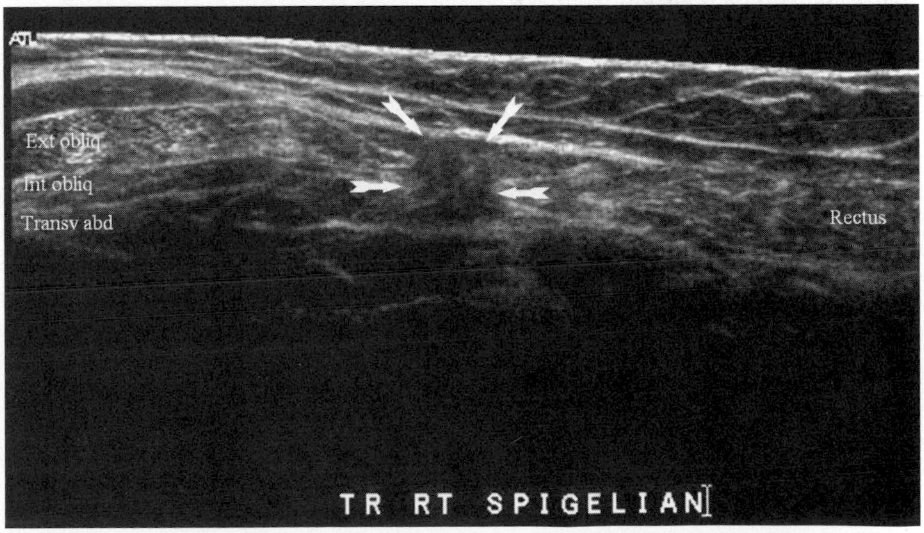

Figure 13-8. ■ *Transverse image demonstrating a right fat-containing Spigelian hernia* (arrows). *The semilunar line is found between the rectus muscle and the oblique muscles.*

MIDLINE HERNIAS

Midline hernias include linea alba and umbilical hernias. Linea alba hernias are protrusions of properitoneal fat or peritoneal contents though the linea alba (Fig. 13-9). Linea alba hernias that lie superior to the umbilicus are classified as epigastric and those inferior to the umbilicus are hypogastric. The linea alba is widest in the epigastric area, making these hernias more common than hypogastric hernias. Umbilical hernias are the most common ventral hernia. They are usually congenital and result from incomplete closure of the abdominal wall after ligation of the umbilical cord. The diagnosis of an umbilical hernia can usually be made clinically, unless the hernia sac is small or if obesity interferes with adequate palpation.

All midline hernias can be acquired or congenital. Acquired hernias can be traumatic but are more often the result of prolonged increased intra-abdominal pressure and distention, secondary to conditions such as pregnancy, ascites, and morbid obesity.

The majority of midline hernias have relatively small necks and are therefore prone to incarceration and/or strangulation (Fig. 13-10).

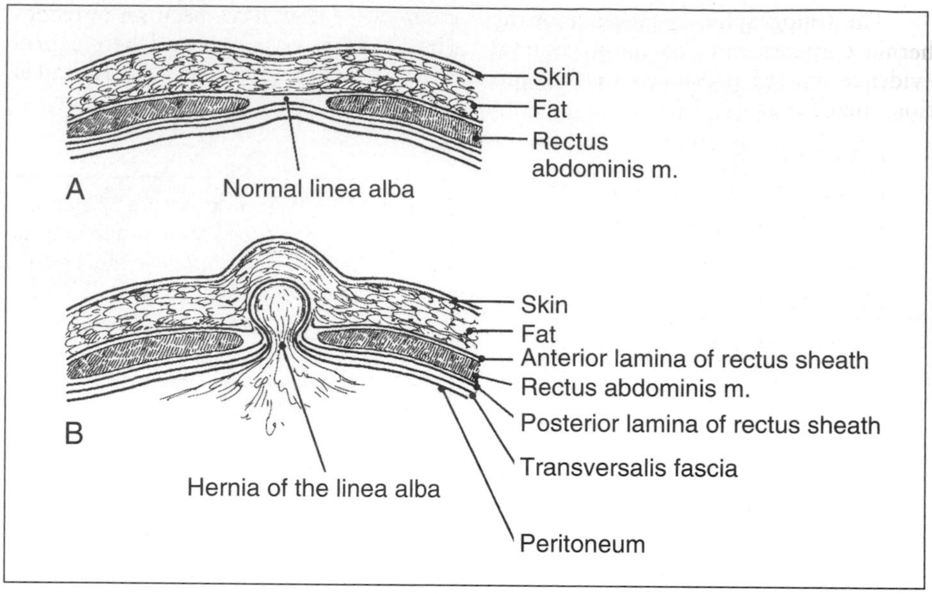

Figure 13-9. ■ *Diagram showing (A) normal linea alba and peritoneal membrane.* ***B.*** *Midline hernia through the peritoneal membrane and linea alba.*

INCISIONAL HERNIAS

Incisional hernias occur through surgical scars. They are most common in midline or paramedian incisions but can be seen with incisional scars in any location and of any size. Even laparoscopy trocar sites and bowel stomal sites may develop incisional hernias.

Predisposing factors include obesity and wound infection with subsequent dehiscence. Large, visible, or palpable incisional hernias pose no diagnostic dilemma; however, small hernias that do not extend through the full thickness of the abdominal wall are more difficult to diagnose clinically.

The mechanism of herniation may be thinning and stretching of the scar, resulting in a broad hernia neck, or a localized complete disruption of the scar, which results in a narrow hernia neck. As is the case for other hernia types, the hernia's neck size dictates the risk of incarceration and/or strangulation.

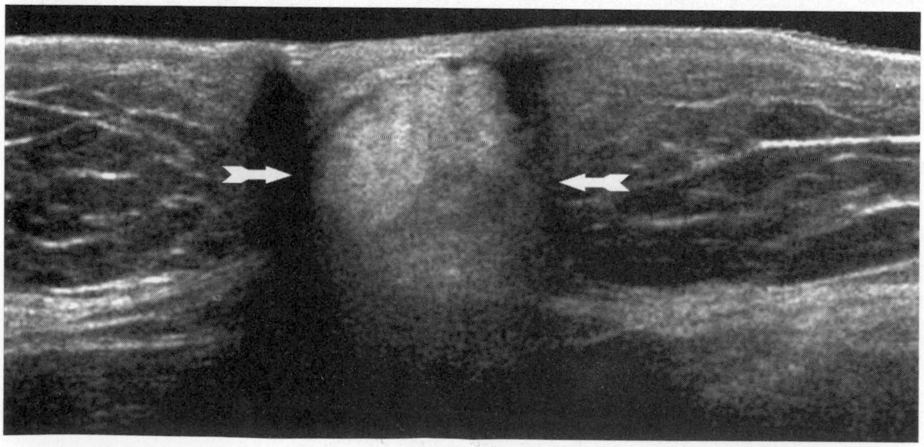

Figure 13-10. ■ *Transverse image demonstrating an incarcerated (nonreducible) and strangulated umbilical hernia* (arrows). *The presence of echogenic fat may be a sonographic key to the diagnosis of strangulation. It is important to use color Doppler and show that no flow is demonstrable to assist in the diagnosis of strangulation.*

INTERSTITIAL (INTRAPARIETAL) HERNIAS

Interstitial (intraparietal) hernias do not represent a distinct type of hernia. Rather, they are hernias that dissect between tissue planes in the abdominal wall. Any type of hernia that passes through multiple layers of fascia or aponeurosis (indirect inguinal, Spigelian, and incisional) can develop an interstitial component. Interstitial dissection can mask outward signs of hernia and can complicate surgical repair. Preoperative knowledge of interstitial components helps minimize the chances of bowel injury.

STRANGULATION OF HERNIAS

A strangulated hernia is defined as "an irreducible hernia in which the circulation is arrested." Without prompt treatment, gangrene will occur. It is important to recognize as well as predict the future risk of strangulation. Strangulated hernias are:

- nonreducible
- tender

The sonographic appearance of the hernia contents can provide additional evidence for the presence of strangulation, including:

- echogenic, edematous fat
- thickening of the hernia sac wall
- loss of normal bowel peristalsis
- bowel wall thickening
- absent blood flow on color Doppler

Of these sonographic findings, hyperechoic, edematous fat is most frequently demonstrated.

RECURRENT HERNIAS

Recurrent or residual pain after hernia surgery is a common dilemma. In the early postoperative period, pain is usually due to hematoma, seroma, or abscess. Later, recurrent hernia is more likely. Although recurrent hernias may be identical in type and appearance to the original hernia, more often, they are not. For example, it is difficult to classify recurrent inguinal hernias as either direct or indirect because the normal anatomic landmarks are altered by surgery. Additionally, repairs that use tension may predispose toward development of other types of hernias. When mesh is used for repair, recurrent hernias occur along the edges of the mesh. In some cases, there may have been an unrecognized asymptomatic second hernia present at the time of surgery. Ultrasound is helpful in sorting out these problems.

MULTIPLE HERNIAS

Patients who have one hernia are at increased risk for additional synchronous hernias as well as for developing additional hernias in the future (Fig. 13-11). It appears that some patients have a generalized connective tissue weakness. Additionally, bilateral hernias are relatively common, particularly for some hernia types, such as direct inguinal. For these reasons, patients should always be scanned bilaterally. Additionally, in patients with groin pain, a search for direct and indirect inguinal hernias as well as femoral hernias should be undertaken.

HEMATOMAS

The sudden appearance of a mass in the abdominal wall is quite suggestive of a hematoma in the correct clinical setting, for example, in a patient taking blood thinners or after trauma. Figure 54-1 demonstrates a large iatrogenic rectus sheath hematoma following an attempted paracentesis where the IEA was inadvertently lacerated.

INFECTION

An abscess may present as an abdominal wall mass, particularly in the patient who presents late to medical care. The clinical setting (fever, tenderness, and abnormal laboratory values) generally suggests the correct diagnosis, but ultrasound may be used to guide needle aspiration of infected fluid for diagnostic and therapeutic purposes.

SOFT-TISSUE TUMORS

The most common soft-tissue tumor is the benign lipoma, a fatty mass that generally causes no problems other than its cosmetic effects. Ultrasound may suggest this diagnosis (Fig. 13-12), but characterization is far from definite. Another benign mass that may be seen on ultrasound is the subcutaneous sebaceous cyst. The rare malignant tumor may present as an abdominal wall mass. The presence of Doppler flow within a mass should suggest a soft-tissue tumor, since hematomas and abscesses generally do not have detectable internal blood flow. Note that old hematomas with ingrowth of granulation tissue, or hematomas that dissect along normal tissue planes, may occasionally have internal flow and thus may be confused with soft-tissue tumors. Suspected malignant tumors should be

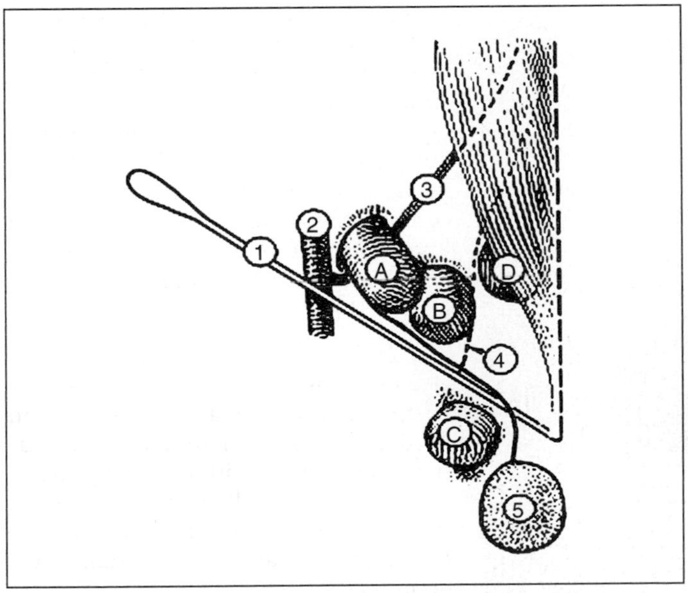

Figure 13-11. ■ *Diagram showing the multiple locations of possible hernias: (A) indirect inguinal hernia; (B) direct inguinal hernia; (C) femoral hernia; (D) supravesical hernia; 1, inguinal ligament (not visualized sonographically); 2, external inguinal artery; 3, IEA; 4, medial umbilical ligament (not visualized sonographically); 5, testis.*

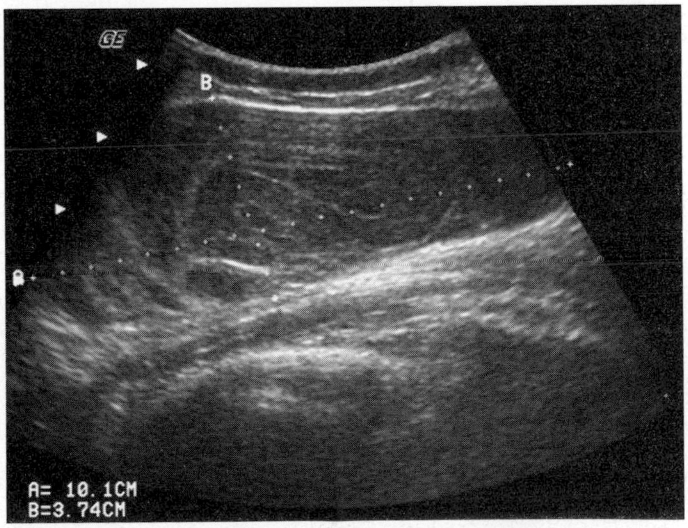

Figure 13-12. ■ *Anterior abdominal wall lipoma. Ultrasound shows a large mass (between cursors, measuring ~10 cm) that corresponded to the palpable lump noted by the patient.*

referred to the appropriate specialist for further evaluation, and biopsy should be deferred until the specialist evaluates the patient.

Pitfalls

1. Lymph nodes. Bumps in the groin may not represent hernias. Other causes for palpable masses in this region include lymphadenopathy, lipomas, cysts of the tunica vaginalis, pseudoaneurysms, and round ligament varices, among others. Ultrasound is usually very accurate at distinguishing a hernia from other entities.
2. Failure to thoroughly understand types of hernias and surrounding anatomical landmarks may result in hernias being missed.
3. Patients should be scanned erect to identify hernias that may not be seen in a supine position, and in some cases to exacerbate symptoms.

Where Else to Look

1. If a hernia is seen on the symptomatic side, the contralateral side should also be evaluated.
2. If a hernia is not found, look for other causes of the patient's symptoms (epididymitis, diverticulitis, appendicitis, ectopic, etc.).
3. If evaluating a patient for scrotal pain and if no scrotal or testicular cause can be found, check for a hernia.

SELECTED READING

Crespi G, Giannetta E, Mariani F, et al. Imaging of early post-operative complications after polypropylene mesh repair of inguinal hernia. *Radiol Med* 2004;108(1-2):107–115.

Inampudi P, Jacobson JA, Fessell DP, et al. Soft-tissue lipomas: accuracy of sonography in diagnosis with pathologic correlation. *Radiology* 2004;233:763–767.

Miller PA, Mezwa DG, Feczko PJ, et al. Imaging of abdominal hernias. *Radiographics* 1995;15:333–347.

Nguyen KT, Sauerbrei EE, Nolan RL, Lewandowski BJ. The abdominal wall. In: Rumack CM, Wilson SR, Charboneau JW, eds. *Diagnostic Ultrasound*, vol. 1, 3rd ed. St. Louis: Elsevier Mosby; 2004:489–501.

Rettenbacher T, Hollerweger A, Macheiner P, et al. Abdominal wall hernias: cross-sectional imaging signs of incarceration determined with sonography. *AJR Am J Roentgenol* 2001;177(5):1061–1066.

Shadbolt CL, Heinze SB, Deitrich RB. Imagining of groin masses: inguinal anatomy and pathologic conditions revisited. *Radiographics* 2001;Oct 21 Spec No:S261–271.

van den Berg JC. Inguinal hernias: MRI and ultrasound. *Magn Reson Imaging Clin N Am* 2004;12(4)689–705.

van den Berg JC. Inguinal hernias: MRI and ultrasound. *Semin Ultrasound CT Mr* 2002;23(2):156–173.

Wechsler R, Kurtz AB, Needleman L, et al. Pictorial essay: cross-sectional imaging of abdominal wall hernias. *AJR Am J Roentgenol* 1989;153:517–521.

Midabdominal Mass: Possible Ascites

14

TERESA BIEKER

SONOGRAM ABBREVIATIONS

Ab	Abscess
Ao	Aorta
Bl	Bladder
Ca	Celiac artery
GBl	Gallbladder
Ia	Iliac artery
Ip	Iliopsoas muscle
IVC	Inferior vena cava
K	Kidney
L	Liver
N	Nodes
P	Pancreas
Ps	Psoas muscle
QL	Quadratus lumborum muscle
RA	Rectus abdominis muscle
SMA	Superior mesenteric artery
Sp	Spleen

KEY WORDS

Adenopathy. Abnormally enlarged lymph nodes.

Aneurysm. Dilatation of an artery, usually the abdominal aorta. There are several types of aneurysms:

True Aneurysm. Enlargement of all three layers of the aorta.

False Aneurysm. Leaking of blood through all three layers of the vessel into surrounding tissues that contain it.

Dissecting Aneurysm. An aneurysm that occurs when the intima layer of the vessel wall separates from the media layer, secondary to bleeding.

Fusiform Aneurysm. A spindle-shaped dilation of an artery.

Saccular Aneurysm. A sac-like dilatation of an artery.

Ascites. Abnormal accumulation of fluid in the abdomen or pelvis.

Exudate. Free fluid that seeps out from blood vessels. Characterized by a high protein and cellular content.

Transudate. Free fluid that passes through membranes, causing protein and cellular content to be filtered out.

Abdominal Aortic Bifurcation. The abdominal aorta divides into the right and left common iliac arteries at approximately the level of the umbilicus.

Crohn's Disease. Chronic inflammatory bowel disease that causes ulcers along the inner surface of the bowel. Infection and bowel obstruction are common symptoms.

Haustra. Normal sacculations of the colon's wall.

Hernia. Protrusion of bowel, fat and/or membranes through an abnormal opening. Hernias are classified according to location. (See Chapter 13.)

Intussusception. Telescoping of a portion of the intestine into an adjacent portion. Most common in children (see Chapter 35).

Ischemic Colitis. Inflammation of the colon resulting in a decreased blood supply. The bowel wall is thickened and does not demonstrate peristalsis.

Lymphoma. Malignancy of the lymph system.

Mechanical Obstruction. Obstruction of the bowel secondary to an extrinsic process, resulting in dilated fluid-filled loops.

Mesenteric Sheath. Membranous fold that attaches the bowel to the dorsal (back or posterior) body wall.

Paracolic Gutter. Area lateral to the ascending and descending colon where fluid may accumulate.

Paralytic Ileus. Paralysis of the intestine, usually occurring secondary to surgery, injury, certain drugs, or illness.

Peristalsis. Rhythmic contraction of the bowel used to propel contents through it. Visible with ultrasound.

Psoas Muscles. Paired muscles that lie lateral to the spine and posterior to the kidneys.

Rectus Abdominus Muscles. Paired, anterior, midline muscles that extend the length of the abdomen.

The Clinical Problem

Midabdominal masses can either originate in the midabdomen or extend from an extrinsic location. Masses that originate in the midabdominal region typically arise from the abdominal aorta, bowel, lymph nodes, or the abdominal wall. Most midabdominal masses can be visualized by ultrasound; however, air within the bowel may interfere in some cases.

AORTIC ANEURYSM

Ultrasound is a useful method for evaluating the abdominal aorta (Fig. 14-1). Information regarding size and location of the aneurysm can aid the surgeon in providing appropriate treatment. Descriptive terms such as *saccular* or *fusiform* may also be helpful (Fig. 14-2). In the case of large body habitus, other imaging modalities such as computed tomography (CT) or magnetic resonance imaging may be necessary.

The abdominal aorta is considered aneurysmal if the anteroposterior diameter measures greater than 3 cm. Surgery is indicated, however, when the diameter is greater than ~5.5 cm. Evidence of significant expansion between sequential sonograms may indicate the need for surgical intervention.

An aneurysm that has ruptured, forming a false aneurysm, is an acute emergency.

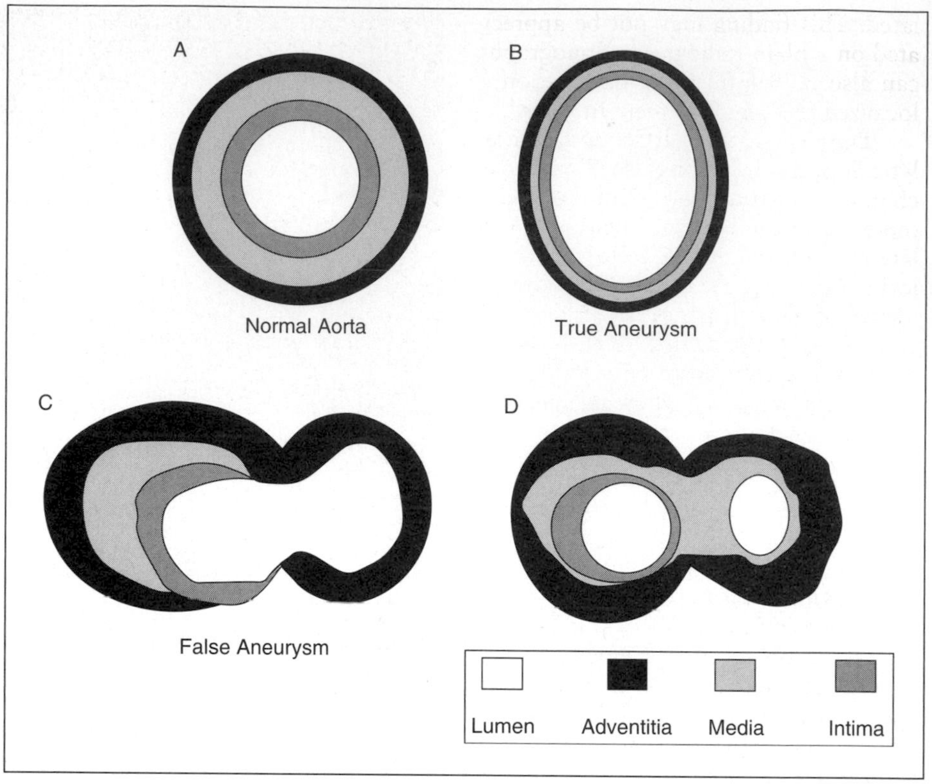

Figure 14-1. ■ *A. Normal aorta showing the three components of the wall—the intima* (gray), *media* (hatched), *and adventitia* (black). *B. True aneurysm. Diffuse swelling of the three layers. C. False aneurysm. Blood is released through all three layers into surrounding tissues. D. Dissection. There is a defect in the intima, with blood between the intima and media. (Adapted and reprinted with permission from Downey D. The retroperitoneum and the great vessels. In Rumack CM, Wilson SR, Charboneau JW, eds.* Diagnostic Ultrasound, *2nd ed. St. Louis: Mosby; 1998:453–486.)*

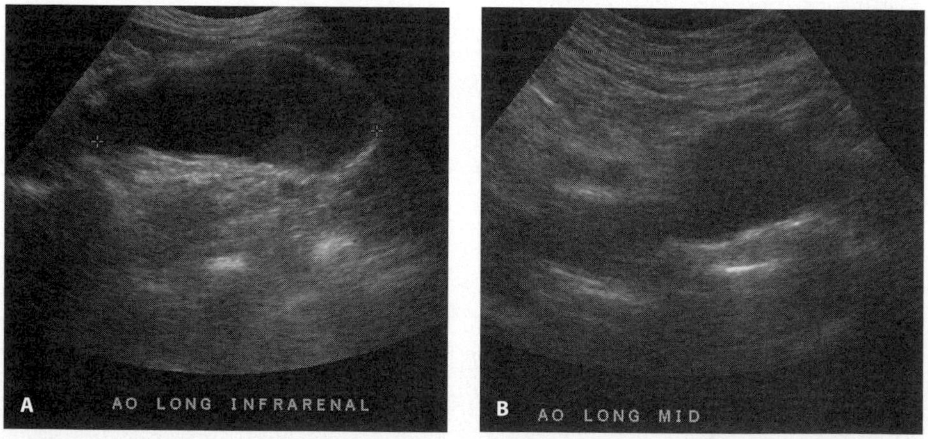

Figure 14-2. ■ *(A) A fusiform aneurysm that has a gradual change in diameter from superior (left caliper) to inferior (right caliper), whereas (B) a saccular aneurysm changes abruptly from normal to abnormal.*

LYMPH NODES

Enlarged lymph nodes may be visualized around the aorta and its branches. Adenopathy usually occurs due to an inflammatory or neoplastic process. Detection of nodal enlargement in the midabdomen should prompt an evaluation for the extent of lymphomatous spread. CT is typically the imaging modality of choice.

BOWEL MASSES

The clinician may palpate large masses arising from the bowel. Sonography is usually not the modality of choice when evaluating for bowel masses due to interference from overlying bowel gas.

Some masses may be incidentally found by ultrasound. Secondary signs of a mass, including thickened bowel wall or dilated fluid-filled loops of bowel due to an obstruction, may be seen by ultrasound.

BOWEL OBSTRUCTION

Another cause of overall abdominal distention is intestinal obstruction or paralytic ileus. With these conditions, the abdomen can be extremely distended. Dilated bowel usually contains a mixture of air and fluid; therefore, an ultrasound exam may not provide an adequate evaluation. If the bowel is entirely fluid-filled and if air is not present, the sonogram can help by showing that the bowel is dilated. This finding may not be appreciated on a plain radiograph. Sonography can also be helpful if the obstruction is localized to a small segment of bowel.

During real-time ultrasound, a paralytic ileus can be distinguished from mechanical obstruction. With an ileus, there will not be peristalsis within the dilated bowel, whereas with early mechanical obstruction, the bowel will show evidence of marked peristalsis. These two conditions are treated differently: high-grade mechanical obstruction is an indication for surgery, whereas paralytic ileus is treated conservatively.

ASCITES

If the entire abdomen appears enlarged, the clinical question of ascites is raised—this is assessed relatively easily by ultrasound. Discovery of ascites is important because aspiration of the ascitic fluid can assist in patient management. Causes of ascites include congestive heart failure, liver disease, nephrotic syndrome, infection, and malignancy. Blood may also appear as simple fluid within the abdomen. This finding may be due to a recent ruptured aneurysm or trauma.

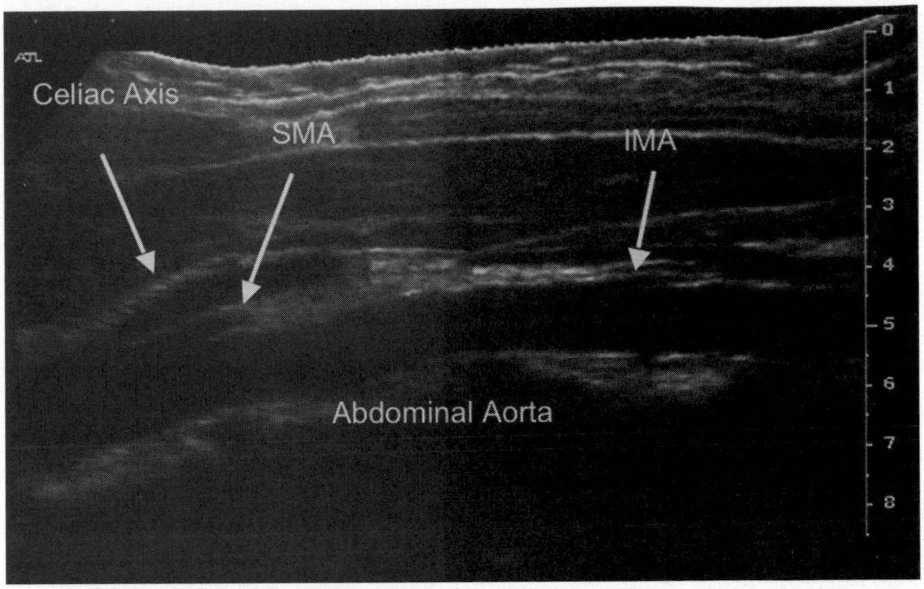

Figure 14-3. ■ *Longitudinal scan of a normal aorta and its branches.*

Anatomy

For information regarding anatomy, see Chapter 6, Sonographic Abdominal Anatomy.

AORTA

All vessels, including the aorta have three wall layers: the adventitia, media, and intima (Fig. 14-1).

In the optimal patient, the aorta can be traced as far as the level of the bifurcation into the right and left common iliac arteries. The celiac axis, SMA, renal arteries, and inferior mesenteric artery arise from the aorta. Although sometimes obscured by overlying bowel gas, most branches can usually be visualized by ultrasound (Fig. 14-3).

The aorta lies midline directly anterior to the spine and to the left of the inferior vena cava (IVC).

MESENTERIC SHEATH

The mesenteric sheath (mesentery, mesenteric root) is a fibrous membrane that attaches the small and large bowel to the abdominal wall. The SMA and the superior mesenteric vein are contained within it. It is not visible by ultrasound unless it is surrounded by enlarged nodes.

BOWEL

Bowel is not well evaluated by ultrasound due to overlying bowel gas. When visualized, however, cross-sectional views through normal empty bowel show an echogenic center surrounded by a thin, echo-free wall. Bowel that is dilated, filled with fluid, or has a thickened wall is much easier to appreciate with ultrasound.

PSOAS MUSCLES

The psoas muscles can be seen on either side of the spine, posterior to the kidneys. The psoas muscles join with the iliacus muscles to form the iliopsoas muscles, which coat the anterior aspect of the iliac crest, just above the true pelvis.

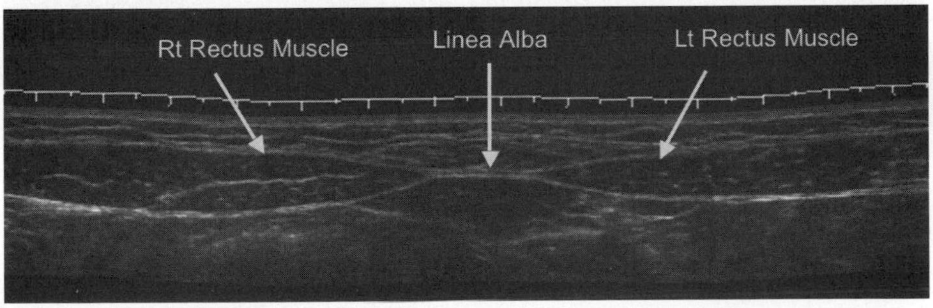

Figure 14-4. ■ *Transverse scan of normal rectus muscles. The linea alba is located in the midline.*

RECTUS SHEATH MUSCLE

The two segments of the rectus muscle lie on either side of the midline in the anterior abdominal wall. They are seen well in the upper abdomen but are not readily visualized below the umbilicus (Fig. 14-4).

ABDOMINAL WALL

The diaphragm marks the superior aspect of the abdominal wall. Inferiorly, it is continuous with the pelvic cavity. The anterior aspect of the abdominal wall is composed of several layers of muscle, including the rectus abdominus, external oblique, internal oblique, and transverse abdominus muscles. The right and left oblique and transverse abdominus muscles come together to form a fibrous band known as the *linea alba*. Posteriorly, the abdominal wall is formed by the spine. The lateral aspects consist of the 12 ribs, psoas muscles, quadratus lumborum muscles, and the iliac crests.

The abdominal wall may be the site of an abdominal mass. Hence, the various layers of the abdominal wall should be identified anterior to the peritoneal line. The subcutaneous tissue contains mainly fat and appears more hyperechoic than the muscular layers. A strong linear echo represents the peritoneal fascial line. The intraperitoneal structures are posterior to this line.

Technique

PALPATION

When a mass is palpated during a physical exam, ultrasound can be used to determine whether the mass is superficial within the abdominal wall or located deep in the abdomen. The peritoneal fascial line is used as a landmark.

COMPRESSION

Midabdominal pathology may be obscured by bowel gas. The transducer can be used to compress overlying gas and to displace the bowel so that the anatomy and pathology can be visualized.

DOCUMENTATION

Once an abnormality has been identified, the relationship between the mass and the abdominal wall, surrounding organs, and vessels should be documented.

Documentation includes:

1. The relationship to surrounding structures
2. Sonographic characteristics: cystic or solid, smooth or irregular borders
3. Mobility
4. Size in three dimensions
5. Vascularity: Color and/or pulsed Doppler should be utilized to determine the presence, location, and resistance of flow.

A high-frequency linear array transducer will also be helpful to evaluate superficial abdominal wall pathology. A lower-frequency, curved linear array transducer can be used to evaluate deeper structures within the abdomen.

AORTA

If an aneurysm is identified, its location and relationship to surrounding structures must be determined (e.g., the origin superior or inferior to the renal arteries). When bowel gas obscures the aorta, pressure with a curved linear array transducer may displace the gas and allow visualization. Also, placing the patient in the left or right decubitus position, or utilizing the liver or spleen as a window, will allow partial visualization of the aorta. Total gain compensation, focus, and dynamic range need to be optimized so clot is not missed or technically created.

The bifurcation of the aorta into the common iliac arteries may be visualized with the patient supine or in a right lateral decubitus (coronal approach) position. The coronal approach will usually allow visualization of both iliac arteries simultaneously (Fig. 14-5). When an aneurysm is identified, anterior-posterior dimension and width should be measured from the outer wall to outer wall. Additionally, the extent of the aneurysm should be determined. When an aneurysm is identified, color and pulsed Doppler should be utilized to document the presence of blood flow and to access the size of the true lumen. Because

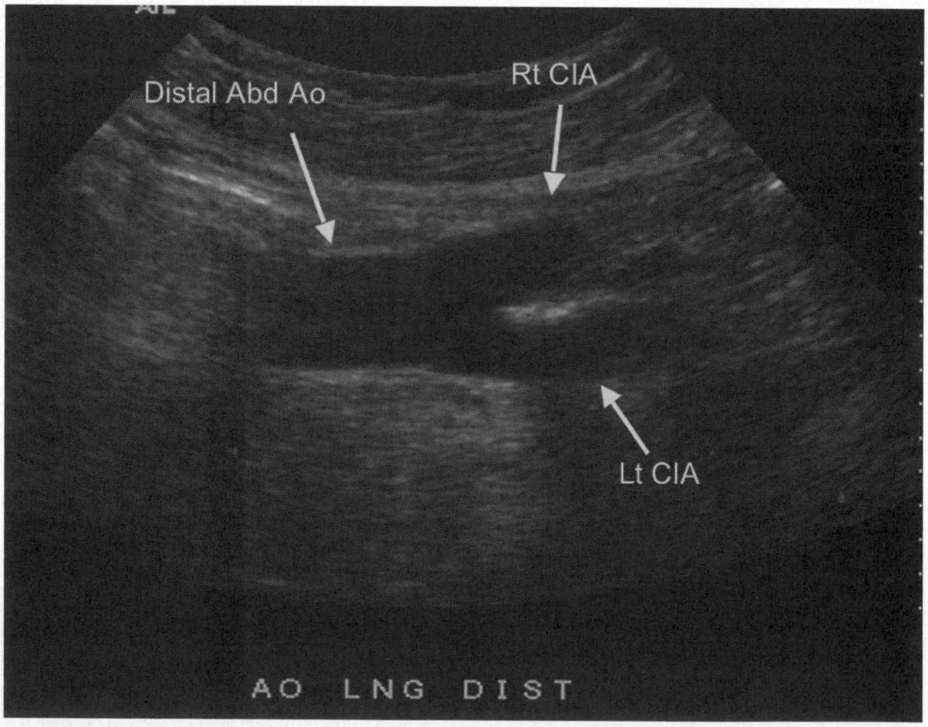

Figure 14-5. ■ *Coronal image at the aortic bifurcation. Note both the right and left common iliac arteries can be demonstrated in this plane.*

an aneurysm is often tortuous, evaluating the entire aorta may be difficult (Fig. 14-6).

MESENTERIC MASSES

If a mass is anterior to the aorta within the mesentery, the relationship of the mass to the superior mesenteric vein and artery should be evaluated. This is the primary site for visualizing lymphadenopathy.

In a right or left lateral decubitus position, use the liver or the spleen as a window to visualize the para-aortic nodes. If gas obscures para-aortic nodes when the patient is in a supine position, he or she can be repositioned.

Peristalsis and visualization in all three planes will differentiate bowel from nodes.

ASCITES

If the clinical issue is to determine the presence or absence of ascites, the paracolic gutters as well as the Morison pouch on the right and the lesser sac on the left should be scanned with the patient in a supine position. These are the areas where small amounts of free fluid can first be identified.

If fluid appears to be complex, loculated ascites, abscess, malignancy, or hematoma should be suspected (Fig. 14-7). Confusion between a pleural effusion

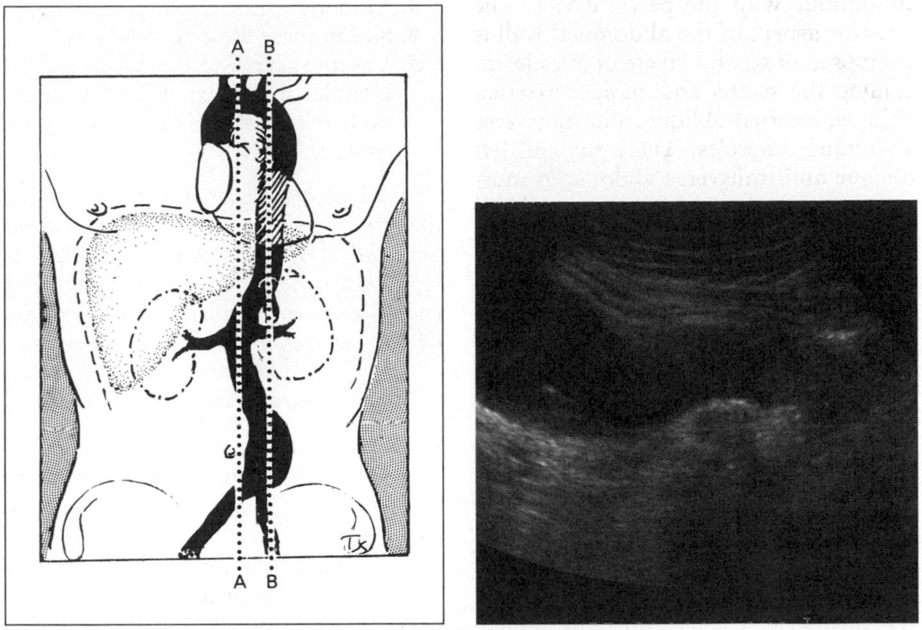

Figure 14-6. ■ *Because the aneurysmal aorta is often tortuous, complete longitudinal sections through the aorta and the aneurysm may be technically difficult.*

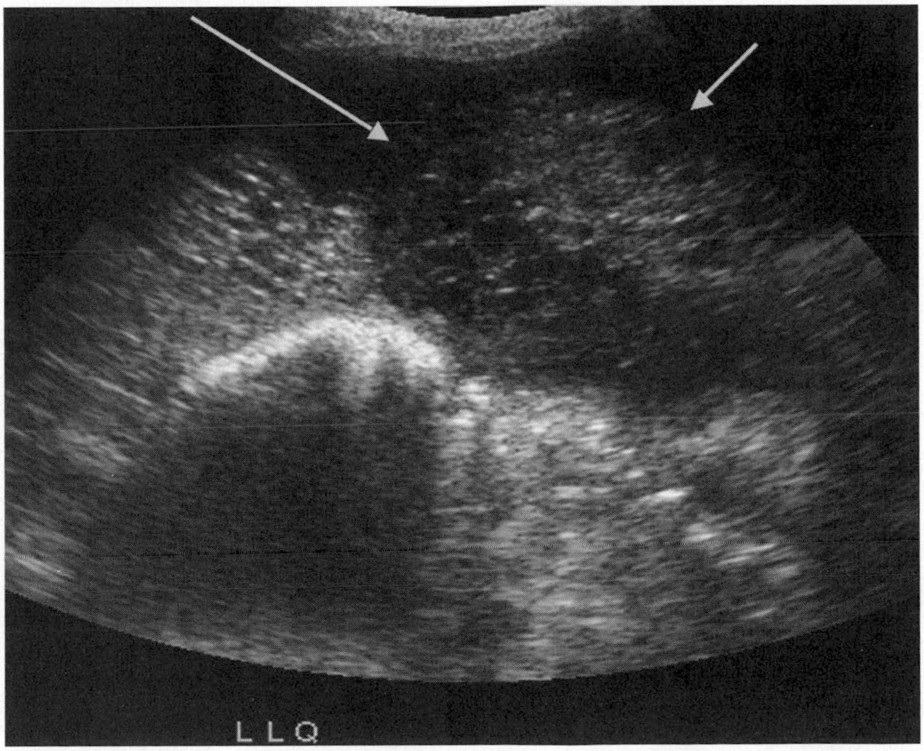

Figure 14-7. ■ *Complex ascites in the paracolic gutter. This appearance can represent an abscess, hematoma, or in this case, malignant fluid.*

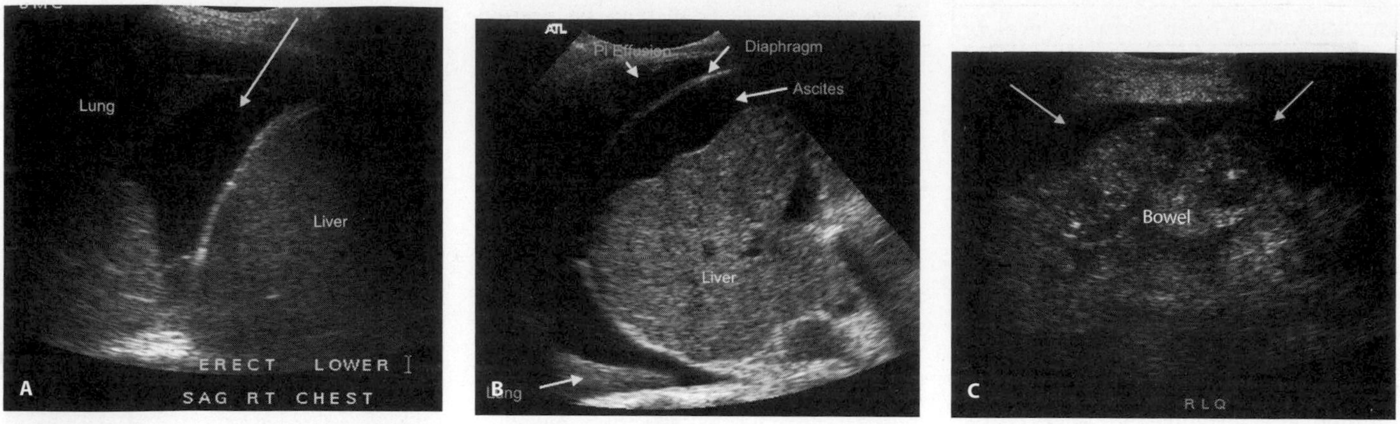

Figure 14-8. ■ *Pleural effusion and ascites. A. Pleural effusion superior to the diaphragm. B. Pleural effusion and ascites outlining the diaphragm. C. Ascites only. Note the irregular outline to the gut where it is outlined by ascites.*

and ascites can occur if the diaphragm is not defined (Fig. 14-8). Pelvic ascites can be distinguished from the bladder by the following:

1. Free fluid will be present in the anterior and/or posterior cul-de-sac.
2. Bowel can be seen within free fluid.
3. The borders of the bladder are smooth.

Pathology

ANEURYSM

Aneurysms are pulsatile dilations of the aorta. The majority are located between the origin of the renal arteries and the aortic bifurcation into the common iliac arteries.

The aorta should be evaluated in both transverse and longitudinal planes. Anterior-posterior and transverse measurements of the aorta and/or aneurysm should include the vessel as well as the wall (Fig. 14-9). Plaque can often be seen in the abdominal aorta.

Features to Look for in Aneurysms

Size. In order for an aortic dilation to be considered an aneurysm, a diameter of greater than 3 cm must be seen. An aneurysm requires surgical intervention if the measurement is 5 to 6 cm or greater.

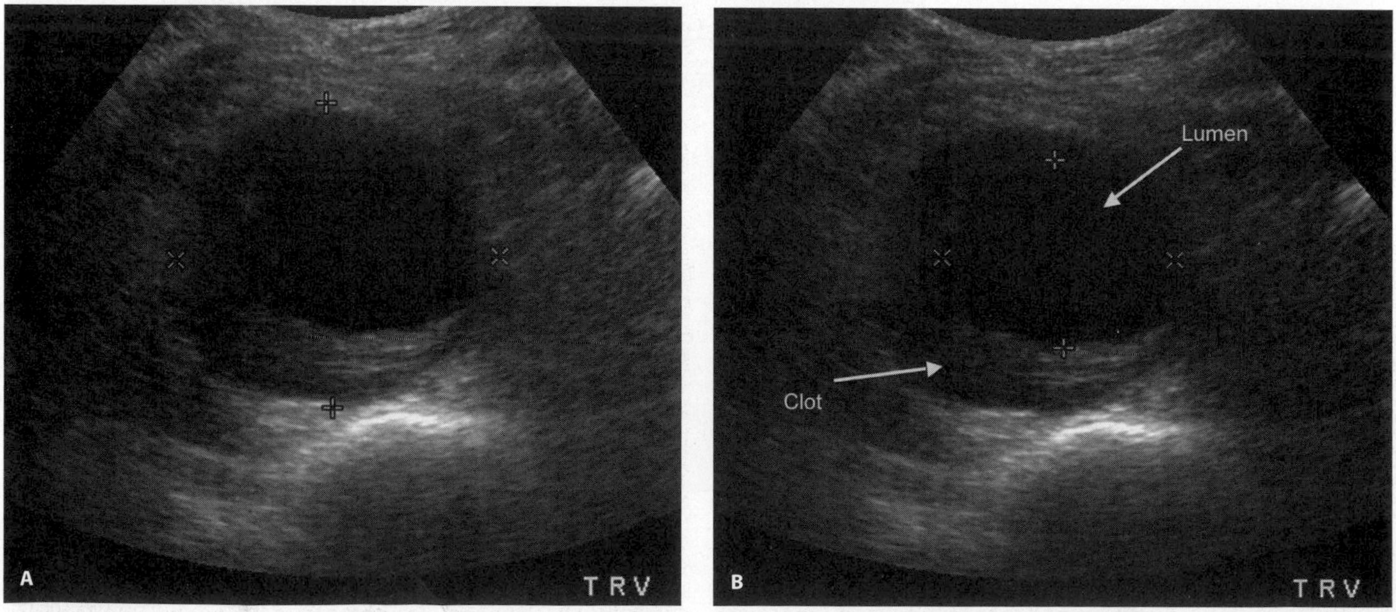

Figure 14-9. ■ *A. An abdominal aneurysm, as well as the normal abdominal aorta, is measured from outer wall to outer wall. B. Because they often contain clot, there may be a relatively small patent lumen.*

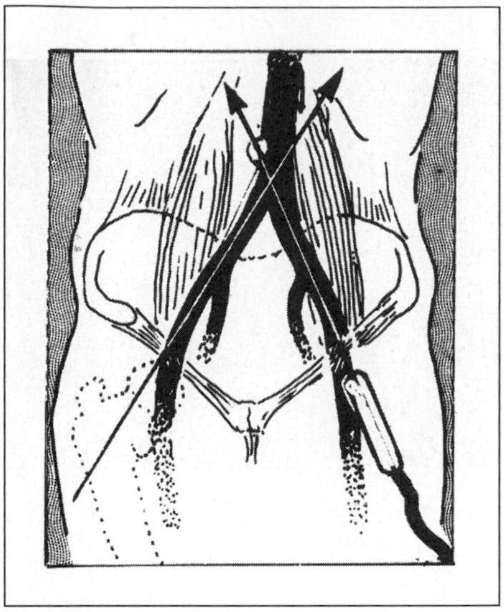

Figure 14-10. ■ *Attempt to show the iliac arteries by finding the bifurcation of the aorta and the femoral arteries in the groin by palpation. Align the transducer along this axis.*

Iliac Arteries. Lower abdominal aneurysms often involve the iliac arteries. Attempt to show involvement of the iliac arteries by scanning in an oblique plane between the bifurcation and the palpated femoral artery in the groin (Fig. 14-10). An iliac artery is considered aneurysmal if its diameter is greater than 2 cm.

Thrombus. Thrombus may be present within an aneurysm. Use appropriate gain settings to ensure that reverberation artifact is not mistaken for an aneurysm, thrombus, or clot (Fig. 14-9B). Conversely, if the gain is set too low, it can mask clot or thrombus within the lumen.

Color Doppler can assist in determining whether or not clot is present. Thrombus may become partially detached from the aneurysm wall and simulate a dissection. This situation is emergent because thrombus can embolize to the lower extremities.

Involvement of Major Vessels. Aneurysms of the superior abdominal aorta may involve the celiac axis as well as the superior mesenteric and renal arteries. An effort should be made to image these vessels, as their involvement can alter surgical management.

Dissection. An abdominal aneurysm dissection is unusual but can occur. The sonographic characteristics include an echogenic septum that pulsates, obliquely aligned in the middle of an aneurysm (Fig. 14-11). A dissection can extend from the chest into the abdomen.

Leaking or Ruptured Aneurysm. If an aneurysm has ruptured, a fluid collection may be seen adjacent to the aorta. A common location for this fluid is at the junction of a graft and the patient's native aorta or iliac artery. When clot or tissue surrounds leaking blood, the appearance is of a false aneurysm. Flow between the aneurysmal collection and the aorta may be visualized at Doppler.

Grafts. Grafts can be recognized by the presence of linear parallel echoes within the aorta and iliac vessels. A baseline study following graft placement is helpful to evaluate for flow within and distal to the graft, as well as possible fluid collections.

False Aneurysms. False aneurysms are aneurysms that do not have a wall but are contained by clot or surrounding tissues. They appear as a mass extending from the vessel (Fig. 14-1C).

Color Doppler may demonstrate flow in and out of the aneurysm during systole and diastole.

LYMPHADENOPATHY

Most lymph nodes are lobulated, hypoechoic masses. Benign nodes have an echogenic hilum and are bean-shaped. Malignant nodes typically do not have an echogenic hilum and are more round in shape.

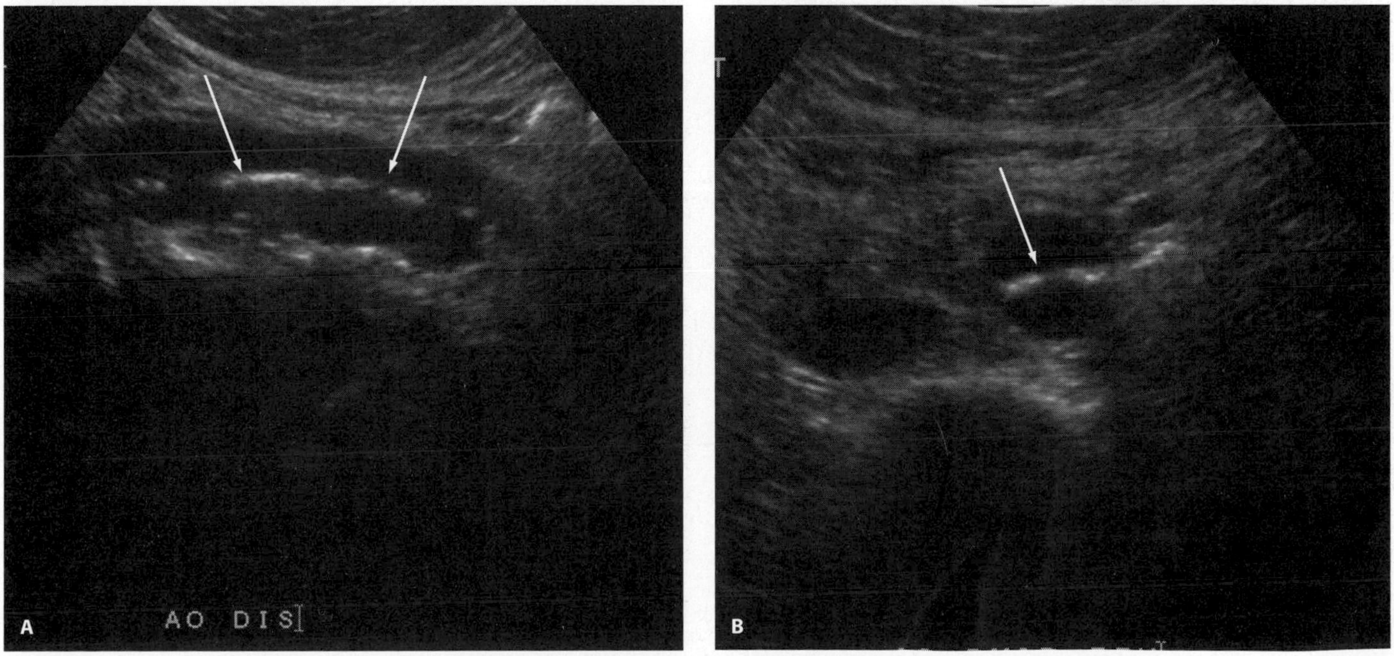

Figure 14-11. ■ *Longitudinal (A) and transverse (B) views of a dissecting aneurysm. Note the line from the intima* (arrow) *that represents one border of the dissection.*

CT is superior to ultrasound for locating and characterizing lymph nodes within the retroperitoneum.

Para-aortic Nodes

Para-aortic nodes can be lobulated or smooth-walled. The aorta and IVC are often displaced anteriorly by enlarged nodes. Lymph nodes may also be seen between the aorta and the IVC. In addition, nodes may be identified between the aorta and the left kidney as well as the aorta and the SMA. Lymph nodes within the abdomen are considered normal if measuring less than 1 cm in short axis (Fig. 14-12).

Celiac Axis Nodes

Celiac axis nodes are sometimes termed *porta hepatis nodes* because they extend into the porta hepatis. The majority of celiac axis nodes lie posterior to the celiac axis and superior to the pancreas.

Mesenteric Nodes

Nodes in the mesentery are characteristically located longitudinally anterior and posterior to the SMA and vein and along the mesenteric sheath. They have an ovoid shape and are usually anechoic. Nodes in the mesentery may be mistaken for bowel.

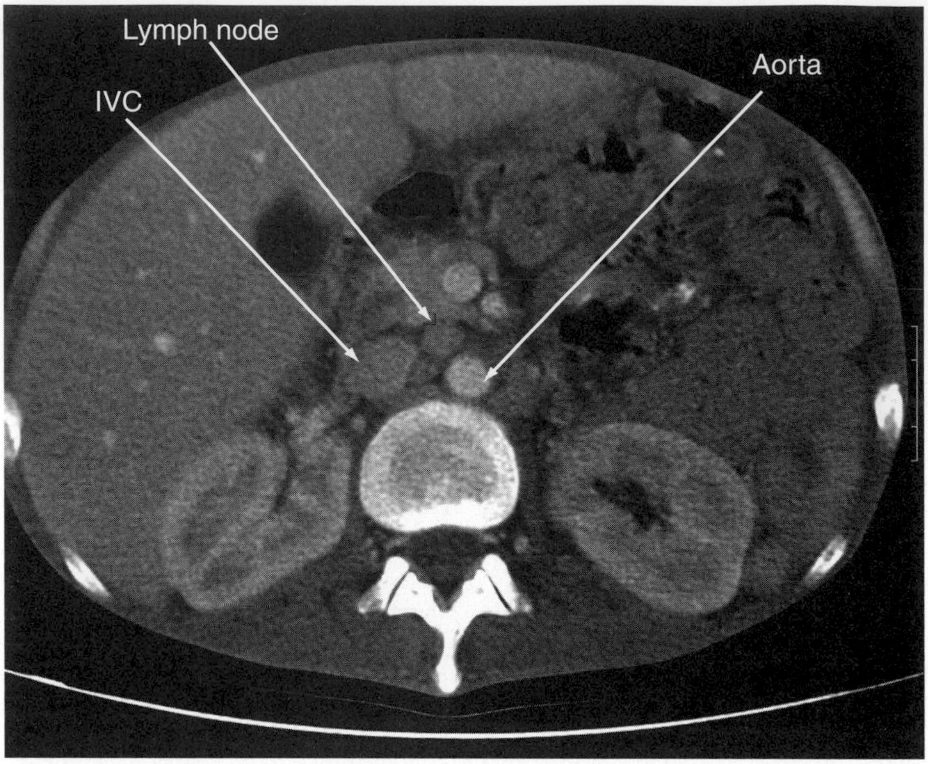

Figure 14-12. ■ *Para-aortic node by CT. This enlarged lymph node lies adjacent to the aorta.*

Pelvic Nodes

Pelvic nodes are located on the lateral walls of the pelvis along the iliopsoas muscles near the iliac vessels. When enlarged, they may compress the bladder. Pelvic lymph nodes are normal if they measure less than 10 mm (Fig. 14-13).

Inguinal Nodes

Inguinal nodes are not usually large but can be easily palpated. They lie adjacent to the inguinal ligament in the groin (Fig. 14-14).

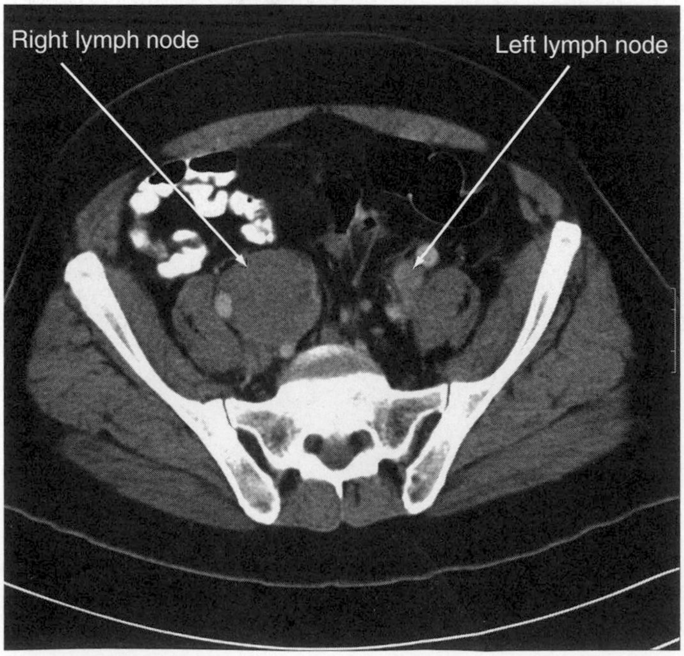

Figure 14-13. ■ *Enlarged pelvic lymph nodes in the right and left pelvis in a patient with prostate cancer.*

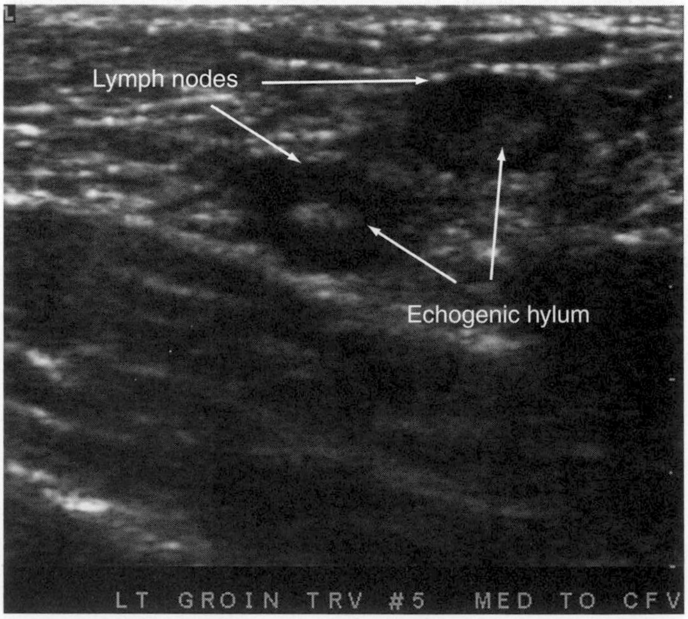

Figure 14-14. ■ *Paired nodes located in the groin, which can be palpated and easily evaluated by ultrasound.*

FLUID-FILLED LOOPS OF BOWEL

Bowel loops filled with fluid rather than air are usually easily seen by ultrasound (Fig. 14-15). In this setting, it is often possible to see the detailed structure of the bowel wall, including the haustral markings.

No peristalsis within the dilated loop of bowel indicates that paralytic ileus or long-standing obstruction has occurred.

BOWEL MASS

A palpable mass may originate from the bowel demonstrating a bull's eye appearance. In the abnormal segment of bowel, the mass will consist of an echogenic center surrounded by a thick sonolucent rim measuring greater than 4 mm in width (Fig. 14-16). This appearance is characteristic of carcinoma of the stomach or colon. Other causes include a variety of nonneoplastic conditions in which there is bowel wall thickening, such as Crohn's disease, ischemic colitis, or intussusception (see Chapter 15).

All masses, except those related to ischemic bowel disease, will typically show arterial flow on pulsed Doppler. In Crohn's disease and other types of inflammatory bowel disease, hyperemia may be present.

OTHER MESENTERIC MASSES

Intramesenteric masses within the peritoneum can usually be distinguished from retroperitoneal masses by the absence or distortion of the psoas muscles, kidneys, or quadratus lumborum muscles. Mesenteric masses can be moved from side to side on palpation. The fat line that runs in front of the retroperitoneal tissues will not be displaced anteriorly by the mass. Other than lymph nodes, most intramesenteric masses are benign, including mesenteric cysts, which are large, fluid-filled, asymptomatic masses that contain septa. These masses are seen mainly in children. Lipomas may also be seen. Sonographically, lipomas appear as large, asymptomatic masses that are evenly heterogeneous.

ASCITES

With large amounts of ascites, bowel loops can be seen floating within the fluid. Small amounts of fluid accumulate first in the subhepatic space (Morison pouch) as well as the paracolic gutters.

It is important to determine whether the ascites is simple or loculated. (Figs. 14-7 and 14-8). Internal echoes in fluid may suggest infection or malignancy.

ABDOMINAL WALL PROBLEMS

Masses that occur in the abdominal wall are usually easily palpated. Optimize

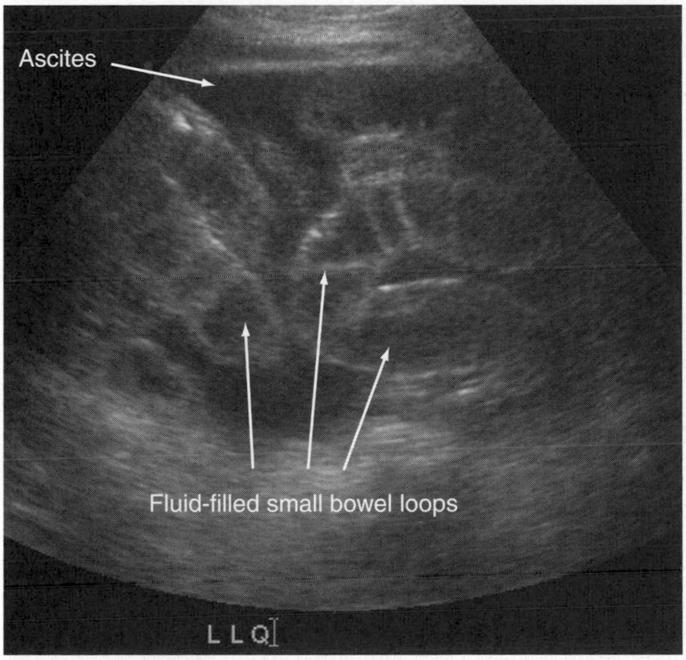

Figure 14-15. ■ *Fluid-filled bowel loops are easily seen by ultrasound.*

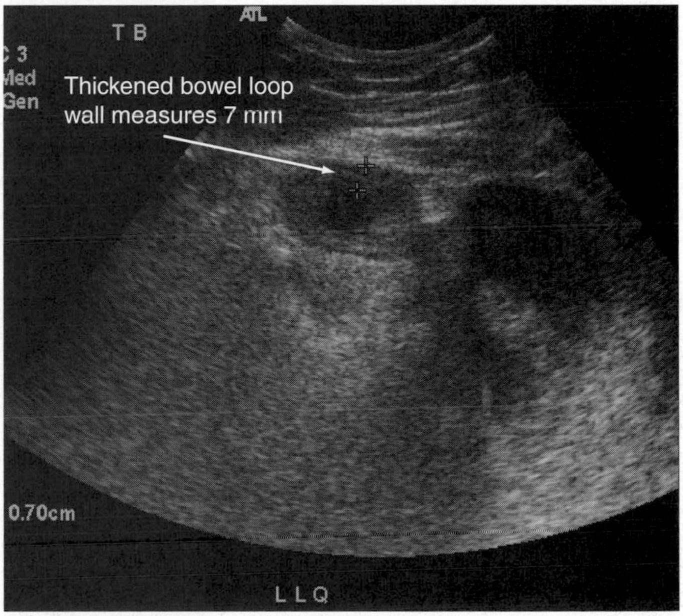

Figure 14-16. ■ *Target sign of intestinal wall thickening. If the wall is more than 3- to 4-mm thick, it is abnormal.*

gain settings, focusing, and transducer selection to concentrate on this superficial area. Abdominal wall masses lie anterior to the fascial/peritoneal echoes (Fig. 14-17).

Rectus Sheath Hematoma

A rectus sheath hematoma causes enlargement of the rectus sheath muscles along the abdominal wall. Most rectus sheath hematomas are more hypoechoic than the normal muscle.

Abscesses

Abscesses may involve both the rectus sheath as well as the area superficial to the muscle. Most abscesses appear complex and hypoechoic with an irregular wall by sonography. Abscesses often have increased blood flow secondary to hyperemia around their periphery, which can be confirmed by color Doppler.

Neoplasm

Neoplasms can involve muscle, subcutaneous tissue, or intramesenteric areas. They are usually better demarcated and more homogeneous than abscesses. Color or pulsed Doppler should show internal vascularity within the tumor.

Lipoma

Lipomas are benign masses that often occur in the abdominal wall. Sonographically, they appear as echogenic structures within the subcutaneous tissues. Lipomatous masses do not extend through the tissue planes of the abdominal wall (Fig. 14-18).

Hernia

An intermittently palpable abdominal mass may be caused by a hernia. Ventral hernias are often associated with a previous incision and are found in the midline. Spigelian hernias are found more laterally. Femoral and inguinal hernias are found in the groin. At the site of a hernia, the peritoneal line is interrupted between the abdominal wall and the contents of the abdomen. The hernia can contain bowel or fat. Hernias may be intermittent and become visible with a change in the patient's position or when the patient performs a Valsalva maneuver. See Chapter 13.

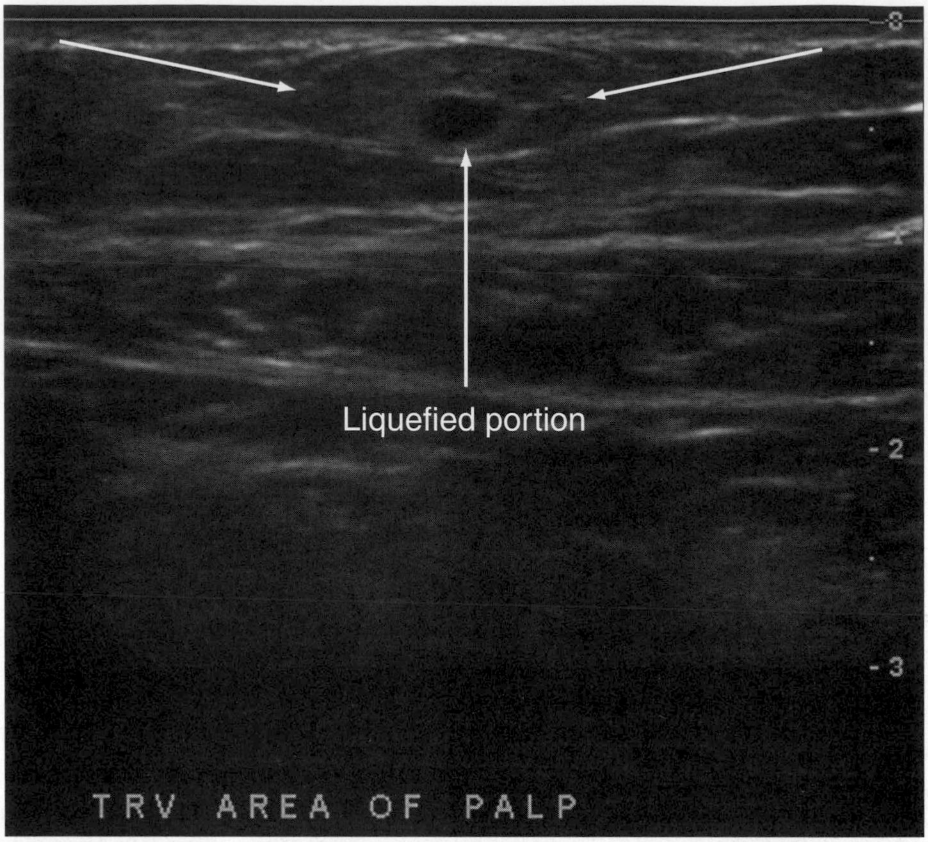

Figure 14-17. ■ *Abdominal wall hematoma* (arrows). *This palpable area lies anterior to the fascial plane.*

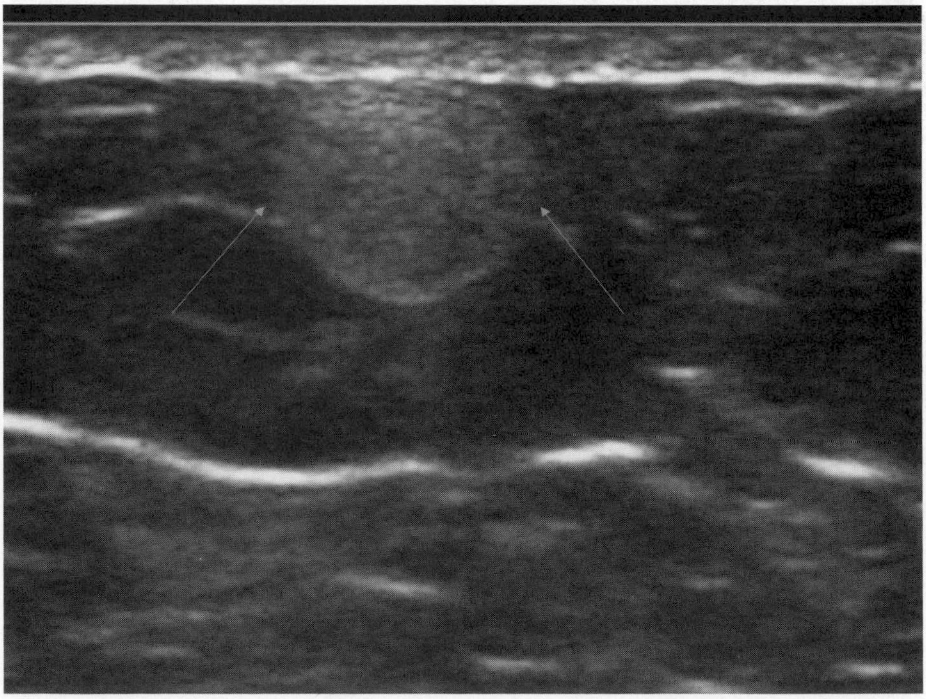

Figure 14-18. ■ *Lipoma* (arrows). *Lipomas are echogenic, well-defined masses that lie anterior to the abdominal wall.*

Pitfalls

1. Abdominal fat. In obese people, fat appears as a sonolucent area posterior to the peritoneum. It can be confused with ascites; however, muscles will have striations and will not be gravity-dependent.
2. Ovarian cystic masses. Ovarian cystic masses can become very large and extend into the abdomen. Unlike ascites, an ovarian cyst will be contained and arise from the ovary. Cystadenomas are the most common ovarian mass to extend into the abdomen (Fig. 14-19).
3. Nodes versus aneurysm. Para-aortic nodes may be confused with a partially clot-filled aortic aneurysm. Color and pulsed Doppler as well as evaluation in all three dimensions will differentiate the two.
4. Bowel loops versus nodes. Nodes can resemble loops of fluid-filled bowel. Real-time scanning will demonstrate bowel peristalsis.
5. Ascites versus peritoneal dialysis. When ascites is present, determine if the patient has had fluid introduced recently for peritoneal dialysis.
6. Pleural effusion versus ascites. Determine the diaphragm's location. On a transverse view, ascites lies between the diaphragm and the liver. A pleural effusion will be superior to the diaphragm (Fig. 14-8).

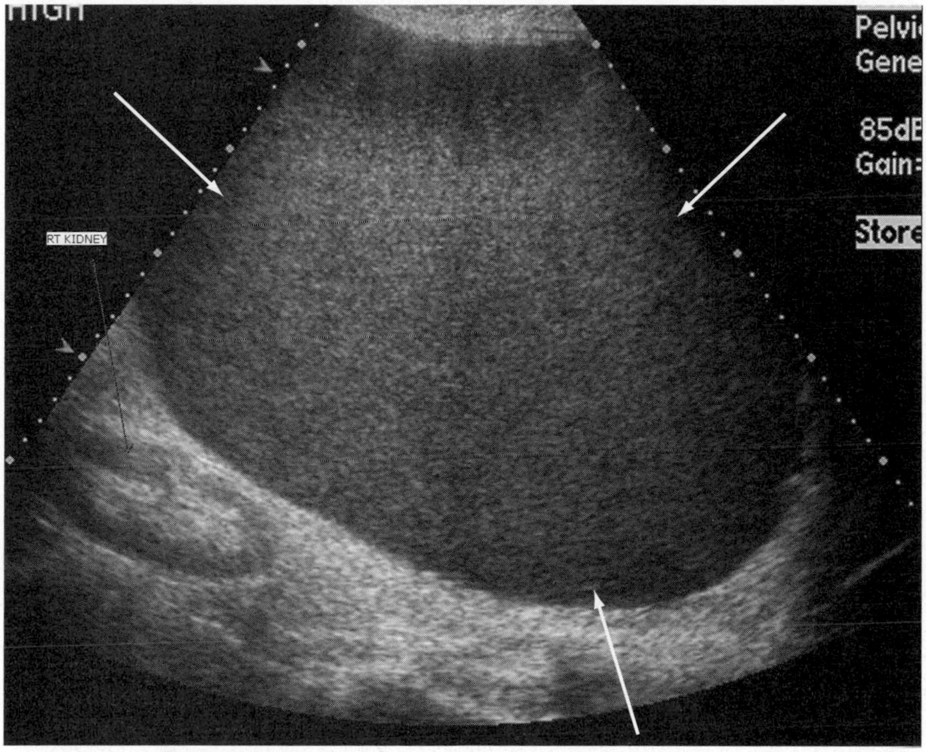

Figure 14-19. ■ *Ovarian cystadenoma* (arrows). *When large, a cystadenoma may extend into the abdomen; however, they are contained and extend from the ovary.*

Where Else to Look

1. Lymph nodes. If nodes are found, evaluate for splenomegaly. It supports the diagnosis of lymphoma.
2. Loculated ascites. If loculations within free fluid are seen, it is worth looking for evidence of peritoneal metastases adherent to the abdominal wall.
3. Ascites. Examine the IVC and hepatic veins for dilation (i.e., congestive heart failure). Evaluate the liver size, echogenicity, and texture for any evidence of cirrhosis.
4. Aneurysm. If an aortic aneurysm is present, the iliac arteries should also be evaluated for aneurysm.
5. The presence of a bowel mass with a thickened wall suggests a gastrointestinal neoplasm such as a carcinoma of the colon. Evaluate the liver for metastases and perform a node search.

SELECTED READING

Choi MY, Lee JW, Jang KJ. Distinction between benign and malignant causes of cervical, axillary, and inguinal lymphadenopathy: value of Doppler spectral waveform analysis. *AJR Am J Roentgenol* 1995;165:981–984.

Downey D. The retroperitoneum and the great vessels. In: Rumack CM, Wilson SR, Charboneau JW, eds. *Diagnostic Ultrasound*, 2nd ed. St. Louis: Mosby; 1998:453–486.

Lederle FA, Walker JM, Reinke DB. Selective screening for abdominal aortic aneurysms with physical examination and ultrasound. *Arch Intern Med* 1988;148:1753–1756.

Right Lower Quadrant Pain

15

GRETCHEN M. DIMLING
ROGER C. SANDERS

KEY WORDS

Adenopathy. Enlarged lymph nodes.

Appendicolith (Fecalith). A calculus that may form around fecal material associated with appendicitis. Sonographically appears as an intraluminal echogenic focus with a varying degree of shadowing.

Bacterial Ileocecitis. Infection of the ileum and cecum.

"Bull's Eye" (Target Sign, Reniform Mass, or Pseudokidney). A characteristic sign of gastrointestinal wall thickening consisting of an echogenic center and a sonolucent rim.

Carcinoid. A yellow, circumscribed tumor occurring in the gastrointestinal tract.

Chronic Intestinal Ischemia. Stenosis or occlusion of the splanchnic (mesentery) arteries. Symptoms may present late in the disease and include upper abdominal pain, which intensifies after a meal and weight loss.

Crohn's Disease. A recurrent bowel inflammatory disease usually involving the terminal ileum but may affect any part of the gastrointestinal tract. Onset usually occurs between 20 and 40 years of age.

Diverticulitis. Occurs when a herniated outpouching of the intestinal lining becomes inflamed. May perforate and form an abscess.

Fistula. An abnormal communication between the gastrointestinal tract and other internal organs or to the body surface.

Malabsorption Syndrome. Impaired intestinal absorption of nutrients that results in deficiency of vitamins, electrolytes, iron, calcium, etc.

McBurney's Point. The site of maximum tenderness in the right iliac fossa with appendicitis.

Mesentery. The connective tissue attaching the intestine to the posterior abdominal wall.

Mesoappendix. The layer of connective tissue attaching the appendix to the mesentery of the ileum.

Mesocolon. The layer of connective tissue that attaches the various portions of the colon to the posterior abdominal wall.

Neutropenia. Decreased white blood cell count.

Neutropenic Typhlitis. Inflammation of the cecum that develops in the setting of severe neutropenia when a patient is immunosuppressed.

Peritonitis. Infection of the abdomen's inner lining.

Rebound Tenderness. Most severe abdominal discomfort when pressure is released quickly rather than when the abdomen is compressed.

Septicemia. Infection involving the bloodstream.

Vasodilation. Increased blood flow in an inflamed organ and the surrounding tissues. Associated with increased heat and redness.

The Clinical Problem

A number of entities can cause right iliac fossa pain—notably appendicitis. The pathology may be linked to the bowel found in this location (i.e., cecum, terminal ileum, and appendix) or the adjacent organs (i.e., right kidney, right ureter, bladder, ovary, uterus, or gallbladder) (see Fig. 15-3). A rapid and accurate diagnosis can be critical for a patient with acute abdominal pain. Ultrasound is a helpful tool to lead the physician to the correct diagnosis.

Not all intestinal problems require surgery. In approximately 25% of appendectomies, a misdiagnosis of appendicitis results in the removal of a normal appendix and a delay of appropriate treatment for the patient. Some conditions, such as bacterial ileocecitis, call for nonsurgical treatments. A thorough history followed by a targeted sonogram will spare the patient unnecessary procedures and point to the proper treatment.

APPENDICITIS

Although appendicitis is most common in children and young adults, it can occur at any age with a lifetime risk of 7%. The cause of appendicitis is obstruction of the appendix followed by infection. If the obstruction is not relieved spontaneously, inflammation and increased intraluminal pressure cause midabdominal pain, which later localizes over the appendix. When surgical intervention is delayed, bacteria may invade the appendiceal wall, and perforation may occur.

At this stage, the patient's life is in danger. When the appendix perforates into the abdominal cavity, peritonitis occurs, followed by abscess formation, and occasionally death.

In most cases, the spread of infection after perforation is contained by mesentery and intestine in the appendix region. This collection is called an *appendical phlegmon* or an *appendical abscess* if there is pus within. Although an appendical phlegmon may resolve and reabsorb on its own, further infections may follow with the development of fistulous tracts to surrounding bowel, the bladder, the skin, or the vagina. If the infection becomes more widespread, death may result from septicemia or peritonitis.

Patients with classic symptoms of appendicitis may be sent straight to surgery. Atypical cases may be referred to ultrasound to rule out pelvic, renal, or gallbladder pathology. A prompt diagnosis is required to avoid perforation of the appendix.

The presenting symptoms include one or more of the following features:

1. Pain that starts in the periumbilical region, then localizes to the right lower quadrant (McBurney's point)
2. Rebound tenderness (tenderness that is most severe when pressure is released)
3. Poor appetite, nausea, vomiting, and/or diarrhea
4. Fever
5. Leukocytosis—white blood cell count of 10,000 to 18,000/mL

BACTERIAL ILEOCECITIS

Bacterial ileocecitis is inflammation of the terminal ileum, cecum, and surrounding nodes caused by a bacterial infection. The most common culprits are *Yersinia enterocolitica*, *Campylobacter jejuni*, *Salmonella enteritidis*, and rarely *Y. pseudotuberculosis* and *Salmonella* Typhi. In this condition, the appendix may be affected, but is not obstructed. Therefore, perforation is not a threat, and surgery is not indicated.

Bacterial ileocecitis is often confused with acute appendicitis. A meal containing chicken in the patient's history may be a clue. Diarrhea may be present and can be bloody.

CROHN'S DISEASE

The cause of this inflammatory process of the gastrointestinal tract is yet unknown. Most patients with Crohn's are young adults. Although this disease may affect any part of the gastrointestinal tract, the terminal ileum is the most common site. The undiagnosed patient may present with the following:

1. A painful mass in the right iliac fossa
2. Crampy abdominal pain
3. Intermittent diarrhea
4. Weakness, fever, increased white blood cell count, weight loss, or malabsorption syndrome

Patients with Crohn's disease are occasionally followed with ultrasound during therapy to monitor bowel wall thickness or abscesses.

DIVERTICULITIS

Clinically similar to appendicitis, although usually on the left, diverticulitis is not often life-threatening. It involves herniated outpouches of large bowel wall and diverticula that become infected and inflamed. Similar to appendicitis, the neck of the diverticulum becomes obstructed and infection accumulates within the diverticulum (Fig. 15-1, stage 1). Usually, the pressure builds until the pus is released into the bowel lumen (Fig. 15-1, stage 2). Despite the abscess, the bowel often functions normally (Fig. 15-1, stage 3). Although not common, perforation may occur followed by fecal peritonitis.

Sigmoid diverticulitis is the most common cause of acute left lower quadrant pain and is referred to as *left-sided appendicitis*. Cecal diverticulitis can be clinically indiscernible from appendicitis.

MESENTERIC ADENITIS

Mesenteric adenitis is often the cause of enlarged mesenteric nodes. It is seen mostly in young children. Presenting symptoms are a painful right lower quadrant mass and possibly positive stool cultures.

INTUSSUSCEPTION

Patients with intussusception are usually children (see Chapter 35, Pediatric Abdominal Masses). Most children present with a painful abdominal mass, often with vomiting or bloody-mucous diarrhea.

NEUTROPENIC TYPHLITIS

Neutropenic typhlitis occurs in immunosuppressed patients. Symptoms include severe neutropenia and right lower quadrant pain. Fever, nausea, vomiting, and bloody diarrhea may also be present.

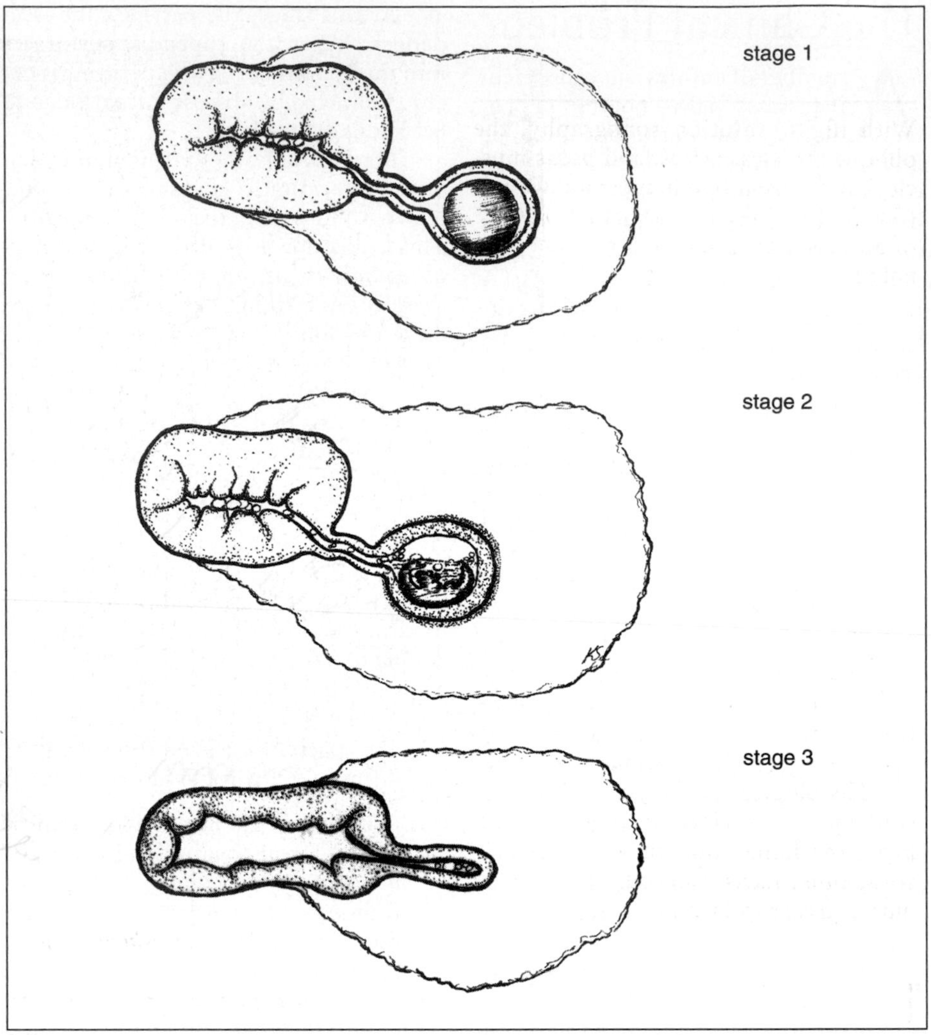

Figure 15-1. ■ *Illustration demonstrating the stages diverticulitis may follow. (Adapted and reprinted from Puylaert JB. Acute appendicitis: ultrasound evaluation using graded compression.* Radiology *1986;158:355–360, with permission.)*

INTESTINAL TUMORS

Intestinal tumors may be seen at any age. Colorectal cancer is the second most frequent cause of cancer-related death in the United States. Lymphoma is a disease of young adults. Leiomyosarcoma occurs in the fifth to sixth decades, and most carcinomas are seen in older patients. Gastrointestinal stromal tumor is a newly described malignancy of the gastrointestinal tract that is similar to leiomyomas and leiomyosarcomas. The clinical signs from any of these entities may include a painful abdominal mass, bloody stool, anorexia, diarrhea, constipation, and weight loss.

Anatomy

MUSCLE

With high-resolution sonography, the oblique muscles, rectus, and psoas muscles can be visualized in most individuals (Fig. 15-2). These muscles can be the site of abscesses or mistaken for an abdominal mass.

INTESTINE

The bowel encountered in the right lower quadrant may include the ascending colon, cecum, appendix, and terminal ileum (Fig. 15-3). With the proper technique, the ascending colon and cecum are usually visualized filled with echogenic bowel gas, feces, or hypoechoic fluid. By following the cecum caudally and medially, the terminal ileum may be seen entering the large bowel with active peristalsis. A normal appendix is rarely identified extending from the cecum. The normal appendix has a diameter of less than 6 mm.

Histologically, the gastrointestinal wall may be divided into five layers. From the lumen out, they are the mucosa, muscularis mucosa, submucosa, muscularis propria, and serosa or fat sur-

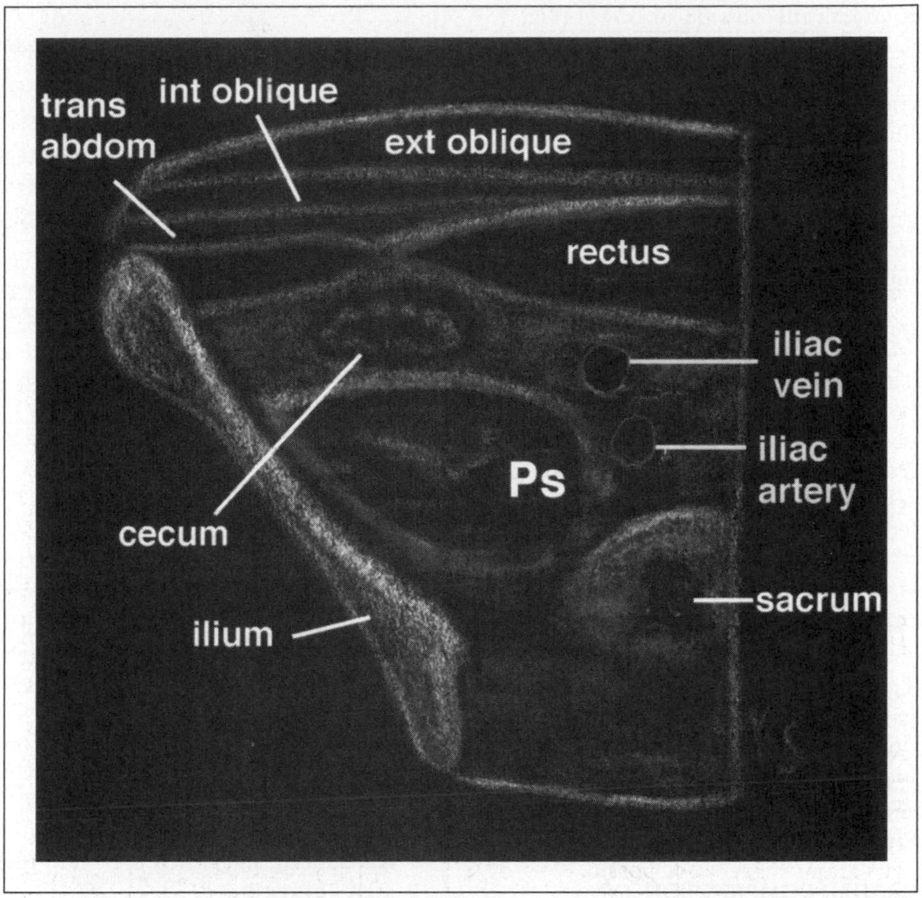

Figure 15-2. ■ *Transverse right lower quadrant.*

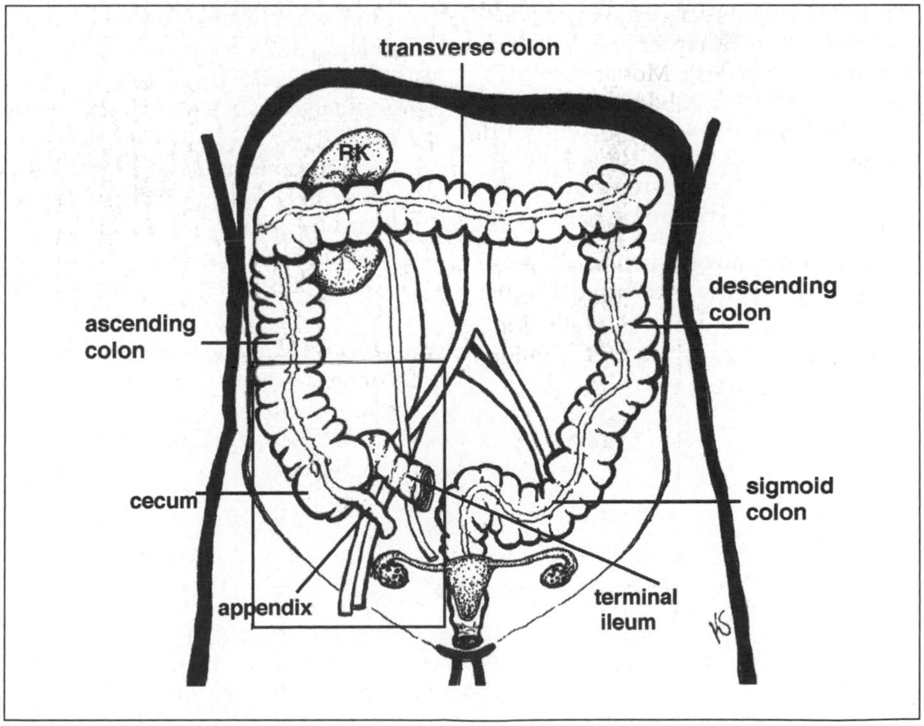

Figure 15-3. ■ *Diagram of the large intestine. The box delineates the right lower quadrant. Notice the numerous potential origins of right lower quadrant pain: the right ureter, the right ovary, the terminal ilium, cecum, and the appendix.*

rounding the outside of bowel (Fig. 15-4). On lower-frequency ultrasound, only three layers are usually discernible—mucosa (mixed echogenicity depending on luminal contents), submucosa (hyperechoic), and muscularis propria (hypoechoic). The echogenic echoes of the outer serosa or fat cannot be distinguished from the bright echoes of the surrounding tissue.

VESSELS

The external iliac artery and vein should be identified traveling in the medial aspect of the right iliac fossa (Fig. 15-2). During pregnancy, enlarged uterine vessels may occupy most of the right and left iliac fossas.

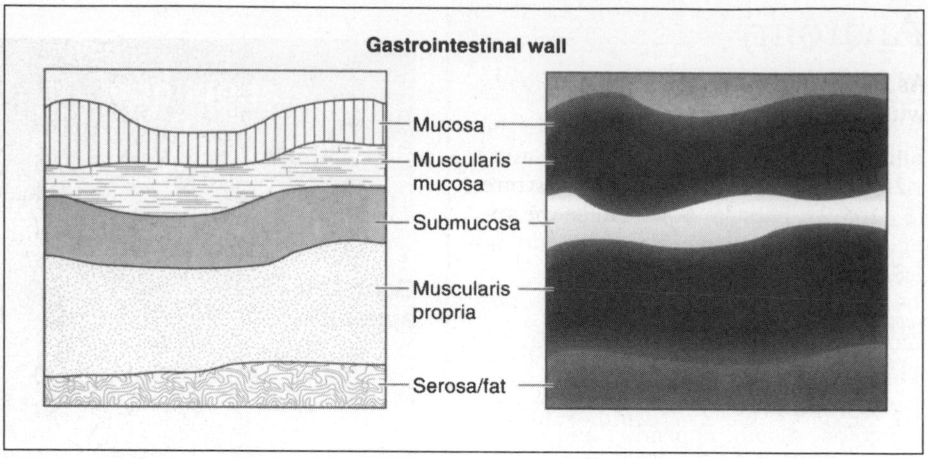

Figure 15-4. ■ *Diagram showing the components of the intestinal wall with the associated appearance on ultrasound.*

Technique

To evaluate the right lower quadrant, no patient preparation is necessary. For optimal visualization, use a 5- to 7.5-MHz linear transducer. A linear-array transducer provides a wide field of view and is best for bowel compression.

GRADED COMPRESSION

Although first described for acute appendicitis, graded compression can be used to evaluate any part of the gastrointestinal tract. As the compression is applied with the transducer, bowel gas and contents are displaced, and intra-abdominal structures are brought closer to the transducer and into the focal zone. By applying and releasing pressure gradually, the patient's discomfort is lessened.

1. After obtaining the patient's history, have the supine patient point to the area of maximum tenderness with one finger. Keeping in mind there may be rebound tenderness, carefully palpate the area for masses.
2. Begin the ultrasound examination holding the transducer transversely at a level slightly above the umbilicus. Gradually start to compress the transducer, and slowly slide it to the area of interest.
3. Ask the patient to indicate when the transducer is over the area of maximum tenderness, and carefully examine this region. Pathology most likely will be identified under this area. Be sure to release pressure gradually while removing the transducer.
4. After demonstrating the normal and abnormal right lower quadrant anatomy in the transverse plane, place the transducer longitudinally just lateral to the ascending colon and gradually compress. Slowly slide the transducer over the area of interest while moving medially.
5. Repeat this technique in oblique planes if that will best demonstrate the pathology.
6. Upward compression of the appendix area may be necessary if the appendix is sliding into the pelvis. Posterior manual compression and moving the patient into a left oblique lateral decubitus position may be helpful in some cases.
7. In larger patients, a lower-frequency curved linear transducer (e.g., 3.5 to 5 mHZ) may be needed.

Endovaginal imaging, with the use of a high-frequency transducer in close proximity to the abnormal bowel, may be very useful in detecting or evaluating intestinal abnormalities (see Figs. 15-8, 15-10, 15-12, and 15-13).

Pathology

As a rule, bowel inflammation presents with the following features:

1. Noncompressible abdominal mass.
2. The bowel wall may demonstrate three layers, giving a bull's-eye appearance in cross section
3. Little or no peristalsis.
4. The surrounding tissue (fat and connective tissue) is edematous, with increased echogenicity and a texture resembling normal thyroid tissue.
5. Color Doppler will demonstrate vasodilation. Spectral analysis may show decreased arterial resistance and increased velocity. In some cases, the venous flow may be continuous (no respiration phasicity) and even pulsatile.
6. Power Doppler will show increased vascularity.

APPENDICITIS

Appendicitis diagnosis may be separated into three categories.

Acute Appendicitis

The graded compression technique will reveal a reproducible, noncompressible, sausage-shaped structure without peristalsis originating from the base of the cecal tip at the site of maximal discomfort. The classic bull's-eye sign of gut should be visualized transversely with the total diameter measuring 0.6 to 1.0 cm (Fig. 15-5 and Color Plate 15-1). There is marked hypervascularity of the inflamed appendix wall. The hyperechoic surrounding edematous connective tissue provides another sonographic sign (Fig. 15-6 and Color Plate 15-1). Because of the similarity to the homogeneous, echogenic appearance of the thyroid, this sign is referred to as the "thyroid in the belly." There is usually no fluid within the appendix lumen.

Gangrenous Appendicitis

As the disease progresses, the appendix lumen distends with fluid and an appendicolith may be identified (Figs. 15-5 and 15-6). The inflamed appendix and its fluid-filled lumen will not compress when pressure is applied. An appendicolith is usually calcified, so shadowing will be seen originating within the appendix (Fig. 15-6). The transverse diameter ranges from 1.1 to 1.9 cm as the muscular wall thickens (Fig. 15-5B,C).

Perforated Appendicitis

Because of delay in the diagnosis, the appendicular wall may rupture. An abscess or fluid collection will develop in the right lower quadrant, the pelvis, or both. The appendix may be difficult to identify, but if it is seen, it will have asymmetric wall thickening and will appear as a hyperechoic, finger-like projection sur-

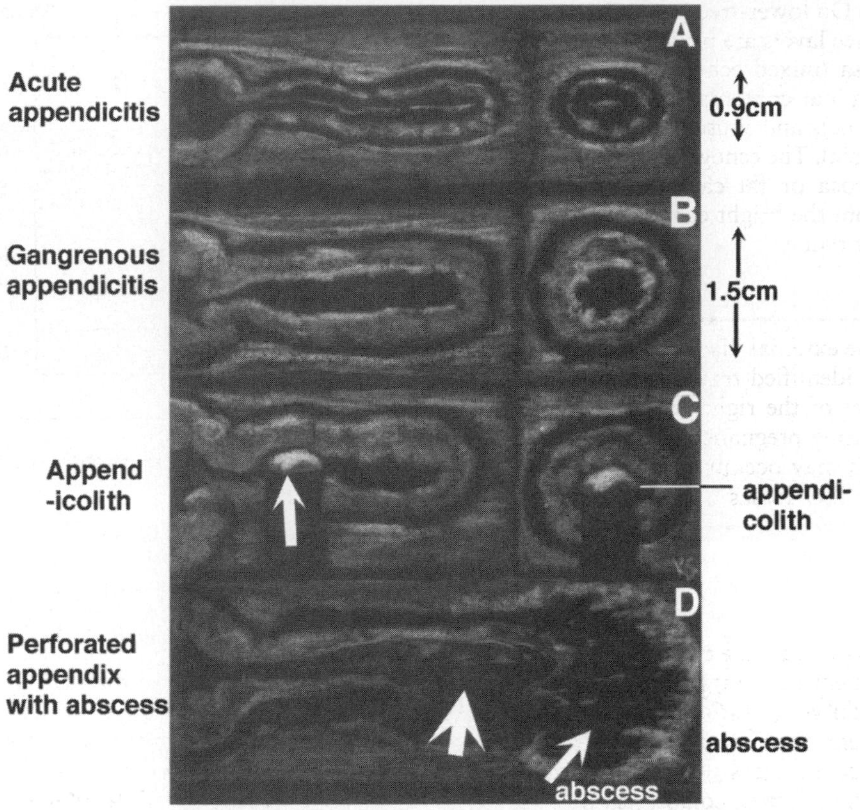

Figure 15-5. ■ *Illustration demonstrating possible sonographic appearances of appendicitis. A. Acute appendicitis. B. Fluid appears in the lumen. C. An appendicolith (fecalith) may be present, with shadowing. D. The perforation site is shown to attach over a perforated appendix. Abscess is delineated by* small arrow.

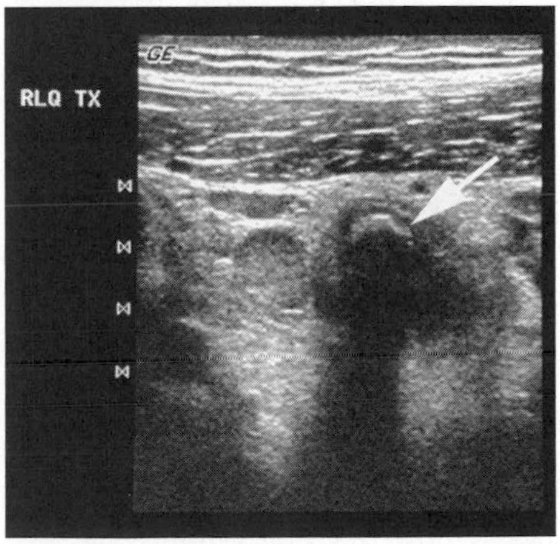

Figure 15-6. ■ *Transverse view of inflamed appendix. The appendix has a round rather than ovoid shape and contains a fecalith* (arrow).

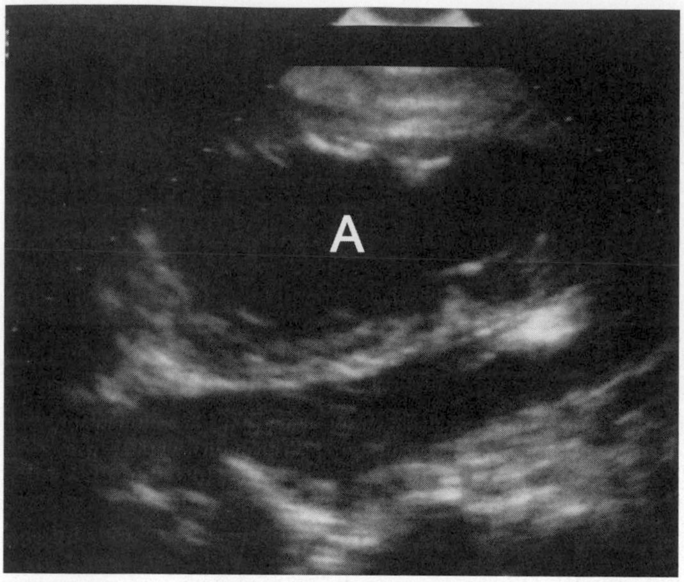

Figure 15-7. ■ *Appendiceal abscess. A painful fluid collection* (A) *in the right iliac fossa was the result of a ruptured appendix.*

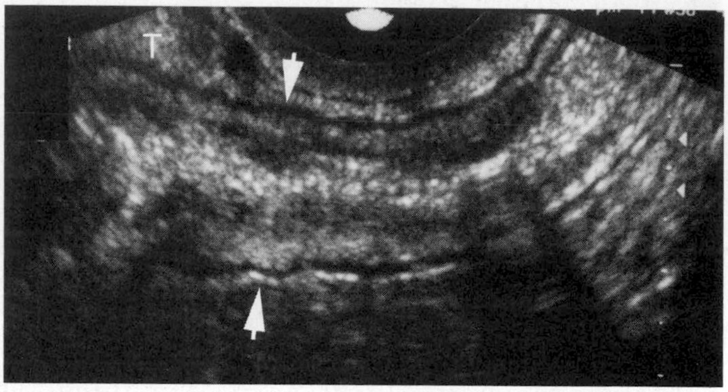

Figure 15-8. ■ *Crohn's disease. A 25-year-old woman with acute pelvic pain and rectal bleeding. The gut wall (between arrows) is markedly thickened and represents a focal area of ileum inflamed by Crohn's disease. The abnormal bowel is surrounded by edematous fat, with the homogeneous graininess of thyroid tissue* (T).

rounded by fluid or an abscess (Figs. 15-5D and 15-7). Abscesses are usually fluid-filled, possibly loculated, and may have debris within. Inflamed mesenteric nodes may be identified in the adjacent right lower quadrant.

CROHN'S DISEASE AND ULCERATIVE COLITIS

Crohn's disease usually affects the terminal ileum, although other bowel segments may be involved. The inflamed intestinal wall thickens to 0.6 to 1.6 cm, and the intestinal lumen is narrowed (Fig. 15-8). The involved area will have reduced peristalsis, but vigorous peristalsis may be seen in the unaffected bowel. There may be many bowel loops involved, congregating together to create a solid abdominal mass. Mesenteric lymphadenopathy is often present. Above the affected area, fluid-filled gut may be seen due to partial obstruction. The affected bowel is noncompressible and lacking haustra. The entire gastrointestinal tract should be evaluated for the previously mentioned characteristics. Color flow will show much vascular activity in involved loops of bowel.

Complications of Crohn's disease include abscess (Fig. 15-9), fistula formation, obstruction, and perforation. Abscesses may be seen adjacent to matted bowel loops and may extend into the psoas or rectus muscles. An abscess will appear as a complex, fluid-filled mass. If the muscles are involved, they will appear swollen on ultrasound when compared to the same muscle on the patient's other side, and the patient will have discomfort sitting up or with leg movement. Fistulous tracts may form between adjacent loops of bowel, bowel to skin, or bowel to bladder. These tracts are difficult to discern with ultrasound; a 7.5- to 10-MHz transducer may be helpful. With fistulae to the bladder, gas may be seen in the bladder with shadowing. Adenopathy is usually present in these complicated cases.

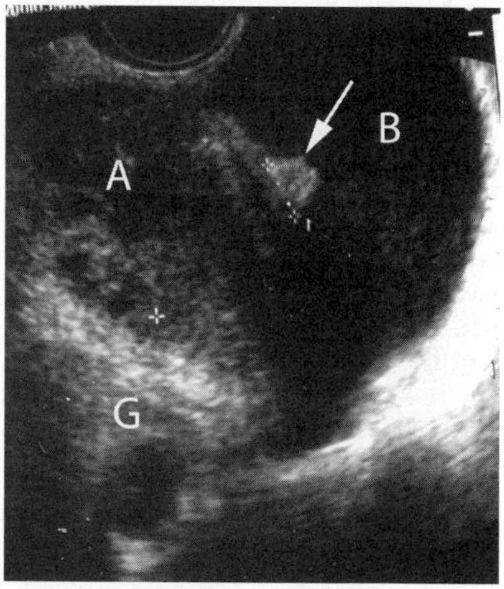

Figure 15-9. ■ *Abscess* (A) *located between the uterus and bladder due to Crohn's disease. The bladder* (B) *contained debris related to pus. The cone-shaped mass* (arrow) *was a connection between the abscess and the bladder. The inflamed bowel* (G) *can just be seen posterior to the abscess.*

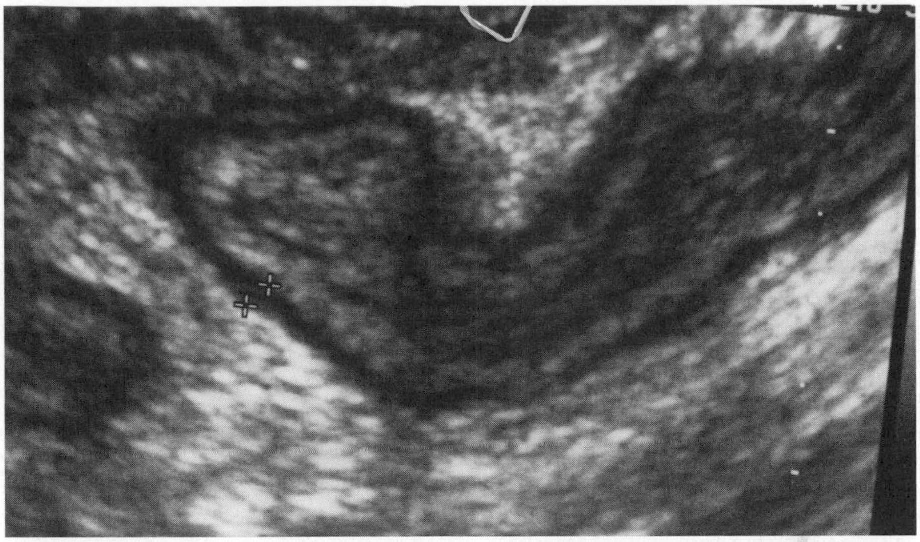

Figure 15-10. ■ *Ulcerative colitis has thickened the bowel wall of this area of actively diseased colon examined with the vaginal probe.*

Ulcerative colitis only affects the colon and does not cause fistula formation. The affected bowel wall is thickened and hypervascular with similar but less severe appearances to those in Crohn's disease (Fig. 15-10).

ISCHEMIC COLITIS

In older patients, particularly those who are hypertensive or who have had heart attacks, loss of blood supply to the small bowel or colon can lead to ischemic colitis. The bowel wall will be thickened and the gut will be inert. Bloody discharge and abdominal pain may develop. Appearances are similar to those seen in Crohn's disease; however, little or no flow will be seen on color flow in the involved segment (Fig. 15-11). Gas bubbles (pneumatosis coli) may form in the wall of the affected gut creating echogenic areas, which may or may not shadow (Fig. 15-11).

DIVERTICULITIS

Diverticulitis is more common in the left lower quadrant than around the appendix, and it occurs in older patients. It occurs in one third of the American population over 45 and in two thirds of those over 85 years of age. Thickened colon wall of greater than 2 mm is seen at the point of tenderness. Echogenic areas are seen within the thickened bowel wall (Fig. 15-12). The surrounding mesocolon will be inflamed and echogenic. In diverticulitis of the cecum, there are fewer but larger diverticula.

MESENTERIC ADENITIS

An enlarged mesenteric lymph node appears as a sphere with a hypoechoic peripheral zone and a hyperechoic center. The anteroposterior diameter is greater than 0.4 cm, and the average dimensions are 1.1 × 1.3 × 1.5 cm. The number of nodes varies from three to 20, and they are usually located deep with respect to the oblique or rectus muscles.

INTUSSUSCEPTION

Intussusception is described as a section of bowel "telescoping" into the lumen ahead of it. Sonographically, a thick hypoechoic ring surrounding one or more thick hypoechoic rings should be seen on transverse views of the affected bowel (see Chapter 35, Pediatric Abdominal Masses). An intestinal mass may be found in addition, because intussusception in the adult is usually caused by a mass invaginating into the bowel lumen ahead of it.

Color Doppler evaluation is helpful to detect blood flow in all of the layers of

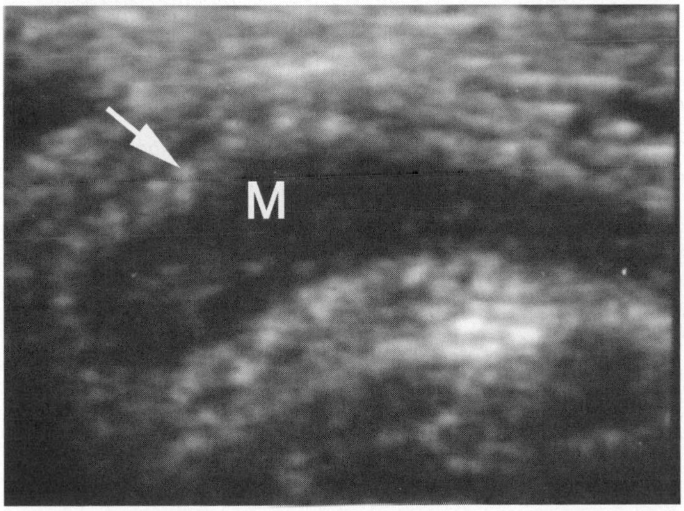

Figure 15-11. ■ *Infarcted bowel. Segment of ischemic bowel. There are small foci of gas in the wall* (arrow) *(pneumatosis coli) insufficiently large to cause subtle shadowing. The mucosal layer of the wall* (M) *is markedly thickened and edematous.*

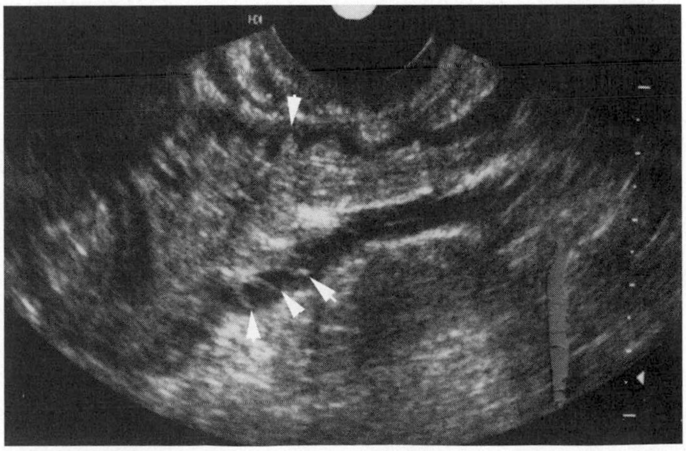

Figure 15-12. ■ *Loop of colon extensively involved with diverticulitis. Each of the echogenic areas* (arrows) *represents an outpouching related to a diverticulum. The colon wall is markedly thickened.*

the affected bowel. Lack of perfusion indicates bowel gangrene and the need for surgical intervention.

NEUTROPENIC TYPHLITIS

Limited usually to the terminal ileum, cecum, and ascending colon, neutropenic typhlitis appears on ultrasound as a homogeneously thickened bowel wall ranging from 1.0 to 2.5 cm in the area of abdominal pain.

INTESTINAL TUMORS

Lymphoma

This neoplasm appears sonographically as a hypoechoic, lobulated mass. The intestinal wall may be quite thickened due to tumor infiltration.

Leiomyosarcoma

Leiomyosarcoma is a large, solid subserosal or intramural mass located in the upper gastrointestinal tract, commonly found in the ileum. This large, irregular mass may be hyperechoic or hypoechoic with anechoic areas that have good, thorough transmission. A central necrotic area may be identified with a fluid level.

Carcinoma

Carcinomas can be located anywhere in the gastrointestinal tract, although they are most common in the stomach or colon. Sonographically, they appear as a circular or ovoid hypoechoic mass contiguous with normal bowel wall. The center, which is echogenic, may have acoustic shadowing. Depending on the degree of infiltration, the bowel wall thickness can range from 1 to 8 cm (Fig. 15-13). Evaluate for enlarged mesenteric nodes and liver metastases.

Carcinoid

This lesion may arise anywhere in the gastrointestinal tract, but it normally appears in the appendix, small bowel, or rectum. It usually measures less than 1.5 cm and sonographically appears as a sharply marginated, hypoechoic, lobulated mass with a strong back wall and lack of acoustic enhancement.

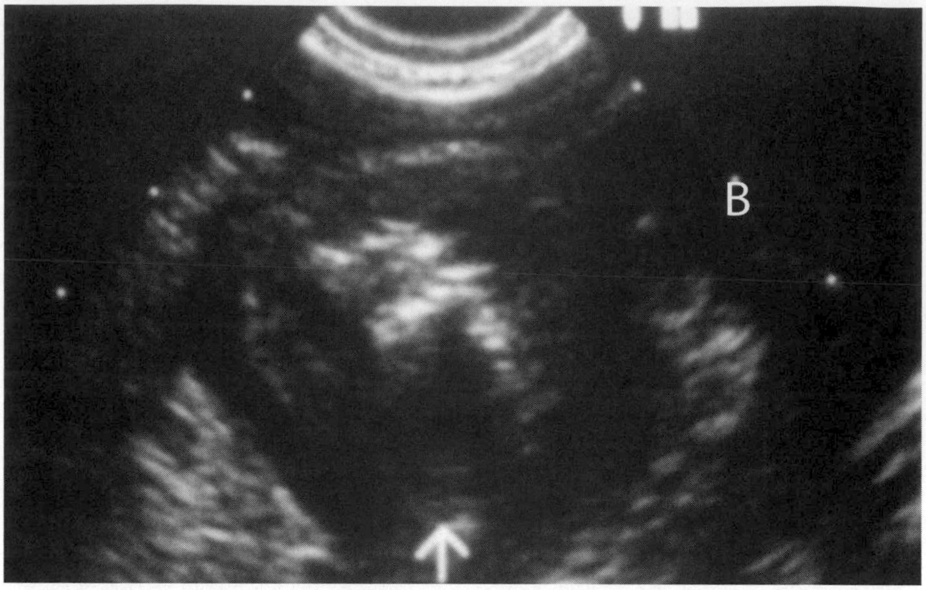

Figure 15-13. ■ *Colon cancer. A mass with shadowing air at the center and thick walls* (arrow) *(the cancer) lies superior to the bladder* (B).

Pitfalls

1. Nondiagnostic examinations. In patients with marked tenderness and guarding, excessive gaseous distention, or ascites, or with obese patients, it may be impossible to apply adequate compression to the bowel in order to make a diagnosis of appendicitis or diverticulitis.
2. False negatives. An inflamed appendix may not be visualized if it lies behind the gaseous shadows of the cecum.
3. Appendix versus terminal ileum. An inflamed appendix will have a blind end and no peristalsis, whereas an inflamed terminal ileum will widen into small bowel and may have some peristalsis.
4. Bowel loops. Fluid-filled loops of bowel can be recognized by watching for peristalsis and by demonstrating compressibility.
5. Mesenteric nodes. Nodes should not be mistaken for an inflamed appendix. They will appear as smooth, solid, ovoid structures with an echogenic center. They are not fluid-filled.
6. Blood vessels. Be careful not to identify the external iliac artery or vein as an inflamed appendix. The transducer should be rotated on any suspicious area. Blood vessels will have an elongated shape and will be pulsatile if an artery, or compressible if a vein. Doppler is helpful to demonstrate flow.
7. Mass mimickers. Fecal formations and spastic thickening of the bowel wall may appear as intestinal tumors. If uncertain, recheck the suspicious area at a later time to see whether there has been a change. In problematic cases involving the colon, examining the area of concern during a water enema may prove useful. Also be alert to an ectopic kidney, which may be mistaken for a mass.

Where Else to Look

1. A pelvic ultrasound should be performed on all female patients. Gynecologic pathology often mimics appendicitis symptoms, which is why ovulating women have the highest negative appendectomy rate. The pelvis should be evaluated for infection, ovarian cysts, ovarian torsion, hemorrhagic corpus luteum cysts, endometriosis, ectopic pregnancy, uterine wall rupture, abruptio placentae, and necrotic fibroids.
2. If tumor or adenopathy is found in the right lower quadrant, search the liver and other nodal sites for further disease.
3. If the findings are negative for intestinal pathology, the right upper quadrant should be scanned to rule out biliary obstruction or disease and renal pathology.
4. If a ruptured appendix or abscess is discovered in the right lower quadrant, the pelvis as well as the right and left gutters should be checked for fluid collections.
5. If a mass or an abscess is seen, scan through the abdomen for mesenteric nodes.
6. If an intestinal tumor is suspected, scan the liver and spleen for metastasis. Evaluate adjacent organs for infiltration or compression (i.e., hydronephrosis). Scan the gastrointestinal tract for other masses and for indications of bowel obstruction. Check for periaortic nodes.
7. In the case of Crohn's disease, the entire gastrointestinal tract should be scanned for other affected bowel segments, fluid-filled bowel loops, abscesses, or evidence of fistula formation.

SELECTED READING

Haber HP, Busch A, Ziebach R, et al. Ultrasonographic findings correspond to clinical, endoscopic, and histologic findings in inflammatory bowel disease and other enterocolitides. *J Ultrasound Med* 2002; 21(4):375–378.

Kessler N, Cyteval C, Gallix B, et al. Appendicitis: evaluation of the sensitivity, specificity and predictive values of US, Doppler US and laboratory findings. *Radiology* 2004;230:472–478.

Kori TM, Nemoto M, Maeda M, et al. Sonographic features of acute colonic diverticulitis: the "dome sign." *J Clin Ultrasound* 2000;28(7):340–346.

Lee HJ, Jeong KJ, Park KB. Operator-dependent techniques for graded compression sonography to detect the appendix and diagnose acute appendicitis *AJR Am J Roentgenol* 2005;184:91–97.

Lim JH. Colorectal cancer: sonographic findings. *AJR Am J Roentgenol* 1996;167:45–47.

Puylaert JB. Acute appendicitis: ultrasound evaluation using graded compression. *Radiology* 1986;158:355–360.

Puylaert JB. Mesenteric adenitis and acute terminal ileitis: ultrasound evaluation using graded compression. *Radiology* 1986;161: 691–695.

Puylaert JB, van der Werf J, Ulrich C, et al. Crohn disease of the ileocecal region: ultrasound visualization of the appendix. *Radiology* 1988;166:741–743.

Rettenbacker T, Hollerwager A, Macheiner P, et al. Ovoid shape of the vermiform appendix: a criterion to exclude acute appendicitis—devaluation with US. *Radiology* 2003; 226;95–100.

Ripolies T, Simo L, Martinez-Perez MJ. Sonographic findings in ischemic colitis in 58 patients. *AJR Am J Roentgenol* 2005;184: 777–758.

Teefey SA, Roarke MC, Brink JA, et al. Bowel wall thickening: differentiation of inflammation from ischemia with color Doppler and duplex US. *Radiology* 1996;198:547–551.

16 Possible Adrenal Mass

TOM WINTER

SONOGRAM ABBREVIATIONS

Ad	Adrenal gland
Ao	Aorta
Ca	Celiac artery
Cr	Crus
IVC	Inferior vena cava
K	Kidney
L	Liver
LRa	Left renal artery
LRv	Left renal vein
Pv	Portal vein
RRa	Right renal artery
RRv	Right renal vein
S	Spine
SMA	Superior mesenteric artery
Sp	Spleen
Spv	Splenic vein

KEY WORDS

Adenoma. Benign tumor of the adrenal cortex seen on computed tomography (CT) in 1% to 3% of the population.

Adrenal Cortical Carcinoma. Large malignant adrenal tumor with very poor prognosis.

Cortex. Outer portion of adrenal gland that secretes steroid hormones.

Cushing's Syndrome. Caused by hypersecretion of cortisol hormones from the adrenal cortex. An adrenal tumor (30%) or excess stimulation by the pituitary (70%) may be responsible.

Hyperplasia. Diffuse enlargement of adrenal glands.

Medulla. Central portion of adrenal gland that secretes adrenalin-related hormones—under the control of the sympathetic nervous system.

Myelolipoma. Benign adrenal tumor that contains fat and bone marrow tissue.

Neuroblastoma. Malignant adrenal mass occurring in children.

Pheochromocytoma. Medullary adrenal tumor that secretes hormones that elevate blood pressure.

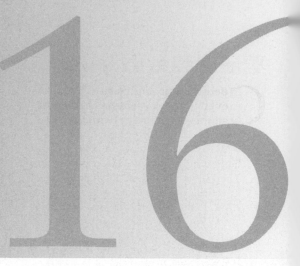

The Clinical Problem

Conditions that should direct the examiner's attention to the adrenal glands are the following:

1. Intermittent hypertension, flushing, and increased sweating—symptoms of pheochromocytoma.
2. Lung cancer. Thirty percent of lung cancer patients have metastatic disease in the adrenal glands.
3. Abnormal laboratory test results. Some adrenal pathology, such as pheochromocytoma, may be suggested by laboratory studies. Ultrasound can help by determining whether one or both glands are diseased.
4. Neuroblastoma. Children with neuroblastoma often present with a palpable abdominal mass.

Except in children (whose adrenal glands are more prominent than those of adults) and in thin adults, ultrasound is not the primary imaging modality for suspected adrenal pathology; CT is generally the most useful and most commonly employed modality for evaluating these structures. Incidental discovery of enlargement of one or both adrenal glands can be a significant contribution to a patient's workup, however ultrasound is also useful in areas that do not have ready access to a CT scanner.

Anatomy

Both glands are normally pyramidal in shape (Fig. 16-1). They are located in the retroperitoneum superior and anteromedial to the upper pole of the kidneys. The right gland lies posterior to the inferior vena cava (IVC) and anterior to the crus

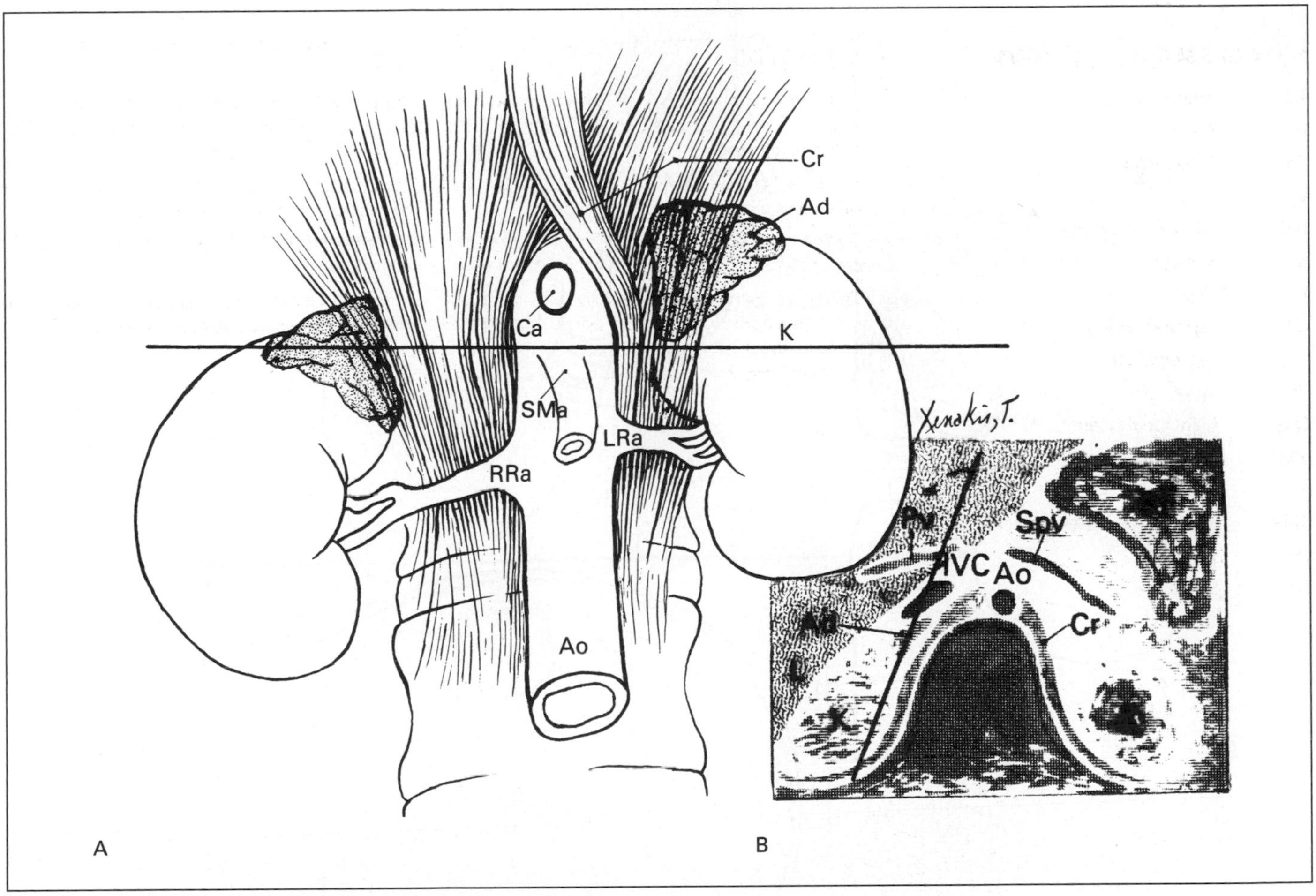

Figure 16-1. ■ *Adrenal glands. A. The adrenals are pyramidal glands located superior and anteromedial to the kidneys. B. The line illustrates the transducer angle used to show the right adrenal gland through the inferior vena cava* (IVC).

of the diaphragm (Fig. 16-2). The left gland lies between the spleen, the upper pole of the kidney, and the aorta and behind the tail of the pancreas.

Adrenal glands can be found in 80% to 95% of neonatal patients, with a lower success rate later in life. Neonatal glands are approximately one third as large as the infant kidney. In the neonate, there is an echogenic center to the gland, which persists to a lesser extent throughout the individual's life. The lack of perinephric fat and the small size of the neonatal patient allow the use of a higher-frequency probe.

Technique

Normal adrenal glands in adults are not easy to see. Their small size (approximately 4 cm × 2.5 cm × 0.5 cm; 4 grams each) and their acoustic texture make the glands difficult to differentiate from surrounding tissue. Using the liver as an acoustic window with current high-resolution ultrasound equipment, the right adrenal gland can be imaged in 90% of patients. The success rate on the left is reduced to approximately 75%, owing to the proximity of the stomach and bowel.

LEFT ADRENAL GLAND

The left adrenal is best approached with the patient in the right lateral decubitus

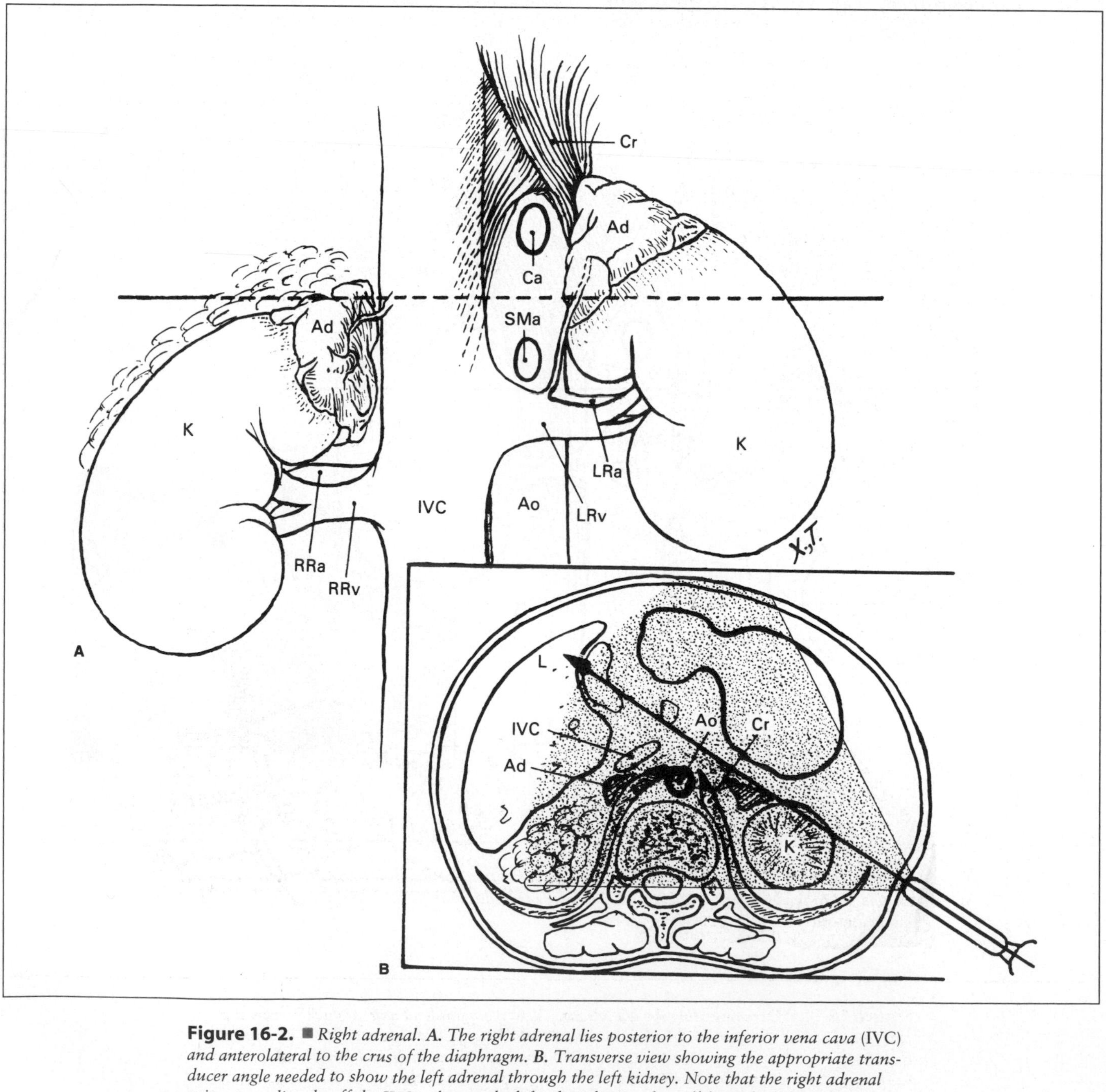

Figure 16-2. ■ *Right adrenal. A. The right adrenal lies posterior to the inferior vena cava* (IVC) *and anterolateral to the crus of the diaphragm. B. Transverse view showing the appropriate transducer angle needed to show the left adrenal through the left kidney. Note that the right adrenal vein comes directly off the IVC, whereas the left adrenal vein takes off from the left renal vein.*

(left-side-up) position (Fig. 16-3). Longitudinal views are most helpful.

1. Select the highest-frequency transducer that can be used.
2. Adjust the gain and/or power output controls to obtain good acoustic texture in the spleen. It is extremely important to avoid an overgained image.
3. Scanning longitudinally, locate the intercostal space that allows visualization of the upper pole of the left kidney and the spleen.
4. Maintain that longitudinal orientation, and rock the transducer in an anterior-posterior fashion until the

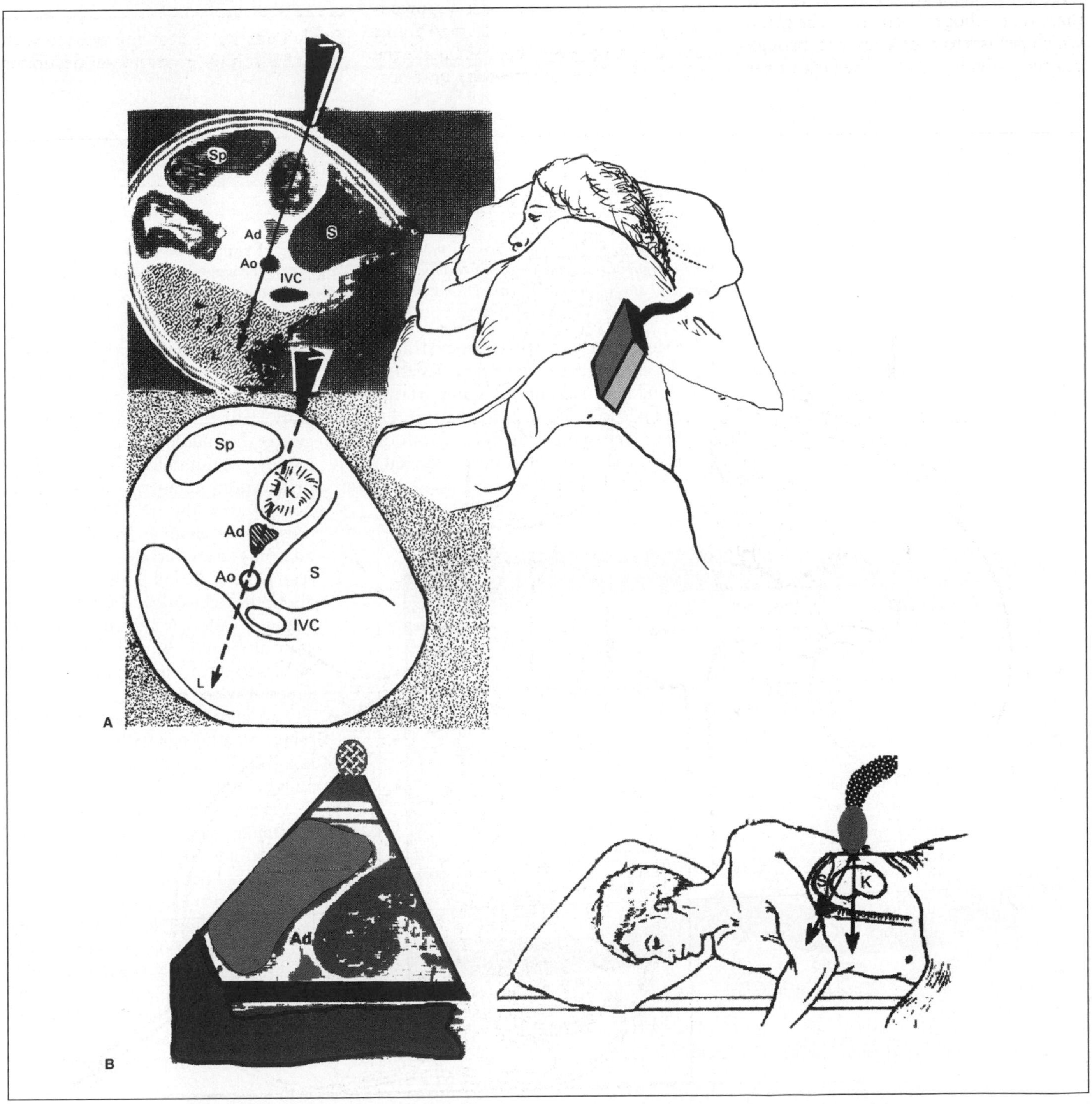

Figure 16-3. ■ *Demonstrating the left adrenal. A. In a longitudinal axis, adjust the scanning plane to align the upper pole of the left kidney with the long axis of the aorta. B. Then, angle the transducer slightly in an anterior-to-posterior fashion to visualize the left adrenal gland. The resulting longitudinal section should show the adrenal at the junction of the spleen, aorta, and upper pole of the left kidney.*

aorta can also be viewed longitudinally.

5. The left adrenal should appear as a triangular area where the spleen, the upper pole of the left kidney, and the aorta can be imaged simultaneously. Set the electronic focus at this level. The normal gland has concave or straight margins.

RIGHT ADRENAL GLAND

The right adrenal can usually be imaged in the traditional transverse and longitudinal views with the patient supine, using the liver as an acoustic window. If this method is unsuccessful because of liver size or position, you may reverse the technique described for the left adrenal.

1. Initiate scanning transversely from a right lateromedial approach perpendicular to the medial borders of the liver and kidney and the right margin of the spine (Fig. 16-4).
2. Enlarge the field size to allow visualization of small structures at the level of the adrenal.

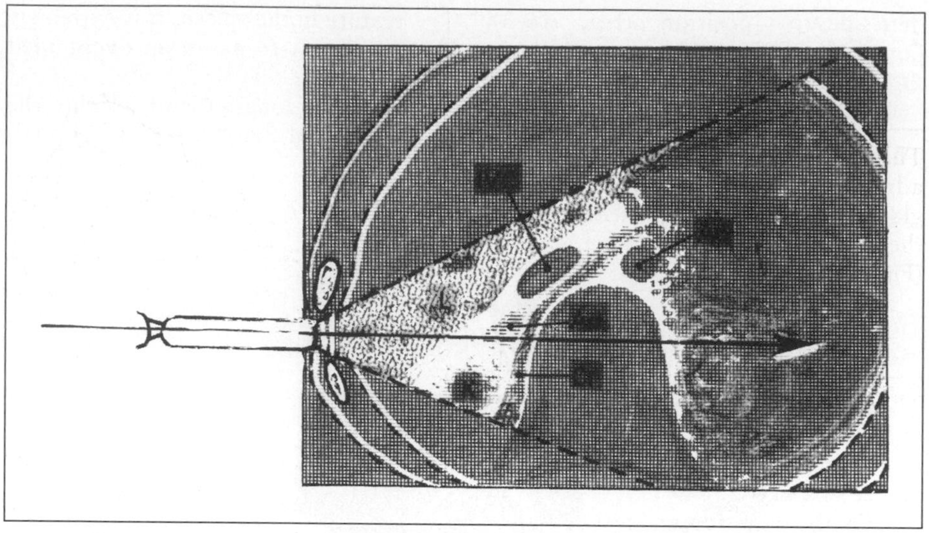

Figure 16-4. ■ *The right adrenal is most effectively imaged by scanning perpendicular to the right margin of the spine in an area bounded by the inferior vena cava* (IVC), *medial margin of the liver, and crus of the diaphragm. Do not confuse the crus with the adrenal gland.*

3. Select the highest-frequency transducer possible for adequate penetration. Fine resolution is important, but you must be able to penetrate the liver well. Adjust the focal depth of the probe to the level of the adrenal.
4. Adjust the gain or output controls so that liver texture is uniform throughout the field.
5. Start scanning transversely in the region of the middle to upper pole of the kidney. Maintaining the transverse orientation, identify the pertinent normal anatomy (i.e., kidney, liver, crus of the diaphragm). Image the anatomy transversely, moving the scan head cephalad until you are just above the right kidney. Be prepared to change to another intercostal space if your ultrasound beam is not perpendicular to the medial liver margin just superior to the kidney.
6. Try to confirm the presence or absence of pathology with longitudinal images. (Transverse scans will probably be more helpful.)
   a. Longitudinal sections can be obtained by angling laterally in the midline to show an enlarged adrenal behind the IVC (Fig. 16-5; see also Fig. 16-1).
   b. Longitudinal sections with medial angulation (approximately 30 degrees) aligning the right kidney and IVC may show the adrenal superior to the kidney. This technique is similar to that described for the left adrenal.

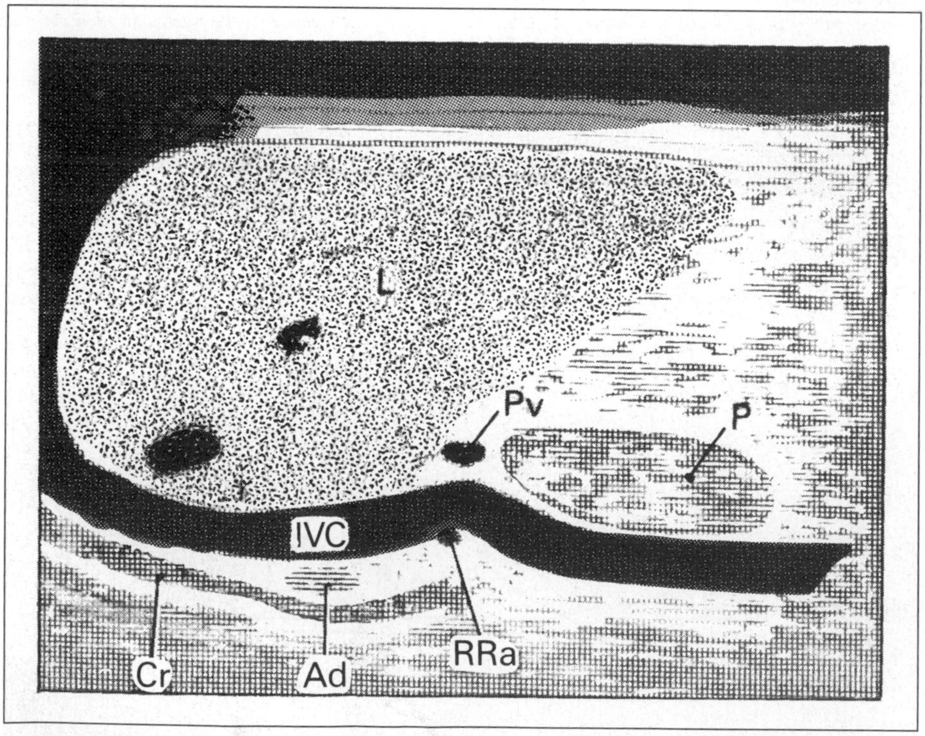

Figure 16-5. ■ *The right adrenal can be imaged longitudinally in the abdominal midline by using a medial-to-lateral angulation through the inferior vena cava* (IVC) *(see also Fig. 16-2).*

Pathology

EARLY SIGNS OF ADRENAL ENLARGEMENT

The normally concave margins of the adrenal gland become convex as the gland enlarges. The larger the gland is, the more rounded the outline becomes (Fig. 16-6).

CHANGES IN POSITION OF ADJACENT ORGANS

The changes in position of adjacent organs or structures may assist the sonographer in recognizing the adrenal as the source of a mass.

On the right side, changes caused by an enlarged adrenal include the following:

1. Anterior displacement of the retroperitoneal fat line, which lies in front of the kidneys and adrenal and behind the liver (see Fig. 8-3).
2. Anterior displacement of the IVC by the mass. It is important to examine this appearance transversely, as a slightly malrotated right kidney may also cause anterior displacement of the IVC.
3. Posteroinferior displacement of the kidney.
4. Draping of the right renal vein over the mass.

On the left side, changes indicative of an enlarged adrenal include anterior displacement of the splenic vein and posteroinferior displacement of the kidney.

CAUSES OF ENLARGEMENT

The following conditions are possible causes of enlargement:

1. Adenomas. Smooth, rounded, homogeneous masses (Fig. 16-7). These are often incidentally discovered and are of little clinical consequence as a rule.

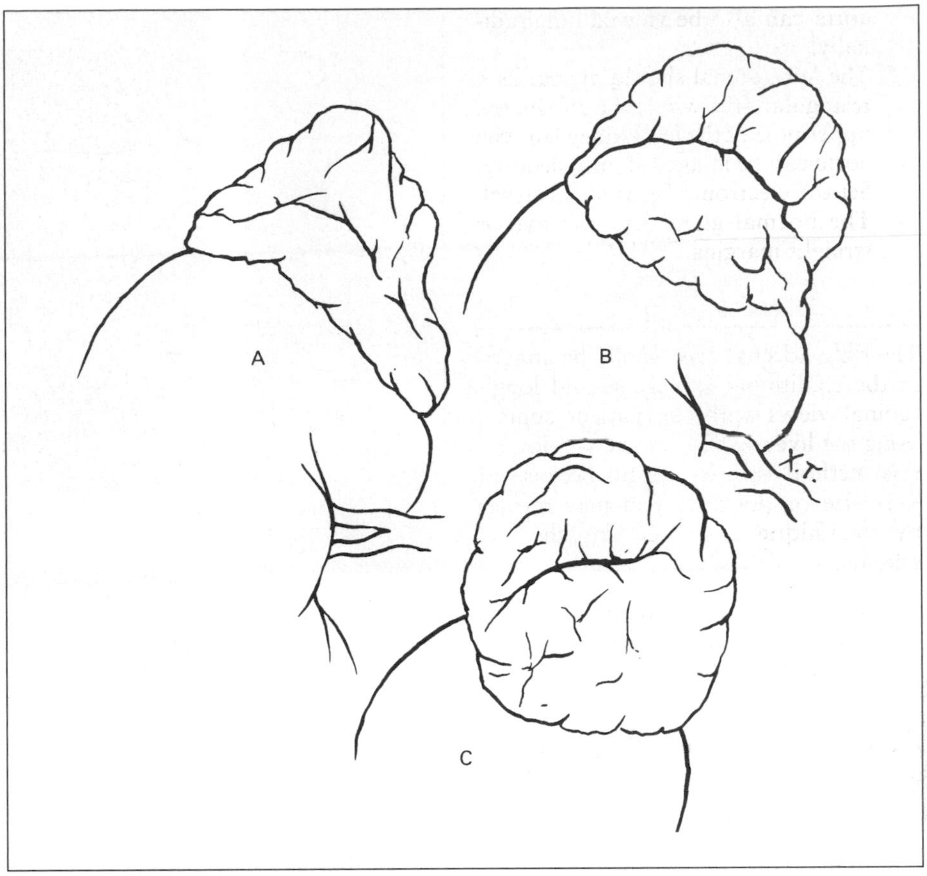

Figure 16-6. ■ *Progressive signs of adrenal enlargement. A. Normal concave margins. B. Convex margins of the slightly enlarged gland. C. The larger the gland is, the more rounded the contour will be.*

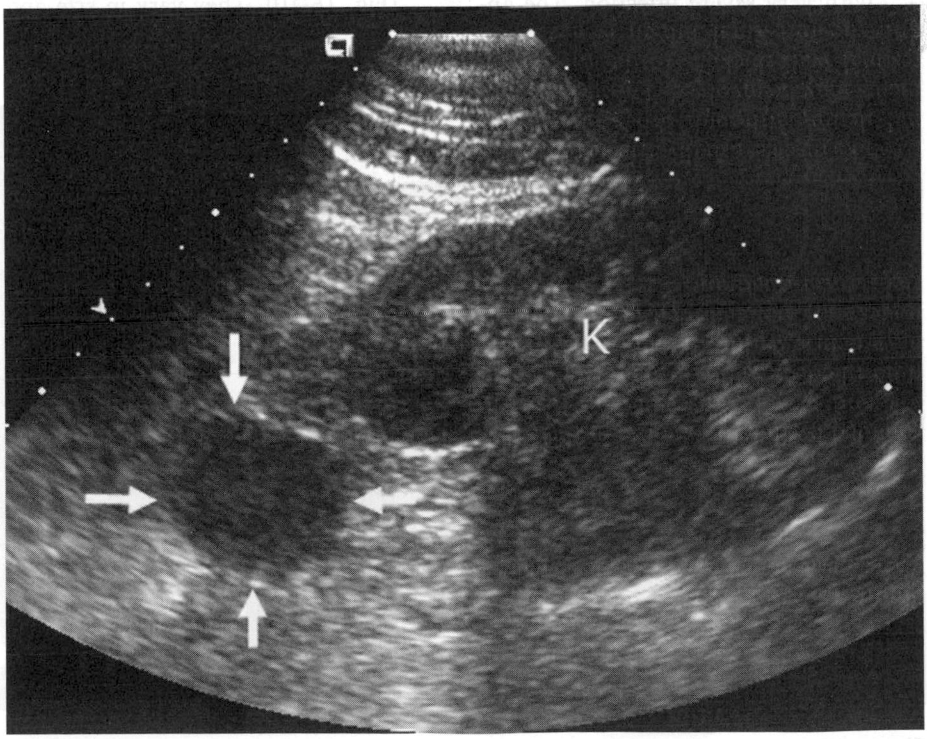

Figure 16-7. ■ *Adrenal adenoma* (arrows). *Round, homogeneous mass in the left adrenal.*

Renal Failure

BARB VANDERWERFF
TOM WINTER

17

SONOGRAM ABBREVIATIONS

C	Calculus
IVC	Inferior vena cava
K	Kidney
L	Liver
P	Pelvis of the kidney
Ps	Psoas muscle
R	Rib
RRV	Right renal vein
S	Spine
Sp	Spleen

KEY WORDS

Acute Tubular Necrosis (ATN). Acute renal shutdown, often after an episode of low blood pressure (hypotension). Spontaneous and fairly rapid recovery is usual, but the condition can be fatal.

Anuria. No urine production.

Azotemia. Renal failure.

Benign Prostatic Hypertrophy (BPH). As men age, the prostate enlarges. If the prostate gets too big, it may obstruct the urethra and cause renal failure.

BUN. Blood urea nitrogen. See Serum Urea Nitrogen.

Calyx. A portion of the renal collecting system adjacent to the renal pyramid in which urine collects. The calyx is connected to an infundibulum.

Central Echo Complex (CEC, Sinus Echo Complex). The group of central echoes in the middle of the kidney that are caused by fat and the collecting system.

Column of Bertin. A normal renal variant in which there is enlargement of a portion of the cortex between two pyramids. Can mimic a tumor on pyelography or ultrasound.

Cortex. The more peripheral segment of the kidney tissue. Surrounds medulla and sinus echoes.

Creatinine. See Serum Creatinine.

Dehydration. If a patient does not drink enough fluid, the skin becomes lax and the eyes sunken. Renal obstruction may be present but may be missed sonographically because the kidneys are not producing much urine.

Dialysis. Technique for removing waste products from the blood when the kidneys do not work properly. The two common types are hemodialysis and peritoneal.

Hemodialysis. Used in long-term renal failure. The patient's blood is circulated through tubes outside the body that allow the exchange of fluids and removal of unwanted substances.

Peritoneal Dialysis. A tube is inserted into the abdomen. Fluid containing a number of body constituents is run into the peritoneum, where it exchanges with waste products. A sonogram shows evidence of apparent ascites.

Dysplasia. Condition resulting from obstruction in utero characterized by echogenic kidneys with cysts. Such kidneys function poorly or not at all. Dysplasia is untreatable.

Glomerulonephritis. Medical condition with acute and chronic forms in which the kidneys function poorly owing to inflammation. Usually it is a self-limiting condition if acute, but if chronic, it may require long-term treatment with dialysis or transplantation.

Hydronephrosis. Dilatation of the kidney collecting system due to obstruction at the level of the ureter, bladder, or urethra.

Hydroureter (Ureterectasis). Distension of the ureter with urine, often due to a blockage of the ureter.

Infundibulum (Major Calyx). A tube connecting the renal pelvis to the calyx.

Medulla. Portion of the kidney adjacent to the calyx, also known as a pyramid. It is less echogenic (hypoechoic) than the cortex.

Nephrostomy or Percutaneous Nephrostomy. Tube inserted through the skin into the kidney to drain an obstructed kidney.

Nephrotic Syndrome. Type of medical renal failure, often due to renal vein thrombosis, in which excess protein is excreted by the kidney.

Oliguria. Decreased urine output.

Polyuria. Increased urine output.

Pyelonephritis (Chronic). Repeated infections destroy the kidneys, which become small with some parenchymal areas narrowed by scar formation.

Pyonephrosis. Hydronephrotic collecting system filled with pus.

Pyramids. See Medulla.

Reflux. A backward (retrograde) flow of urine between the urinary bladder and the kidney.

Serum Creatinine. Waste product that accumulates in the blood when the kidneys are malfunctioning.

Serum Urea Nitrogen (SUN) (Blood Urea Nitrogen [BUN]). Waste products that accumulate in the blood when the kidneys are malfunctioning.

Sinus Echo Complex. See Central Echo Complex.

Staghorn Calculus. Large stone located in the center of the kidney.

Ureterectasia. Dilatation of a ureter.

Ureterocele. Congenital partial obstruction of the ureter at the place where it enters the bladder. A cobra-headed deformity of the lower ureter is seen on a pyelogram.

Urinalysis (UA). Laboratory test that evaluates the patient's urine for a variety of factors. Used in patients with suspected renal failure, urinary tract infections, diabetes, and many other diseases.

RELEVANT LABORATORY VALUES

Blood urea nitrogen: 7 to 20 mg/dL

Creatinine (Cr): 0.6 to 1.3 mg/dL

Oliguria: For an adult, the excretion of less than 400 or 500 mL of urine in a day

Polyuria: For an adult, the excretion of more than ~2,500 mL of urine in a day

Urinalysis:

- Protein: Negative to trace
- 0 to 5 white blood cells per high power field
- 0 to 2 red blood cells per high power field
- Specific gravity: 1.005 to 1.030
- Glucose: Negative

The Clinical Problem

Renal failure occurs when the kidneys are unable to remove waste products from the bloodstream. Waste products used as a measure of the severity of renal failure include the serum creatinine level and serum urea nitrogen (or blood urea nitrogen [BUN]) level. Loss of 60% of the functioning parenchyma can exist without elevation of the BUN or creatinine levels, so these laboratory tests are not very sensitive for the early detection of renal failure.

The onset of renal failure is often insidious. The patient may have the condition for months before seeking medical attention with anemia, nausea, vomiting, and headaches. Other symptoms include increased or decreased urine frequency. Renal failure may be the result of either kidney disease or lower genitourinary tract disease within the ureter, bladder, or urethra with obstruction of urine excretion.

MEDICAL RENAL DISEASE

Kidney disease can either be an acute process or a chronic and irreversible one, treatable only by dialysis or transplant. In potentially reversible, short-term renal failure (e.g., acute tubular necrosis or acute glomerulonephritis), the kidneys are normal in size or large. In patients with long-standing renal failure (e.g., chronic glomerulonephritis or chronic pyelonephritis), the kidneys are small and often abnormally echogenic. Many drugs, particularly the aminoglycoside type of antibiotic, can cause medical renal failure.

HYDRONEPHROSIS

By far the most important diagnosis to exclude in patients with renal failure is hydronephrosis. If hydronephrosis is the cause of renal failure, both kidneys are likely to be obstructed unless the patient has some other renal disease coincident with obstruction. Occasionally, obstruction of one kidney may precipitate renal failure if the other kidney is absent or damaged. If obstruction is the sole cause of renal failure, the level of the obstructive site is probably in the bladder or urethra, because bilateral ureteral obstruction is very unusual. Once renal obstruction has been documented, a drainage/decompressive procedure such as bladder catheterization, nephrostomy, or prostatectomy is urgently required to relieve obstruction. If a drainage procedure is not performed and obstruction persists, kidney function will be permanently impaired. Because of its accuracy, ease of use, lack of risk, and lack of ionizing radiation, sonography has replaced retrograde pyelography as the screening procedure of choice for hydronephrosis in renal failure.

DYSPLASIA

In children, the kidneys may function poorly as a result of obstruction in utero. Such damaged kidneys are seen with posterior urethral valves or the prune belly syndrome.

Anatomy

SIZE AND SHAPE

The normal adult kidney as measured by ultrasound is approximately 11 cm in length (see Appendix 29), with the left being slightly larger than the right. The parenchyma is 2.5 cm thick, and the kidney is approximately 5 cm wide.

The kidneys have a convex lateral edge and a concave medial edge called the hilum. The arteries, veins, and ureter enter the hilum.

LOCATION

The kidneys are located retroperitoneally in the lumbar region, between the 12th thoracic and 3rd lumbar vertebrae. The left kidney lies 1 to 2 cm higher than the right. The kidneys rest on the lower two thirds of the quadratus lumborum muscle, on the posterior and medial portion of the psoas muscle, and laterally on the transverse abdominis muscle.

1. The lower pole is more laterally located than the upper pole.
2. The lower pole is more anteriorly located than the upper pole owing to the oblique course of the psoas muscle.
3. The renal hilum is situated in the center of the medial side.

SINUS AND CAPSULAR ECHOES

The kidney is surrounded by a well-defined echogenic line representing the capsule in the adult (Fig. 17-1). This line may be difficult to see in the infant or lean people owing to the sparse amount of perinephric fat. At the center of the kidney are dense echoes (the central sinus echo or sinus echo complex) due to renal sinus fat (Fig. 17-1). In the infant or emaciated patient, these echoes may be virtually absent.

PARENCHYMA

The renal parenchyma has two components. The centrally located pyramids, or medulla, are surrounded on three sides by the peripherally located cortex. The medullary zone or pyramid is slightly less echogenic than the cortex (Fig. 17-1). In infants or thin people, a differentiation of medulla from cortex may be very obvious, but in other healthy adults, this separation may be undetectable.

Organ echogenicity from greatest to least in the healthy patient is as follows: renal sinus, pancreas, liver, spleen, renal cortex, and renal medullary pyramids. In healthy adults, the renal cortex should be hypoechoic, or at most isoechoic, to the liver.

SHAPE VARIANTS

The spleen may squash the left kidney, causing a flattened outline or distorted outline so that the lateral border bulges, creating what is termed a dromedary hump (see Fig. 17-9). The renal border may show subtle indentations known as fetal lobulations.

VASCULAR ANATOMY

See Figures 17-1, 17-4, and 22-1.

Renal Veins

The renal veins, which are large, connect the inferior vena cava with the kidneys and lie anterior to the renal arteries. The left renal vein has a long course and passes between the superior mesenteric artery and the aorta (see Fig. 6-12).

Renal Arteries

The renal arteries lie posterior to the renal veins. They may be multiple and too small to visualize, but if only one artery is present, visualization is relatively easy. The right renal artery is longer than the left and passes posterior to the inferior vena cava. The main renal artery gives rise to a dorsal and a ventral branch. These branch first into the interlobar arteries, then into the arcuate arteries (see Fig. 22-1), and finally into the tiny interlobular (cortical) arteries. Typical arterial flow patterns in the renal artery are shown in Figure 22-4.

URETERS

See Chapter 20.

URINARY BLADDER

See Chapter 20.

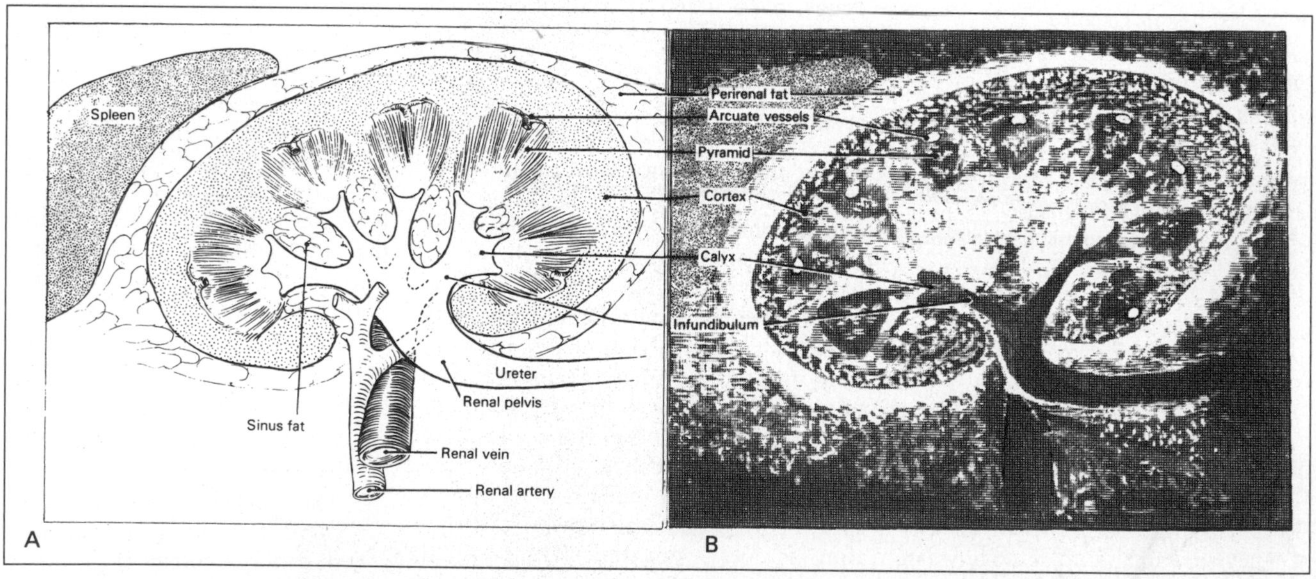

Figure 17-1. ■ *Major structures of the left kidney. A. Coronal anatomic view. B. Sonogram. Echogenic area at the center of the kidney is the result of renal sinus fat. The pyramids are less-echogenic areas adjacent to the sinus. The cortex is slightly more echogenic, and the capsule (perirenal fat) is an echogenic line.*

Technique

RIGHT KIDNEY

The right kidney is best examined in the supine position through the liver (Figs. 17-2–17-4). Angle the transducer obliquely if the liver is small. A coronal and lateral approach can also be used if the liver is small (Figs. 17-4 and 17-5). It is often helpful to have the patient take in and hold a deep breath to see the kidney in a subcostal (under the ribs) approach. If bowel gas obscures visualization of the lower pole, it may be necessary to roll the patient into the right-side-up decubitus position and scan from a lateral approach. The harmonic and compound imaging technologies available on newer ultrasound machines can enhance the renal outline and improve corticomedullary differentiation.

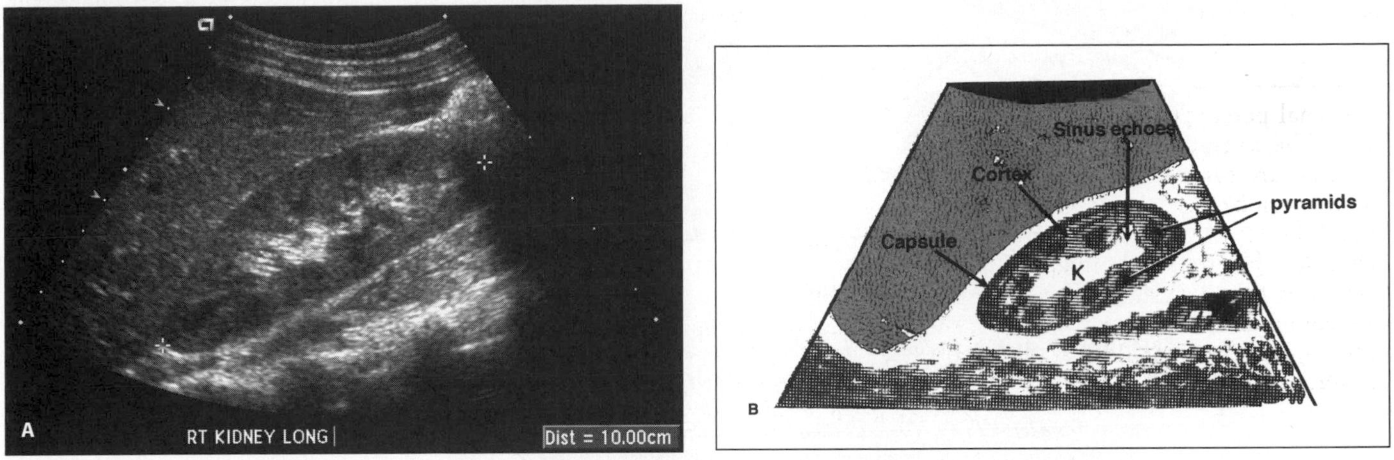

Figure 17-2. ■ *Normal right kidney demonstrated on supine longitudinal views. Sinus echoes are surrounded by pyramids which are less echogenic than the neighboring cortex. A. Sonogram. B. Diagram.*

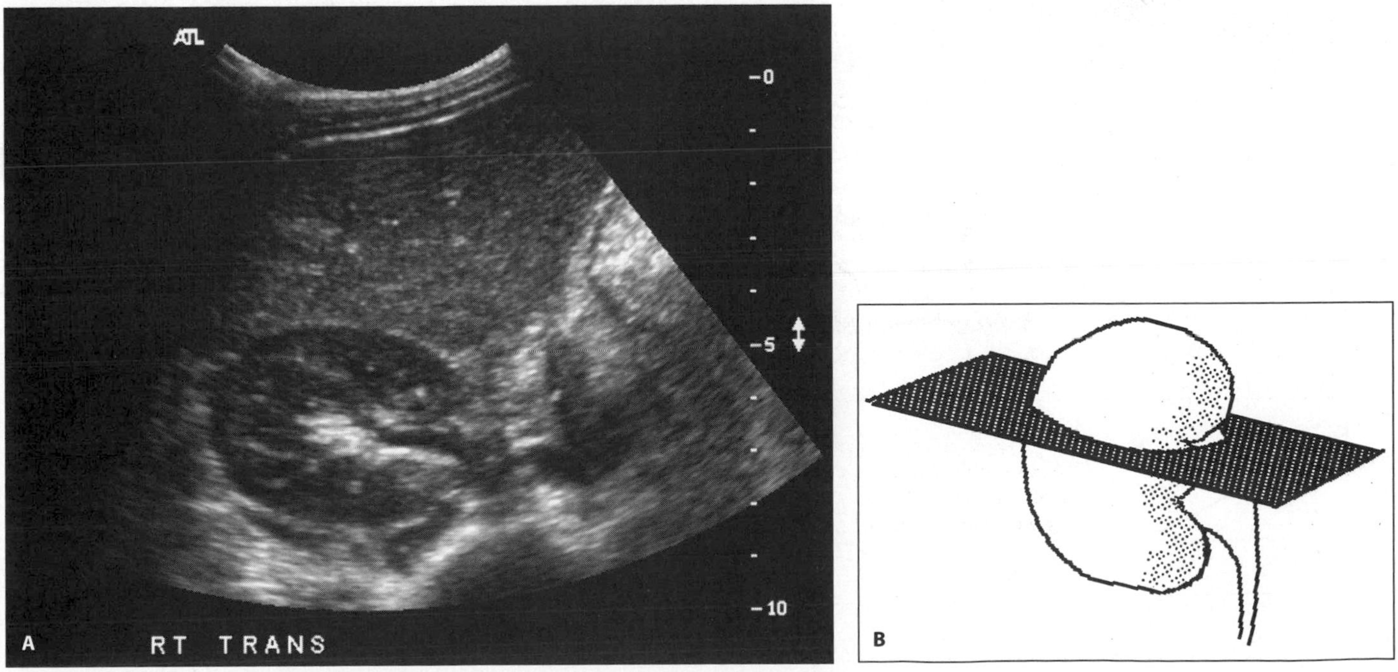

Figure 17-3. ■ *Transverse view of right kidney with diagram showing how the view was obtained. A. Sonogram. B. Diagram.*

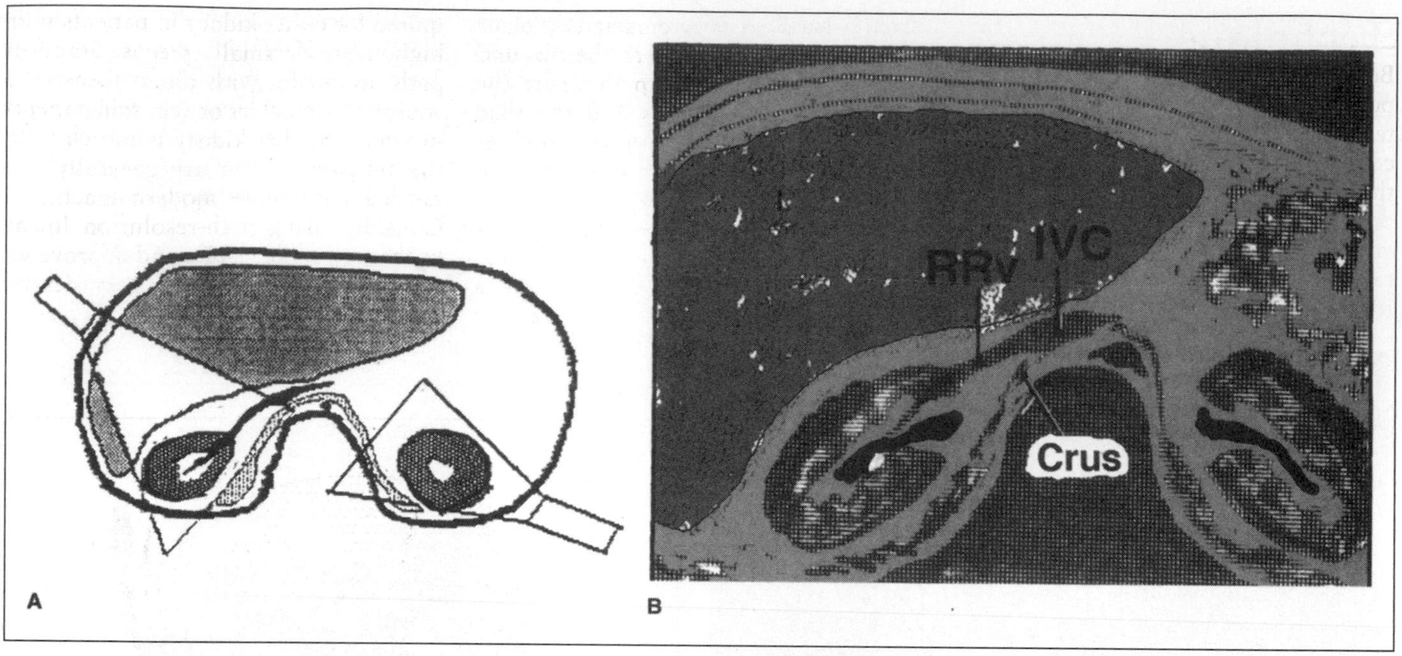

Figure 17-4. ■ *A. Technique diagram. The right kidney is examined with the transducer held obliquely through the liver, which acts as an acoustic window. The left kidney is examined from a posterolateral approach. It may be necessary to put the patient in the left-side-up position for ideal views of the left kidney. The crus (diaphragm) lies behind, posterior to the inferior vena cava and anterior to the aorta. B. Transverse view of both kidneys.*

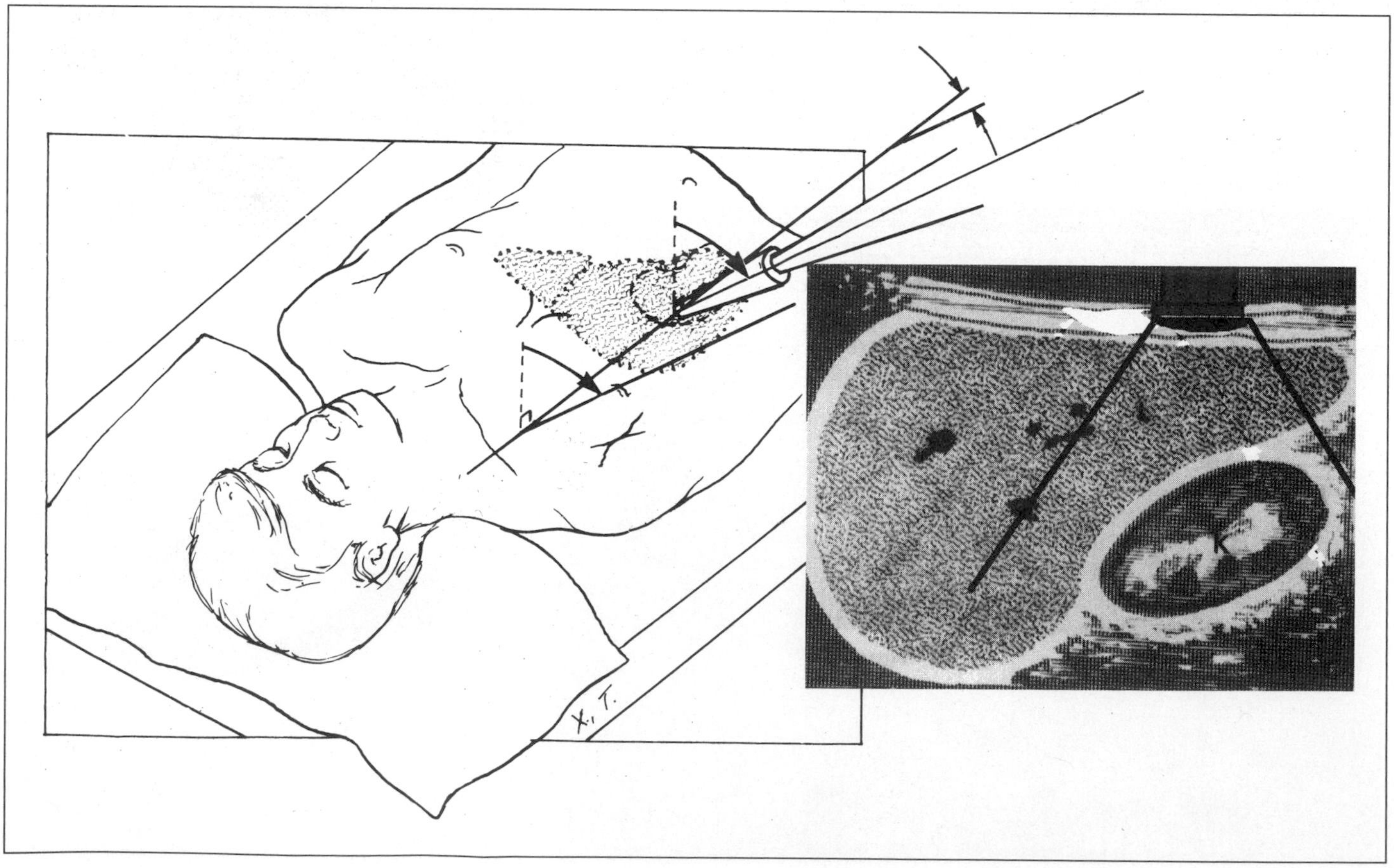

Figure 17-5. ■ *A helpful technique for viewing the right kidney is to place the transducer on an oblique longitudinal axis but still use the liver as an acoustic window.*

LEFT KIDNEY

Begin with the patient in the left-side-up position. With the patient's left arm extended over his or her head, and using a coronal approach, scan intercostally through the spleen (Fig. 17-6). Vary the decubitus and oblique positions until you can see the kidney. Suspended inspiration is usually necessary. Use as high a frequency transducer as you can.

If the patient is emaciated, place supportive pillows between the ribs and iliac crest. This will help eliminate the cavity between the ribs and the iliac crest. The prone position gives good results in children, but ribs interfere with this view in adults.

Separate views of the lower and upper poles may be needed. If the lower pole is hidden by the iliac crest, try an expiration view. Erect views may be required for either kidney in patients with high livers or small spleens. Standoff pads are useful with older ultrasound equipment in babies or very thin patients in whom the left kidney is too close to the transducer, but are generally not needed with more modern machines. Consider using high-resolution linear probes to problem solve and improve visualization in pediatric or very slender patients.

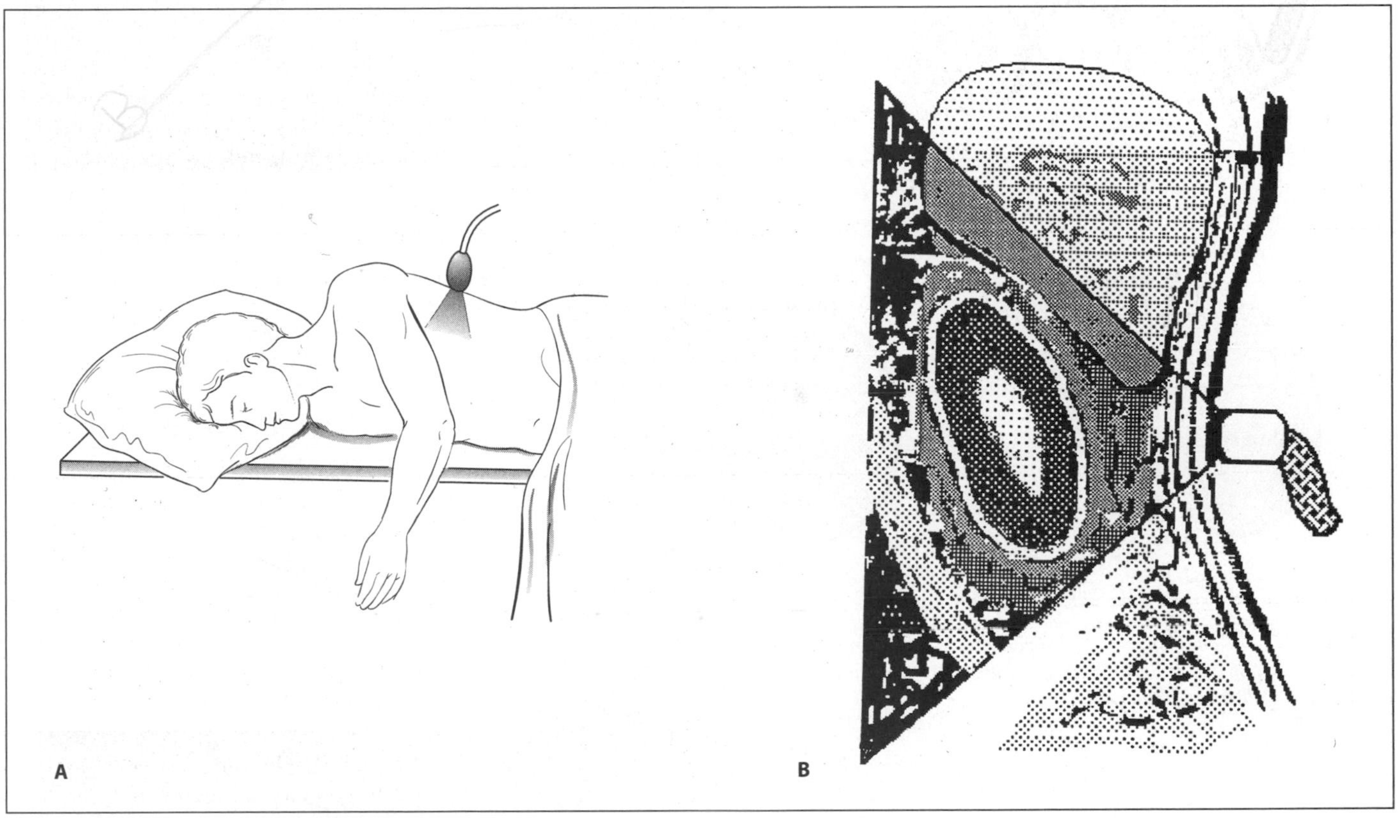

Figure 17-6. ■ *Viewing the left kidney. A. Technique diagram. B. Sonographic view. The usual technique for viewing the left kidney is to place the patient in the left-side-up (coronal) position using the spleen as a partial window. The same technique can be used on the right.*

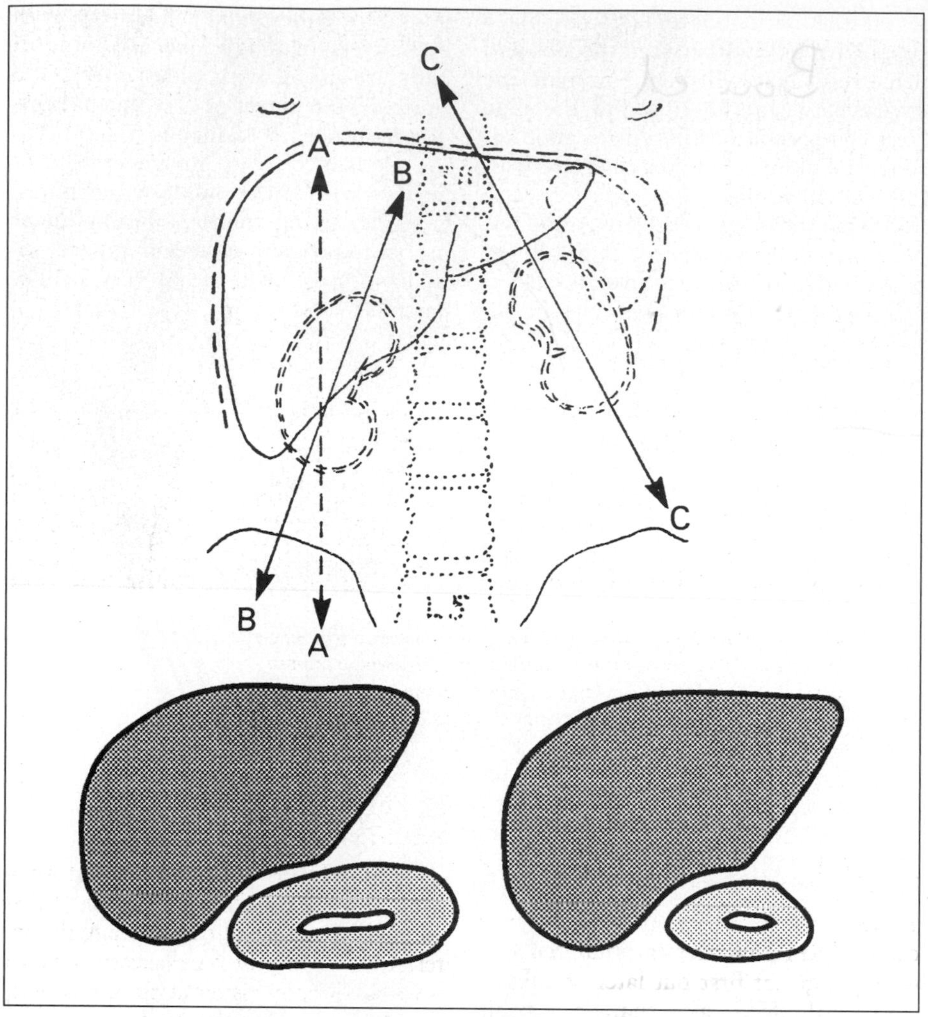

Figure 17-7. ■ *Renal length. The longest renal length (lines* B *and* C*) should be obtained. A length taken along a standard longitudinal view of the kidney (line* A*) is too short. The kidneys usually have a slightly oblique axis.*

LENGTH

Make sure you have found the longest length of the kidney by trying various oblique views to see which yields the largest value (Fig. 17-7).

Ideally, there should be an even amount of cortical tissue around the sinus echoes, except on the medial aspect. Be sure not to foreshorten the true kidney length. (Sometimes, the lower pole is obscured by bowel gas; try a more coronal or lateral approach.) For large kidneys, a curved linear array is preferred; the large field of view is needed. It may be necessary to take a rather "unsonogenic" image to be accurate; try angling through the lower pole to the upper pole (Fig. 17-7). This will give you poor detail at the upper pole because the beam is not perpendicular to it, but allows for an accurate measurement without extrapolating. This is especially effective on the left side.

Pathology

ACUTE MEDICAL RENAL DISEASE

The kidneys are normal in length or enlarged with acute medical renal disease. Parenchymal echogenicity is generally increased compared with the liver. The degree of parenchymal echogenicity can be graded as follows:

Grade I. The renal parenchymal echogenicity equals that of the liver.

Grade II. The renal parenchymal echogenicity is greater than that of the liver.

Grade III. The echogenicity of the renal parenchyma is equal to the renal sinus echoes.

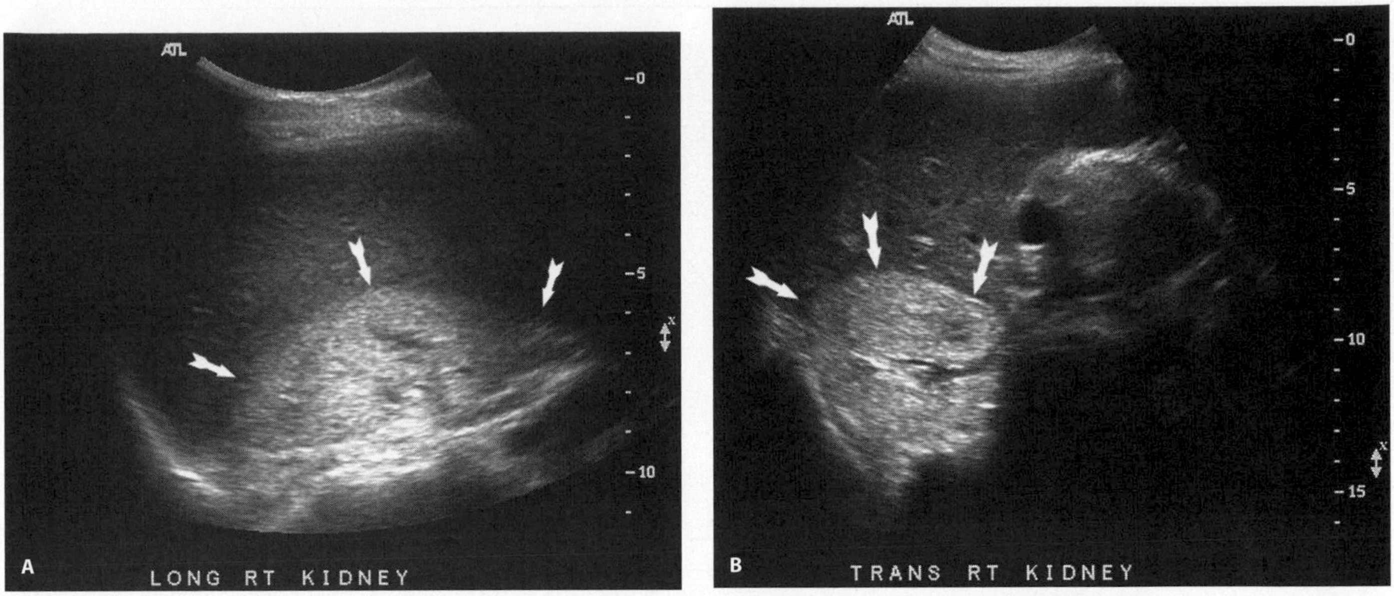

Figure 17-8. ■ *Longitudinal (A) (obliqued through peripheral cortex) and transverse (B) images through right kidney* (arrows) *affected with classic sonographic manifestations of human immunodeficiency virus nephropathy. Renal length was borderline large (12.3 cm) in this small female patient. Note striking increased echogenicity of the cortex when compared with the adjacent normal liver. Left kidney appeared similar.*

In patients with human immunodeficiency virus (HIV) and kidney disease, very bright and very normal appearances to the kidney have diagnostic value in respectively establishing or excluding HIV-associated nephropathy (Fig. 17-8).

SMALL END-STAGE KIDNEY (CHRONIC MEDICAL RENAL DISEASE)

With end-stage kidney disease, both kidneys are small—5 to 8 cm in length—but renal sinus echoes are visible. The amount of renal parenchyma is usually shrunken. Focal loss of parenchyma indicates chronic pyelonephritis or a renal infarct (Fig. 17-9).

The renal parenchyma may show evidence of increased echogenicity. However, if only one kidney is small and diseased (e.g., in recurrent unilateral pyelonephritis), the kidney may be extremely small. In fact, the kidney may be almost impossible to visualize, even though the patient is asymptomatic. Even when an end-stage kidney measures only 2 to 3 cm in length, an echogenic center and some renal parenchyma will sometimes still be visible. The parenchyma may show evidence of focal narrowing due to scars (Fig. 17-9).

VASCULAR DISEASE

Renal Artery Occlusion

Bilateral renal artery occlusion can be a cause of renal failure. An infarcted kidney enlarges at first but later shrinks in size. Focal infarcts are usually echopenic at first but may later become echogenic.

Hemorrhagic infarcts may be echogenic. Color or power Doppler can be helpful in showing no flow to the involved kidney or area.

Renal Artery Stenosis

Drinking fluids for 6 hours before a sonogram for renal artery stenosis (RAS) enhances image quality. Although the arterial narrowing of renal artery stenosis is rarely directly visible with ultrasound, there may be Doppler evidence of narrowing. At the site of stenosis, there is little or no flow in diastole, much turbulence, and an abnormally high velocity. Significant controversy attends the use of

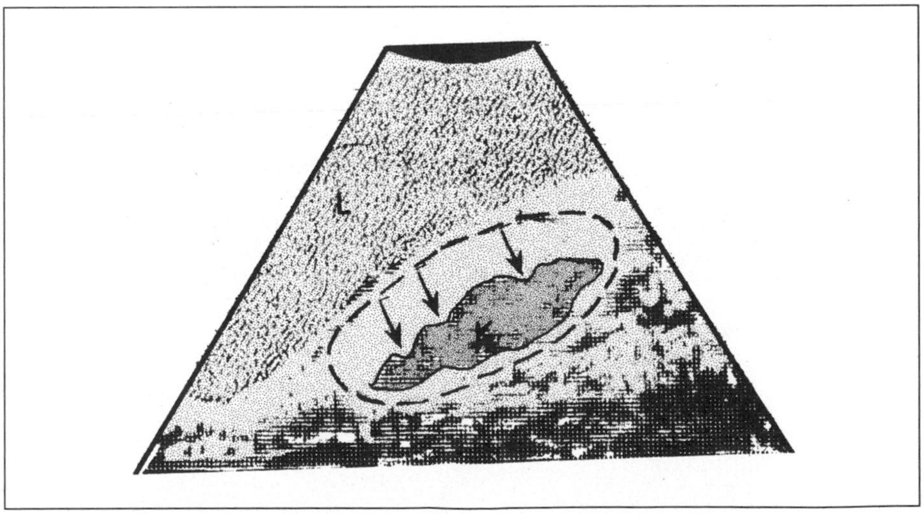

Figure 17-9. ■ *A small, shrunken, misshapen kidney* (arrows) *is usually a long-term consequence of chronic pyelonephritis. Original kidney size* (dotted lines). L, *liver.*

Doppler in diagnosing RAS, but two direct measurements worrisome for stenosis include a peak systolic velocity of greater than 180 cm/sec and a greater than 3.5 ratio between the peak velocity in the stenotic renal segment and the aorta. The stenotic site is usually at the junction of the renal artery and the aorta. This area is difficult to see owing to overlying intestinal gas. Distal to the stenotic area, Doppler shows a small peak coupled with a long upswing and slow descent in systole (Fig. 17-10).

The acceleration time—the duration of the ascent segment in systole—is a widely used method for assessing renal artery stenosis. This pattern is assessed distal to the narrowed region and is known as the parvus and tardus pattern (see Chapter 4).

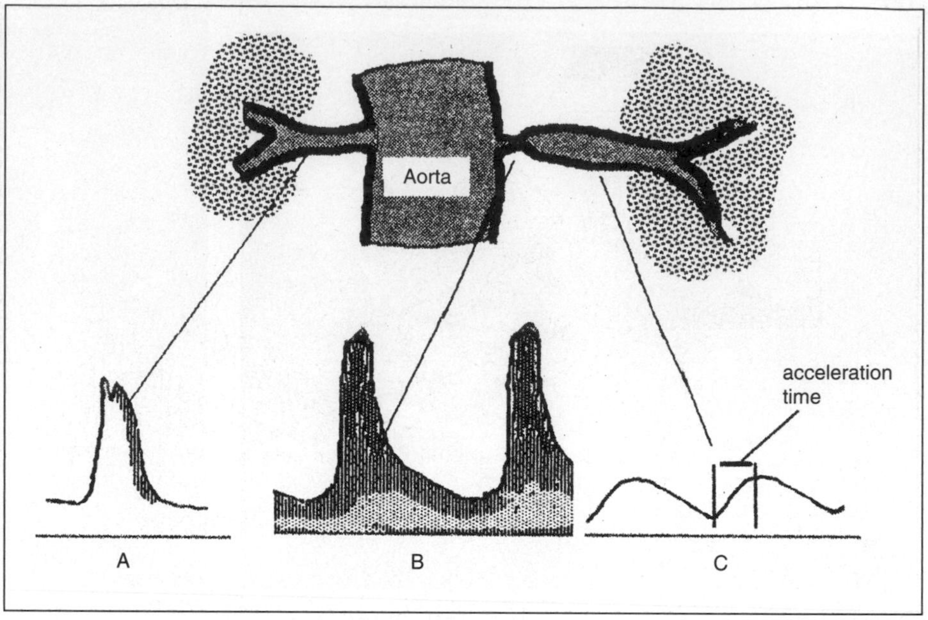

Figure 17-10. ■ *Doppler flow pattern changes with renal artery stenosis. A. Normal appearance. B. Left main renal artery is narrowed so that there is increased peak systolic flow and much turbulence at the site of stenosis. C. Beyond the stenosis, the systolic peak is lower and longer than normal.*

Renal Vein Thrombosis

Renal vein thrombosis occurs in both acute and chronic forms. In the acute form, the kidney swells and the central sinus echoes usually become more prominent, although this is a variable phenomenon. Sometimes, thrombosis can be visualized within the renal vein. Clot expands the renal vein and inferior vena cava.

Absence of the main renal vein flow may be seen using color Doppler, although all of the clot may be located in the peripheral vessels, so the presence of main renal vein flow does not exclude peripheral vein clot. Reversal of arterial flow in intrarenal arteries is a useful indirect indicator of renal artery thrombosis.

In the chronic form, the kidney is small and somewhat echogenic.

HYDRONEPHROSIS

In hydronephrosis, the sinus echoes surround a fluid-filled center because the calyces, infundibula, and renal pelvis are dilated. Usually, the renal pelvis is more distended than the calyces. The calyces and infundibula can be traced to the

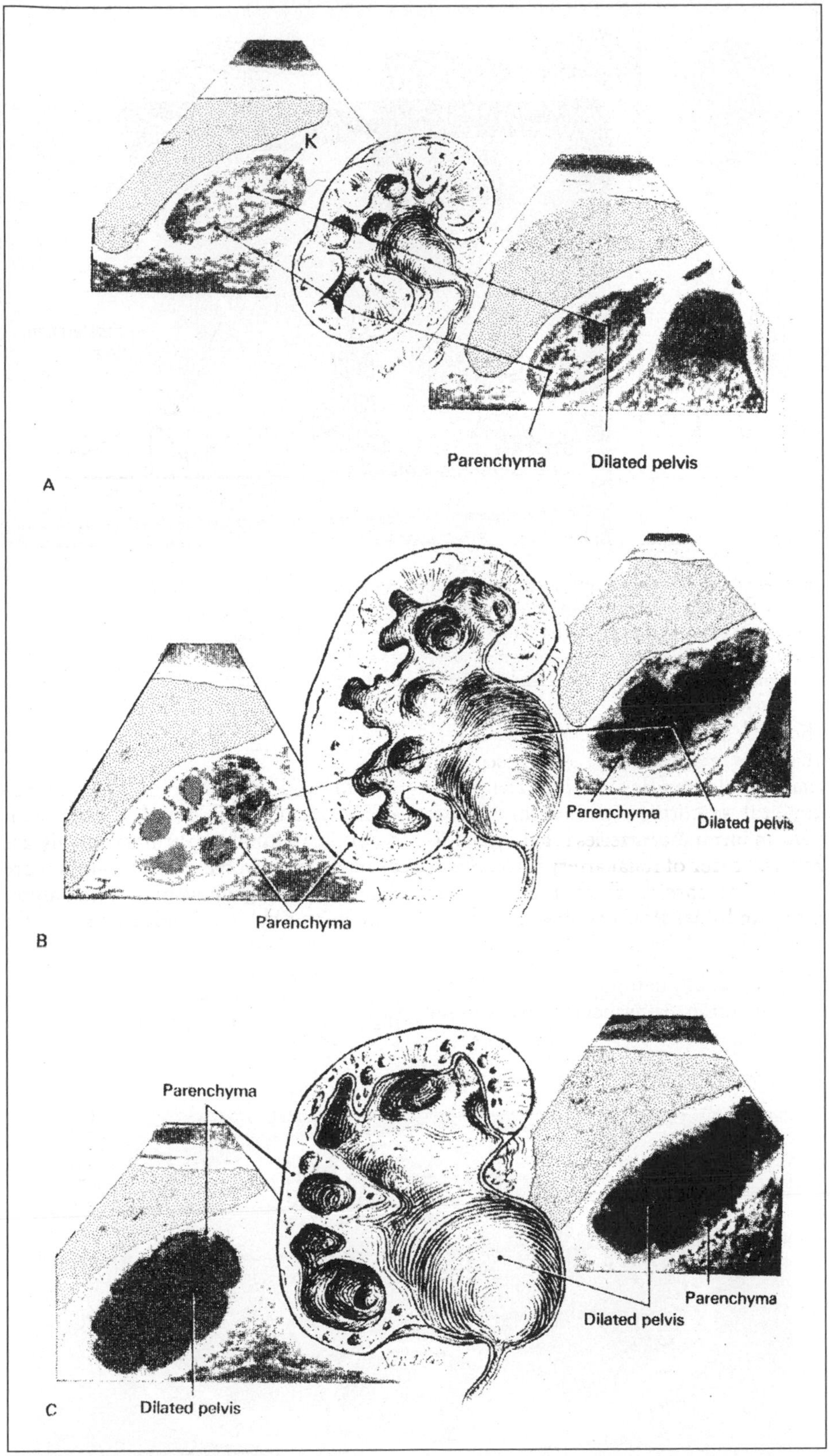

Figure 17-11. ■ *Varying degrees of dilatation of the renal pelvis caused by hydronephrosis. Note the decreased parenchyma as hydronephrosis becomes more severe. The renal parenchyma may shrink to such an extent that only septa are seen between dilated calyces. Note the dominant renal pelvic cystic area (C).*

pelvis with real-time analysis (Figs. 17-11 and 17-12). The calyces may be so effaced that only a single large sac is seen. However, multiple cystic structures due to dilated calyces usually dominate the sonographic picture.

The amount of renal parenchyma may be thinned depending on the severity and duration of hydronephrosis. The normal parenchymal width is approximately 2.5 cm in the adult.

The ureter can sometimes be traced toward the pelvis or seen behind the bladder, indicating that the obstruction is not at the ureteropelvic junction.

If the hydronephrosis is longstanding, the pelvis and calyces may remain dilated when the obstruction is relieved. It is then difficult to follow recurrent obstruction by the sonographic appearances. Doppler interrogation of the renal arteries is of some help in detecting recurrent obstruction. The resistive index in the renal artery increases when obstruction is present. The normal resistive index is 0.64. It increases to 0.72 or

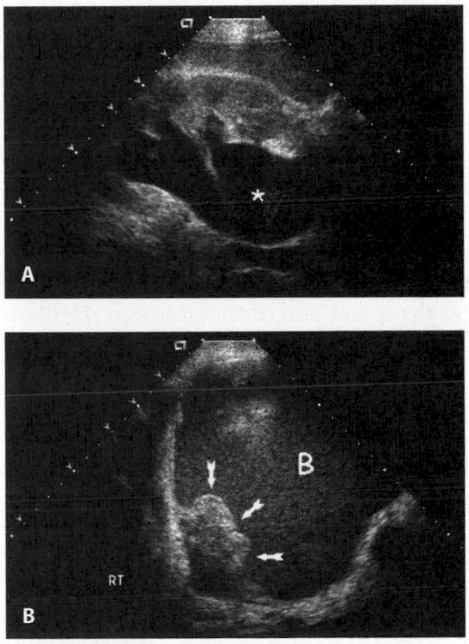

Figure 17-12. ■ *A. Longitudinal image through the right kidney showing severe hydronephrosis (*). Although no obvious internal echoes were seen within the dilated right renal collecting system, frank pus was drained from the right kidney when a percutaneous nephrostomy was placed (pyonephrosis).* ***B.*** *Oblique image through the urinary bladder showing tumor (transitional cell carcinoma, arrows) that obstructed the right ureteral orifice. Low-level echogenic debris within the bladder (B) represented more pus when a Foley catheter was placed.*

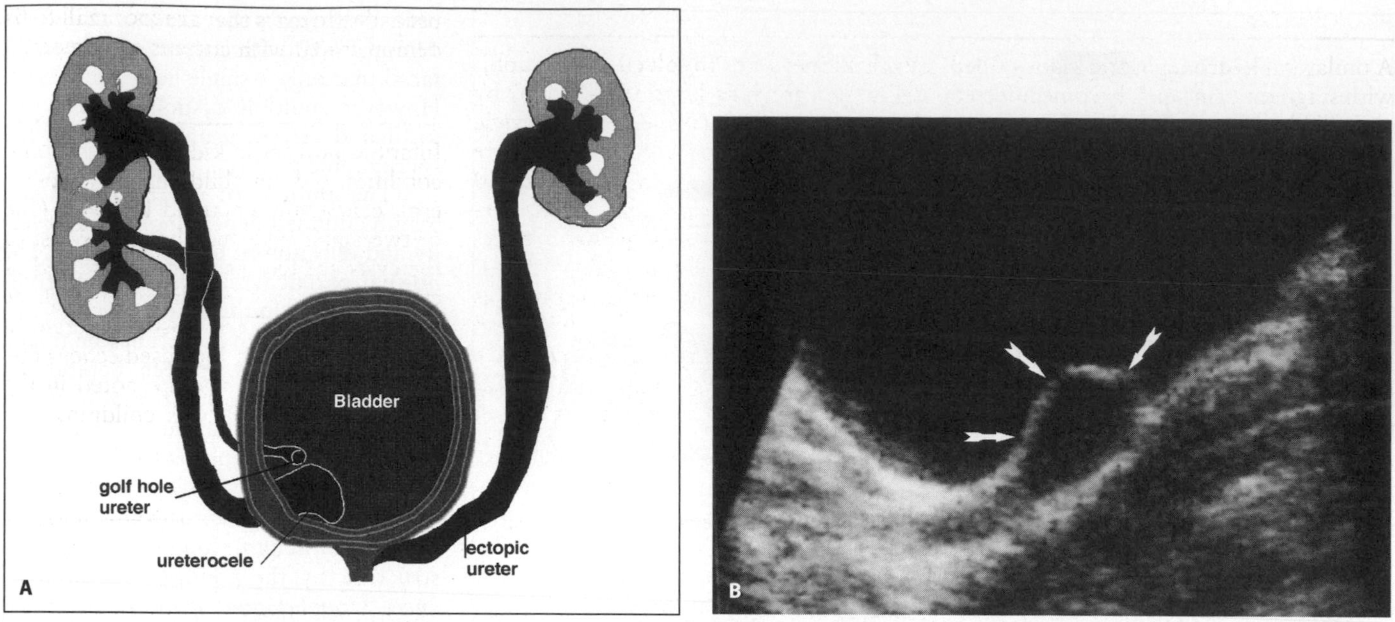

Figure 17-13. ■ *A. Diagram showing ureterocele on the right with secondary dilation of the ureter up to the level of the kidney. The lower pole of the kidney in this double collecting system is also dilated because of reflux caused by a "golf-hole" ureter. On the left, an ectopic ureter inserts into the proximal urethra, with secondary dilation of the ureter and collecting system. B. Sonogram showing typical "cobra-head" appearance of ureterocele* (arrows) *protruding into the urinary bladder.*

more with obstruction. However, due to the marked variability in resistive index measurements, the clinical utility of this parameter is less than optimal.

URETEROCELE

On some occasions, the hydronephrosis and renal obstruction are due to a block at the lower end of the ureter in the bladder. Sometimes, a stone is impacted at this narrowed site. Alternatively, a ureterocele may be present. A ureterocele is a cobra-headed expansion of the lower ureter as it enters the bladder (Fig. 18-3B), which is particularly well seen using the vaginal probe. Sometimes, only the ureter at the entrance to the bladder is dilated. On other occasions, the whole ureter is dilated back into the kidney.

Ureteroceles are often seen in patients with a double collecting system. In this situation, the upper pole of the kidney is obstructed even though the ureter enters inferior to the ureter from the lower segment of the kidney. The lower pole ureter often enters the bladder at an abnormal angle so that reflux occurs and a wide "golf-hole" ureter develops (Fig. 17-13A). A similar type of obstruction occurs when the ureter is ectopically inserted into the proximal urethra, rather than the bladder (Fig. 17-13). The ureter can be traced down lateral to the bladder to a point inferior to its usual insertion into the bladder.

XANTHOGRANULOMATOUS PYELONEPHRITIS

Xanthogranulomatous pyelonephritis, a rare infection, is associated with renal calculi and hydronephrosis. A large staghorn calculus is usually present with secondary hydronephrosis and echogenic changes in the parenchyma. A rare focal form in which there is a mass lesion with increased echogenicity due to fat may occur. Typically, the renal pelvis is shrunken and contains a stone. The dilated calyces may be seen radiating from the renal pelvis (Fig. 17-14).

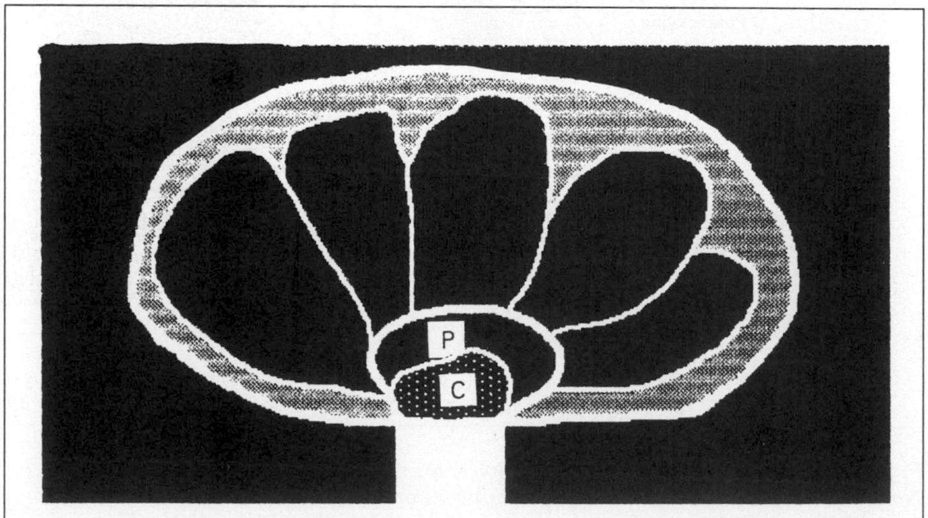

Figure 17-14. ■ *Xanthogranulomatous pyelonephritis. A stone* (C) *is present in the center of the pelvis* (P) *with acoustic shadowing. There are large dilated calyces, but the pelvis is small.*

PYONEPHROSIS

A unilateral hydronephrotic kidney filled with stagnant urine may become infected and filled with pus. This life-threatening condition can rapidly lead to death if it is not discovered and treated rapidly. Sometimes a kidney with pyonephrosis is indistinguishable from ordinary noninfected hydronephrosis (Fig. 17-12). More often, low-level echoes occur throughout the pus-filled renal pelvis. A fluid-fluid level may even develop. Percutaneous nephrostomy under ultrasonic control may be lifesaving.

ADULT POLYCYSTIC KIDNEY

Both kidneys are involved sonographically and are very large (15–18 cm) by the time a patient with adult polycystic kidney disease presents with renal failure (usually between the ages of 40 and 50 years). Multiple cysts with lobulated irregular margins and variable size are present throughout the kidney (Fig. 17-15).

The central sinus echo complex is not easy to see and is markedly distorted by cysts. In areas where no cysts are sonographically apparent, the renal parenchyma will be more echogenic than usual due to cysts that are too small to be demonstrated with current equipment.

INFANTILE POLYCYSTIC KIDNEY

Infantile polycystic kidney, a congenital condition seen in children, causes bilateral, echogenic, enlarged kidneys. One or two small cysts may be seen. Most of the cysts are too small to be resolved as cystic spaces but are large enough to cause echoes and are most prominent in the medullary area. Increased echoes due to hepatic fibrosis may be noted in the liver parenchyma of older children.

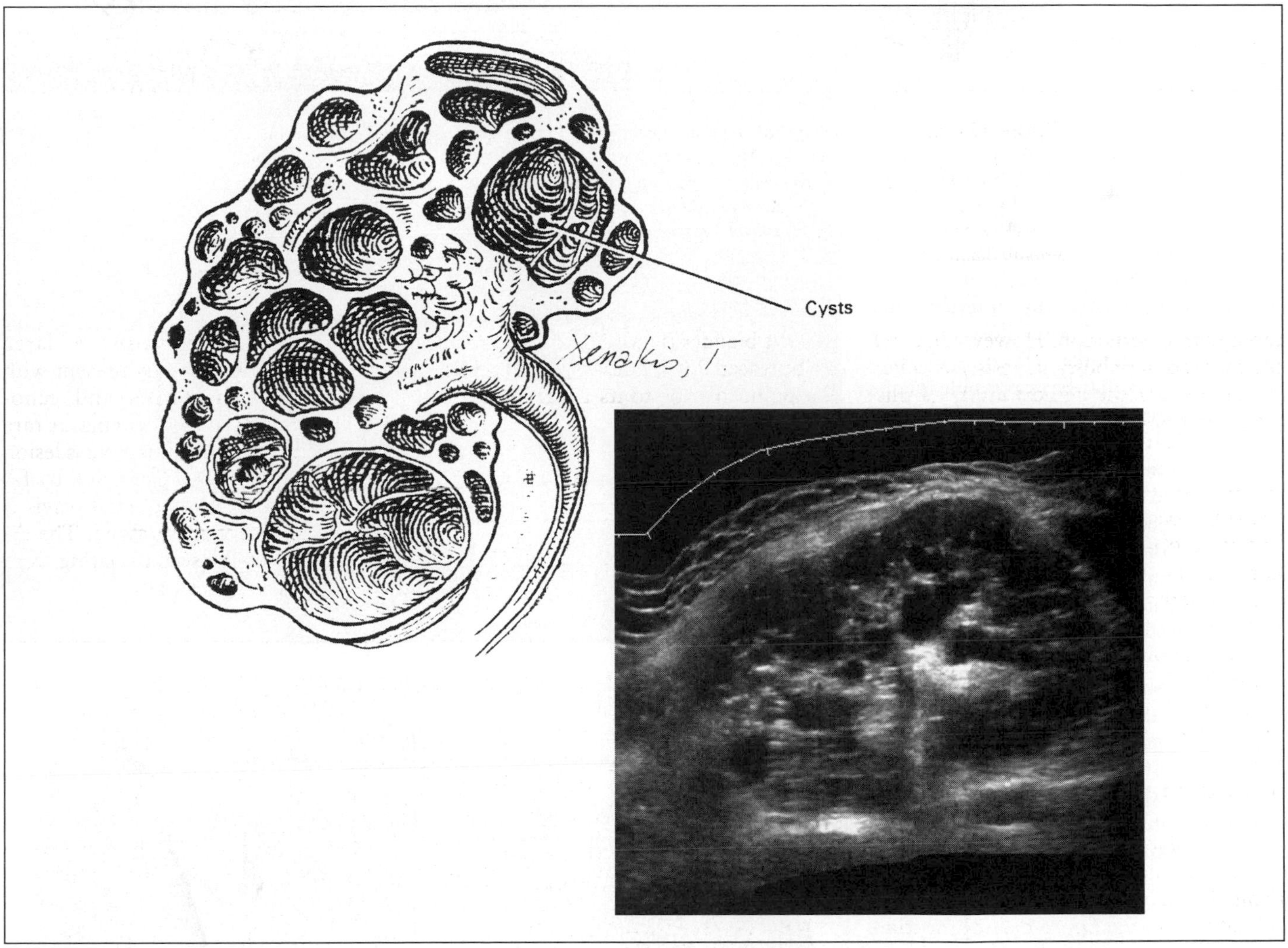

Figure 17-15. ■ *Adult polycystic disease causes the kidneys to enlarge and develop cysts of differing shapes and sizes. The liver is involved in polycystic disease in 40% of cases.*

Pitfalls

1. Pseudohydronephrosis
   a. Make sure that the bladder is empty before hydronephrosis is diagnosed definitively. In children and in patients with renal transplants, a full bladder can provoke apparent hydronephrosis, which disappears when the bladder is empty.
   b. Try to ensure that apparent hydronephrosis is not caused by a parapelvic cyst. In general, parapelvic cysts do not have as dense an echogenic margin as do dilated calyces. They usually occupy only a portion of the renal sinus echoes.
   c. An extrarenal pelvis may mimic hydronephrosis because it is a large cystic structure at the renal hilum. Dilated infundibula may also be seen normally, but connecting calyces will be delicately cupped (if they can be seen).
   d. The renal vein can be mistaken for a dilated pelvis but can be connected to the inferior vena cava and shows flow on color flow Doppler.
   e. Reflux may be responsible for apparent hydronephrosis; it disappears on standing and changes with voiding.
2. Possible missed hydronephrosis
   a. Be cautious about excluding hydronephrosis in the presence of renal calculi, which may obscure dilated calyces.
   b. Make sure that the patient is not dehydrated with lax skin and sunken eyes. Dehydration can mask hydronephrosis. Reexamination when hydrated may be worthwhile.
3. Calculi. In the presence of severe hydronephrosis, a staghorn calculus can be confused with a normal renal pelvis but will show evidence of shadowing (Fig. 17-16).

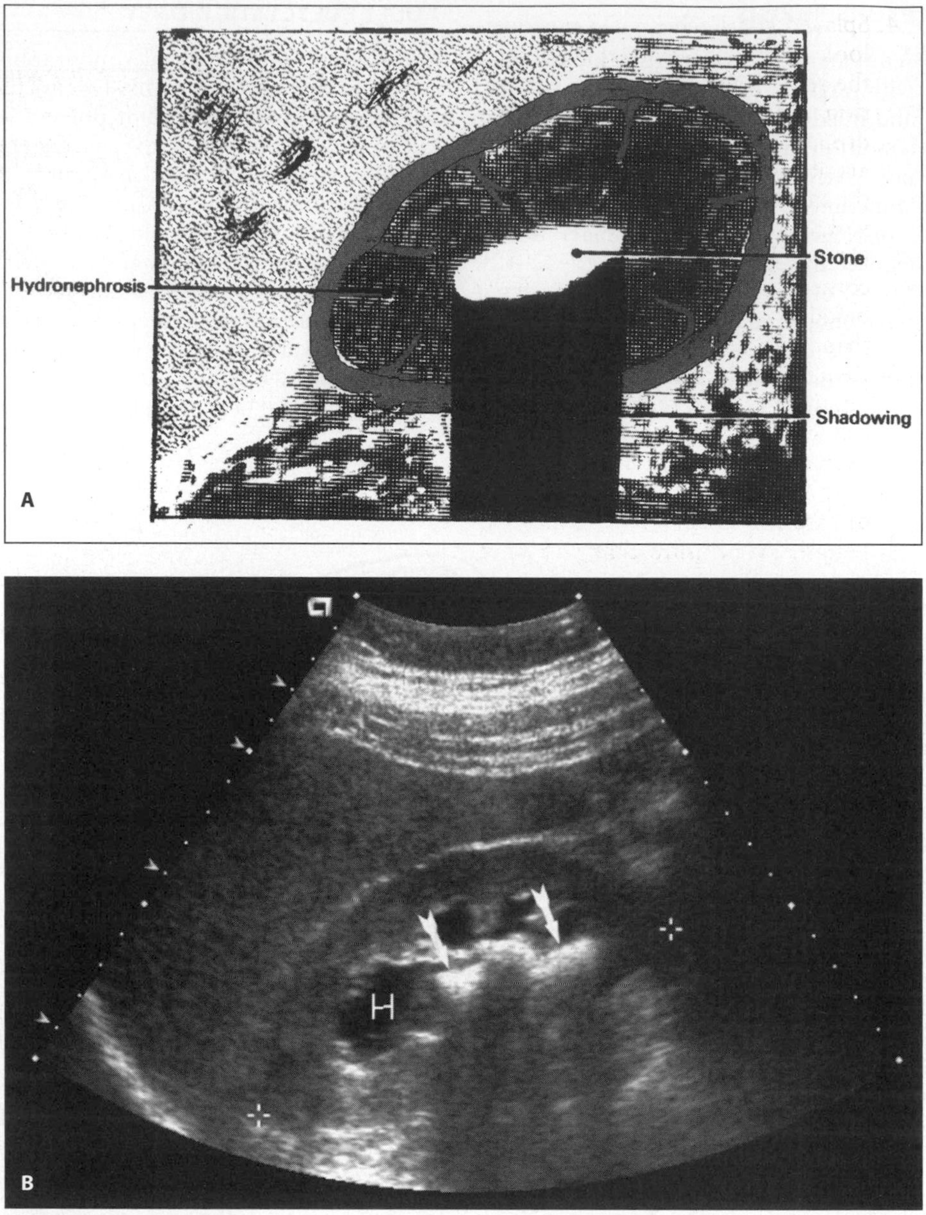

Figure 17-16. ■ *A. Diagram of gross hydronephrosis with large staghorn stone in the center. The staghorn could be mistaken for the renal pelvis, but note the shadowing. Note that almost no renal parenchyma remains after long-term obstruction. B. Sonogram of right kidney (between cursors) showing hydronephrosis* (H) *and large central staghorn calcification* (arrows).

4. Splayed sinus echoes. Do not overlook relatively mild separation of the renal sinus echoes. The correlation between the severity of hydronephrosis and the degree of separation is not good. Separation of the sinus echoes may be (1) a normal variant due to an extrarenal pelvis; (2) due to a parapelvic cyst; (3) a consequence of overdistention of the bladder; or (4) due to reflux rather than renal obstruction.
5. Renal parenchyma. If you are assessing the degree of renal parenchymal echogenicity in comparison with the liver, make sure you think that the liver is normal. Patients with liver disease are prone to renal failure.
6. Length. Make sure that you have obtained the longest renal length. Careless technique can make the kidney appear shorter than it really is (Fig. 17-7).
7. Sinus fat. Excess fat within the renal sinus (fibrolipomatosis) can have a confusing sonographic appearance, sometimes appearing more extensive than usual (Fig. 17-17) and at other times appearing less echogenic than normal and mimicking hydronephrosis.
8. Column of Bertin. The cortex between pyramids may be unduly large as a normal variant called a "column of Bertin." The parenchymal texture will not be altered in the suspect area, which is usually toward the upper pole.
9. Pseudokidney sign. Normal empty colon can mimic a kidney, especially if the patient has no kidney. The colon then lies at the site where the kidney usually lies.
10. Small end-stage kidney. A very small end-stage kidney can easily be mistaken for the target sign seen with loops of bowel. Conversely, make sure that an apparently small kidney is not a relatively empty colon by a prolonged look with real-time analysis.

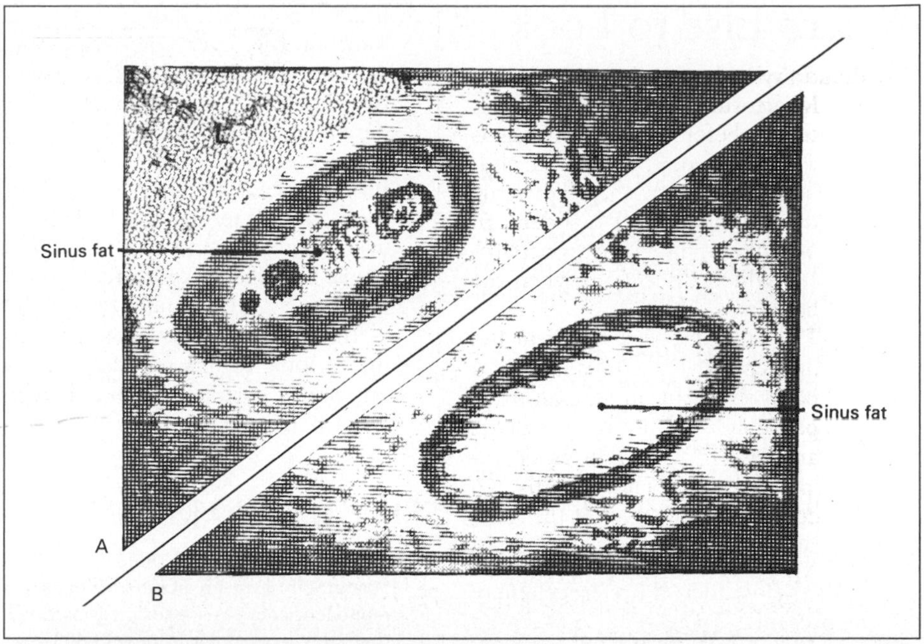

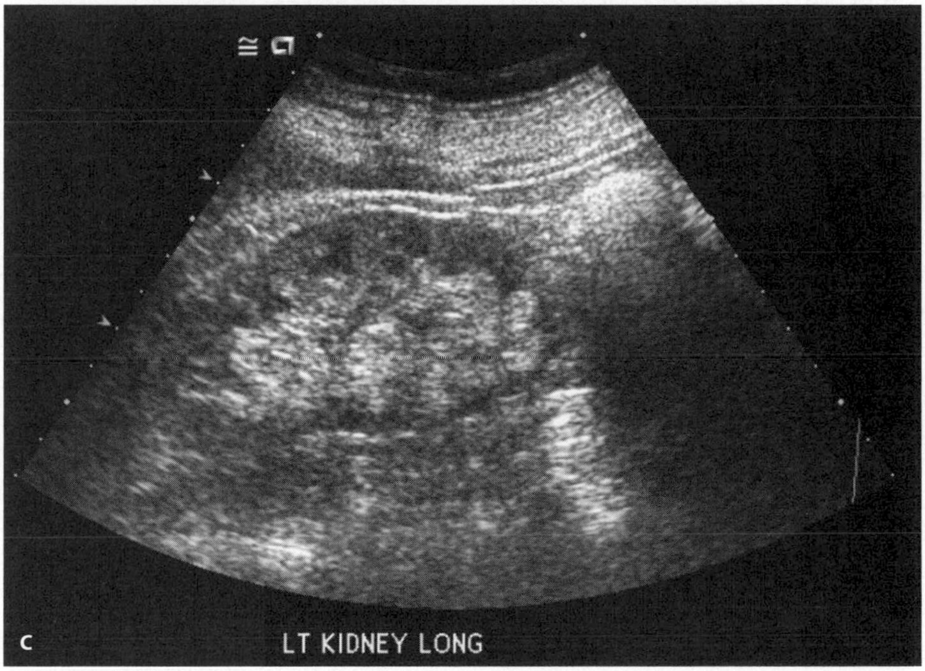

Figure 17-17. ■ *Fibrolipomatosis. A. Diagram: the less-echogenic appearances can be mistaken for hydronephrosis or transitional cell cancer. B. Diagram: excess fat in the renal sinus usually causes enlargement of the echogenic center of the kidney. C. Sonogram: excess echogenic fat in the renal sinus, corresponding to diagram (B).*

Where Else to Look

The discovery of hydronephrosis should prompt an effort to identify the site of obstruction.

1. Look within the kidney and bladder for renal calculi (see Chapter 20). Look for an impacted stone at the ureterovesical junction that may be associated with edema of the bladder wall.
2. Look along the course of the ureter and in the pelvis for masses.
3. Examine the true pelvis to see whether the bladder is distended. If it is, look for evidence of bladder neoplasm or prostatic hypertrophy (see Chapter 20).
4. Follow the course of the ureter behind the bladder; a ureterocele may be present.
5. If adult polycystic kidney is present, look in the liver, pancreas, and spleen; 40% of patients will have liver cysts, 10% (allegedly) will have pancreas cysts, and 1% will have spleen cysts.
6. If no kidney is seen in the renal bed, look in the pelvis. Pelvic kidneys usually lie close to the midline, just above the bladder or uterus.
7. If a congenital anomaly or absence of the kidney is discovered in a female, look for associated uterine anomalies, such as uterus didelphys (see Chapter 29).

SELECTED READING

Atta MG, Longenecker JC, Fine DM, et al. Sonography as a predictor of human immunodeficiency virus-associated nephropathy. *J Ultrasound Med* 2004;23:603–610; quiz 612–603.

Halpern EJ, Needleman L, Nack TL, et al. Renal artery stenosis: should we study the main renal artery or segmental vessels? *Radiology* 1995;195:799–804.

Mallek R, Bankier AA, Etele-Hainz A, et al. Distinction between obstructive and nonobstructive hydronephrosis: value of diuresis duplex Doppler sonography. *AJR Am J Roentgenol* 1996;166:113–117.

Qanadli SD, Soulez G, Therasse E, et al. Detection of renal artery stenosis: prospective comparison of captopril-enhanced Doppler sonography, captopril-enhanced scintigraphy, and MR angiography. *AJR Am J Roentgenol* 2001;177:1123–1129.

Stavros T, Harshfield D. Renal Doppler, renal artery stenosis, and renovascular hypertension: direct and indirect duplex sonographic abnormalities in patients with renal artery stenosis. *Ultrasound Q* 1994; 12(4):217–263.

Tublin ME, Bude RO, Platt JF. The resistive index in renal Doppler sonography: where do we stand? *AJR Am J Roentgenol* 2003;180: 885–892.

Possible Renal Mass

TIM WALKER
TOM WINTER

18

SONOGRAM AI

Ao	Aorta
Bl	Bladder
K	Kidney
L	Liver
Sp	Spleen

Berx oll-1 -400
Kofte-1 -250
Birre-3 -1350
Sallat M-1 -350
Patate-11 -300

2650

(AML). Unusual (1%), benign, kidney that is usually seen in en. AML also occurs in approxi- ents with tuberous sclerosis.

ulum. Postinflammatory fluid- acent to a pyramid.

f the renal collecting system ad- pyramid in which urine collects ted to an infundibulum.

Sometimes the calyces and the from the pelvis in two groups. ormal parenchyma can falsely a tumor and is known as a col-

). A bulge off the lateral margin -a normal variant.

. Excess fat deposition in the y; seen with aging.

Dilatation of the pelvic collect- obstruction.

nnel-shaped tube connecting al pelvis. Also known as a major

ogram (IVP, IVU, EU). Classic ing the genitourinary tract. A y examination of the kidneys, bladder after the injection of a trast agent ("dye"). Rapidly be- computed tomography.

tosis. An abnormal persistence ic tissue into infancy and child- nt tissue can be diffuse, multi- and can behave along a spec- l variant to malignant tissue

(Wilms' tumor). Nephroblastoma is a synonym for Wilms' tumor.

Polycystic Kidney Disease. A relatively common hereditary disease in which multiple cysts develop on each kidney. There are two forms relating to the mode of heredity and time of onset.

Pseudotumor. Overgrowth of a portion of the cortex indenting the sinus echoes and simulating a tumor.

Renal Cell Carcinoma (RCC) (also known in the past as hypernephroma or Grawitz Tumor). Adenocarcinoma of the kidney that accounts for almost 90% of all primary malignant renal parenchymal tumors.

Renal Pelvis. Centrally located sac into which the various infundibula drain. The pelvis drains into the ureter.

Transitional Cell Carcinoma (TCC). A tumor of the kidney, collecting system, ureter, or bladder lining cells that often recurs in another site in the genitourinary tract after removal. TCC accounts for approximately 7% of all primary malignant renal parenchymal tumors.

Tuberous Sclerosis (TS). A disease whose triad is characterized by skin lesions, epileptic seizures, and mental deficiency. AMLs associated with TS are classically small, multiple, and bilateral. TS is also associated with renal cysts, and uncommonly, renal cell carcinoma (RCC).

Uric Acid Calculus. A renal stone that is invisible on plain radiographs.

von Hippel-Lindau (VHL) Disease. A hereditary syndrome that has a greatly increased risk for a variety of cancers, including RCC in approximately 40%.

Wilms' Tumor. Most common malignant renal lesion seen in children.

The Clinical Problem

Although the intravenous pyelogram (IVP) was a common method of detecting renal masses in the past, it does not effectively aid in deciding whether such a mass is fluid filled (a cyst) or solid tissue—a decision that can generally be made easily with ultrasound. Cysts are managed by benign neglect (or rarely cyst puncture), whereas tumors require surgical resection or ablation (radiofrequency or cryoablation).

In the United States, computed tomography (CT) is often used in the further investigation of renal masses, but the nature of some renal masses may be confusing on CT and may be clarified by ultrasound and Doppler. Clinical symptoms related to the kidney may include pain, fever, urinary frequency and urgency, a palpable mass, hematuria, pyuria, white cells, and protein in the urine. With the increased frequency of imaging today, tumors may be clinically silent and discovered incidentally when the study is being performed for other reasons.

Anatomy

See Chapter 17.

Technique

See Chapter 17.

Do not perform a sonogram without first examining the report and images of the IVP or CT scan (if available), so you know what you are looking for. Doppler is helpful for examining the inferior vena cava and renal vein to detect tumor involvement. Be alert for stones, their posterior acoustic shadowing, and the associated "twinkle artifact" on color Doppler (see Chapter 20). With the use of these techniques, stones sometimes are readily visible on ultrasound when hard to see on plain films.

Pathology

FLUID-FILLED MASSES

Renal Cysts

Renal cysts are rare in children, gradually becoming more frequent with age. In the elderly, they are very common. They may be single (Fig. 18-1) or multiple (Fig. 18-3). The sonographic features of a cyst are as follows:

1. Acoustic enhancement (good through transmission with a strong back wall) (Fig. 18-1)
2. Usually a smooth spherical outline with thin walls
3. Usually fluid filled with no internal echoes

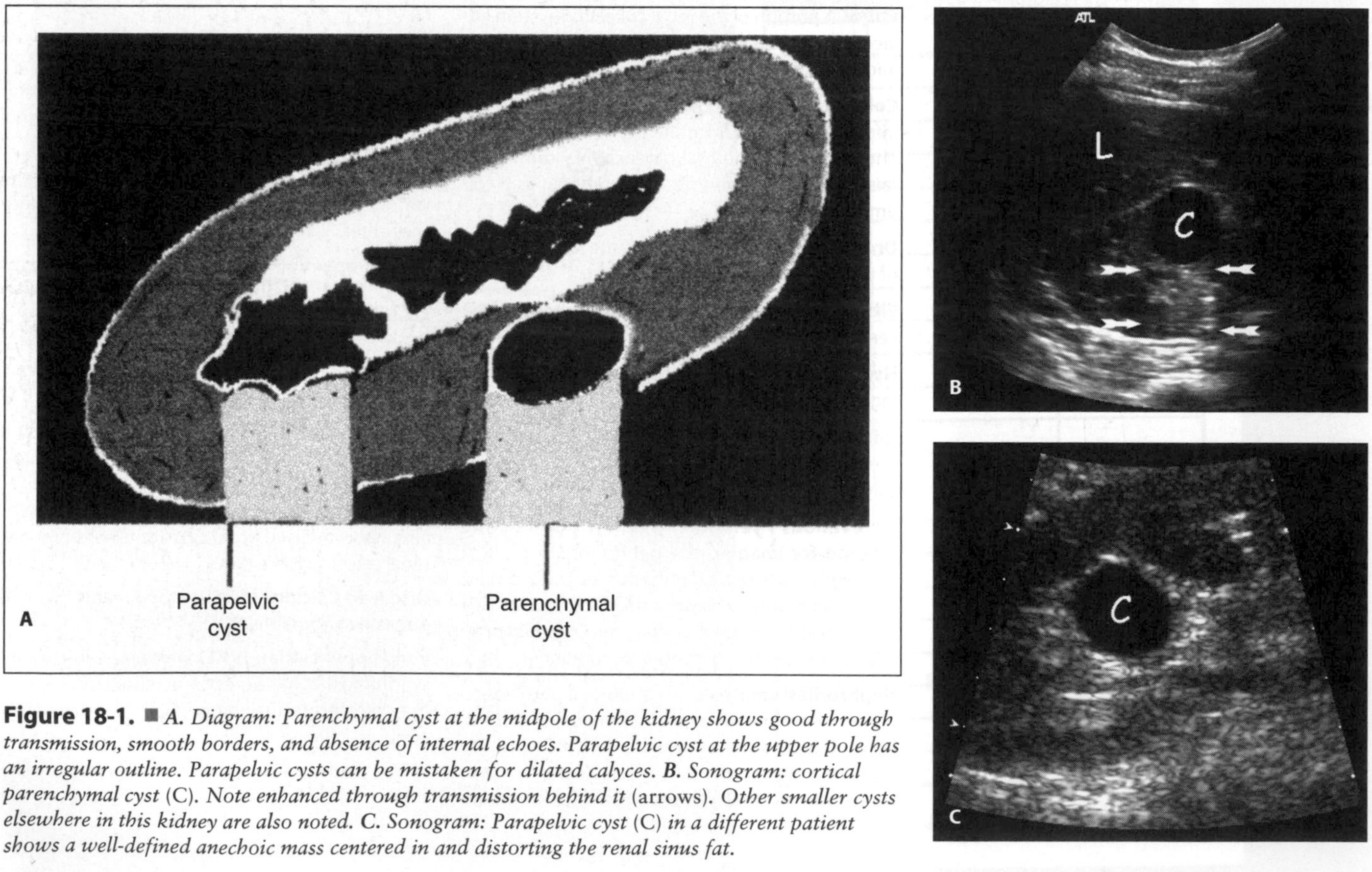

Figure 18-1. ■ *A. Diagram: Parenchymal cyst at the midpole of the kidney shows good through transmission, smooth borders, and absence of internal echoes. Parapelvic cyst at the upper pole has an irregular outline. Parapelvic cysts can be mistaken for dilated calyces. **B.** Sonogram: cortical parenchymal cyst* (C). *Note enhanced through transmission behind it* (arrows). *Other smaller cysts elsewhere in this kidney are also noted. **C.** Sonogram: Parapelvic cyst* (C) *in a different patient shows a well-defined anechoic mass centered in and distorting the renal sinus fat.*

Unusual cysts may have irregular walls and may contain low-level echoes in a dependent position owing to debris. Debris may be confused with spurious echoes related to the slice thickness artifact (Fig. 18-2; see also Chapter 57).

Septa dividing a cyst into compartments may be seen (Fig. 18-2). Such septa prove that a cyst is fluid filled but may be difficult to visualize completely and may be mistaken for a mural mass.

Irregular borders, septations, or debris should raise the question of malignancy or necrosis and require further investigation, usually by CT.

Peripelvic cysts may be centrally located and hard to distinguish from a dilated pelvis or calyx (Fig. 18-1). Their shape is often irregular.

The Bosniak classification of renal cysts is a grading system originally developed for CT but is now commonly used in magnetic resonance imaging. It uses morphologic criteria to divide cystic masses along a spectrum from benign (Category I) to obviously malignant (Category IV), allowing one to decide whether a lesion can be ignored, requires follow-up, or requires surgery. However, because the system relies on the assessment of both calcifications and soft-tissue enhancement within the mass, its usefulness has not been rigorously evaluated when cystic masses are imaged by ultrasound. Perhaps when ultrasound contrast agents are widely available in the United States, this system will be reevaluated; regardless, it is useful to be familiar with the general Bosniak concept because radiologists and urologists commonly use the terminology.

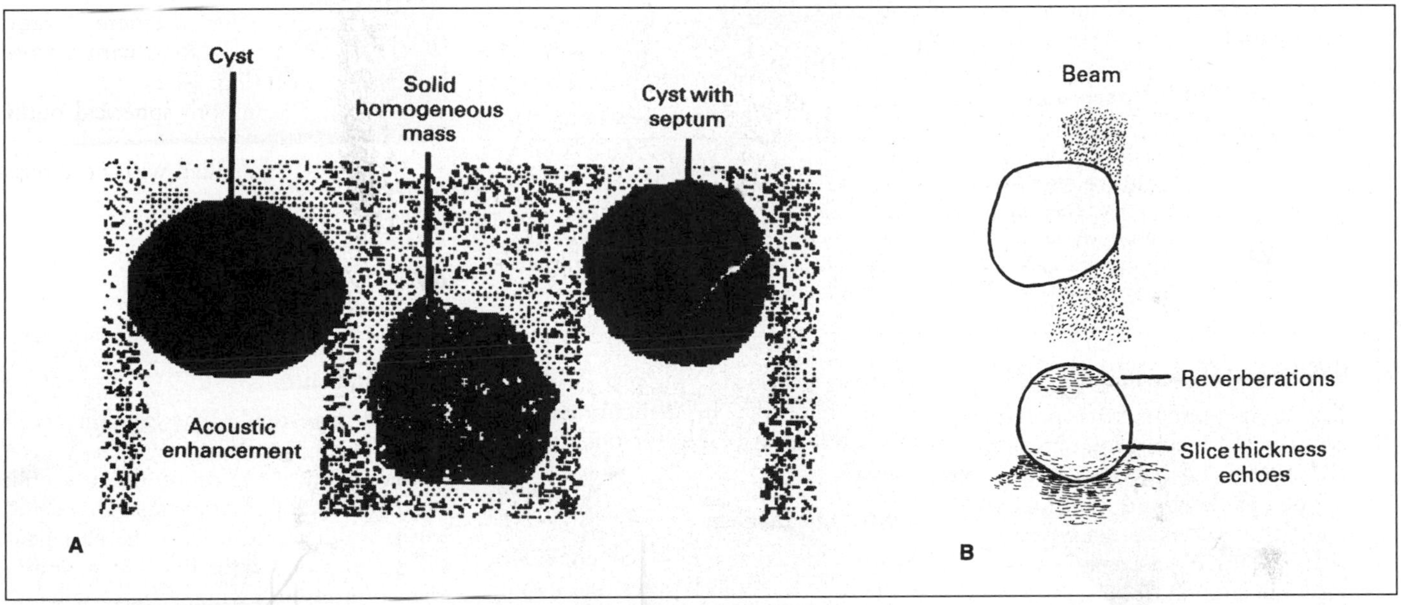

Figure 18-2. ■ *Cyst versus solid homogeneous mass.* ***A.*** *Diagram showing the difference between a cyst and a solid homogeneous mass. Through transmission beyond a solid homogeneous mass is limited, although there will be a back wall, and there are usually a few internal echoes. Septa within a cyst are incompletely seen unless they are at right angles to the acoustic beam.* ***B.*** *Artifactual echoes caused by reverberations and slice thickness effect. (For details of how these artifacts develop, see Chapter 57.)*

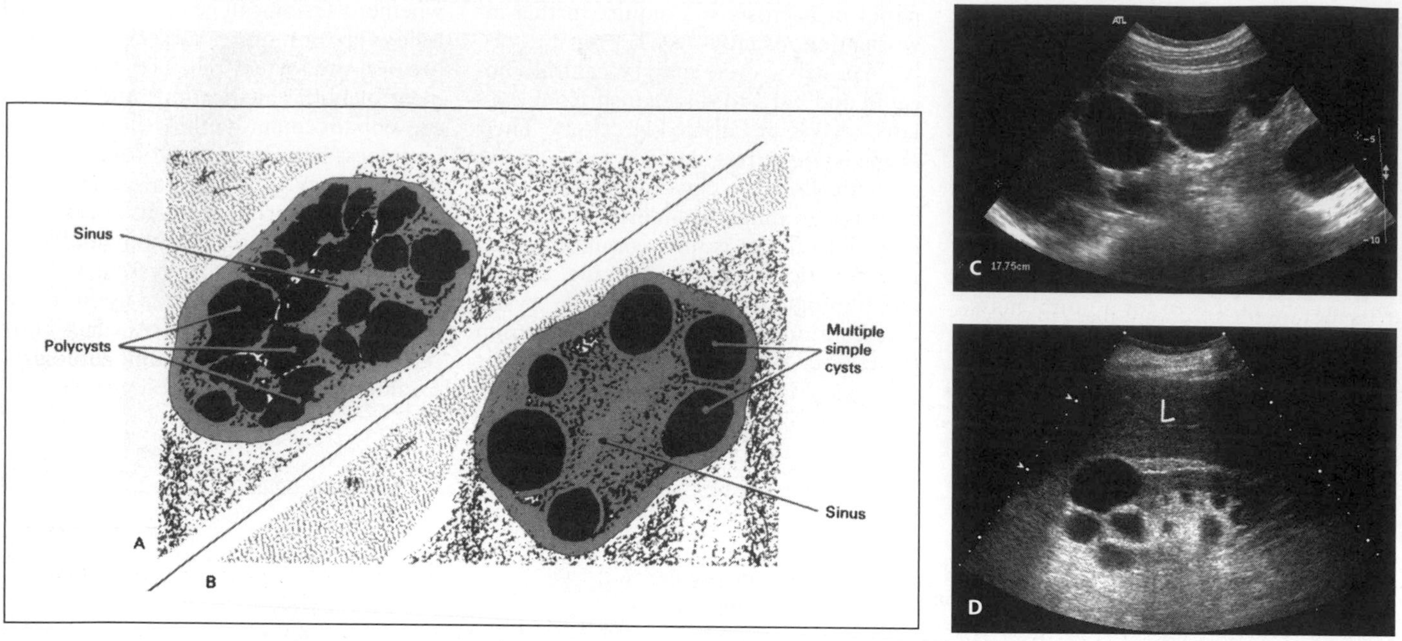

Figure 18-3. ■ *Multiple cysts. A. Cysts in polycystic disease have irregular walls and are variable in size. They distort the renal sinus echoes. B. Multiple simple cysts have smooth walls, are not nearly as numerous, and vary less in size. C. Classic sonogram for hereditary autosomal dominant polycystic kidney disease. Note multiple cysts and large size (~18 cm). The opposite kidney appeared the same. D. Multiple simple cysts in a different patient.*

Adult Polycystic Disease

Renal cysts in patients with polycystic disease usually have an irregular outline and are of markedly varied size (Fig. 18-3A). The background parenchymal echogenicity is often increased in polycystic disease owing to small cysts that are not large enough to be seen as fluid-filled structures but are large enough to cause echoes. This is always a bilateral process, although one side may be more severely affected than the other.

Multiple Simple Cysts

Multiple simple cysts can occur but are fewer in number, more equal in size, and smoother in outline than the cysts seen in polycystic disease (Fig. 18-3B). Although definite distinction between multiple simple cysts and adult polycystic kidney disease may occasionally be problematic, enlarged kidneys bilaterally with multiple cysts favor the latter diagnosis. Family history is also helpful, because polycystic kidney disease is often inherited; in difficult cases, a DNA test is available for definitive diagnosis.

Multicystic Disease

Multicystic disease is a congenital process that involves only one kidney. The entire kidney, which is small, is filled with multiple adjacent cysts (see Chapter 35). In adults, these cysts may develop a calcified shell, also known as multicystic dysplastic kidney.

Calyceal Enlargement

Calyceal diverticula and locally obstructed calyces look like cysts but connect with the pelvicaliceal system. They are generally surrounded by an echogenic border owing to sinus fat.

Milk of Calcium

Calyceal diverticula may contain "milk of calcium." An echogenic focus is seen in the region of the calyx. Because milk of calcium is liquid, it changes shape and forms a fluid-fluid level if the patient is placed in a decubitus or erect position. Usually nonshadowing, milk of calcium may be mistaken for a small calculus.

Duplex Collecting System

An upper pole, congenitally duplicated hydronephrotic collecting system may look like a cyst but usually has septa separating the duplicated calyces. Duplication is associated with complete or partial duplication of the ureter. There is often a ureterocele obstructing the upper of the two collecting systems. One may be able to trace the ureter from the upper kidney toward the true pelvis, where it will insert medial and inferior to the orifice for the ureter for the lower kidney (see Fig. 17-13).

Abscess and Focal Pyelonephritis

Although abscesses are fluid-filled, they are rarely totally echo-free (Fig. 18-4). They may even occasionally contain a number of internal echoes. Local infection without abscess formation causes an area of decreased echoes with swelling and local tenderness. Such local infection is known as focal pyelonephritis or, in older terminology, lobar nephronia. One may be unable to distinguish an abscess with drainable pus from an area of inflammation.

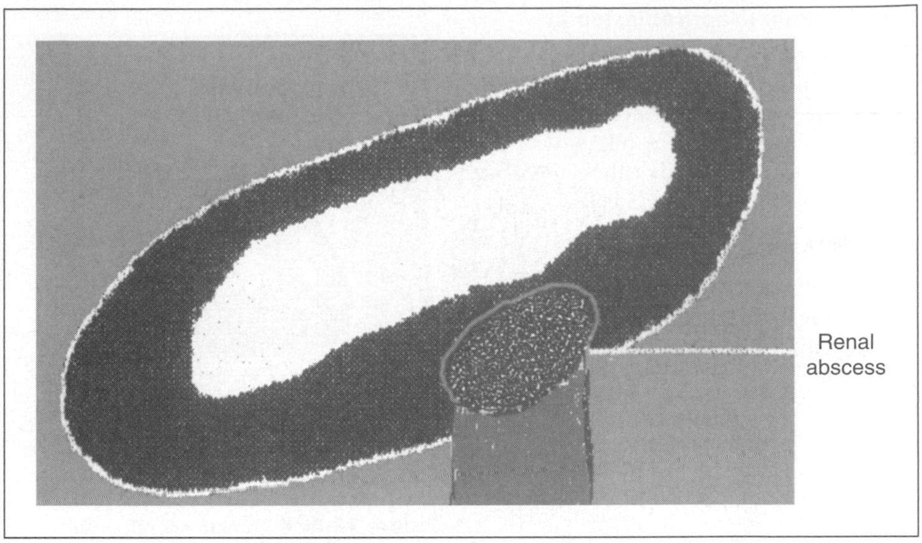

Figure 18-4. ■ *Abscesses in the kidney tend to have some internal echoes and irregular walls.*

Hematoma

Hematomas have a varied sonographic appearance. They may be echo-free or evenly echogenic, or they may contain clumps of echoes. Hematomas usually develop around, rather than within, a kidney. Hematomas are a consequence of trauma, surgical procedure, or abnormal bleeding conditions.

Urinoma

Urinomas may be seen, usually after a surgical procedure. These fluid collections are echo-free. They most often surround the kidney (i.e., they are peri-renal). They are particularly common in transplant kidneys.

Renal Artery Aneurysm

A centrally placed cystic structure may represent a renal artery aneurysm. Providing the aneurysm is not clot filled, flow will be seen with color flow Doppler. There is often calcification in the wall of aneurysms.

TUMOR MASSES

Adenocarcinoma (Hypernephroma or Renal Cell Carcinoma)

Adenocarcinomas contain internal echoes, do not show good through transmission, and usually have an irregular border that expands the outline of the kidney. Most renal cell carcinomas (RCCs) are hypoechoic or isoechoic to the adjacent renal parenchyma (Fig. 18-5). Smaller RCCs (<3 cm) may be more echogenic than the remaining kidney. RCC is, by far, the most common renal neoplasm.

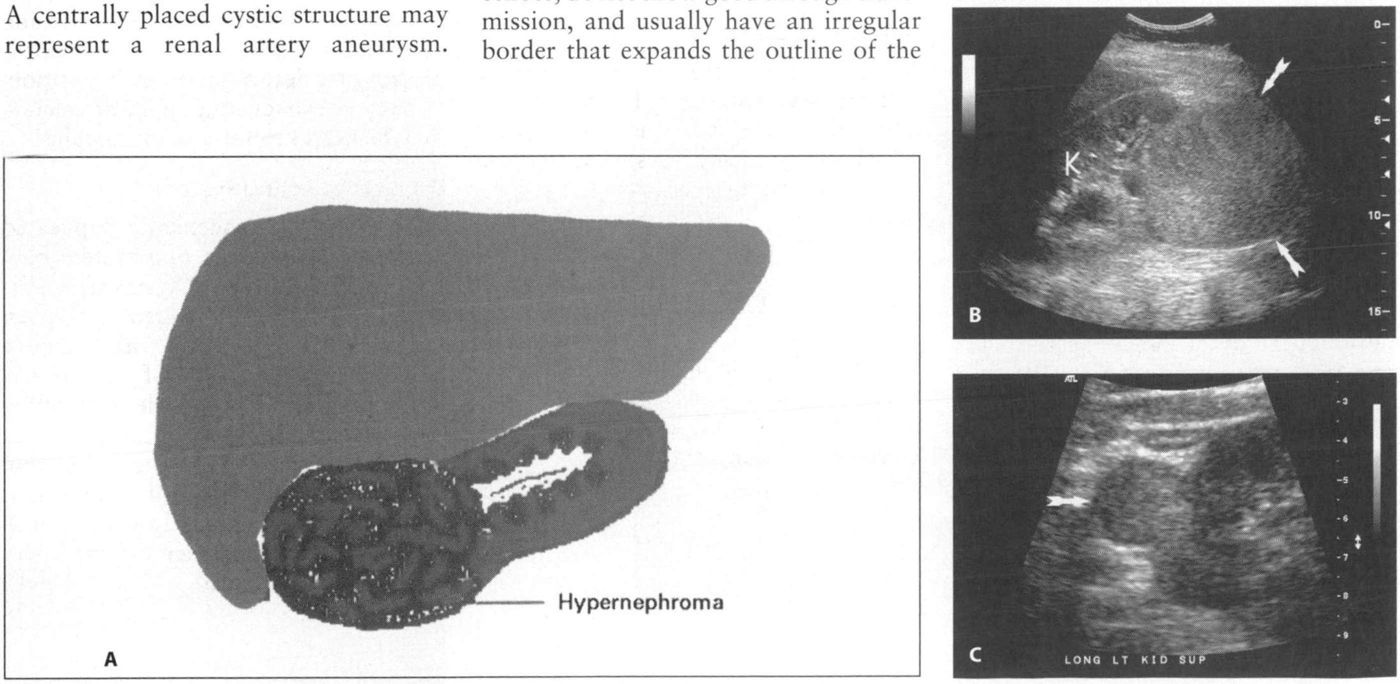

Figure 18-5. ■ *A. Diagram of a large renal cell carcinoma* (RCC) *expanding the upper pole of the kidney. Notice that it is slightly more echopenic than the renal parenchyma. RCCs are frequently relatively hypoechoic but show poor through transmission. B. Sonogram depicting a large* RCC (arrows) *arising from the lower pole of the right kidney. C. Small* RCC (arrow) *arising from the upper pole of another kidney.*

Wilms' Tumor (Nephroblastoma)

Wilms' tumor is a malignant lesion affecting children. The tumor is usually unilateral, occupying only part of the kidney. Ten percent are bilateral. They appear as a large, evenly echogenic mass (see Chapter 35 and Fig. 35-9).

Transitional Cell Tumors

Renal transitional cell carcinomas (Fig. 18-6) generally occur in the renal pelvis and are difficult to distinguish from fibrolipomatosis or normal sinus fat. A small, evenly echogenic mass slightly less echogenic than the sinus echoes is seen within the renal sinus. Hematuria often presents clinically when no mass is visible sonographically.

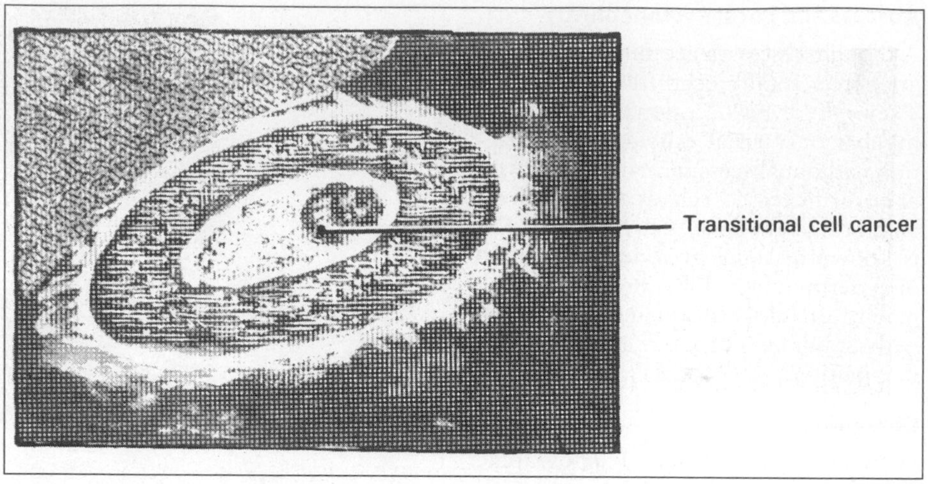

Figure 18-6. ■ *Transitional cell cancer involving the sinus of the kidney, causing a hypoechoic area.*

Tumors in Cysts

Tumors may infrequently occur within cysts. There is focal irregularity of the cyst wall at one site. However, the irregularity may be due to a septum. A cyst with an irregular wall and internal echoes is usually subjected to contrast-enhanced CT scan to rule out neoplasm.

Lymphoma

Renal lymphoma may have three different appearances in the kidney:

1. A local echopenic mass
2. Diffuse sonolucency of the entire kidney with loss of the sinus echoes
3. Large kidneys that may have reduced echogenicity

Adenoma

Adenomas are small, solid, echogenic tumors that measure less than 1 cm. They are usually located in the renal cortex and may cause a bulging of the renal capsule but are seldom visible.

Angiomyolipoma

A highly echogenic tumor with a smooth, round outline is suggestive of angiomyolipoma (AML) (Fig. 18-7), but be careful because small RCCs may be hyperechoic. A noncontrast CT is generally a quick and simple test to confirm the internal fat diagnostic of AML. AMLs are benign and composed of blood vessels, muscle, and fat. They may bleed when large (>4 cm), causing symp-

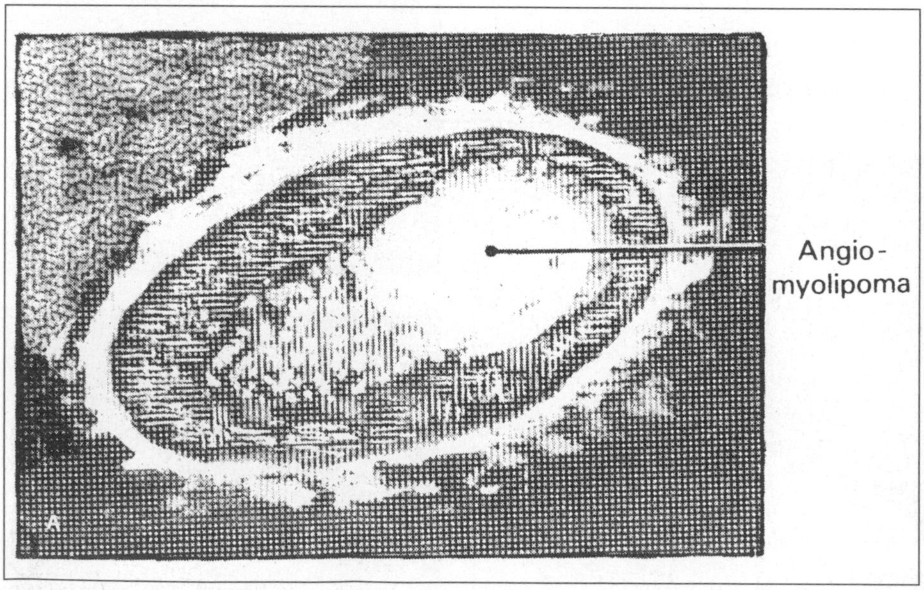

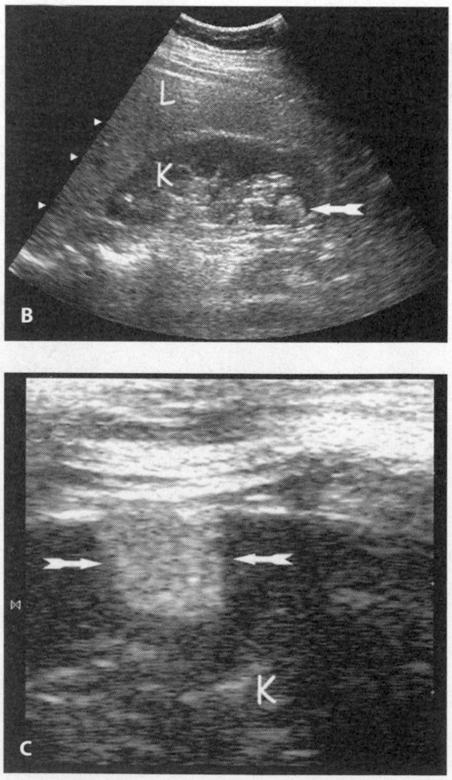

Figure 18-7. ■ *Angiomyolipoma* (AML) *at the lower pole of the kidney. AMLs are almost always densely echogenic. A. Diagram. B. Sonogram depicting spherical echogenic AML* (arrow) *at lower pole of right kidney. C. Note that using a linear transducer on the kidney can dramatically increase the resolution of selected structures. In this case, the AML* (arrows) *from (B) is shown in much better detail.*

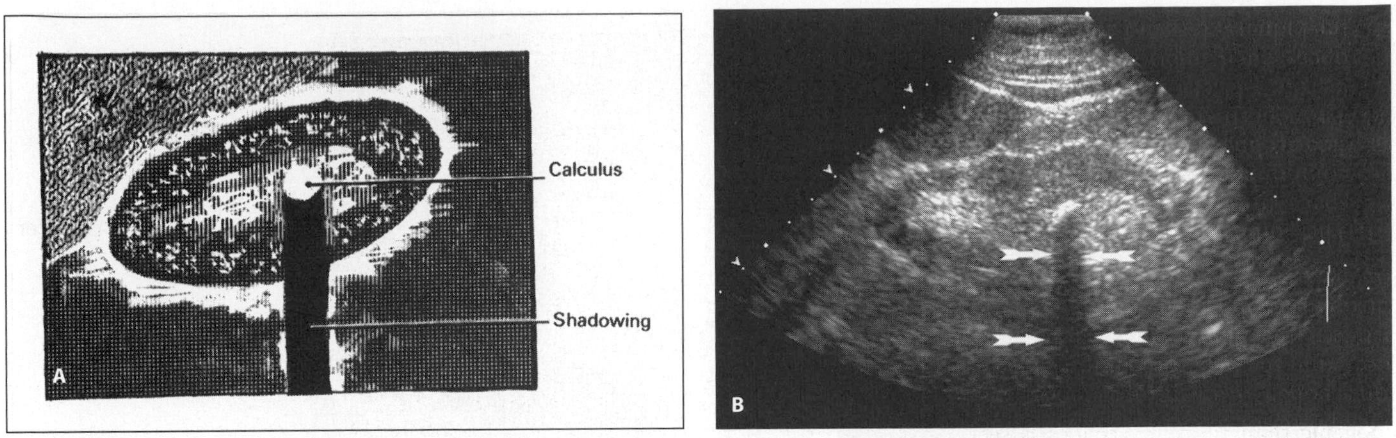

Figure 18-8. ■ *Renal calculus with acoustic shadowing. Calculi do not cause shadows if they are small (less than 5 mm). Diagram (A) and sonogram (B) (shadowing =* arrows*).*

toms and areas of decreased echogenicity in or around the mass.

Filling Defects in Renal Pelvis (Calculi)

A small filling defect in the renal pelvis on IVP has a number of possible causes, including transitional cell cancer. Some are due to radiolucent uric acid stones. Stones can be recognized on sonography by an acoustic shadow arising from the renal pelvis echoes (Fig. 18-8).

Pitfalls

NORMAL VARIANTS VERSUS PSEUDOLESIONS

Normal variants or congenital abnormalities may create the impression of a mass.

1. An enlarged spleen or liver can compress the kidney, causing an apparently abnormal IVP appearance (Fig. 18-9).
2. The left kidney often has a hump on its lateral aspect known as a dromedary hump (Fig. 18-10). This is

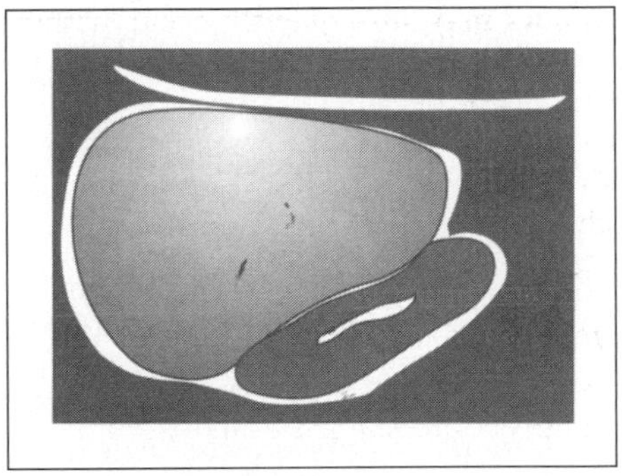

Figure 18-9. ■ *The left kidney is squashed by an enlarged spleen. Splenomegaly can cause an apparent mass on intravenous pyelogram* (IVP).

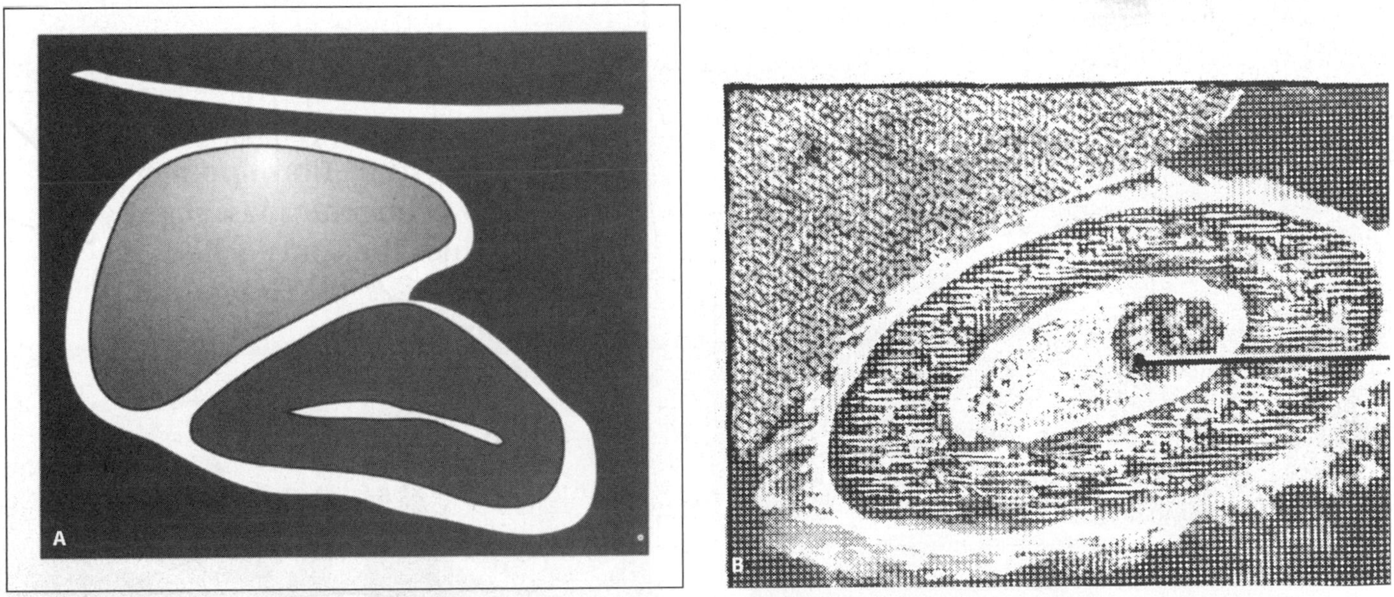

Figure 18-10. ■ *Bulge at the lateral border of the left kidney shown as a dromedary hump, a normal variant. It is thought to be a consequence of compression by the spleen. Diagram (A) and sonogram (B).*

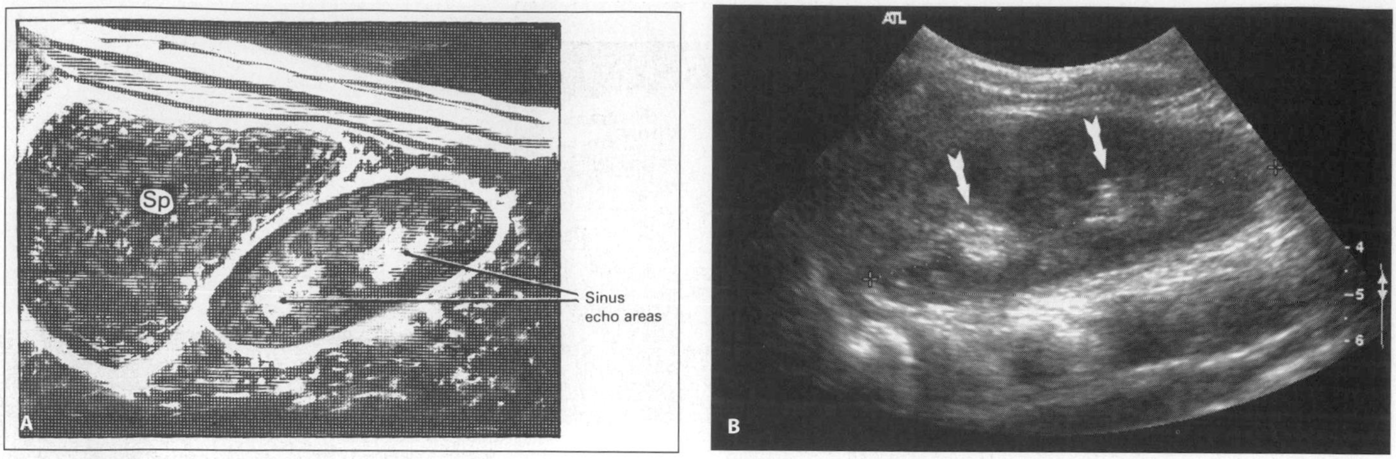

Figure 18-11. ■ *Bifid pelvicaliceal system; the sinus echoes are separated into two groups. A similar appearance is seen with a double collecting system. Diagram (**A**) and sonogram (**B**).*

thought to be due to normal renal tissue being compressed by the spleen.

3. A bifid pelvicaliceal pattern may suggest a central mass on IVP. The intervening tissue between the two portions of the collecting system appears sonographically normal (Fig. 18-11). Pseudomasses and the column of Bertin have a similar location and appearance. Angle medially and obtain transverse views to see whether the sinus echoes join at the pelvis. In a bifid pelvicaliceal system, the sinus echoes will join, whereas with a double collecting system, they will be separate.
4. Ectopic renal locations are common:
   a. A pelvic kidney (Fig. 18-12) is located in the pelvis. Malrotation and pelvic dilatation occur often in pelvic kidneys.
   b. A thoracic kidney, in which the kidney lies partially or completely in the chest, is a rare variant.
   c. In crossed ectopia without fusion, both kidneys are located on one side of the body. The kidney is very long, with two sinus echo groups.
5. Malrotated kidneys often look abnormal on IVP but are normal, except for an unusual axis on the sonogram (Fig. 18-13).
6. Fibrolipomatosis (excessive fatty infiltration of the renal pelvis) is often a consequence of aging. The sonographic appearances are variable and include (1) an enlarged central echogenic complex; (2) fat that may be relatively sonolucent, giving the impression of mass lesions or hydronephrosis (use higher gain settings to see low-level echoes); and (3) fat that may be densely echogenic. Confusion with transitional cell carcinoma is possible; transitional cell carcinoma has a more irregular outline and will not be present in the other kidney.

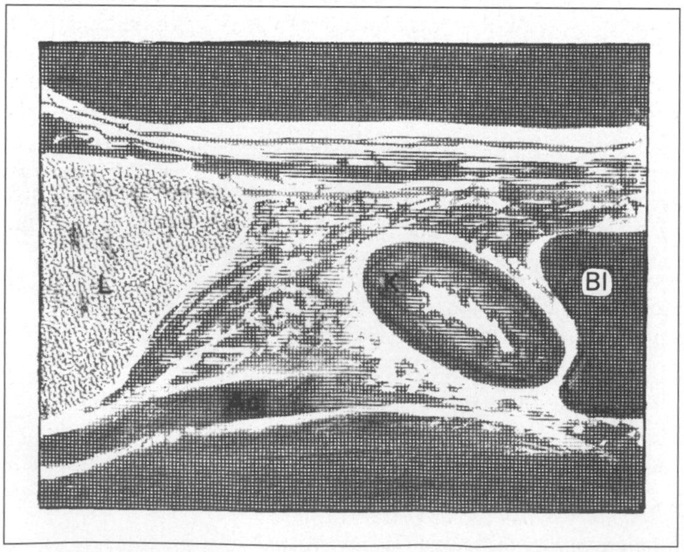

Figure 18-12. ■ *Pelvic kidney. Sonographically normal kidney is located in the pelvis.*

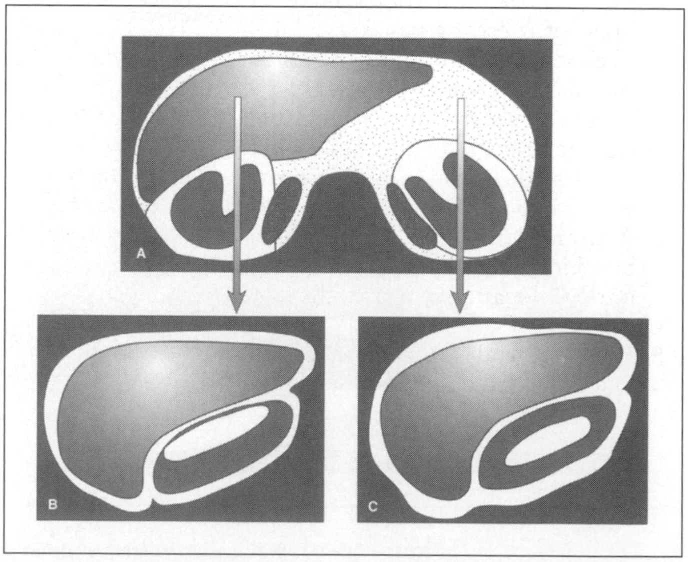

Figure 18-13. ■ *A. Kidney positions. B. Malrotated kidney. In the right kidney, the axis of the kidney is rotated so that the sinus echoes exit anteriorly. C. Normal kidney position.*

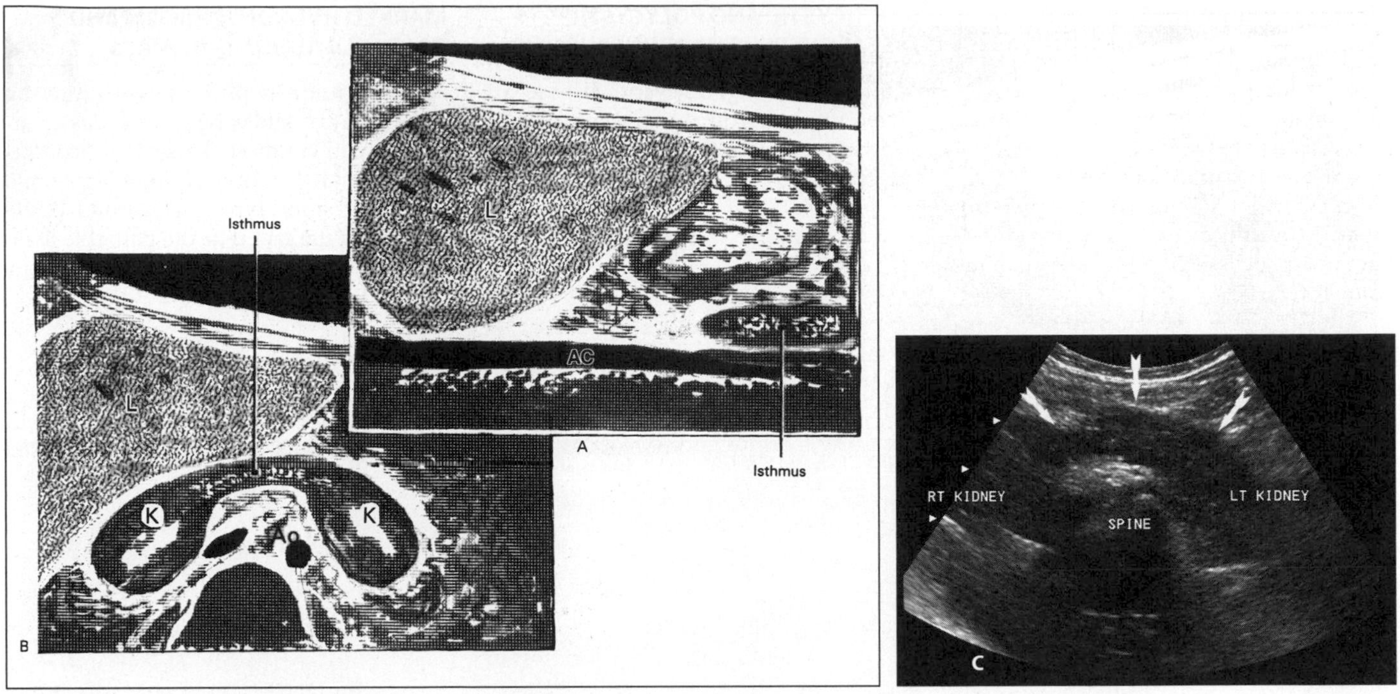

Figure 18-14. ■ *Horseshoe kidney. A. The isthmus can be mistaken for nodes on longitudinal section. B. Horseshoe kidneys are located more centrally than other kidneys and are connected by an isthmus. C. Transverse midline sonogram showing the isthmus of a horseshoe kidney* (arrows) *crossing the midline in front of the spine. As in (A), be careful to recognize this appearance and not mistake it for abnormally enlarged lymph nodes surrounding the aorta.*

7. Horseshoe kidneys are bilateral, low-lying, medially placed kidneys with partial or complete fusion of the lower poles. An isthmus of tissue connects the two kidneys, passing anterior to the aorta and inferior vena cava. The kidneys are often difficult to see on a supine view because of overlying gas (Fig. 18-14). The inferior pole of the kidney is angled medially and may be obscured by gas. A short kidney should precipitate a search for a horseshoe kidney. Use the isthmus as an acoustic window to see the renal pelvis.
8. A ptotic kidney is an unusually mobile kidney that descends from its normal location toward the true pelvis.
9. Persistent fetal lobulation may result in a lobulated outline to the kidney. It is without pathologic consequence. Indentations separated by an equal distance are seen. The lobulated pattern with focal infarcts or scarring is more random.
10. Supernumerary (extra) kidney is rare. Both a pelvic kidney and two normally placed kidneys are seen.
11. A triangular echogenic area on the anterior superior aspect of the kidney, particularly the right one, is probably a junctional fusion defect. This fat-filled area is an embryologic remnant of the site of fusion between the upper and lower components of the kidney.

CYST VERSUS NEOPLASM

A cyst may be difficult to distinguish from a solid homogeneous mass (Fig. 18-2). Use of a higher-frequency transducer may help determine whether the lesion is solid. Use a broad footprint probe, rather than a narrow sector or vector transducer, whenever possible. Find the best acoustic window (i.e., through the liver and spleen) and set the focal zone for the center of the cyst. Look at the inner wall of the cyst from different angles so that wall irregularities can be clearly differentiated from artifact. Echoes on the transducer side of the cyst may be due to reverberations, and on the far side, by the "slice thickness" effect (Fig. 18-2B; see also Chapter 57). If ultrasound contrast agents are available at your location, they may be very helpful in distinguishing between cystic and solid masses.

"BLOWN" CALYX VERSUS CYST

Look at the IVP if available, because a cystic lesion in the kidney might be a focally dilated portion of the renal collecting system.

Subtle textural changes can be enhanced by switching to a higher-frequency transducer and by trying different postprocessing features, such as color filters.

ARCUATE VESSELS

Calcification in the wall of the arcuate vessels may give rise to some subtle acoustic shadowing and mimic the appearance of a stone. Calcified arteries may also occur in the renal sinus echoes. Arteries can usually be distinguished from calculi by the appearance of two walls: Two parallel echogenic lines are seen. Check for pulsation with Doppler.

MULTICYSTIC AND POLYCYSTIC DISEASE VERSUS HYDRONEPHROSIS

Multicystic and polycystic disease are differentiated from hydronephrosis by showing the lack of connection between the cysts.

MARKED HYDRONEPHROSIS AND PALPABLE ABDOMINAL MASS

Marked hydronephrosis is a common cause of a palpable abdominal mass, particularly in children. This often prompts the clinician to worry about a large solid tumor of some type. Ultrasound easily diagnoses the fact that the palpable mass is simply hydronephrosis (Fig. 18-15).

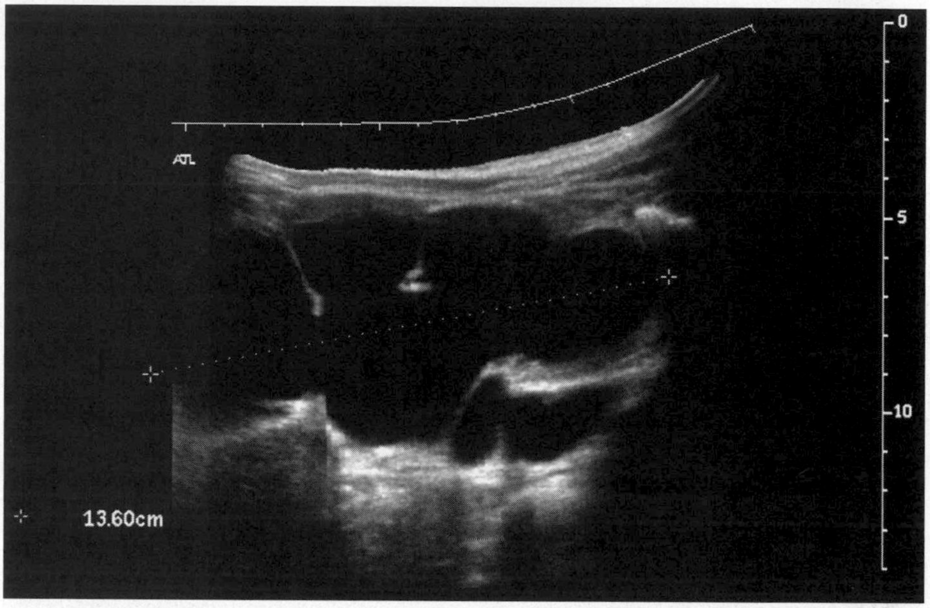

Figure 18-15. ■ *Extended field-of-view ultrasound depicting massive hydronephrosis presenting as a palpable abdominal mass that was referred to "rule out" a large renal cell carcinoma* (RCC).

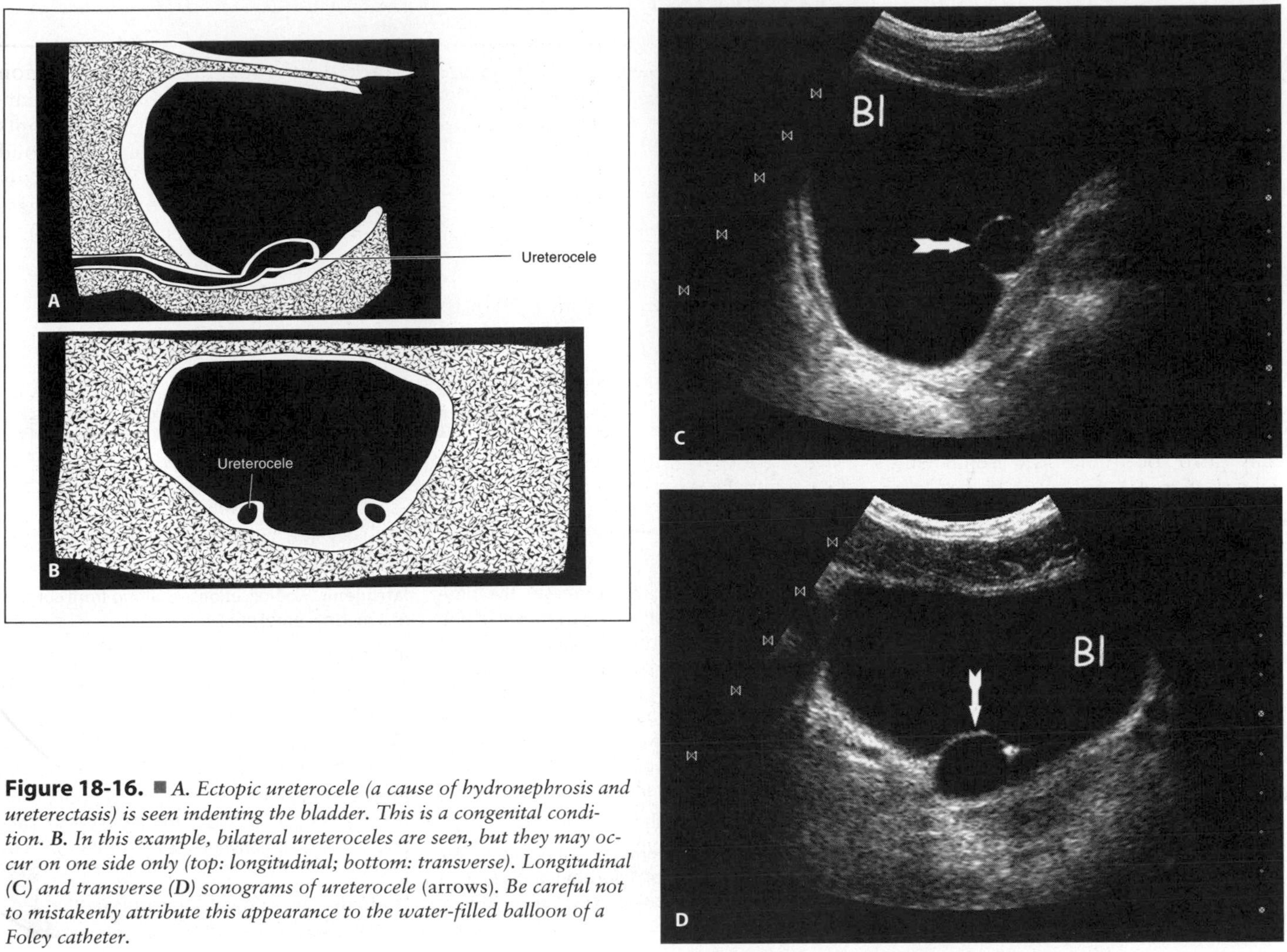

Figure 18-16. ■ *A. Ectopic ureterocele (a cause of hydronephrosis and ureterectasis) is seen indenting the bladder. This is a congenital condition. B. In this example, bilateral ureteroceles are seen, but they may occur on one side only (top: longitudinal; bottom: transverse). Longitudinal (C) and transverse (D) sonograms of ureterocele* (arrows). *Be careful not to mistakenly attribute this appearance to the water-filled balloon of a Foley catheter.*

Where Else to Look

1. With any renal tumor, examine the renal vein and the inferior vena cava for tumor extension or clot. Look for para-aortic nodes and liver metastases.
2. With polycystic disease of the kidney, examine the liver, pancreas, and spleen for associated cysts. Approximately 40% of patients with polycystic disease have liver cysts.
3. With a more or less echo-free mass, think of lymphoma and look for evidence of splenomegaly and para-aortic adenopathy.
4. With a tumor in the renal pelvis, examine the bladder and opposite kidney. There may be a synchronous transitional cell tumor at these sites as well.
5. With localized hydronephrosis of the upper pole of the kidney, look in the bladder for an ectopic ureterocele into which the duplicated ureter inserts (Fig. 18-16).

SELECTED READING

Einstein DM, Herts BR, Weaver R, et al. Evaluation of renal masses detected by excretory urography: cost-effectiveness of sonography versus CT. *AJR Am J Roentgenol* 1995; 164:371–375.

Israel GM, Hindman N, Bosniak MA. Evaluation of cystic renal masses: comparison of CT and MR imaging by using the Bosniak classification system. *Radiology* 2004;231:365–371.

Jamis-Dow CA, Choyke PL, Jennings SB, et al. Small (= 3-cm) renal masses: detection with CT versus US and pathologic correlation. *Radiology* 1996;198:785–788.

Robbin ML, Lockhart ME, Barr RG. Renal imaging with ultrasound contrast: current status. *Radiol Clin North Am* 2003;41: 963–978.

Siegel CL, Middleton WD, Teefey SA, et al. Angiomyolipoma and renal cell carcinoma: US differentiation. *Radiology* 1996;198: 789–793.

Unexplained Hematocrit Drop

Rule Out Perinephric Hematoma; Possible Perinephric Mass

BARB VANDERWERFF
TOM WINTER

19

SONOGRAM ABBREVIATIONS

Ao	Aorta
Du	Duodenum
IVC	Inferior vena cava
K	Kidney
L	Liver
P	Pancreas
Ps	Psoas muscle
QL	Quadratus lumborum muscle

KEY WORDS

Anticoagulant. Drug that increases the time needed for blood to clot; used in treatment of pulmonary emboli and myocardial infarcts. Control of dosage is not always easy, and bleeding may ensue if there is overdosage. Examples include warfarin (Coumadin), heparin, the new low-molecular weight heparin derivatives, and, to a lesser extent, platelet-inhibiting drugs like aspirin and nonsteroidal anti-inflammatory drugs.

Contralateral. Opposite side of the body.

FAST. Focused abdominal sonography for trauma. The use of a quick, focused ultrasound in an emergent setting to detect free intraperitoneal fluid in blunt trauma.

Gerota's Fascia. Tissue plane around the kidney that includes the adrenals and much fat; important in the localization of hematomas and abscesses.

Hematocrit (HCT or "Crit"). A measurement of blood concentration; indicates the amount of blood in the body.

Hemophilia. Hereditary bleeding disorder seen in males. Those affected have a particular tendency to bleed into joints and the muscles in the retroperitoneum.

Iatrogenic. Complications resulting from surgery or a medical procedure.

Ipsilateral. Same side of the body.

Lymphocele. Lymph fluid accumulation usually resulting from surgery.

Morrison's pouch. Space between the liver and the right kidney.

Retroperitoneum. Part of the body posterior to the peritoneum; includes the kidney and pancreas, as well as many muscles in the paraspinous area.

Urinoma. Collection of urine outside the genitourinary tract.

White Blood Cell Count. Number of leukocytes (white blood cells) in the blood. An elevated count can indicate an infectious process.

RELEVANT LABORATORY VALUES

HCT (Hematocrit): For adult males, 40 to 52 mL/dL. For adult females, 34 to 46 mL/dL.

White blood cell count: 3,800 to 10,500/μL

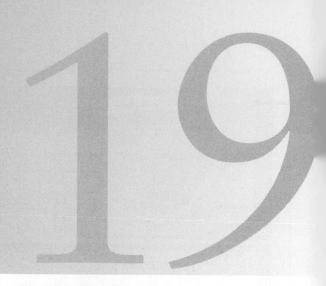

The Clinical Problem

The retroperitoneum is a clinically silent area where large fluid collections that cannot be readily diagnosed by conventional radiographic techniques (plain films) may accumulate. Such collections include hematomas (trauma, anticoagulation, surgery), abscesses (infection), lymphoceles (surgery), and urinomas (trauma, surgery). Common sites of bleeding include the psoas muscle and the perinephric space. Computed tomography (CT) is generally preferable to ultrasound because it is more sensitive and specific in identifying the presence and extent of the collection, but ultrasound may be used for diagnosis when CT is not available or applicable (remote areas, patients too sick to go to CT). Acute retroperitoneal hemorrhage is a potentially lethal condition that may have a variety of sonographic characteristics, ranging from complex fluid to mimicking a focal mass.

HEMATOMAS

An unexplained hematocrit drop may indicate that a patient has bled internally. Often the site of the bleed is unclear to the clinician. Patients at risk for unexplained hematocrit drop are those who (1) have recently undergone an operation or medical procedure; (2) are taking anticoagulants (e.g., warafin, heparin, aspirin); (3) have had a recent injury such as a car or bicycle accident, or trauma such as stabbing; (4) have bleeding or clotting problems, such as hemophiliacs or leukemics; or (5) have spontaneous or traumatic vascular rupture (ruptured abdominal aortic aneurysm, bleeding tumor).

The following are the most likely sites of asymptomatic hematomas:

1. In the abdominal wall around an incision
2. Deep to an incision
3. In a site where fluid collects adjacent to a surgical site (e.g., in the cul-de-sac, paracolic gutters, or subhepatic space)
4. Around the spleen (perisplenic), liver (perihepatic), or kidney (perinephric)
5. In the retroperitoneum (this site is particularly likely in patients with no previous injury, such as those taking anticoagulants or with bleeding problems)
6. In the iliopsoas or rectus muscles, particularly in hemophiliacs

Hematomas may develop into abscesses; they are good culture media for bacteria. Expansion of a hematoma on subsequent sonograms suggests that the lesion is infected or that there has been rebleeding. Normal hematomas slowly retract.

URINOMAS

A urinoma is a walled-off collection of extravasated urine. Urine usually collects around the kidney or under the ureter in the perinephric space. Urinomas develop mainly in patients who have had trauma, who have passed a renal stone, or who have undergone operations such as a renal transplant. Urinomas may be asymptomatic and may be found years after the original process that caused them occurred. It is useful to follow the progress of urinomas that occur after an operation because they usually resolve spontaneously. Generally, the collection is anechoic unless it has become infected.

LYMPHOCELES

Lymphoceles are collections of lymph fluid and are common after surgical procedures. Most are small, develop within 10 to 21 days after surgery, and resolve spontaneously. Treatment of larger lesions includes surgery, sclerosis, or percutaneous drainage. Most are anechoic and resemble simple cysts. Lymphoceles frequently are septated and occasionally contain debris or loculations, making them difficult to differentiate from a hematoma, urinoma, or abscess.

ABSCESSES

Abscesses are pockets of purulent fluid and commonly occur in the retroperitoneum. They may be relatively asymptomatic, particularly in the psoas muscle, presenting with fever rather than with localized symptoms. These infections may be a primary complication of surgery, septicemia, or trauma, or may be caused by spread from an adjacent organ, such as the kidney, bowel, or spine. A preexisting fluid collection such as a pancreatic pseudocyst may also become secondarily infected. Percutaneous ultrasound-guided aspiration is an important diagnostic test, as are clinical symptoms such as elevated white count, fever, chills, localized tenderness, and increasing size. The appearance on ultrasound is rarely specific, so distinguishing abscesses from other collections or masses is challenging and usually a needle aspiration is an integral part of the examination.

VASCULAR ABNORMALITIES

Vascular pathologic conditions can develop after surgery, trauma, or a medical condition. They include arteriovenous fistulas, aneurysms, and varices. They can be confused with simple fluid collections. Color flow imaging and Doppler spectral analysis can define whether the abnormality is vascular or not and are essential before inserting a needle into any "fluid" collection to prevent inadvertent puncture of a vascular abnormality.

OTHER MASSES AND PSEUDOMASSES

Benign masses and pseudomasses—such as horseshoe kidneys, ptotic kidneys, dromedary hump, double collecting system, bowel duplication cysts, and adenopathy—should be considered as possible explanations for a retroperitoneal mass. Perhaps the most frequent problem occurs when a loop of aperistaltic bowel mimics a true mass or fluid collection. Changing the patient's position during the examination and watching the area while the patient drinks can usually make the distinction.

Anatomy

RETROPERITONEUM

In practice, the retroperitoneum is a term used to describe the area that includes the kidneys, ureters, adrenal glands, pancreas, aorta, and inferior vena cava; the psoas, iliacus, and quadratus lumborum muscles; and the presacral area (Fig. 19-1). The ascending colon, descending colon, and most of the duodenum are also situated in the retroperitoneum, as are the abdominal lymph nodes and somatic nerves.

SPACES AROUND THE KIDNEY

The area around the kidney is traversed by several fibrous sheaths that form natural barriers to the passage of fluid and act as a guide for the site of origin of a collection. First, the kidney is covered with a tough, fibrous capsule. Second, a layer of perirenal fat surrounds the encapsulated kidney and is continuous with the fat in the renal sinus. The third layer, the renal fascia, surrounds the kidney and perirenal fat. Another term for the renal fascia is Gerota's fascia. Gerota's fascia is surrounded by yet another layer of fat, called pararenal fat. The latter is especially thick posterior to Gerota's fascia. Morrison's pouch is an intraperitoneal space located in the hepatorenal fossa and lies between the kidney and the liver. The retroperitoneum is divided into the following areas:

1. The anterior pararenal space. A space in front of the kidney that communicates with the opposite side around the pancreas.
2. The perinephric space within Gerota's fascia. This space may be open-ended inferiorly and encloses the kidneys, fat, and adrenal glands.
3. The posterior pararenal space. This space extends behind the kidney into the lateral aspects of the abdominal wall. The fascial planes can be seen on a good-quality sonogram in an obese patient when they are outlined by fat.
4. The psoas muscles. These muscles lie lateral to the spine and widen inferiorly (Fig. 19-2). They eventually join the iliacus muscles that arise on the anterior aspect of the iliac crest to form a joint muscle (the iliopsoas) in the pelvis.

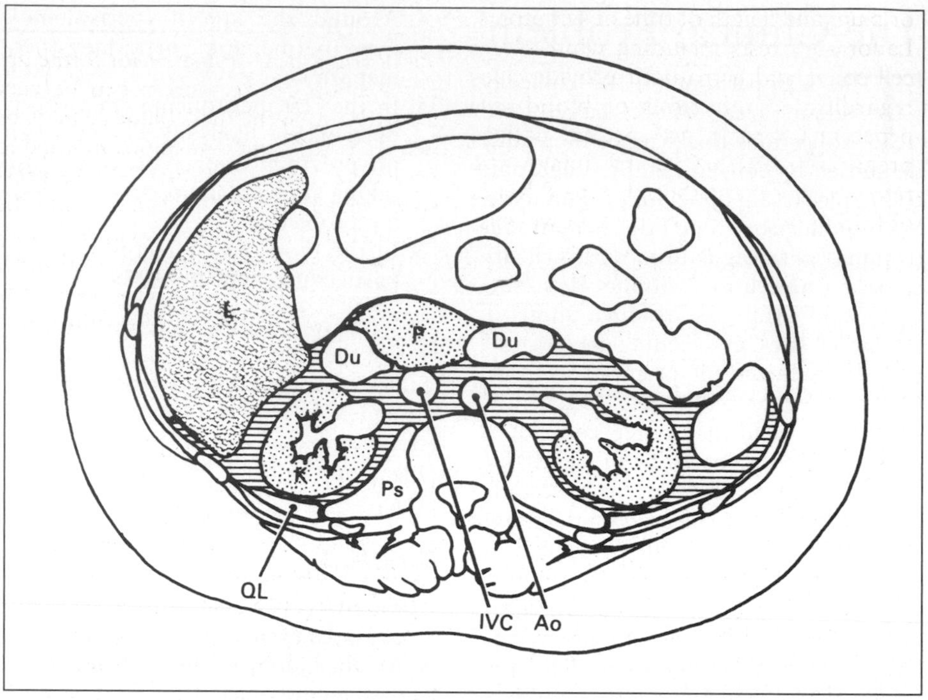

Figure 19-1. ■ *Retroperitoneum* (cross-hatched area). *Large structures in the retroperitoneum include the psoas muscles, quadratus lumborum muscles, kidneys, and pancreas.*

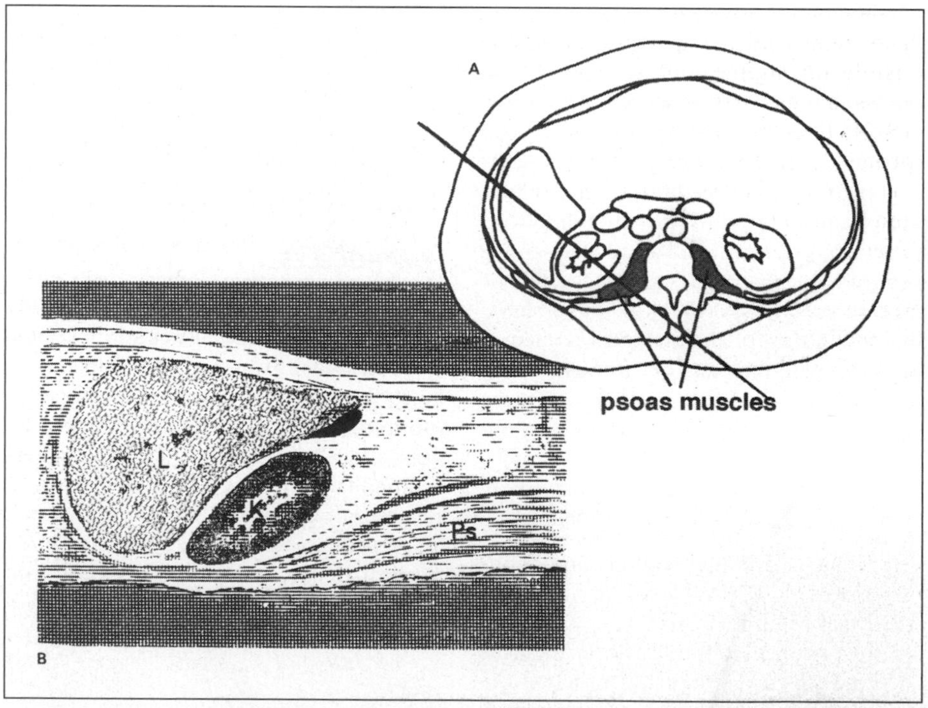

Figure 19-2. ■ *Psoas muscles are usually shown best by an oblique view through the liver.*

5. The quadratus lumborum muscles. These muscles lie posterior to the kidney (Fig. 19-1) and are often surprisingly sonolucent, giving the impression that a collection is present. If one looks on the opposite side, a similar sonolucent area will be seen.

Technique

By asking the patient a few clinical questions, you can tailor your examination and improve your diagnosis. Pertinent areas to cover include any recent trauma, medical procedures, or surgeries; fever or pain; and length of time of symptoms. Laboratory tests including white blood cell count and hematocrit provide clues regarding an infectious or blood loss process. There is no specific patient preparation necessary to image the retroperitoneum, although 6 to 8 hours of fasting may help to reduce bowel gas.

PERINEPHRIC AREA

As a rule, the prone or decubitus position gives the best view of the retroperitoneal areas around the kidneys down to the level of the iliac crest. By using a coronal approach and having the patient take in a breath, the kidneys and the area surrounding them can be visualized without overlying bowel gas or rib shadowing. Occasionally, scanning between the ribs is necessary. If the patient puts the ipsilateral arm overhead in the decubitus position, it can open up the rib spaces for easier visualization. The liver can be used as the acoustic window for the right kidney and the spleen for the left kidney.

PSOAS MUSCLES

The psoas and iliacus muscles may be visible on supine and supine oblique views, but gas may obscure the area (Fig. 19-2). It is usually best to perform a prone oblique decubitus view looking through the kidneys at the psoas muscles and at the area between the aorta and the inferior vena cava. This view is similar to the one used to look at the adrenal glands. When evaluating a muscle, it should lengthen on a longitudinal view.

PRESACRAL AREA

Visualizing the region anterior to the upper portion of the sacrum can be very difficult. A fluid-filled bladder may be helpful in the supine position and used to provide a "sonic window." Deep pressure using a linear array can displace the gut away from this area and allow views of the lower aorta and presacral area. For an evaluation of a deeper collection, transvaginal or endorectal scanning may be helpful.

FOCUSED ABDOMINAL SONOGRAPHY FOR TRAUMA

Performed emergently by properly trained and credentialed staff, focused abdominal sonography for trauma (FAST) allows timely diagnosis of potentially life-threatening hemorrhage and triage of the patient. The FAST examination's only objective is the detection of free intraperitoneal fluid in blunt abdominal trauma.

The FAST examination can be performed by using six views:

1. Morrison's pouch: Visualization of the right upper quadrant at the interface between the liver and Gerota's fascia of the kidney.
2. Perisplenic view: Visualization of the left upper quadrant at the left kidney and spleen interface.
3. Pelvic view: Visualization of the rectovesicular pouch in males and the cul-de-sac in females. This is the most sensitive of the abdominal views with less than 200 mL of fluid sometimes seen. Sensitivity for free fluid is increased if one scans through a distended bladder.
4. The right and left paracolic gutters.
5. The pericardium: Visualization outside the peritoneum to evaluate for pericardial effusion; the probe is placed just to the right of the patient's xiphoid. The ultrasound beam is then focused through the liver to visualize the interface of the right ventricle and pericardium.

Additional views are often obtained. One should not forget the limitations of this study and that significant injuries can be missed even in the hands of the most experienced sonographer. If time and resources allow, CT is a better test to evaluate the abdomen and pelvis in the trauma setting; however, when time is crucial or resources limited, FAST may be a useful adjunct.

Pathology

HEMATOMA

Sonographic Appearances

Solid or cystic mass-like areas are the most common sonographic findings. Cystic lesions may vary from being entirely sonolucent to being markedly echogenic and indistinguishable from adjacent fat or soft tissue (Fig. 19-3). Cellular debris may layer dependently in a hematoma, making its differentiation from an abscess difficult. Fluid–fluid levels may be seen. The character of clot-

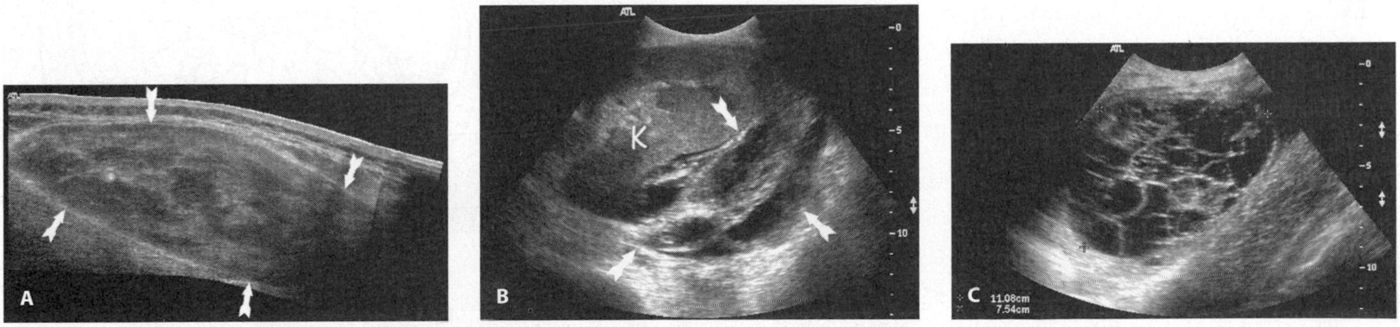

Figure 19-3. ■ *Patterns of hematoma. Some hematomas are evenly echogenic, whereas others contain clumps of echoes. Fluid–fluid levels may be seen when bleeding occurs into a fluid-filled structure (e.g., a renal or ovarian cyst).* **A.** *Solid-appearing hematoma. A 30-year-old man with decreasing hematocrit after snowboard accident. Extended field-of-view sonogram shows a large solid mass* (arrows) *in the right gluteal region.* **B.** *Cystic and solid-appearing hematoma. A 56-year-old woman with decreasing hematocrit after renal transplant. Ultrasound shows a large complex mixed cystic and solid mass* (arrows) *surrounding the transplant kidney.* **C.** *More cystic-appearing hematoma: A 16-year-old, with trisomy-21 and increasing creatine after renal transplant, was found at surgery to have a 11 × 7.5-cm liquefied perinephric hematoma* (cursors).

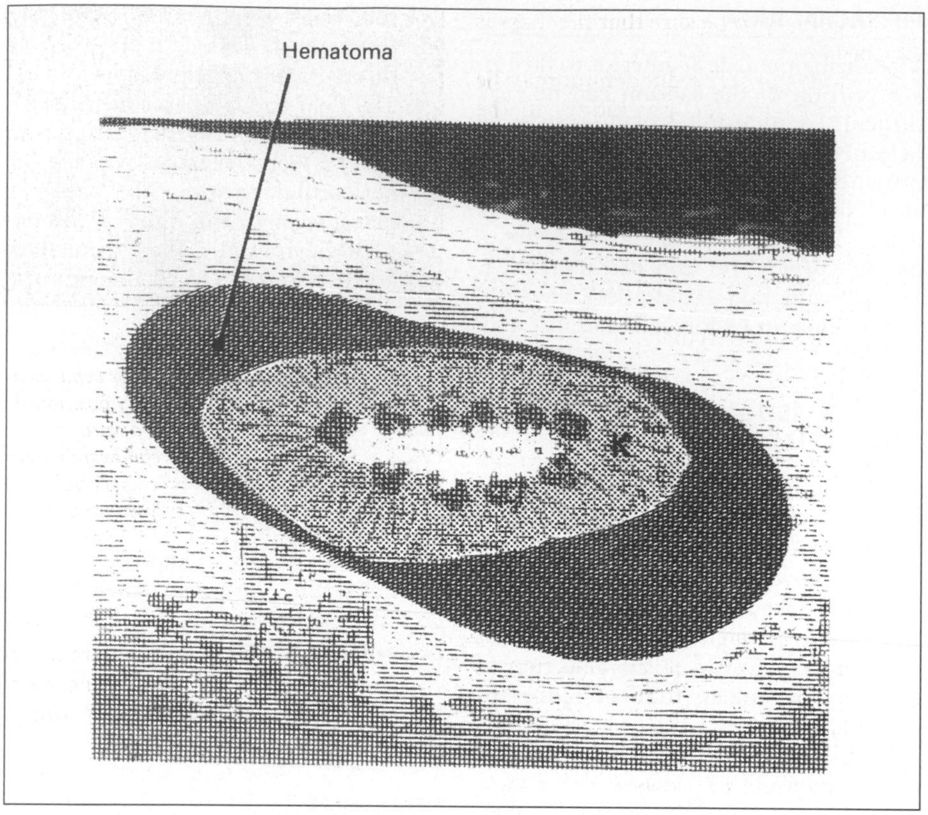

Figure 19-4. ■ *A subcapsular hematoma may be suggested when the border of the kidney is flattened and the capsular echogenic line is absent.*

ted blood changes over time. Fresh hematomas present as sonolucent areas, whereas organized thrombus with clot formation can show a more solid component within the mass. Calcification may be seen in longstanding hematomas. If the hematoma occurs after a penetrating injury, there may be visible distortion of an organ, for example, the kidney outline.

Location

- Subcapsular. If the hematoma is adjacent to the kidney in the subcapsular location, it will have circular superior and inferior margins, and the shape of the kidney will be flattened (Fig. 19-4).
- Perinephric. If the hematoma is in Gerota's fascia, it will usually be located posteromedially and will extend above and well below the level of the kidney.
- Posterior pararenal. A hematoma in the posterior pararenal space extends up the lateral walls of the abdomen and displaces the kidney anteriorly.
- Anterior pararenal. Hematomas in the anterior pararenal space lie anterior to the kidney and may extend medially into the region of the pancreas.
- Intramuscular. A hematoma in the psoas muscle forms an asymmetric bulge within that muscle, displacing the kidney laterally. It tracks down into the pelvis toward the iliacus muscle and inguinal ligament (Fig. 19-5).
- A hematoma secondary to deep cutting trauma (e.g., a stab wound) does not necessarily confine itself to the tissue planes described above. Scan the opposite side to check for symmetry.

ABSCESSES

Abscesses develop in the same areas as hematomas and are difficult to distinguish from them sonographically. They may bulge more because they are not as well confined by the tissue planes, and evidence of a septum and loculation is more apparent. The borders of abscesses are usually more irregular. The abscess usually has a complex pattern with thick irregular walls, septa, and layering de-

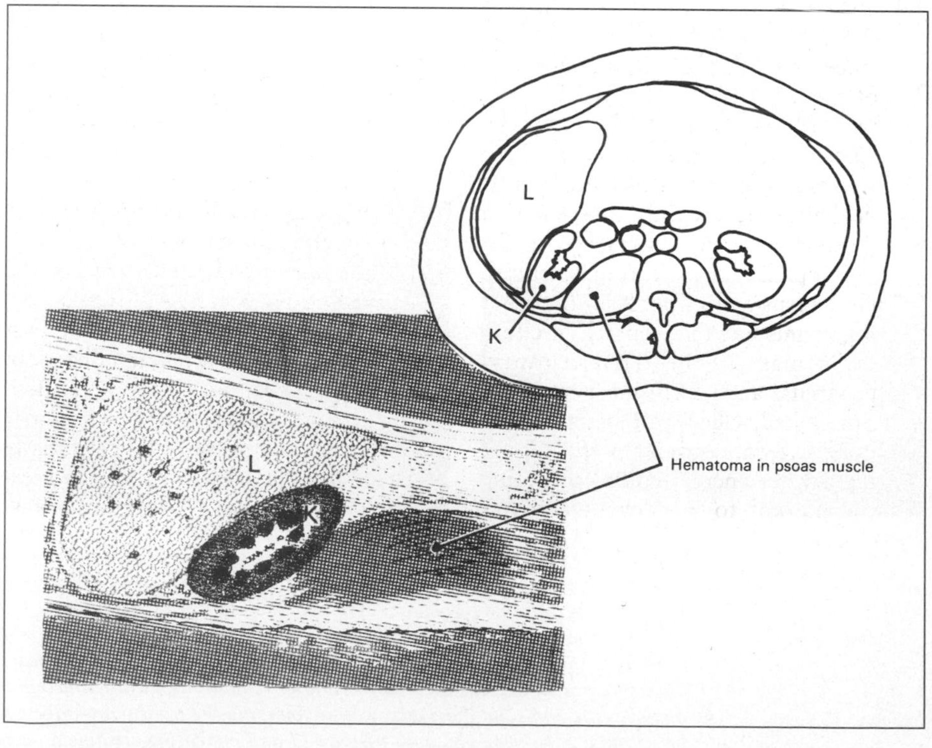

Figure 19-5. ■ *Sonolucent area that expands the psoas muscle owing to a hematoma.*

bris. Gas within the abscess is reflective and casts an acoustic shadow. The sonographer should be careful not to misdiagnose a gas-containing abscess for a loop of bowel.

OTHER FLUID COLLECTIONS

Urinomas may develop around the kidney, usually within Gerota's fascia. These are anechoic collections.

Pitfalls

1. Collection versus shadowing. Particularly in the prone position, it may be hard to distinguish between a true collection and rib shadowing. Attempts to view the suspect area in either the erect or the decubitus position are important. Alteration of the phase of respiration can help to clarify the issue.
2. Echogenic hematoma. At some stages in the course of its evolution, a hematoma may be markedly echogenic. Do not miss it by scanning at too high a gain.
3. Quadratus lumborum muscles. The quadratus lumborum may be much less echogenic than other muscles and may mimic an abscess or hematoma. Comparison with the other side will show its true nature.
4. Spleen versus collection. It may be difficult to distinguish between the spleen and a mass at the upper pole of the left kidney. This is especially true in the case of an accessory spleen. The interface between these two organs may be seen better with a decubitus view or with the patient in an erect position. Angling up at a different phase of respiration is helpful.
5. Gut versus collection. It is important not to mistake the stomach or colon for a mass in the retroperitoneal pararenal area. Such masses will be fluid filled. Check for peristalsis; if none is seen, consider performing a high-water enema (colon) or asking the patient to sip degassed water (stomach) to be sure that the mass is not gut.
6. Duodenum. The duodenum may lie anterior to the right kidney in the subhepatic space, mimicking a perinephric collection. Real time will show peristalsis when fluid is administered by mouth.
7. Malrotated kidney versus collection. The pelvis of a malrotated kidney lies anterior to the right kidney and may mimic a collection in the subhepatic space. Careful real-time and color Doppler analysis will show that the renal vein, renal artery, and ureter enter the supposed collection. The crossing isthmus of a horseshoe kidney may mimic a retroperitoneal mass or hematoma in front of the aorta (Fig. 19-6).
8. Psoas versus masses. In young patients or athletes, the psoas muscles may be exceptionally prominent and may be mistaken for a mass; the psoas muscles will be symmetrically enlarged.
9. Perinephric fat versus mass. In obese patients, considerable perinephric fat may be present, forming a relatively echogenic rim around the kidneys. Do not mistake this for a pathologic process. It will be bilateral.
10. A large fluid-filled collection in the pelvis can be mistaken for a distended urinary bladder. Having the patient void and meticulous scanning techniques help to prevent this.
11. Harmonic imaging may help to define the region of interest, especially in the near field. This will aid in clearing up artifactual echoes within a simple cyst or fluid collection and help define the walls.
12. Make sure to identify whether the pathology is projecting from an organ such as an exophytic renal cyst versus an associated fluid collection.
13. Doppler imaging can quickly identify a potential collection as vascular in origin and prevent the potentially catastrophic mistake of inadvertently aspirating or draining a vascular malformation. Be aware of using the correct transducer and technical settings to optimally image slow flow.

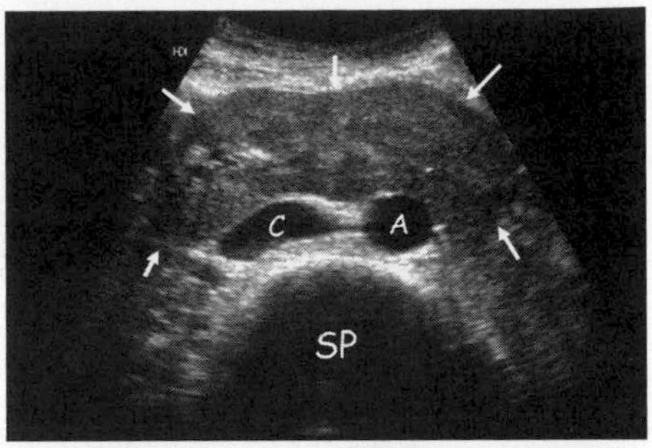

Figure 19-6. ■ *Horseshoe kidney* (arrows) *lies in front of the aorta* (A), *inferior vena cava* (C), *and spine* (SP); *this abnormally positioned renal tissue may be mistaken for a retroperitoneal hematoma or mass. Careful examination of the kidneys, showing that the lower pole of each kidney connects with this pseudomass, will prevent this mistake.*

Where Else to Look

Psoas abscesses may track along the muscles into the hip (Fig. 19-5). A subtle collection in the hip may be seen near the femoral head.

SELECTED READING

Cosgrove DO, Dubbins PA. The peritoneum and retroperitoneum. In: *Clinical Ultrasound: comprehensive text*, 2nd ed. Eds Meire HB, Cosgrove D, Dewbury K, et al. Edinburgh: Churchill Livingstone; 2001:447–477.

Hermann G, Gilbert MS, Abdelwahab IF. Hemophilia: evaluation of musculoskeletal involvement with CT, sonography, and MR imaging. *AJR Am J Roentgenol* 1992; 158:119–123.

McGahan JP, Richards J, Gillen M. The focused abdominal sonography for trauma scan: pearls and pitfalls. *J Ultrasound Med* 2002; 21:789–800.

Molmenti EP, Balfe DM, Kanterman RY, et al. Anatomy of the retroperitoneum: observations of the distribution of pathologic fluid collections. *Radiology* 1996;200:95–103.

Hematuria

LISA PARSONS
TOM WINTER

20

SONOGRAM ABBREVIATIONS

Bl	Bladder
Pr	Prostate gland

KEY WORDS

Benign Prostatic Hypertrophy. Enlargement of the glandular component of the prostate. The true prostate forms a shell around the enlarged gland.

Cystitis. Infection or inflammation of the wall of the bladder.

Hematuria. Blood in the urine.

Hydroureter. Dilated ureter.

Nephrocalcinosis. Multiple small calculi deposited in the renal pyramids. Found in association with renal tubular acidosis and medullary sponge kidney.

Pyelonephritis. Infection of the kidney without abscess formation.

Pyonephrosis. Pus-filled hydronephrosis.

Staghorn Calculus. A stone that occupies most of the renal pelvis and infundibulum.

Trigone. Base of the bladder. Area between the insertion of the ureters and the urethra.

Urethra. Urinary outflow tract below the bladder.

RELEVANT LABORATORY VALUES

Microscopic hematuria: More than two to three red blood cells per high-power field prompts a full diagnostic workup, whereas one to three red blood cells per high-power field may warrant a workup in patients at risk for urologic malignancy.

The Clinical Problem

Hematuria is an important sign of genitourinary tract problems. The abnormality may be located within the kidneys, ureter, bladder, or urethra. The segments of the genitourinary tract that can be visualized by ultrasound (i.e., the kidney, upper and lower portions of the ureter, bladder, and upper part of the urethra) should be carefully examined. A specialized computed tomography (CT) scan (so-called CT-intravenous pyelogram [IVP]) is the gold standard, gradually replacing the older excretory urogram (IVP or intravenous urogram [IVU]), for evaluating patients with hematuria. Ultrasound, however, particularly when combined with a plain film, offers a safe and less-expensive method for evaluation of patients with suspected stone disease who cannot have contrast or who do not have access to modern CT. Good sonographic scanning technique is essential because the responsible lesions, such as calculi or tumors, are often relatively minute.

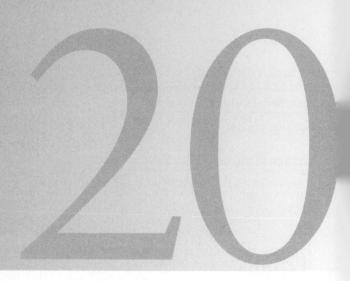

Anatomy

KIDNEYS

See Chapter 17.

BLADDER

The bladder has a muscular wall whose thickness can be discerned with ultrasound. It is usually symmetric and is more or less square on transverse section. The base of the bladder where the ureters enter is known as the trigone (Fig. 20-1).

The bladder wall is proportionately thicker in infants than in other age groups. The bladder wall is approximately 3 mm thick when distended and 5 mm thick when empty in individuals other than infants.

The normal bladder in an adult contains approximately 150 to 400 mL and empties nearly completely.

URETERS

The ureters are the small tubes that convey urine from the kidney to the bladder. Each begins where the renal pelvis narrows (ureteropelvic junction) and travels anterior to the psoas muscle into the true pelvis. They insert into the trigone region of the bladder (ureterovesicular junction). The normal ureter measures less than 8 mm wide and is difficult to see with ultrasound under normal conditions. In hydroureter, the entire length of the ureter may be seen.

Two small bumps on the posterior aspect of the bladder on either side of the midline represent the ureteric orifices (see Fig. 18-1). The jet phenomenon may be seen when the ureteric orifices open and allow the emptying of urine from the ureters into the bladder. Color Doppler is a useful tool to demonstrate ureteral jets. The normal ureter can be seen as a subtle echopenic tube leading obliquely superiorly from the ureteric orifice. It distends with peristalsis.

URETHRA

The urethra is the tube that conveys urine from the bladder to the outside of the body. Ultrasound evaluation is generally limited to the posterior urethra above the external sphincter. In the male, the posterior urethra is surrounded by the prostate. The anterior urethra in the male can be scanned with a specialized technique in which aqueous gel is injected into the urethra and a linear transducer is placed parallel to the urethra on the penile shaft.

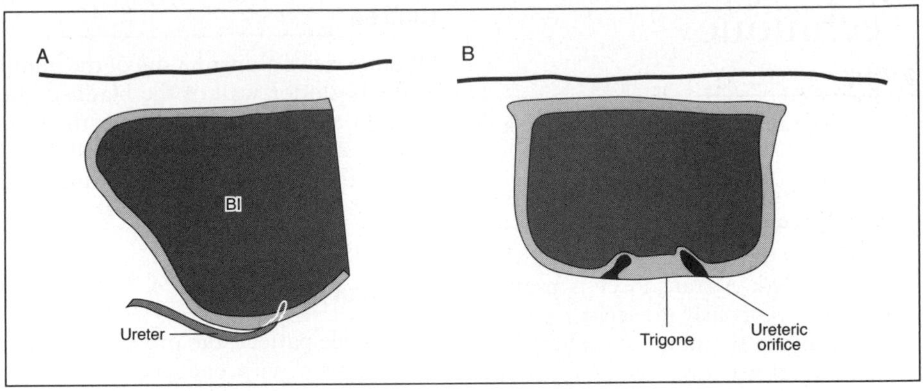

Figure 20-1. ■ *Ureteric orifices can be seen as two small buds in the trigone. Ureters can be traced through the wall to the ureteric orifice.* ***A.*** *Sagittal.* ***B.*** *Transverse.*

MALE ANATOMY

There are two major parts of the urethra, the posterior (most of which lies within the prostate gland) and the anterior (which courses through the penis). Posterior to the lower bladder lie the mustache-shaped seminal vesicles. The prostate lies posterior to the symphysis pubis and inferior to the bladder and seminal vesicles. It is more or less round. Sometimes a line of echoes from the urethra can be seen at its center.

FEMALE ANATOMY

In the female, the uterus and vagina lie posterior and inferior to the bladder (Fig. 20-2). The vagina and lower segment of the uterus are normally never separated from the bladder. A tissue similar to the prostate in the male lies around the female urethra (Fig. 20-2) and can occasionally be mistaken for a mass in the base of the bladder.

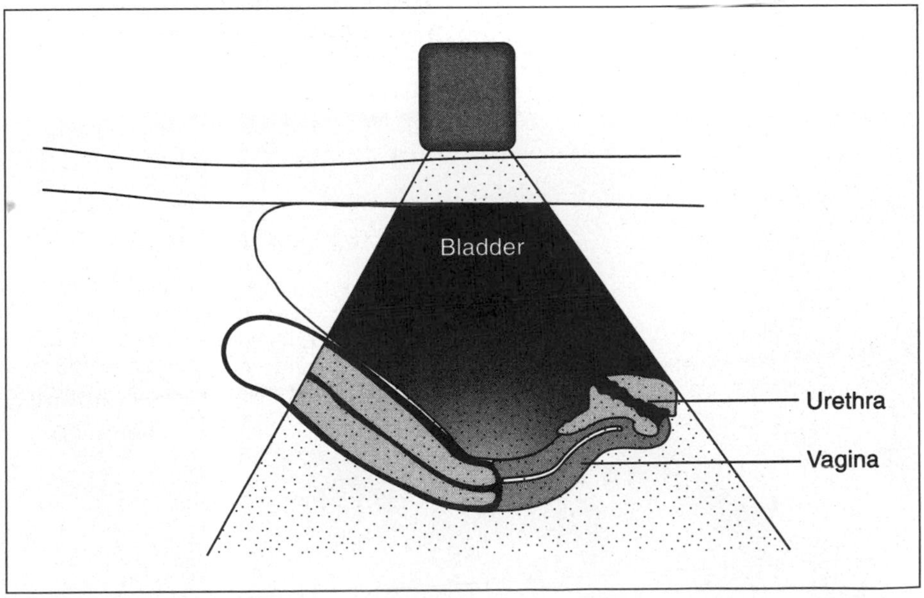

Figure 20-2. ■ *In the female, the uterus and vagina lie posterior and inferior to the bladder. The posterior urethra is seen as a mass at the inferior aspect of the bladder.*

Technique

KIDNEY

The sonographic examination of the kidney is reviewed in Chapter 18.

BLADDER

The bladder can be examined only when it is distended. A transducer is pressed, somewhat vigorously if necessary, into a site just above the pubic symphysis and angled superiorly to show the upper portions of the bladder wall. The bladder normally has a smooth, curved surface and is surrounded by an echogenic line that represents the wall. Some have used a transrectal or endovaginal transducer to examine the anterior bladder wall if it is not well seen due to reverberation artifact. If the patient has a Foley catheter in place, the bladder can be examined by either clamping the Foley and waiting for the bladder to distend, or by instilling in sterile retrograde fashion approximately 200 mL (in adults) of sterile normal saline solution.

Bladder volume can be calculated by multiplying width, height, and length together and halving the result.

Postvoid views should be obtained because significant residual urine may indicate urethral obstruction or neurogenic bladder and may result in urinary tract infection.

URETER

Oblique views along the site of the bump in the posterior wall of the bladder (the trigone) angling laterally show the normal ureter within the bladder wall. In females, the ureteric insertions into the bladder can be well seen with the endovaginal probe.

URETHRA

In the male patient, the prostatic urethra may be seen with endorectal imaging, and the anterior urethra may be seen using a high-frequency probe along the shaft of the penis.

In the female patient, the urethra may be seen with endovaginal imaging.

CATHETERIZATION

It may be necessary to insert a catheter to fill the bladder adequately. One cannot perform a satisfactory transabdominal ultrasonic examination of the bladder unless it is well distended. Care must be taken not to introduce air into the bladder if the patient is catheterized because this will cause scattering of the ultrasound waves and provide an unsatisfactory image.

CALCULI

The highest possible frequency should be used to search for renal calculi because the acoustic shadowing is emphasized by a high frequency, and stones can be subtle. It is best to use a single focal point when demonstrating a stone, because this will maximize the shadowing characteristic. Place the focal zone at the expected location of the stone.

Pathology

CALCULI

Renal Calculi

Ultrasound can be a more sensitive method of detecting calculi than an intravenous pyelogram. Some calculi cannot be seen on an intravenous pyelogram because they are not radiopaque or because they are concealed by gas or feces. If calculi are more than 3 or 4 mm in size, acoustic shadowing can be seen beyond a dense echo (Fig. 20-3).

Smaller calculi appear as densely echogenic structures within the renal sinus echoes; decreasing the gain makes them stand out more against the background echogenicity of the renal sinus.

In nephrocalcinosis, the calculi are often too small to cast shadows. Instead, calculi can be seen as symmetric echogenic areas located where the pyramids normally lie (Fig. 20-4).

Calculi, whether due to uric acid, cysteine, or calcium mixtures, cause echogenic areas with shadowing if they are large. Smaller calculi may not demonstrate shadowing, or shadowing may be seen only fleetingly with real time. Asso-

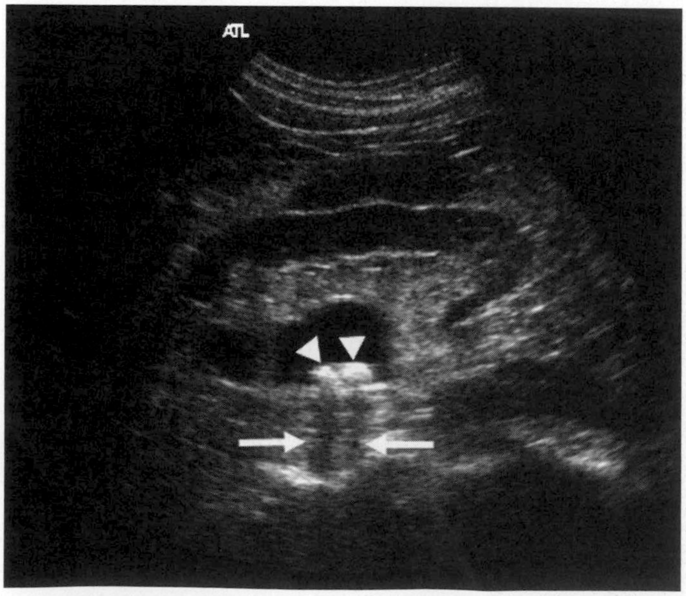

Figure 20-3. ■ *Two adjacent stones* (arrowheads) *with posterior acoustic shadowing* (arrows) *in a dilated extrarenal pelvis.*

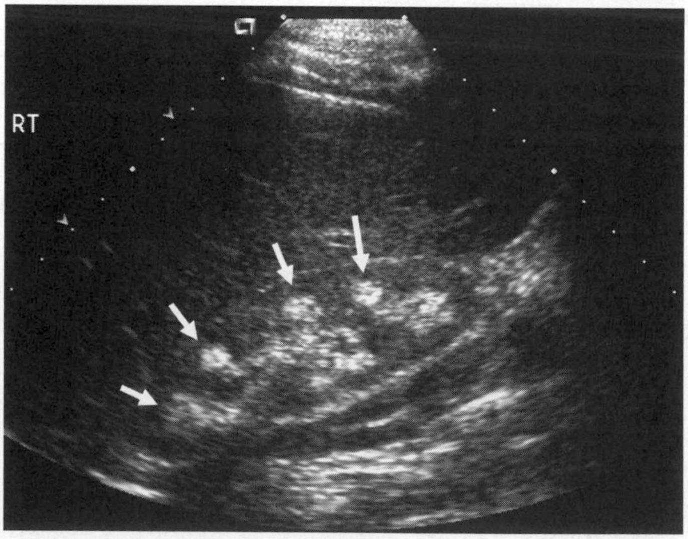

Figure 20-4. ■ *In nephrocalcinosis, the pyramids* (arrows) *are filled with small stones. Echogenic areas are seen in the pyramids, although the stones are usually too small to create shadows. Remember that normal pyramids should be hypoechoic.*

ciated cystic areas adjacent to the calculi may represent dilated calyces. Staghorn calculi in the renal pelvis can be mistaken for the renal sinus echoes.

A rapidly fluctuating mixture of Doppler signals, both red and blue pixels, occurring behind a stone at color Doppler imaging is a very characteristic feature of calculi. This so-called twinkle artifact occurs in approximately 80% of urinary tract calculi and may be a very helpful sign in detecting calculi that are not well seen on grayscale imaging (Color Plate 20-1).

If there is hydronephrosis or hematuria, make a specific effort to see calculi in the distal ureter or within the bladder wall. Usually, the ureter is dilated superior to the calculus; with good technique, shadowing from the calculus can be seen (Fig. 20-5). Subtle calculi may be seen in the distal ureter as it enters the bladder with rectal (in men) or vaginal (in women) probes (Fig. 20-6) when they cannot be seen with a transabdominal approach.

Grayscale, or even better, Doppler detection of ureteric jets is a useful but not infallible observation when searching for ureteral obstruction. Jet frequency should be symmetric on both sides in healthy individuals, although the frequency of jet occurrence may vary considerably depending on the patient's state of hydration. In obstruction, jets on the affected side may be completely absent or show continuous low-level flow. However, patients with low-grade obstruction may have normal jets, so a normal jet flow pattern does not exclude the possibility of ureteral calculi.

Bladder Calculi

Bladder calculi may be missed on IVP because they can be confused with phleboliths. They are particularly easy to see with ultrasound because they are surrounded by fluid (Fig. 20-7) Movement

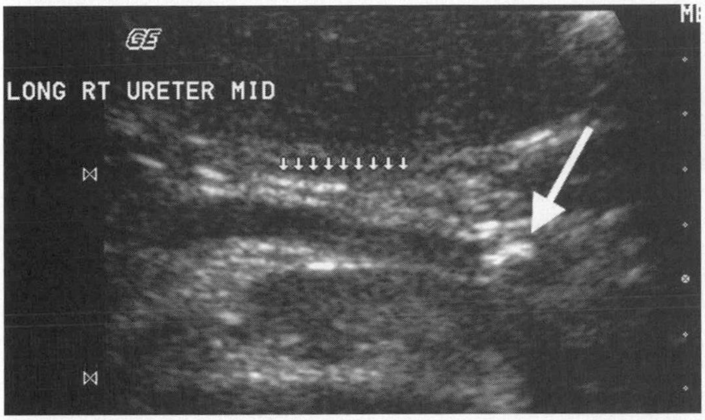

Figure 20-5. ■ *A midureteral stone* (large arrow) *is seen just below the mildly dilated proximal ureter* (multiple small arrows).

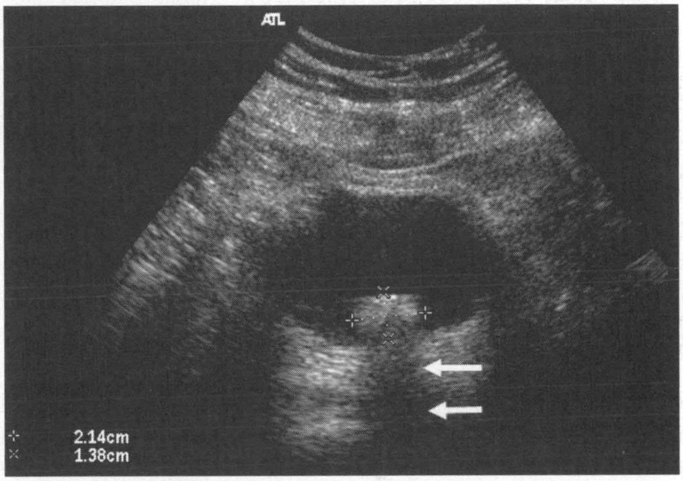

Figure 20-7. ■ *Bladder calculi usually cause acoustic shadowing* (white arrows). *This transabdominal scan shows a 2.1- × 1.4-cm stone* (cursors) *on the posterior wall of the urinary bladder.*

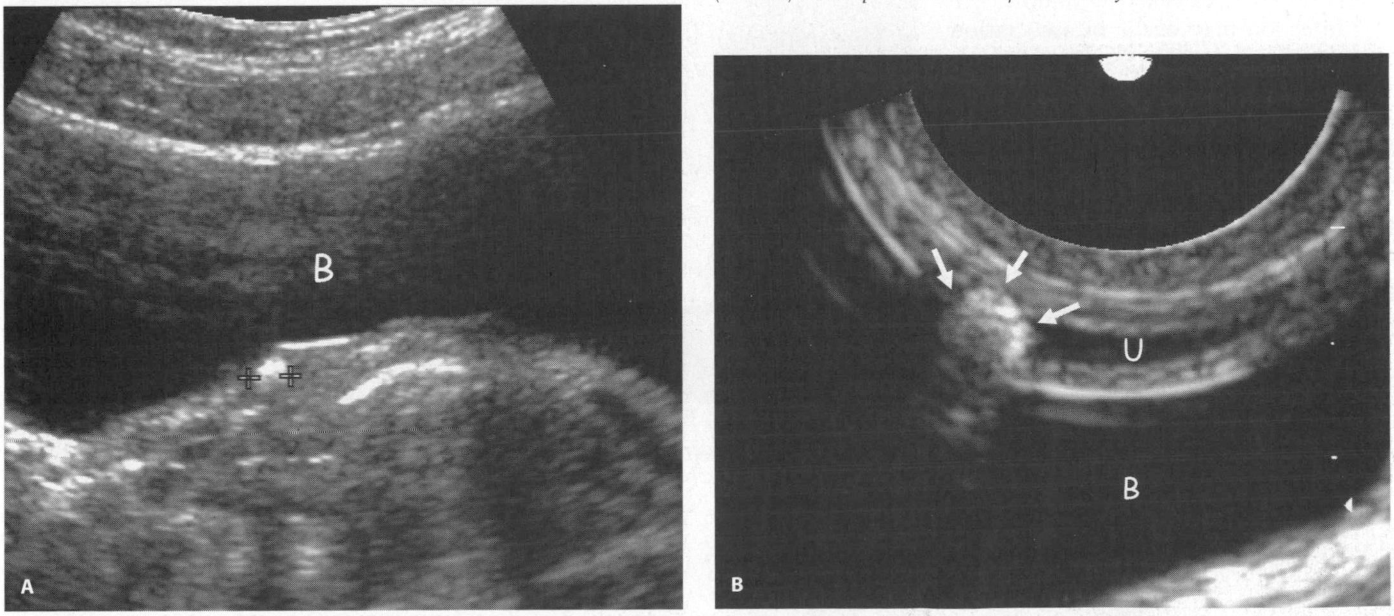

Figure 20-6. ■ *A. A 4.5-mm stone* (cursors) *is seen in the right ureteral orifice of a transabdominal scan through a partially filled urinary bladder* (B). *B. Transvaginal imaging much better delineates the stone* (arrows) *and the dilated ureter proximal to it* (U).

of a bladder calculus can be demonstrated by turning the patient to an oblique or decubitus position.

Distal ureteral calculi may be associated with bladder wall edema.

TUMORS

Tumors in the kidney and bladder may be seen first with ultrasound and may be responsible for hematuria. Tumor appearances in the kidney are described in Chapter 17. Tumors in the bladder are usually small, relatively echogenic structures adjacent to the bladder wall but occasionally can be quite large (Fig. 20-8). The extent of invasion of the bladder wall can be assessed with ultrasound. The echogenic line around the bladder is absent when a tumor has invaded the wall. The degree of bladder wall invasion affects the staging and therefore the therapy of a bladder tumor.

A bladder tumor protruding into the true pelvis through the bladder wall is unresectable; therefore, a cystectomy, the preferred treatment for bladder tumor, cannot be performed.

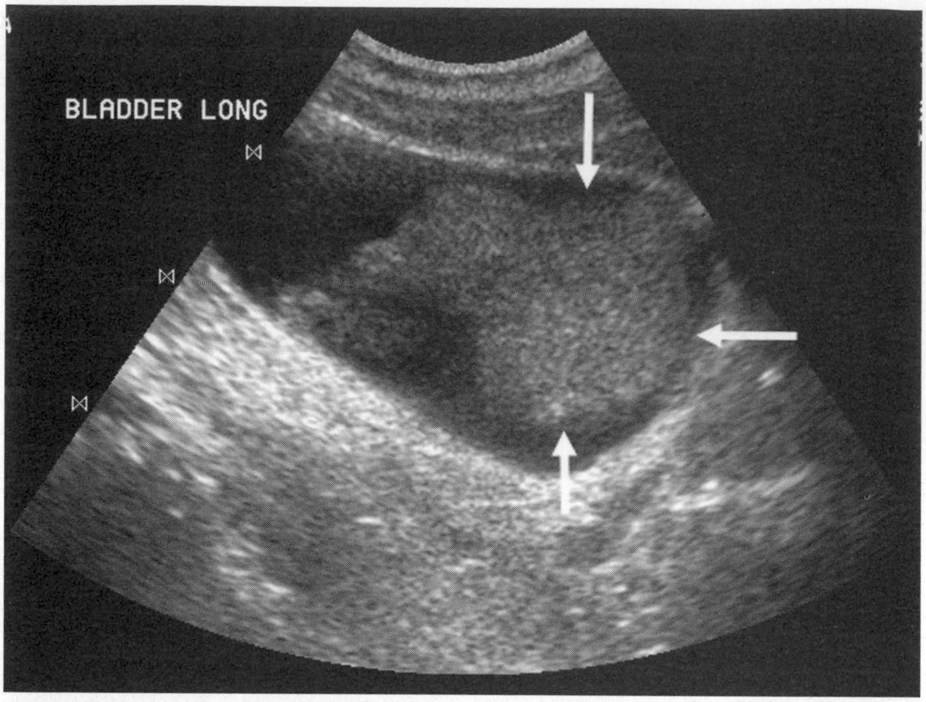

Figure 20-8. ■ *Tumors are echogenic areas within the bladder lumen. If they extend through the bladder wall, the echogenic line around the bladder is disrupted. Large transitional cell carcinoma* (white arrows) *partially filling the bladder.*

INFECTION

Infection can be responsible for hematuria. In the kidney, infection looks like an abscess (see Chapter 11) or pyelonephritis. In the bladder, infection may cause generalized or local thickening of the bladder wall (cystitis). If localized, such thickening may be indistinguishable from thickening caused by a tumor.

Infection may occur in association with a diverticulum, a cystic bud arising from a bladder that is chronically obstructed (Fig. 20-9). The neck of a diverticulum is easy to see with ultrasound. To be sure which is the bladder and which is the diverticulum, watch with real-time analysis as the patient voids. The diverticulum will enlarge as the bladder contracts.

Tumors occur more frequently in diverticuli than on the normal bladder wall.

Fluid debris levels may occur due to infection. They change when the patient's position is changed.

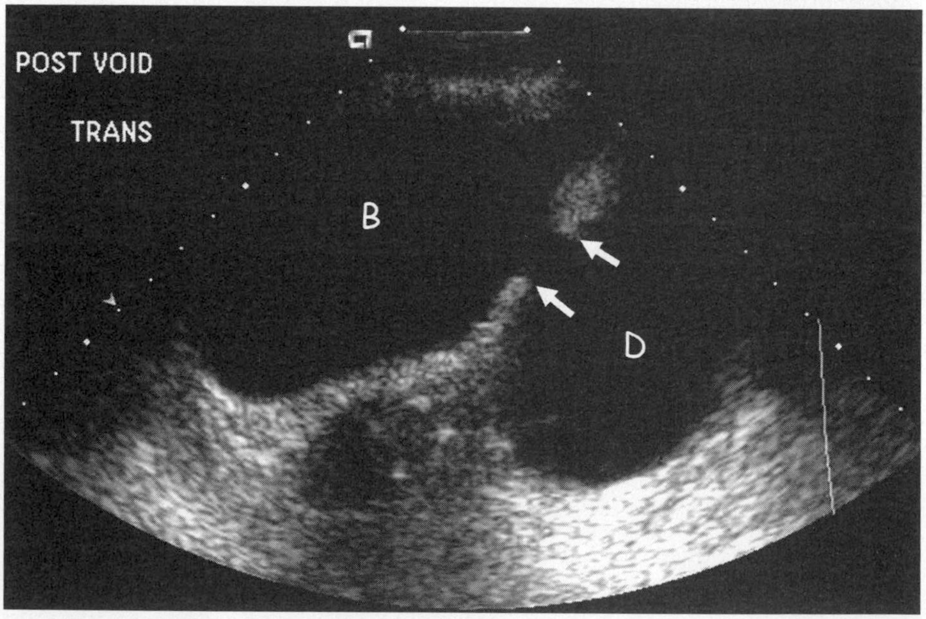

Figure 20-9. ■ *Bladder diverticula* (D) *appear as pedunculated extensions to the bladder* (B). *They generally have a relatively small connection or mouth* (arrows) *to the bladder.*

TRAUMATIC CHANGES

Traumatic damage to any site in the genitourinary tract will produce hematuria. When the kidney has had trauma, a localized area of altered echogenicity, possibly fluid filled, may indicate a blood clot or a laceration of the kidney. A distorted outline and a line through the kidney may indicate a kidney fracture. A perinephric hematoma will almost certainly develop at the site of the laceration. Bladder trauma is revealed by the presence of a perivesical hematoma—a collection of blood lying outside the bladder. The actual site of a bladder wall tear is usually not visible with ultrasound.

A Foley catheter that has been in place for some time often causes traumatic damage to the superior wall (dome) of the bladder. Local bulging and irregularity are seen at the site of the traumatic cystitis.

PROSTATIC HYPERTROPHY

Prostatic hypertrophy may be responsible for hematuria. The engorged veins that run along the surface of an enlarged prostate bleed easily. Enlargement of the prostate is detected by impingement of a prostatic soft tissue mass on the bladder or by extension of the prostate toward the rectum.

The prostate is considered in detail in Chapter 26.

Pitfalls

1. Do not mistake air in the kidney or bladder for calculi. Air lies in the most nondependent aspect of the organ being examined even when the patient's position is changed.
2. Do not mistake blood clot for tumor within the bladder. Changing the patient's position usually alters the blood clot configuration and position but does not change tumor appearances. Blood clot should not have detectable flow within it, whereas tumor may show vessels at color Doppler imaging.
3. Renal calculi versus arterial calcification. In older patients, arterial calcification in the renal sinus is common. Areas of arterial calcification may resemble multiple small calculi in the renal sinus (an unusual site for true small calculi). Calcification may occur in the two walls of an artery and a "tramline" (double) calcification will occur, typical of arterial calcification. It may be impossible to decide whether there is a small calculus or a small arterial calcification if the tramline sign is not seen, but it is worth watching for pulsations in the vessel on a magnified real-time image. In general, tiny calculi not associated with obstruction are clinically irrelevant anyway.
4. When searching for and demonstrating stones, it is best not to use the spatial compound imaging feature available on many newer ultrasound systems. This software option may minimize posterior acoustic shadowing, which is an important artifact when searching for stones.
5. Do not mistake a pelvic fluid collection for a normal bladder. For example, a large cystic ovarian cancer may be mistaken for a normal urinary bladder if the bladder happens to be empty. Look for the echogenic wall line and the ureteric buds on the posterior wall of the bladder. When in doubt, have the patient void and observe for the expected change in size of the bladder.

Where Else to Look

1. If the prostate is found to be enlarged or a mass is found in the bladder, examine the kidneys to be certain there is no secondary hydronephrosis.
2. If a renal calculus is seen, evaluate the bladder for calculi, debris, and wall thickening.
3. If a bladder calculus or tumor is found, look in the kidney for additional calculi or tumor.
4. If an irregular bladder wall is found, look in the patient's chart for a history of infections before dictating a list of differentials.

SELECTED READING

Burge HJ, Middleton WD, McClennan BL, et al. Ureteral jets in healthy subjects and in patients with unilateral ureteral calculi: comparison with color Doppler US. *Radiology* 1991;180:437–442.

Haddad MC, Sharif HS, Shahed MS, et al. Renal colic: diagnosis and outcome. *Radiology* 1992;184:83–88.

Laing FC, Benson CB, DiSalvo DN, et al. Distal ureteral calculi: detection with vaginal US. *Radiology* 1994;192:545–548.

Lee JY, Kim SH, Cho JY, et al. Color and power Doppler twinkling artifacts from urinary stones: clinical observations and phantom studies. *AJR Am J Roentgenol* 2001;176:1441–1445.

Vrtiska TJ, Hattery RR, King BF, et al. Role of ultrasound in medical management of patients with renal stone disease. *Urol Radiol* 1992;114:131–138.

Yoon DY, Bae SH, Choi CS. Transrectal ultrasonography of distal ureteral calculi: comparison with intravenous urography. *J Ultrasound Med* 2000;19:271–275.

Rule Out Pleural Effusion and Chest Mass

21

MIKE LEDWIDGE
TOM WINTER

SONOGRAM ABBREVIATIONS

Ao	Aorta
D	Diaphragm
K	Kidney
L	Liver
S	Spine
Sp	Spleen

KEY WORDS

Atelectasis (Collapsed Lung). Collapse of part of the lung due to volume loss; atelectasis is caused by either extrinsic compression (pneumothorax or pleural effusion) or intrinsic obstruction of a central bronchus.

Consolidation. An infected segment of the lung filled mainly with fluid instead of air.

Empyema. Pus in the pleural cavity.

Hemothorax. Blood in the pleural cavity.

Paradoxical Motion. Opposite from normal motion of the diaphragm. Specifically, downward motion of the diaphragm with expiration and upward motion on inspiration due to hemidiaphragm paralysis.

Pleura. A thin membrane that lines the thorax and diaphragm and surrounds the lungs. It has two layers:

> **Parietal (Costal) Pleura.** Extends from the inferior aspect of the lungs and covers the sides of the pericardium to the chest wall and backward to the spine. The outer layer of the pleura.
>
> **Visceral Pleura.** Lines the lungs and the interlobar fissures; it is loose at the borders to allow for lung expansion. The inner layer of the pleura.

Pleural Cavity. The space between the two layers of the pleura, where pleural fluid accumulates.

Pleural Fibrosis. Fibrous tissue thickening the pleura; results from chronic inflammatory diseases of the lungs such as tuberculosis.

Pneumothorax. Air within the pleural cavity outside the lung—a possible complication of thoracentesis. Hydropneumothorax implies both fluid and air within the pleural space.

Subpulmonic. Inferior to the lungs, above the diaphragm.

Thoracentesis. Puncture of the chest to obtain pleural fluid.

The Clinical Problem

Because of the air in the lungs, chest sonography is limited to assessing pathology adjacent to the pleura. Fluid accumulates in the pleural space as a reaction to underlying pulmonary or upper abdominal disease, or as a consequence of systemic disease such as heart failure. Effusions are usually detected by chest radiography. Fluid that is free follows gravity and falls to the base of the chest; however, loculated fluid, which is the result of adhesions or malignancy, does not layer on chest radiograph. The distinction is easily made using ultrasound, providing the pocket lies adjacent to the ribs.

Obtaining a fluid sample can be important for diagnostic purposes or may be a palliative measure to alleviate shortness of breath. Clinicians customarily localize for thoracentesis in the patient's room by percussing the chest ("thumping" with their fingers) and listening for dullness. In obese or muscular patients, clinical localization may fail. In cases like these, ultrasound is helpful in guiding thoracentesis. Ultrasound is also helpful in determining the nature of an opaque hemithorax on the chest radiograph. Such an opacification may indicate tumor, fluid, collapsed lung, or a combination of these entities.

Diaphragmatic movement can be detected by ultrasound. This demonstration is especially helpful in ruling out paradoxical motion due to diaphragmatic paralysis.

Ultrasound is being used more and more, particularly in trauma settings, as a rapid, easily obtained tool to diagnose pneumothorax.

Anatomy

NORMAL CHEST

When no fluid or mass is present, the tissues within the chest do not conduct sound. There are alternating bands of echogenicity due to reverberations from air and the rounded, bright reflectors seen due to the bone. Between the skin and ribs are subcutaneous fat and muscles; the soft tissue between ribs is mostly muscle. Because the intercostal vessels lie under the lower lip of each rib, they are poorly seen; however, remember their location when deciding on needle placement. All thoracentesis needle placements should be just on top of the rib to avoid these vessels.

The pleural space is that potential space between the parietal and the visceral pleura, which normally contains only a few millimeters of a lubricating secretion. The surface of the lung can be seen moving up and down with respiration, and the ventilated lung produces a reverberation artifact in the intercostal spaces (Figs. 21-1 and 21-2).

DIAPHRAGM

The diaphragm is seen as an echogenic, curved line above the liver and spleen. The diaphragm can be difficult to demonstrate, especially on the left, because it lies along virtually the same axis as the ultrasonic beam. The spleen provides less of a window to angle through than does the liver.

Technique

For masses or loculated effusions, position the patient so the pathology site is easily accessible and so he or she is comfortable enough not to move during the procedure.

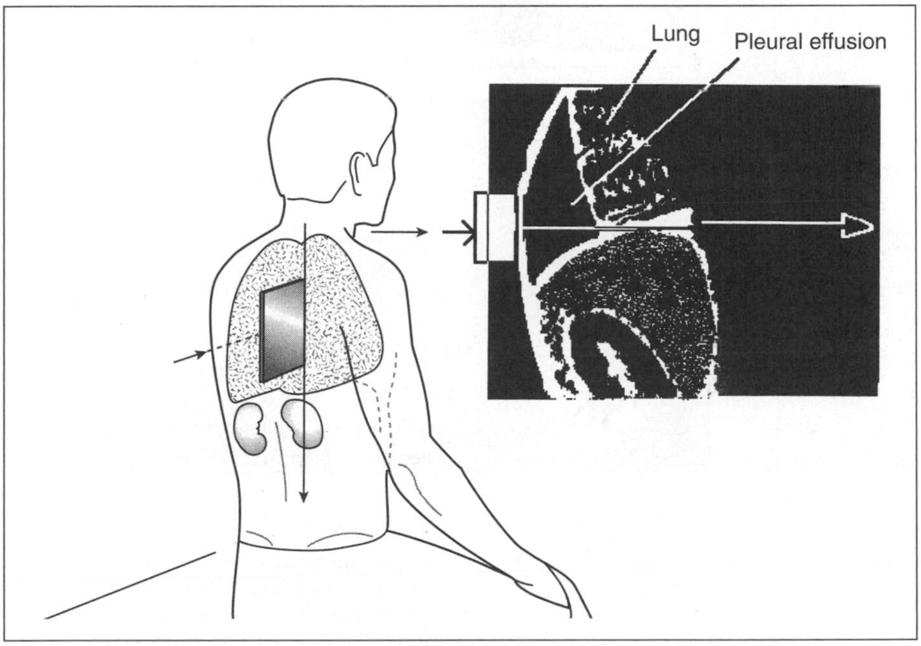

Figure 21-1. ■ *Usual position used when scanning a pleural effusion. The ultrasonic appearance of a pleural effusion and lung* (inset). *Note the alternating pattern of reverberations from the air and absent transmission from bone in the lung area.*

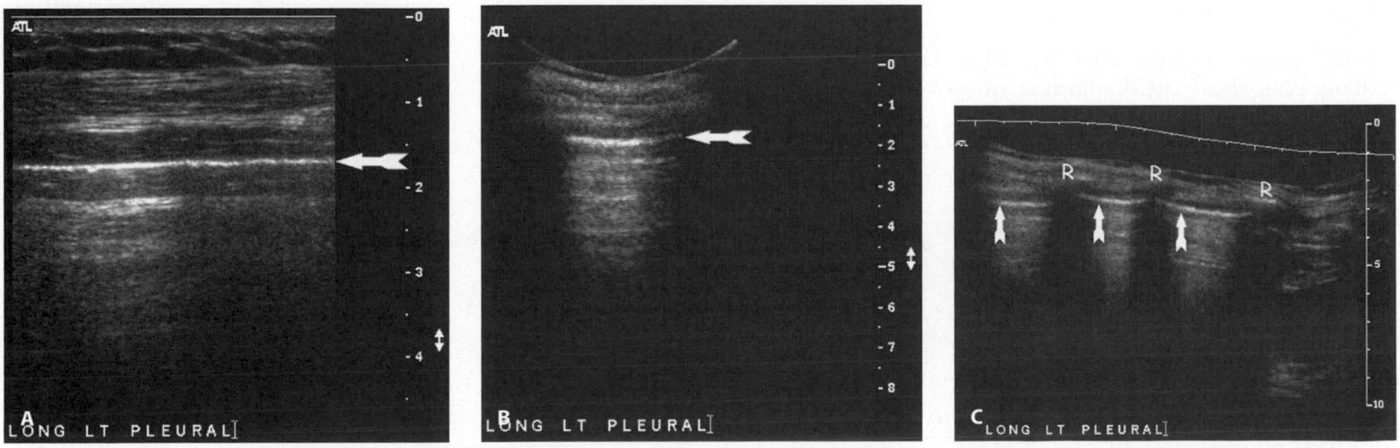

Figure 21-2. ■ *Longitudinal sonogram of the chest wall in a healthy patient without pneumothorax. Note ribs* (R) *with posterior acoustic shadowing, and reverberation artifact found in normal lung. A. Linear transducer for best resolution. B. Curved linear transducer. C. Extended field-of-view technology with linear transducer showing several interspaces. Pleural margin* (arrow).

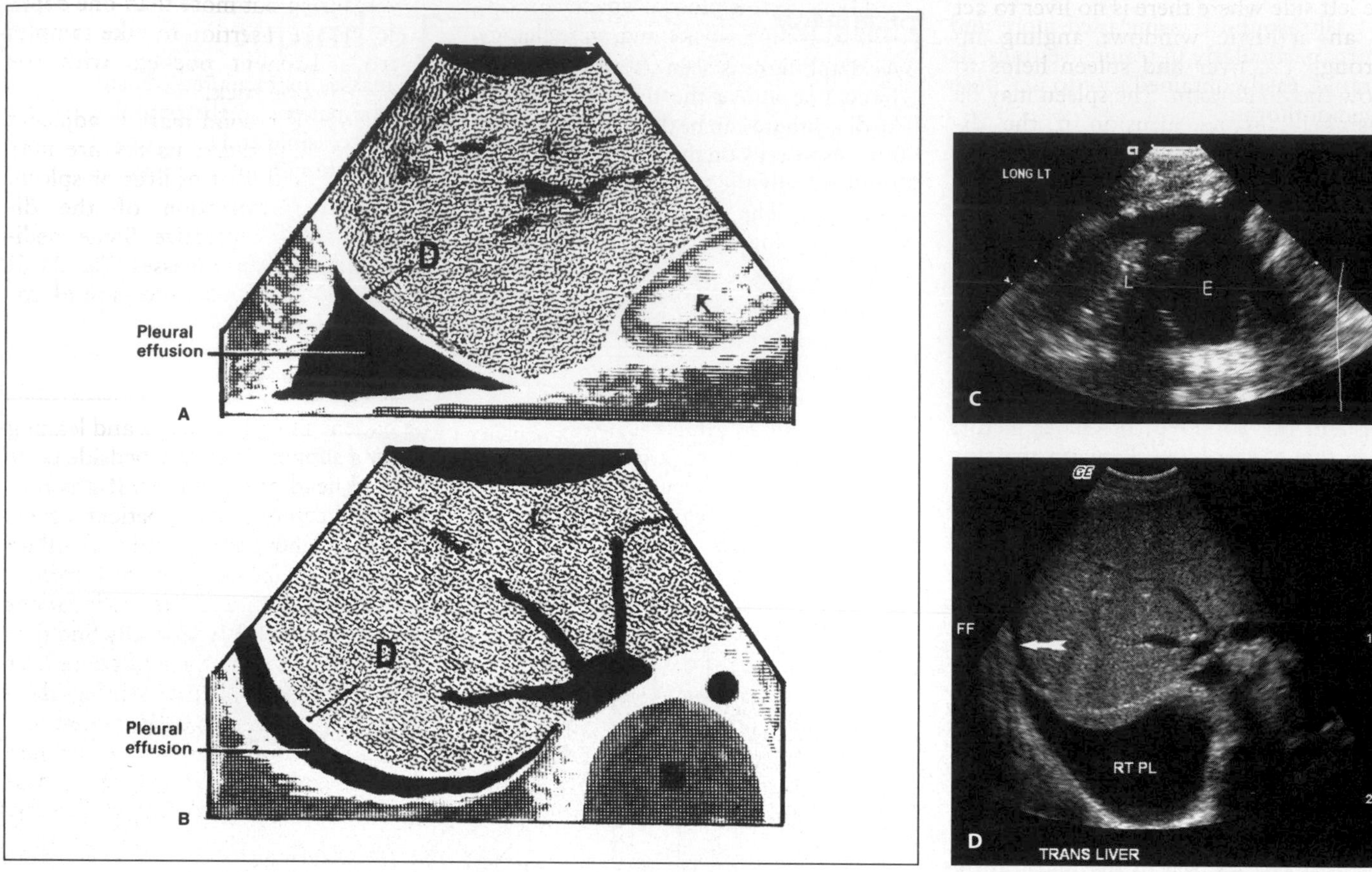

Figure 21-3. ■ *Diaphragmatic representation of a pleural effusion above the diaphragm* (D) *on a supine longitudinal view (A) and supine transverse view (B). Note that the fluid extends to the spine on transverse views. Longitudinal sonogram (C) showing left-sided pleural effusion* (E) *in a premature neonate who was born with a complex cardiac defect. L, collapsed lung surrounded by the pleural fluid. Transverse sonogram (D) through the base of the right lung showing an anechoic (simple) right pleural effusion ("RT PL") above the hemidiaphragm and a tiny amount of ascites* (arrow) *under the hemidiaphragm.*

PLEURAL EFFUSION

Pleural effusions (Figs. 21-1 and 21-3) usually pool above the diaphragm along the posterior chest wall. It is sometimes necessary to scan along the axillary line to check for fluid laterally. Loculated effusions can be found in any location (Fig. 21-4). Plan the search by examining the chest radiograph or computed tomography (CT).

The patient is scanned upright, sitting on a stool without a back, or a stretcher with his or her legs dangling from the sides, thus affording ready access from all sides (Fig. 21-1). For ill patients, it is helpful to have a sturdy table or stand in front of the patient to rest his or her chest on during the procedure. If looking in the posterior chest, one can better visualize the area behind the scapulae by having the patient cross his or her arms, rotating the scapulae outward. Scanning in the supraclavicular fossa will allow access to the superior sulcus to look for loculated effusions or apical tumors. Subpulmonic masses or empyema may be best seen by scanning from the abdomen.

A 3.5- to 5-MHz transducer is usually an appropriate frequency to display the chest wall and the distance to the lung. A curved, linear transducer with a wide footprint is best for the initial search, whereas changing to a smaller sector is helpful in evaluating deeper structures, where the near field is less important. For small collections, scanning with a linear transducer may be helpful in obtaining optimal visualization and localization.

The diaphragm should be shown well. This can be difficult, especially on

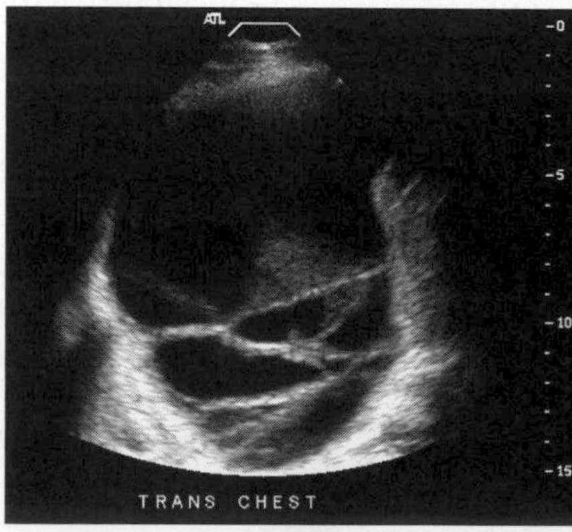

Figure 21-4. ■ *Ultrasound of a complex loculated pleural effusion, a postoperative infected hemothorax after removal of a malignant mesothelioma.*

the left side where there is no liver to act as an acoustic window; angling up through the liver and spleen helps to show the diaphragm. The spleen may be mistaken for an effusion if the diaphragm is not demonstrated, so find the upper pole of the left kidney if necessary to localize the spleen and diaphragm.

SUPINE VIEWS

Right-sided pleural effusions can be easily assessed on a supine view looking through the diaphragm and liver (Fig. 21-3). Effusions on the left are more difficult to see in the supine position but can sometimes be seen with an oblique scan through the spleen.

THORACENTESIS (PLEURAL EFFUSION ASPIRATION) OR CHEST MASS ASPIRATION

Obtaining fluid by percutaneous puncture may be necessary either to determine the nature of the fluid or as a therapeutic maneuver to relieve shortness of breath. Large pleural effusions may be tapped without imaging guidance. A site is chosen after percussing the chest and listening for dullness. A short needle is routinely used.

Thoracentesis without ultrasonic guidance has potential pitfalls. The effusion may be in a location different from the one that was percussed or may not be present at all. In an obese or muscular patient, a deeper penetration than is possible by a short needle is often required. If a tap is unsuccessful when attempted "blindly," the patient is often referred to ultrasound so that the puncture can be attempted again with the aid of ultrasound.

INITIAL LOCALIZATION OF PATHOLOGY

Look at the most recent chest radiograph or CT to see whether the fluid is mobile or loculated. If the fluid is free-flowing, a blunted costophrenic angle on chest x-ray film means there are at least 200 mL of fluid present. If it is loculated, a CT scan may be better for characterizing the position of the loculations. Often ultrasound alone may be all that is necessary, but sometimes loculated fluid in a fissure (pseudotumor) is impossible to detect on ultrasound because it is obscured by air; however, this will be readily detectable on a chest x-ray (CXR) film or CT.

Fluid in the pleural space, as opposed to pleural thickening, will change shape with respiration. This can be characterized by a "flash" of color on color Doppler. Serous fluid may also exhibit thin septations that will float gently on respiration.

1. *Free-moving fluid.* Free-moving fluid will flow to a dependent site in the chest, just above the diaphragm, if the patient is upright, which is the preferred position for aspirating free collections. The best sites are usually along the posterior chest wall or in the axillary line. Look for the biggest pocket. Identify the diaphragm by finding the kidneys and moving superiorly.
2. *Loculated fluid.* A lateral chest radiograph or CT will help decide whether fluid is anterior or posterior. Scan the entire chest, including the anterior chest wall, before ruling out a loculated effusion. Collections in the left anterior chest may be cardiac in origin, such as pericardial effusions or pericardial cysts. If the loculation contains septa, consider measuring out more than one depth for needle insertion to take samples from different pockets with the same needle stick.
3. *Tumor.* If a solid mass is adjacent to the diaphragm, its texture may be similar to that of liver or spleen. Careful localization of the diaphragm is imperative. Some mediastinal or pleural masses (Fig. 21-5) are localized with ultrasound for core biopsy.

PATIENT POSITION

The patient should be sitting and leaning against a support such as a bedside table or raised head of a stretcher. If it is necessary to keep one of the patient's arms raised throughout the procedure, pull up the edge of the hospital gown to form a kind of sling that will keep the patient from getting tired. We generally find that sick patients tolerate the procedure best if they sit on the stretcher, their legs dangling off the side, and curl their chest forward to lean on a high stand placed just next to the stretcher. This position provides maximum comfort and stability,

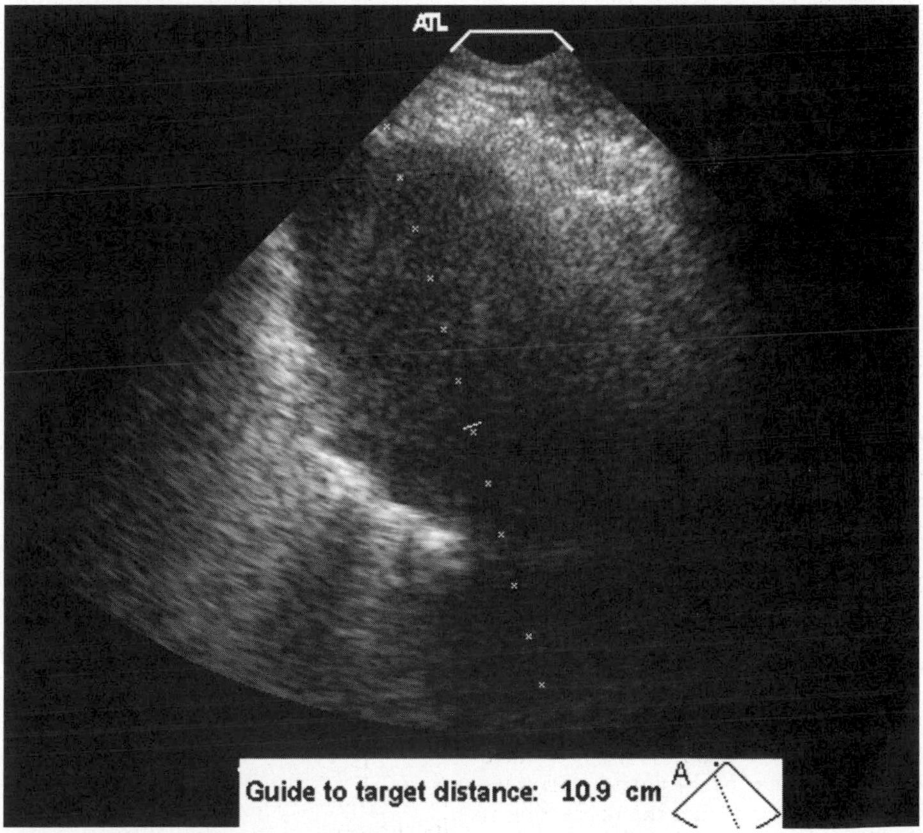

Figure 21-5. ■ *Ultrasound-guided biopsy of a pleural-based metastasis from non–small-cell lung cancer. Biopsy guide planned path* (dotted line) *of the core biopsy needle into this solid mass.*

and opens up the intercostal spaces between the ribs posteriorly, allowing for easier needle placement.

LOCALIZATION OF PATHOLOGY AND ASPIRATION

To visualize the pleura, use a transducer with a low enough frequency to penetrate the patient's chest wall and the pathology to visualize the pleura. Broad-bandwidth curved linear transducers generally do a very nice job. Although a linear array gives a "picket-fence" appearance from shadowing ribs that may obscure a small collection, it can be preferable to a small footprint transducer because its larger field of view makes diaphragmatic and pleural effusion movements easier to see, and more of the superficial tissues can be seen.

A small footprint transducer will fit well between the ribs, but the angle must be carefully calculated because the slightest angulation of the transducer throws the beam into an entirely different plane. Biopsy guides are more difficult to use in the chest than the abdomen because of rib interference. If a biopsy guide is used, line the transducer up with the curved axis of the rib interspace so that the needle entry site under the biopsy guide is in the same interspace as the beam from the transducer; if this is not done, one will often have a beautiful image of the effusion but the needle entry site will be over a rib.

The aspiration may be performed (1) "blindly" after localization and marking with ultrasound if the pocket is large or (2) alongside a sterilely draped transducer if the pocket is small.

1. Ensure patient comfort. Locally infused lidocaine and a calm, concerned manner are generally all that is necessary for most pleural fluid aspirations, but if a large tube is going to be placed and left in place, further medication, including formal moderate sedation, may be desirable.
2. Demonstrate the diaphragm. This is particularly important on the left side where the spleen can look cystic, and the upper pole of the left kidney can simulate a curved diaphragm in a large patient.
3. Watch respiration. If the pocket is small, watch on real-time imaging to see which phase of respiration best shows the effusion; have the patient practice holding his or her breath at that point so he or she can reproduce it for the needle insertion.
4. Know a safe depth of insertion. Use a needle stop if you like. This is especially important in the chest. If the needle enters too deeply, the lung may be pierced and pneumothorax may result. Use a 20-gauge needle in most patients for simple diagnostic aspirations. Even better may be commercially available kits, which include an 18-gauge sheathed needle, such as an Angiocath, to prevent laceration as the fluid is removed and the lung re-expands. Larger gauges may be necessary if the fluid is thick.
5. Prepare for laboratory tests. The most commonly ordered laboratory tests for pleural effusions require the following fluid containers: tubes, cytopathology tubes, heparinized tubes (if the tap is bloody), and an anaerobic culture bottle (one can use a sealed syringe instead). Check with your local laboratory personnel to determine their preference for containers to transport various samples; remember that the tubes required depend on what the clinical service is investigating, so plan ahead of time.
6. Use a one-way valve attached to a drainage bag for removal of large volumes of fluid. Alternatively, wall suction or vacuum bottles may be used. Remember to ensure that the needle or catheter in the patient's back is never opened to room air. In other words, never let room air be sucked into the patient's pleural space. This can cause a large pneumothorax. Generally, no more than 1,500 mL is removed at any one time to prevent the possible complication of reexpansion pulmonary edema. A postprocedure chest radiograph should be obtained to exclude pneumothorax. Although a CXR obtained in expiration is more sensitive to small volumes of pneumothorax, some cardiothoracic surgeons believe that the extra sensitivity of an expiration CXR is not warranted because a tiny pneumothorax that is only seen on an expiration CXR is not clinically relevant.

Pathology

PLEURAL EFFUSION

Pleural effusions (Figs. 21-1 and 21-3) are usually echo-free, wedge-shaped areas that lie along the posterolateral inferior aspect of the lung. Occasionally they contain internal echoes, sometimes indicating the presence of a neoplasm (malignant implants). Internal echoes may be due to blood or pus (empyema) (Fig. 21-4), especially when the collection is loculated. Loculated effusions do not necessarily lie adjacent to the diaphragm and may be located anywhere on the chest wall. Subpulmonic effusions lie between the lung and the diaphragm.

PLEURAL FIBROSIS

Pleural fibrosis can be confused with pleural fluid on a radiograph. There are some subtle sonographic differences between the two (Fig. 21-6):

1. A simple effusion is echo-free, whereas pleural fibrosis should contain low-level echoes.
2. Free fluid appears wedge-shaped as it fits between the lung base and the diaphragm (Figs. 21-1 and 21-3).
3. Pleural fluid changes shape when the patient breathes, and usually flashes on color; pleural fibrosis does not (see Pitfalls).
4. Pleural effusions taper sharply at the upper end, whereas pleural fibrosis tends to be the same width throughout (Fig. 21-6).
5. Fluid exhibits more through transmission than fibrosis, but this is difficult to assess; the air-filled lung forms a strong interface, whether it be fluid or fibrosis.

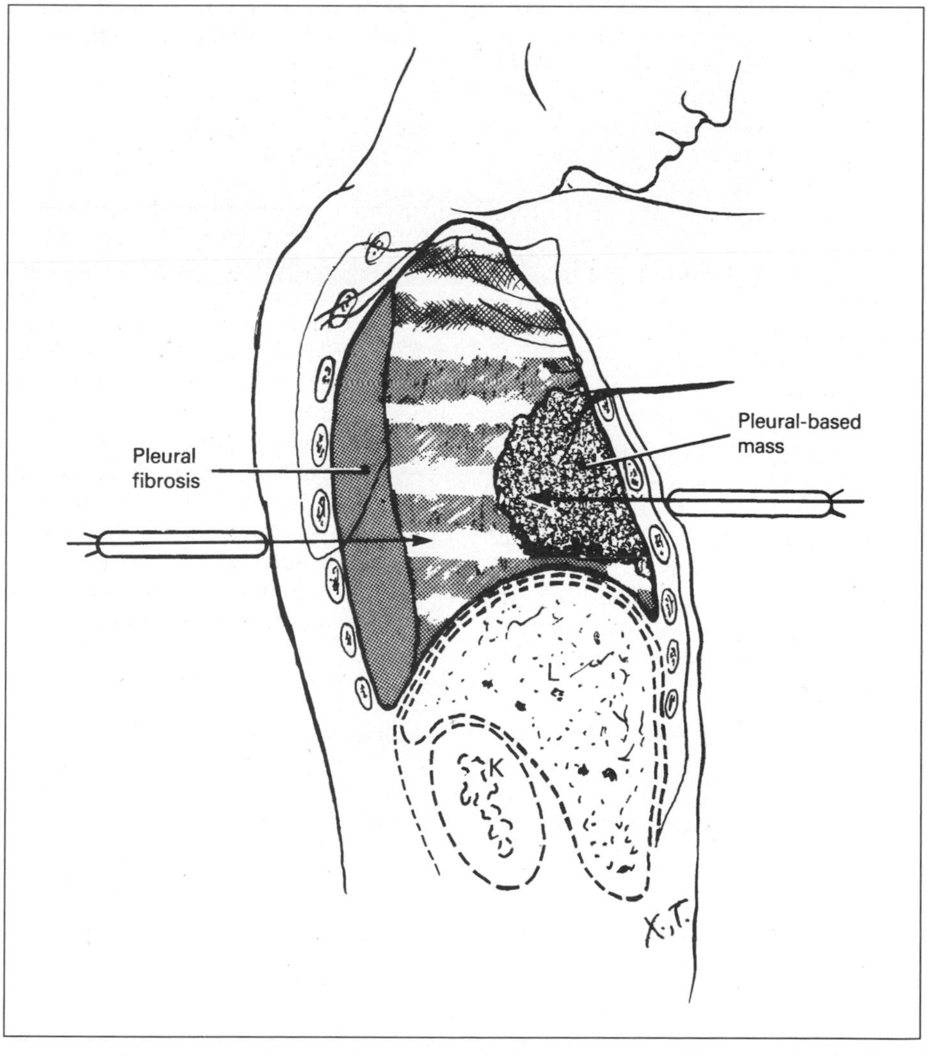

Figure 21-6. ■ *Usual shape of pleural fibrosis (posterior lesion). There will be some internal echoes. Pleural-based solid mass is shown on the anterior aspect of the chest.*

SOLID MASS

If a lesion seen on x-ray film or CT touches the pleura, ultrasound is a good place to continue the workup. If there are numerous internal echoes within a mass when compared with a known fluid-filled structure such as the heart, one can be fairly confident that the lesion is a mass (Fig. 21-5). Solid, homogeneous masses with few internal echoes are more difficult to distinguish from fluid because they simulate a cystic collection. They may have strong back walls and appear to have no echoes at low gain settings. Because the lung lies beyond the lesions and does not conduct sound, through transmission is not easy to evaluate. The presence of definite internal flow on Doppler imaging strongly suggests a solid mass. Mass analysis is greatly simplified if there is a coincidental pleural effusion. Peripheral tumors often obliterate the pleural parenchymal line as they spread into the chest wall.

PNEUMOTHORAX

Probably the most important observation for identifying a pneumothorax is the absence of the "gliding" or "sliding" lung. This refers to the bright hyperechoic line of the visceral pleura, which is attached to the lung and moves with it during respiration. The absence of lung sliding is greater than 90% accurate in diagnosing a pneumothorax. Also absent in pneumothorax is the normal reverberation artifact of aerated lung. Instead, there is only the bright, specular reflection of air in the pleural cavity, which does not move and produces what has been called a comet tail, ring-down, or free-air artifact. This artifact can be distinguished from the reverberation artifact found in normal lung by its greater brightness. In addition, the distance between the repeating bands of comet tail artifact is less than the distance between the skin-to-lung interface, whereas the distance between these repeating bands matches the distance of the skin-to-lung interface in the reverberation artifact of normally aerated lung. Although pneumothorax is usually a radiographic diagnosis, recognizing this appearance can be helpful when scanning a patient too ill to be moved from the intensive care unit, when using ultrasound as an adjunct to an invasive procedure that could result in a pneumothorax, or in the trauma setting.

CONSOLIDATION

A consolidated lung contains a lot of fluid and may conduct sound, even though there will be a number of internal echoes with a radiating linear pattern due to small pockets of air in bronchi. The appearance of consolidated lung can be similar to that of liver or spleen. Coincident pleural effusion is often present and makes the diagnosis much more simple.

PASSIVE ATELECTASIS

If pleural effusion is present, a wedge-shaped mass is seen. An increase in the size of the mass on inspiration may be seen if bronchial obstruction is incomplete. With complete lung collapse, no change with inspiration will be seen and there will be no echogenic air bronchogram pattern within the mass. Tubular vascular structures will be seen with color flow with both veins and arteries visible.

DIAPHRAGMATIC PARALYSIS

Assessment of diaphragmatic motion is helpful in a variety of clinical scenarios. Although this evaluation has traditionally been done using fluoroscopy, ultrasound is readily available, uses no radiation, and can easily be performed bedside. Ultrasound can document paradoxical, diminished, or normal mobility. Compare the degree and direction of movement with that on the contralateral side.

Pitfalls

1. Reverberation versus effusion. At times there may be doubt about whether an "effusion" is real on decubitus or supine views, or just a mirror artifact (Fig. 21-7 and Color Plate 21-1; see also Chapter 57). Place the patient in a sitting position when scanning for fluid to change the angle of the transducer to the area in question and eliminate this artifact.
2. Spleen versus effusion. The spleen may be mistaken for an effusion in a large patient if the position of the kidney in relation to the spleen is not documented and the diaphragm is not seen adequately.
3. Mass versus effusion. A solid mass may be mistaken for a loculated effusion if the contents of the mass are particularly homogeneous. Watch for the fluid to change shape on respiration. Usually soft tissue masses adjacent to the pleura do contain internal echoes. Use Doppler to look for internal flow.
4. Consolidation versus liver or spleen. Consolidation can be confused with

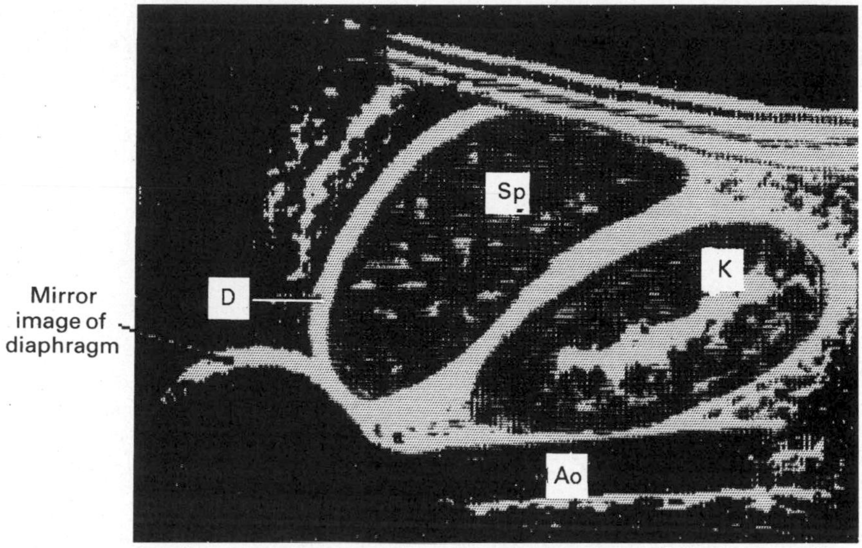

Figure 21-7. ■ *Diagram of mirror artifact of the diaphragm above the spleen. This artifact is seen when the patient is scanned from an oblique axis through the spleen. See Color Plate 21-1.*

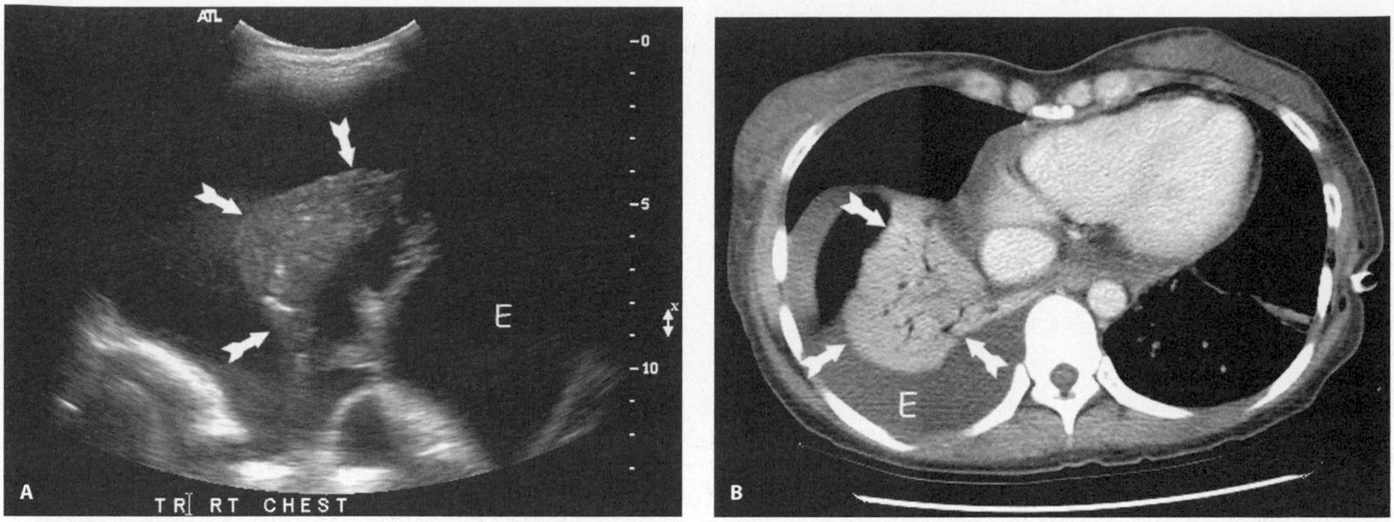

Figure 21-8. ■ *Ultrasound (A) and computed tomography* (CT) *(B) of consolidated lung* (arrows) *surrounded by pleural effusion* (E). *Note how consolidated lung on the ultrasound might be easily mistaken for liver or spleen in the absence of the surrounding pleural fluid.*

liver or spleen (Fig. 21-8). In consolidation, there will be a linear pattern to the bronchi with small pockets of air; just make sure the area of concern is superior to the diaphragm.

5. False-positive fluid color sign. It is possible to have color signals appear in areas adjacent to an anechoic fluid collection, or even potentially in hypoechoic pleural thickening, if the color gain is set inappropriately high or the wall filter is set inappropriately low.

SELECTED READING

Chan SS, McGahan JP, Richards J, et al. The comet tail artifact in the diagnosis of pneumothorax. *J Ultrasound Med* 2002;21: 1060; author reply 1060–1062.

Civardi G, Fornari F, Cavanna L, et al. Vascular signals from pleura-based lung lesions studied with pulsed Doppler ultrasonography. *J Clin Ultrasound* 1993;21:617–622.

Dodd GD III, Esola CC, Memel DS, et al. Sonography: the undiscovered jewel of interventional radiology. *Radiographics* 1996;16:1271–1288.

Dulchavsky SA, Schwarz KL, Kirkpatrick AW, et al. Prospective evaluation of thoracic ultrasound in the detection of pneumothorax. *J Trauma* 2001;50:201–205.

Ferrari FS, Cozza S, Guazzi G, et al. Ultrasound evaluation of chest opacities. *Ultrasound Int* 1995;1:68–74.

Kantarci F, Mihmanli I, Demirel MK, et al. Normal diaphragmatic motion and the effects of body composition: determination with M-mode sonography. *J Ultrasound Med* 2004;23:255–260.

Lomas DJ, Padley SG, Flower CDR. The sonographic appearances of pleural fluid. *Br J Radiol* 1993;66:619–624.

Targhetta R, Chavagneux R, Bourgeois JM, et al. Sonographic approach to diagnosing pulmonary consolidation. *J Ultrasound Med* 1992;11:667–672.

Wu RG, Yang PC, Kuo SH, et al. "Fluid color" sign: a useful indicator for discrimination between pleural thickening and pleural effusion. *J Ultrasound Med* 1995;14:767–769.

Yang PC. Ultrasound guided transthoracic biopsy of the chest. *Radiol Clin North Am* 2000;38:323–343.

Transplants: Renal, Liver, Pancreatic

CAROL MITCHELL
TOM WINTER

22

Renal Transplants

SONOGRAM ABBREVIATIONS

Bl	Bladder
D	Diastole
K	Kidney
R	Reversed flow
S	Systole

KEY WORDS

Acute Tubular Necrosis (ATN). Acute renal shutdown, usually due to abrupt decrease of blood pressure.

Anuria. Total absence of urine production.

Creatinine. A waste product excreted in the urine. Elevated values may indicate that the patient is in renal failure.

Cyclosporine. Drug given to transplant recipients to prevent rejection; may cause a clinical picture resembling rejection.

Iliac Fossa. Area on either side of the lower part of the abdomen. Usual location of a transplanted kidney.

Immunosuppression. Suppression of host's immunologic defenses.

Infarct. Dead tissue due to lack of blood supply.

Ischemia. Decrease in blood supply. Prolonged ischemia may result in an infarct.

Lymphocele. A collection of lymphatic fluid. Usually a postoperative complication.

Oliguria. Decreased urine production.

Rejection. Reaction of the body's immune system to the presence of a foreign kidney.

Steroids. Drugs similar to the hormones produced by the adrenal glands. Steroids lead to a suppression of the immunologic response.

Urinoma. A collection of extravasated urine, usually a postoperative or ischemic complication.

RELEVANT LABORATORY VALUES

Creatinine (serum): Normal is less than 1.5 mg/dL.

Urine output: Less than 200 mL in adults (<15–20 mL/kg in children) per 24 hours is abnormally low.

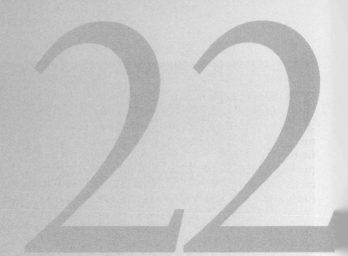

The Clinical Problem

Renal transplantation has been performed since the 1950s and has become the usual long-term treatment for end-stage chronic renal failure. In the last few years, results have improved considerably with the development of effective immunosuppressive medication and better tissue typing, decreasing the risk of rejection. Often these patients will present with symptoms of worsening renal failure. It is helpful to obtain as much clinical history from the patient before starting the ultrasound examination. Obtaining information such as date of transplant, location of transplant, type of transplant, and relevant laboratory value information can help the sonographer and sonologist to tailor the ultrasound examination to answer the clinical question.

Indications for renal transplant ultrasound include worsening renal failure, decreased urine output, elevated serum creatinine, suspected rejection, fever, bruit, flank pain, and fluid leaking from wound. The most common indication to examine a renal transplant is worsening renal failure. Possible explanations include obstruction, rejection, acute tubular necrosis (ATN), and vascular problems such as infarct or venous thrombosis. Renal transplant rejection, the usual cause of fever and increasing serum creatinine levels, has a typical although far from diagnostic ultrasonic appearance. Hydronephrosis and vascular problems can be diagnosed by ultrasound. Computed tomography and nuclear medicine are other imaging modalities that may be used, but ultrasound is generally the most useful first test for most patients.

Another common clinical problem in a renal transplant recipient is postoperative fever, which may be due to an infected fluid collection. Types of collections are hematomas, lymphoceles, and urinomas. All of these collections are easily localized by ultrasound and can be drained or aspirated under ultrasound guidance. Because transplant recipients are immunosuppressed, serious infections may produce few warning signs and infection may spread rapidly.

Ultrasound is also a useful tool to guide renal biopsy. This procedure is usually done when there is difficulty in distinguishing rejection, ATN, and cyclosporine toxicity.

The site for placement of a transplant kidney is determined by several factors, including presence of a previous transplant graft, asymmetry in peripheral vasculature, presence of polycystic kidney disease, and preference to perform the transplant in a fashion that does not require crossing of the renal artery and renal vein. This can be done by transplanting the kidney to the same side that it was removed from. However, if the internal iliac artery is used for the arterial anastomosis, the artery and vein do not cross when situated in the contralateral iliac fossa. The renal artery is attached to either the internal or the external iliac artery. The ureter is inserted into the bladder above the ureteral orifice through a submucosal tunnel in the bladder wall. This tunnel creates a valve in the distal end of the ureter to prevent reflux into the renal transplant. Because operative procedures and recipient shape and size vary, the transplanted kidney may have a large renal pelvis or an unusual axis. A baseline ultrasound scan after surgery is therefore sometimes worthwhile to document renal size, pelvicaliceal pattern, and any perirenal fluid collection. Other variations on the surgical procedure include pediatric en bloc transplants (paired kidneys and aorta donated from a young child, with the two kidneys compensating for the fact that the kidneys are smaller than usual) and transplanting two somewhat poorly functioning adult kidneys into an adult, one in each iliac fossa, to compensate for the decreased function of each kidney with an extra kidney.

Anatomy

The kidney parenchyma has two main components: the cortex, in which arteries, veins, convoluted tubules, and glomerular capsules are found; and the medulla, which contains the renal pyramids. These are conical masses with papillae projecting into cuplike cavities in the renal pelvis. The main renal artery is located at the hilum, the segmental artery lies adjacent to the medulla, the interlobar artery runs alongside the pyramids, and the arcuate arteries are found at the apex of the pyramids. The interlobular (or cortical) arteries carry blood from the apex of the pyramid to the cortex. The veins parallel the arteries. Arterial anatomy must be understood before undertaking Doppler investigation of the kidneys because this is a very important part of the renal transplant ul-

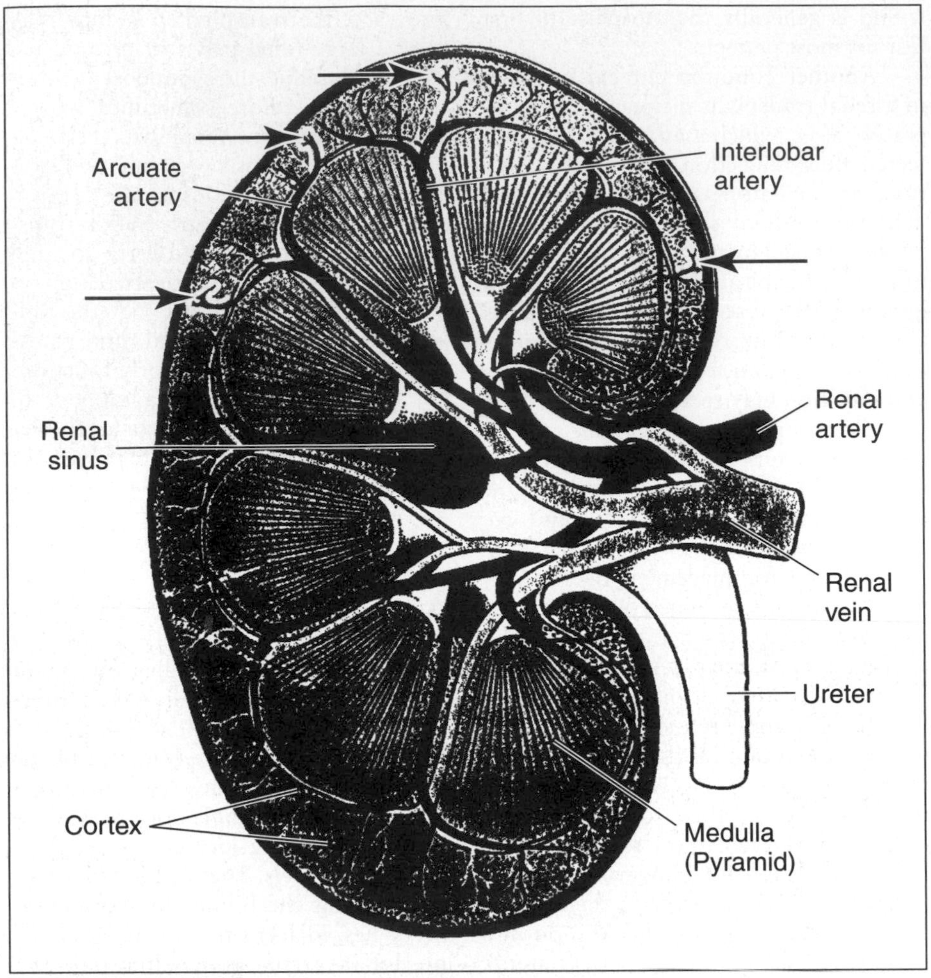

Figure 22-1. ■ *Details of renal arterial flow. Doppler is usually performed at the main renal artery, interlobar artery, and arcuate artery. Interlobular (cortical) arteries* (arrows without labels).

trasound examination (Fig. 22-1). In renal transplant recipients, often the kidney is placed in the right iliac fossa. In cases in which a pancreas is also transplanted or if this is a second renal transplant for the patient, the renal transplant may be located in the left iliac fossa.

Technique

Begin by selecting the transducer with the highest frequency that allows for adequate depth penetration. Most renal transplants can be imaged with a 5-MHz transducer. A curved linear transducer will provide a large field of view in the near zone, so that accurate length measurements may be made without cutting off part of the kidney on either end of the image. Newer developments such as extended field-of-view technology or sector width extension make it even easier to accurately measure large kidneys. Once the transducer has been selected, begin scanning along the long axis of the scar. The scar provides a landmark for beginning to look for the transplant kidney. The long axis of the kidney is usually oriented along the long axis of the scar and the transverse kidney images will sit at right angles to the scar (Fig. 22-2). The transplant kidney should be imaged from lateral to medial in the longitudinal plane, paying close attention to note any fluid collections. After the longitudinal survey of the kidney is completed, the kidney should be imaged in the transverse plane and surveyed from superior to inferior pole, again evaluating for any evidence of fluid collections while in the survey mode. Fluid collections may represent hematomas, abscesses, or lymphoceles. The kidney should be measured in both longitudinal and transverse planes (length, height, and width), because size increase is a potential sign of rejection (although in clinical practice this is generally not too useful). Also, while imaging the kidney the sonographer/sonologist should be evaluating the kidney's echogenicity (cortex, medulla, sinus), the shape of the kidney, and any evidence of urinary obstruction (i.e., dilated renal pelvis).

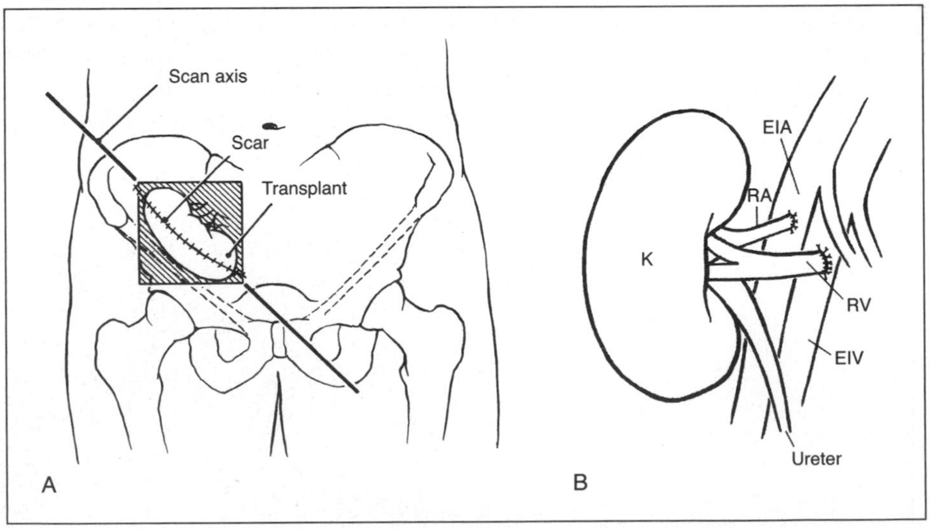

Figure 22-2. ■ *A. Usual placement site of the renal transplant. As a rule, the renal transplant is best shown by scans that are parallel to the scar. The transplant can be in either iliac fossa.* ***B.*** *One of the many types of vascular anastomoses.* (**B** from Jaques BC. Renal transplant surgery. In: *Ultrasound of abdominal transplantation.* Sidhu PS, Baxter GM, eds. New York: Thieme, 2002:24, Fig. 3-2.)

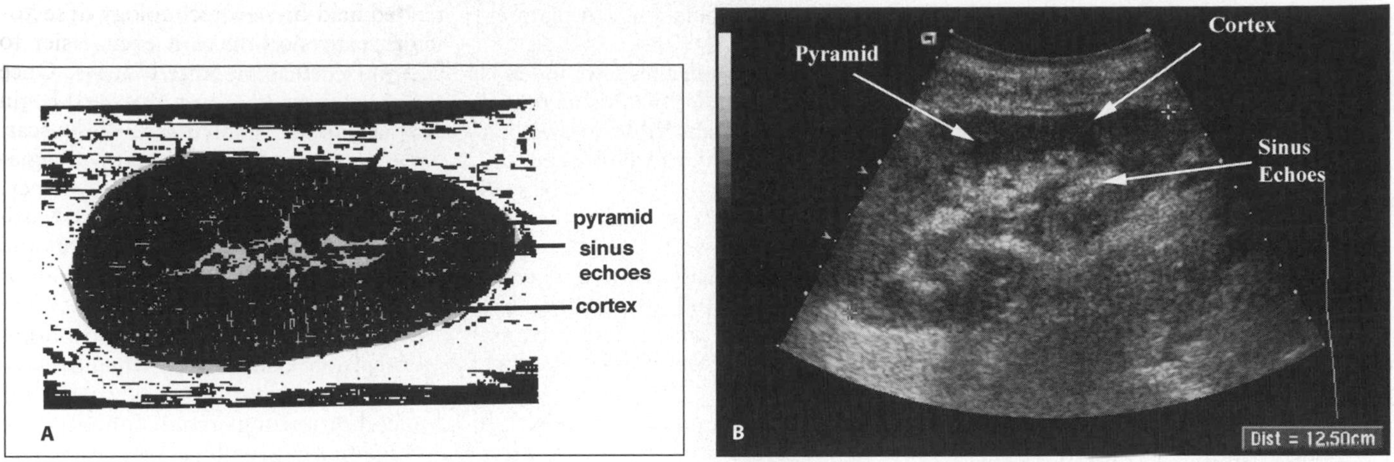

Figure 22-3. ■ *Ultrasound image of a transplant kidney showing the principle anatomic structures. A, diagram; B, sonogram.*

The urinary bladder should be scanned; if it is filled with urine and there is evidence of urinary obstruction in the kidney, the scan should be repeated with an empty bladder. Hydronephrosis, if present with a full bladder, may disappear with voiding. Doppler signals are obtained in the main renal vein and in the main, segmental, interlobar, and arcuate arteries (Figs. 22-1 to 22-4). The arcuate arteries are sampled in the upper pole, interpolar, and lower poles of the kidney. Color Doppler is helpful in determining the best position and angle in which to place the Doppler gate. Many machines offer a preset for "low flow" states. This setting is helpful to optimize the color Doppler imaging of the kidney. Once a spectral Doppler signal is obtained, the resistive index can be measured. The resistive index should be

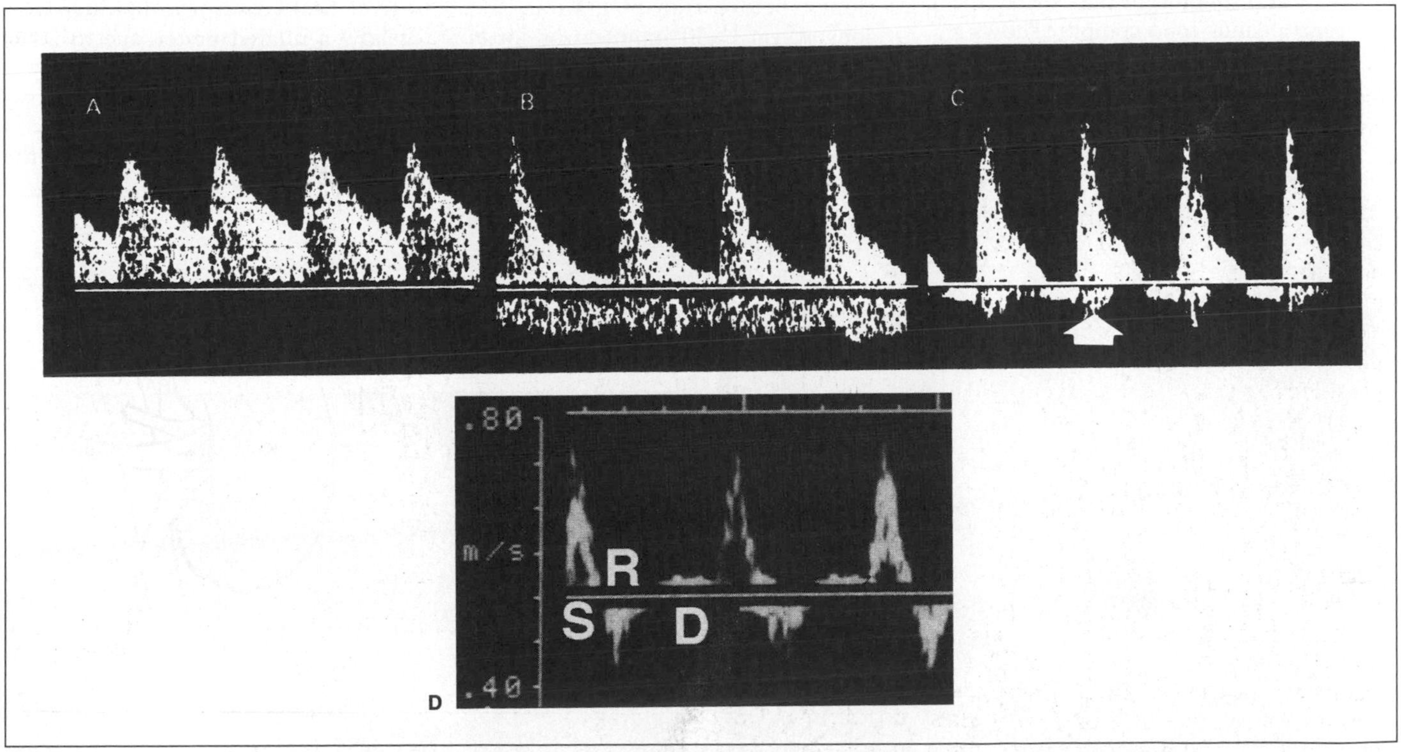

Figure 22-4. ■ *Renal artery Doppler flow pattern. A. Ultrasound image of a normal transplant kidney and main renal artery Doppler. B. Moderate rejection, little diastolic flow; venous flow also seen below the baseline. C. Severe rejection. Reversal of flow in diastole* (white arrow). *D. Normal iliac artery showing systolic phase* (S), *reversal phase* (R), *and diastolic phase* (D).

measured in the arcuate arteries and is calculated from the signal as follows:

$$\frac{\text{Peak Systolic Velocity} - \text{End Diastolic Velocity}}{\text{Peak Systolic Velocity}}$$

If the baseline scan is performed, the incision will be fresh and sterile technique should be used. See Chapter 55 for a discussion of how to scan with a gel-film skin barrier or how to cover the transducer.

POWER DOPPLER IMAGING

This technology is particularly helpful in the assessment of renal and pancreatic transplants. It is less dependent on beam angle and is free from aliasing. Perfusion of the transplant can be assessed so infarcts with no flow can be seen. Slower flow can be seen to enable investigation of the venous structures.

Pathology

1. Acute rejection. Acute rejection can occur hours or days after transplantation and has a typical sonographic appearance. The kidney is swollen and the pyramids are more prominent and sonolucent than usual; the central sinus echo complex shows a decrease in both size and echogenicity (referred to as loss of the cortical/medullary junction) (Fig. 22-5). Volumetric changes in renal size can be followed by using the following formula: length × width × height × 0.52 (the formula for a prolate ellipse).

   If the Doppler resistive index is greater than 0.75, there is increased vascular resistance due to swelling of the parenchyma. This generally means rejection but can also be seen with other processes that can cause tissue swelling, such as ATN and cyclosporine toxicity, as well as tense perinephric fluid collections, hydronephrosis, or excessive transducer pressure pushing on the kidney.
2. Chronic rejection. Chronic rejection develops months to years after transplantation as a consequence of repeated episodes of acute rejection. This disease results in vascular compromise of the transplant and decrease in renal function. In chronic rejection, the renal parenchyma becomes echogenic and the kidney decreases in size. The vascular resistive index increases. Eventually, the kidney fails.
3. Acute tubular necrosis (ATN). ATN is the most common complication in the first 48 hours after transplantation. Risk factors for ATN include cadaveric graft, hypotension in the donor before transplantation, or long warm (>30 minutes) or long cold (>24 hours) ischemic time periods. Clinically, ATN is difficult to diagnose because it mimics rejection. On ultrasound, the kidney may appear normal or enlarged (enlargement seen with severe disease). If edema is present, the cortex may appear hypoechoic with loss of the normal cortical/medullary interface. If the disease is severe, the renal sinus may appear small due to being compressed by the swollen cortex. With severe ATN, the Doppler resistive index may be greater than 0.75; however, clinically significant ATN may be associated with a normal resistive index as well.
4. Cyclosporine toxicity. Cyclosporine nephrotoxicity occurs when the levels of cyclosporine are elevated, thus compromising renal function. A sonogram usually shows no change in renal size or resistive indices, although resistive indices may be elevated.
5. Hydronephrosis. Obstruction can occur at any time, but commonly occurs in the first few weeks after surgery. There are similar symptoms to rejection. The sonographic characteristics of hydronephrosis (Fig. 22-6) are discussed in Chapter 18. Obstruction may be due to a fluid collection or a poor-quality ureteral anastomosis. A baseline comparison study is important because some pelvic dilatation may be postoperative. Scans over the bladder may show a dilated ureter due to kinking. If the bladder is full, empty it because apparent hydronephrosis may be caused by an overdistended bladder causing kinking of the ureter or reflux.

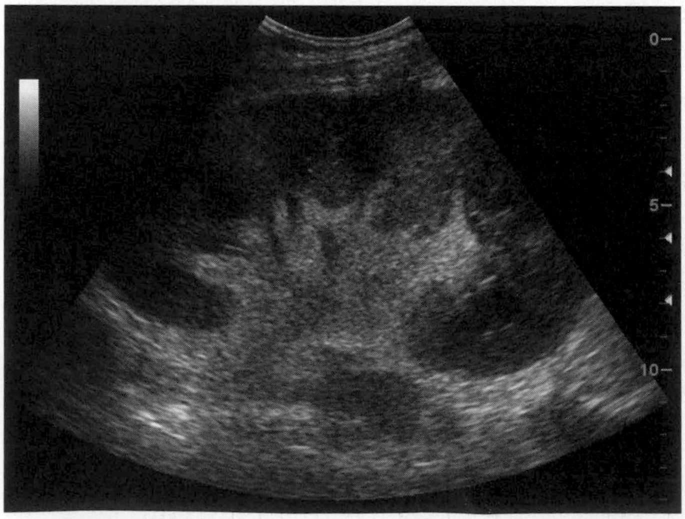

Figure 22-5. ■ *Swollen echogenic kidney associated with acute rejection.*

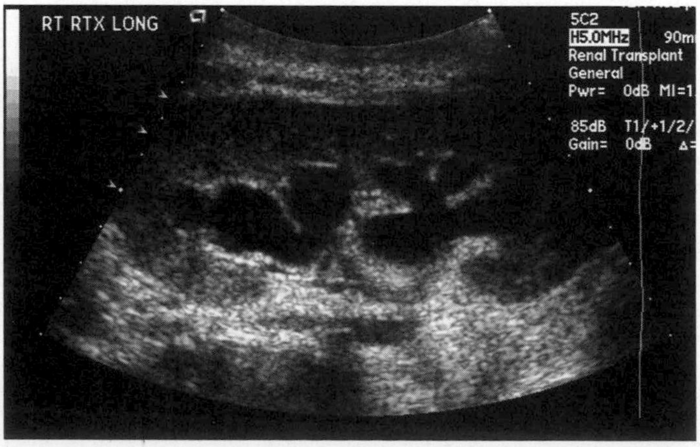

Figure 22-6. ■ *Transplant kidney demonstrating anechoic fluid-filled calyces as seen with hydronephrosis.*

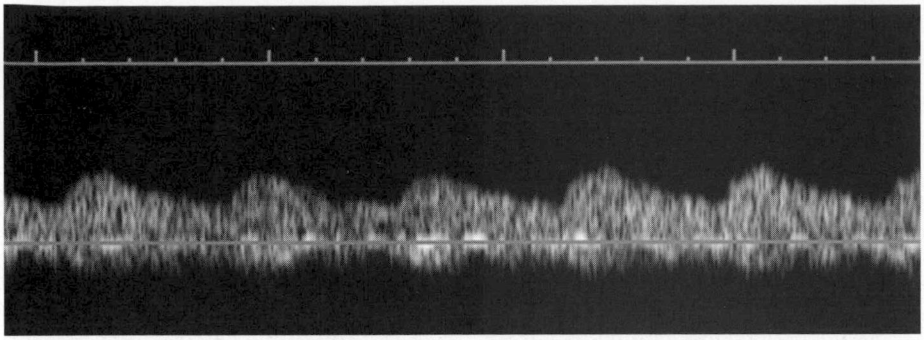

Figure 22-7. ■ *Tardus parvus signal in the arcuate artery distal to a stenosis.*

6. Vascular problems.
   a. Renal artery stenosis (RAS). RAS is the most common vascular complication and affects renal function. RAS usually occurs within 1 cm of the anastomosis; therefore, it is important to try and see the anastomosis site. This is done by locating the iliac artery and its communication to the main renal artery. The iliac artery will demonstrate a high-resistance Doppler signal (Fig. 22-4D). After the anastomosis site is located, scan the main renal artery thoroughly using both duplex and color Doppler. If the renal artery is stenosed, the Doppler signal will show increased velocity at the site of stenosis (Color Plate 22-1) and a slow increase in systole with delayed acceleration to peak velocity distal to the stenotic site (Fig. 22-7). This waveform is referred to as a tardus parvus waveform (see Renal Artery Stenosis in Chapter 18). Color Doppler may demonstrate aliasing at the site of narrowing, indicative of elevated velocities. After interrogating the main renal artery, sample the arcuate arteries. Obtain a sample in the upper pole, mid-kidney, and lower pole. Again, note any evidence for a tardus parvus waveform, possibly indicating a proximal stenosis.
   b. Renal artery thrombosis. Renal artery thrombosis is an unusual complication that sometimes happens in the early postoperative period. Patients often present with anuria and hypertension. Duplex and power Doppler show absent arterial and venous flow within the kidney or a portion of the kidney (an infarct). Angiography may be used to confirm the diagnosis.
   c. Renal vein thrombosis (RVT). RVT is a rare complication that usually occurs in the first week after surgery. RVT usually occurs due to extrinsic compression or kinking of the renal vein due to mobility of the graft. These patients usually present with oliguria or anuria and elevated creatinine in the early postoperative period. There will be an enlarged hypoechoic kidney. Both duplex and color Doppler show absent venous flow in the kidney and in the main renal vein and a high-resistance arterial flow with reversed diastolic flow (resistive index >1.00) (Fig. 22-8). If the thrombus is in only the peripheral veins, it will not be seen with ultrasound. Sometimes, the renal sinus echoes are more prominent than usual because of hemorrhage.
   d. Renal vein stenosis. Renal vein stenosis can be detected with ultrasound if it occurs in the main renal vein. In most cases, the kidney is enlarged and the renal sinus echoes are more prominent than usual. Doppler analysis reveals increased velocity—three to four times greater than that of the prestenotic vein. Color Doppler shows aliasing at the site of stenosis.
   e. Intrarenal arteriovenous (AV) fistulas. Both intrarenal AV fistulas and pseudoaneurysm complications result from biopsy. These are generally benign and usually resolve spontaneously. AV fistulas are easily detected with duplex and color Doppler. Color Doppler shows a localized region of disorganized color that extends outside the normal renal vessels (Color Plate 22-2). Doppler shows a high-velocity, turbulent mass with low resistant arterial and pulsatile venous flow within.

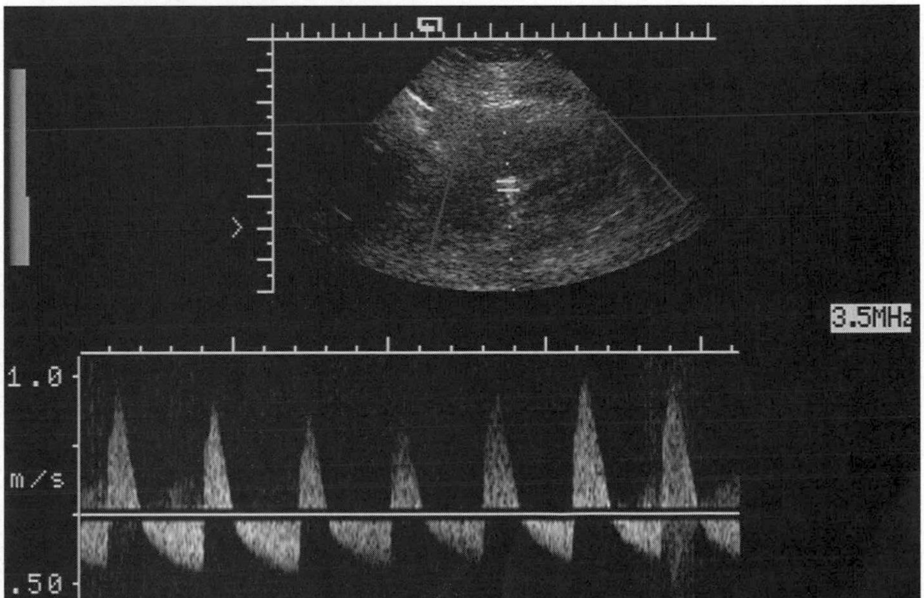

Figure 22-8. ■ *Classic reversed diastolic flow in the intrarenal arterial signal in a patient with renal vein thrombosis* (RVT).

f. Pseudoaneurysm. A pseudoaneurysm on grayscale looks like a complex or simple cyst; however, color interrogation of the structure demonstrates arterial flow within the cyst. Spectral Doppler will demonstrate to and fro flow in the neck and disturbed flow in the pseudoaneurysm.

g. Renal infarcts. These are usually focal but may involve all of the kidney. Fresh infarcts present as hypoechoic, wedge-shaped areas within the kidney. Power Doppler shows absent flow in the infarcted areas. Occasionally, there may be a focally echogenic area that relates to hemorrhage into the infarct. Eventually, the infarcts decrease in size and a scar develops at the infarct site.

7. Fever or local tenderness of renal transplant. Fever in the posttransplant period may be due to an abscess, hematoma, or, usually, rejection. Because such patients are treated with steroids, they are immunosuppressed, and local tenderness over a collection may be relatively trivial. Whenever hydronephrosis is found, a collection should be sought as its cause.

8. Fluid collections (Fig. 22-9).
   a. Hematomas commonly occur in the postoperative patient and are usually located either in the

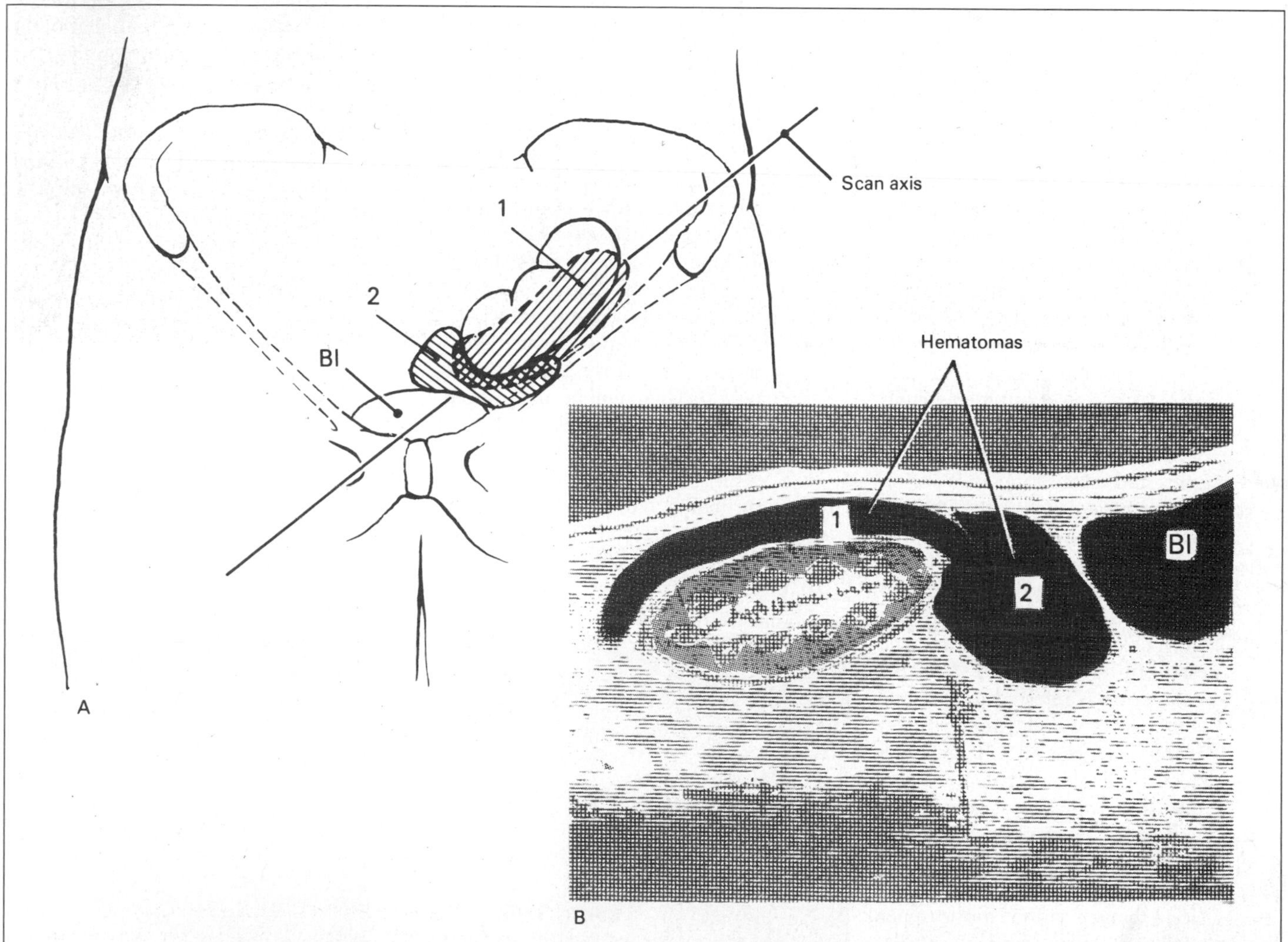

Figure 22-9. ■ *Collections, generally hematomas, are common with renal transplants. Collection 1 is in the usual site of hematoma accumulation. Collection 2 is in a site where urinomas or lymphoceles commonly occur. The axis along which the "sonogram" was performed is shown in (A).*

subcutaneous tissues or around the transplant. The sonographic characteristics vary with age; acute (Fig. 22-10A) or chronic hematomas are echogenic and typically hard to distinguish from neighboring structures, whereas intermediate ones (Fig. 22-10B) are complex. The borders are usually well defined. They are often aligned along the renal capsule. Some hematomas are fluid-filled and resemble a urinoma (Fig. 22-10C).

b. Abscesses are suspected when the patient presents with fever and increased white blood count. They can be found in any location and can vary sonographically from an echo-free to a complex echo pattern. They are difficult to distin-

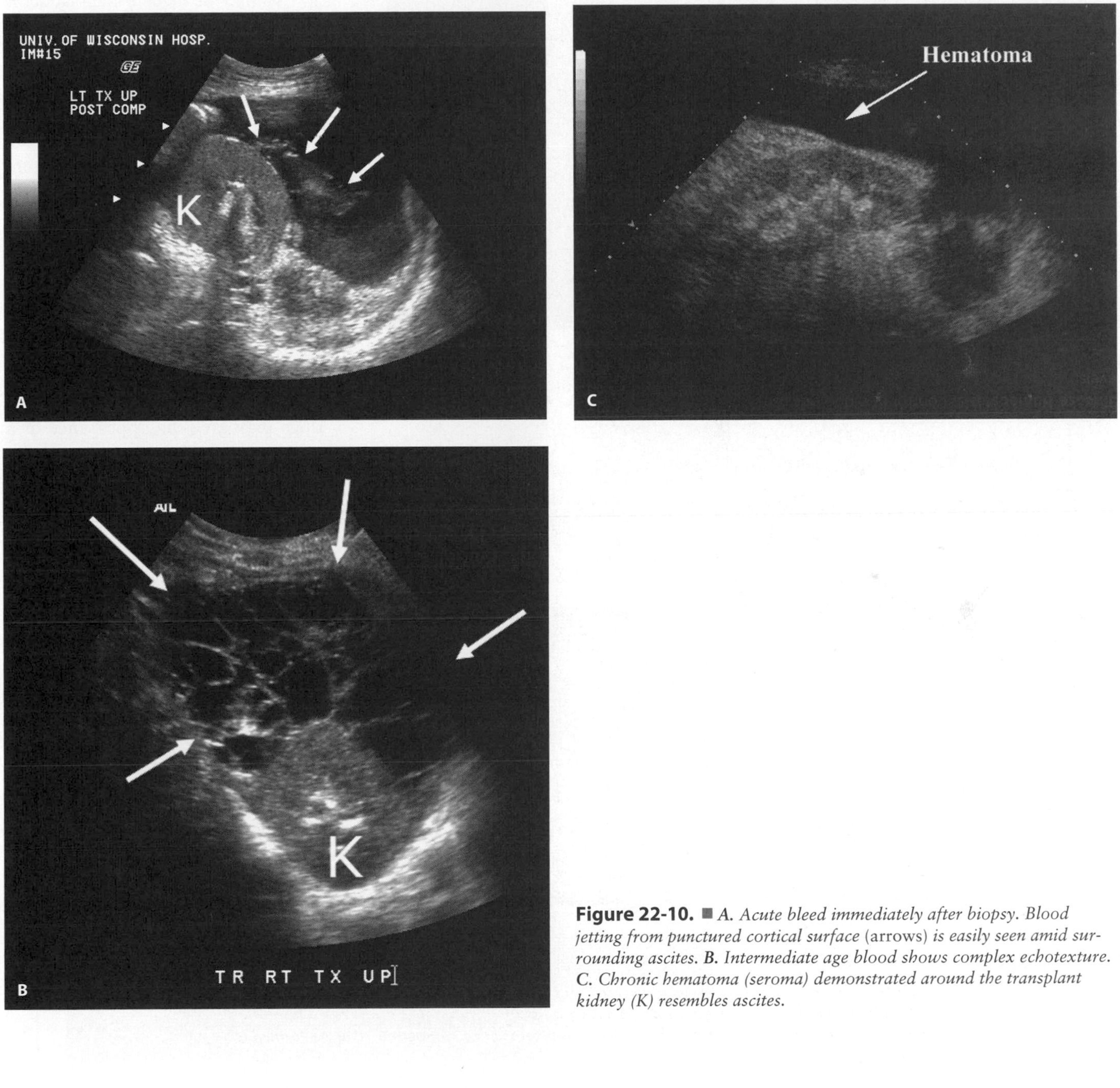

Figure 22-10. ■ *A. Acute bleed immediately after biopsy. Blood jetting from punctured cortical surface* (arrows) *is easily seen amid surrounding ascites. B. Intermediate age blood shows complex echotexture. C. Chronic hematoma (seroma) demonstrated around the transplant kidney (K) resembles ascites.*

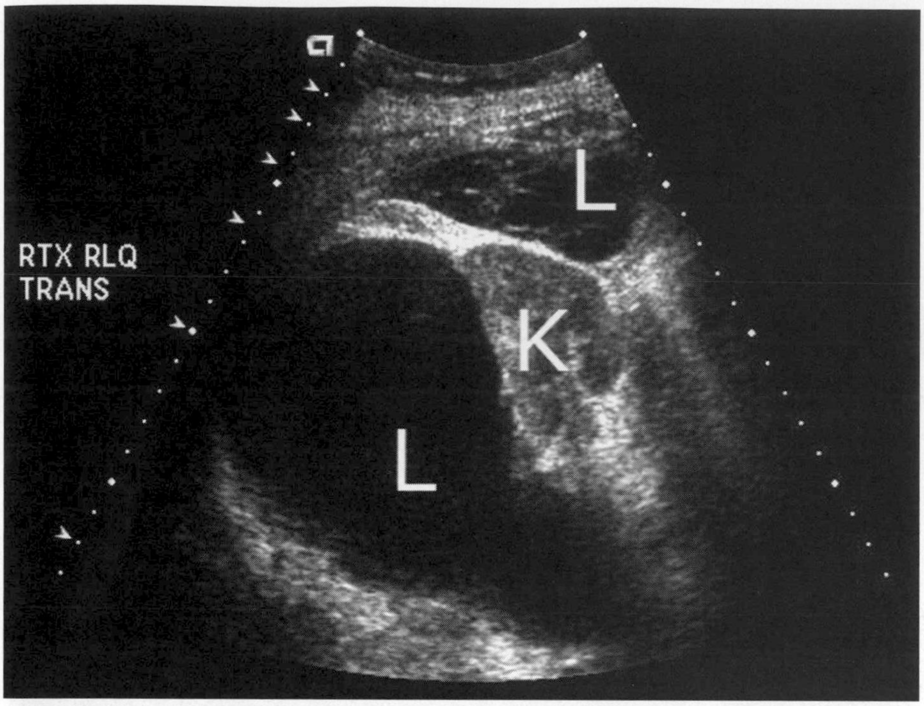

Figure 22-11. ■ *Two well-defined cystic masses, one of which is anechoic and the other of which is slightly complex, representing lymphoceles* (L) *surrounding the transplant kidney (K).*

guish from hematomas by their sonographic appearance.

c. Lymphoceles (Fig. 22-11) can occur after surgery, especially when there is a blockage or damage of the lymphatic channels. On ultrasound they are usually well-defined, anechoic cystic areas; a majority tend to have septations. Such collections are usually located between the bladder and the kidney. Hydronephrosis due to obstruction by the lymphocele may develop.

d. Urinoma is a serious complication, and it is most commonly caused by an ischemic or surgical problem at the ureteropelvic, ureteroureteral, or ureterovesical anastomosis. Patients usually present with a decrease in urine output, pain, and swelling around the transplant. This type of collection is usually echo-free. Its location is variable, although it is more commonly seen around the lower pole. As always in the presence of a fluid collection, a percutaneous aspiration can determine the cause of the collection. Urinomas, however, can be diagnosed by a nuclear medicine study in a noninvasive fashion.

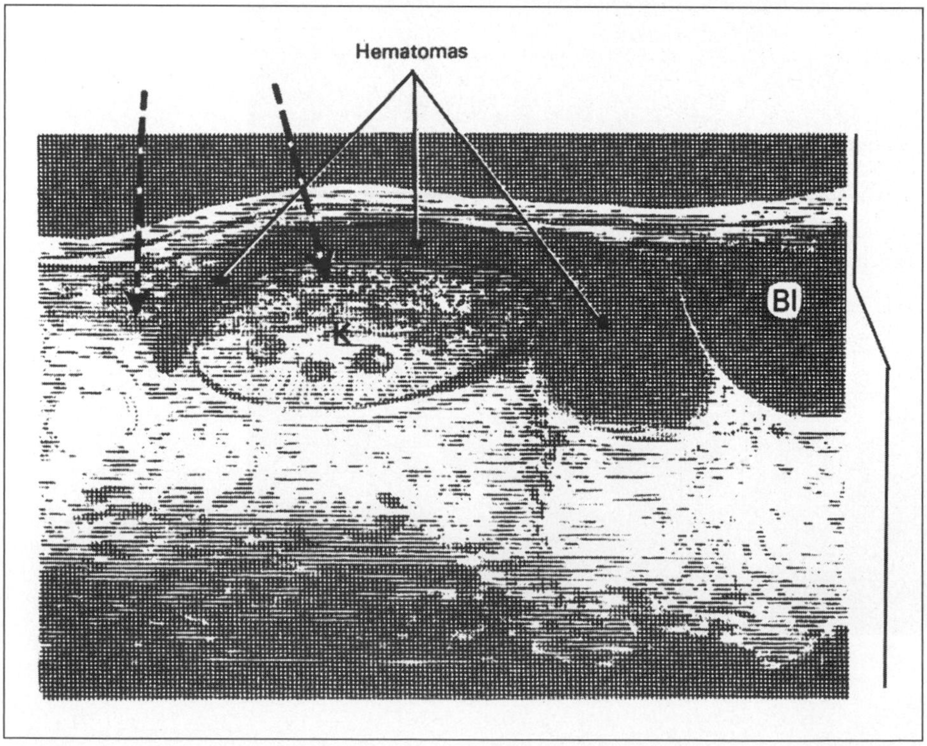

Figure 22-12. ■ *Unsatisfactory time-gain compensation* (TGC) *settings may prevent assessment of the anterior aspect of the kidney. This hematoma is hard to distinguish from the neighboring tissues because the TGC was too steep* (right). *TGC artifact is apparent* (broken arrows).

Pitfalls

1. Pseudohydronephrosis.
   a. Bladder overdistention. An erroneous diagnosis of hydronephrosis may be made if the bladder is full. Make sure that a postvoid view is obtained if hydronephrosis appears to be present. Sometimes the apparent hydronephrosis disappears when the bladder is empty.
   b. Baseline sinus distention. An incorrect diagnosis of hydronephrosis may be made if a baseline study has not been performed because many transplanted kidneys show some apparent renal pelvic fullness. Long-standing renal transplants often demonstrate a mildly dilated collecting system.
2. Time-gain compensation problems. Poor time-gain compensation settings may give the appearance of a

collection anterior to the kidney or even an anterior infarct if the time-gain compensation is too steep (Fig. 22-12).

3. Echogenic collections. Hematomas and abscesses may be missed unless their occasional high echogenicity is kept in mind. If bowel is around, look for peristalsis to differentiate fluid-filled bowel from an abscess or hematoma.
4. Bladder versus other fluid collection. Make sure that an apparent collection below the kidney is not the bladder; ask the patient to void or fill the bladder. Conversely, do not mistakenly attribute an abnormal fluid collection as the urinary bladder. Voiding or placement of a Foley catheter is helpful in this situation.
5. Iliac artery. Do not confuse the iliac artery with the main renal artery. The iliac artery will be outside the confines of the transplant kidney and will show a high-resistance flow pattern (Fig. 22-4D).
6. Sample gate angle. Be sure to set the sample gate at an angle less than 60 degrees to the vessel. Patterns suggestive of rejection may be seen if the sample gate is at a wrong angle (i.e., >60 degrees).
7. Because of surgical technique and body habitus, the transplant may be placed in a vertical position, which affects the pulsed and color Doppler signal. One may not be able to examine this type of transplant with ultrasound.

If a patient presents with fever of unknown origin and no collections are found around the transplanted kidney, look at the native kidneys or other areas where abscesses may develop (see Chapter 11). Intrahepatic or perihepatic abscesses may occur. Occasionally, transplant recipients develop pancreatitis due to steroid overadministration.

SELECTED READING

Bruno S, Ferrari SK, Remuzzi G, et al. Doppler ultrasonography in posttransplant renal artery stenosis: a reliable tool for assessing effectiveness of revascularization? *Transplantation* 2003;76(1):147–153.

Jacques BC. Renal transplant surgery. In: *Ultrasound of abdominal transplantation.* Sidhu PS, Baxter GM, eds. New York: Thieme; 2002:23–26.

Little AF, Dodd GD III. Postoperative sonographic evaluation of the hepatic and renal transplant patient. *Ultrasound Q* 1995;13: 111–119.

Pozinak MA. Doppler ultrasound evaluation of renal transplantation. In: *Clinical Doppler ultrasound.* London: Churchill Livingstone; 2000:191–201.

Patel U, Haw KK, Hughes NC. Doppler ultrasound for detection of renal transplant artery stenosis-threshold peak systolic velocity needs to be higher in a low-risk surveillance population. *Clin Radiol* 2003; 58(10):772–777.

Radermacher J, Mengel M, Ellis S, et al. The renal arterial resistance index and renal allograft survival. *N Engl J Med* 2003;349(2): 115–124.

Liver Transplants

SONOGRAM ABBREVIATIONS

CBD	Common bile duct
Ha	Hepatic artery
IVC	Inferior vena cava
Pv	Portal vein

KEY WORDS

Allograft. The newly transplanted liver.

Bacteremia. Blood stream infection.

Ischemia. Impaired blood supply.

Seroma. A fluid collection composed of blood products.

The Clinical Problem

In the last decade, hepatic transplantation has become a successful treatment for many patients with end-stage liver disease. Improvements in organ preservation, surgical technique, and immunosuppressive therapy have led to increased survival. Actuarial survivals at 1, 10, and 18 years were 79%, 57%, and 48%, respectively, in a series of 4,000 recipients between 1981 and 1998. The most common causes of death among all recipients were infection (28%) and recurrent or new cancer (12%).

Common indications for liver transplantation include biliary cirrhosis, chronic hepatitis (viral or autoimmune), sclerosing cholangitis, fulminant hepatic failure, hepatocellular carcinoma, and metabolic disorders in adults; and extrahepatic biliary atresia and metabolic disorders in children.

Ultrasound is used both in preparation for transplantation and to look for complications after the transplantation has been performed. The preoperative assessment should include evaluation of native vascular anatomy, vascular patency, identification of vascular collaterals secondary to portal hypertension, and evaluation of the liver for evidence of intrahepatic malignancy; and evaluation of the surrounding anatomy to identify extrahepatic malignancy. The postoperative assessment should include evaluation of the organ for rejection, vascular stenosis or thrombosis, biliary obstruction or leak, and malignant disease. Postoperative liver transplant complications are often related to problems with the hepatic vasculature and biliary tree. Typical indications for sonograms are fever, pain, jaundice, abnormal liver function tests, and vascular complications. Possible pathology seen with ultrasound includes biliary obstruction, liver parenchymal abnormalities, malignancy, biliary leaks, hematomas, abscesses, and thrombosis or stenosis of the hepatic artery, portal vein, or inferior vena cava. The most common vascular problem is hepatic artery stenosis or thrombosis.

Anatomy

The liver transplant takes the place of the native liver. There is an end-to-end anastomosis of the portal vein and generally a "piggy-back" connection to the inferior vena cava. The hepatic arteries are sewn together. Either an end-to-end biliary duct anastomosis is performed or the bile duct is connected to the jejunum (Fig. 22-13). It is important to note, however, that variations of the previously described surgical techniques may occur. Living split-liver donation is becoming more common as surgical procedures improve and the organ shortage worsens. Other variations include segmental or reduced size transplantation, especially in children. Also, if the vascular anatomy is anomalous, variations of the arterial and

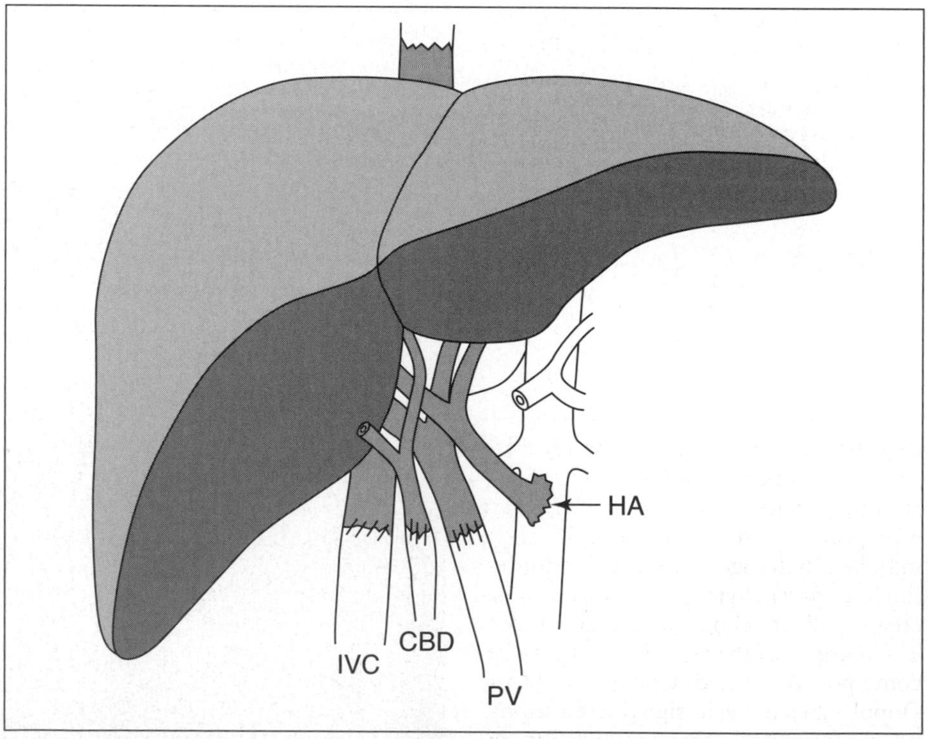

Figure 22-13. ■ *Usual way in which the portal vein and bile ducts are connected after liver transplant. Note that variations are common; in particular, the donor hepatic artery is often anastomosed to the recipient hepatic artery, and a "piggy-back" anastomosis is often used for the inferior vena cava.*

venous anastomoses may be present. Always review the patient's chart to see what has been done surgically.

Technique

When using ultrasound for screening pretransplant, examine the extrahepatic portal vein with care. If it is severely narrowed or thrombosed, transplantation may not be possible.

For both pre- and posttransplant evaluations, the liver is examined with the same techniques as described in Chapter 8 using a 3.5-MHz transducer (higher frequencies are generally beneficial in thinner patients). Particular attention should be paid to the following after transplant:

1. Defining the biliary and portal structure with pulsed and color Doppler.
2. Carefully examining the anastomosis, looking for any areas of narrowing or irregularity (Color Plates 22-3 and 22-4). Doppler will normally show mild to moderate turbulence and an increased flow velocity at the anastomotic site. A normal portal vein should demonstrate flow toward the liver (hepatopetal), showing slight variation with breathing (Color Plate 22-5). Flow is in the same direction as the intrahepatic artery. The normal inferior vena cava demonstrates variation in flow with the cardiac and respiratory cycles. The hepatic veins also vary flow depending on the cardiac pulsations and should demonstrate flow away from the liver (Color Plate 22-6).

Pathology

REJECTION

Rejection occurs in approximately 50% to 70% of liver transplants. With acute rejection, the ultrasonic findings are nonspecific and often normal. There may be a heterogeneous echo texture to the liver parenchyma, and an overall decrease in liver echogenicity may be seen. The margins of the hepatic veins may become poorly defined. Conversion of the Doppler hepatic vein signal from triphasic to monophasic suggests rejection, although this is far from specific. Biopsy is still the best way to identify acute graft rejection. In chronic rejection, there may be an increase in periportal echogenicity.

BILIARY COMPLICATIONS

Most biliary complications will occur within 3 months of transplantation. If there is a bile leak, patients usually present with fever, pain, and increasing liver function tests. Leaks occur at the biliary anastomosis most often. Intrahepatic bile ducts may also leak secondary to arterial infarcts or liver biopsy. Typically, fluid collects in the region of the porta hepatis.

Many obstructions relate to a stricture at the anastomosis, but bile duct strictures may also occur when hepatic artery stenosis or thrombosis leads to ischemia. Biliary sludge or stones can occlude the duct system, but are uncommon. Biliary duct dilation to the level of the anastomosis may be seen.

VASCULAR PROBLEMS

Thrombosis or stenosis usually takes place within 3 months of transplantation. Patients may be asymptomatic or present with hepatic failure.

Hepatic Artery Thrombosis

This is the most common vascular complication. Patients present with infection of the biliary tree or a biliary leak. Typical features of both are abnormal bilirubin, pain, and fever. No arterial signals at the porta hepatis will be detected with color or pulsed Doppler. Because this diagnosis is based on the absence of flow, great care should be taken to make sure that Doppler settings are optimized and not set too high to create a false-positive diagnosis. Although the hepatic artery may thrombose, it is important to remember that collaterals can form with this complication. These collaterals are often not enough to sustain the liver, but may give detectable arterial flow from within the liver. Assessment of the arterial waveform (tardus parvus) is therefore important.

Abnormal Doppler waveforms with absence of diastolic flow (but with appropriate rapid early systolic increase times) are commonly seen in the first few days after surgery and do not indicate thrombosis or stenosis. This high-resistance spectral Doppler pattern is thought to occur due to anoxia and traumatic insult occurring during harvesting, handling, and surgery.

Focal, blotchy, hepatic hypoechoic liver lesions occur with arterial thrombosis if arterial collaterals do not develop. Usually such infarcts are at the liver edge. Eventually, the infarcted area liquefies and becomes cystic.

Hepatic Artery Stenosis

This usually occurs at an anastomotic site. Thrombus may be a secondary finding. Duplex Doppler shows high-velocity flow that is greater than or equal to 2 m/sec at the anastomosis and turbulence distally (spectral broadening of the waveform). Also noted distal to the site of a stenosis is a tardus parvus arterial signal (Fig. 22-14). The tardus parvus

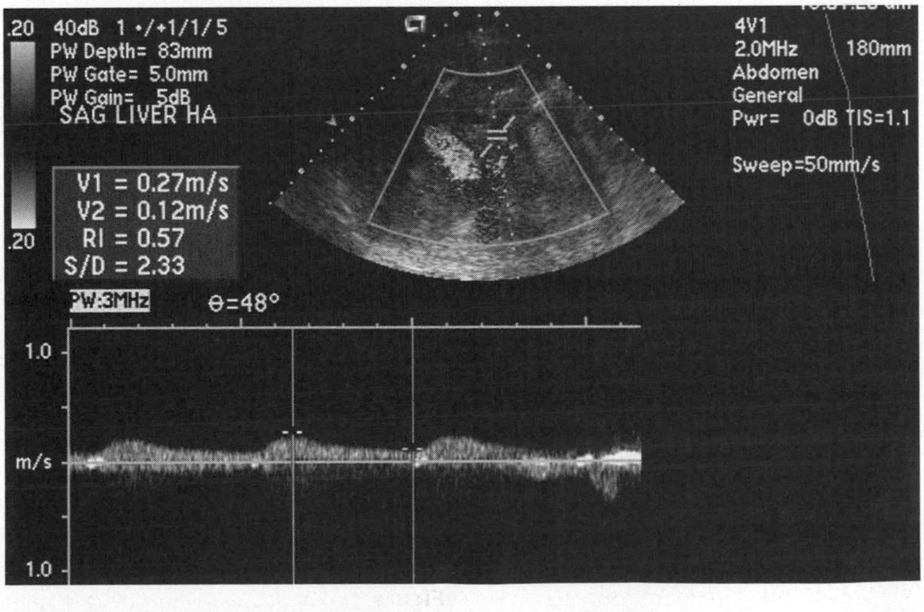

Figure 22-14. ■ *Tardus parvus Doppler signal in the proper hepatic artery of a liver transplant recipient. This signal demonstrates that the stenosis is proximal in location. Note slow increase in systolic acceleration and delayed time to peak systole.*

signal is an arterial Doppler signal that is described as an arterial signal with a rounded, late-arriving peak and a low resistive index. If the sonographer finds a signal like this in the liver, he or she should search back and map the arterial signal from proximal to the anastomosis site to distal to the anastomosis site. If there is severe stenosis, the parenchyma may be diffusely inhomogeneous, indicating ischemia. Sometimes the stenotic area and the region of the porta hepatis are not visible owing to overlying bowel gas, in which case the tardus-parvus pattern, with reduced arterial flow amplitude and low acceleration pattern in the hepatic arterial vessels distal to the stenosis, is helpful (see Chapter 18). If normal waveforms are detected in the right and left hepatic arteries, this is adequate to determine that the proper hepatic artery is patent.

Portal Vein or IVC Thrombosis (Rare)

The portal vein and inferior vena cava should normally be echo-free postsurgery. The normal portal vein has a luminal diameter of 8 to 12 mm and has flow into the liver in the same direction as the hepatic artery. If the walls are thick, the lumen is small (<4 mm), and there are internal echoes, angiography is usually performed. Thrombosis usually causes echogenic material within the vessel lumen (Fig. 22-15 and Color Plate 22-7). However, thrombus may be isoechoic with blood. Power Doppler is helpful in determining whether blood is flowing in the vein. To make sure that the vein is truly occluded, the sonographer should make sure that the Doppler settings are optimized for slow flow and reevaluate the vessel with slow-flow settings. If there still appears to be no flow with color Doppler, one can use power Doppler to again interrogate the vessel for slow flow. After portal vein thrombosis occurs, collaterals may develop. Venous collaterals appear as small tubular pulsatile structures in the porta hepatis. Some describe this as the "bag of worms" appearance.

Portal Vein or IVC Stenosis

Focal narrowing of the vessels is seen normally at the anastomosis site. In true stenosis, Doppler assessment will show high-velocity flow and distal turbulence. There will be a loss of the normal pulsation seen in the inferior vena cava. Internal echoes may be seen due to clot.

Pseudoaneurysm

This problem occurs at the arterial anastomosis and is most often the result of vascular reconstruction or a complication after a biopsy. A hypoechoic fluid collection in an anastomotic site with arterial flow within a pseudoaneurysm will be seen.

FLUID COLLECTIONS

Distinguishing between the various types of fluid collections often requires a diagnostic puncture, which is done under ultrasound control (see Chapter 54). It is important not to confuse the more common fluid collections with a solid mass such as a posttransplant lymphoma (Fig. 22-16).

Hematomas

Hematomas are usually found around the liver, particularly in a subphrenic location, but they may be seen in the abdomen. Very common immediately posttransplant, these collections have varying degrees of echogenicity depending on the amount of liquefaction.

Abscesses

Abscesses have varying degrees of echogenicity, similar to hematomas. The patient may or may not be tender or febrile because the patient is immunosuppressed. Some abscesses contain gas (see Chapter 11). They may occur in an intrahepatic or extrahepatic location.

Biloma

Sonolucent collections of bile seen alongside the biliary tree, bilomas are a result of a bile leak. These leaks usually occur at the anastomosis, but they may be seen elsewhere since they may be caused by hepatic artery thrombosis and subse-

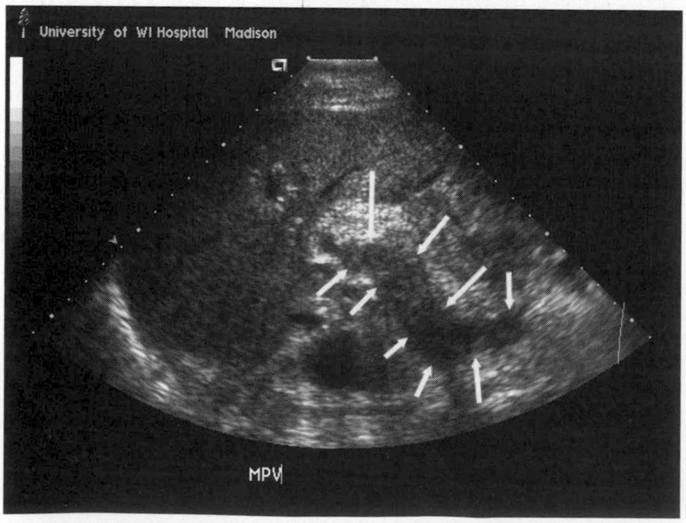

Figure 22-15. ■ *Portal vein thrombosis in a patient status-post liver transplant. Gray-scale image shows clot* (arrows) *as intermediate level echoes filling expected location of portal vein.*

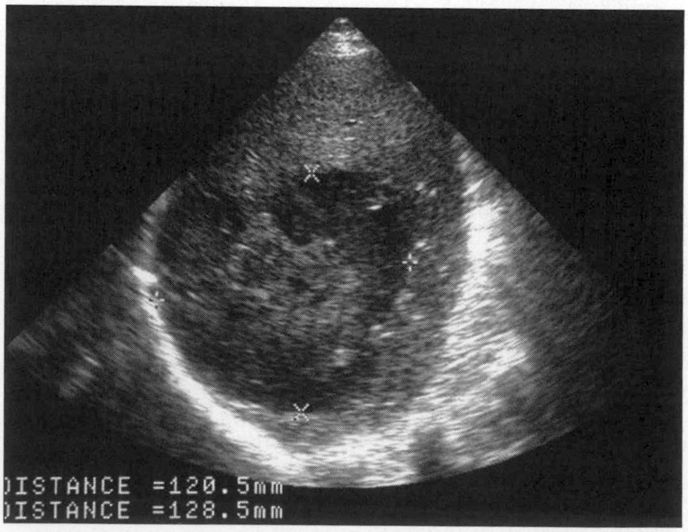

Figure 22-16. ■ *Large solid mass in the liver representing posttransplant lymphoproliferative disorder* (PTLD).

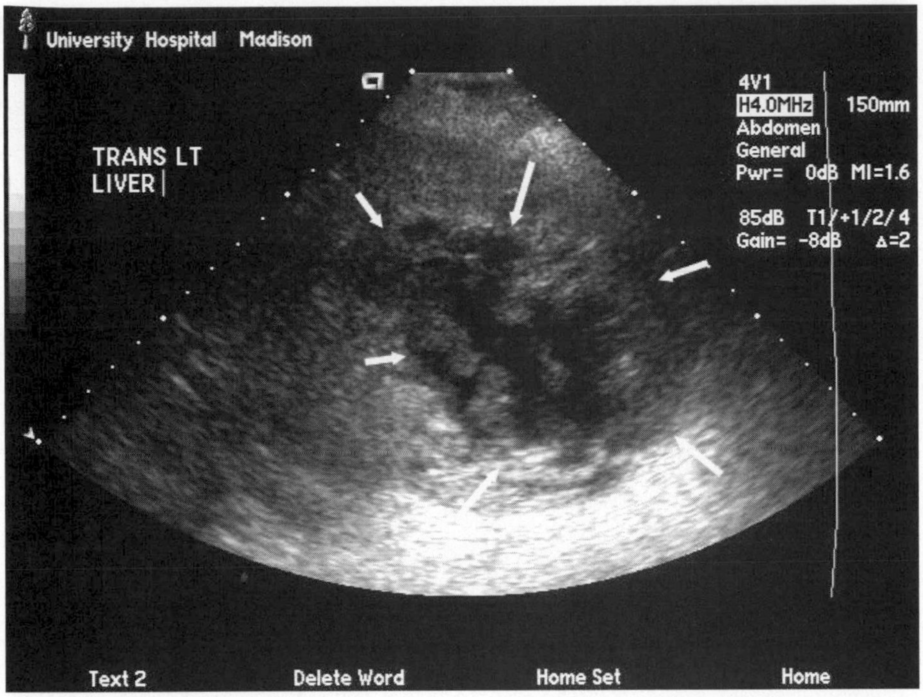

Figure 22-17. ■ *Classic biloma. Grayscale image shows biloma* (arrows).

quent infarction (Fig. 22-17 and Color Plates 22-8 and 22-9).

Ascites

Anechoic free fluid may be seen anywhere in the abdomen or pelvis and is common in the early postoperative course after transplantation.

Seromas

As sonolucent collections adjacent to the liver, seromas are common in the early postoperative period.

Pitfalls

1. A slight narrowing or irregularity of the portal vein or IVC at the anastomosis is a normal finding in the transplanted liver.
2. Biliary duct air or sludge may obscure the biliary duct lumen, making determination of biliary dilation difficult; try scanning coronally with the patient supine or turning the patient.
3. Respiration. Doppler may be difficult in these sick patients because of breathing motion. Have the patient suspend respiration when possible.
4. Bowel gas. Overlying bowel may obscure anatomy. Rolling the patient into an oblique or decubitus position may be helpful.
5. In the early postoperative period, a right pleural effusion is almost always present. Scan above the diaphragm to look for hypoechoic fluid in the chest.
6. Right adrenal gland. Liver transplant recipients are at risk for right adrenal hemorrhage. A suprarenal mass with varying echogenicity, depending on the age of the hemorrhage, will be seen in the right adrenal gland.

SELECTED READING

Nghiem HV, Tran K, Winter TC III, et al. Imaging of complications in liver transplantation. *Radiographics* 1996;16:825–840.

Pozniak MP. Doppler ultrasound of the liver. In: *Clinical Doppler ultrasound*. Allan PL, Dubbins PA, Pozniak MA, McDicken WN, eds. Churchill Livingstone: London; 2000.

Sidhu PS, Baxter GM. *Ultrasound of Abdominal Transplantation*. Thieme: New York; 2002.

Shaw As, Ryan SM, Beese RC, et al. Ultrasound of non-vascular complications in the post liver transplant patient. *Clin Radiol* 2003; 58(9):672–680.

Vit A, De Candia A, Como G, et al. Doppler evaluation of arterial complications of adult orthotopic liver transplantation. *J Clin Ultrasound* 2003;31(7):339–345.

Pancreatic Transplants

SONOGRAM ABBREVIATIONS

Ao	Aorta
Bl	Bladder
IVC	Inferior vena cava

KEY WORDS

Glucose Homeostasis. Control of blood glucose levels.

The Clinical Problem

Pancreatic transplantation is used as a treatment for severe (Type I) diabetes. This technique is used when there is multiorgan failure—as occurs in many long-term, insulin-dependent diabetic patients—as a means to achieve glucose homeostasis. A pancreas may be transplanted at the same time as a kidney (simultaneous pancreas and kidney), after a kidney transplant (pancreas after kidney), or alone (pancreas transplant alone) (in patients without end-stage renal disease).

Many of the complications after pancreatic transplantation may be seen with ultrasound:

1. Pancreatic failure, usually due to rejection. Unfortunately, the ultrasound findings of rejection are usually minimal or nonspecific. Ultrasound is used to guide biopsy to make the definitive diagnosis of rejection.
2. Peripancreatic fluid collections
3. Vascular problems
4. Arteriovenous fistulas
5. Pancreatitis and pseudocysts

Anatomy

Surgical techniques for pancreatic transplantation are variable. An entire pancreas may be transplanted from a cadaver or a living related donor. Most commonly, a whole cadaver pancreas is removed from the donor along with the duodenum, which is then anastomosed to the urinary bladder or loop of small intestine of the recipient (Fig. 22-18). This allows for direct elimination of pancreatic secretions into the patient's urine or bowel. Early diagnosis of rejection by monitoring levels of urinary amylase can be performed if a urinary bladder anastomosis is present. The arterial supply to the pancreatic transplant is from the donor superior mesenteric artery and celiac/splenic artery, which is then anastomosed to the iliac artery or sometimes the aorta. Venous drainage is accomplished by anastomosis of the portal vein to the external iliac vein or superior mesenteric vein. The pancreas is placed in the iliac fossa or upper abdomen. Patients with combination renal and pancreatic transplants have the kidney placed on the opposite side.

Technique

STANDARD SCAN

1. Know what was done surgically! Surgical techniques vary widely. If the pancreas is transplanted in the most common way, one may begin the scan by finding the iliac vessels in the iliac fossa. This can be accomplished simply by using color flow. The transplant allograft is located superficially just medial to the iliac vessels.

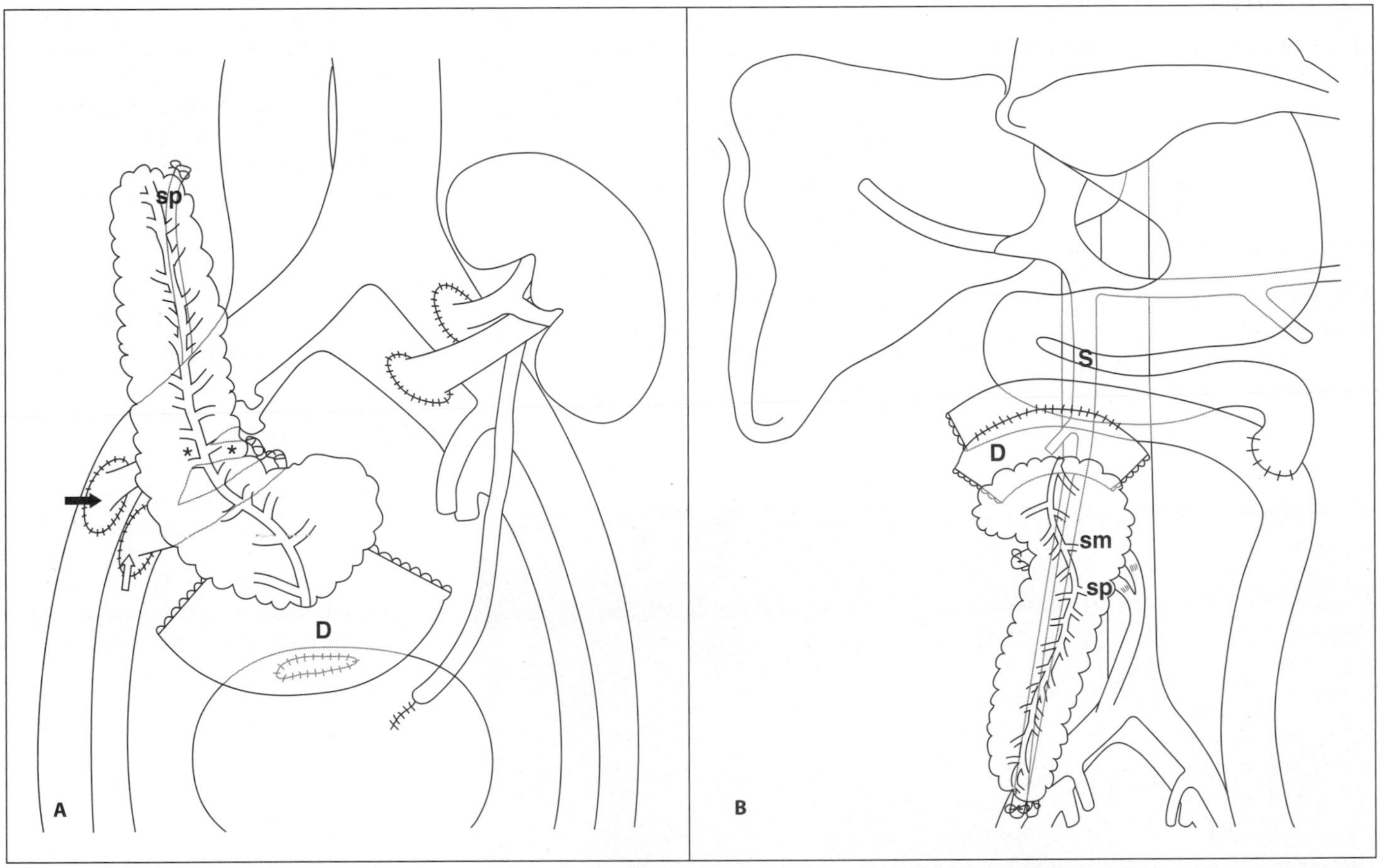

Figure 22-18. ■ *Two of the more common surgical procedures used to place a pancreatic transplant. A. Bladder drainage. B. Enteric drainage.* Black arrow, *celiac artery;* white arrow, *external iliac vein;* S, *SMV;* D, *donor duodenum;* sp, *splenic artery;* sm, *SMA. Chen PC, Nikolaidis P, Amin RS, et al. Role of sonography in pancreatic transplantation.* Radiographics *2003;23:939–949.*

2. Examine the texture and anatomy of the pancreas. The gland is usually fairly well defined, with a homogeneous echo texture similar to a native pancreas in the normal location (Fig. 22-19). An anechoic or hypoechoic graft is often seen immediately postoperatively and may be a sign of rejection, pancreatitis, or a normally functioning gland. The pancreatic duct should be less than 2 to 3 mm in diameter, and the anterior-posterior diameter of the pancreas should measure from 1.5 to 2 cm.
3. The vascular connection to the pancreas may be found by first scanning longitudinally over the iliac vessels, then rotating the transducer to visualize the anastomosis of the celiac axis and superior mesenteric artery to the iliac artery and the takeoff of the portal vein from its origin at the external iliac vein. The splenic artery and vein are along the posterior portion of the transplant.

COLOR FLOW/DUPLEX DOPPLER

Doppler is helpful in identifying anatomy and vascularity in the pancreatic transplant (Color Plate 22-10). Color flow Doppler is used to show vascular patency and to determine whether a vessel is an artery or a vein. Color flow is helpful in determining whether a peripancreatic structure is vascular or is a fluid collection, and to see whether there is adequate flow within the vessels.

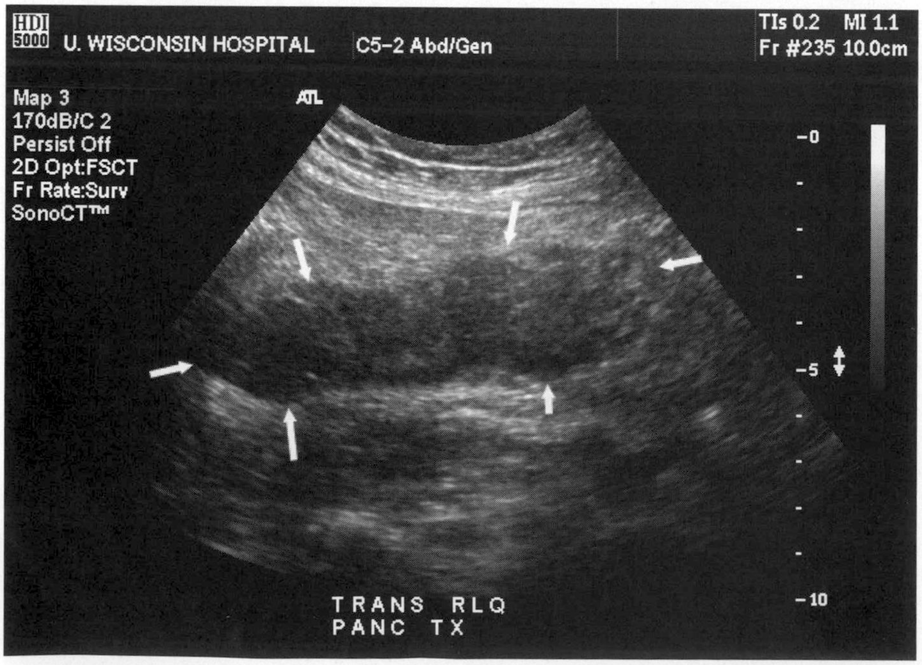

Figure 22-19. ■ *Ultrasound image of the transplant pancreas. Note the homogeneous echotexture of the transplant pancreas* (arrows).

Pathology

REJECTION

1. Acute rejection. An inhomogeneous parenchyma may be seen with acute rejection. However, this finding is nonspecific.
2. Chronic rejection. Sonographic signs may include the following:
   a. An increase in the parenchymal echogenicity of the pancreas
   b. A decrease in the size of the gland
   c. Calcifications—echogenic foci with posterior acoustic shadowing

PANCREATITIS

Findings are similar to pancreatitis in the native gland. These include edema with enlargement, heterogeneous echo texture, and dilatation of the pancreatic duct.

VASCULAR COMPLICATIONS

Graft Thrombosis

Clinical presentation. Patients may present with back, flank, or abdominal pain; increased serum glucose; and decreased urine amylase levels. Graft thrombosis is the most common postoperative vascular complication and usually occurs within the first few days or weeks after surgery. Ultrasound examination shows inhomogeneous echo texture or enlargement of the gland. Documentation of blood flow within the pancreas itself, as well as within the vascular pedicle (at the anastomosis site), proves patency of the graft vasculature. Absence of flow will be seen with graft thrombosis. Knowledge of the vascular construction of a pancreatic transplant is crucial in performing this part of the examination. Another helpful technique to evaluate the perfusion of the pancreas gland is to use power Doppler and to optimize settings for low flow states.

Venous Thrombosis

Elevated resistive index, often greater than 1.0, is seen in the spectral Doppler signal of gland arteries (Color Plate 22-11).

Pseudoaneurysms

Pseudoaneurysms develop from a disruption of arterial continuity. Extravasation of blood occurs resulting in the development of a fibrous capsule that enlarges due to arterial pressure. Doppler examination will show arterial flow within a perianastomotic fluid collection.

Anastomotic Strictures

Turbulent color flow suggests a stenosis at the anastomosis site.

FLUID COLLECTIONS

Hematomas

Hematomas are usually seen immediately postoperatively in close proximity to the pancreatic transplant. The ultrasound appearance will vary from anechoic to complex.

Abscesses

The patient may or may not be tender or febrile. Sonographically, abscesses will appear similar to a hematoma and may require aspiration for differentiation. An abscess may contain gas.

Urinomas

These collections are usually found at the medial aspect of the pancreas. Urinomas are caused by an anastomotic leak at the duodenal-bladder junction. They appear anechoic unless they contain leaked pancreatic enzymes, in which case they will be complex.

Pseudocysts

Occasionally associated with pancreatitis, these anechoic to complex collections are found within or adjacent to the pancreas.

Ascites

Anechoic free fluid may be seen anywhere in the pelvis. Always look for free fluid elsewhere in the patient's abdomen to help confirm the diagnosis of ascites. This free fluid may be related to previous dialysis.

Pitfalls

1. Obesity. Blood flow in the transplanted pancreas of an obese patient may be difficult to detect with color flow and duplex Doppler.
2. Ill-defined borders. The pancreas may blend in with surrounding bowel, making identification difficult.
3. Duodenum. Do not mistake the transplanted duodenum for a complex fluid collection. Watch for peristalsis and use color flow Doppler to rule out vascularity.
4. Bladder versus collection. Same as for renal transplants.
5. Time-gain compensation problems. Same as for renal transplants.
6. Echogenic collections. Same as for renal transplants.

What Else to Consider

1. If the patient is febrile, look elsewhere in the abdomen for abscesses (see Chapter 11).
2. Scan the native pancreas if there is clinical pancreatitis and the transplant appears normal.

SELECTED READING

Nelson NL, Largen PS, Stratta RJ, et al. Pancreas allograft rejection: correlation of transduodenal core biopsy with Doppler resistive index. *Radiology* 1996;200:91–94.

Nikolaidis, P, Amin RS, Hwang CM, et al. Role of sonography in pancreatic transplantation. *Radiographics* 2003:23(4):939–949.

Possible Invasive Rectal Wall Mass or Anal Sphincter Break

BEVERLY E. HASHIMOTO

23

KEY WORDS

External Sphincter. Concentric muscle group deep to the internal sphincter.

Fistula in Ano. Track that extends from the skin near the anus to the muscles surrounding the anus.

Fecal Incontinence. Involuntary leakage of fecal material through the anus.

Internal Sphincter. Ring of muscle that surrounds the anus and lies under the mucosa and submucosa.

Puborectalis Muscle. Muscle extending from the rectal wall to the pubic symphysis.

Villous Adenoma. Benign tumor of the rectal wall.

RELEVANT LABORATORY VALUES

Serum carcinoembryonic antigen (CEA). CEA is a colorectal tumor marker. The normal range is less than 2.5 ng/mL in an adult nonsmoker and less than 5.0 ng/mL in a smoker. Abnormal values are not specific for colon cancer or malignancy. CEA determination may have prognostic value for patients with colon cancer and may be used to monitor treatment, but fails to detect recurrent disease in more than 50% of patients. CEA usually returns to normal within 1 to 2 months of surgery.

The Clinical Problem

The anus and rectal wall are best imaged with a transducer in the rectum (transrectal sonography). Rectal neoplasms may be locally excised if the tumor is contained within the rectal wall. However, if the tumor extends into the perirectal fat or adjacent organs, local excision is not possible. Transrectal ultrasound has been found to be an excellent method to determine whether the tumor extends beyond the rectal wall. Because transrectal transducers extend approximately 10 to 12 cm into the rectum, tumors beyond this range cannot be examined.

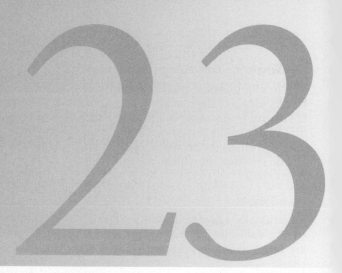

When the muscles of the anus are damaged, patients experience fecal incontinence. Transrectal ultrasound can assess tears in the internal sphincter that may be the cause of fecal incontinence.

Finally, for inflammatory processes, transrectal and transvaginal ultrasound may be useful to define fistulous tracks and abscesses around the rectum.

Anatomy

RECTUM

The rectal wall consists of five alternating echogenic and echopenic layers (Fig. 23-1):

1. Transducer interface and mucosa: mildly echogenic, most superficial layer
2. Muscularis mucosa: echopenic ring deep to mucosa
3. Submucosa: brightest echogenic layer of rectal wall
4. Muscularis propria: deepest echopenic ring that is generally slightly thicker than muscularis mucosa
5. Perirectal fat: echogenic area surrounds rectal wall

Anterior to the rectum are the cervix and vagina in the female and prostate and seminal vesicles in the male.

ANUS

The anus is dominated by the two sphincter muscles (Fig. 23-2):

1. Transducer and mucosa interface: mildly echogenic, superficial layer.
2. Internal sphincter: well-defined echopenic ring deep to the mucosa.
3. External sphincter: ill-defined area of heterogeneous echogenicity deep to the internal sphincter.
4. Puborectalis muscle: forms a sling that wraps around the anus and blends into the external sphincter approximately 2 cm from the anal margin. It attaches to the symphysis pubis.

Technique

RECTAL APPROACH

The rectal approach is generally superior to the vaginal approach in imaging the rectum and anus. Ideally, one should have a 360-degree transverse transducer and a longitudinal linear transducer. Because the rectal and anal walls are thin and superficial, high frequencies (>7.5 MHz) are preferable. However, most commercial transrectal transducers are 7.5 or 5 MHz. The patient is instructed to lie left-side down (left lateral decubitus). The imager then feels the rectum to identify the location of the tumor. The transducer is inserted into the anus. For rectal tumors, the water bath round the transducer is filled to better visualize the mass. In the anus, the luminal diameter is too small to accommodate the water bath. Once the transducer is in the rectum, one should be aware of one's orientation. To address this problem, most transducers have grooves that indicate where the transducer face is located. The images should be unambiguously labeled regarding position of the abnormality relative to the posterior rectal wall, anterior rectal wall, patient's left side, and patient's right side. One convention is to use the surgical rectal "clock" terminology: 12:00, posterior rectal wall; 3:00, patient's right side; 6:00, anterior rectal wall; 9:00, patient's left side.

TRANSVAGINAL APPROACH

In females, rectal abnormalities may be imaged by placing a transducer in the vagina. In general, this is a less accurate method to determine the extent of the tumor within the wall. However, this method may be useful for extremely large tumors that extend into the perirectal fat or adjacent organs or for pelvic abscesses. To image the rectum, point an end-fire transducer posteriorly to initially image the rectum transversely and then sagittally.

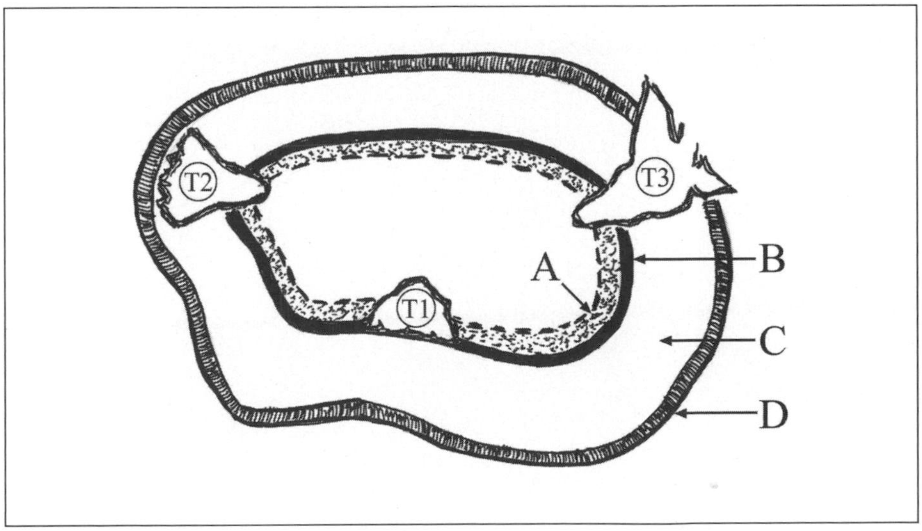

Figure 23-1. ■ *Schematic view of the rectal wall. There are four layers of the rectal wall. The mucosa/transducer interface (A) is echogenic. The muscularis mucosa (B) and muscularis propria (D) are echopenic. The submucosa (C) is the most hyperechoic layer of the wall. The tumors are classified by their location. T1 tumors are confined to the mucosa and submucosa. T2 tumors extend into the submucosa but do not invade the muscularis propria. T3 tumors breach the muscularis propria and extend into the subserosal fat.*

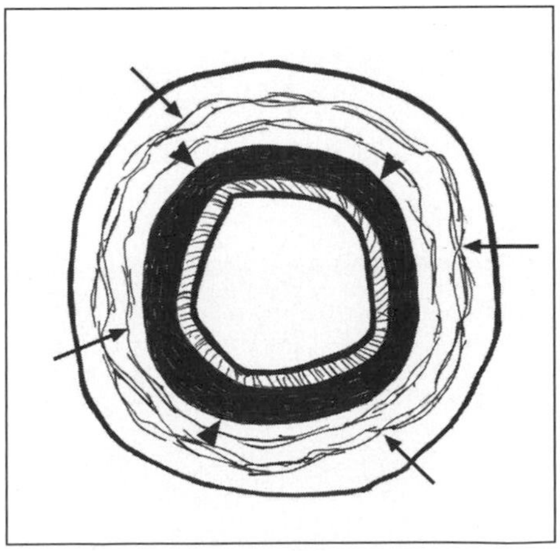

Figure 23-2. ■ *Schematic transverse view of the anus. The internal sphincter is the well-defined echopenic layer adjacent to the lumen* (arrowheads). *The external sphincter is an ill-defined structure of heterogeneous echogenicity adjacent to the internal sphincter* (arrows).

Pathology

RECTUM

Cancer of Rectum

Rectal tumors are echopenic masses that extend irregularly from the mucosa into the deeper layers of the rectal wall. With progressive invasion, the layers become echopenic and thickened and the borders between the affected layers become obliterated. Ultrasound is important in staging the tumor. When the tumor is confined to the mucosa and echogenic submucosa, it is classified as a T1 tumor. If the tumor does not extend beyond the muscularis propria, then it is still contained within the rectal wall (T2). The muscularis/fat interface will be sharp, and the border will be smooth. If the tumor extends beyond the muscularis propria into the perirectal fat, then it is considered to be beyond the rectal wall (T3) (Fig. 23-3). The border between the rectal wall and the perirectal fat will be irregular. Color flow Doppler may show low resistance within the malignant tumor. Limited study has found that three-dimensional rectal sonography is more accurate than two-dimensional sonography in tumor staging.

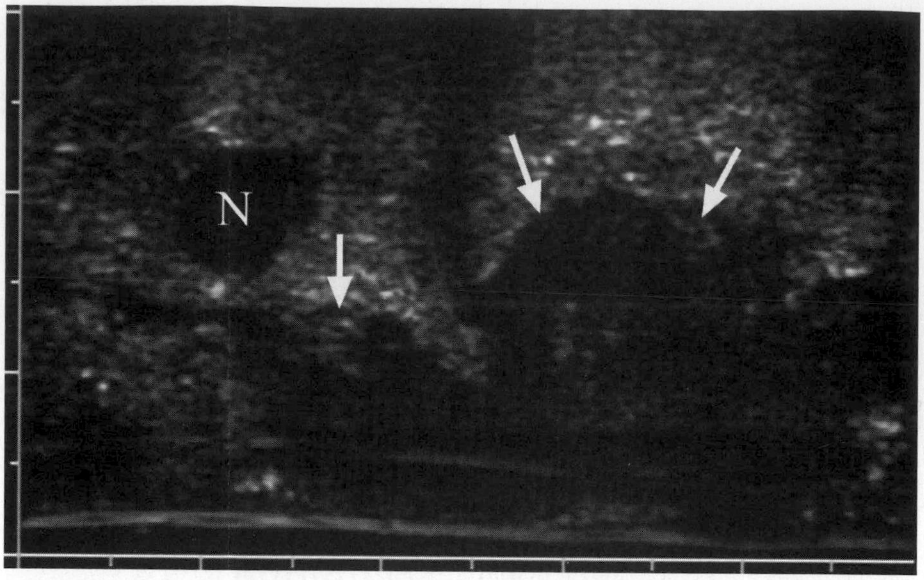

Figure 23-3. ■ *Longitudinal sonogram of rectal tumor. The bulky T3 tumor* (arrows) *extends beyond the muscularis propria. Adjacent to the tumor is an abnormal echopenic lymph node* (N).

Lymph Nodes

Perirectal lymph nodes are commonly identified. Normal lymph nodes are oval and have echogenic centers. Malignant or inflammatory nodes are round, echopenic, and without the echogenic center. Size does not differentiate malignant from benign lymph nodes.

Villous Adenomas

Villous adenomas are the most common rectal tumors. Even when they are large, they generally do not extend beyond the rectal wall. However, their sonographic appearance is similar to malignant rectal cancers.

ANUS

Anal Sphincter Break

The external sphincter is difficult to evaluate sonographically because it is ill defined. Therefore, ultrasound evaluation of the anal sphincter consists of mainly examining the internal sphincter. When the internal anal sphincter has been torn, the echopenic muscular ring will be ruptured on the transverse view and absent on the corresponding longitudinal view

(Figs. 23-4 and 23-5). Although the external sphincter is more important in maintaining continence, when the internal sphincter is broken, the external sphincter is also generally ruptured. Injury to the anal sphincter is common with childbirth associated with vaginal deliveries.

Anal Fistula

Anal fistulas and abscesses are common and may be associated with underlying diseases such as inflammatory bowel disease, rectal neoplasms, diabetes, trauma, and disorders affecting the immune system. The tracks form between the internal and external anal sphincter muscles and may spread vertically, horizontally, or circumferentially. The tract appears as an echopenic line parallel to the internal sphincter. Although it is clinically important to determine the location and extent of the track, it may be difficult to assess the relationship of the track to the sphincter because they are both echopenic. If incision of the track is through the sphincter muscle, then the patient may develop fecal incontinence.

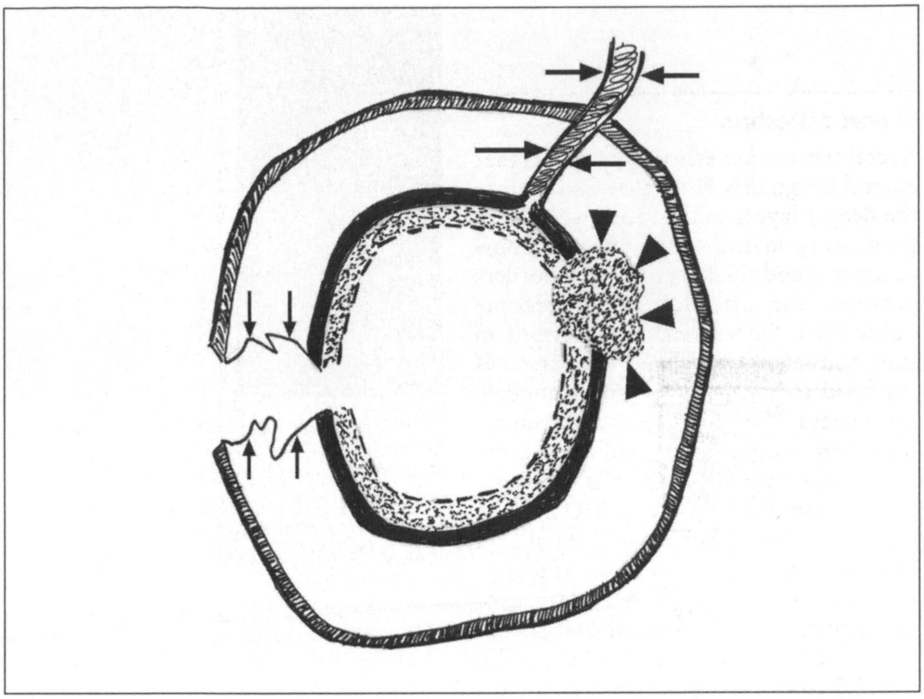

Figure 23-4. ■ *Schematic transverse view of the rectal wall. An abscess* (arrowheads) *is located between the internal and external sphincters. Anal fistulas may form horizontally between the internal and external sphincter (fistula in ano) or spread vertically* (large arrows). *Trauma may produce a tear* (small arrows) *in the external and internal sphincters and result in fecal incontinence.*

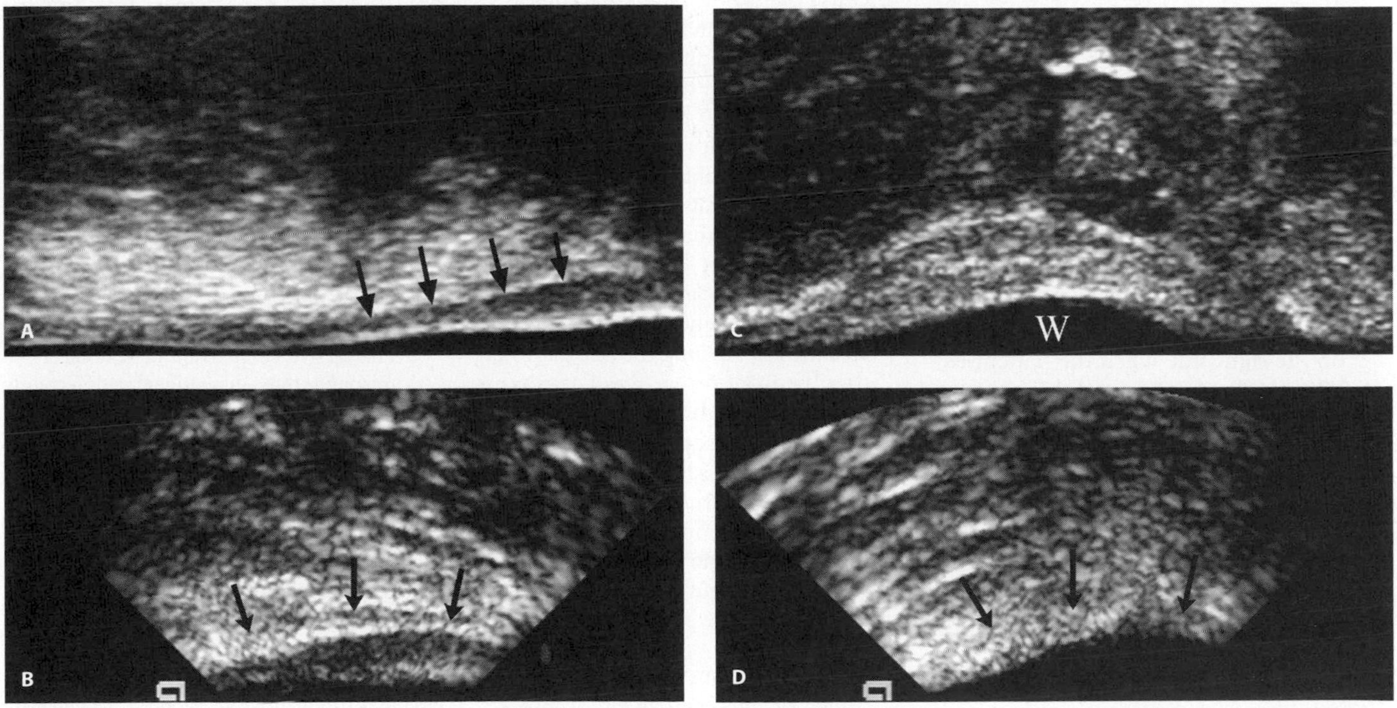

Figure 23-5. ■ *A. Longitudinal sonogram of anal sphincter, imaged at intact region. The normal echopenic internal sphincter* (arrows) *is present at the 12:00 position of the anus. External sphincter is the ill-defined streaky layer of heterogeneous echogenicity deep to the internal sphincter.* ***B.*** *Transverse sonogram of anal sphincter in same patient, imaged at intact region.* ***C.*** *Longitudinal sonogram of anal sphincter (same patient as in A), imaged at site of tear. At the 6:00 position of the anus, the internal and external sphincters are absent. The anechoic layer next to the transducer* (W) *is the water bath surrounding the transducer.* ***D.*** *Transverse sonogram of anal sphincter (same patient as in B), imaged at the site of tear.*

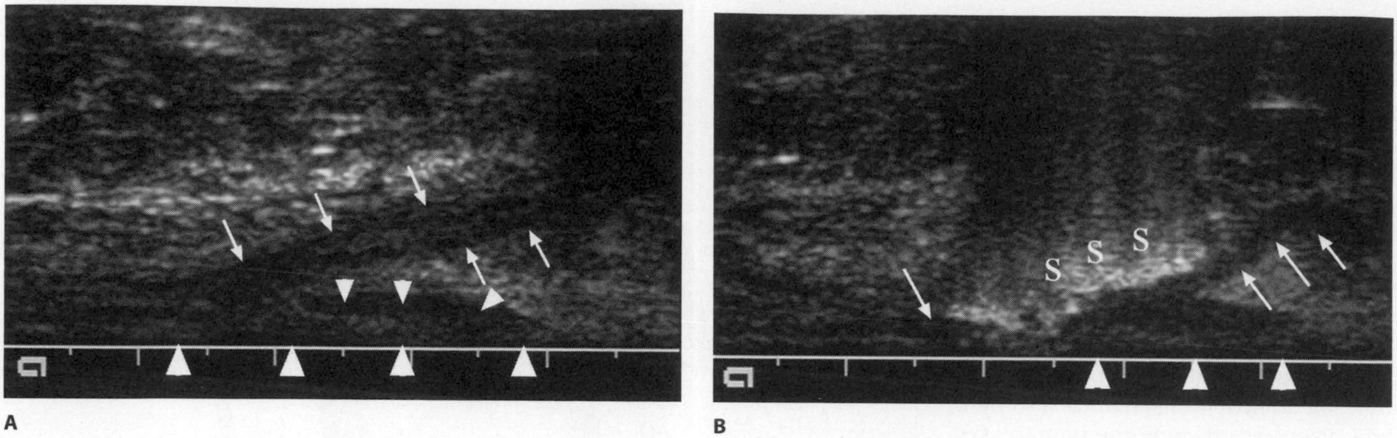

Figure 23-6. ■ *A. Longitudinal sonogram of anal sphincter. The patient has a buttock fistula* (arrows) *that extends to the anal sphincter. However, because the fistula is echopenic, one is unable to determine whether the fistula passes through the anal sphincter or dissects in a parallel path next to the sphincter. Internal sphincter* (arrowheads). ***B.*** *Longitudinal sonogram of anal sphincter (same patient as in A). Peroxide was injected into the buttock fistula with simultaneous real-time imaging of the anal sphincter. Shadowing* (S) *from the peroxide air artifact was identified within the perianal track* (arrows). *The track extended through the internal sphincter* (arrowhead). *Because the track extended through the sphincter, the surgeon did not incise the track. Incision of the track may produce fecal incontinence.*

Recently, we found that 1 to 2 mL of sterile peroxide or ultrasound contrast injected into the track may define the extent of the fistula (Figs. 23-4 and 23-6).

Pitfalls

1. Large rectal tumors commonly have irregular surfaces so ultrasound images are distorted by fecal gas. Pressure on the tumor or inflation of the water bath may reduce the artifact from air. Air artifact may also result from air within the transducer water bath. If the tumor is located on the right side when the patient is left-side down, then roll the patient to his or her back or right side.
2. The most common error in grading rectal tumors is labeling a tumor contained within the rectal wall (T2) as being invasive beyond the wall (T3). This error is called "overstaging."
3. Inflammation may simulate tumor invasion.
4. If one is not careful when performing transverse imaging of the rectum, oblique coronal images may be produced. Oblique images of the rectal tumor exaggerate the invasive appearance of the tumor and may cause one to overstage the tumor.
5. Transvaginal imaging is useful when the tumor produces severe narrowing, preventing the transducer from passing through the lumen and imaging the entire tumor.
6. When the patient is in the left lateral decubitus position, the structures on the right side may not appear symmetric compared with those on the left side. This asymmetry may be due to the dependent position of the structures. Turning the patient to either the front or back will cause this asymmetry to disappear.
7. The anal sphincter may be difficult to image because it is located a short distance from the edge of the anus. To adequately image the anus, one must anchor one's scanning hand on the patient's buttocks so the transducer does not slip deeper into the rectum.
8. Anal sonography may miss fistulous tracks or abscesses in the ischiorectal fossa or supralevator region.

Where Else to Look

If the tumor extends beyond the rectal wall, consider looking in the upper abdomen for liver metastases or paraortic nodes.

SELECTED READING

Elmas N, Killi RM, Sever A. Colorectal carcinoma: radiological diagnosis and staging. *Eur J Radiol* 2002;42:206–223.

Hashimoto BE, Kramer DJ, Wiitala L. Applications of ultrasound of the rectum and anus. *Ultrasound Q* 1996;13:179–196.

Hunerbein M, Pegios W, Rau B, et al. Prospective comparison of endorectal ultrasound, three-dimensional endorectal ultrasound, and endorectal MRI in the preoperative evaluation of rectal tumors. *Surg Endosc* 2000;14:1005–1009.

Kumar A, Scholefield JH. Endosonography of the anal canal and rectum. *World J Surg* 2000;24:208–215.

Ogura O, Takebayashi Y, Sameshima T, et al. Preoperative assessment of vascularity by color Doppler ultrasonography in human rectal carcinoma. *Dis Colon Rectum* 2001; 538–548.

Pricolo VE, Potenti FM. Modern management of rectal cancer. *Dig Surg* 2001;18:1–20.

24 Neck Mass

SARA BAKER
TOM WINTER

SONOGRAM ABBREVIATIONS

CCa	Common carotid artery
IJv	Internal jugular vein
PTh	Parathyroid gland
Th	Thyroid gland

KEY WORDS

Adenoma

(Thyroid). Benign solid tumor of the thyroid gland.

(Parathyroid). Benign solid tumor of the parathyroid gland that secretes parathyroid hormone, resulting in inappropriately high levels of serum calcium.

Branchial Cleft Cyst. Congenital cystic mass located close to the angle of the mandible.

Cervical Adenopathy. Enlargement of lymph nodes in the neck.

Cold Nodule. A region of the thyroid where radioisotope has not been taken up on a nuclear study. The area of decreased uptake may correspond to a palpable mass. The risk of malignancy in a cold nodule is approximately 5% to 15%.

Goiter. Diffuse enlargement of the thyroid gland due to iodine deficiency.

Hashimoto's Disease. Inflammatory disease of the thyroid gland usually characterized by diffuse enlargement and echopenic texture, often accompanied by marked hyperemia.

Major Neurovascular Bundle. A tubular structure that includes the common carotid artery, jugular vein, and vagus nerve.

Microcalcifications. Tiny hyperechoic foci that are sometimes present within a thyroid nodule. The presence of microcalcifications within a thyroid nodule significantly increases the risk for malignancy, with some sources quoting a 70% positive predictive value for cancer.

Minor Neurovascular Bundle. A tubular structure that contains the inferior thyroid artery and the recurrent laryngeal nerve.

Parathyroid Hormone (PTH). A hormone produced by the parathyroid glands that adjusts the amount of calcium and phosphorus in the body.

Photon-Deficient Area. See Cold Nodule.

Thyroglossal Duct Cyst. A developmental fluid-filled space variably extending from the base of the tongue to the isthmus of the thyroid.

Thyrotropin. A hormone secreted by the pituitary gland that stimulates the activity of the thyroid gland. Also called thyroid-stimulating hormone (TSH).

Thyroid Hormones

Thyroxine (T4). A hormone produced by the thyroid to regulate metabolism.

Triiodothyronine (T3). Another hormone produced by the thyroid that regulates metabolism.

Traumatic Pseudocyst. A fluid collection that is a response to damage to the salivary duct.

RELEVANT LABORATORY VALUES

Calcium, Total Serum: 8.5 to 10.2 mg/dL

Parathyroid Hormone Intact Molecule: 15 to 65 pg/mL

Thyroxine, Free: 0.71 to 1.85 ng/dL in adults

Triiodothyronine, Free: 2.4 to 4.2 pg/mL

Thyrotropin: 0.5 to 4.7 uIU/mL

The Clinical Problem

THYROID MASS

The three most common indications for an ultrasound examination of the neck are as follows:

1. A palpable neck mass
2. A cold nodule or photon-deficient area on a nuclear medicine study
3. Elevated serum calcium levels suggesting parathyroid disease

Thyroid masses are common and are seen by ultrasound in approximately half of elderly patients. The decision to proceed to biopsy is based on a combination of factors including clinical history, whether the lesion is palpable, physical examination of the neck, and sonographic features. Some patients are sent for a nuclear medicine study.

A cold nodule on a nuclear medicine study indicates a nonfunctioning area within the thyroid gland. Because all cysts and most malignancies do not take up radioisotope, an ultrasound study may then be performed to differentiate a solid from a cystic lesion. Of the lesions that are detected by nuclear scan, approximately 20% are cysts, 60% are benign, and 20% are malignant.

An increasing trend is to go straight to biopsy with or without ultrasound guidance if the mass is felt or revealed by ultrasound.

Clinical management is influenced by the ultrasonic differentiation of cystic from solid lesions. The diagnosis of a cystic lesion is followed by either observation or aspiration of the cyst, whereas the management of a solid mass may involve a surgical procedure, biopsy, thyroid medication, or watchful waiting. If follow-up ultrasound studies or clinical examination show that the lesion continues to enlarge, despite administration of thyroid hormone to suppress thyroid activity, surgical intervention may be recommended. If no increase in size occurs, a conservative clinical approach may be appropriate (thyroid carcinomas are slow-growing neoplasms).

A high-resolution, high-frequency transducer (12–15 MHz) is essential because its fine resolution will indicate whether multiple rather than single nodules are present. Compound imaging (see Fig. 24-8) allows the sonographer to create a smooth, well-defined image. Electronic beam steering is a nice feature that enables the sonographer and radiologist to better view a biopsy needle for fine-needle aspiration (FNA). A single solid nodule should be biopsied, preferably under ultrasound guidance if the lesion is either nonpalpable or difficult to feel. Although classic teaching was that multiple nodules are usually managed by medical follow-up because multiple nodules were thought to carry a benign prognosis, more recent research indicates that the risk of malignancy may not be decreased in the setting of multiple nodules; therefore, biopsy of one or more suspicious nodules in this setting may be warranted.

NECK MASS OF UNKNOWN ORIGIN

When a mass is found by physical examination in the neck, the organ of origin may not be obvious—it may arise from the thyroid, enlarged lymph nodes, salivary glands, or other structures adjacent to the thyroid. Abscess and hematoma are possibilities if fever or trauma is included in the patient's history. Two congenital anomalies, thyroglossal duct cyst and branchial cleft cyst, cause cystic masses outside the thyroid. Recognition of the anatomic structures in the neck and their sonographic appearance is necessary to determine the origin of the neck mass.

PARATHYROID MASS

A persistently high blood calcium level may suggest a diagnosis of parathyroid adenoma or cancer even though the gland cannot be felt. Surgery is difficult in this area because of the small size of the abnormal gland and the overlying thyroid; thus, the surgeon is greatly assisted by knowing which of the four parathyroid glands are enlarged.

Anatomy

THYROID GLAND

The thyroid consists of right and left lobes connected by a narrow bridge of tissue anterior to the trachea called the isthmus (Fig. 24-1). The common carotid artery and the internal jugular vein are important landmarks that lie posterior and lateral to the thyroid and define its lateral margins.

The sternocleidomastoid, sternohyoid, and sternothyroid muscles can be imaged anterior and lateral to the more homogeneous texture of the normal thyroid gland (Fig. 24-1).

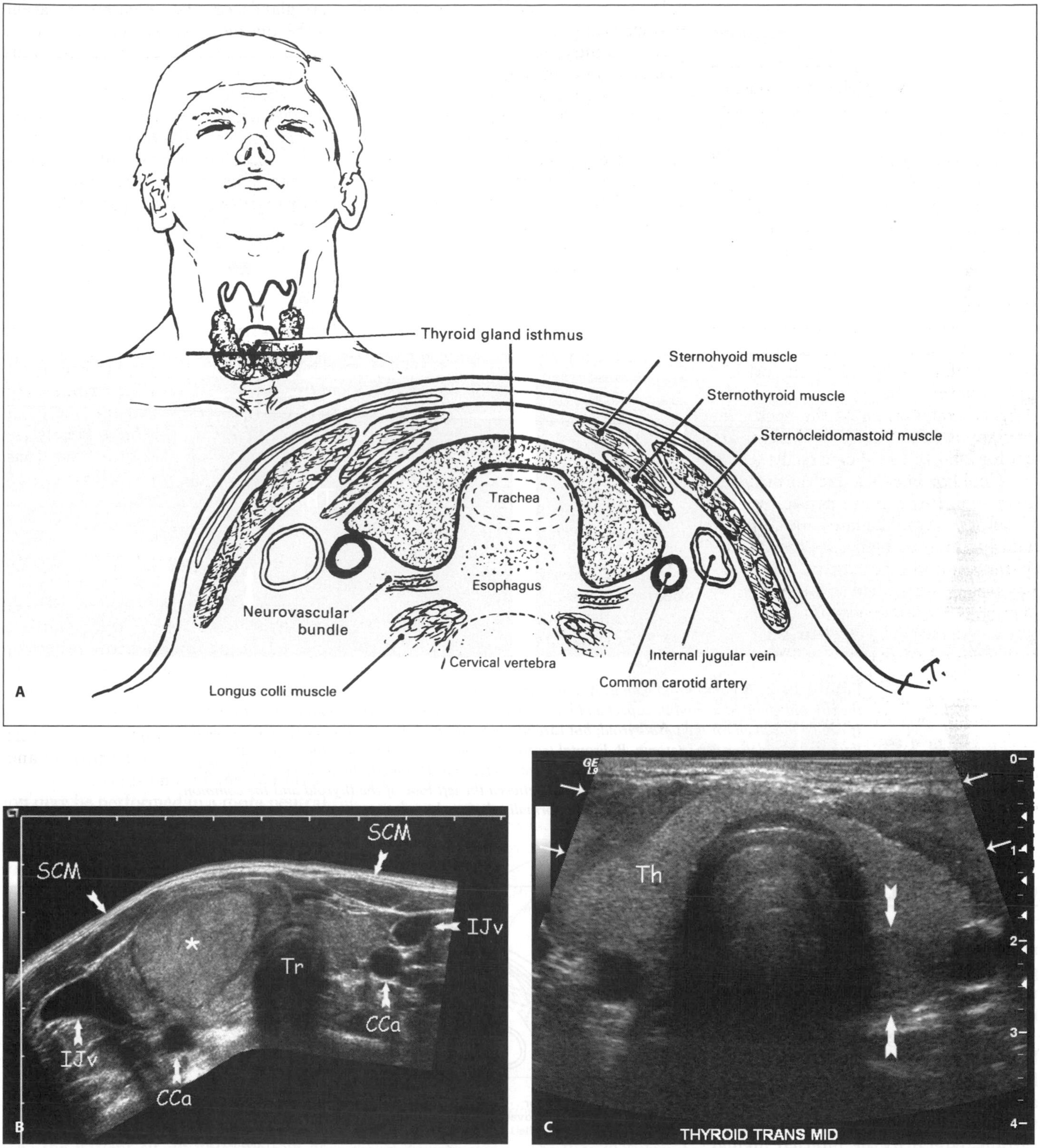

Figure 24-1. ■ *A. The thyroid gland consists of right and left lobes joined anteriorly by a narrow band of tissue called the isthmus. The common carotid artery and internal jugular vein are important landmarks.* ***B.*** *Extended field-of-view image oriented similarly to* (***A***)*. Dominant mass in the right lobe of the thyroid (*) was biopsied and shown to be a manifestation of Hashimoto's thyroiditis. SCM, sternocleidomastoid muscle; Tr, trachea. Trapezoidal field-of-view image* (***C***) *(virtual convex) oriented similarly to* (***A***)*. An ~1-cm indeterminate mass* (block arrows) *is seen just posterior to the midportion of the left lobe of the thyroid. Note how virtual convex imaging technology* (line arrows) *improves the width of the scan field of view for this linear probe.*

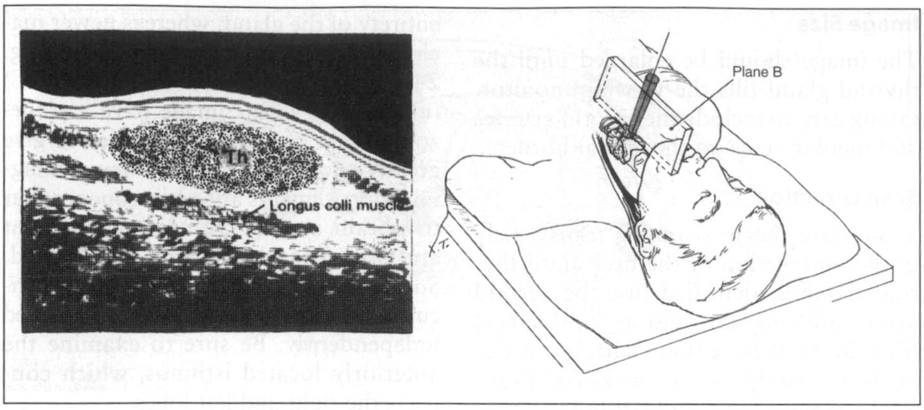

Figure 24-5. ■ *Longitudinal sections through the thyroid can best be obtained by using a 10- to 20-degree medial angle for maximum contact. Note the longus colli muscle posterior to the thyroid.*

(Figs. 24-5 and 24-7B). Determining the intrathyroidal or extrathyroidal nature of a neck mass is an excellent first step toward sorting out its origin. Most extrathyroidal masses displace the carotid artery and jugular vein medially. Mark the site of any palpable mass or textural changes with calipers to draw attention to the changes when the images are reviewed later.

Scan Technique

1. Apply acoustic couplant (gel) to the neck. The higher-viscosity (thicker) couplants are preferable because they remain on the skin surface longer. For humanitarian reasons, invest in a gel warmer so it is not ice-cold on patient contact.
2. Place the transducer directly on the skin surface in the transverse plane (Fig. 24-4). Adjust the electronic focus to the level of the thyroid tissue. Additional adjustments in focal depth will probably be needed to image the isthmus adequately. Care must be taken not to obliterate the texture of the isthmus, which may be hidden in near-field reverberations.
3. It is important to be light-handed. Excessive pressure on the tissue may make imaging difficult by compressing tissue planes, or it may displace a small lesion from the imaging field.

Color Flow

Both benign and malignant thyroid lesions are vascular. Color or power Doppler imaging is of help, however, when the lesion is isoechoic and when one is uncertain whether it is real, because the mass may be outlined with color. Color flow can also be used to appreciate the color flow within each thyroid lobe.

Pathology

INTRATHYROIDAL MASSES

Cysts

Thyroid cysts resemble those in other parts of the body except that their walls may be irregular and they may contain internal echoes from hemorrhage (Fig. 24-6). Predominantly cystic lesions within the thyroid are generally benign.

Adenomas

The most common thyroid masses are adenomas. They have several sonographic manifestations. Typical appearances are (1) a halo of echopenic tissue surrounding a more echogenic mass with echoes that are more dense than the remainder of the gland; (2) a solid homogeneous mass with very few internal echoes that can easily be confused with a cyst; and (3) a densely echogenic lesion. Larger (eggshell) foci of calcification may be seen. Although older literature stated that the halo appearance was diagnostic of a benign adenoma, we now know that this is not true and that cancers may have this appearance as well.

The presence of a comet-tail artifact (see Chapter 57) is a sign that the lesion

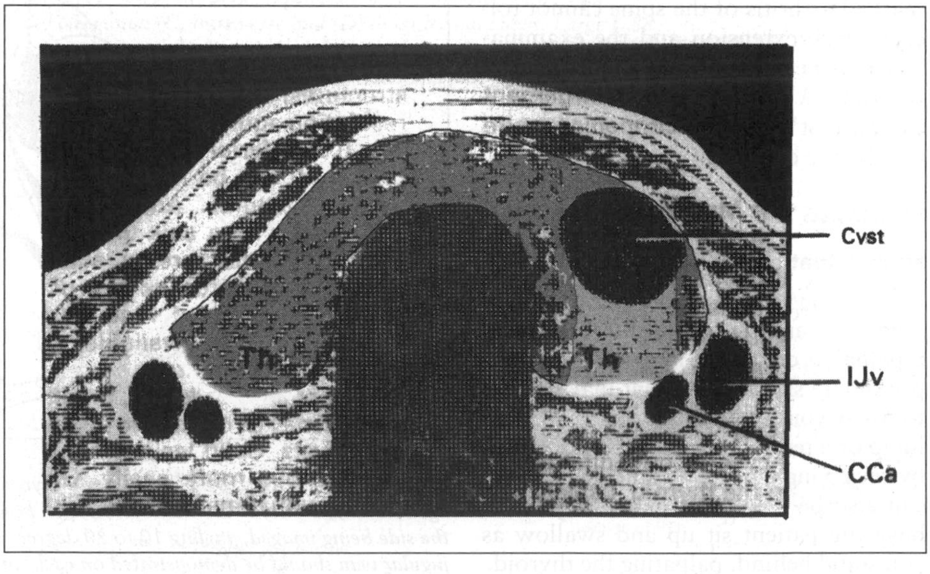

Figure 24-6. ■ *Thyroid cyst, showing the typical characteristics of smooth borders, lack of internal echoes, and increased through transmission.*

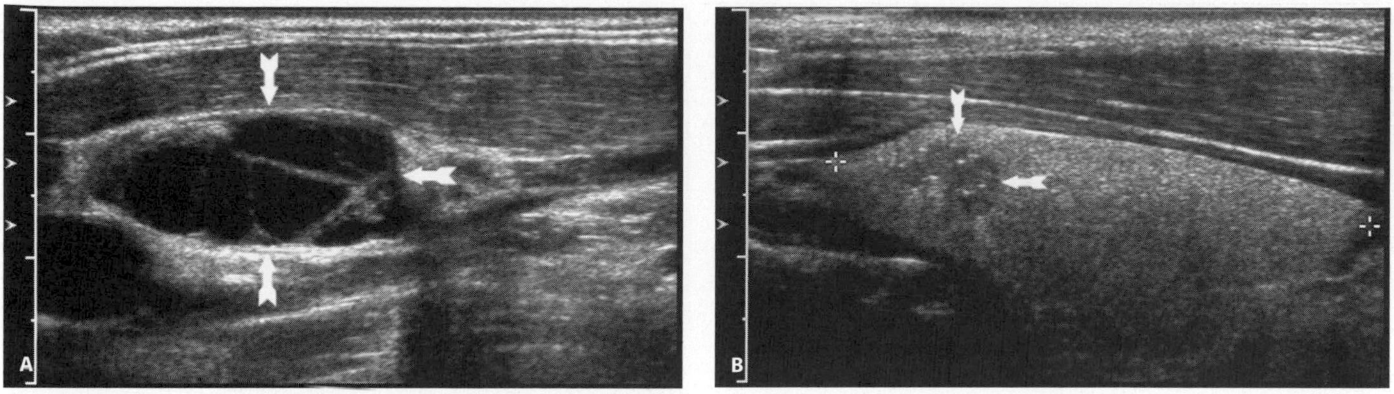

Figure 24-7. ■ *Thyroid cancer and cystic neck adenopathy. This 30-year-old otherwise healthy man was noted to have a palpable neck mass on a routine physical examination. Longitudinal sonogram **(A)** lateral to the right lobe of his thyroid demonstrated a 28-mm complex cystic mass* (arrows), *which corresponded to his palpable mass. Longitudinal sonogram of the right lobe of the thyroid **(B)** found a 7-mm mass* (arrows) *with tiny microcalcifications within the gland. Top and bottom* (cursors) *of the right lobe. Fine-needle aspiration (FNA) of this small mass yielded papillary thyroid carcinoma. The patient then underwent surgery, and the 28-mm cystic extrathyroidal mass was removed and shown to be a malignant node. Note that thyroid cancer nodes in the neck are often partially cystic, whereas cystic masses within the thyroid itself are usually benign.*

is benign because the calcific origin of the comet effect is large. Unlike carcinomas, adenomas are almost invariably multiple.

Carcinomas

Carcinomas (Figs. 24-7B and 24-8) of the thyroid are suggested by the following features: (1) an echopenic mass with an irregular border; (2) tiny foci of calcification (microcalcification); (3) a single nodular lesion; and (4) the development of nodes in neighboring structures. Peak systolic velocity has been reported to be increased in malignancy, but this sign is generally of little practical use. There is currently a great deal of controversy over how accurate ultrasound is at characterizing thyroid masses as malignant or benign. Most everyone agrees, however, that the presence of microcalcifications within a mass is a strong predictor for malignancy. When the question of cancer needs to be answered definitively, FNA of a thyroid nodule is performed (Fig. 24-8). Thyroid FNA is a very safe and relatively painless procedure that can be performed with just local anesthesia. A 25-gauge needle is easily placed under ultrasound guidance into any suspicious nodules for tissue analysis. See also Chapter 54.

Goiters

Goiters are a diffuse, asymmetric expansion of the thyroid with a coarse acoustic texture. Multiple nodules are usually present.

Hashimoto's Thyroiditis

In Hashimoto's thyroiditis, an inflammatory condition, there is diffuse, mild enlargement of the thyroid with multiple small echopenic nodules. Fibrous interfaces between the nodules will be evident. Increased blood flow is often seen.

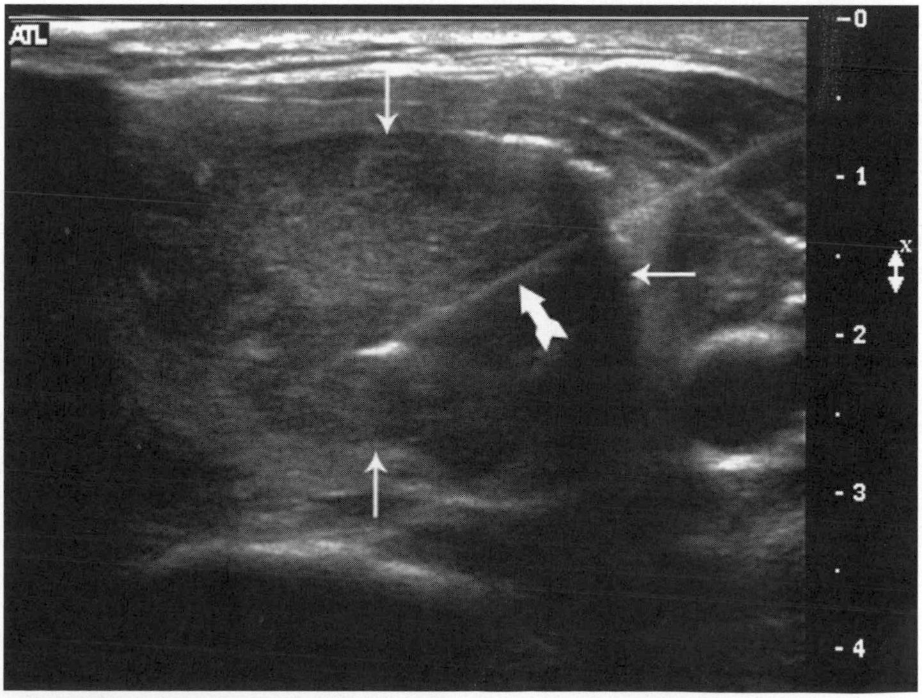

Figure 24-8. ■ *Thyroid FNA. FNA needle* (block arrow) *is visualized as it is placed into an 8-cm follicular neoplasm* (line arrows) *of the thyroid. Spatial compound imaging technology helps to depict this tiny 25-gauge needle.*

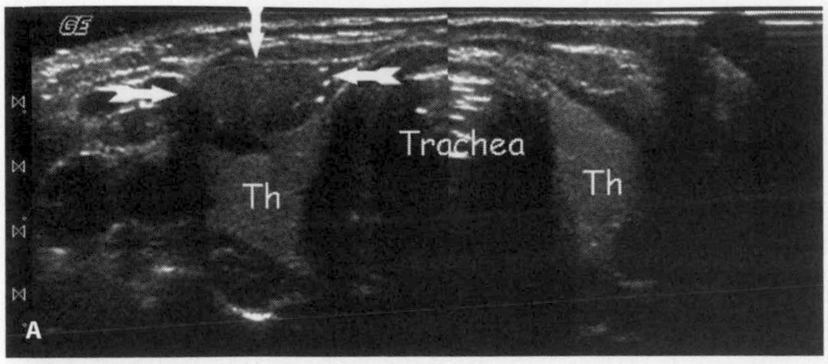

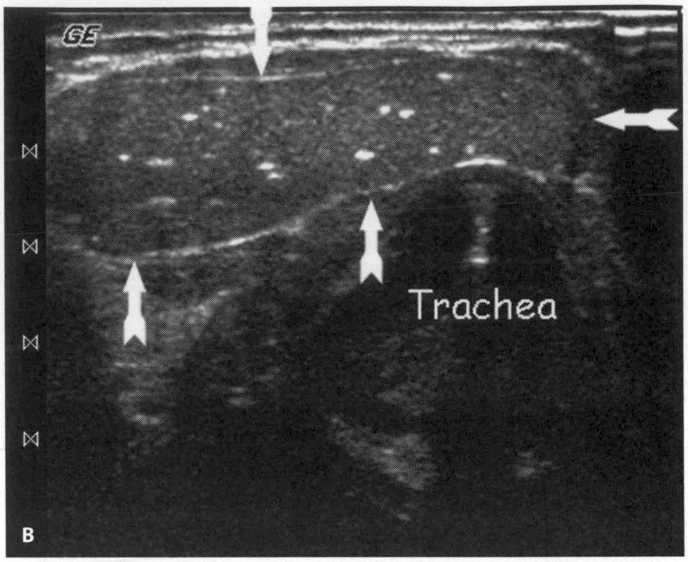

Figure 24-9. ■ *Thyroglossal duct cyst. A complex fluid collection* (arrows) *is seen anterior to the superior right side of the thyroid gland on these two transverse views:* ***A.*** *Dual split-screen of the entire thyroid.* ***B.*** *Image obtained above the thyroid. At surgery, this thyroglossal duct cyst containing thick proteinaceous debris was found to be involving the hyoid bone.*

Hemorrhage

With hemorrhage, there is sudden onset of pain with development of a mass associated with intrathyroidal clot. This clot is similar in appearance to clot in other parts of the body.

Subacute Thyroiditis

Subacute thyroiditis is a painful condition exhibiting diffuse, mild enlargement of the thyroid with an echopenic texture but no focal nodules. It may be a prelude to Hashimoto's thyroiditis.

EXTRATHYROIDAL MASSES

Thyroglossal Duct Cyst

A thyroglossal duct cyst is an embryologic remnant. It has the appearance of a cyst, but can contain either simple or complex fluid, and is found in the midline high in the neck above the thyroid (Fig. 24-9).

Branchial Cleft Cyst

A branchial cleft cyst is congenital and found lateral to the thyroid and anterior to the sternocleidomastoid muscle, usually at a higher level than the thyroid.

Nodes

Enlarged lymph nodes occur commonly in the neck and can be difficult to distinguish clinically (by palpation) from the thyroid gland. Sonographically, they lie lateral to the major vessels. Their echo texture is homogeneous, but less echogenic than normal thyroid texture. Most enlarged nodes are benign and have an echogenic center, but extrathyroidal masses in the neck may represent metastases or malignant nodes (Figs. 24-10 and 24-7A).

Abscess

Abscesses may develop in the neck. They have the typical ultrasonic features of abscesses in other parts of the body and similarly are associated with pain, fever, and focal swelling.

Carcinoma Invasion

Carcinoma (e.g., of the tongue) may invade the neck; the extent of the tumor can be seen with ultrasound.

Parathyroid Enlargement

Enlarged parathyroids can be difficult to distinguish from an intrathyroidal mass or normal anatomy of the neck; they appear as echopenic masses adjacent to the posterior aspect of the thyroid, close to

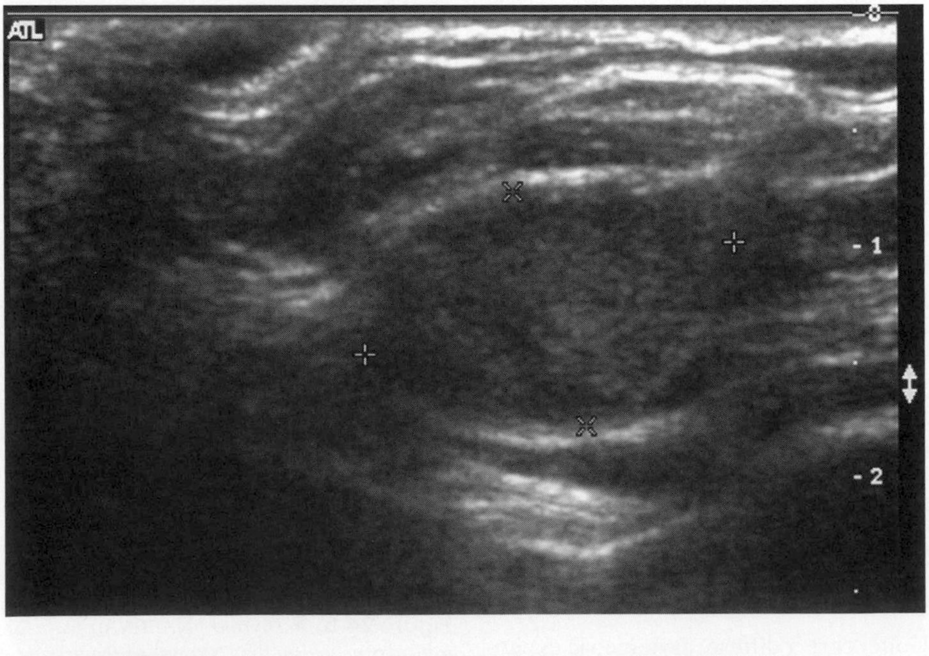

Figure 24-10. ■ *Palpable soft tissue mass in the neck. A 17- × 11-mm solid mass* (cursors) *at the left sternoclavicular joint, well away from the thyroid, was biopsy proven to be a metastasis from thyroid cancer.*

the carotid artery. Carefully sort out normal anatomic structures (Fig. 24-2). A parathyroid gland is considered abnormal if it measures more than 5 mm.

Pitfalls

1. Cyst versus solid lesion. Small solid lesions may be difficult to distinguish from cysts. Solid lesions should fill with echoes more easily. Observe the through transmission.
2. Identifying the mass. Small lesions may be displaced by the transducer and may never actually be imaged. Therefore, use very light pressure on the neck while scanning to keep the mass under the transducer. If the mass is palpable, immobilize it with your fingers and scan over the area of interest.
3. Isthmic mass. An anterior mass may be overlooked because of near-field artifact (reverberation) and contact problems.
4. Parathyroid adenoma. This type of adenoma may be mimicked by the following structures:
   a. The minor neuromuscular bundle. This structure has a longitudinal axis, unlike the ovoid parathyroid (Fig. 24-3).
   b. The esophagus. Scan while asking the patient to swallow water drunk through a straw to rule out the normal esophagus mimicking apparent left parathyroid enlargement or other pseudomass (Fig. 24-2).
   c. The longus colli muscle. This muscle is seen on both sides of the neck. Turning the probe to scan longitudinally will often easily show that the suspected mass seen in transverse plane is simply this muscle.
   d. Intrathyroidal adenoma. It may be impossible to distinguish an intrathyroidal adenoma from parathyroid gland enlargement (Fig. 24-3). Both are very vascular.

Where Else to Look

1. If a mass outside the thyroid could represent an enlarged lymph node, look for other adenopathy or a primary neoplasm in the abdomen.
2. An enlarged parathyroid gland, usually caused by an adenoma, causes hypercalcemia; check for renal calculi.

SELECTED READING

Frates MC, Benson CB, Charboneau JW, et al. Management of thyroid nodules detected at US: Society of Radiologists in Ultrasound Consensus Conference statement. *Radiology* 2005;237:794–800.

Hegedus L. Clinical practice. The thyroid nodule. *N Engl J Med* 2004;351:1764–1771.

Iannuccilli JD, Cronan JJ, Monchik JM. Risk for malignancy of thyroid nodules as assessed by sonographic criteria: the need for biopsy. *J Ultrasound Med* 2004;23:1455–1464.

Khati N, Adamson T, Johnson KS, et al. Ultrasound of the thyroid and parathyroid glands. *Ultrasound Q* 2003;19:162–176.

Lewis BD, Hay ID, Charboneau JW, et al. Percutaneous ethanol injection for treatment of cervical lymph node metastases in patients with papillary thyroid carcinoma. *AJR Am J Roentgenol* 2002;178:699–704.

Reading CC, Charboneau JW, Hay ID, et al. Sonography of thyroid nodules: a "classic pattern" diagnostic approach. *Ultrasound Q* 2005;21:157–165.

Titton RL, Gervais DA, Boland GW, et al. Sonography and sonographically guided fine-needle aspiration biopsy of the thyroid gland: indications and techniques, pearls and pitfalls. *AJR Am J Roentgenol* 2003;181:267–271.

Possible Testicular Mass: Pain in the Testicle

25

MIKE LEDWIDGE
CHRIS LABINSKI
TOM WINTER

SONOGRAM ABBREVIATIONS

E, EP	Epididymis
H	Hydrocele
M	Mass
MT	Mediastinum testis
S	Spermatocele
T	Testis
V	Varicocele

KEY WORDS

Appendix Epididymis. Embryologic remnant projecting off of the epididymis.

Appendix Testis. Embryologic remnant of the Müllerian duct. Small ovoid structure seen just beneath the head of the epididymis. Both the appendix testis and the appendix epididymis are best seen in the presence of a hydrocele.

Cryptorchidism (Undescended Testicle). Condition in which the testes have not descended and lie either in the abdomen or in the groin. The latter is the site in 95% of cases. The cryptorchid testicle and, to a lesser extent, the normally descended opposite testicle have an increased risk of malignancy.

Epididymis. "C"-shaped organ that lies posterolateral to the testicle in which the spermatozoa accumulate before passing out the vas deferens. It has three parts, the head (globus major), body (corpus), and tail (globus minor).

Epididymitis. Inflammation of the epididymis. Often associated with orchitis, inflammation of the testicle.

Hematocele. Blood filling the sac that surrounds the testicle.

Hydrocele. Distention of the sac that encloses the testicle with straw-colored fluid.

Mediastinum Testis. Linear fibrous structure in the center of the testicle.

Pampiniform Plexus. Group of veins that drain the testicle. They dilate and become tortuous when a varicocele is present.

Rete Testis. The tubules at the hilum of the testicle may become so large that they are visible as cylinders or cysts. This is a normal variant finding.

Scrotum. Sac in which the testes and epididymides lie.

Seminal Vesicles. Paired comma-shaped organs located posterior to the bladder that add fluid necessary for reproduction to the sperm arriving from the vas deferens.

Serous. Term used to describe thin, straw-colored fluid present within a cyst regardless of location (e.g., renal, thyroid, or ovarian cysts or hydrocele).

Spermatic Cyst (Spermatocele). Cyst along the course of the vas deferens containing sperm.

Testicle (Testis). Male gonad enclosed within the scrotum; it produces hormones that induce masculine features and spermatozoa.

Tunica Albuginea. White membrane surrounding the testicle within the scrotum; may be the source of a cyst or adenoma.

Tunica Vaginalis. Membrane skirting the inner wall of the scrotum. It has two parts: the inner or tunica vaginalis, and the outer or tunica albuginea. Hydroceles form between the two layers of the tunica vaginalis.

Varicocele. Dilated veins caused by obstruction of the venous return from the testicle. Varicoceles may be associated with infertility or tumors in the renal hilar regions.

Vas Deferens. Tube that connects the epididymis to the ejaculatory duct.

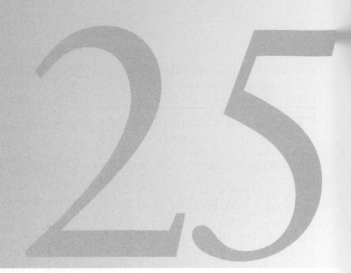

The Clinical Problem

MASS

The testicle is superficial and therefore easily examined with high-frequency ultrasound. The detection of a small mass within the testicle is important because such a mass may be malignant. Most intratesticular masses should be considered to represent cancer until proven otherwise; however, benign masses in the testicle occur. Although fluid within the scrotal sac is usually easily detected clinically, identification is difficult if the scrotal wall is thickened. An additional mass may be missed on palpation but revealed by ultrasound.

TESTICULAR PAIN

Ultrasound helps in the differential diagnosis of acute pain in a testicle. One can reliably differentiate between the two most common causes: epididymo-orchitis and associated complications (abscess), and testicular torsion. Doppler and color flow are particularly useful in making this distinction. Acute epididymitis is often followed by infection of the testicle (orchitis). Infarction of the testicle can also occur after severe epididymitis.

TESTICULAR TRAUMA

Trauma to the testicle is an ultrasonic emergency—rupture of the testicle requiring surgical repair has to be distinguished from a paratesticular hematoma (a hematocele). An unrepaired ruptured testicle atrophies and will not function.

INFERTILITY

A common cause of male infertility is a varicocele. Most varicoceles are palpable, but if a man has unexplained infertility, a sonogram to exclude a varicocele that cannot be felt is worthwhile.

UNDESCENDED TESTICLE

Most testicles descend from the abdomen into the scrotum by 28 weeks of fetal life. If descent is arrested in the abdomen or the groin, there is an increased chance of tumor development. Surgeons move the undescended testicle into the scrotum in the first few years of life. Ultrasound can be of help in locating a testicle that cannot be felt within the groin, although those that lie deep in the abdomen cannot be detected with ultrasound; magnetic resonance imaging or computed tomography may be necessary in those cases.

Anatomy

TESTICLE

The testicle is an ovoid, homogeneous, mildly echogenic structure (Fig. 25-1). The adult testicles are normally symmetric and approximately 3 to 5 cm in length, 2 to 4 cm in width, and 3 cm in anteroposterior dimension. A central line within each testicle is termed the "mediastinum testis."

A series of tubules radiate from the mediastinum testes into the testicle. Sometimes a vague hypoechoic region is seen. On other occasions, visible tubules or even cysts can form in this area as a benign normal variant, known as "rete testis" or tubular ectasia.

EPIDIDYMIS

The tubular, slightly sonolucent structure lying posterosuperior to the testicle

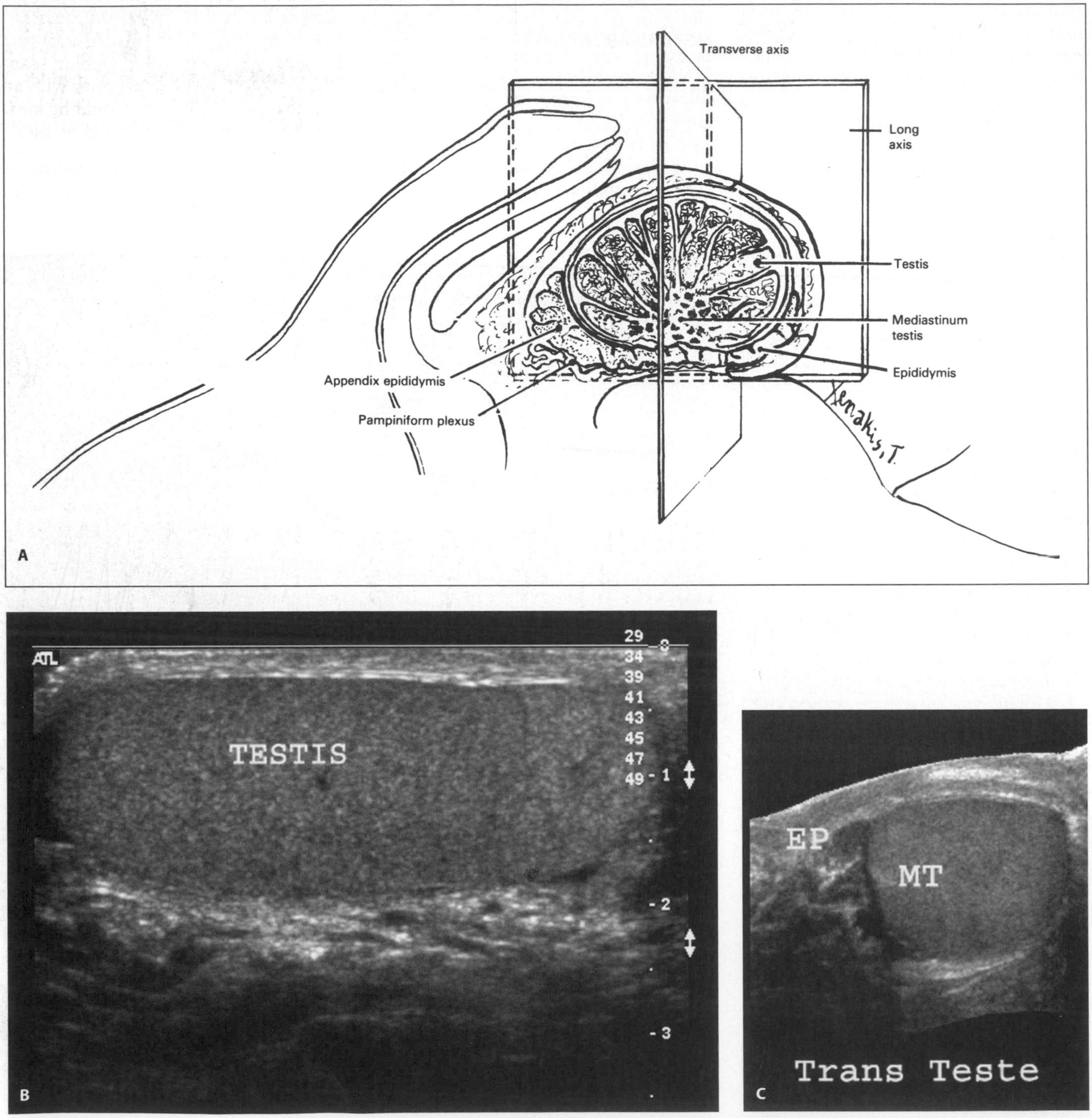

Figure 25-1. ■ *Diagram showing the normal structures visible within the scrotum. The mediastinum testis is only occasionally seen as an echogenic line. A. Diagram of imaging planes. B. Longitudinal axis view. C. Transverse axis view.*

at the proximal end is termed the "head of the epididymis." The body of the epididymis varies in its position and generally lies posterolateral to the testicle. The testicular artery and the veins of the pampiniform plexus run along the lateral and posterior aspect of the testicle in the region of the epididymis and are not normally visible. The epididymis is an echopenic structure.

SCROTAL WALL

The scrotal wall is an echopenic structure that surrounds the testicle and epididymis. The wall thickens with edema and infection. The two layers of the tunica vaginalis form a double layer around the testicle. Fluid can accumulate between these two layers forming a hydrocele. A small amount of serous fluid here is a common normal variant of no significance, but pus accumulating here ("pyocele") is a serious problem.

Technique

A high-frequency, broad-bandwidth, 7- to 14-MHz, linear-array transducer gives excellent resolution of superficial structures and yields superior axial and lateral resolution compared with other probes. The testicles and scrotum are optimally imaged with such a probe. Occasionally a curved array probe with a larger field of view can be used if the scrotum or testicular mass is too large to fit on the linear image due to intrinsic mass, swelling, or fluid collection. Current state of the art ultrasound machines have an extended field-of-view (XFOV) option that allows the full field of view to be imaged with a linear transducer. Some machines also have a virtual convex option that allows a slightly greater field of view while using a linear transducer. Support the testicles and scrotum with a towel under the scrotum or with the examiner's hand. By tucking the towel under the thighs, the scrotum is immobilized and elevated. Have the patient use another towel to retract and cover the penis. Then move the transducer smoothly and slowly along the anterior aspect of the scrotum. Image the testicles in the longitudinal axis from lateral to medial, measuring both the length and anteroposterior dimension. Transverse imaging is performed from superior to inferior measuring the maximum transverse axis. XFOV technology is an elegant way of demonstrating anatomic relationships and is helpful in showing differences in size and echogenicity between the two testicles. If this technology is not available, a coronal view from the side can often accomplish the same goal. Color Doppler images should be obtained in each testicle, and findings should be compared from side to side (using the same color settings) to demonstrate any asymmetry suggestive of torsion or inflammation. A spectral Doppler should be included of each testicle to prove definite arterial blood flow to each testicle. The epididymal head, body, and tail should be imaged with color flow Doppler to assess for the abnormal hyperemia suggestive of epididymitis.

If a mass is palpable, it must always be identified on the image. This may require placing a finger on the posterior aspect of the mass while performing a scan from an anterior approach, or having the patient localize the palpated mass between his fingers to ensure accurate imaging (Fig. 25-2). A posterior scanning approach may be necessary with an anterior mass. The mass should be measured and color Doppler used to assess the mass's vascularity.

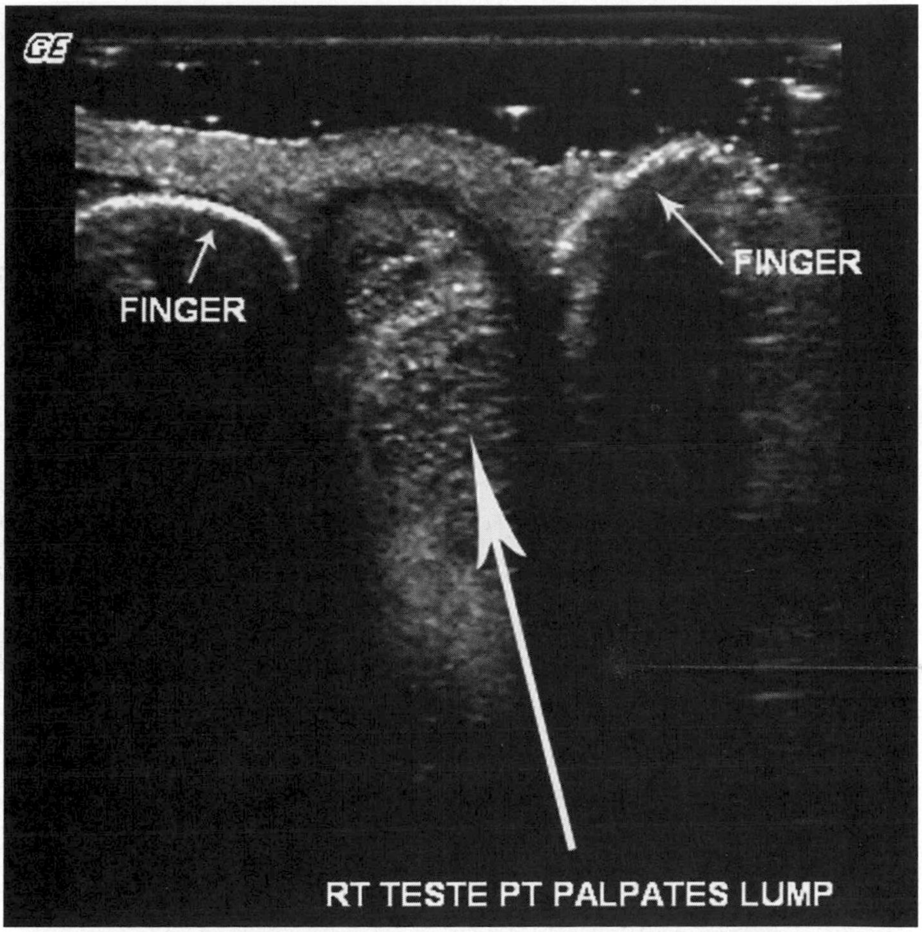

Figure 25-2. ■ *Sonogram obtained while the patient isolated the suspected mass between his fingers. In this case, the worrisome mass turned out to be the head of the epididymis (globus major), a normal structure. The ultrasound examination was immensely reassuring to this patient.*

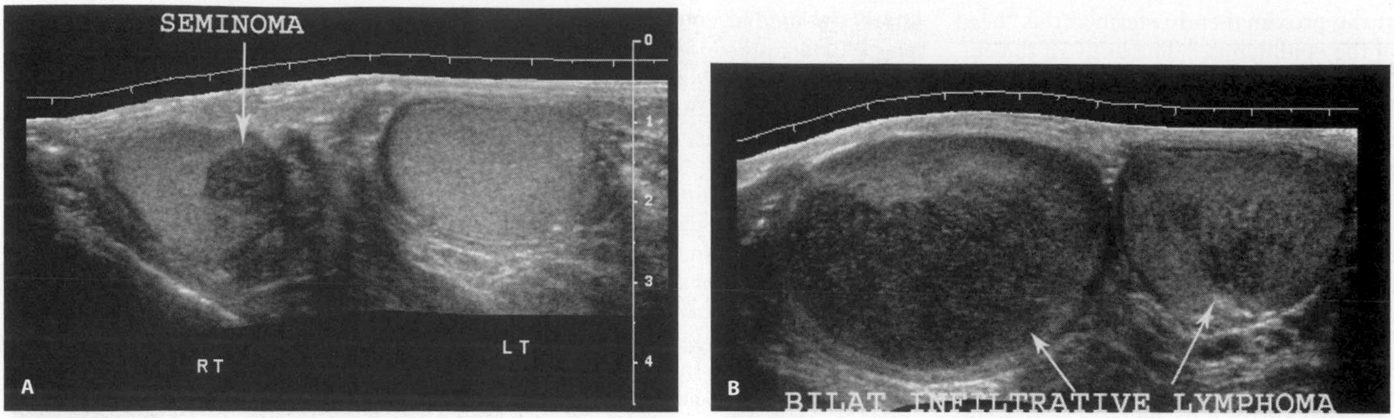

Figure 25-3. ■ *A. Extended field-of-view* (XFOV) *image shows an intratesticular mass caused by a seminoma in the right testis, and a normal left testicle. B.* XFOV *of bilateral infiltrative lymphoma of the testicle.*

Pathology

TUMORS

Normally, the testicle is of uniformly homogeneous echogenicity. The most common testicular tumor, a seminoma, is usually hypoechoic compared with the remaining testicular parenchyma. The tumor can be as small as 2 to 3 mm (Fig. 25-3A). Seminoma may be unifocal or multifocal. Mixed germ cell tumors (including embryonal, yolk sac, choriocarcinoma, and teratocarcinoma) are the second most common type of tumor and are typically much more heterogeneous than seminomas and may contain cystic regions. Metastases may occur to the testicles, generally in advanced cancer.

Lymphoma and leukemia may persist in the testicle when they have been eliminated elsewhere because chemotherapy often does not reach the testicle. Recurrence in the testicle may appear as either focal masses or enlarged, hypoechoic, hyperemic testicles (Fig. 25-3B).

BENIGN TESTICULAR MASSES

Cysts may be seen within or adjacent to the testicle. Small anechoic cysts on the border of the testicle are the common benign cysts of the tunica albuginea. Small, hard, echogenic mobile structures within the tunica vaginalis may be palpable but are of no importance. These scrotal calculi ("scrotal boulders" or "scrotal pearls") may show shadowing (Fig. 25-4).

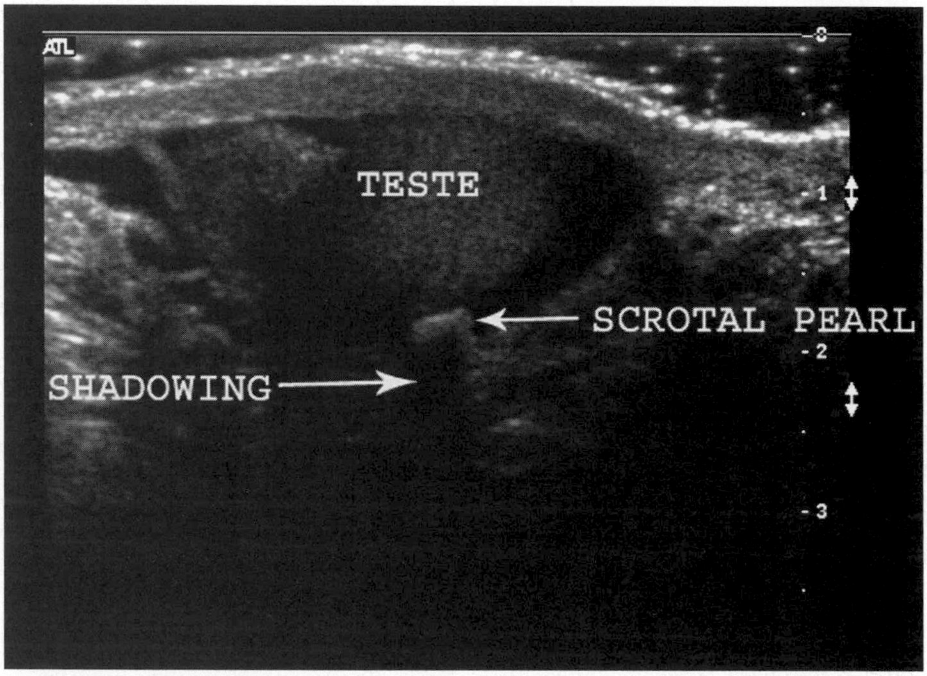

Figure 25-4. ■ *Benign "scrotal pearl." Note posterior acoustic shadowing from this calcified structure.*

EPIDIDYMITIS

Acute

The epididymis in acute epididymitis is enlarged, hypoechoic, and often heterogeneous. Comparison with the opposite, presumably unaffected, side is very useful (Fig. 25-5). Color flow may show increased blood flow in the epididymis due to inflammation. The epididymis is generally focally tender.

Chronic

A chronically inflamed epididymis becomes thickened and focally echogenic and may contain calcification.

ORCHITIS

Orchitis (infection of the testicle) may involve the entire testicle or rarely be focal. The testicle is isoechoic to hypoechoic depending on the severity of the disease.

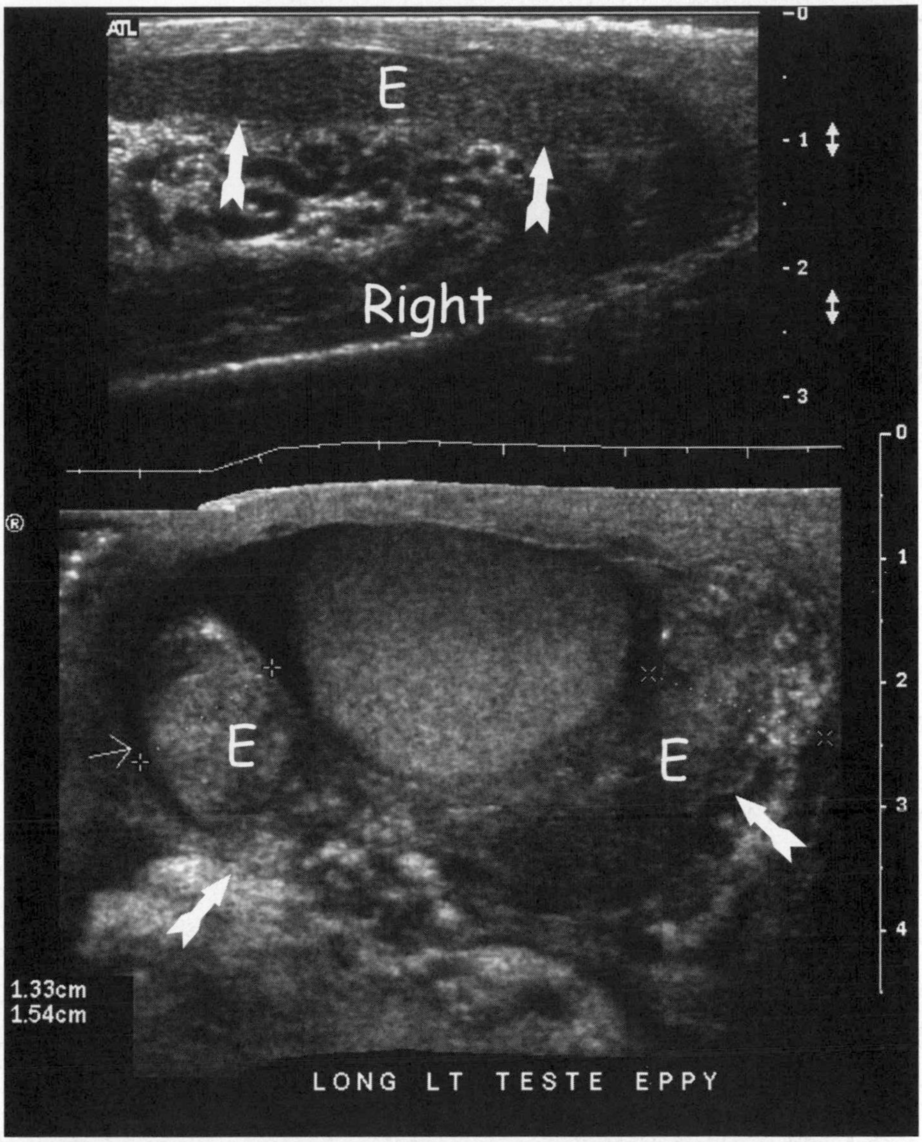

Figure 25-5. ■ *Acute epididymitis. Grayscale sonogram of the body of the normal right epididymis* (arrows, top) *shows normal size and internal architecture. Note how modern high-resolution ultrasound machines are capable of denoting the fine tubular structures of the normal epididymis. Contrast this appearance with the affected, painful left side. Here the left epididymis* (arrows, bottom) *is grossly enlarged with loss of the normal internal echotexture. This left epididymis was also markedly hyperemic at color Doppler imaging (not shown) when compared with the right side.*

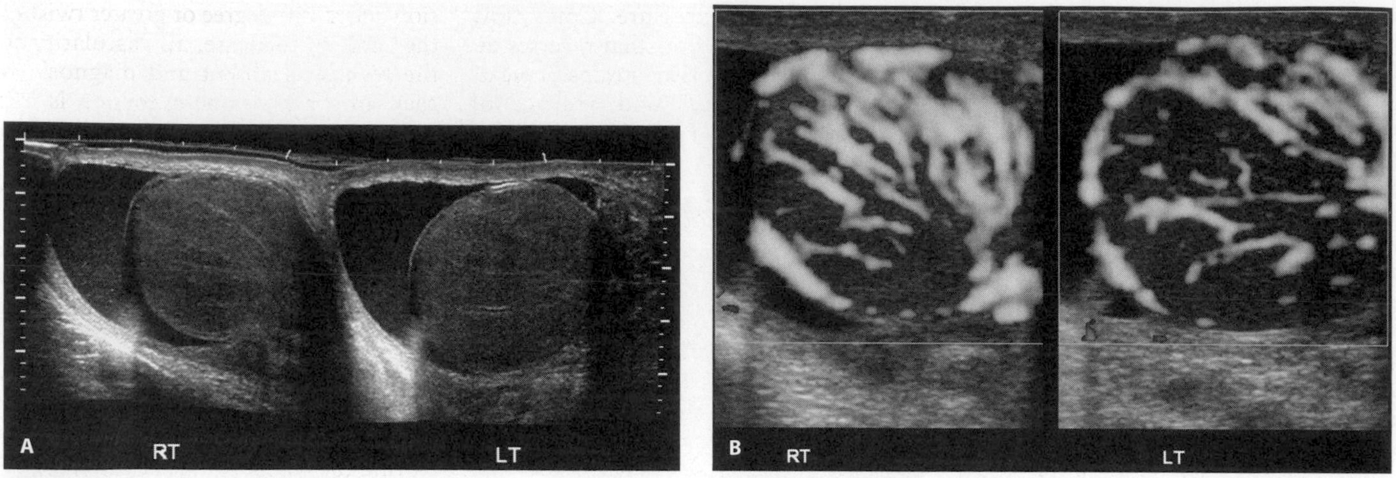

Figure 25-6. ■ *A. XFOV sonogram of a patient with bilateral orchitis and the typical hypoechoic appearance of the testicles. B. Power Doppler image of the same patient showing the expected marked hyperemia bilaterally.*

Infarction and some tumors may have a similar appearance. The scrotal wall is thickened with epididymitis and orchitis. Color flow may show increased vascularity in the testicle, epididymis, and scrotal wall (Fig. 25-6).

HYDROCELE

In hydrocele, the testicle and epididymis are surrounded by fluid, which is usually sonolucent, unless blood (hematocele) is present (Fig. 25-7A). Occasionally hydroceles have a proteinaceous composition and are evenly echogenic. If septa are present and the wall of the fluid-filled area is thickened, the collection may be infected and pus filled (pyocele). Pyoceles are very tender (Fig. 25-7B).

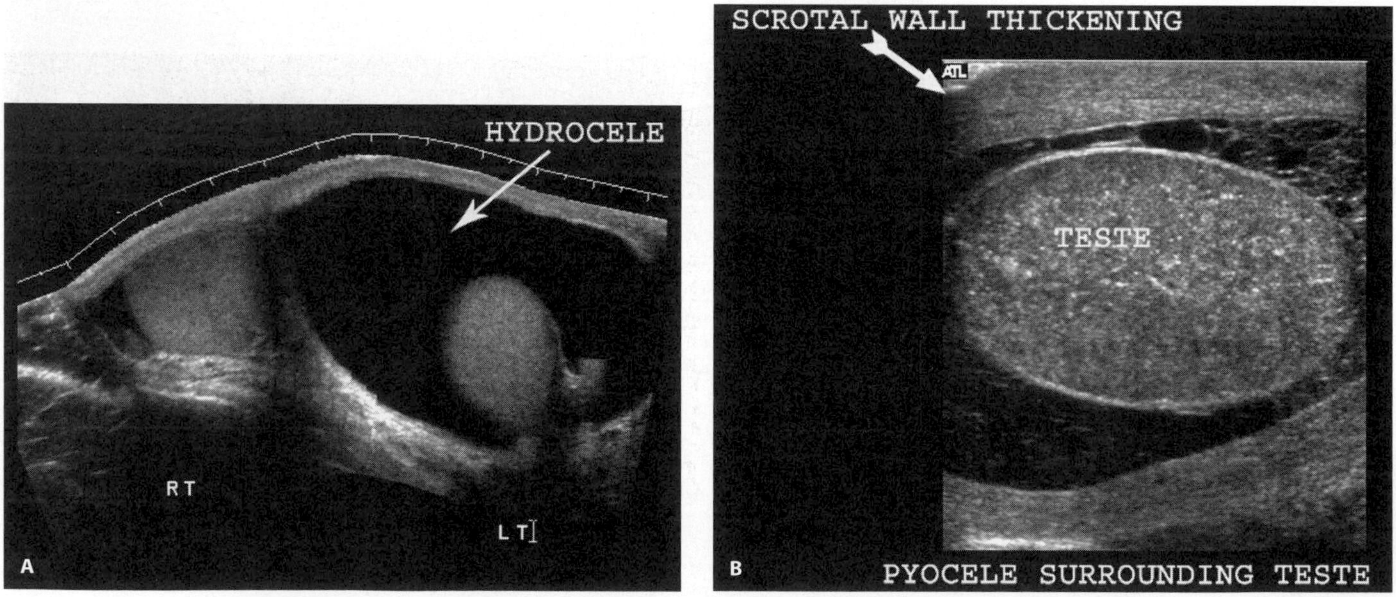

Figure 25-7. ■ *Fluid collections around the testicle. A. XFOV sonogram demonstrating a large left hydrocele and a normal right hemiscrotum. B. Pyocele surrounding the testicle in another patient. Note septations and thickening of scrotal wall.*

VARICOCELE

Varicoceles are numerous tortuous curvilinear venous structures in the region of the epididymis that extend superior to the testicle toward the pubic symphysis (Fig. 25-8 and Color Plate 25-1). They are much more common on the left side than the right side because the left gonadal vein empties into the left renal vein before coursing into the inferior vena cava (IVC), whereas on the right the gonadal vein goes directly to the IVC. A sizeable or sudden onset varicocele, especially on the right, raises the possibility of a renal tumor or obstructing hilar mass blocking the gonadal vein. Our protocol is to change to an abdominal transducer and to perform a brief examination of the ipsilateral renal hilum whenever a varicocele is detected, especially on the right side.

To demonstrate the dilated veins that form a varicocele, venous pressure must be increased by a Valsalva maneuver. Examination in the erect position also helps increase venous pressure (although we rarely perform this anymore due to improvements in ultrasound Doppler technology, relying instead on a Valsalva). The veins increase in size with increased venous pressure. Color flow and Doppler show flow that reverses direction when the patient strains, indicating "incompetence" and absence of valves in the vein (Fig. 25-8 and Color Plate 25-1).

TESTICULAR TORSION

Acute pain occurring in the testicle is most likely due to twisting (torsion) of the testicles or acute infection with epididymitis and orchitis. The distinction between these two problems is crucial because torsion is relieved by emergency surgery, whereas epididymitis is treated with antibiotics (Color Plates 25-2 and 25-3).

The window of opportunity to treat torsion is relatively small (8–12 hours). The testicle maintains a normal grayscale appearance acutely with torsion. If the testicle is normal on grayscale but shows no flow by color Doppler, the chance of successful surgical detorsion is high. With time, the torsed testicle enlarges and develops a mottled grayscale texture; an abnormal grayscale appearance in torsion carries a much less optimistic prognosis for successful surgical repair. Commonly, there is complete torsion and a 360-degree or greater twist of the cord. In this case, all vascularity to the testicle is absent and diagnosis is easy. In some instances, torsion is not complete, so some vascularity may be maintained, but comparison with the opposite testicle and the clinical scenario allows for accurate diagnosis.

If torsion is untreated (chronic torsion), the texture of the testicle changes, becoming more hypoechoic and mottled. Secondary enlargement of the epididymis can occur.

UNDESCENDED TESTICLES

During the embryologic development of the genitourinary tract, the testicles descend from the region of the kidneys into a normal location. Arrested development may occur at any point. However, the usual "sticking point" occurs when the testicles are in the region of the inguinal ligament and pubic symphysis in an extra-abdominal location. At this site, undescended testicles can be visualized by ultrasound. They can look like normal, malpositioned testicles, but may have a somewhat distorted shape or can be confused with lymph nodes.

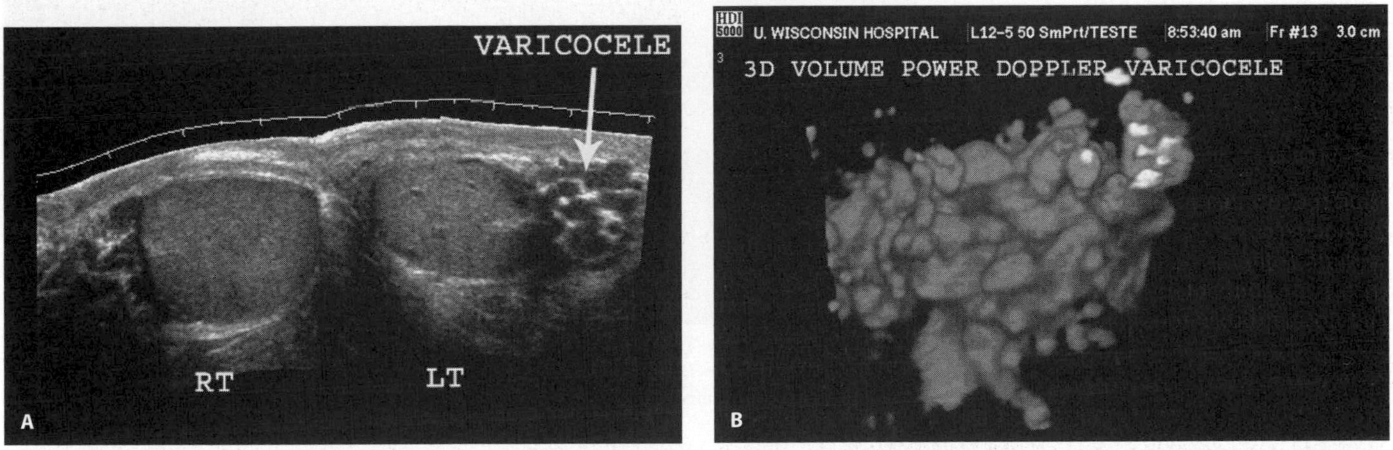

Figure 25-8. ■ *Varicocele. A. Varicocele, composed of numerous veins with a diameter of at least 3 mm, is seen lateral to left testicle on this XFOV image. B. Three-dimensional power Doppler image of this varicocele shows classic appearance of a "bag of worms" from dilated veins.*

SPERMATOCELE AND EPIDIDYMAL CYST

A cystic structure found along the course of the vas deferens superior to the testicle or in the epididymis, a spermatocele is of little clinical significance (Fig. 25-9). Spermatoceles may be multiple. They are sonolucent and have smooth walls. Epididymal cysts may be seen in the epididymis and appear identical to spermatoceles but are likewise of no clinical significance.

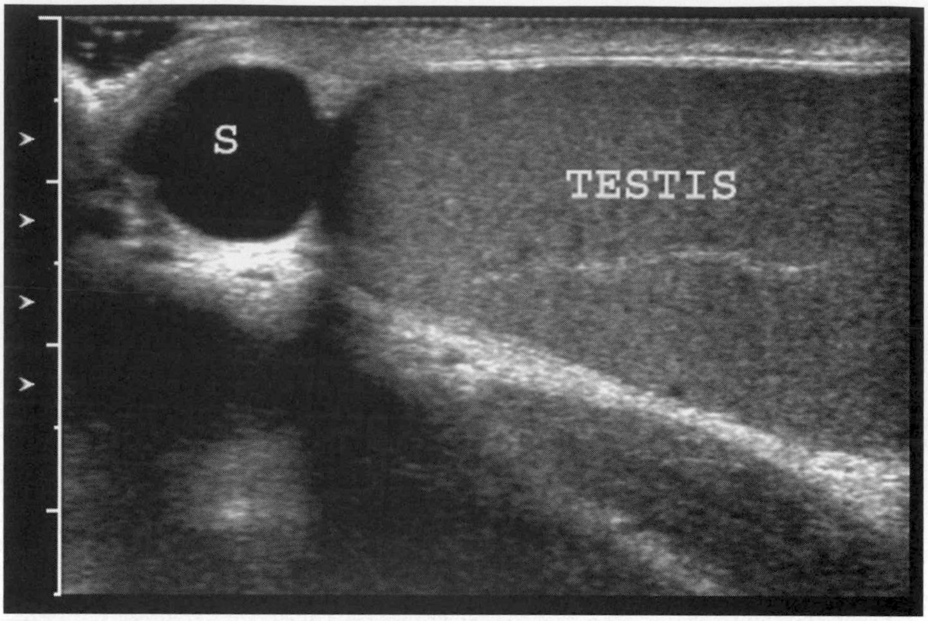

Figure 25-9. ■ *Spermatocele lying superior to the testicle.*

ATROPHIC TESTICLE

An infarcted testicle becomes small and echogenic. Color flow shows no vascularity within an atrophic testicle. Atrophy may occur after trauma, torsion, or infection.

ABSCESS

Abscesses may develop in the testicle or epididymis and are sonolucent with an echogenic, irregular border.

HERNIAS

A normal connection between the peritoneal cavity in the abdomen and the scrotal sac, known as the processus vaginalis, exists in every male fetus. This connection may persist after birth, allowing abdominal contents such as gut or properitoneal or omental fat to descend into the scrotum. Hernias are recognized by the presence of peristalsis on real-time imaging, by shadowing from air in the gut within the apparent mass or by the characteristic appearance of fat (Fig. 25-10). All hernias tend to move with Valsalva maneuver.

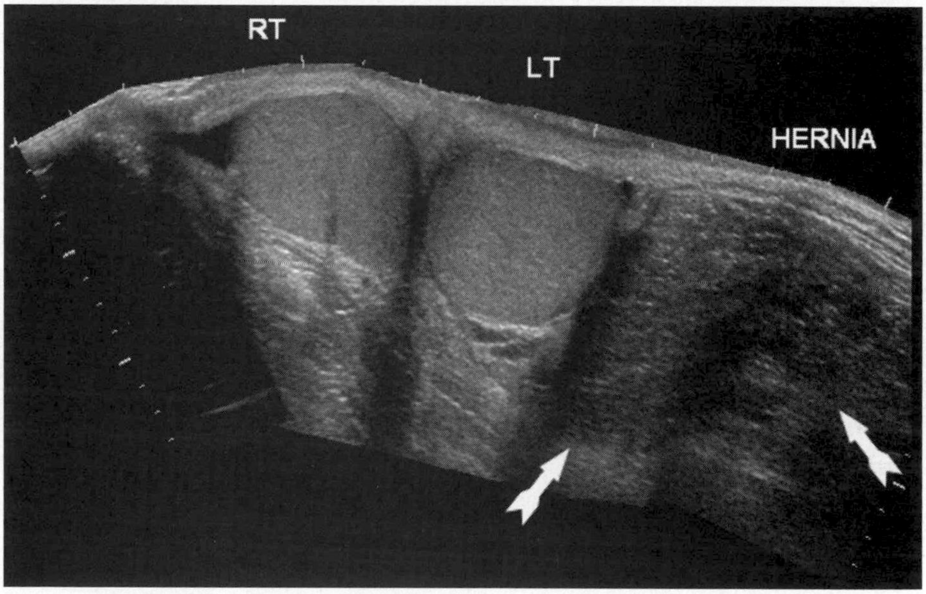

Figure 25-10. ■ *Hernia. Transverse extended field-of-view sonogram through the scrotum shows a normal right side and a large fat-containing hernia* (arrows) *lateral to the left testicle.*

TESTICULAR TRAUMA

A damaged scrotum almost always contains blood. Blood is generally echogenic with several different patterns. There are usually both echogenic and echo-free areas. The normal testicle has a smooth ovoid border. When the testicle is ruptured, the outline is irregular and there may be echopenic areas within. Sometimes a fracture line divides the testicle (Fig. 25-11). If not directly examined at surgery, any potential hematomas within the testicle must be followed with serial ultrasound to ensure that a small testicular tumor did not predispose the testicle to rupture.

TESTICULAR MICROLITHIASIS

Testicular microlithiasis (TM) refers to the presence of multiple small (1–3 mm) nonshadowing hyperechoic foci within

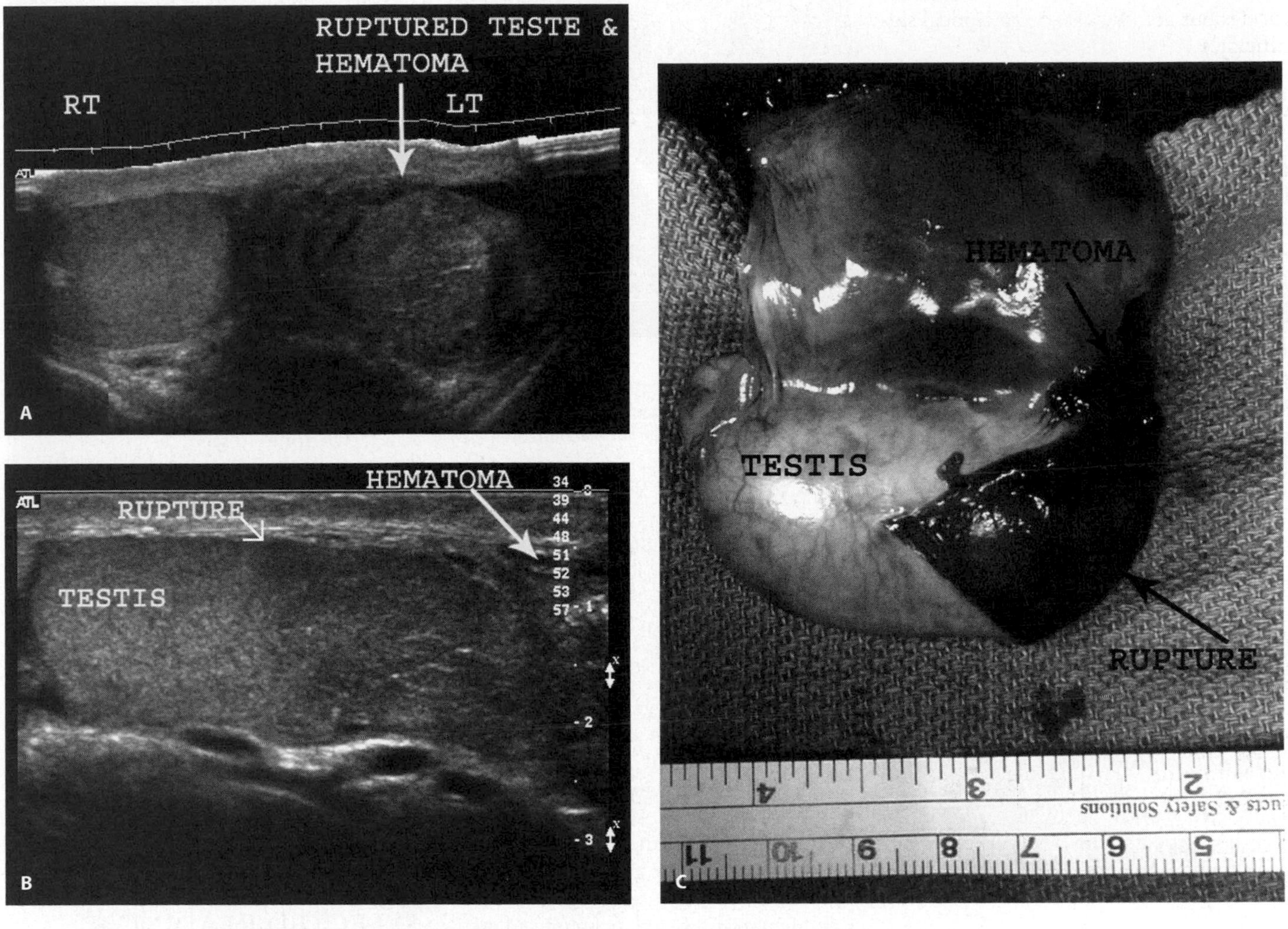

Figure 25-11. ■ *A. Fractured testicle after trauma (gunshot wound). XFOV sonogram shows a normal right testicle. The outline of the left testicle is irregular, caused by fluid (blood) surrounding the left testicle (i.e., a hematocele). **B.** Longitudinal image of this left testicle. The (subtle) fracture plane* (thin arrow) *and surrounding hematocele* (thick arrow). *Note the inhomogeneous echotexture of the testicle within the fracture. **C.** Intraoperative image of same testicle demonstrating gross pathology corresponding to the sonogram.*

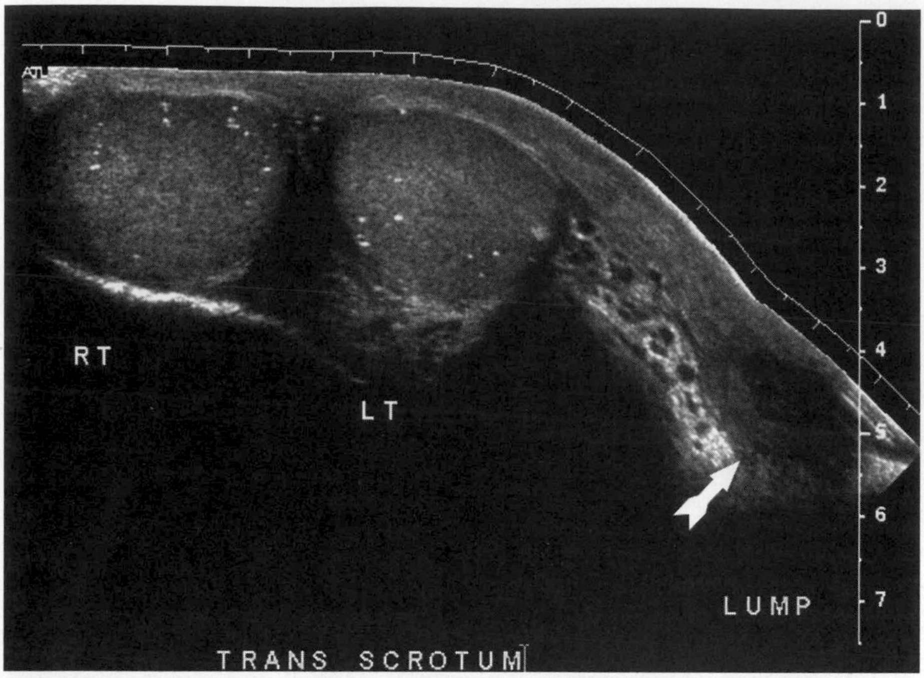

Figure 25-12. ■ *Testicular microlithiasis* (TM). *XFOV sonogram demonstrates multiple* (≥*5 per image*)*, bilateral, punctate, nonshadowing, echogenic foci within each testicle. This diagnosis was made incidentally; the patient presented for evaluation of a palpable scrotal mass* (arrow), *which turned out to be an infected hair follicle.*

the testicle (Fig. 25-12). The process is usually bilaterally symmetric. This entity is not as rare as once thought, approaching a prevalence of approximately 4% for the classic definition (five or more microliths in one image). TM is associated with germ cell neoplasm, but the strength of this association with malignancy is controversial. Any mass found in association with TM should be assumed to be malignant until proven otherwise, whereas patients with TM without mass should undergo periodic follow-up.

Pitfalls

1. Scanning technique. Scanning the testicle evenly and symmetrically can be difficult. Be sure that an apparent diminution in testicular size is not due to poor scanning technique, or that an apparent area of heterogeneous echotexture is not simply due to the intrinsically better resolution of current state-of-the-art transducers.
2. Mediastinum testis versus echogenic mass. Do not mistake the mediastinum testis for an echogenic mass.
3. Node versus undescended testicle. It is easy to confuse a benign inflammatory node with an undescended testicle. Benign nodes have an echogenic center due to fat deposition.
4. Position change for varicocele. Varicoceles can be overlooked unless the patient is stood up or a Valsalva maneuver is performed. Although varicoceles usually lie superior to the left testicle, they may lie lateral to the testicle and can occur on the right side.
5. Hematoma versus traumatized testicle. Some blood collections can resemble testicles. Identify the two testicles by noting these features:
   a. Smooth ovoid outline.
   b. Presence of mediastinum testis.
   c. Even echogenic texture. Carefully use the gain control to allow distinction between the testicle and hematoma.
   d. Subtle vessels in the normal testicle, seen with power Doppler.
6. Infarct versus focal orchitis versus seminoma. All three conditions can look similar. Color flow will show increased vascularity around areas of orchitis. Seminoma may contain flow within the center of the lesion. Infarcts show no flow.
7. Previous surgery for varicocele. When previous surgery has been performed, the varicocele does not disappear. However, the reversal of flow seen on Doppler with Valsalva maneuver is no longer present.
8. Rete testis (tubular ectasia). The tubules that collect at the mediastinum testes may be so dilated that they appear as a group of cysts. This normal variant can be confused with an echopenic tumor if a low-quality system is used. High-quality machines will show that the tubules are all interconnected. Tubular ectasia is often bilateral.
9. Cleft versus fracture. A prominent vessel often normally traverses the testicle. Flow will be evident on real-time imaging. This vessel could be mistaken for a fracture after testicular trauma, and it can cause shadowing over a portion of the testis that could suggest a carcinoma (the "two-tone" testis).

Where Else to Look

1. If a testicular tumor is found, look in the abdomen around the region of the renal hilum for possible nodal metastases.
2. If a varicocele is found on the right, look in and around the kidney for a tumor blocking the draining gonadal vein. Although left-sided varicoceles are usually isolated, a quick look in the left renal hilar area will occasionally discover pathology.

SELECTED READING

Dogra VS, Gottlieb RH, Oka M, et al. Sonography of the scrotum. *Radiology* 2003;227:18–36.

Kim, BI, Winter TC, Ryu J. Testicular microlithiasis: clinical significance and review of the literature. *Eur Radiol* 2003:13(12): 2567.

Middleton WD, Teefey SA, Santillan CS. Testicular microlithiasis: prospective analysis of prevalence and associated tumor. *Radiology* 2002;224:425–428.

Ragheb D, Higgins JL Jr. Ultrasonography of the scrotum: technique, anatomy, and pathologic entities. *J Ultrasound Med* 2002;21: 171–185.

Winter TC. Ultrasonography of the scrotum. *Appl Radiol* 2002;31(3):9–18.

Prostate

Prostate Carcinoma, Benign Prostatic Hypertrophy

TERESA BIEKER

26

SONOGRAM ABBREVIATIONS

AFMS	Anterior fibromuscular zone
Bl	Bladder
CZ	Central zone
ED	Ejaculatory duct
Ip	Iliopsoas muscle
NVB	Neurovascular bundle
Ob	Obturator muscle
Pr	Prostate gland
PZ	Peripheral zone
SP	Symphysis pubis
SV	Seminal vesicle
TZ	Transitional zone
UR	Urethra

KEY WORDS

Anterior Fibromuscular Stroma. Smooth muscle that forms the anterior surface of the prostate.

Apex. Inferior region of the prostate.

Base. Superior region of the prostate.

Benign Prostatic Hypertrophy (BPH). Nonmalignant enlargement of the glandular component of the prostate. The true prostate forms a shell around the enlarged gland. Common in older men.

Central Zone. Portion of the prostate that surrounds the urethra and encases the ejaculatory ducts. It is located at the prostatic base. It is typically the site of BPH but is rarely affected by prostate cancer. Accounts for 20% to 25% of the prostate glandular tissue.

Corpora Amylacea. Calcification within the prostate.

Ejaculatory Ducts. Paired ducts that connect the seminal vesicle and the vas deferens to the urethra at the verumontanum.

Neurovascular Bundle. Grouping of nerves, veins, and arteries located on the posterolateral aspect of the prostate at the junction of the seminal vesicles. Sonographically they appear hyperechoic.

Peripheral Zone. Comprises the posterior, lateral, and apical aspects of the prostate. The peripheral zone is the most common site for prostate cancer. It accounts for 70% of the prostate.

Prostate-Specific Antigen (PSA). A protein produced by the prostate gland. PSA levels may become elevated in the blood secondary to prostate cancer, BPH, or prostatitis.

Prostatitis. Inflammation of the prostate.

Seminal Vesicles. Paired glands that lie posterior and lateral to the base of the prostate. Responsible for producing fluid in which sperm move and are nourished.

TNM Classification. Staging technique for prostate cancer. "T" refers to tumor size, "N" refers to lymph node involvement, and "M" refers to the presence of metastasis.

Transitional Zone. Two small glandular areas located on either side of the proximal urethra. Comprises approximately 5% of the gland. It cannot be distinguished from the central zone by ultrasound.

Transurethral Resection of the Prostate (TURP). Surgical procedure most often used to treat men with BPH. A portion of the prostate is removed by a cystoscope to relieve pressure on the urethra.

Urethra. Canal through which urine is drained from the bladder. The urethra passes through the center of the prostate.

Vas Deferens. The ducts that convey sperm from the epididymis to the urethra.

Verumontanum. Junction of the ejaculatory ducts with the urethra.

RELEVANT LABORATORY VALUES:

PSA (Prostate-Specific Antigen)

Less than 4 ng/mL is normal.

More than 10 ng/mL increases the risk of prostate cancer by 67%.

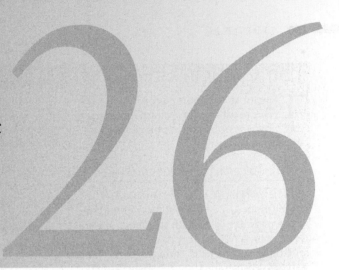

The Clinical Problem

The most common diseases to affect the prostate are benign prostatic hypertrophy (BPH), prostatic cancer, and prostatitis.

BENIGN PROSTATIC HYPERTROPHY

BPH is common in older men. As the name implies, it is a benign hypertrophy of the prostate. Although the exact cause is not completely understood, diminished androgen secretion is thought to be involved. Histologically, the transitional and central zones of the prostate undergo hypertrophy, resulting in an increase in fibromuscular stroma. The enlarged prostate obstructs the outflow of urine by compressing the prostatic urethra. Symptoms include a poor urinary stream and frequent urination. Hydronephrosis may occur secondary to urethral obstruction. Ultrasound can be used to determine:

1. the size of the prostate, which determines the type of treatment.
2. the amount of postvoid residual urine in the bladder.
3. the presence of hydronephrosis.

PROSTATE CANCER

Prostate cancer is the second most common cancer in American men. More than 70% of prostate cancers are diagnosed in men over 65 years of age. The disease is much more common in African-American men then in white men. It is less common in Asian and American Indian men. A man's risk of developing prostate cancer is elevated if he has an affected father or brother. Prostate-specific antigen (PSA) is a blood test that is usually elevated in the presence of prostate cancer, but may also be elevated by BPH or prostatitis. PSA levels also increase with age. Many unsuspected cancers are found when a PSA is performed on a screening basis. If symptoms are present, they usually include difficult or painful urination. In the setting of an increased PSA or an enlarged prostate by digital rectal examination, ultrasound can be used to identify the presence of a prostatic mass. However, not identifying a focal mass does not decrease the risk of prostate cancer being present. Ultrasound is also used to:

1. aid in the biopsy of patients with increased PSA.
2. attempt to stage periprostatic spread.
3. guide radiotherapy treatment.

PROSTATITIS

Prostatitis is defined as inflammation or infection of the prostate gland. Prostatitis is usually classified as acute, chronic, or noninfectious. Acute and chronic infectious prostatitis are caused by bacteria and treated with antibiotics. Noninfectious prostatitis is a chronic condition not caused by bacteria. Causes are not fully understood but may include mechanical or chemical trauma, or an autoimmune process. The role of sonography in acute prostatitis may be limited. In many cases, the patient may not be able to tolerate the transrectal ultrasound secondary to pain.

Anatomy

SEMINAL VESICLES AND VAS DEFERENS

The two paired seminal vesicles lie posterior to the bladder and superior to the prostate (Figs. 26-1 and 26-2). Typically, they are symmetric in size, homogeneous, and hypoechoic. The internal fluid is usually simple, but complex fluid may also be visualized. The size of the seminal vesicles is variable.

The vas deferens inserts on the medial aspect of the seminal vesicle to form the bilateral, paired ejaculatory ducts (Fig. 26-1).

PROSTATE

The prostate is a pear-shaped organ with the urethra running through the center. The base is the superior end closest to the bladder. The inferior margin is the apex. At the apex of the prostate lies a thin

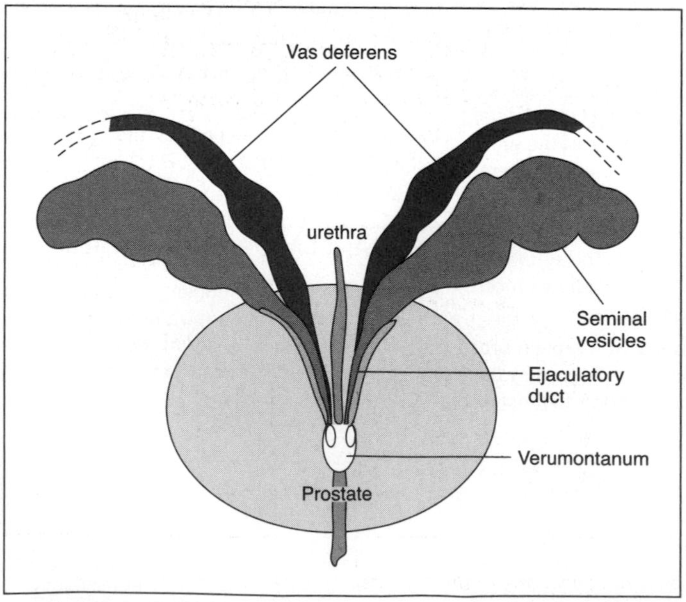

Figure 26-1. ■ *Diagram showing the relation of the seminal vesicles to the vas deferens. Both structures empty into the ejaculatory duct that ends at the verumontanum.*

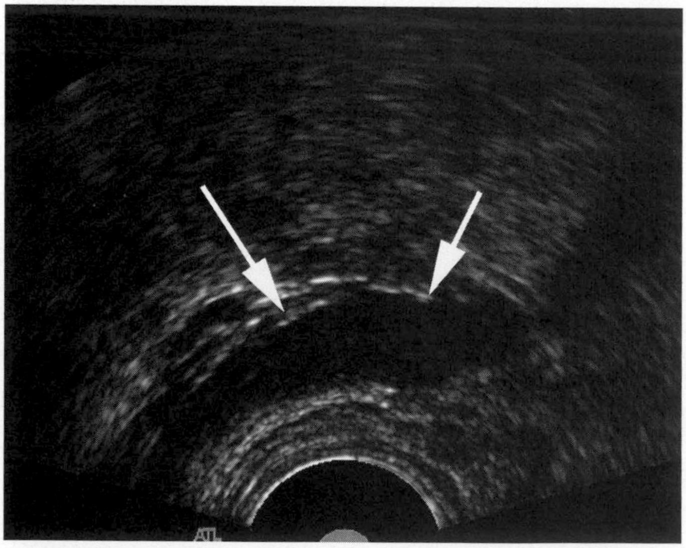

Figure 26-2. ■ *Normal view of a seminal vesicle* (arrows) *by transrectal ultrasound imaging.*

muscular structure, the urogenital diaphragm, separating the prostate from the penile structures. Sonographically, the normal prostate gland is homogeneous, with the fibromuscular stroma appearing slightly more hypoechoic.

The central and transitional zones surround the urethra. Cupping the central and transitional zones posteriorly is the peripheral zone. The peripheral zone is relatively larger at the apex. The peripheral zone is typically isoechoic to the central and transitional zones.

EJACULATORY DUCTS

The ejaculatory ducts run alongside the peripheral zones within the prostate, from the seminal vesicles to the verumontanum. They are normally quite small but are visible by ultrasound (Figs. 26-1 and 26-3).

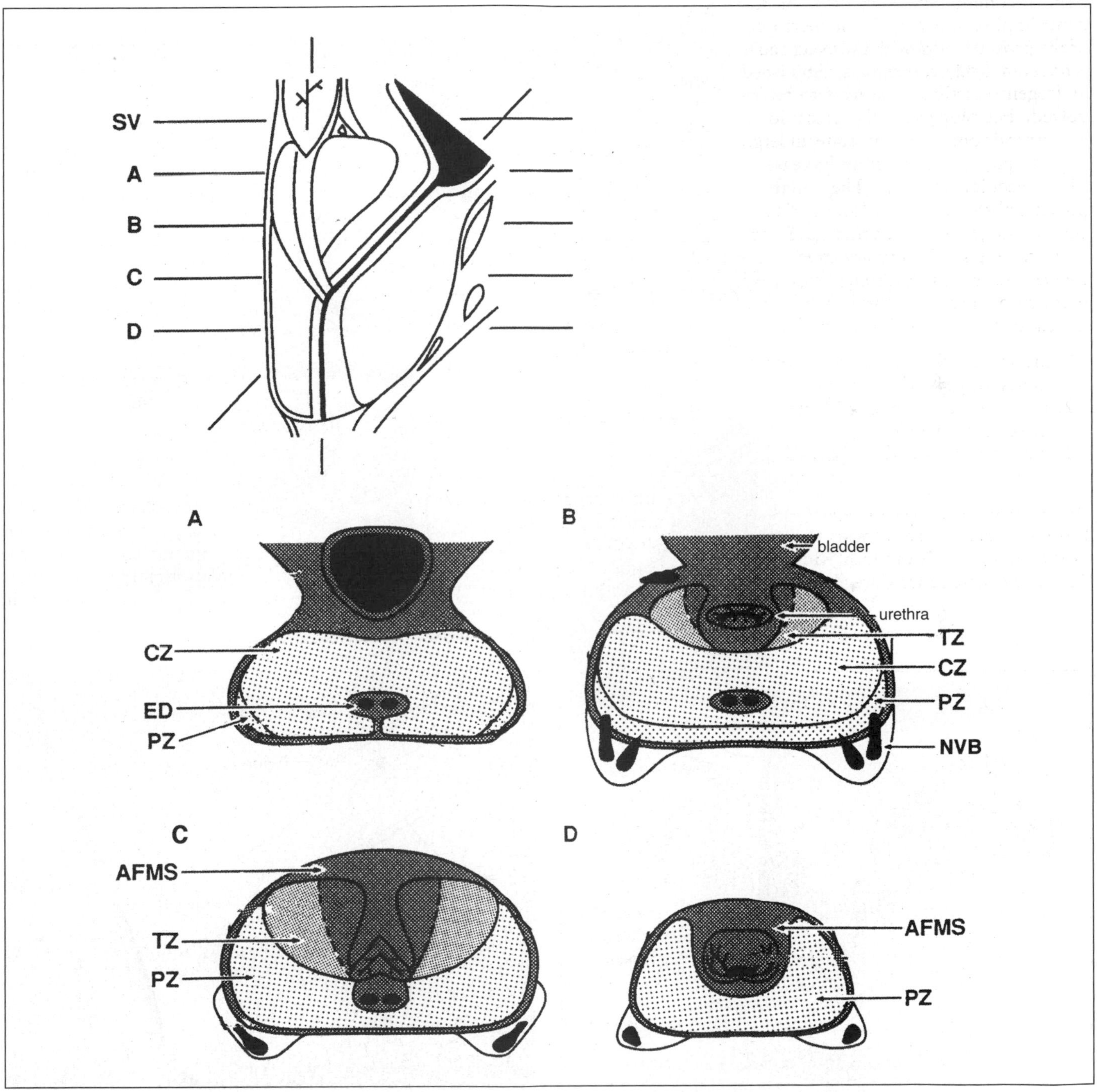

Figure 26-3. ■ *Diagram of the longitudinal and transverse anatomy of the prostate, showing the location of the central* (CZ), *transitional* (TZ), *peripheral* (PZ), *and fibromuscular zones* (AFMS). *The neurovascular bundles are seen at the posterolateral aspect* (NVB). *(Adapted from Villers A, Terris MK, McNeal JE, et al. Ultrasound anatomy of the prostate.* J Urol *1990;143:732–738, with permission.)*

PROSTATE VOLUME

The normal prostate volume is less than 20 mL in younger men. In older men, prostate volumes greater than 40 mL are considered enlarged. Volume is calculated using the formula for a prolate ellipse:

$$\text{Length} \times \text{Width} \times \text{Height} \times 0.523$$

Because the specific gravity of the prostate is approximately 1, a direct translation to grams can be made from volume. This formula may also be used to estimate volume of a prostate mass.

Technique

TRANSABDOMINAL APPROACH

Although an enlarged prostate may be visualized transabdominally, this approach is generally not considered adequate to evaluate the prostate (Fig. 26-4). By using

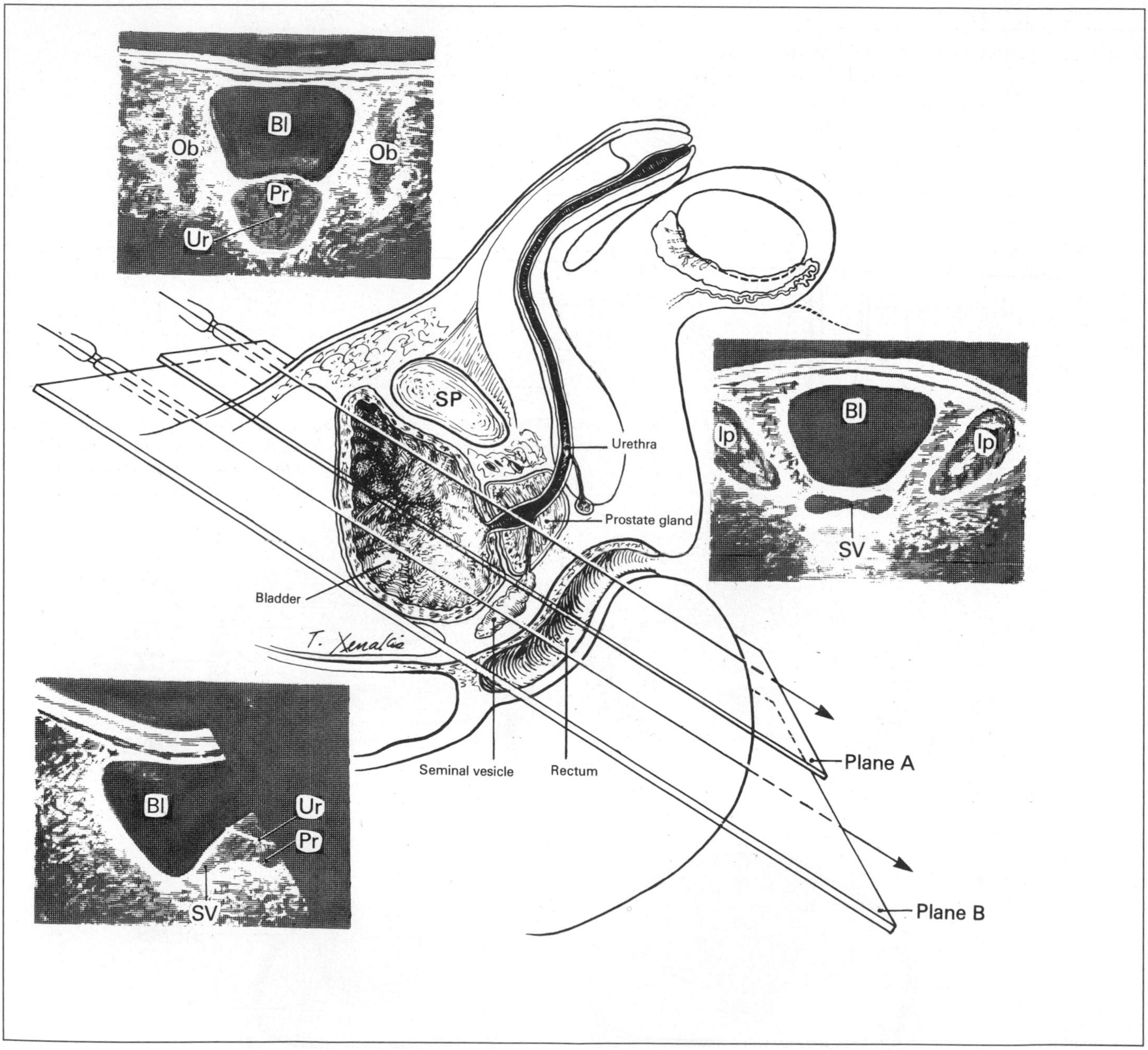

Figure 26-4. ■ *Prostate and bladder. Diagram showing the prostate being examined in an oblique axis through the bladder acoustic window.* Top left: *Section taken at plane A through the prostate. Note the obturator muscles.* Right: *Section taken at plane B at a higher level showing the seminal vesicle posterior to the bladder.* Bottom left: *Longitudinal section showing the urethra, prostate, and seminal vesicles.*

a 3.5- to 5-MHz transducer and a full bladder, the prostate may be identified by angling slightly inferior. Longitudinal and transverse images and measurements may be obtained; however, a thorough evaluation of prostate tissue is not possible. A transabdominal approach allows postvoid residual within the bladder to be determined (length × width × height × 0.523).

TRANSPERINEAL APPROACH

Imaging the prostate from an abdominal approach may be difficult if the bladder cannot be adequately filled (Fig. 26-5). A perineal approach can be used, scanning between the legs posterior to the scrotum. Again, this is not an ideal way to evaluate the prostate by ultrasound. Both transverse and longitudinal images can be obtained and the prostate volume can be calculated; however, internal architecture may not be well appreciated. This approach can be used for biopsy if the patient has had a surgical removal of the rectum.

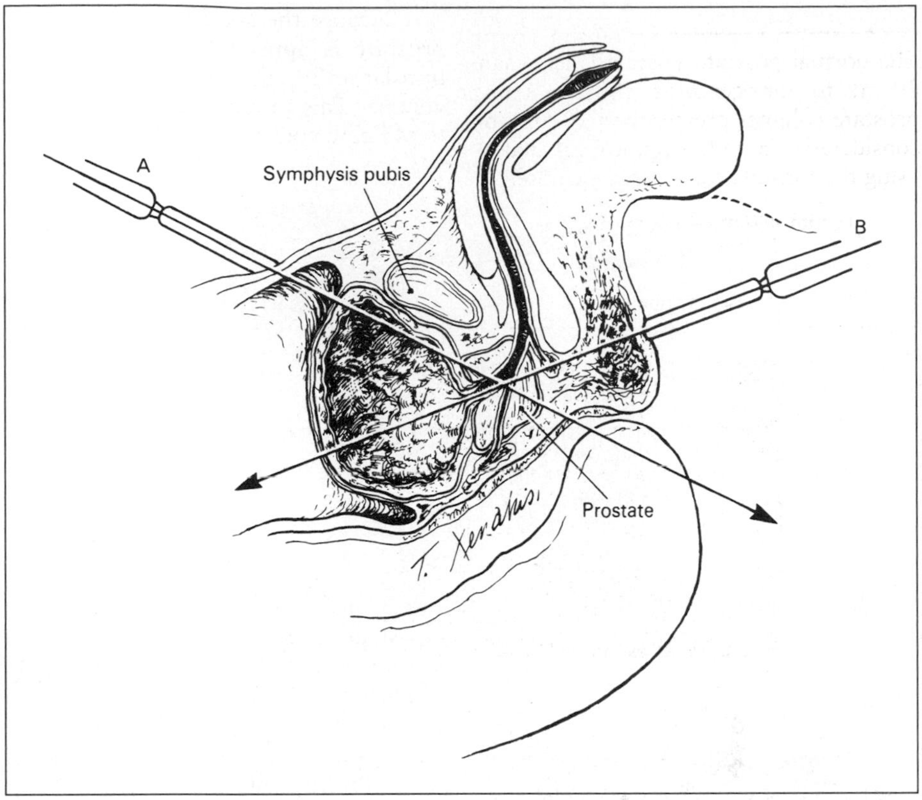

Figure 26-5. ■ *Diagram showing two approaches used to avoid the bone in the symphysis pubis when scanning the prostate. From an abdominal approach (**A**), the transducer is tilted toward the feet at an angle of 15 to 30 degrees; the beam passes through the acoustic window of the bladder to the prostate. A second approach (**B**) uses the perineum as a window for viewing the prostate. The sonographer scans through a site posterior to the scrotum.*

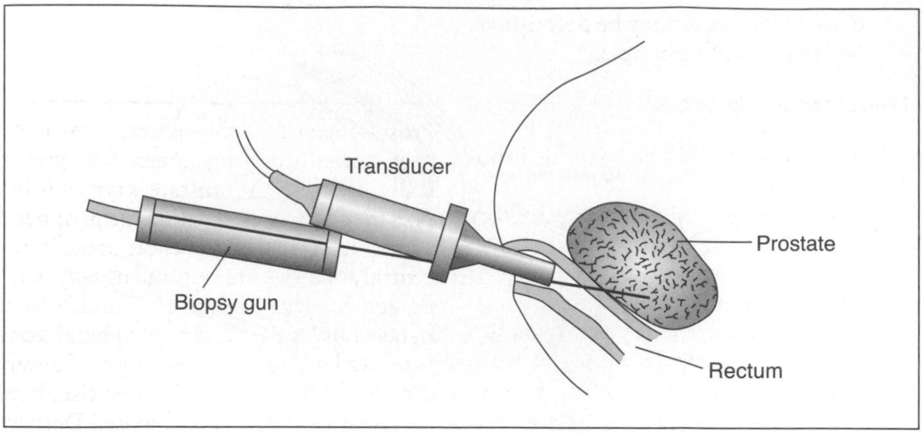

Figure 26-6. ■ *Transrectal biopsy technique. The needle is inserted alongside the transducer with the transducer inside the rectum.*

TRANSRECTAL APPROACH

Transrectal ultrasound is the most accepted scanning approach when evaluating the prostate (Figs. 26-6 and 26-7).

Probe Preparation and Patient Position

Ultrasound transducers best suited for transrectal visualization are 5- to 9-MHz endocavitary transducers. The probe should be covered with a condom or protective sheath. The patient is placed in a left lateral decubitus position with the knees bent.

Probe Insertion

Insert the probe and then angle slightly posterior, following the curve of the rectum. Continue to insert until the prostate is visualized. Performing a digital rectal examination before inserting the probe is often useful in excluding any potential obstructing masses and determining the appropriate angle for probe insertion to lessen the discomfort of the procedure.

Performing the Scan

Transrectal prostate scanning is performed in transverse and longitudinal planes.

Transverse plane. Start above the base of the prostate at the level of the seminal vesicles. The symmetry of the seminal vesicles should be documented. Multiple images of the prostate from the base to the level of the apex should also be documented. A transverse measurement of the prostate at its widest point should be obtained.

Longitudinal plane. Multiple longitudinal images should be obtained from one lateral aspect of the prostate to the other. Images should be appropriately labeled "left," "right," or "midline." A midline image of the prostate using the distal urethra at the apex and the proximal urethra at the base as landmarks should be used to obtain measurements in both the longitudinal and anterior-posterior planes.

Problems with Bowel Gas

If gas obstructs views of the right lobe of the prostate, place the patient in the right decubitus position. This may allow bowel gas to rise to the left side. In addition, in older probes equipped with a water path, more water can be injected to displace bowel gas.

Probe Care

After a prostate ultrasound, remove the sheath and soak the probe in a suitable disinfectant, such as Cidex for the time period suggested by the manufacturer (see Chapter 55).

BIOPSY

Two methods of prostate biopsy may be used: transrectal and transperineal. The

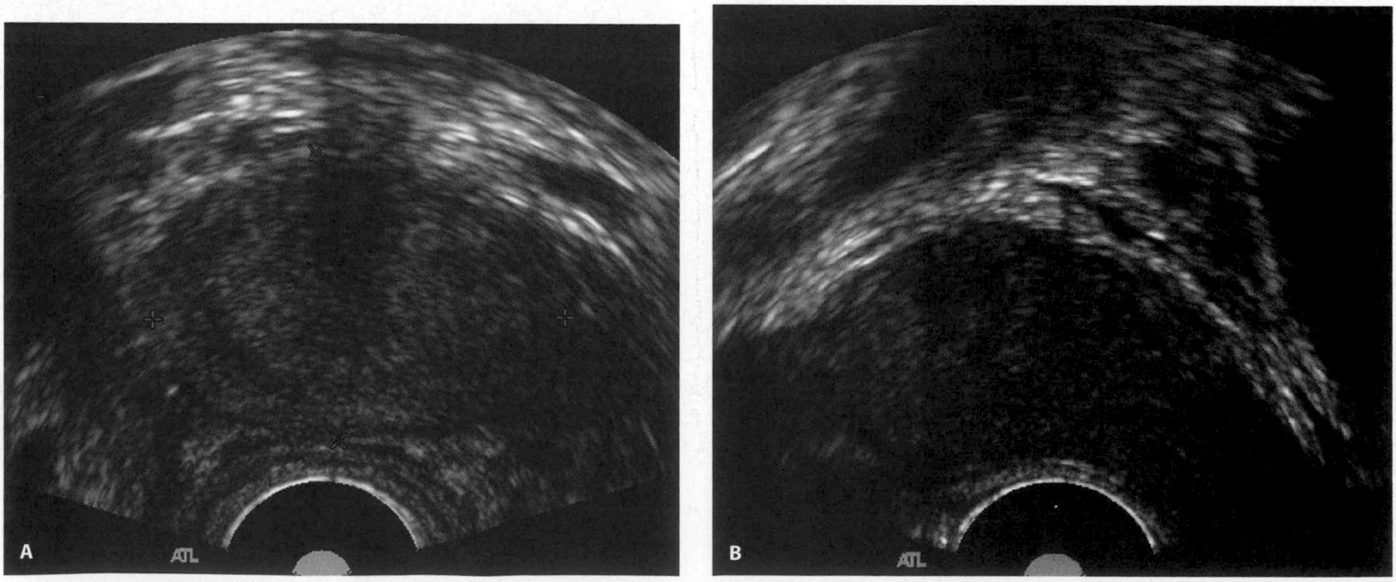

Figure 26-7. ■ *Coronal (A) and sagittal (B) transrectal views demonstrating a normal prostate.*

transrectal approach is more common and less painful but carries a greater risk of infection. The transperineal approach is generally only used for radiotherapy seed placement or if the rectum is absent.

Transrectal Technique

(See Figure 26-6.)

1. Informed consent is obtained by the physician.
2. The patient is prepared by giving an antibiotic 24 hours before the performance of the biopsy.
3. The needle guide is placed alongside the transrectal transducer. The guide and transducer are covered with a sterile condom.
4. The transducer is inserted, and the biopsy guide marks are displayed on the screen.
5. Lidocaine may be injected into the neurovascular bundle at the confluence of the seminal vesicle and prostate bilaterally as well as at the apex of the prostate. A wait time of 5 to 10 minutes is used to allow the anesthetic to take affect. In addition, moderate (conscious) sedation may be administered under Joint Commission on Accreditation of Healthcare Organizations guidelines (generally, a combination of fentanyl and midazolam, although there are a variety of anxiolytics and analgesics that can and have been used).
6. The biopsy device, usually a biopsy gun, is inserted until it can be seen at the edge of the prostate or mass. The gun is then fired. If a specific mass is visualized, the biopsy needle can be directly aligned with the mass.
7. Additional random passes are made in the superior, central, and inferior portions of each side of the gland. The specific number of biopsies varies by physician, but current literature recommends 12 to 18 passes (6 to 9 on each side). Several different systems are in use for describing the portions of the gland, but two of the more common use "1" or "A" for the right superior gland (base); "2" or "B" for the right middle gland; "3" or "C" for the right inferior gland (apex); "4" or "D" for the left superior gland; "5" or "E" for the left middle gland; and "6" or "F" for the left inferior gland. When in doubt, given the variety of nomenclatures in use, simply be descriptive, for example, "right apex."

Transperineal Approach

1. The patient is placed in the lithotomy position.
2. A side- or end-viewing endocavitary transducer is placed within the rectum until the lesion can be seen. If the rectum is absent, a linear transducer is placed on the peritoneum.
3. The perineal area is cleansed with antiseptic, and local anesthesia is injected. Premedication or moderate sedation is useful.
4. When the lesion has been identified and biopsy guide markers have been placed on the screen, a needle is inserted through the perineum until it can be seen within the mass.
5. Either an aspiration or biopsy technique for obtaining tissue is used.

After either procedure, blood pressure and pulse are taken because hemorrhage is a possible complication. Infection on a delayed basis may occur after a transrectal biopsy, but it is uncommon. It is expected that blood may be seen within stool, urine, or sperm after the procedure, for up to 48 hours. Severe bleeding is extremely rare.

Pathology

PROSTATE CANCER

Prostate cancer is the second most common cancer occurring in men. Sonographically, cancer of the prostate is typically hypoechoic and located within the peripheral zone (Fig. 26-8). Hypoechoic areas in the central zone are common and usually of little significance. Between 10% and 20% of hypoechoic areas in the peripheral zone prove to be carcinoma on biopsy. Cancers can also be isoechoic and not be visualized on ultrasound. Color and pulsed Doppler may show increased blood flow within a prostate cancer; however, this finding can also be seen with prostatitis or after ejaculation for at least 24 hours.

A deformed prostatic outline at the site of the presumed cancer is indicative of capsular invasion. Involvement of the seminal vesicles is less likely to be visualized but is important in predicting inoperability and poor prognosis. Seminal vesicle invasion is likely if the tumor extends to the edge of the seminal vesicle.

Carcinoma of the prostate may spread to pelvic or para-aortic lymph nodes. Enlargement of these nodes can occasionally be seen with ultrasound. Other common sites for metastases include the lungs, bones, and brain.

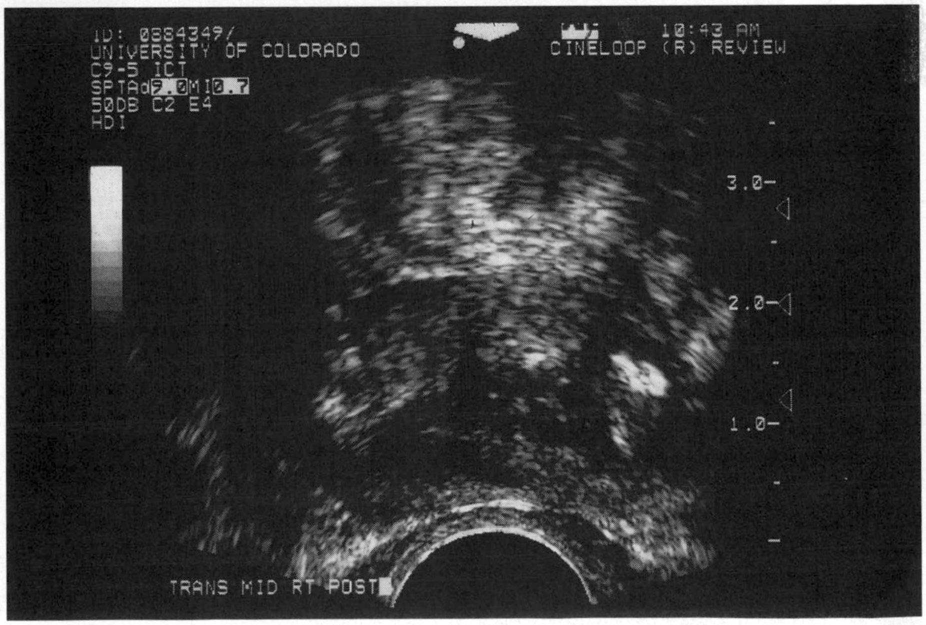

Figure 26-8. ■ *Coronal image of prostate cancer. Note the hypoechoic regions within the peripheral zone.*

lateral kidney. Seminal vesicle cysts have also been associated with autosomal dominant polycystic kidney disease.

PROSTATE CYST

The differential diagnosis for a prostatic cyst includes Müllerian duct cysts, utricle cysts, prostatic retention cysts, and ejaculatory duct cysts. An ejaculatory duct cyst is suggested when a cyst is seen posterior to the prostatic urethra, just lateral to midline. Müllerian duct cysts and utricle cysts are midline cystic structures that do not contain sperm when aspirated. Müllerian duct cysts often extend above the prostate and may manifest as large pelvic masses. Utricle cysts vary in size, but are usually smaller than Müllerian duct cysts and do not extend above the prostate. Prostatic retention cysts occur as a result of BPH and are usually 2 to 6 mm in size. They can be scattered within the central zone or the junction of the central and peripheral zones.

INFERTILITY

Absence of sperm (azoospermia) has various causes including blockage of the ejaculatory ducts or congenital absence of the seminal vesicles and vas deferens. Transrectal ultrasound can often show the cause of an ejaculatory duct obstruction, a cyst or calcification, dilatation of the ejaculatory ducts, or dilatation of the seminal vesicles. In addition, agenesis of the seminal vesicles or vas deferens may be appreciated by ultrasound.

Pitfalls

1. The lateral border of the peripheral zone on the dependent side may have a hypoechoic rim suggestive of neoplasm or infection. Because this can be artifactual, when the patient is turned onto the opposite side, this appearance changes.
2. A small posterolateral hypoechoic area is present adjacent to the peripheral zone on either side. This represents the neurovascular body and is a normal structure (Fig. 26-3). Color flow will show venous structures within.
3. Increased gain settings or reverberation artifact may cause a hypoechoic neoplasm to be overlooked. Optimize overall gain and time-gain compensation or alter the position of the probe in relation to the rectal wall to change the position of the reverberation artifact.
4. Peripheral zone calcifications can obscure hypoechoic areas located more centrally.
5. Prostate cancer can be present even if no focal lesions are detected within the prostate; therefore, prostate ultrasound cannot be used as a screening tool.
6. Use a generous volume of lubricant on your gloved finger for the digital rectal examination and on the ultrasound probe to minimize patient discomfort.
7. It is easy to confuse right and left while scanning the patient in the left lateral decubitus position. Double check your labeling while scanning the patient.

Where Else to Look

1. If the prostate is enlarged due to BPH:
   a. Evaluate the kidneys to exclude obstructive hydronephrosis.
   b. Evaluate the bladder size before and after voiding. Calculate the postvoid residual by using the following formula: length $\times$ width $\times$ height $\times$ 0.523.
2. If carcinoma of the prostate is suspected, evaluate for:
   a. Evidence of capsular or seminal vesicle invasion.
   b. Pelvic and para-aortic adenopathy.
3. If a seminal vesicle cyst is seen, evaluate for ipsilateral renal agenesis.

SELECTED READING

Berger AP, Gozzi C, Steiner H, et al. Complication rate of transrectal ultrasound guided prostate biopsy: a comparison among 3 protocols with 6, 10, and 15 cores. *J Urol* 2004;171(4):1478–1481.

Bree RL, Ioi A. The prostate. In: Rumack CM, Wilson SR, Charboneau JW, eds. *Diagnostic ultrasound, 3rd ed.* St. Louis: Mosby; 2005: 395–424.

Bulbul MA, Haddad MC, Khauli RB, et al. Periprostatic infiltration with local anesthesia during transrectal ultrasound-guided prostate biopsy is safe, simple and effective. *Clin Imaging* 2002;26(2):129–132.

Dahnert WF, Hamper UM, Eggleston JC, et al. Prostatic evaluation by transrectal sonography with histopathologic correlation: the echopenic appearance of early carcinoma. *Radiology* 1986;158:97–102.

Inal G, Yazici S, Adsan O, et al. Effect of periprostatic nerve blockade before transrectal ultrasound-guided prostate biopsy on patient comfort: a randomized placebo controlled study. *Int J Urol* 2004;11(3): 148–151.

Kuligowska E, Barish MA, Fenlon HM, et al. Predictors of prostate carcinoma: accuracy of gray-scale and color Doppler US and serum markers. *Radiology* 2001;220(3): 757–764.

Neumaier CE, Martinoli C, Derchi LE, et al. Normal prostate gland: examination with color Doppler US. *Radiology* 1995;196: 453–457.

Penile Problems

Impotence, Penile Pain, and Abnormal Curvature

MIKE LEDWIDGE
TOM WINTER

27

KEY WORDS

Cavernosal Artery. Bilateral arteries centrally placed within the corpus cavernosum. Flow in the artery is measured to detect arterial insufficiency.

Corpora Cavernosum. Two paired tubular structures of erectile cavernous tissue in the penis that become filled with blood during an erection.

Corpus Spongiosum. Third tubular structure of erectile cavernous tissue that lies in front (anterior) and between the paired corpora cavernosa. The urethra lies in the center of it.

Flaccid. Relaxed and without muscle tone.

Fossa Navicularis. Focally dilated portion of the urethra within the glans penis.

Glans Penis. Head of the penis.

Impotence. The inability of the male patient to achieve or maintain erection.

Peyronie's Disease. A painful curvature of the penis during erection due to fibrous plaques.

Papaverine. A substance that causes an erection by dilating blood vessels when injected directly into the penis.

Priapism. Abnormal persistent erection of the penis, accompanied by pain and tenderness.

Prostaglandin. A hormone that causes an erection when injected directly into the penis.

Sildenafil, Tadalafil, and Vardenafil. Enzyme inhibitors that may be taken orally to cause an erection ("Viagra").

Sonourethrography. Ultrasound of the urethra while injecting fluid into the urethra.

Stricture. The narrowing of a tube or opening, in this case involving the urethra.

Tunica Albuginea. A fibrous coat around the penis that surrounds the corpora cavernosa.

Urethra. The tubular canal that extends from the bladder to the tip of the penis, through which urine passes.

Venous Incompetence. When referring to a failed erection, a problem caused when blood leaks out of the penis faster than normal, thereby leading to an inability to sustain an erection.

The Clinical Problem

The penis is easy to examine with ultrasound because its internal anatomy is superficial, thereby permitting use of a high-resolution, high-frequency transducer. Four main clinical problems are encountered for which sonography may be of help:

1. Peyronie's disease. Calcified or fibrous tissue is deposited in the dorsal (Fig. 27-1) portion of the penis so that the organ deviates and is painful when it is erect. The extent of the disease may be defined by ultrasound.
2. Stricture. The length of a stricture and the width of the stricture walls may be determined when the urethra is distended with fluid (the patient's urine, iatrogenically introduced saline, or gel) while imaging with a linear array transducer over the relevant area.
3. Impotence due to poor penile arterial flow. Arterial flow can be calculated using pulsed Doppler studies. An inadequate systolic flow indicates arterial insufficiency.
4. Impotence due to venous leak. An inadequate erection occurs because venous blood "leaks" out during attempted erection.

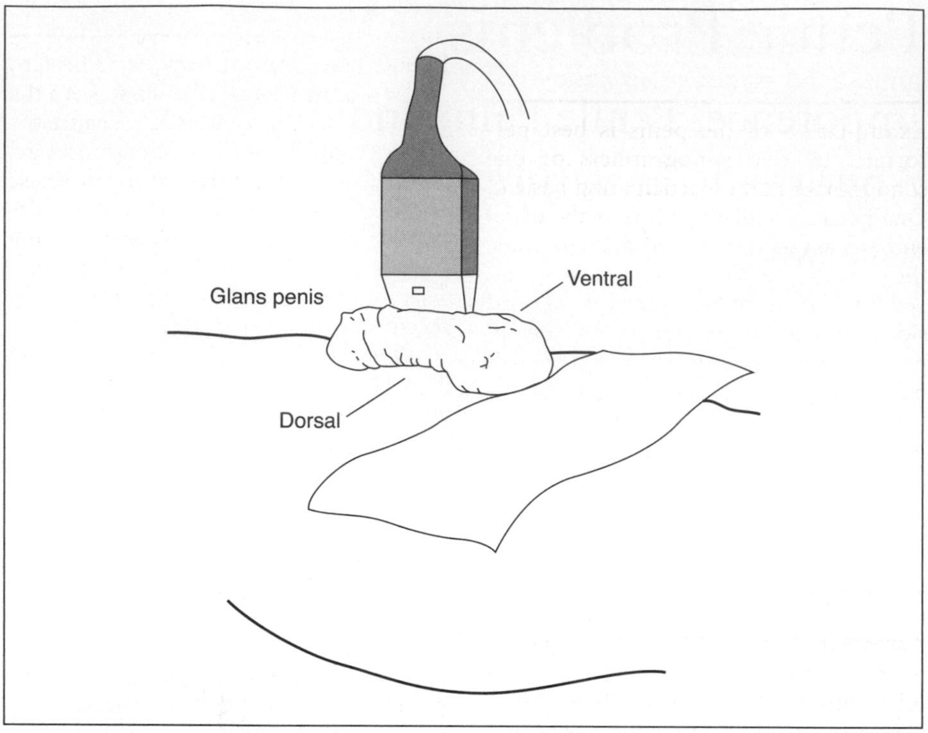

Figure 27-1. ■ *Position used for examining the penis in penile flow studies. It is also a good position for evaluating the penis for Peyronie's disease. The penis is in the anatomic position.*

Anatomy

The penis is considered in correct anatomic position when the dorsum lies against the abdomen, exposing the ventral side (Fig. 27-1). The penile portion of the urethra is midline, ventral, and surrounded by the corpus spongiosum. Posterior and lateral to the urethra are two vascular structures called the corpora cavernosa. All three components are surrounded by fibrous tissue called the tunica albuginea. Contained within each corpora cavernosum is erectile tissue and a cavernosal artery. In the dorsal portion of the penis are the deep dorsal artery and vein, and the superficial dorsal vein (Fig. 27-2).

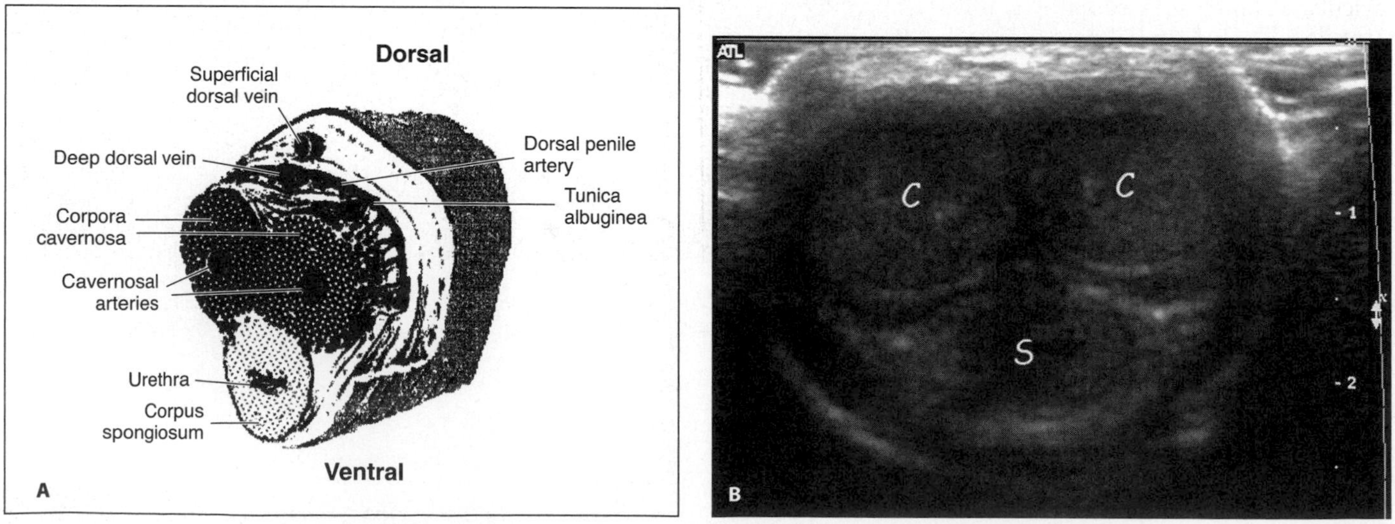

Figure 27-2. ■ *A. View showing the position of the cavernosal arteries within the corpora cavernosa and of the urethra within the corpus spongiosum. Note the tunica albuginea surrounding the corpora. B. Corresponding transverse sonogram showing the paired corpora cavernosa* (C) *and corpus spongiosum* (S).

Technique

EVALUATION OF PEYRONIE'S DISEASE

Examination of the penis is best performed by two sonographers or one sonographer and a participating patient. One person holds the penis at the distal end (glans) against the abdomen, while the other performs the sonogram. Scanning from either dorsal or ventral side is acceptable. Scan from the side opposite to the area of interest. A stand-off pad is helpful with older equipment, although newer high-frequency, broad-bandwidth linear transducers generally do not require such a pad.

EVALUATION OF STRICTURE

To perform sonourethrography for evaluation of a stricture, the urethra may be distended with fluid by several mechanisms. Perhaps the most elegant and useful technique is to scan while a patient with a full bladder is instructed to void, using his urine as a natural contrast agent. Once a full stream has been obtained, the patient manually clamps his glans penis with his fingers and ultrasound imaging of the distended urethra is performed. Alternatively, retrograde filling of the urethra with sterile saline (by using a Foley catheter as described below) or viscous lidocaine gel (place a tapered tip syringe into the urethral opening and inject while clamping the distal penis) may be performed. To use a Foley catheter, insert it into the distal urethra with the balloon within the fossa navicularis. Inject approximately 2 mL of sterile saline into the balloon to secure the catheter. It is useful to cut the catheter tip just beyond the balloon of the Foley, thereby allowing visualization of the centimeter of urethral lumen just proximal to the fossa navicularis that would otherwise be obscured by the catheter tip. Longitudinal and transverse views of the urethra are performed while slowly and constantly injecting sterile saline into the open lumen by syringe.

EVALUATION OF ARTERIAL FLOW

To evaluate arterial flow, it is best to scan from the ventral side. First, scan the penis in a flaccid condition. Measure the diameter and flow of the cavernosal arteries. Color flow helps to locate these small arteries, which may not be detectable when the penis is flaccid. Having the patient well hydrated and placing warm compresses along the penis may accentuate these small arteries.

The Doppler angle should be less than 60 degrees and corrected to match the direction of flow. Peak systolic and end-diastolic velocities are measured. Then, a vasodilator like prostaglandin or papaverine is injected into the corpus cavernosum. At 5, 10, 15, and 20 minutes postinjection, the diameter of the vessels and the Doppler velocities (Fig. 27-3) are again obtained until the penis stops being erect. The quality of the erection is then assessed.

Pathology

PEYRONIE'S DISEASE

Peyronie's disease is an uncommon disease that results in a painful curvature of the penis when it is erect. Fibrous thickening may progress to calcification. These calcifications are usually located in the tunica albuginea on the dorsal aspect. A slightly echogenic fibrous plaque is seen on the uncurved side of the penis. The affected area often contains small foci of calcification. This condition is often associated with impotence and poor arterial flow. Intracavernosal calcifica-

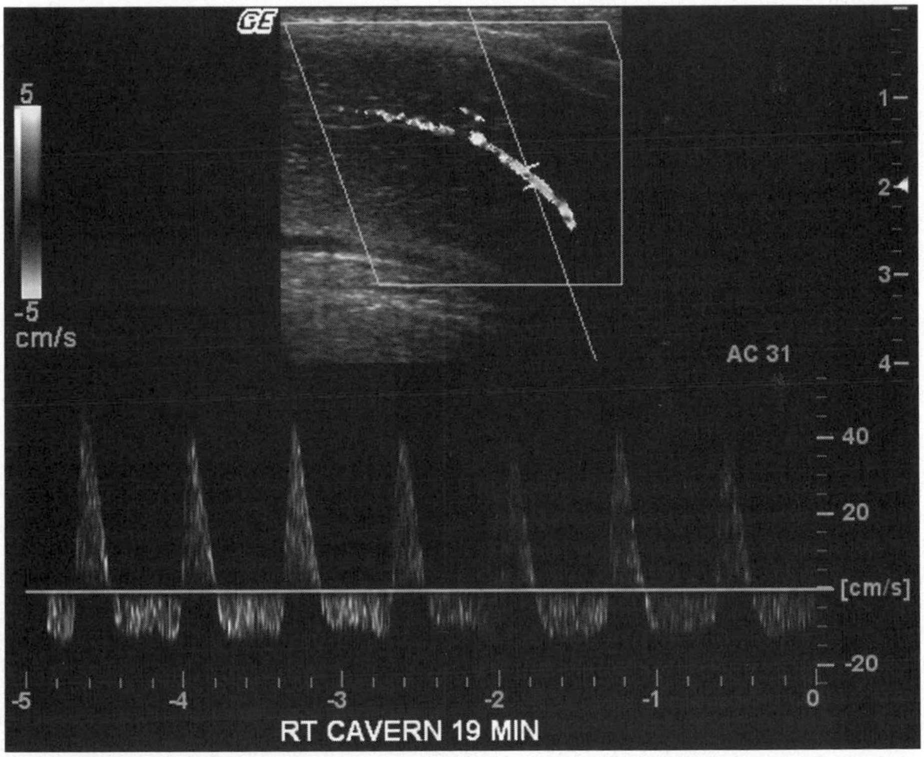

Figure 27-3. ■ *Pulsed Doppler tracing from the right cavernosal artery 19 minutes after papaverine injection showing normal peak systolic velocities of approximately 40 cm/sec.*

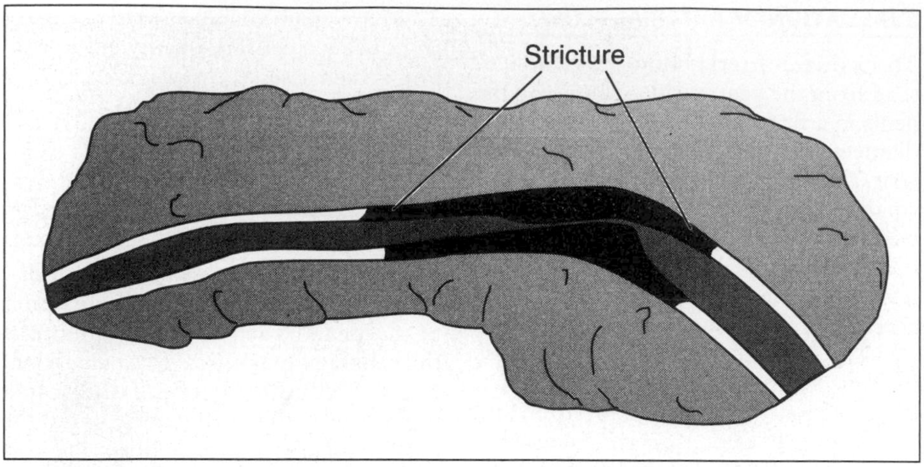

Figure 27-4. ■ *View of a stricture within the penis. Note that at the narrowed segment the walls are much thicker and the wall thickness extends beyond the narrowed urethral portion. The segment with abnormal wall thickness also needs to be excised surgically.*

tion can also be seen in a patient who has repeatedly injected himself with an agent that causes an erection such as papaverine.

URETHRAL STRICTURE

Urethral strictures develop after infection (usually gonorrhea) or trauma. The urethra is narrowed, with a markedly thickened wall at the stricture site. The thickness of the stricture wall and the length of the stricture are measured in an ultrasound evaluation (Fig. 27-4).

IMPOTENCE

For an erection to occur, arterial blood flows through the cavernosal arteries, filling the erectile tissue in the corpora cavernosa. As this process occurs, the veins are compressed so there is a buildup of blood within the corpora cavernosa with resultant rigidity. Cavernosal systolic arterial velocity less than 25 cm/sec after the injection of a vasodilator suggests inadequate arterial inflow to support a good erection, whereas peak systolic velocity greater than 30 cm/sec is normal. If the end-diastolic flow within the cavernosal artery at 15 to 20 minutes after injection is greater than or equal to approximately 5 cm/sec, it is too high and indicative of venous incompetence. The presence of many large collaterals connected to the deep cavernosal artery is abnormal and suggests the diagnosis of venous leak. Venous incompetence is a surgically correctable condition. More recent studies have been performed evaluating erectile dysfunction using oral sildenafil citrate as an erection induction agent, a much more convenient approach for the patient than intrapenile injections of prostaglandin or papaverine.

To supplement the findings, grading the degree of erection with the Doppler values is helpful. The patient stands when the penis is fully rigid, and the angle of the penis with respect to vertical is estimated. If the penile erectile angle is less than 90 degrees, it is considered abnormal.

Sonography may also be used to assess surgical devices implanted to treat impotence (Fig. 27-5).

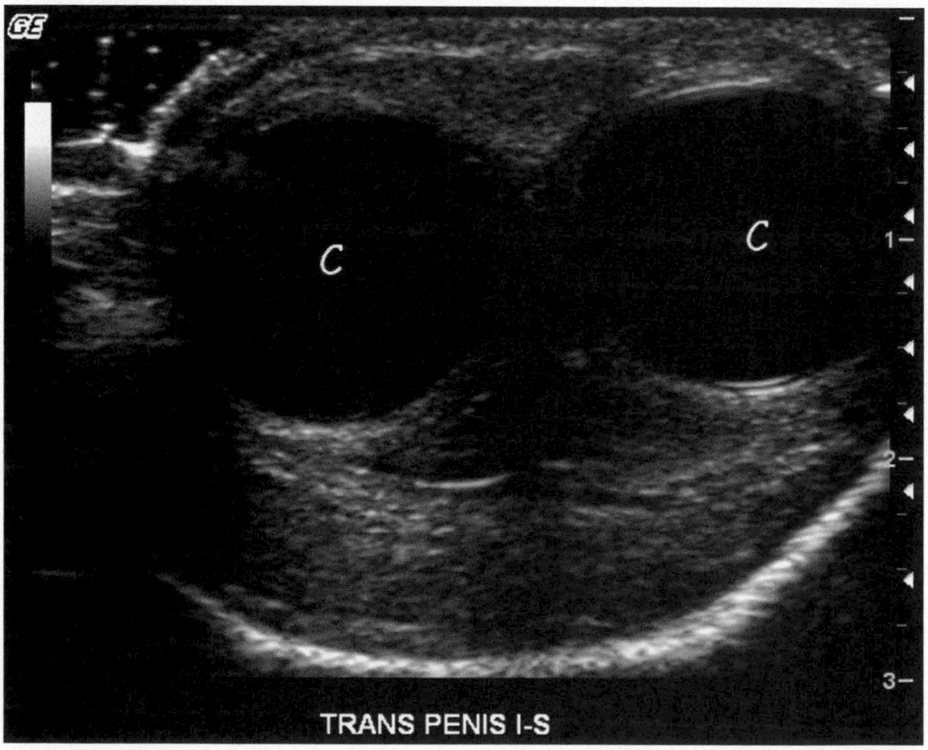

Figure 27-5. ■ *Transverse view through the penile shaft demonstrates the paired, fluid-filled, inflatable cavernosal chambers* (C) *that are surgically implanted to treat impotence.*

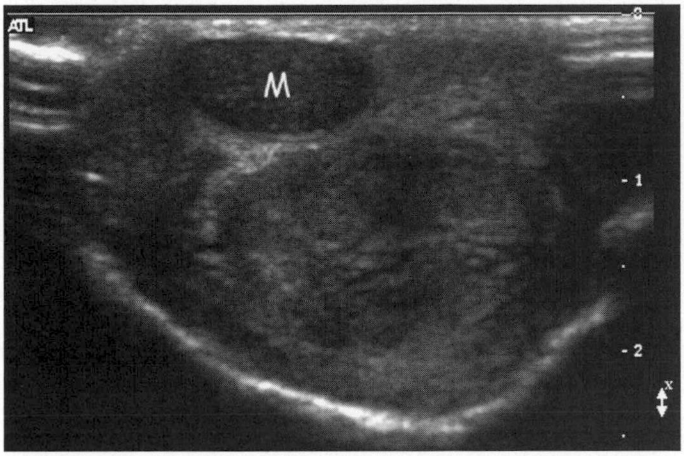

Figure 27-6. ■ *Fibroma: an 11-mm solid avascular mass* (M) *is noted on the dorsal aspect of the glans penis, to the right of midline.*

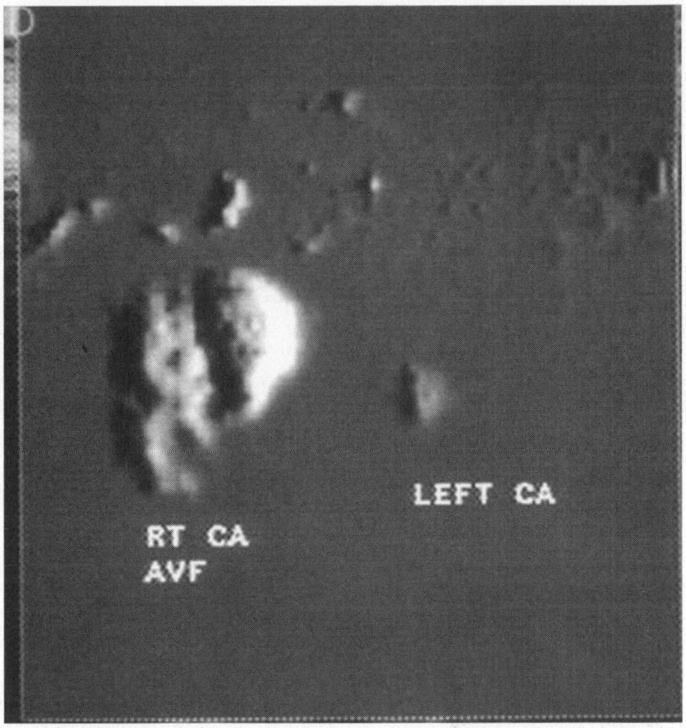

Figure 27-7. ■ *Transverse topographic power Doppler image through the midpenile shaft nicely demonstrates a large posttraumatic (after a skateboard mishap) arteriovenous fistula* (AVF) *of the right cavernosal artery* (CA) *that caused priapism in this teenaged male. Note normal size of the left cavernosal artery.*

MISCELLANEOUS

In addition to morphologic abnormalities like the tunica thickening and calcifications of Peyronie's disease, the penis may be involved with a variety of tumors and cancers. Ultrasound is a useful modality to assess and define these masses (Fig 27-6). Doppler can demonstrate flow abnormalities after traumatic injury (Fig. 27-7).

Pitfalls

1. Excessive near-field gain prevents visualization of Peyronie's plaques. Scanning from the opposite side of the penis or using the stand-off pad may help in showing subtle plaques.
2. The cavernosal arteries can be difficult to find in a flaccid penis. Use the most sensitive settings on Doppler and color flow, with the highest frequency transducer (up to ~15 MHz on the newest machines). Warm compresses along the penis may help. The room temperature should not be too cold.
3. The dorsal artery typically has a high-resistance flow pattern. Be careful that you do not scan toward the dorsal aspect of the penis when obtaining the Doppler velocities, which should be obtained from the deep cavernosal artery.
4. If the patient is evaluated too soon after injection and has not reached full rigidity, a low-resistance sonographic pattern may be obtained, producing a false-positive finding. It is best not to wait any longer than 5 minutes postinjection to obtain the initial Doppler velocities. Scanning both sides several times postinjection and documenting the velocities over the next 20 minutes is a good technique.

SELECTED READING

Benson CB, Aruny JE, Vickers MA Jr. Correlation of duplex sonography with arteriography in patients with erectile dysfunction. *AJR Am J Roentgenol* 1993;160:71–73.

Berman LH, Bearcroft PW, Spector S. Ultrasound of the male anterior urethra. *Ultrasound Q* 2002;18:123–133.

Erdogru T, Usta MF, Ceken K, et al. Is sildenafil citrate an alternative agent in the evaluation of penile vascular system with color Doppler ultrasound? *Urol Int* 2002;68:255–260.

Herbener TE, Seftel AD, Nehra A, et al. Penile ultrasound. *Semin Urol* 1994;12:320–332.

Kadioglu A, Tefekli A, Erol H, et al. Color Doppler ultrasound assessment of penile vascular system in men with Peyronie's disease. *Int J Impot Res* 2000;12:263–267.

Oates CP, Pickard RS, Powell PH, et al. The use of duplex ultrasound in the assessment of arterial supply to the penis in vasculogenic impotence. *J Urol* 1995;153:354–357.

Schwartz AN, Lowe M, Berger RE, et al. Assessment of normal and abnormal erectile function: color Doppler flow sonography versus conventional techniques. *Radiology* 1991; 180:105–109.

28

Breast Ultrasound

CYNTHIA L. RAPP

SONOGRAM ABBREVIATIONS

AX	Axilla
CA	Carcinoma
CC	Craniocaudal
DCIS	Ductal carcinoma in situ
FCC	Fibrocystic change
IDC	Invasive ductal carcinoma
MLO	Medial lateral oblique
SA	Subareolar
TDLU	Terminal ductolobular unit

KEY WORDS

Antiradial. Is 90 degrees to the radial plane.

Benign. Refers to a condition, tumor, or growth that is NOT cancerous; it does not spread to other parts of the body or invade nearby tissue. Benign tumors usually grow slowly.

DCIS. Ductal carcinoma in situ, or DCIS, is the most common kind of noninvasive breast cancer. It is *ductal* because the cancer is confined to the milk ducts.

Fibroadenoma. A benign tumor that represents a hyperplastic or proliferative process in a single terminal ductal unit.

Fibrocystic Change. Common, benign changes involving the tissues of the breast. Formerly the term "fibrocystic disease" was used; because this is misleading, many providers prefer the term " fibrocystic change." The condition is so commonly found in normal breasts that it is believed to be a normal variant. Other related terms include "mammary dysplasia," "benign breast disease," and "diffuse cystic mastopathy.

Fremitus. A thrill of the chest wall. The tissues surrounding a lesion will vibrate and fill in with echoes, whereas the lesion itself will be void of power Doppler signal.

Invasive. Invasive ductal carcinoma (IDC) accounts for approximately 80% of all breast cancers. *Invasive* means that it has "invaded" or spread to the surrounding tissues.

Radial. Scan plane running the same direction as the ducts, similar to the spokes on a bicycle wheel.

TDLU. Terminal duct lobular unit, terminal ductolobular unit. The functional unit of the breast.

Clinical Problem

Breast ultrasound is a valuable tool in the diagnosis of breast disease. Most often it is used as a diagnostic rather than a screening procedure. It is targeted to a specific clinical or focal mammographic finding in the majority of patients. Breast ultrasound should be performed on palpable lumps when the mammogram in the area of the lump is negative or nonspecific.

In addition, it should be born in mind that breast ultrasound is extremely operator-dependent, and therefore it is essential to receive appropriate training and use the appropriate equipment.

Anatomy

SONOGRAPHIC APPEARANCE

Sonographically, the skin is hyperechoic and approximately 2 mm thick. Subcutaneous fat is seen anterior to the premammary fascia. Cooper's ligaments may be seen as hyperechoic bands coursing through the subcutaneous fat. The mammary zone is where the majority of breast cancers detectable by ultrasound are located. Posterior to the mammary zone is the retromammary fascia and fat. The most posterior structures are the

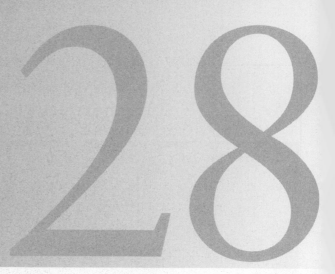

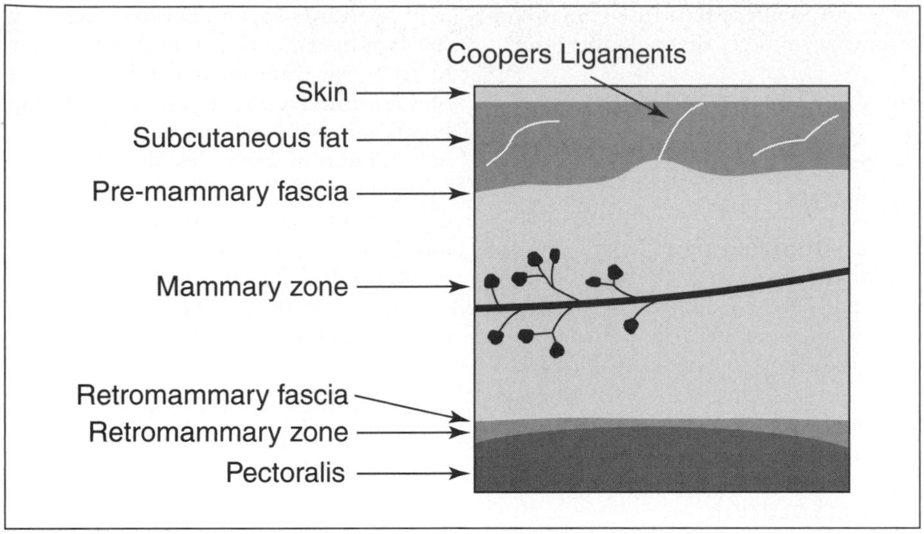

Figure 28-1. ■ *Layers of breast tissue visualized by ultrasound. (Adapted from Stavros AT.* Breast Ultrasound. *Philadelphia: Lippincott Williams & Wilkins; 2004, with permission.)*

pectoralis muscle and then the lung (Fig. 28-1).

NORMAL DEVELOPMENT

During the fifth week of human development, the embryo develops a milk line that extends from the armpit to the groin. Most of the ridge involutes, leaving an upper portion that remains to form the breast bud. If there is failure of involution along any portion of this "milk line," accessory breast tissue may form. The most common sites for accessory breast tissue are just below the breast and the axilla. By birth, the breast bud has developed a network of small branching ducts. At puberty, the ducts elongate and proliferate, and mature lobules form. Over the next several years, the process continues with growth of connective tissue and the deposition of fat. With the onset of menarche, normal cyclic breast changes begin, stimulated by estrogen and progesterone. These changes are characterized by premenstrual changes in the lobar acinar cells and stromal elements, breast edema, and venous congestion. The hormones of pregnancy cause marked proliferation of both ductal and lobular elements. Normal age-related involutional changes occur at variable rates and can begin before menopause. This change is characterized by atrophy of the ducts and lobules.

BREAST COMPOSITION

The breast is composed of fibroglandular and ductal tissue that is surrounded by and intermixed with fat. It is completely surrounded by superficial and deep fascia and covered by skin. Cooper's ligaments are supportive fibrous bands that course between the superficial and deep fascial layers. Breast tissue extends from the second to seventh rib but can extend as far superiorly as the clavicle. The sternum and anterior axillary lines mark the medial and lateral boundaries, but breast tissue can extend into the axilla. The glandular parenchyma is composed of approximately 15 to 20 lobes, each with its own excretory duct that terminates in the nipple. Montgomery's glands are small oil glands that are located around each areola. They release a lubricant that protects the nipples during nursing. Each excretory duct branches into multiple segmental ducts, terminating as the extralobular terminal ducts. It is from this portion of the duct that most breast cancers arise. This duct continues as the intralobular terminal duct and branches into 10 to 100 blind ending ductules called acini. The intralobular terminal duct and acini are surrounded and contained by loose fibrous connective stromal tissue; this unit is called the lobule. There are approximately 20 to 40 lobules per lobe. Connective tissue is present within and surrounding the lobular units (Fig. 28-2).

BLOOD SUPPLY

The arterial supply to the breast is composed of the lateral mammary branch of the lateral thoracic artery, the anterior cutaneous or perforating branches of the internal mammary artery, and the branches derived from the second to the sixth intercostal arteries. The veins describe an anastomotic circle around the base of the nipple, the so-called "circulus venosus." From the circulus, small veins take the blood to the circumference of the gland before terminating in the axillary and internal mammary veins.

BREAST LYMPHATICS

The lymphatic drainage is particularly important because it is by this route that the spread of malignant disease may occur. There is both a superficial and a deep plexus of lymphatic vessels. The superficial plexus lies beneath the skin anterior to the gland. It receives afferent vessels from the gland and sends its efferent lymph to lymph nodes in the pectoral and infraclavicular chains; other vessels pass to the deep plexus that lies in the deep fascia on which the mammary gland rests. It is this plexus that directly receives most of the lymphatic drainage of the breast.

MISCELLANEOUS ANATOMIC POINTS

Age-Related Changes

In the prepubertal child, the breast contains a few small ducts scattered throughout the fibrous stroma without formation of lobules. With the onset of estrogen secretion by the ovaries, glandular tissue enlarges quickly (thelarche). This breast development occurs before

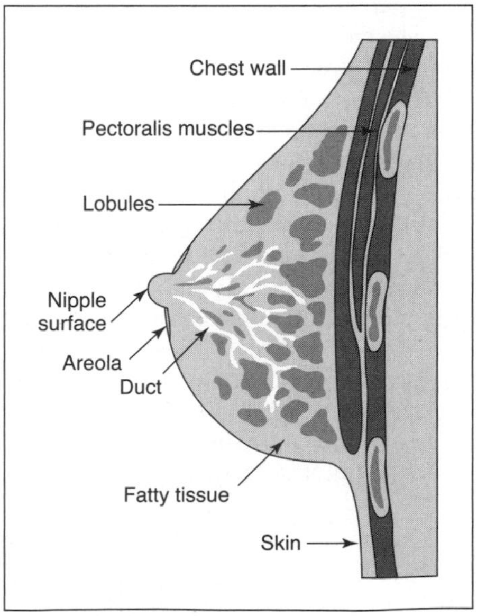

Figure 28-2. ■ *Normal breast anatomy.*

menarche. Occasionally, asymmetric development may simulate a hard subareolar nodule; one should not mistake this for a tumor because excision will remove all of the glandular tissue and prevent the development of the breast.

In the young woman, glandular tissue is relatively thick and the subcutaneous and retromammary fat areas are small.

During pregnancy and lactation, there is considerable increase in the size and numbers of the terminal ductolobular units (TDLUs) at the expense of the breast stroma and epithelial elements. This breast has very little fatty tissue. Occasionally, asymmetric secretory changes may occur in the breast resulting in a palpable abnormality.

Involutional changes occur after full-term pregnancies with progressive thinning of the mammary zone. The parenchymal and stromal atrophy is most pronounced in the area between Cooper's ligaments. In extreme involution, the parenchymal elements are almost absent and only strands of connective tissue are seen, appearing as echogenic bands between the isoechoic fat.

Anomalies

Amastia, complete absence of one or both of the breasts, absence of breast tissue or the nipple, or a rudimentary mammary gland, is rare.

Accessory or supernumerary breasts occur in approximately 1% to 2% of patients and may involve any of the three components of the breast: the fibroglandular parenchyma, areola, or nipple.

The most common anomaly is an accessory nipple (polythelia), which can occur in both male and female patients. This nipple can develop anywhere along the milk line, but the most common location is just below the normal breast.

Congenital nipple flattening or inversion needs to be differentiated from retraction of the nipple that can be caused by a carcinoma or ductal ectasia.

Accessory breast tissue is often asymmetric from left to right. The axillary segment is most often involved, but accessory breast tissue can occur anywhere along the milk line. Accessory breast tissue can be the cause of mammographic asymmetry or a palpable lump.

Technique

EQUIPMENT

Breast ultrasound must have excellent spatial and contrast resolution. Both the axial and lateral components of spatial resolution must be good. Broadband, high-frequency linear electronically focused probes currently offer the best combination of spatial and contrast resolution for breast ultrasound.

AXIAL RESOLUTION

Excellent axial resolution is important in identifying normal structures that course parallel to the skin (such as the mammary ducts and fascial planes surrounding the mammary zone) and in identifying the characteristics of the capsules around cysts and solid nodules.

LATERAL RESOLUTION

Lateral resolution at all depths within the breast is important to minimize volume averaging of surrounding normal breast tissues with pathologic lesions. Such volume averaging may cause mischaracterization of small cystic lesions as solid and may even cause small solid lesions to be indistinguishable from surrounding tissues. Lateral spatial resolution is also a complex subject. For linear probes, there are two planes that determine lateral resolution, the long axis and short axis (elevation plane focus).

The long axis of the linear probe can be electronically focused. Continuous electronic focusing may be done on receive or transmit phases. The degree of electronic focusing on receive depends on many factors, including the following:

- Number of channels
- Aperture size
- Number of elements
- Number of scan lines

In general, lateral resolution improves with increasing number of channels, aperture size, number of elements in the transducer, and scan lines. Electronic focusing on transmit depends on many of the same factors as receive focusing but is more limited. It depends on the number of transmit zones. In general, the more transmit zones, the better the lateral resolution. However, increasing the number of transmit zones decreases the frame rate. In general, multiple transmit focal zones in the first 2 cm are very beneficial in breast sonography.

ELEVATION PLANE

The elevation plane (short axis) of the probe cannot currently be electronically focused. The elevation plane is focused at a fixed depth by an acoustic lens. The manufacturer decides how deeply to focus this plane before the probe is built. Elevation plane focal lengths are usually decided by the application for which the probe will primarily be used. Dedicated small parts or near-field probes should be focused at approximately 1.5 cm or even more superficially (Fig. 28-3).

Five-megahertz linear array probes were designed with peripheral vascular applications in mind and are focused in the elevation plane at approximately 3 to 4 cm. This is too deep for most breast imaging, because the elevation plane for these probes would correspond to the

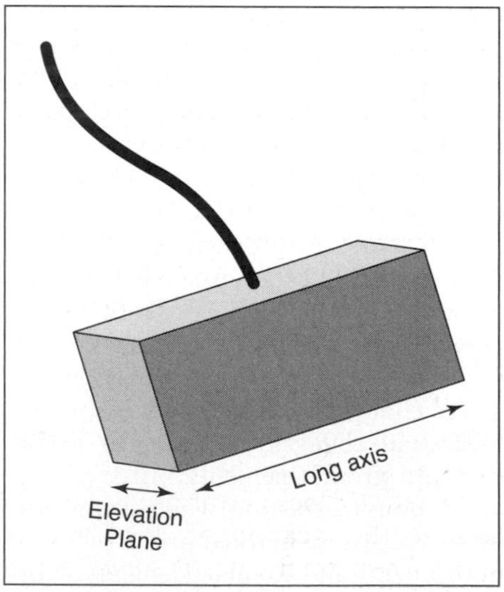

Figure 28-3. ■ *Relationship of elevation plane to the long axis of the transducer.*

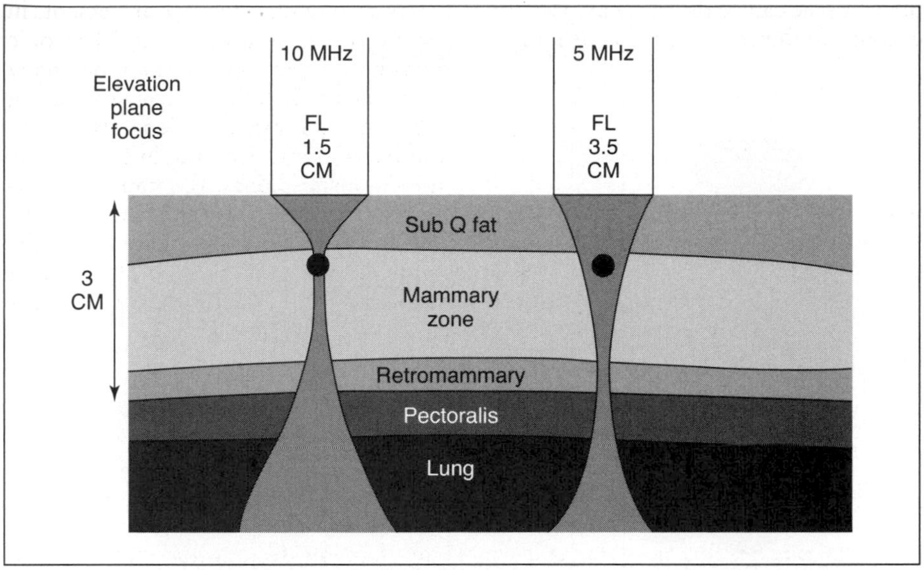

Figure 28-4. ■ *If a 5-MHz transducer is used and the lesion of interest is small and superficial, volume averaging of adjacent normal tissues will be a problem. Cysts may fill in and be misclassified as solid. Small solid lesions may be completely missed. (Adapted from Stavros AT.* Breast Ultrasound. *Philadelphia: Lippincott Williams & Wilkins; 2004, with permission.)*

pectoralis muscle in most patients. In general, a 7.5- to 13-MHz transducer, with an elevation plane of approximately 1.5 cm, is the best breast ultrasound transducer currently available (Fig. 28-4).

If a palpable nodule is very small and near the skin, even optimally focused transducers may have difficulty resolving and characterizing the lesion. In such circumstances, a 1-cm standoff pad or a large "glop" of gel should be used to move the elevation plane focus closer to the skin.

ANNOTATION

Most ultrasound departments use the clock method to label breast images. In addition, ABC and 123 notation is helpful to label the exact location of a lesion.

If a lesion is being labeled for the purpose of biopsy, distance from nipple to lesion should also be included.

First a clock position is stated. Second, the location of the lesion is noted. There are five possible choices for the 123 location. One through 3 is divided into 3 concentric rings. A lesion near the nipple is location 1, a lesion midway out in the breast is 2, and a lesion in the periphery is 3. If a lesion is under the nipple, it should be labeled SA for subareolar; lesions in the axilla are labeled AX.

ABC notation: A is used if a lesion is near the surface or close to the transducer. B is used if a lesion is midway down and represents the mammary zone in the breast. C is used in the setting of lesions located against the chest wall (Fig. 28-5).

POSITIONING

The patient should be positioned in a supine position with the ipsilateral hand raised above the head. Lesions in the medial quadrants may be scanned in a straight supine position. The patient is then rolled into a contralateral posterior oblique position, which minimizes breast thickness in the lateral quadrants. Generally, greater degrees of obliquity are required for larger breasts. By positioning a patient in this manner, two things can be accomplished:

- First, the breast is thinned to the greatest extent possible so that the high-frequency, near-field probe used may adequately penetrate to the chest wall while preserving the optimal focusing characteristics of the probe.
- Second, the tissue planes of the breast, which are conical in the upright and prone positions, are pulled into a plane that is parallel to the skin line. This minimizes critical angle shadowing, improves penetration, and prevents degradation of focusing characteristics.

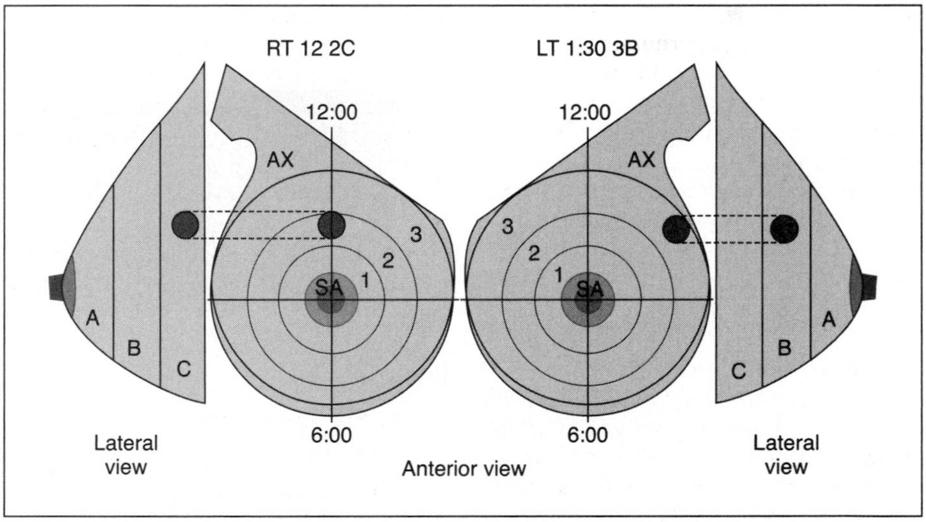

Figure 28-5. ■ *Right breast lesion, approximately 4 cm directly superior to the nipple and near the chest wall, that was scanned in a radial plane, which would be described as* ***"RT 12 2C RAD"*** *(RAD, radial). The left breast lesion in the upper outer quadrant, approximately 6 cm from the nipple and 3 cm deep, that was scanned in an antiradial plane, would be labeled* ***"LT 1:30 3B AR"*** *(AR, anti-radial). (Adapted from Stavros AT.* Breast Ultrasound. *Philadelphia: Lippincott Williams & Wilkins; 2004, with permission.)*

SCAN PLANE: RADIAL AND ANTIRADIAL

All solid lesions should be scanned in the plane of the ductal system (radial and anti-radial) to demonstrate subtle projections that course toward the nipple or branch outward in the breast (Fig. 28-6).

If a nodule is scanned using only the conventional methods of true longitudinal and transverse sections, subtle findings may be missed, lesions may falsely appear spheroid or ellipsoid, and lesions may be misclassified as probably benign.

SYSTEM OPTIMIZATION

System optimization is essential in breast imaging. If the gain is not set correctly, solid lesions can look cystic or a cyst may look solid. Before starting to scan the area of interest, find an area in the breast with fatty tissue. Most patients have some fat, usually in the inner aspect of the breast. Set your gain so the fat is medium gray.

Compare all lesions in the breast with fat. If the gain is set correctly and fat is medium gray, glandular tissue and most benign lesions, such as fibroadenomas, appear isoechoic to mildly hypoechoic compared with fat. Malignant lesions can be mildly hypoechoic to markedly hypoechoic and cysts are markedly hypoechoic to anechoic compared with fat. The structures that are hyperechoic compared with fat are skin, fibrous tissue, and calcifications (Fig. 28-7).

MAMMOGRAPHIC VERSUS SONOGRAPHIC CORRELATION

When the main indication for breast ultrasound is a palpable lump, it is imperative that the lump be palpated while scanning. A breast biopsy can be avoided if it can be shown that the lump is due to a simple cyst or normal fibroglandular tissue. Both can cause palpable lumps. Simple cysts are so common in some age groups that they are virtually a variant of normal. Fibroglandular tissue is present in at least some part of the breast in the majority of all women, especially those who are within the reproductive years, and even in postmenopausal women who are undergoing hormonal replacement therapy.

When the primary indication for breast ultrasound is a mammographic nodule, mass, or focal asymmetric density, it is essential that the size, shape, lo-

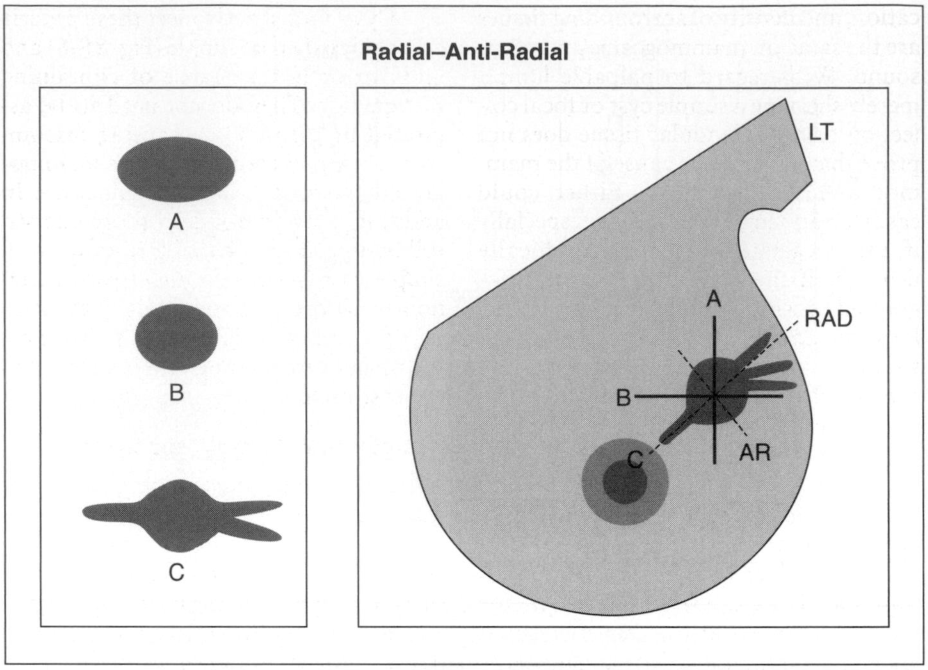

Figure 28-6. ■ *Radial and antiradial scan planes. (Adapted from Stavros AT.* Breast Ultrasound. *Philadelphia: Lippincott Williams & Wilkins; 2004, with permission.)*

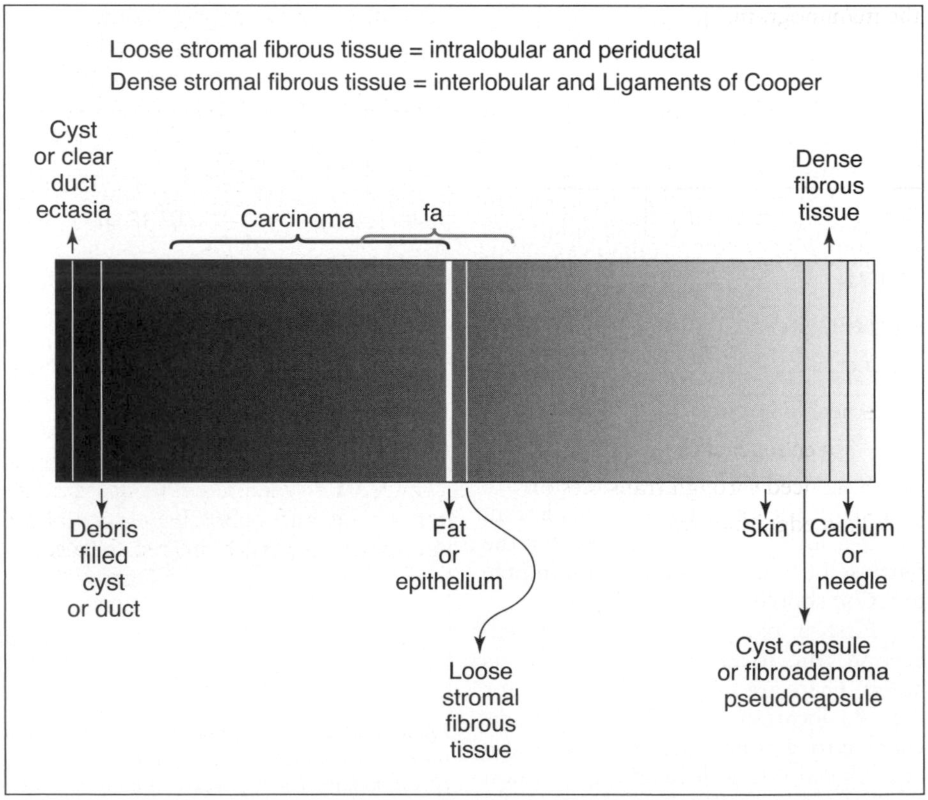

Figure 28-7. ■ *Echogenicity relationships of different structures and lesions within the breast. (Adapted from Stavros AT.* Breast Ultrasound. *Philadelphia: Lippincott Williams & Wilkins; 2004, with permission.)*

cation, and density of surrounding tissues are the same on mammograms and ultrasound. With regard to palpable lumps, merely showing a simple cyst or focal collection of fibroglandular tissue does not prove that either is the cause of the mammographic abnormality. Either could easily be an incidental finding, especially if the breasts are mammographically dense or if there are multiple mammographic densities. Only if the size, shape, location, and density of surrounding tissues are similar on mammography and sonography can you be sure that a simple cyst or fibrous pseudo-tumor is the cause of the mammographic abnormality.

When correlating breast ultrasound with mammography, one should compare the craniocaudal view of the mammogram with the transverse view on ultrasound. The shape of a mammographic lesion will be easier to reproduce sonographically if the scan plane is identical to the projection plane of the mammogram. The medial lateral oblique (MLO) view of the mammogram may vary from 30 to 60 degrees. It is difficult to reproduce the exact degree of obliquity on the ultrasound that was used on the MLO view of the mammogram.

Pathology

CYSTS

Breast cysts are usually classified as simple, complex, or complicated, depending on internal echogenicity.

Simple Cysts

Strict criteria for a simple cyst include:

- Anechoic center
- Thin echogenic capsule
- Enhanced through transmission
- Thin edge shadows

Cysts that strictly meet these criteria can be classified as simple (Fig. 28-8) and have virtually no chance of containing malignancy. They do not need to be aspirated unless they are causing discomfort or are preventing adequate mammographic compression and evaluation. In addition, they do not need short-interval follow-up. Although malignancy inside a simple cyst is virtually unknown, carcinoma can occur in the immediate vicinity of a cyst, so it is necessary to survey the tissues surrounding the cyst as well as the cyst itself.

Complex and Complicated Cysts

Cysts that do not meet strict criteria for a simple cyst are classified as either complex or complicated cysts. However, the term "complicated breast cyst" does not carry the significance of a complex cyst of the kidney or liver. It is important to understand that complicated cystic breast malignancies are extremely rare and usually have other features that are obviously malignant. The majority of nonsimple cysts fall within the broad spectrum of fibrocystic change. For these reasons, the majority of nonsimple breast cysts are not worrisome and do not need to be aspirated or biopsied. Cysts that have some potential to be associated with malignancy have been designated complex cysts, distinguishing them from those that have little likelihood of harboring malignancy, which have been designated complicated cysts. Complex cysts demonstrate at least one of three findings: thick walls, thick septations, or mural nodules.

With the improved resolution of current high-end equipment, a large percentage of breast cysts no longer appear simple. This is because they contain internal debris consistent with fibrocystic change. With older equipment, these internal cells and debris were not visible; therefore, the cysts appeared simple.

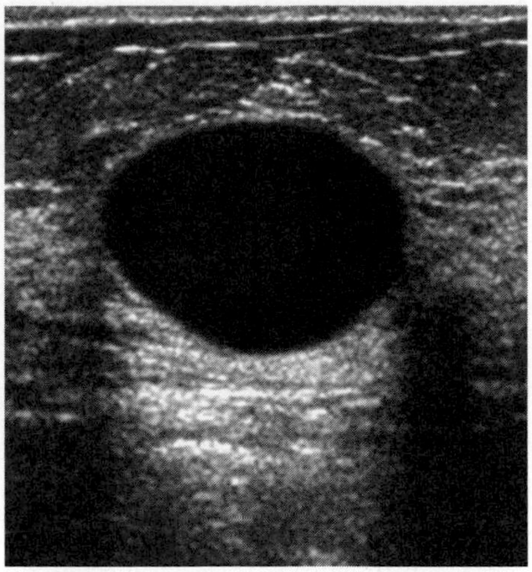

Figure 28-8. ■ *Sonogram of a simple cyst: anechoic, thin echogenic capsule, enhanced through transmission, and thin edge shadows.*

Internal contents within breast cysts are part of the spectrum of fibrocystic change and include:

- Protein globs
- Cellular debris
- Cholesterol crystals
- Foam cells
- Apocrine cells

Therefore, it is necessary to have a method of evaluating the relative risk of an individual complex or complicated breast cyst for two complicating factors:

- Infection
- Malignancy

Categorizing complex and complicated cysts into categories can help assess their risk of infection or neoplasm. Complex breast cyst categories include:

- Diffuse low-level internal echoes
- Fluid-debris levels
- Septations
- Eccentric wall thickening

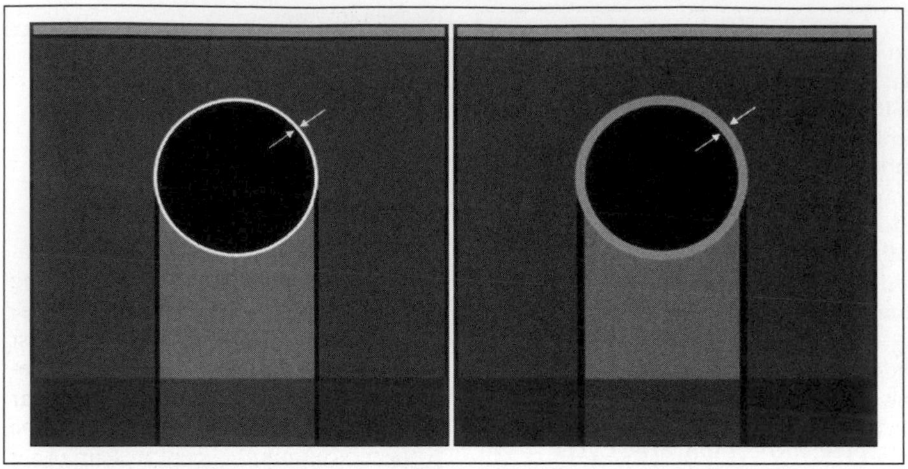

Figure 28-9. ■ *Low-level internal echoes and wall thickness. Left, thin and echogenic wall. Right, thick and isoechoic wall. (From Stavros AT.* Breast Ultrasound. *Philadelphia: Lippincott Williams & Wilkins; 2004, with permission.)*

Complicated cysts with low-level diffuse internal echoes should be evaluated for wall thickness and particle mobility. Determine whether the cyst has a normal thin, echogenic wall versus a uniformly thickened, isoechoic wall that indicates inflammation (Fig. 28-9). A cyst with a thickened wall should be considered acutely inflamed and potentially infected, and should be aspirated.

If the cyst with low-level internal echoes does not have a thickened wall, then the size of the internal particulate matter should be evaluated. Complicated cysts with diffuse low-level internal echoes can contain either light, subcellular particles or heavier cellular particles; subcellular particles are merely part of the spectrum of fibrocystic change and are not worrisome.

Fluid Debris Level

Cysts with fluid-debris levels also may have a uniformly thickened wall indicating acute inflammation; these cysts are often tender. The position of the debris level within such complicated cysts will shift with changes in patient position in a manner similar to the movement of sludge within a gallbladder. When a fluid debris level is suspected, the cyst should be evaluated in the left lateral decubitus or upright position, as well as in the usual supine position. Complicated cysts with fluid debris levels should be aspirated (Fig. 28-10).

Septations

The majority of thinly septated cysts can be more precisely defined as clusters of simple cysts or as a large simple cyst with normal tissue indenting it. These do not need to be aspirated or even followed. They should be considered simple cysts.

Complex cysts with thick septations should undergo further diagnostic evaluation. Aspiration alone is insufficient because the risk of false-negative cytology is too high. In addition, should the cyst be aspirated and the cytology later found to be atypical or malignant, it may be difficult to find the lesion again for needle biopsy or needle localization unless the fluid reaccumulates. If aspiration is performed, one should be ready to follow aspiration immediately with large-core needle biopsy (Fig. 28-11).

Eccentric Wall Thickening

The appearance of the cyst capsule immediately adjacent to eccentric wall thickening is very important. Complex cysts containing papillomas or papillary carcinoma more frequently have an irregular, angular outer margin and lack the smooth thin echogenic capsule. For the purposes of evaluating surface characteristics, the eccentric wall thickening is assumed to be a solid nodule within a cyst. As in solid nodules, the smooth, thin, echogenic capsule indicates a noninfiltrating leading edge, more typical of benign lesions. The lack of a thin capsule

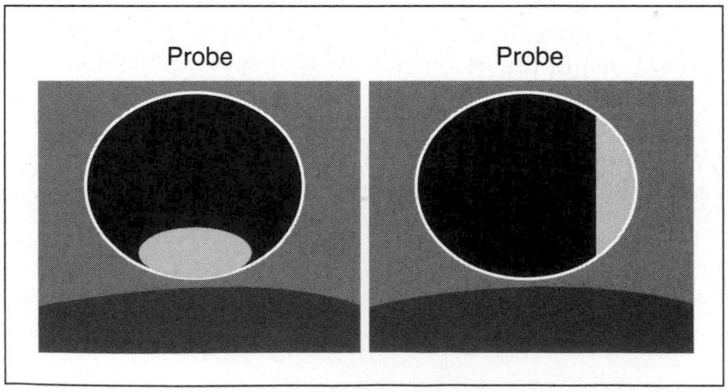

Figure 28-10. ■ *Shifting of fluid-debris level depending on patient position. Left, supine. Right, upright. (Adapted from Stavros AT.* Breast Ultrasound. *Philadelphia: Lippincott Williams & Wilkins; 2004, with permission.)*

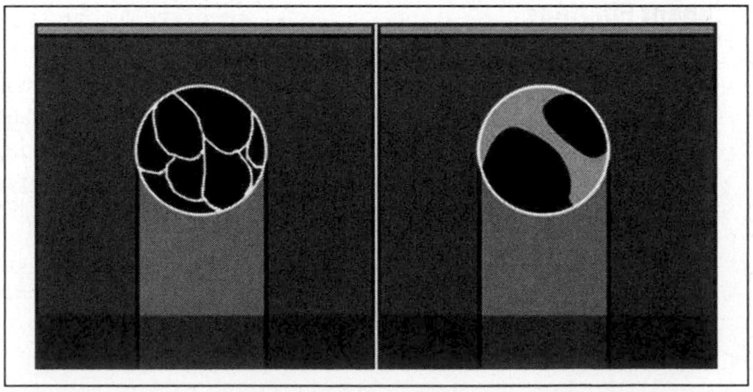

Figure 28-11. ■ *The difference between thin and thick septations within a cystic mass. Left, thin septations. Right, thick septations. (From Stavros AT.* Breast Ultrasound. *Philadelphia: Lippincott Williams & Wilkins; 2004, with permission.)*

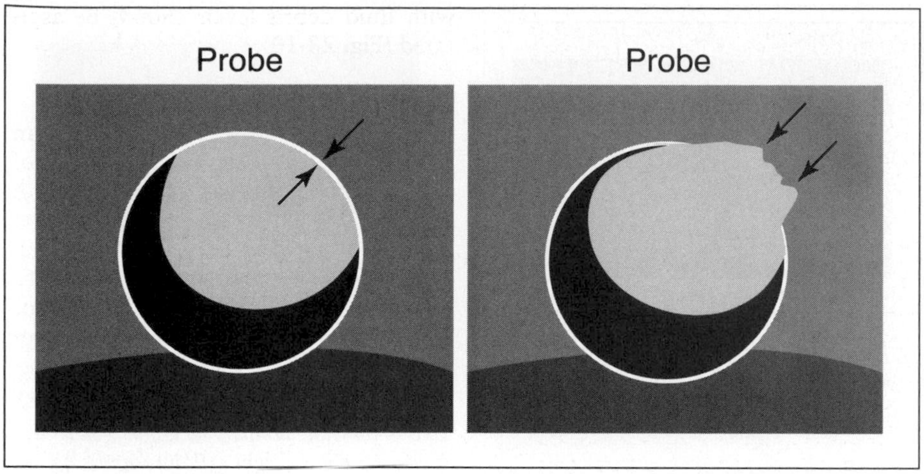

Figure 28-12. ■ *Eccentric wall thickening with an intact capsule* (left) *and extension beyond the capsule wall* (right). *(Adapted from Stavros AT.* Breast Ultrasound. *Philadelphia: Lippincott Williams & Wilkins; 2004, with permission.)*

increases the likelihood of an infiltrating leading edge, a sign of malignancy (Fig. 28-12).

SOLID NODULES

All solid nodules should be considered worrisome and malignant findings sought (Fig. 28-13), with findings recorded as being present or absent. If even a single malignant feature is present, the nodule cannot be classified as benign. If no malignant features are found, specific benign features then need to be sought. Only if benign findings are found, can the nodule then be classified as benign. If specific benign features are not found, the lesion should be classified as indeterminate.

Malignant Findings

Individual sonographic criteria are as follows:

- Spiculation
- Taller-than-wide (larger anteroposterior than transverse dimensions)
- Angular margins
- Markedly hypoechoic (compared with fat)
- Shadowing
- Calcifications
- Duct extension
- Branch pattern
- Microlobulation

Spiculation

Spiculation is a sonographic finding that corresponds to invasion of surrounding tissues and a desmoplastic host response to the lesion. Spiculation may manifest as alternating hypoechoic and hyperechoic lines that radiate out perpendicular to the surface of the nodule, where the hypoechoic components represent either fingers of invasive tumor or ductal carcinoma in situ (DCIS) components of tumor extending into the surrounding tissues, and the hyperechoic components

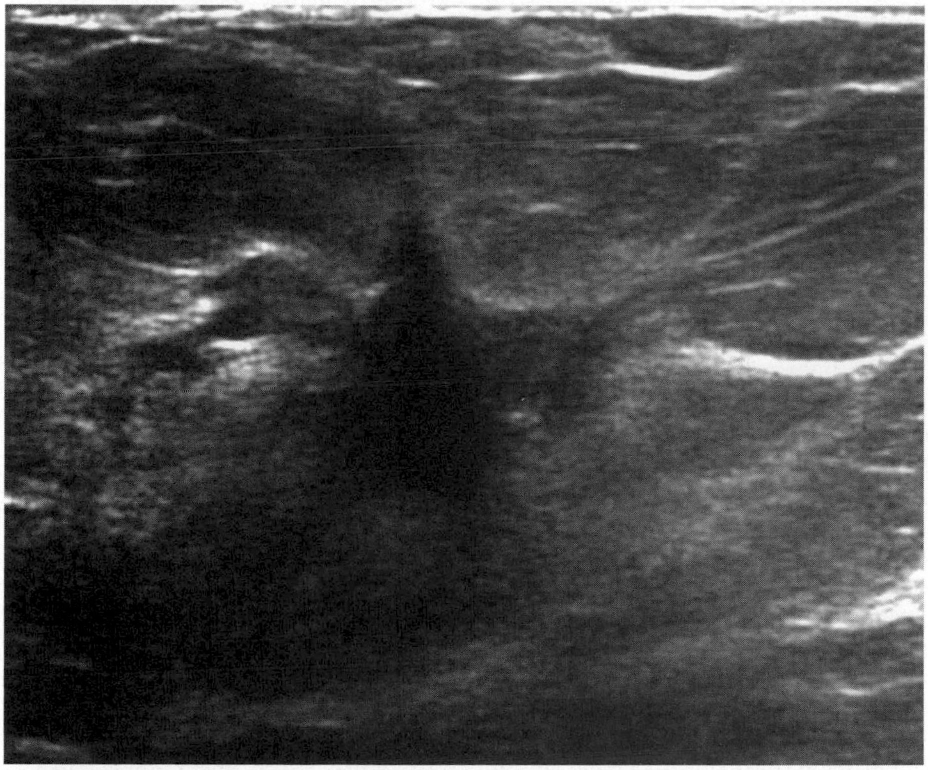

Figure 28-13. ■ *Sonogram of a malignant breast carcinoma: hypoechoic echogenicity, irregular shape, spiculations, angular margins, microcalcifications, and duct extension with architectural distortion.*

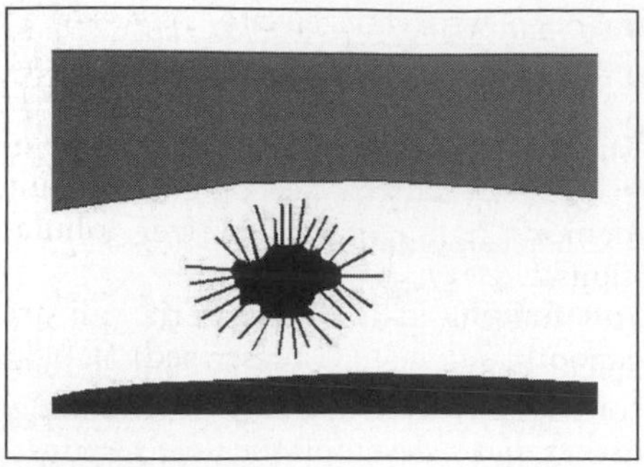

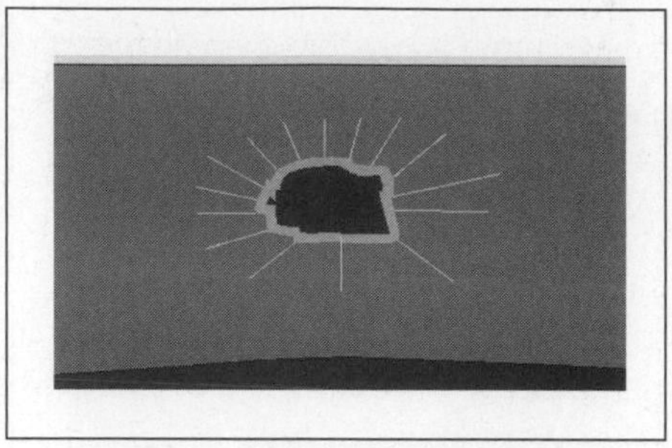

Figure 28-14. ■ *Spiculations surrounded by fibrous tissue* (left) *and fatty tissue* (right). *(From Stavros AT.* Breast Ultrasound. *Philadelphia: Lippincott Williams & Wilkins; 2004, with permission.)*

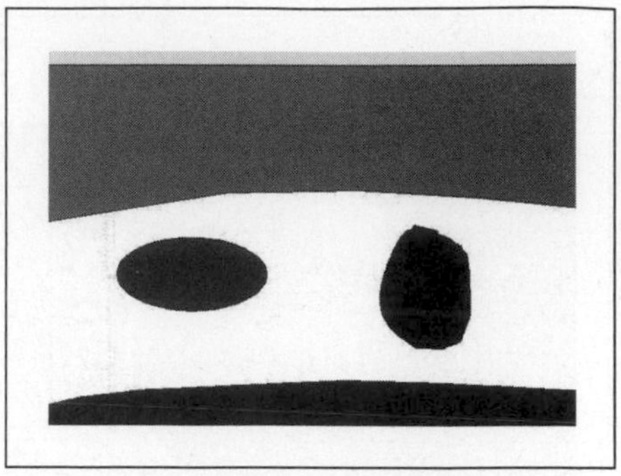

Figure 28-15. ■ *A wider-than-tall parallel lesion* (left), *typical for a fibroadenoma, and a taller-than-wide, nonparallel lesion seen with small carcinomas* (right). *(From Stavros AT.* Breast Ultrasound. *Philadelphia: Lippincott Williams & Wilkins; 2004, with permission.)*

represent the interfaces between the spicules and surrounding breast tissues. However, in most cases, spicules present as purely hyperechoic or purely hypoechoic depending on the echogenicity of the tissue within which the lesion lies (Fig. 28-14).

Taller-Than-Wide (Nonparallel)

Lesions that are larger in the anteroposterior dimension than in any horizontal dimension are suspicious for malignancy. This finding is generally associated with smaller malignancies. As lesions enlarge, they tend to become wider than tall. The shape of small carcinomas is believed to reflect the shape of the TDLU within which the carcinoma arose (Fig. 28-15).

Angular Margins

Angular margins are identical to the jagged or irregular margins seen on mammography. Angular margins represent a sonographic finding indicative of invasion. The angles of the lesion margins can be acute, right angle, or obtuse. A single angle of any type on the surface of the lesion should be considered suspicious and should exclude the lesion from the probably benign. Angles on the surface of the nodule occur in regions of low resistance to invasion (Fig. 28-16).

Markedly Hypoechoic

Marked hypoechogenicity of a solid nodule (compared with fat) is a suspicious sonographic finding for malignancy. As transducer frequency, bandwidth, and system dynamic range have increased, the percentage of malignant nodules that appear markedly hypoechoic has decreased.

Shadowing

Acoustic shadowing is a suspicious finding that suggests the presence of invasive malignancy. Acoustic shadowing occurs in approximately one-third of all solid malignant nodules. The desmoplastic components of the tumor substance and spiculations cause the shadowing. Because breast carcinomas can be internally heterogenous, only part of a solid malignant nodule might give rise to acoustic shadowing (Fig. 28-17).

Calcifications

The presence of calcifications are mammographically suspicious findings that have been applied to sonography. Calcifications occur within the lumen of ducts distended by DCIS and thus are usually associated with other suspicious findings (duct extensions and/or branch pattern). Calcifications shown sonographically are smaller than the ultrasound beam width and therefore do not cast acoustic shadows.

Duct Extension and Branch Pattern

Duct extension correlates with the presence of DCIS components of tumor. It is best demonstrated when the scan plane is oriented parallel to the long axis of the mammary ducts in the region of the nodule. Duct extension is seen as a single projection of solid growth toward the nipple from the main nodule.

Branch pattern manifests as projection of the solid nodule into multiple small ducts away from the nipple. As with duct extension, branch pattern is seen when the scan plane is oriented parallel to the long axis of the mammary

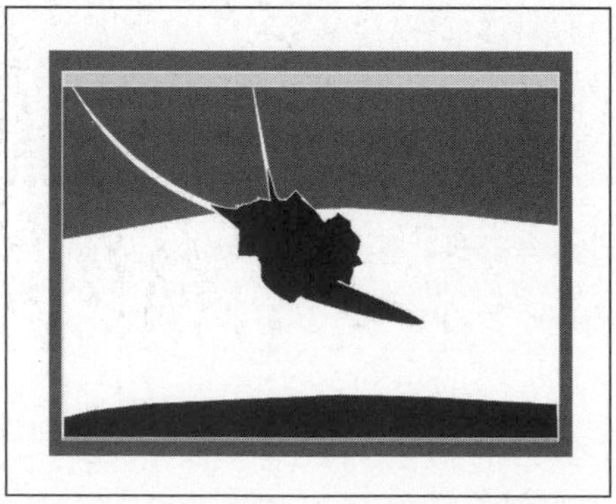

Figure 28-16. ■ *Angular margins. (From Stavros AT.* Breast Ultrasound. *Philadelphia: Lippincott Williams & Wilkins; 2004, with permission.)*

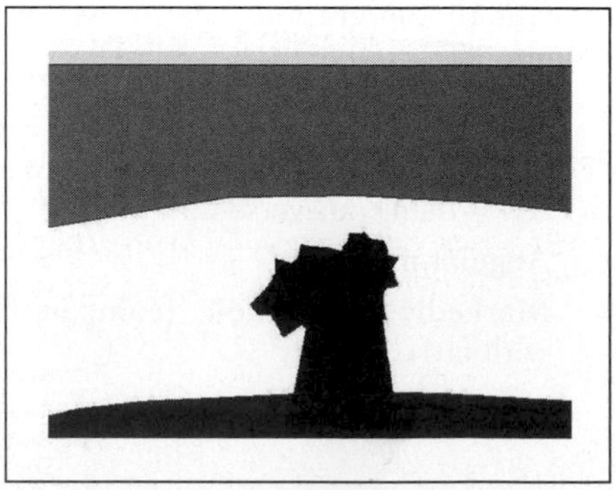

Figure 28-17. ■ *Acoustic shadowing only behind part of the malignant solid nodule. (From Stavros AT.* Breast Ultrasound. *Philadelphia: Lippincott Williams & Wilkins; 2004, with permission.)*

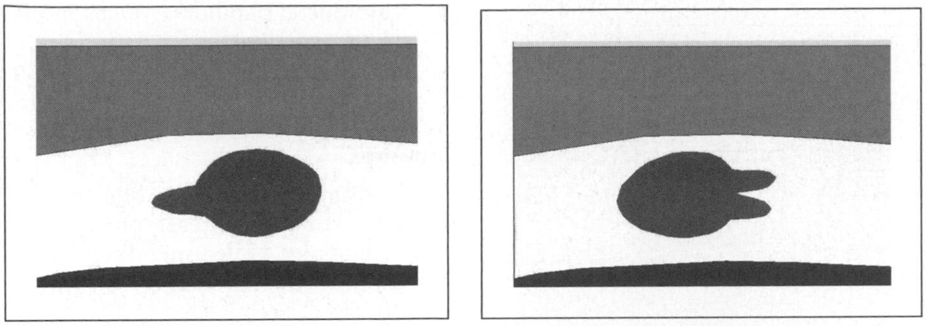

Figure 28-18. ■ *Duct and tumor extension toward the nipple* (left) *and branch pattern tumor growth away from the nipple* (right). *(From Stavros AT.* Breast Ultrasound. *Philadelphia: Lippincott Williams & Wilkins; 2004, with permission.)*

ducts in the region of the nodule (Fig. 28-18).

Microlobulation

Microlobulations are 1- to 2-mm lobulations that vary in number and distribution along the surface and within the substance of a nodule (Fig. 28-19). Microlobulation can be seen with both invasive and DCIS components of tumor. The size of microlobulations correlates with the histologic grade of the tumor. High-grade lesions tend to have large microlobulations, whereas low-grade lesions tend to have very small microlobulations. Intermediate-grade lesions tend to have intermediate-sized microlobulations.

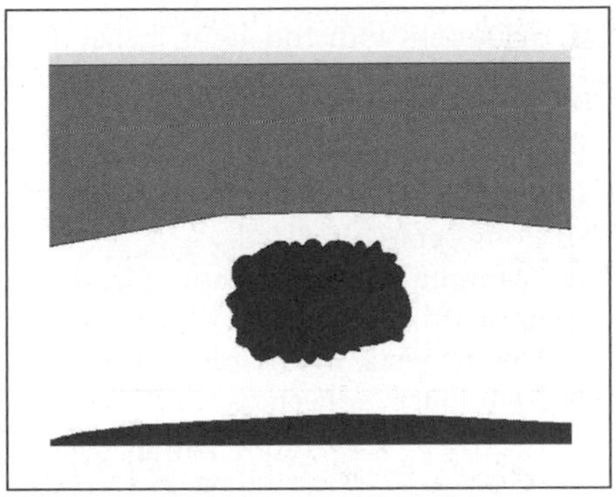

Figure 28-19. ■ *Microlobulated lesion. (From Stavros AT.* Breast Ultrasound. *Philadelphia: Lippincott Williams & Wilkins; 2004, with permission.)*

Benign Findings

Only if no suspicious findings are present should benign findings be sought (Fig. 28-20). These findings are (1) pure and marked hyperechogenicity, representing interlobular stromal fibrous tissue; and (2) an elliptical, wider-than-tall lesion shape with the lesion completely encompassed by a thin, echogenic capsule demonstrating three or fewer lobulations.

Individual benign criteria (all are smooth and well-circumscribed) include

- Markedly hyperechoic (compared with fat)
- Ellipsoid shape
- Three or fewer gentle lobulations
- Thin, echogenic capsule

Purely hyperechoic tissue is normal interlobular stromal fibrous tissue; this can result in either palpable or mammographic abnormalities. To be considered benign, the hyperechoic tissue may contain normal-sized ducts or TDLUs, but should contain no isoechoic or hypoechoic structures larger than the size of normal ducts or lobules (Fig. 28-21).

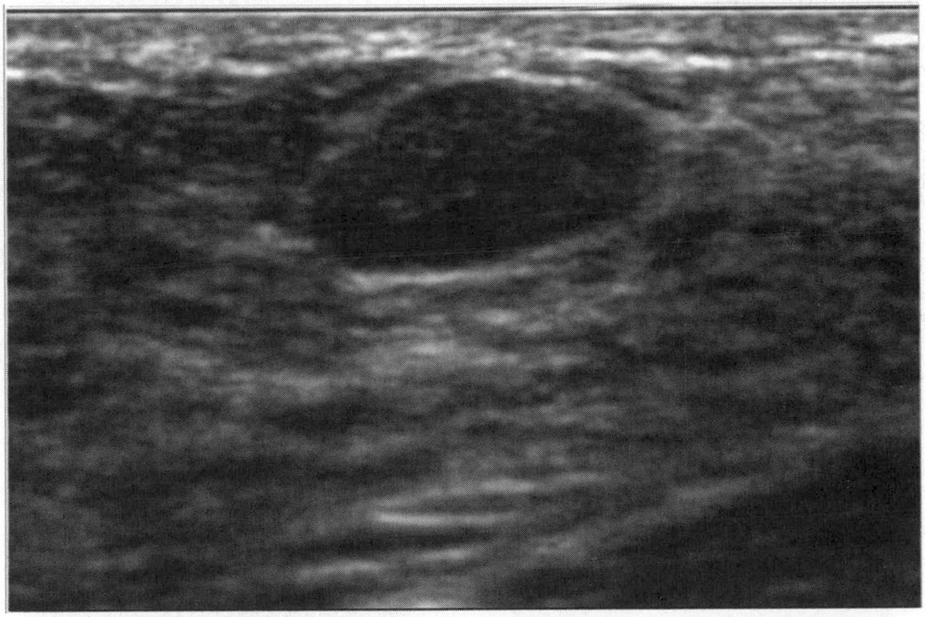

Figure 28-20. ■ *Sonogram of a benign fibroadenoma: elliptical, wider-than-tall lesion shape, and an encompassing thin echogenic capsule.*

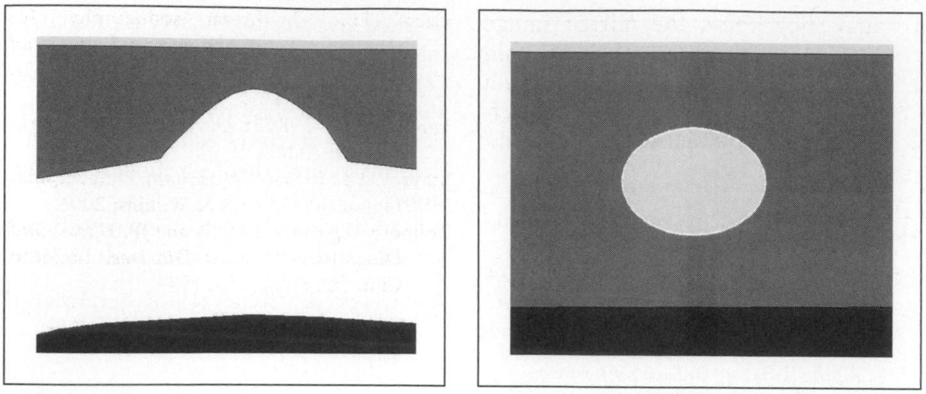

Figure 28-21. ■ *Purely hyperechoic fibrous tissue* (right) *versus palpable ridge of normal fibrous tissue* (left). *(From Stavros AT.* Breast Ultrasound. *Philadelphia: Lippincott Williams & Wilkins; 2004, with permission.)*

Ellipsoid Shape with Thin Echogenic Capsule

An elliptical wider-than-tall shape is the classic shape of fibroadenomas. However, this shape also has to be encompassed completely by a thin, echogenic capsule to meet strict criteria for a probably benign classification. The lesion can be gently lobulated with three or fewer lobulations (Fig. 28-22).

Color Doppler

Color Doppler is often used in breast ultrasound to look for neovascularity. It should not be used to determine benign from malignant nodules. More effectively, color Doppler can be used to help distinguish solid from cystic lesions. If there is a question about a lesion being a complex cyst versus a solid nodule, the presence of flow should be sought (Fig 28-8). Absence of flow does not mean that a lesion is a cyst, but the presence of flow does determine that a lesion is solid. By applying slight pressure with the transducer, all flow in a solid lesion can be temporarily obliterated; remember to scan with very light transducer pressure. Some uses for color Doppler include

- Solid versus cystic, fibrovascular stalk
- Inflamed versus noninflamed
- Anatomic landmark, internal mammary lymph node
- Intraductal papilloma versus inspissated secretions
- Normal from abnormal tissue, fremitus

Fremitus

Vocal fremitus is a technique that involves evaluating breast tissue with power Doppler while using different vocal stimuli, such as having the patient hum or say "eeeee." This will cause the tissues around a lesion to vibrate and create a power Doppler signal. Although there is continuing debate regarding the sensitivity of this technique, the premise is that if the vibration causes color to be displayed in the center of a lesion as well as surrounding tissue, it is considered worrisome for malignancy. If color is only visualized in the surrounding tissue, the lesion is more likely to be benign. Fremitus may also be helpful in distinguishing an isoechoic solid nodule from surrounding fat by enhancing the border of the lesion. This is also useful when determining whether a disease process is unifocal or multifocal. Fremitus is also reported to eliminate artifactual shadowing, thus decreasing the suspicion of calcification associated with malignancy.

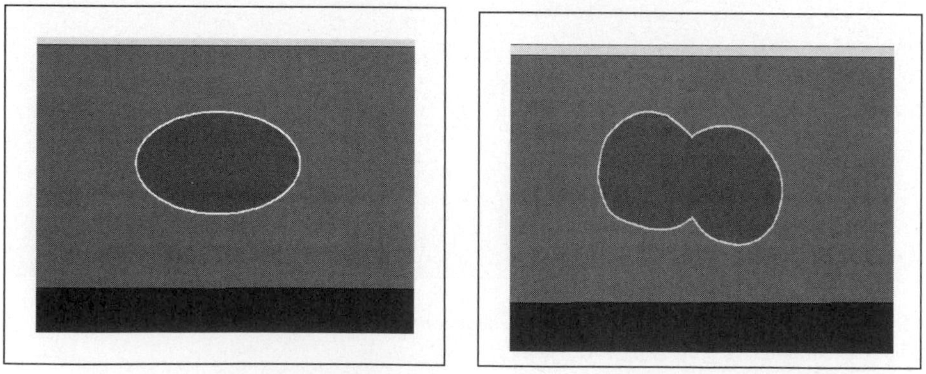

Figure 28-22. ■ *Wider-than-tall thinly encapsulated probably benign lesion* (left) *and gently lobulated lesion* (right). *(From Stavros AT.* Breast Ultrasound. *Philadelphia: Lippincott Williams & Wilkins; 2004, with permission.)*

Pitfalls

1. Scanning with too light transducer pressure may result in artifactual shadowing.
2. Scanning with too heavy transducer pressure may result in underlying lesions being obscured.
3. Scanning with too heavy transducer pressure while using color or power Doppler may ablate blood flow.
4. Scanning a superficial area without the use of a stand-off pad or gel can result in a lesion being missed secondary to partial volume artifact, particularly with older equipment.
5. Using breast ultrasound without performing mammographic correlation may result in nonvisualization of a suspected lesion.

Where Else to Look

1. If a suspicious lesion is seen, the patient's axilla should also be evaluated for the presence of metastatic lesions or abnormal lymph nodes.
2. If a suspicious lesion is identified, the entire breast should be evaluated for the presence of multifocal or multicentric disease.
3. When using ultrasound to evaluate asymmetric tissue density seen on mammography, the mirror image area of the contralateral side should be scanned for comparison. Using a "split screen" image can be very effective in showing this comparison.

SELECTED READING

Cardenosa G. *Breast Imaging Companion.* Philadelphia: Lippincott Williams & Wilkins; 2001.

Carr-Hoefer C. Breast sonography. In: Kawamura D, ed. *Abdomen and superficial structures, second edition.* Philadelphia: Lippincott; 1997.

Lanfranchi ME. *Breast Ultrasound.* New York: Marban; 2000.

Stavros AT. *Breast Ultrasound.* Philadelphia: Lippincott Williams & Wilkins; 2004.

Tohno E, Cosgrove DO, Sloane JP. *Ultrasound Diagnosis of Breast Diseases.* London: Churchill Livingston; 1994.

29

Infertility

ROGER C. SANDERS

SONOGRAM ABBREVIATIONS

FSH	Follicle-stimulating hormone
GIFT	Gamete intrafollicular transfer
hCG	Human chorionic gonadotropin
IVF	In vitro fertilization
LH	Luteinizing hormone
OHS	Ovarian hyperstimulation syndrome
PCO	Polycystic ovary syndrome
PID	Pelvic inflammatory disease
ZIFT	Zygote intrafollicular transfer

KEY WORDS

Adenomyosis. Abnormal endometrial tissue invasion into the uterine myometrium. The abnormally placed endometrial tissue responds to hormonal stimulation and bleeds at the time of periods.

Amenorrhea. Absence of menstrual periods. If periods have never occurred, primary amenorrhea is present. If periods have occurred in the past, there is secondary amenorrhea.

Anovulation. Absence of ovulation. Menstruation and follicle development may still occur.

Asherman's Syndrome. Scarring of the endometrial cavity of the uterus, usually as a consequence of previous infection or surgery.

Chocolate Cyst. Blood-filled cyst associated with endometriosis.

Clomid. Hormone used to stimulate ovulation.

Corpus Albicans. Scar at the site of a previous corpus lutein.

Corpus Luteum (or Corpus Lutein). A progesterone-producing cyst that forms at the site of a burst dominant follicle; persists during the first trimester of pregnancy.

Cuff. The blind sutured end of the vagina after hysterectomy is known as the cuff.

Estrogen. Hormone secreted by growing follicles that stimulates the uterine endometrium to regenerate.

Follicle. Fluid sac containing a developing ovum within the ovary. With each normal menstrual cycle several follicles enlarge: The largest follicle is termed the "dominant" or "graafian" follicle. Ovulation takes place from this large follicle.

Fornix. The upper portion of the vagina surrounds the cervix. A vaginal pouch forms a recess around the cervix known as the fornix (see Fig. 29-2).

Gamete. Unfertilized egg.

Gamete Intrafollicular Transfer (GIFT). Technique whereby ova are removed, fertilized, and then placed within the fallopian tube.

Hirsutism. Excessively hairy.

Human Chorionic Gonadotropin (hCG). Hormone produced by the gestational sac trophoblastic tissue that increases with pregnancy. It can be measured in maternal blood.

In Vitro Fertilization. Technique for fertilizing eggs with sperm outside the body, in a culture dish.

Luteinizing Hormone. Hormone put out by the pituitary that stimulates ovulation.

Luteinized Unruptured Follicle Syndrome (LUFS). Term used for a type of infertility in which a normal follicle fails to rupture and ovulate and continues to grow on a repeated basis.

Nabothian Cyst. A mucous-filled cyst that forms in the cervix; it is a normal finding.

Nulliparous. A woman who has not been pregnant.

Ovarian Hyperstimulation Syndrome (OHS). Stimulation of ovulation by hormonal therapy.

Ovulation Induction (OI). Technique whereby ova are removed, fertilized, and placed within the uterine cavity.

Ovum (Ova). An unfertilized egg (eggs) within a follicle.

Parous. Previously pregnant woman.

Pergonal. Hormone that stimulates follicle growth.

Posterior Cul-de-Sac. Pouch of Douglas space behind the uterus where fluid can collect.

Progesterone. Hormone secreted by the corpus luteum that prepares the endometrium to receive a fertilized egg.

Proliferative. Preovulatory phase of the menstrual cycle, at which time the endometrial cavity echoes form a single thin line (see Fig. 29-7A).

Secretory. Postovulatory phase of the menstrual cycle, at which time the endometrial cavity echoes are thick (see Fig. 29-7C).

Zygote. A fertilized egg.

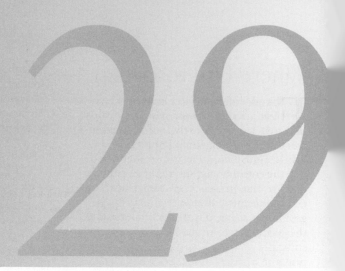

The Clinical Problem

Female infertility is a common problem affecting approximately 10% of couples, partly because many women defer pregnancy until a later age. If conception does not occur after a year or so of unprotected intercourse, couples usually seek advice from a reproductive endocrinologist. One of the first investigations performed is a sonogram. Both the ovaries and the uterus undergo ultrasonically obvious changes during ovulation and menstruation. Normally, one of several follicles becomes the dominant follicle; in midcycle, this follicle bursts and releases an egg. Subsequently, a corpus luteum forms from the remnants of the deflated follicle. In some instances, ultrasound can show that follicle production does not occur (anovulation) or the follicle continues to grow and does not release an egg (luteinized unruptured follicle).

The causes of some types of ovulation failure can be determined only by biochemical assay, but ultrasound has a role in following follicular development so that hormonal intervention, intercourse, or follicular puncture can be performed when the follicle reaches an appropriate size. If the fallopian tube is blocked or absent, the ovum may be retrieved with a needle, fertilized outside the patient, and then placed back in the uterus, a technique known as in vitro fertilization. Ultrasound is used to guide egg retrieval. Replacement of the fertilized ova into the uterus or tube may be monitored with ultrasound. Placement of the fertilized ova into the fallopian tube is known as the GIFT (gamete intrafollicular transfer) or ZIFT (zygote intrafallopian transfer) technique. These techniques are not performed with ultrasonic aid.

At the time of the initial sonogram, the sonographer should also look for structural problems that prevent the process of conception. Look for the following problems:

1. Congenital malformations such as a double uterus, bicornuate uterus, or hypoplastic uterus; uterine anomalies are associated with premature labor and spontaneous abortion.
2. Blockage of the pathway of the sperm and ovum by adhesions or masses secondary to infection or endometriosis (e.g., hydrosalpinx and endometrioma).
3. Distortion of the endometrial cavity by fibroids or polyps.

MENSTRUAL CYCLE PHYSIOLOGY

See Figure 29-1.

An average menstrual cycle lasts 28 days but may vary between 25 and 35 days. Day 1 is the first day of bleeding. The hypothalamic-pituitary-ovarian axis regulates the normal menstrual cycle. Immediately after the onset of menses, the hypothalamus prompts the pituitary gland to secrete follicle-stimulating hormone, which stimulates ovarian follicular growth. As the follicles grow, they produce estrogen, which induces endometrial regeneration. A dominant follicle (Graafian follicle) develops, containing the egg (ovum). Follicles reach a size of 1.5 to 2.7 cm. A large surge of the pituitary-secreted luteinizing hormone causes the graafian follicle to rupture, releasing the ovum. After ovulation, the graafian follicle becomes a corpus luteum, producing progesterone, which prepares the uterine endometrium to receive a fertilized egg (zygote). If the egg is not fertilized, estrogen and progesterone levels decrease, which causes bleeding (menses), and the cycle repeats itself. The corpus luteum degenerates into the corpus albicans, a small white scar on the ovary.

Changes in the endometrium also occur. Shortly after menstruation, the endometrium is inactive and thin. As ovulation approaches, an echogenic rim develops on either side of the thin endometrium. After ovulation has occurred, the area between the echogenic rim and the central line fills in with echoes when the patient is in the secretory phase of the cycle (see Fig. 29-7A–C).

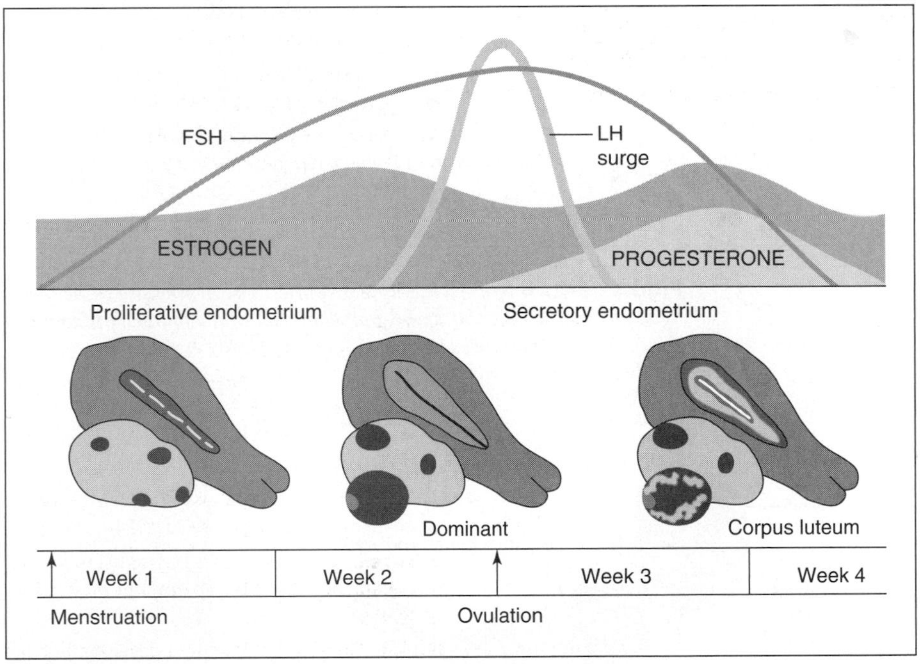

Figure 29-1. ■ *Sequence of events during a normal menstrual cycle. The ovary contains several follicles; one (the dominant follicle) slowly increases in size until it ovulates. At the site where ovulation takes place, the corpus luteum develops. The developing follicle (a sonographic cyst) ovulates when it reaches a size of 15 to 27 mm. A degenerating corpus luteum has an echogenic border with much vascular flow and may contain blood in its center. The uterine endometrium thickens in the secretory phase before menstruation.*

Anatomy

See Figure 29-2.

VAGINA

See Figures 29-2 and 29-3.

A central bright linear echo represents the opposing inner vaginal walls. The surrounding muscular portion is more hypoechoic. After hysterectomy, the blind end of the vagina is sutured to form a fibrous mass, the cuff. The cuff is variable in size depending on surgical technique and is usually not seen but should not normally be more than 2.2 cm long.

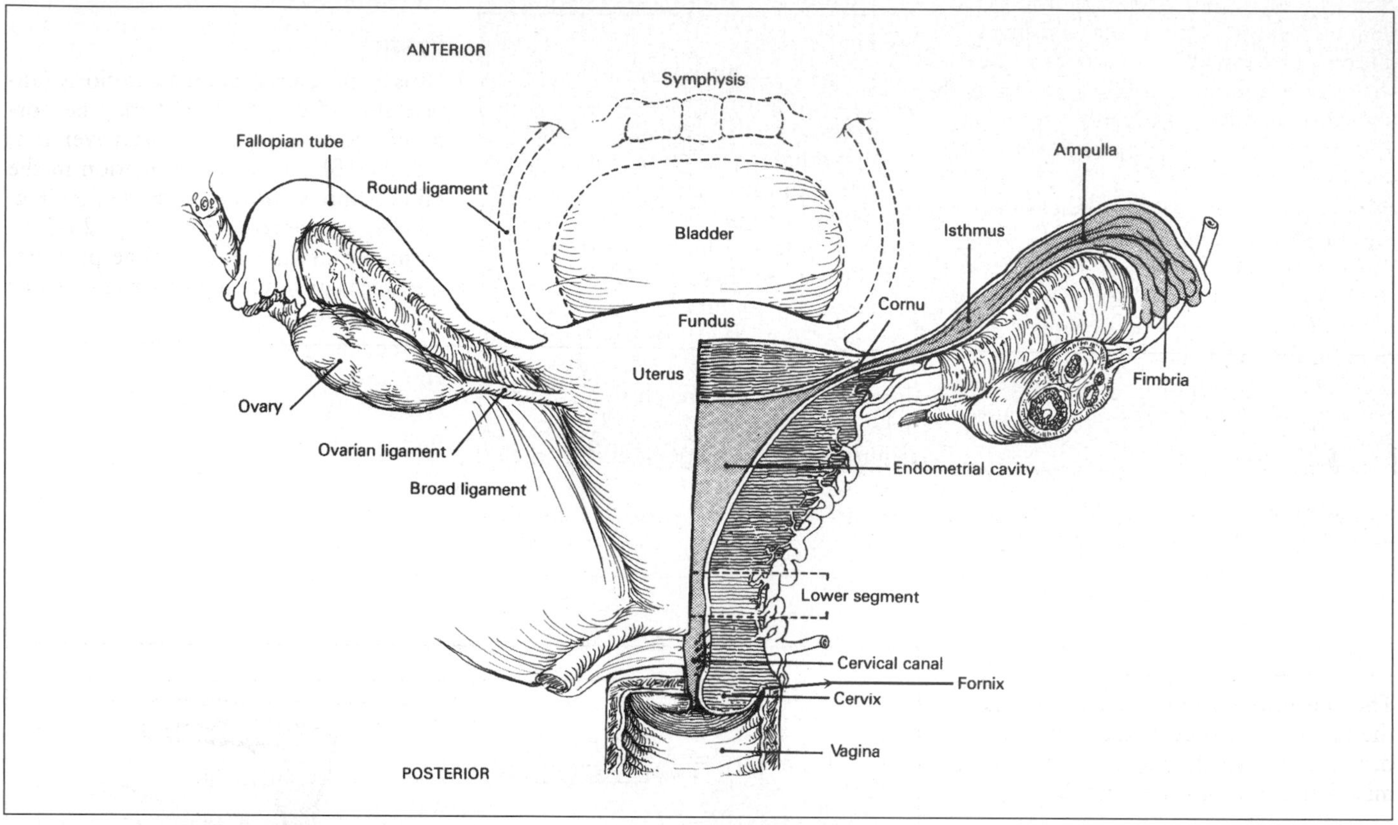

Figure 29-2. ■ *Normal uterus and ovaries. The ovaries are suspended from the utero-ovarian ligament and lie adjacent to the ampullary end of the fallopian tube. The fallopian tube arises from the cornu of the uterus. The tube is sonographically visible when outlined by ascites, but the normal lumen is never seen.*

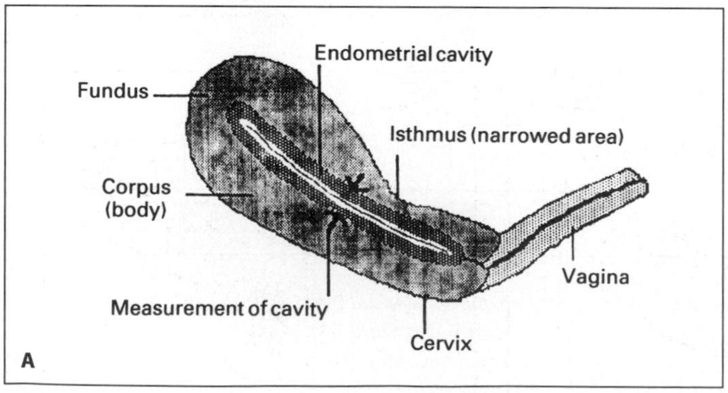

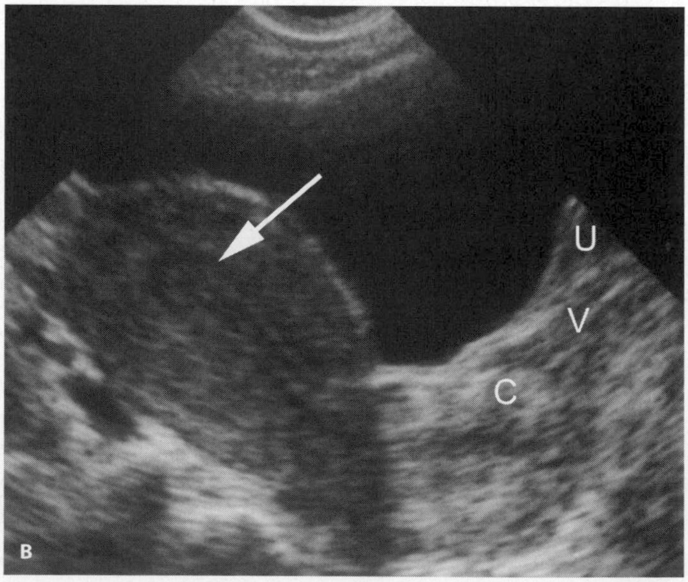

Figure 29-3. ■ *A. Uterus. Normal anteverted uterus with decidual reaction in the cavity. The anatomic components of the uterus, the cervix, corpus, fundus, and isthmus, are shown. The site for measuring the endometrial cavity is indicated. B. Anteverted uterus as seen on abdominal sonogram. Midcycle endometrial cavity can be seen* (arrow). *The urethra* (U) *is visible anterior to the vagina* (V). *The different texture of the cervix* (C) *can be seen.*

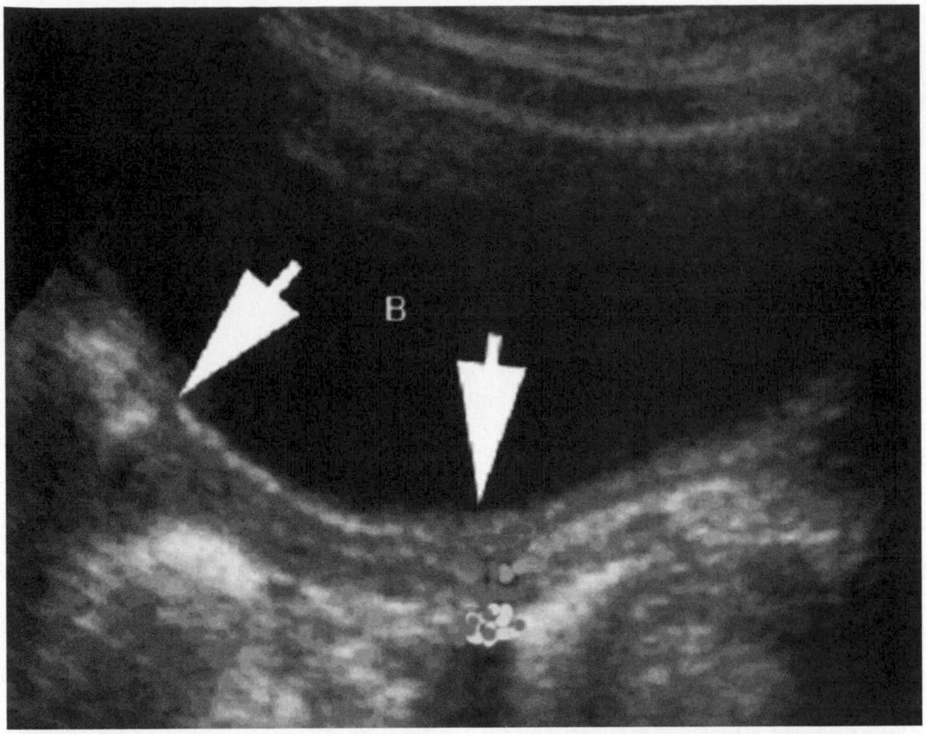

Figure 29-4. ■ *Prepubertal uterus. The uterus extends between the arrows posterior to the bladder (B). Note that the uterus is small and tubular without the fundal expansion seen in an adult.*

URETHRA

The posterior urethra forms a bulge in the posterior aspect of the female bladder, anterior to the vagina, that can be mistaken for a mass (see Fig. 29-3B).

UTERUS

The uterus is a thick-walled, pear-shaped, muscular organ lying posterior to the bladder and anterior to the rectum. A central echogenic line represents the endometrial cavity (Fig. 29-3A,B). Small cysts in the cervical region are a common normal variant and are known as nabothian cysts. The uterus is composed of four parts: the fundus, corpus (body), isthmus, and cervix (Fig. 29-3A).

Size

Normal uterine measurements in nulliparous menstruating women are 6 to 9 cm in length and up to 4 cm in anterior-posterior diameter and width. The uterus of parous women will have larger dimensions depending on the number of pregnancies. Before puberty, the uterus is approximately 3 cm long and more or less tubular in shape (Fig. 29-4). After menopause, the uterus shrinks in size but retains the shape it adopted with the onset of puberty.

Position

Usually the uterus is tilted anteriorly (anteversion; Fig. 29-5A) but may be normally tilted posteriorly (retroversion; Fig. 29-5B). An acute angulation in the midportion is known as anteflexion (Fig. 29-5C) or retroflexion (Fig. 29-5D). Although usually in a midline position, the uterus may lie obliquely to the left or right.

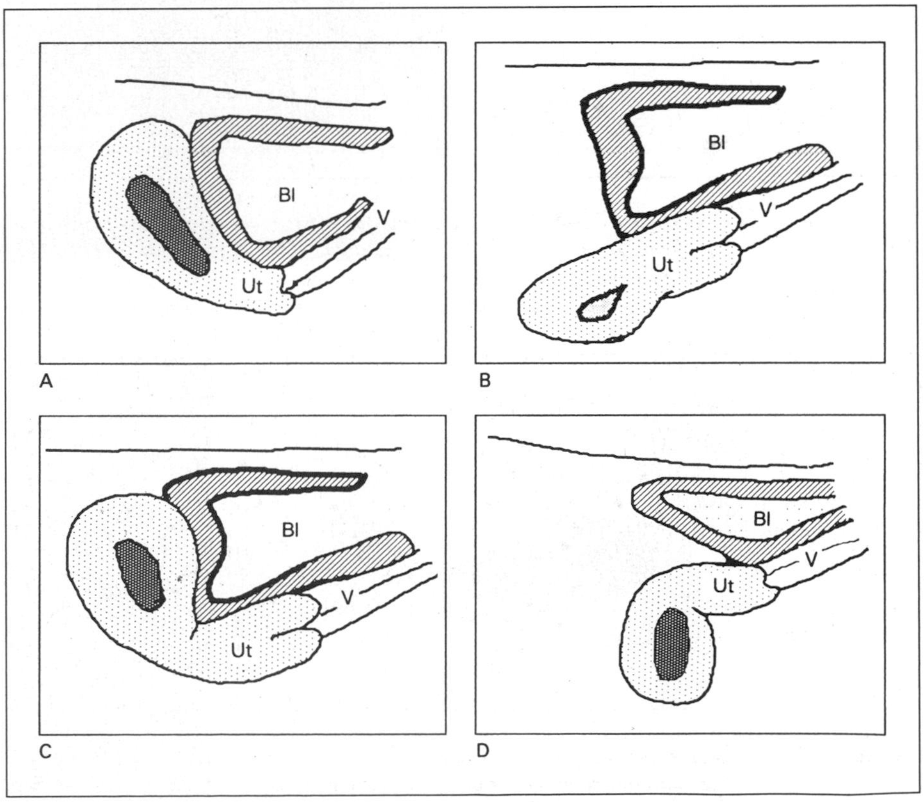

Figure 29-5. ■ *Various uterine positions.* ***A.*** *Anteverted.* ***B.*** *Retroverted.* ***C.*** *Anteflexed.* ***D.*** *Retroflexed. Note the echogenic septum where the uterus folds over on itself.*

Shape

The menstruating uterus widens toward the fundus and the cornu, the bilateral, somewhat triangular regions where the fallopian tubes insert (Fig. 29-6). It is tubular in the part near the vagina known as the cervix.

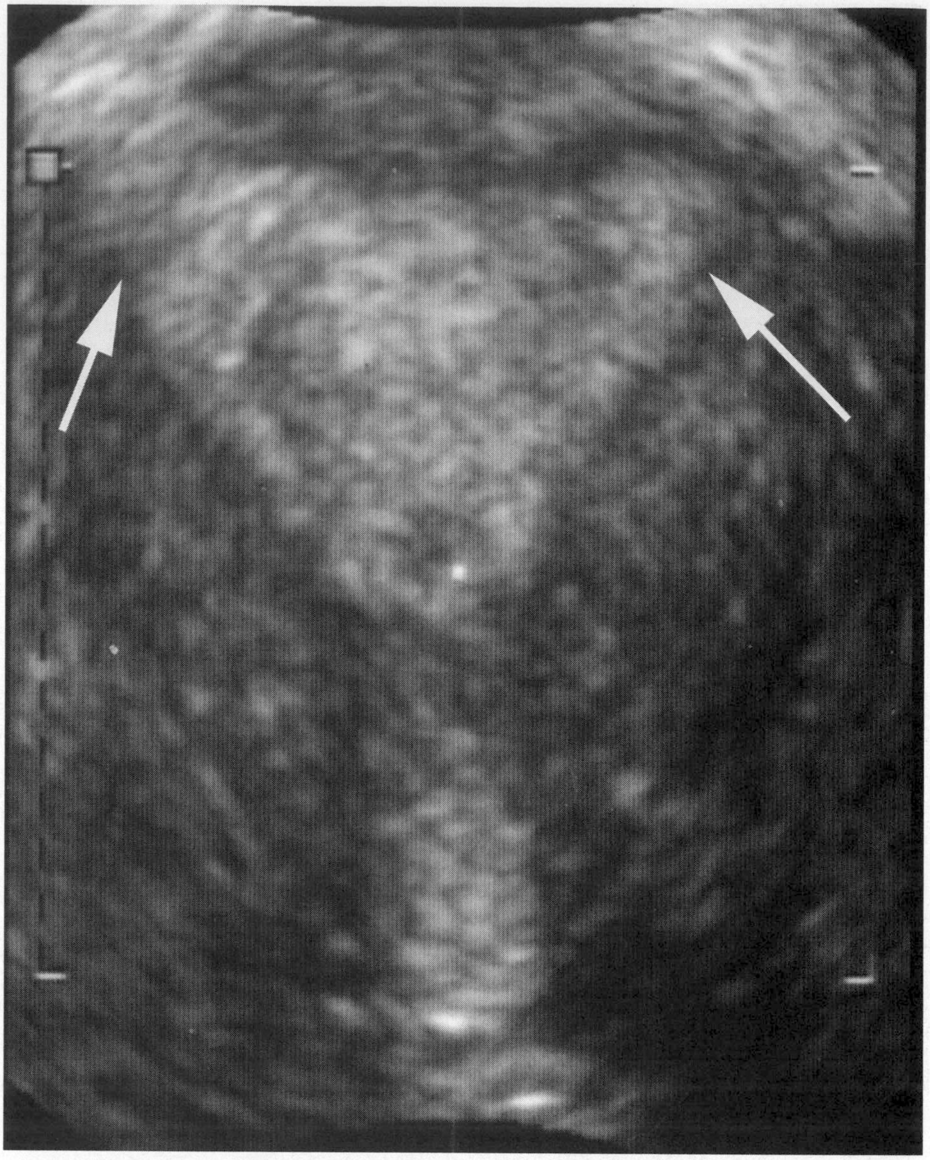

Figure 29-6. ■ *Three-dimensional C scan of the uterus showing the secretory endometrium extending toward the fallopian tubes at the fundus forming the cornu* (arrows).

Changes with Menstruation

The lining of the endometrial cavity is partially shed each month at menstruation, with consequent changes in cavity appearance during the course of the cycle (Fig. 29-7A–C).

During the preovulatory (proliferative) phase, the endometrial cavity echo is only about 3 mm thick and is surrounded by an echopenic halo (Fig. 29-7A). Shortly before ovulation, two additional linear echoes outline the echopenic area (the "three line sign") (Fig. 29-7B). The echopenic area becomes more echogenic so that in the postovulatory (secretory or luteal) phase, the cavity echo becomes brighter and thicker (Fig. 29-7C). At this point, the width of the cavity is between 8 mm and 1.3 cm thick.

FALLOPIAN TUBES

The lumen of the normal fallopian tubes cannot be seen. The fallopian tubes lie within the broad ligament. They can often be traced from the uterine fundus to the ovaries on endovaginal views. This is especially easy if there is cul-de-sac fluid.

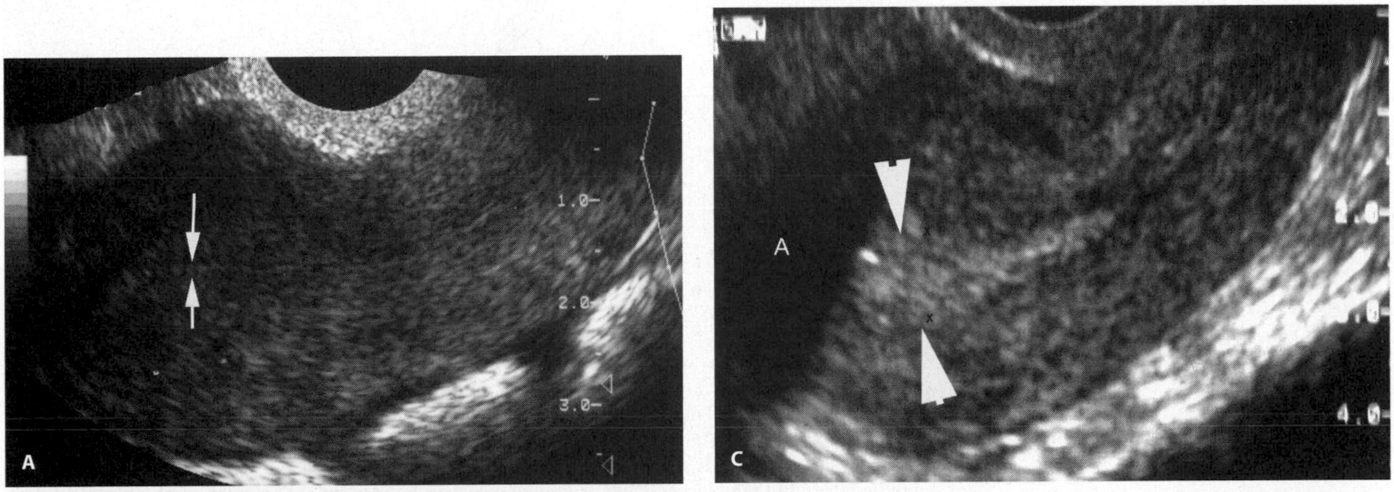

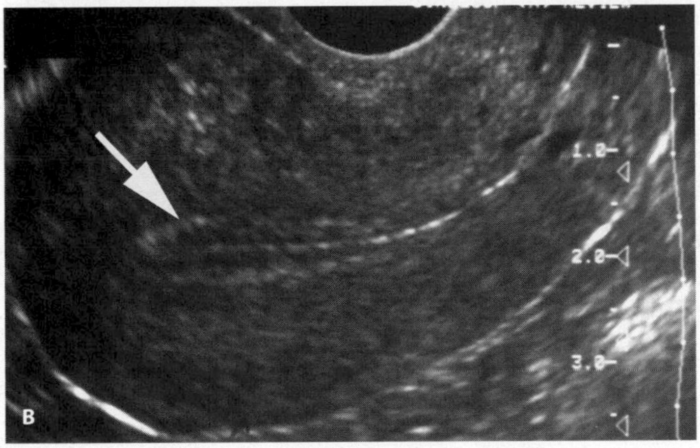

Figure 29-7. ■ *A. Proliferative endometrium. Sagittal endovaginal view of the adult uterus a few days after menstruation has stopped, showing the thin endometrium in the proliferative phase of the cycle* (arrows). *The endometrium is less than 5 mm thick. This is the ideal phase to perform most sonograms because the ovary is quiescent and the endometrium is thin. B. Midcycle endometrium. Sagittal endovaginal view of the adult uterus approximately 14 days after the start of menstruation. When this three-line appearance* (arrow) *is seen in a healthy menstruating women ovulation is imminent. C. Secretory endometrium. Sagittal endovaginal view of the adult uterus in the second half of the cycle showing thick glandular endometrium (between* arrowheads*). Endometrial pathology is difficult to see at this stage of the cycle because the endometrium is so thick and echogenic. Note the artifactual dropout (A) at the fundus of the uterus, a technical problem caused by beam axis to uterine interfaces, spuriously suggesting a fibroid.*

OVARIES

Location

The ovaries are usually found at the level of the uterine fundus where the uterus becomes triangular (the cornu) (Figs. 29-8 and 29-9; see also Fig. 29-2). By using the endovaginal probe, the utero-ovarian ligament (which runs parallel with the Fallopian tubes) can often be traced to the ovary. Do not mistake the ovaries for the internal iliac vein, which lies lateral to the usual site of the ovary (Fig. 29-9).

Size

In a menstruating woman, ovaries normally measure approximately 2 × 2.5 × 3 cm. There is variation, so 5 × 2 × 1.5 cm and 4 × 3 × 1.5 cm, for example, are measurements that may be within normal limits if a dominant follicle or corpus luteum is present. The ovaries are approximately 1 cm^3 in young girls, gradually increasing in size as puberty approaches (see Appendix 24). In menopausal women the size of the ovary gradually decreases.

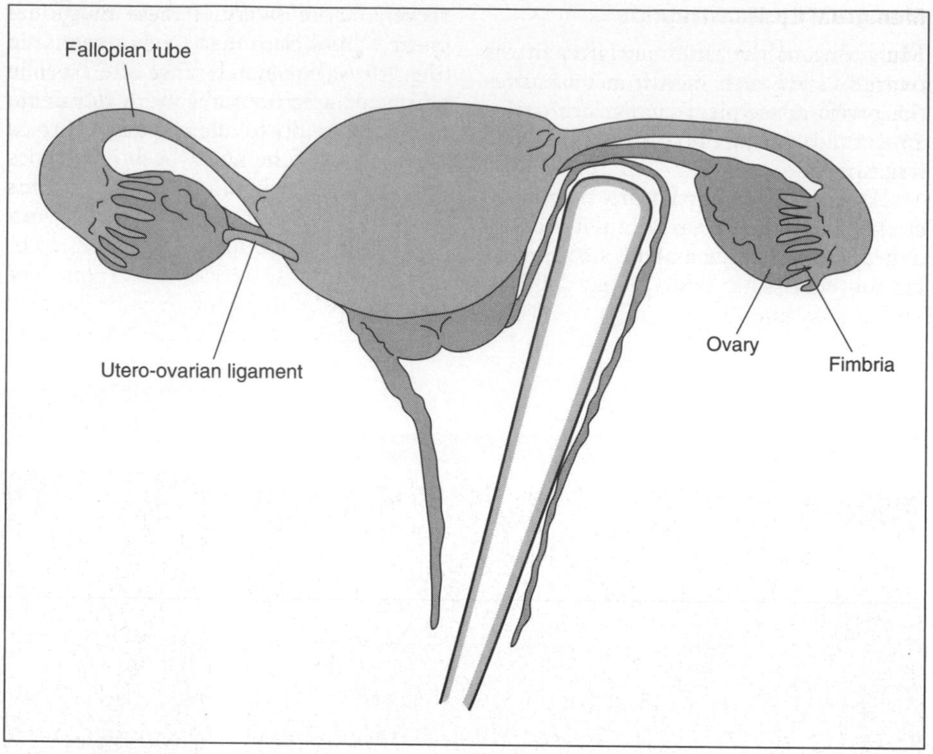

Figure 29-8. ■ *Vaginal probe seeking for pelvic pain. The probe tip is pressing against the utero-ovarian ligament, an important landmark in finding the ovary and the site where the patient is most tender if chronic infection is present. Note how distensible the vagina is. Both the utero-ovarian ligament and the takeoff of the Fallopian tube can be seen on endovaginal ultrasound.*

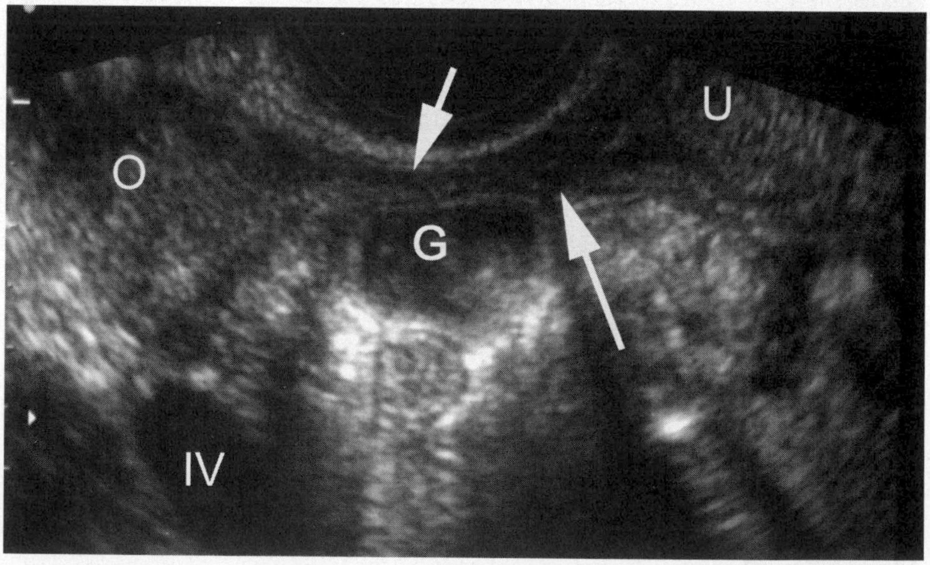

Figure 29-9. ■ *Localized view of the right adnexa showing the ovary* (O), *utero-ovarian ligament* (arrow), *and uterus* (U). *The Fallopian tube* (arrow) *can be traced toward the ovary. G, gut; IV, iliac vein.*

Menstrual Cycle Changes

Multiple small follicles are seen in the ovaries shortly after menstruation ends in the proliferative phase of the cycle (Fig. 29-10A). Normally one follicle grows to a size of between 1.5 and 2.7 cm (Fig. 29-10B), often alternating sides each menstrual cycle. Hormonal stimulation with drugs such as Pergonal or Clomid increases the number of dominant follicles, which may number as many as six or more in each ovary if these drugs are given. Follicles are not seen in menopausal women but are often seen in young girls before puberty. A dominant follicle normally bursts and disappears at midcycle. It is replaced by a corpus luteum (Fig. 29-10C). Typically, a corpus luteum has a thick, slightly echogenic, vascular rim (the rim of fire on color Doppler) and an echopenic center. The central echopenic area may be large if there is much bleeding at the time of ovulation. The corpus luteum will usually disappear within a week or so.

PELVIC MUSCLES AND LIGAMENTS

Bands of muscle tissue play an important role in maintaining the position of the uterus and ovaries. The utero-ovarian ligament extends from the uterus to the ovary. The broad ligament is a filmy structure not visible with sonography. The obturator internus muscles lie

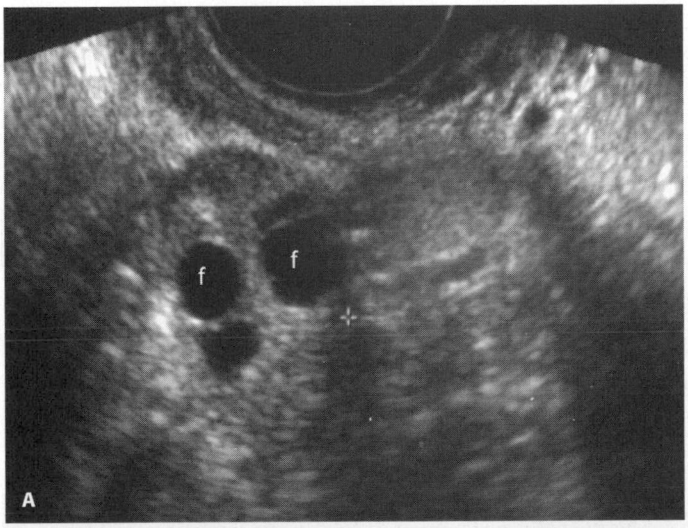

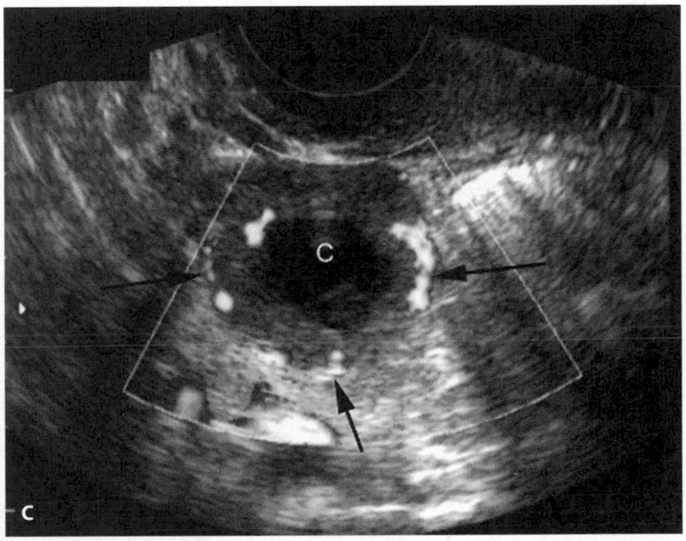

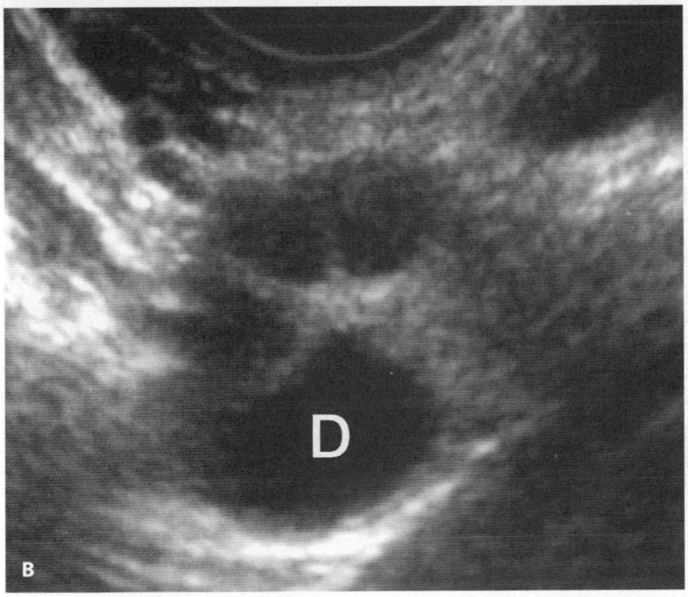

Figure 29-10. ■ *A. Ovary early in the cycle showing several follicles* (f). *B. Dominant follicle* (D) *with several smaller follicles. C. Corpus luteum. An echogenic rim containing vessels* (arrows) *surrounds the cystic center of the corpus luteum* (C). *Some clot is present within the cystic center. Corpus luteum often have hemorrhage within.*

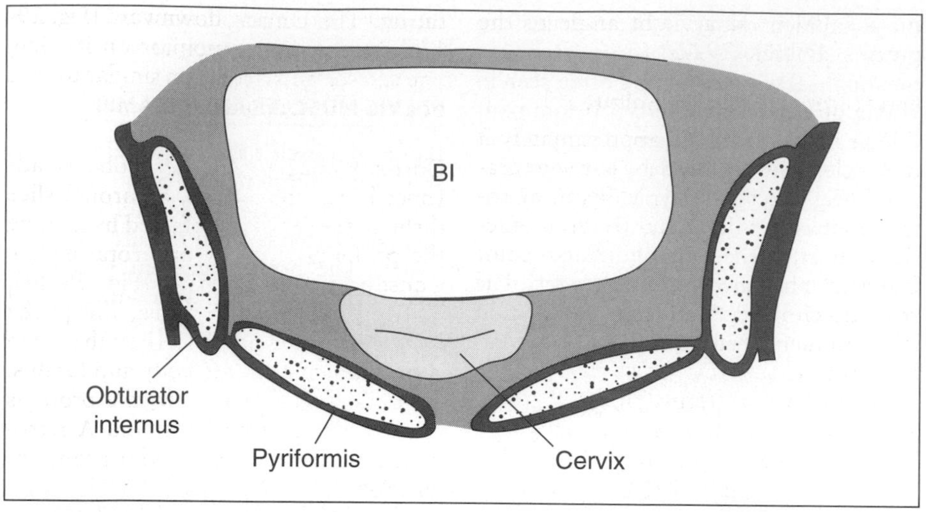

Figure 29-11. ■ *Transverse view at the level of the cervix showing the muscles that form the side walls of the pelvis.*

alongside the bony wall, lateral to the ovaries (Fig. 29-11). The iliopsoas muscles are lateral and anterior to the iliac crest; the femoral nerve sheath is seen as an echogenic area within the muscle. The levator ani, pyriformis, and coccygeus muscles make up the pelvic floor and are located posterior to the uterus, vagina, and rectum.

SPACES SURROUNDING THE UTERUS

Small amounts of fluid may normally collect adjacent to the uterus in the anterior or posterior cul-de-sac, also known as the pouch of Douglas (Fig. 29-12). The fluid may result from normal ovulation. The anterior cul-de-sac is anterior and superior to the uterine fundus, whereas the posterior cul-de-sac is posterior to the cervix.

Technique

ENDOVAGINAL SCANNING (TRANSVAGINAL SCANNING, VAGINAL SCANNING)

Endovaginal scanning has become the dominant technique used for the examination of the female pelvic structures. Detail of the ovaries, endometrium, and myometrium is far superior to that obtained with the transabdominal approach. In addition, the vaginal probe can be used like an examining finger to decide the following:

1. Whether local tenderness is greatest in the ovaries, tubal region, or uterus.
2. Whether the ovaries move freely; if the ovaries cannot be separated from the neighboring bowel or the adjacent uterus, adhesions are the likely cause.
3. Whether a mass is intrauterine or extrauterine.

Endovaginal scanning is essential whenever greater detail is required, for example, in the following entities:

1. Ectopic pregnancy
2. Threatened abortion
3. Follicle monitoring and egg retrieval
4. A questionable adnexal mass
5. Intrauterine pathology (e.g., endometrial polyps or fibroids) and monitoring of endometrial thickness
6. Chorionic villi sampling
7. Early pregnancy

Endovaginal scanning is often used after a brief transabdominal scan unless it is only follicles that are being monitored or it is suspected that the patient has an ectopic pregnancy and the bladder is empty. It is more convenient to perform the transabdominal study first because the bladder can easily be emptied but takes at least 45 minutes to refill. The endovaginal pelvic examination cannot entirely replace the transabdomi-

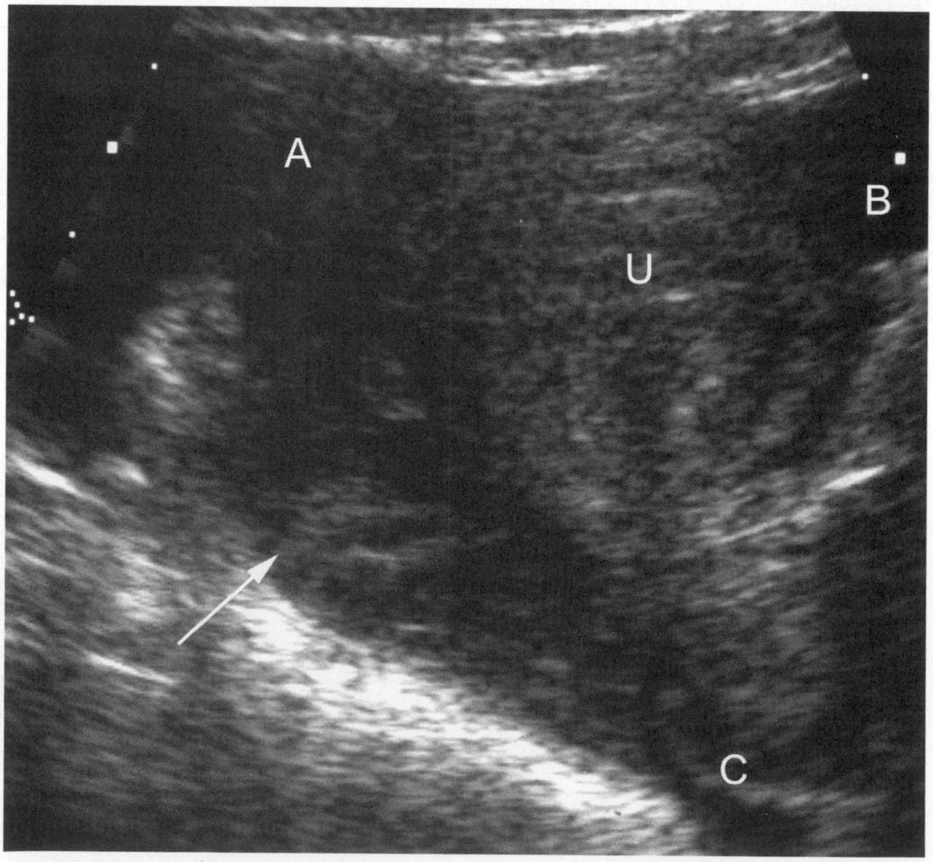

Figure 29-12. ■ *Sagittal view of the uterus in a patient with a ruptured ectopic. Fluid* (arrow) *surrounds the uterus* (U). *The blood lies in the posterior cul-de-sac* (C) *and anterior cul-de-sac* (A). *B, bladder.*

nal pelvic sonogram for the following reasons:

1. It does not show the entire extent of large pelvic masses or midabdominal pathology.
2. It cannot be used in young girls or in some postmenopausal women—it may be too threatening for some sexually inexperienced women, and the older woman's vagina may not accommodate the probe.
3. Some ovaries are located at such a high level they can only be seen with transabdominal views.

Preparation

Because the endovaginal examination is similar to a pelvic examination, the male sonographer should have a chaperone. A clean transducer is covered with a condom after gel has been placed on the transducer tip. The bladder should be as empty as possible because urine in the bladder creates an artifact.

Instrumentation

The endovaginal transducer is a rod-shaped probe or wand approximately 6 to 12 inches in length with a handle at one end and the transducer crystal located in the tip at the opposite end. The ultrasound beam is transmitted from the tip parallel or at a slight angle to the probe shaft (Fig. 29-13).

Endovaginal Probe Technique

The probe is advanced approximately 3 to 4 inches into the vagina. The sonographer then directs the sound beam by rotating and angling the probe from anterior to posterior and sliding it in and out. Use a gynecologic table with stirrups if you can; elevating the hips with a pillow is a poor substitute because you cannot angle the probe posteriorly adequately to see an anteverted uterus. The patient will let you know if she is experiencing discomfort; however, the vagina is very distensible, and angling the probe is usually pain-free unless the patient has a disease process such as a pelvic infection.

Orientation

Sagittal and coronal images of the uterus and ovaries can be obtained transvaginally. Because the probe is inserted into the vagina with the ultrasound beam directed toward the uterus, the vagina itself is not normally visualized. The probe is partially withdrawn to visualizc thc cervix and distal vagina.

Sagittal images. As the probe is advanced into the vagina, the cervix can be seen approaching the top of the screen with the uterus extending downward (Fig. 29-13). By resting the monitor on its side, one can see an orientation similar to that of a transabdominal pelvic scan.

Coronal images. As the probe is advanced into the vagina, a coronal slice through the cervix is obtained by angling the probe posteriorly and rotating the transducer head laterally (Fig. 29-14). With an anteverted uterus, the probe handle is angled posteriorly so the beam is perpendicular to the body and fundus. To obtain a coronal view, the probe is rotated into a lateral position. A retroverted uterus requires anterior probe angulation.

When the probe is angled laterally, the ovaries can usually be seen. If a transverse view through the fundus of the uterus is obtained, the utero-ovarian ligament is usually found. In many women, tracing this structure laterally will lead to the ovary (Fig. 29-9).

TRANSABDOMINAL SCANNING

Distention of the urinary bladder is helpful for a high-quality transabdominal pelvic sonogram. The full bladder displaces bowel and repositions the uterus in a more longitudinal fashion that al-

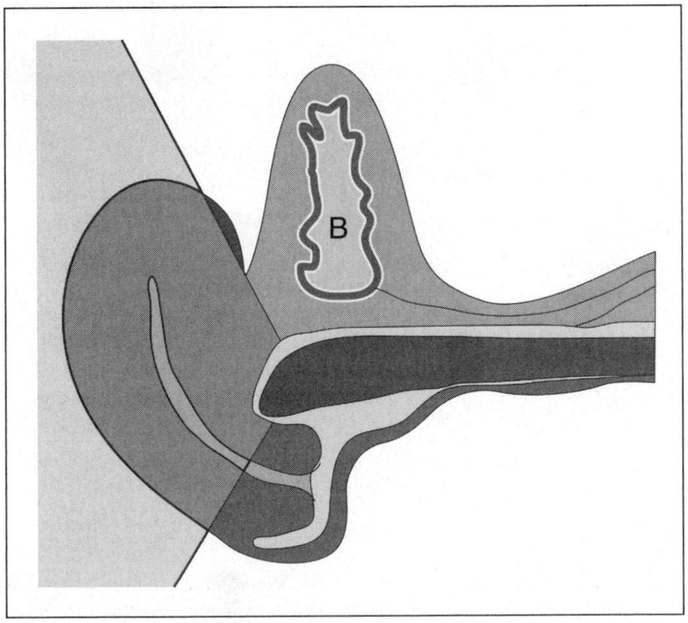

Figure 29-13. ■ *Usual position of the vaginal probe in the anterior fornix when sagittal views of the uterus are obtained. Because the vaginal probe is adjacent to the uterus, one sees very detailed views of the endometrium. B, bladder.*

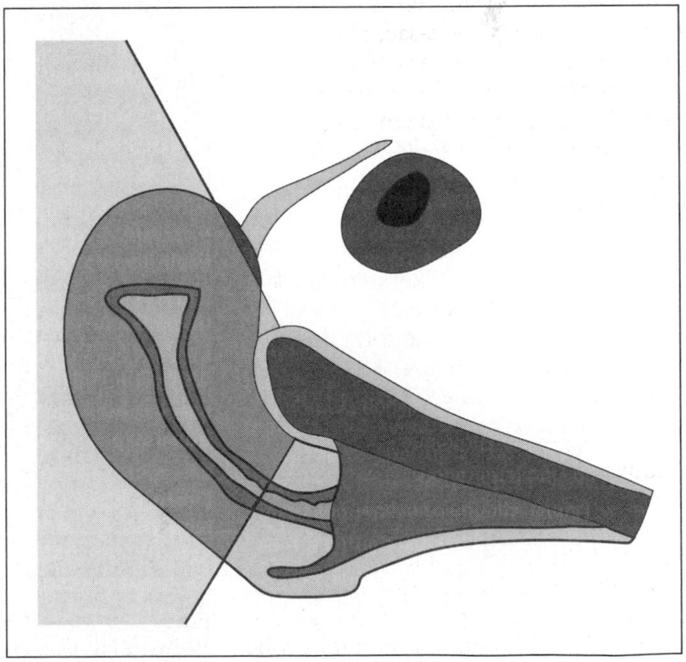

Figure 29-14. ■ *Position of the vaginal probe when coronal views of the uterus are obtained. A minor shift in the angulation of the probe will show the ovary and the utero-ovarian ligament.*

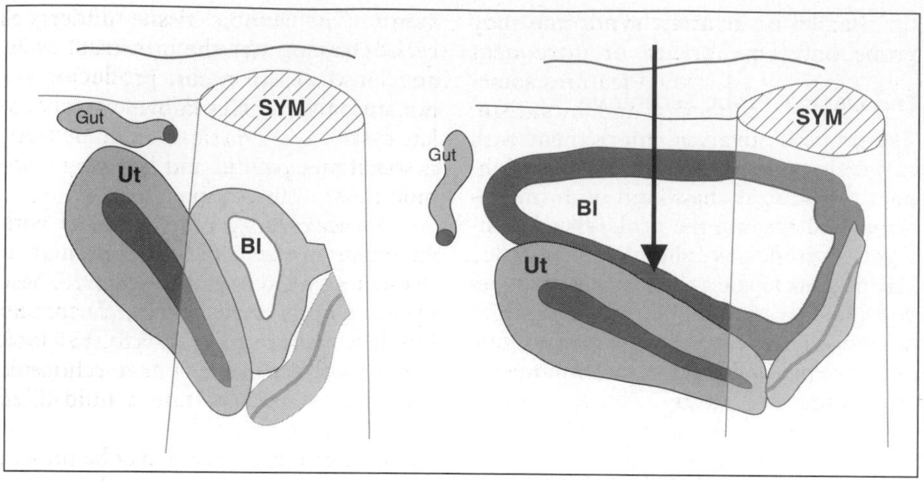

Figure 29-15. ■ *Filling the bladder to alter the uterine axis. When this bladder was filled* (right), *the uterus became less anteflexed, allowing more of the uterus to be seen. A retroverted uterus also adopts a more satisfactory position when the bladder is filled. Note the shadowing from the symphysis* (sym) *partially obscuring the vagina and cervix unless the transducer is angled inferiorly.*

lows the ultrasound beam to transect the uterus perpendicularly. The urinary bladder provides an acoustic window for better visualization of the pelvic structures. Overdistention or underdistention of the bladder can distort or obscure the view. A sufficiently full bladder will extend just over the uterine fundus.

A commonly used approach is to ask the patient not to void for 1 hour before an examination so there is a little urine in the bladder at the time of the abdominal examination. The abdominal approach is then only used to look at large adnexal masses and to discover the uterine axis. Details of the endometrium and ovary are obtained using the vaginal probe.

1. The sonographic examination should begin in a longitudinal fashion by attempting to align the uterus with the vagina. The uterus can be recognized by the central line of the endometrial cavity and by its alignment with the vagina. The vagina is visualized as an echogenic line with relatively sonolucent walls.

   The uterus is normally located in the midline, but it may be deviated to either side in an oblique axis. An anteflexed or retroverted uterus may become more normal in position and shape if the bladder is filled (Fig. 29-15).
2. Scanning at right angles to the axis of the uterus should demonstrate the ovaries. The ovaries are usually close to the triangular cornual regions near the uterine fundus. Caudal angulation is helpful for visualizing the pelvic musculature and retroverted uteri. Cranial or caudal angulation may be necessary to see the ovaries.

Pathology

Female infertility can be a result of the following:

1. Physiologic factors disrupting the hormonal control of ovulation.
2. Structural problems preventing fertilization.

CONGENITAL UTERINE MALFORMATIONS

See Figure 29-16.

Uterine structural defects often cause repeated abortions rather than absence of pregnancy. One to two percent of the female population have some type of structural defect. The most common uterine anomalies are the following:

1. Uterus didelphys: two adjacent cervices with two separate uterine bodies (Fig. 29-16).
2. Septate uterus: there is a partial lack of embryologic fusion that results in a septated uterine body with two separate cavities within a single uterus (Fig. 29-16).

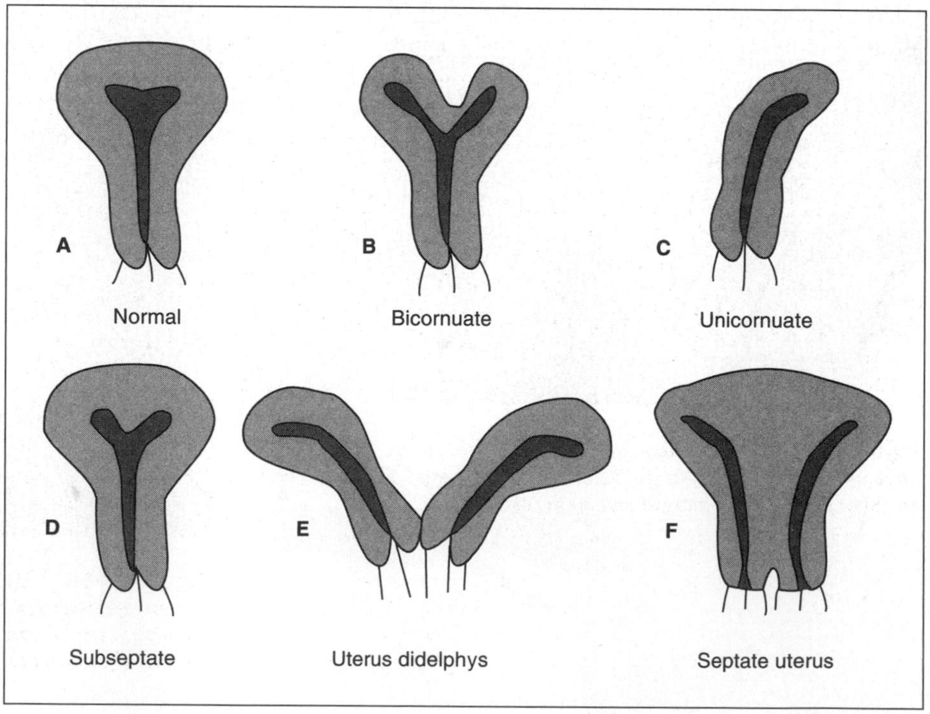

Figure 29-16. ■ *Congenital uterine anomalies. A. Normal. B. Bicornuate uterus. Note the V-shaped indentation in the fundus of the endometrial cavity. C. Unicornuate uterus that has only one horn. D. Uterus subseptate. There is no deformity of the uterine outline, but the two horns of the uterus are split. A milder variation of this deformity in which the indentation at the fundus of the measures between 1 and 1.5 cm is known as an arcuate uterus. E. Uterus didelphys. There are two uteri that are separate, two cervices and two vaginas. F. Septate uterus. Two completely separate uterine cavities are enclosed in a single uterine outline.*

3. Bicornuate uterus: the uterus has a single cavity in the cervix and lower uterine segment. The cavity splits in the fundus into two horns (Fig. 29-16). Only one vagina is present. This is the most common structural defect.
4. Uterus unicornis: there is one uterine horn and cervix, and one vagina (Fig. 29-16).
5. Uterus subseptus: the endometrial cavity bifurcates into two horns, but the uterine outline is unaltered (Fig. 29-16).
6. Hypoplastic uterus: the uterus is normally formed, but is less than 4 cm long. Sometimes the patient can menstruate with a uterus this small.

POLYCYSTIC OVARIES

See Figure 29-17.

Polycystic ovarian syndrome may cause only amenorrhea or infrequent ovulation, but additional features sometimes seen are obesity and hirsutism. There is mild ovarian enlargement with numerous small cysts around the periphery of the ovary, best seen with the endovaginal transducer. The central cyst-free area is increased in size and is called stroma. Such sonographic appearances may be found in apparently healthy women, so a diagnosis of polycystic ovaries is usually made in conjunction with biochemical tests.

ENDOMETRIOSIS

See Figure 29-18.

During the reproductive years, endometrial tissue may become implanted outside the uterine cavity, adhering to any structure, but particularly to the ovaries, fallopian tubes, and broad ligaments. The ectopic tissue undergoes cyclic changes with the menstrual cycle, and bleeding can occur, producing endometriomas, masses known as "chocolate cysts," and adhesions. Endometriosis is sometimes painful and is a very common cause of infertility.

Typical sonographic findings with endometriosis are fluid-filled circular or ovoid masses within the ovary. These masses may (1) be echo-free, (2) contain low-level echoes (Fig. 29-18), (3) look like a solid mass, or (4) have echogenic areas or a septum within a fluid-filled mass.

One or more masses may be present that consist of hematomas. The abnormal endometrial tissue that produces the bleeding is not seen, but there may be evidence of adhesions with an abnormal or fixed ovarian position (see Chapter 32). Occasionally, extraovarian endometrioma develop in the adnexa.

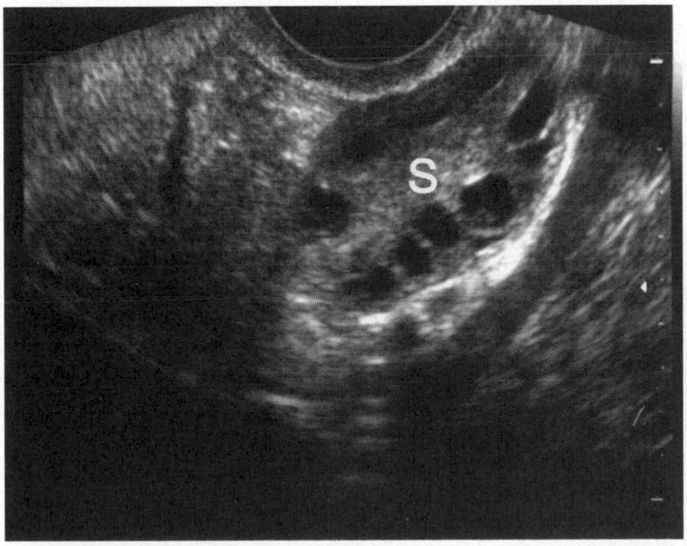

Figure 29-17. ■ *Endovaginal view of polycystic ovary. The ovary is large with many small cysts (follicles) lining the border. The stromal center* (S) *of the ovary is enlarged and more echogenic.*

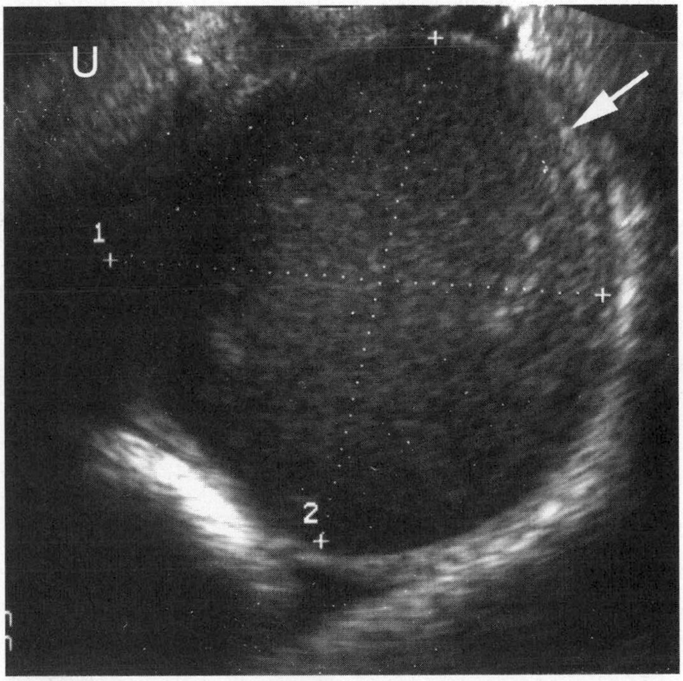

Figure 29-18. ■ *Transverse endovaginal view of the ovary and uterus* (U). *An endometrioma is present within the ovary. A rim of normal ovarian tissue* (arrow) *can be seen around the ovary. Note the typical low-level echoes within the endometrioma.*

PELVIC INFLAMMATORY DISEASE

Pelvic inflammatory disease, when responsible for infertility, is characterized by fluid-filled Fallopian tubes and adhesions of the pelvic structures. Patency of the fallopian tubes is diminished secondary to scarring from infections, so bilateral hydrosalpinx may be seen (Fig. 29-19). The sonographic findings of pelvic inflammatory disease are discussed in detail in Chapter 33. Previous pelvic surgery can also lead to adhesions and blocked fallopian tubes causing infertility due to hydrosalpinx. Tubal patency can be assessed using hysterosonosalpingography with the injection of fluid or ultrasonic contrast. This technique is described in Chapter 34.

FIBROIDS

Large uterine masses can hinder zygote implantation and cause premature labor or spontaneous abortion. Intracavitary fibroids are especially likely to prevent conception (see Chapter 32).

UTERINE SYNECHIAE

Previous intrauterine surgery, such as a dilatation and curettage, may result in fibrous strands across the uterine cavity, known as synechiae. These can prevent egg implantation. If many synechiae are present and the two walls of the endometrial cavity are gummed together, implantation cannot occur; this condition is known as Asherman's syndrome. The endometrial cavity contents can be demonstrated by the use of the saline infusion study (hysterosonogram; see Chapter 34 for a description of this technique). Strands of fibrous tissue will be seen crossing the cavity. In the more severe form, the cavity will be obliterated and it will be impossible to get fluid into the cavity (Asherman's syndrome).

OVULATION DISORDERS

Anovulation is failure to ovulate characterized by poor ovarian follicular development or a dominant follicle that enlarges but never bursts and ovulates (luteinized unruptured follicle syndrome). Serial sonograms during a cycle can reveal abnormal follicle development or even their absence. Unstimulated follicles normally burst when they reach a size of between 1.5 and 2.7 cm. The luteinized unruptured follicle syndrome is diagnosed when serial follow-up views show the follicle size continuing to increase beyond 2.7 cm. Eventually, the unruptured follicle will spontaneously disappear.

Guiding Therapy for Infertility

Several approaches are used to assist infertile couples when anovulation is the problem. Most therapies involve using a pharmacologic agent, Clomid or Pergonal, to stimulate follicular growth. A human chorionic gonadotropin (hCG) injection may then be used to initiate ovulation. Fertilization is planned by one of the following methods: intercourse, artificial insemination, or in vitro fertilization. As a last resort implantation procedures (in vitro fertilization and GIFT) may be performed. An experienced sonographer is a necessary member of the team.

SERIAL SCANNING FOR FOLLICLES

1. A baseline study is performed shortly after the onset of menses to rule out any adnexal pathology or residual cysts from the previous cycle.
2. Serial sonograms are usually started 5 to 8 days after the onset of menses, using the endovaginal route. Multiple small follicles less than 1 cm in size should be visible at this time.

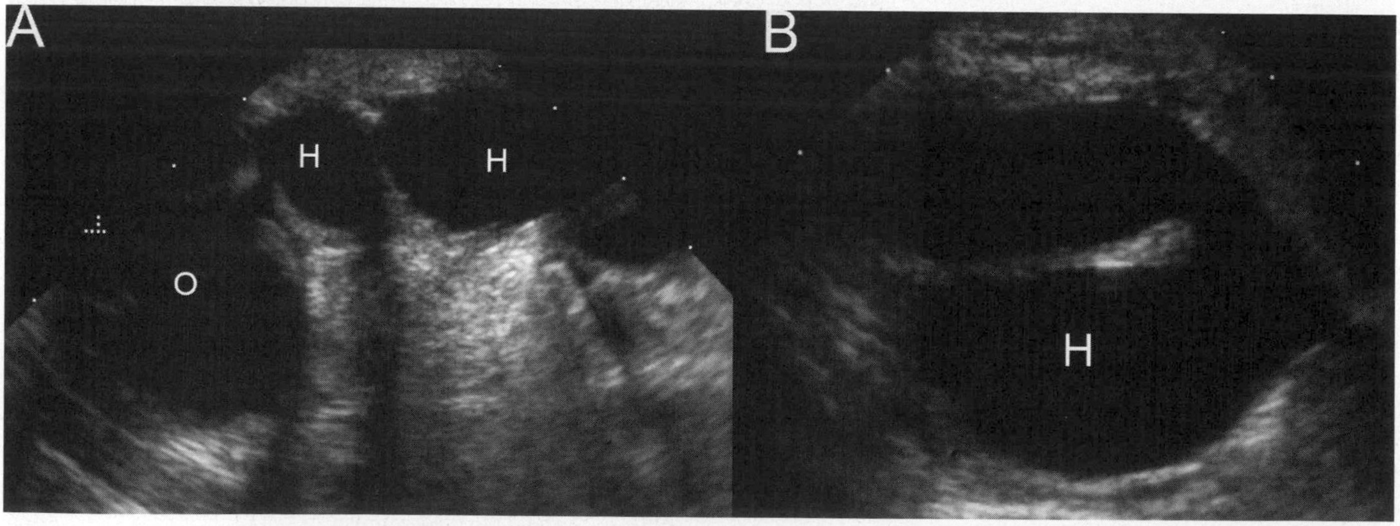

Figure 29-19. ■ *Hydrosalpinx* (H) *transverse (A) and sagittal (B) views. A tubular cystic mass lies alongside the ovary* (O). *On the sagittal view, the components of the hydrocele connect and form the typical retort shape. On the transverse view, the hydrocele seems multilocular. The ovary contains a cysts.*

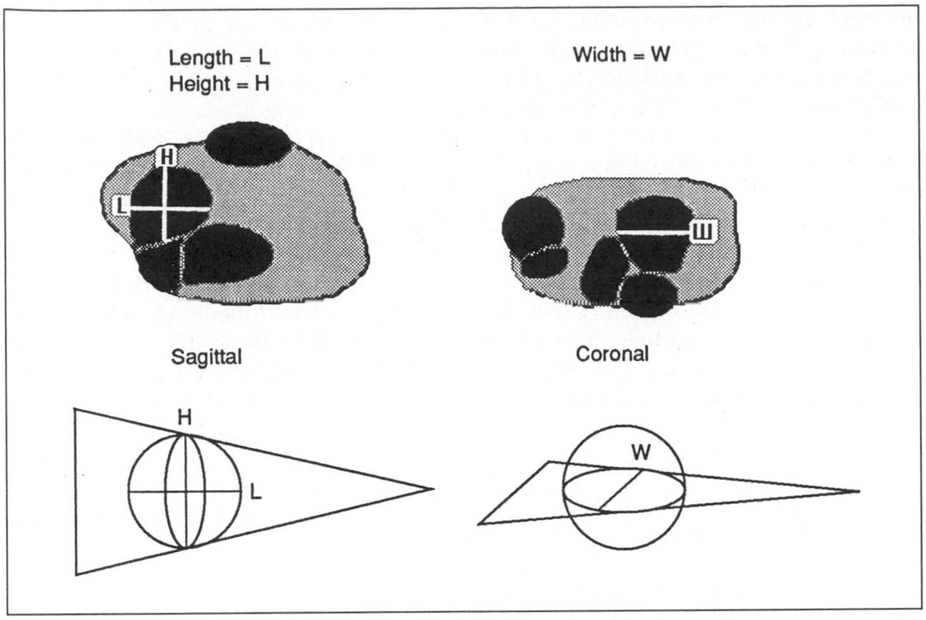

Figure 29-20. ■ *Follicles are measured in both the sagittal and coronal plane so a volume can be calculated. It is very easy to be confused about which follicle you are measuring when you reexamine the patient another day. Be consistent; start at 12:00 and label follicles A,B,C clockwise in each ovary.*

3. Follicles may be measured in three dimensions to produce a volume measurement using the formula length × height × width × 0.5233, or the largest dimension may be used for follow-up (Fig. 29-20). Be consistent in labeling so the growth of two different follicles is not confused.
4. As follicles increase in size, it can be confusing and time-consuming to attempt to measure every follicle. We suggest noting the number of follicles more than 8 mm in each ovary. Only the largest three are then measured.
5. As multiple follicles develop, they may distort and compress adjacent follicles, which is why it is imperative to use all three measurements.
6. For consistent measurements, the same sonographer should examine a patient throughout the cycle.
7. Mature follicular size ranges from 1.5 to 2.7 cm. When stimulated, the follicles may reach a size of 3 cm. When a large size is reached and other biochemical indicators are appropriate, hGC is given to initiate ovulation.
8. Endometrial changes have been used as an indicator of follicular maturity. When the endometrium develops three lines, ovulation is imminent (Fig. 29-7B).
9. Fluid in the cul-de-sac may be a sign of follicular rupture (Fig. 29-12).
10. When the follicle has ruptured, a corpus luteum forms where the follicle used to be. It is sonolucent with a thick, mildly echogenic border and some internal echoes. Color flow performed shortly after ovulation will show a rim of vessels around a corpus luteum (Fig. 29-10C).
11. A sonogram may be performed to prove that ovulation has occurred.

Hyperstimulation Syndrome

A dangerous side effect of inducing follicular development by hormone administration is the ovarian hyperstimulation syndrome (OHS). The features of OHS are the following (Fig. 29-21):

1. Multiple, large, thin-walled cysts in both ovaries that are actually huge follicles; these are known as theca lutein cysts.
2. Ascites.
3. In severe cases, pleural effusions.

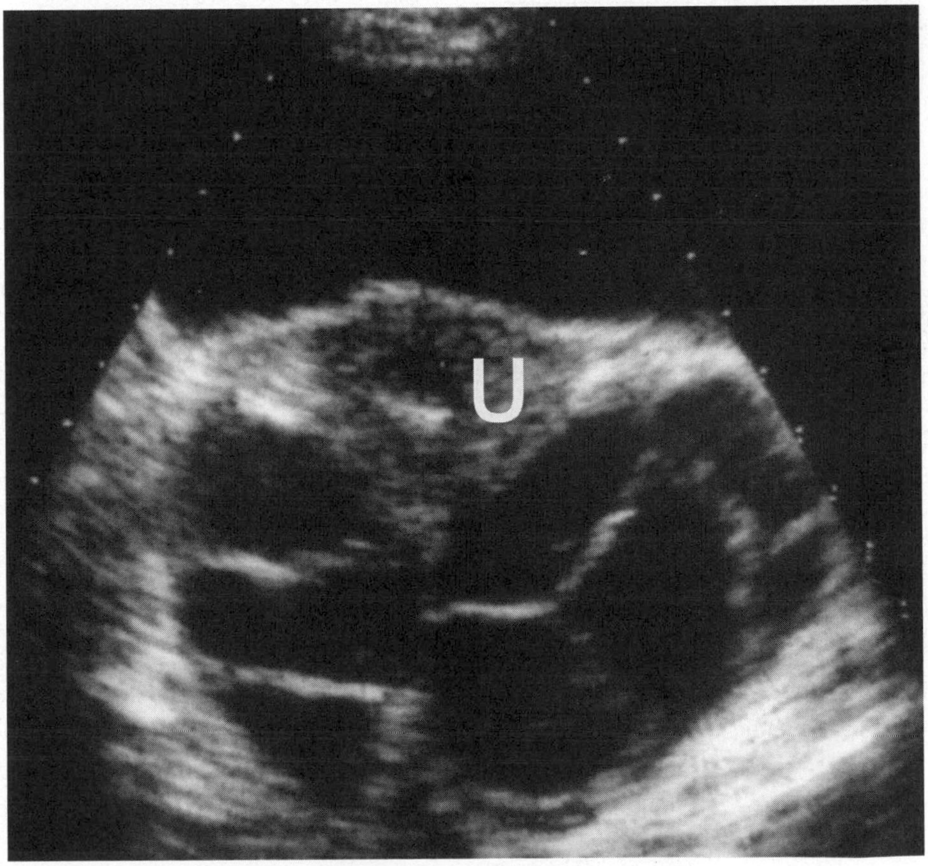

Figure 29-21. ■ *Hyperstimulation of the ovaries. Both ovaries contain multiple large follicles; however, no ascites is present. The uterus* (U) *lies anterior to the ovaries. This degree of hyperstimulation is common in successful pregnancies. Larger cysts with ascites and pleural effusion are hazardous to the patient.*

If the patient fails to become pregnant, the cysts will usually resolve with the next cycle. If pregnancy occurs, the cysts will usually resolve within 6 to 8 weeks.

IN VITRO FERTILIZATION

If the fallopian tubes are absent or blocked, conception cannot occur because the ova cannot reach the uterus. With in vitro fertilization, the mature follicles are aspirated to retrieve the eggs. The retrieval of the eggs is performed either at laparoscopy or under ultrasonic guidance. Ten to twenty-five percent of in vitro fertilization procedures will result in a pregnancy. Egg retrieval is generally guided with ultrasound.

FOLLICULAR ASPIRATION UNDER ULTRASONIC GUIDANCE

Three ultrasonic approaches have been used to aspirate follicles. All use an 18-gauge needle.

1. The needle is directed through the urinary bladder into the follicle through a guidance attachment to the transducer. The needle path is monitored with ultrasound.
2. With the bladder full, the needle is pushed through the vaginal fornix into the ovary, being guided by real-time imaging through the bladder. Sometimes the needle traverses the bladder wall twice on its way to the ovary.
3. The needle is inserted into the follicle alongside a vaginal transducer with the bladder empty (Fig. 29-22). This technique has proven to be the best and is almost universally used. Needle visualization is adequate, and with the bladder empty, the ovary lies very close to the vaginal fornix so the possibility of damaging gut is reduced.

GAMETE INTRAFOLLICULAR TRANSFER

In the gamete intrafollicular transfer technique, follicles are removed from the ovary under sonographic control. They are then fertilized in a petri dish, and a laparoscope is used to replace them within the fallopian tube.

Pitfalls

1. Tampons in the vagina can produce a mass-like effect or can cause shadowing if they do not contain blood on a transabdominal sonogram.
2. The degree of bladder distention will affect the shape of pelvic structures. Overdistention will flatten and distort the ovaries and may make them undetectable, particularly with a vaginal probe. With underdistention, the ovaries may be obscured by gas on a transabdominal examination.
3. The uterus is not always in the midline and may lie in an oblique axis. Suspect adhesions if this is the case.
4. Do not mistake the rectum or sigmoid colon for a mass or fluid. Watch for peristalsis to see movement.
5. Failure to use a gynecologic table or to elevate the hips during an endovaginal study may result in the ovaries not being seen and the urethra being mistaken for a mass.
6. Nabothian cysts in the cervix, a normal variant, can be mistaken for follicles if only a transvaginal approach is used.
7. Compression of a follicle can cause distortions in measurement. This is especially likely if only the longest dimension is used for comparison with previous studies. An overdistended bladder may compress follicles.
8. The muscles of the pelvis, in particular the pyriformis muscle, can be mistaken for ovaries. They lie more posteriorly, are ovoid in shape, and are symmetrical.
9. Failure to empty the bladder completely before an endovaginal study will lead to reverberation artifacts that may hide important structures.
10. Difficulty in seeing the endometrial cavity. Occasionally the endometrial cavity is difficult to see with the endovaginal probe because it is aligned in the same axis as the ultrasonic beam. Placing the patient in the knee-elbow position and reinserting the endovaginal probe sometimes helps under these circumstances.

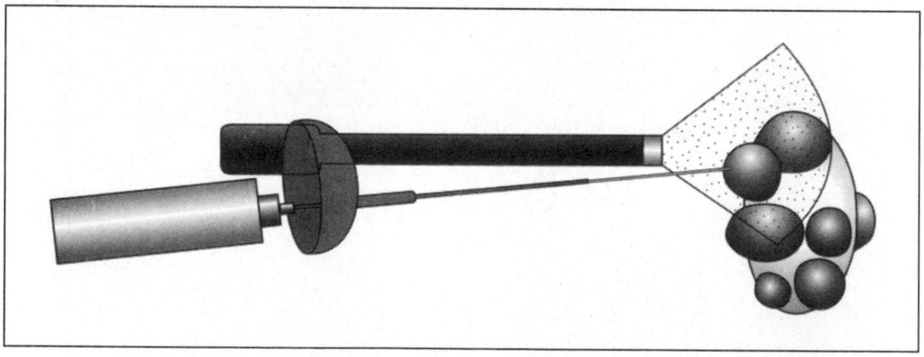

Figure 29-22. ■ *Follicle aspiration performed with a vaginal transducer with a needle guide alongside.*

Where Else to Look

1. Uterine anomaly. If a congenital uterine anomaly is present, such as a double uterus, be sure to check the kidneys because one may well be absent.
2. In patients with repeated miscarriages, check for uterine abnormalities such as bicornuate or septate uterus.
3. Intrauterine pregnancy with pain and bleeding in an infertile patient. Look for a heterotopic pregnancy—an ectopic pregnancy as well as an intrauterine pregnancy—because infertility patients are at risk for ectopic.
4. Hyperstimulation. Check the abdomen for ascites and the chest for pleural effusions, which often occur with hyperstimulated ovaries.

SELECTED READING

Bega G, Lev-Toaff AS, O'Kane P, et al. Three dimensional ultrasonography in gynecology. *J Ultrasound Med* 2003;22:1249–1269.

Botsis D, Kassanos D, Pyrgiotis E, et al. Sonographic incidence of polycystic ovaries in a gynecological population. *Ultrasound Obstet Gynecol* 1995;6:182–185.

Kupesic S. Clinical implications of sonographic detection of uterine anomalies for reproductive outcome. *Ultrasound Obstet Gynecol* 2001;18:387–400.

Pfeifer DG. The role of sonography in diagnosing and treating female infertility. *JDMS* 1995;11:61–66.

Sanders R, Parsons A. *Integrated Gynecological Ultrasound and Management.* Mosby. In press.

Strandell A, Bourne T, Bergh C, et al. The assessment of endometrial pathology and tubal patency: a comparison between the use of ultrasonography and x-ray hysterosalpingography for the investigation of infertility patients. *Ultrasound Obstet Gynecol* 1999;14;200–204.

30 Rule Out Adnexal Mass

ROGER C. SANDERS

KEY WORDS

Chocolate Cyst. Blood-filled mass associated with endometriosis.

Corpus Luteum Cyst. Physiologic cyst developing in the second half of the menstrual cycle and in pregnancy that regresses spontaneously.

Cuff. After hysterectomy, the blind end of the vagina is sutured and forms a fibrous mass, the cuff.

Dermoid. Form of teratoma that is benign and tends to occur in young women.

Endometrioma. Hematoma (chocolate cyst) caused by bleeding from abnormally implanted endometrial tissue.

Endometriosis. Deposits of endometrial tissue on the ovaries, exterior of the uterus, and intestines, among other places. They bleed at monthly intervals, causing hematomas and fibrosis.

Follicle. Developing ovum within the ovary forming a physiologic cyst.

Hydrosalpinx. Blocked fallopian tube that fills with sterile fluid as a consequence of adhesions usually related to a previous infection.

Multiparous. A woman who has been pregnant more than once.

Nulliparous. A woman who has not been pregnant.

Parous. A woman who has been pregnant.

Polycystic Ovary Syndrome (PCO, Stein-Leventhal Syndrome). Multiple cysts developing in both ovaries. The condition is sometimes associated with obesity and masculine distribution of body hair.

Progesterone. Hormone secreted by the corpus luteum that prepares the endometrium to receive a fertilized egg.

Pseudomyxoma Peritonei. Condition that occurs when a mucin-secreting ovarian cystic tumor bursts and its contents spread through the abdomen, forming additional lesions.

Teratoma. Tumor composed of the various body tissues including skin, teeth, hair, and bone, among others. May be malignant but is usually benign in the pelvic area.

Theca Lutein Cysts. Multiple cysts that develop in association with trophoblastic disease because of increased human chorionic gonadotropin levels. May also occur with multiple pregnancy and induced ovulation.

The Clinical Problem

It is often difficult to perform a clinical examination on the female pelvis, especially if the patient is obese, is a child, or has an acute condition such as pelvic inflammatory disease. Sonography is helpful in (1) determining whether a mass is present, (2) deciding whether a mass relates to the uterus or the ovary or the adnexa, and (3) determining whether the mass has a benign appearance or might be malignant.

An adnexal mass may come to light for a number of different reasons:

1. There may be pain on the side of the mass.
2. The mass may be found at a routine clinical examination.
3. Secondary obstruction of the genitourinary or gastrointestinal tract may occur.
4. An alternative imaging technique such as a computed axial tomography (CAT) scan may show a mass.

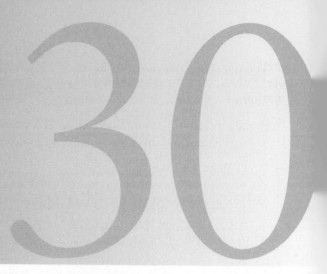

The questions that need to be answered about an adnexal mass are the following:

1. Is a pathologic pelvic mass present or is the supposed mass a normal anatomic variant?
2. Is the mass uterine, adnexal, or neither?
3. Is the mass cystic, complex, or solid? If it is cystic, does it have septa?
4. Is there blood flow to the mass? Is the blood flow high or low resistance?
5. Is the mass involving or invading any other pelvic structure?
6. Are other associated findings such as ascites, metastases, or hydronephrosis present?

By using a combination of the clinical background and the sonographic appearance, a relatively specific diagnosis is usually possible. The sonographer needs the following information to perform a quality sonogram and to make sure that the sonogram is correctly interpreted:

1. What was the date of the first day of the last period (if the patient is still menstruating)?
2. Are menstrual cycles regular, and how long do they last?
3. If the patient has had a hysterectomy, does she know when she ovulates?
4. How long ago did the patient stop menstruating (if she is menopausal)?
5. How many children has the patient had?
6. Has the patient had pelvic surgery? Have any pelvic structures been removed?
7. Has there been pain? If so, where is it located?
8. If the patient is postmenopausal, is she on hormone replacement therapy?

Adnexal mass assessment is helped by sonography in the following situations:

1. Ovarian masses in premenopausal women are usually followed for several weeks to make sure the mass is not a physiologic variant such as a corpus luteum or follicular cyst. However, if the mass is greater than 10 cm in diameter or has typical dermoid appearances, or if there are sonographic features suggestive of malignancy, immediate surgery may be elected.
2. Particularly in obese people, it may be difficult to be certain by pelvic examination whether a pelvic mass is present. Ultrasound can help by definitely showing a mass and determining whether it is uterine or ovarian.
3. Small cysts in postmenopausal women are common, and as long as they are echo-free, most cysts are followed with serial sonograms.
4. Screening for ovarian cancer in at-risk patients may be helpful in women aged more than 40 years because this cancer has few signs and symptoms and usually presents when it has already metastasized. In women with a strong family history of ovarian cancer or of an associated cancer—colon, endometrium, and breast—annual sonograms for early cancer detection may be worthwhile.

Anatomy

See Chapter 29.

Technique

See Chapter 29.

Investigation of masses in the female pelvis hinges on the identification of the ovaries and the uterus. The easiest structure to find is the uterus. Always note the patient's menstrual history. The uterus is recognized:

1. as a structure containing a linear echogenic structure—the endometrial cavity echoes.
2. by tracking the vagina to it; the uterus lies superior to the vagina. On some occasions, the uterus has an oblique axis.

The ovaries are recognized by:

1. their location at the end of the utero-ovarian ligament;
2. the presence of follicles in women who are menstruating;
3. their proximity to the iliac vessels particularly the internal iliac vein.

Features to look for in an adnexal mass include the following:

1. Is the mass cystic or solid? If the mass is cystic, does it contain septa or masses? Are the walls thin or fat? Are the walls smooth or irregular?
2. Is the mass inside or outside the ovary?
3. What is the size of the mass?
4. Is the mass round or some other shape, such as tubular?
5. Is there vascularity within the mass? Is the flow within the mass high or low resistance? Low-resistance flow favors malignancy.

MANEUVERS TO HELP IN THE CHARACTERIZATION OF MASSES

Endovaginal Transducer

The endovaginal transducer is essential

1. to show mass detail—an extraovarian mass, for example, may turn out to have the shape of a dilated fallopian tube;
2. to distinguish the uterus from an ovarian mass;
3. to locate the site of local tenderness—the transducer is pushed toward adnexal structures and the patient reports when and where there is a painful sensation;
4. to see whether the ovary and neighboring gut move well.

Doppler

Doppler analysis of pelvic cystic structures is of some help. Dilated veins in the region of the ovary can mimic ovarian cysts or hydrosalpinx. Malignant masses may show a low-resistance pattern. Doppler may be of assistance in determining whether an ectopic pregnancy is present, because a flow pattern with high diastolic flow (low resistance) is seen with ectopics and corpus luteum cysts. If a solid mass might be ovarian or a fibroid, use color flow to see whether vessels from the uterus enter and surround a fibroid.

Pathology

Adnexal masses can be divided into four basic groups: (1) single cystic masses; (2) multiple cystic masses; (3) complex masses; and (4) solid masses. With the clinical information and a follow-up examination, a relatively specific diagnosis can be made.

CYSTIC MASSES

Cystic masses have well-defined smooth borders, show good through transmission, and are usually spherical.

Single Intraovarian Cysts

Cystic masses may originate in the ovary or may be separate from the ovary. The differential diagnosis is different depending on whether the cyst is within or outside the ovary. Intraovarian cysts are surrounded by a rim of ovarian tissue. If the cyst is single, echo-free, and less than 2.7 cm in diameter, and if the patient is menstruating, a follicle is by far the most likely diagnosis (Fig. 30-1).

Follicular cysts (reproductive age group). Follicular cysts are caused by continued hormonal stimulation of a follicle that does not rupture at ovulation. Such cysts are usually 3 to 5 cm in diameter but can measure up to 10 cm in size. They disappear within a few weeks. Ovulation often takes place on alternate sides, so a repeat study after 3 to 4 weeks is desirable when a mass that could be a follicular cyst is found in a menstruating patient, to document its disappearance. Hemorrhage may occur within a follicular cyst and cause internal echoes, although such cysts are generally echo-free.

Corpus luteum cysts (reproductive age group). Corpus luteum cysts are progesterone-producing cysts or masses that occur after ovulation or in the first 10 to 15 weeks of pregnancy. Their size is variable, and occasionally they become large (up to 10 cm). Although most often containing echoes, owing to hemorrhage, they may be echo-free. Characteristically there is a hyperechoic rim around the cyst. This rim is very vascular on color flow Doppler ("the ring of fire") shortly after ovulation (see Fig. 29-10C).

Cystadenoma (reproductive and postmenarche age groups). The most common benign tumors of the ovary, cystadenomas are large, thin-walled cysts that may have septa within them (Fig. 30-2). They occur most commonly in women between the ages of 20 and 50 years. These cysts may be small, but they are usually large and may grow large enough to occupy most of the abdomen. Approximately 30% are bilateral, but the contralateral cyst may be small. Color flow may show arterial flow in the septa, which is typically high resistance.

Postmenopausal cysts. Small cysts of up to 3 or 4 cm in diameter are commonly encountered in postmenopausal women. Many gynecologists now follow cysts of this type with serial ultrasound studies at 6-month to 1-year intervals. The cyst must be shown by high-quality endovaginal ultrasound to be echo-free and without worrisome Doppler patterns in the wall. Many such cysts disappear spontaneously.

Endometrioma. Endometrioma often occur within the ovary and may occasionally be echo-free (see Extraovarian Cystic Masses for a detailed description of endometrioma).

Dermoid. Although most dermoids contain echogenic structures or calcifications, some are entirely cystic.

Cystadenocarcinoma. Although cystadenocarcinomas are practically never entirely cystic, they may be almost echo-free.

Extraovarian Cystic Masses

Paraovarian cyst. Paraovarian cysts lie between the uterus and the ovary. Thought to represent embryonic remnants, paraovarian cysts are ovoid and echo-free (Fig. 30-3).

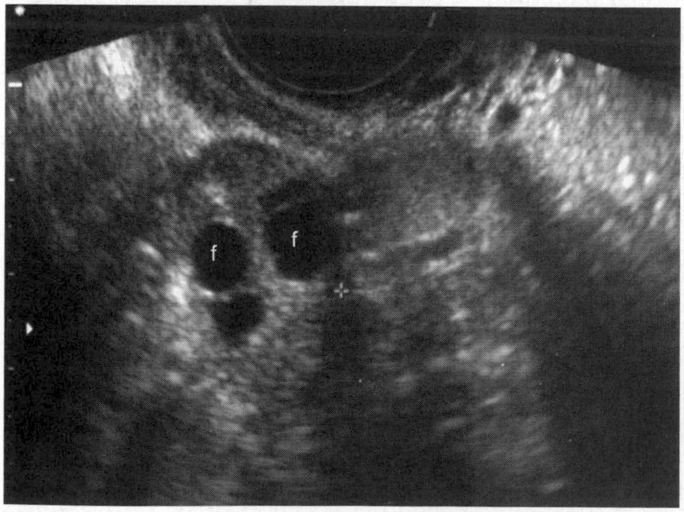

Figure 30-1. ■ *Endovaginal view of the ovary. Three follicles are present in the ovary, one of which is larger than the other two and will become the dominant follicle.*

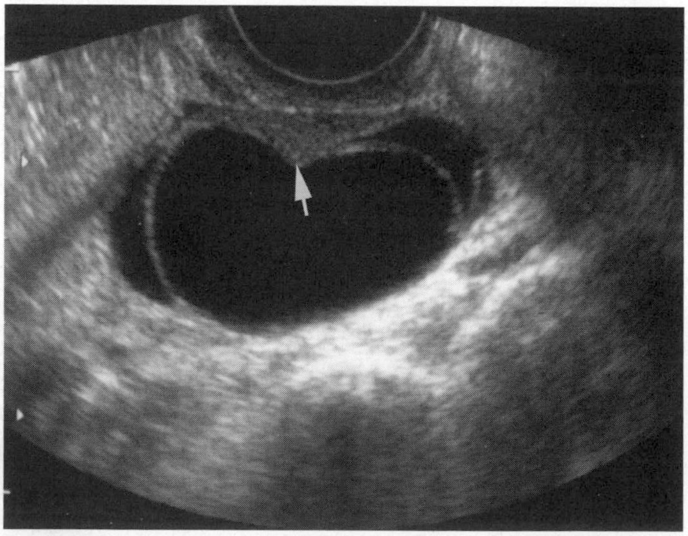

Figure 30-2. ■ *Ovarian cystadenoma. The cyst contains septa. Site* (arrow) *where ovarian tissue bulges into the cystadenoma.*

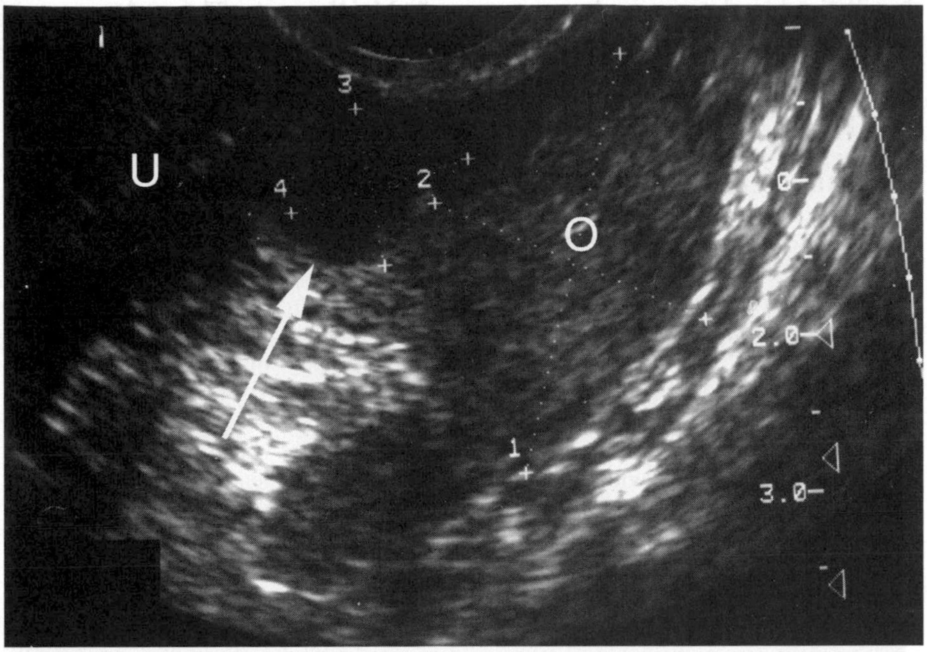

Figure 30-3. ■ *Paraovarian cyst. This echo-free and unimportant cyst* (arrow) *lies between the ovary* (O) *and the uterus* (U).

Peritoneal inclusion cyst. Peritoneal inclusion cysts are a consequence of previous surgery or infection. The peritoneal surfaces become adhesed, and fluid slowly collects. These cysts may be of any shape and may contain septa and debris.

Hydrosalpinx. Hydrosalpinx are usually the sequelae of pelvic inflammatory disease or, less often, of adhesive processes such as endometriosis involving the fallopian tube outlet. The pus in a pyosalpinx resorbs and is transformed into fluid. The sonographic findings may suggest hydrosalpinx when the tube folds over on itself and forms a funnel-shaped or kinked structure (see Fig. 29-19).

Extraovarian Multiple Cystic Masses

Endometriosis. A disease state that occurs during the reproductive years, endometriosis is caused by implantation of endometrial tissue in abnormal locations in the pelvis. This ectopic endometrial tissue responds to cyclic ovarian hormones and bleeds as if it were located within the uterus. Endometrial cysts (endometrioma) may develop in these areas of bleeding. Small cysts are termed blebs, whereas in larger ones, because of their contents (blood) and color, are called chocolate cysts. This type of cyst may occur singly, but more than one are generally seen. Because these cysts contain blood, internal echoes may be present in the form of either many moderate-level echoes or a dense echogenic "blob." Most endometrioma develop within the ovary.

Tubo-ovarian abscesses. Tubo-ovarian abscesses are irregularly shaped, thick-walled, fluid-filled structures in the adnexa that may develop a few internal echoes and even an internal fluid-fluid level (see Chapter 33). Tubo-ovarian abscesses are usually bilateral. These abscesses are usually not an isolated finding; multiple abscesses are often noted elsewhere. They are very tender.

Intraovarian Cystic Masses: Complex

Complex masses in the ovary contain sonolucent and echogenic areas. The walls are generally smooth; the shape is usually spherical.

Mucinous cystadenoma and cystadenocarcinoma of the ovary. These masses, seen in the reproductive or postmenopausal age group, are less common than the serous type of mass. They often have a characteristic sonographic appearance (Fig. 30-4). A spherical cystic mass may be present with many septa;

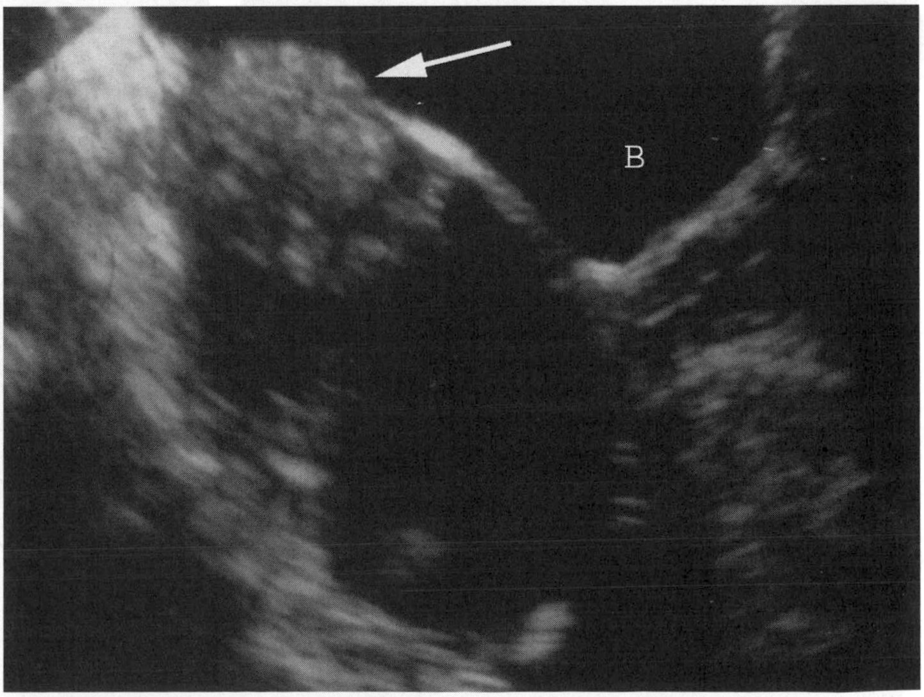

Figure 30-4. ■ *Cystadenocarcinoma of the ovary. Cystic mass lies posterior to the bladder* (B). *A papillary mass within the tumor bulges through the capsule* (arrow) *indicating malignant spread.*

quite the same evenness of texture (Fig. 30-9). If the corpus luteum is examined shortly after ovulation, a ring of vessels will be see with color Doppler, the so-called ring of fire, which disappears after the corpus luteum hemorrhage has been there for a while (see Fig. 29-10C). The corpus luteum hemorrhage will be spontaneously resorbed after some weeks, so distinction between a corpus luteum with hemorrhage and endometrioma is made by performing a follow-up examination in approximately 6 weeks.

Solid Masses

Solid masses contain only low-level echoes, show little or no through transmission, and have irregular or smooth walls. Most solid masses in the ovary have a nonspecific appearance. Nevertheless, the features of malignancy, as described previously, should be sought. Any solid ovarian mass in a postmenopausal woman carries a high probability of malignancy. In menstruating women, an endometrioma should be considered.

Fibroma. Fibromas are solid ovarian masses that affect menopausal and postmenopausal women. They tend to be large and have a sonographic appearance similar to fibroids. Basically echopenic, calcification can occur. Meigs syndrome, in which there is associated ascites and pleural effusion, may be seen.

Pitfalls

1. Gut versus ovary. When no follicles are seen in postmenopausal women, an indolent loop of feces-containing bowel may be confused with an ovary. Watch for a considerable time for peristalsis. Look to see whether the supposed ovary lies close to the utero-ovarian ligament, which can be seen leading from the lateral aspect of the fundus of the uterus to the ovary. Consider performing a water enema, although this is rarely necessary.
2. Fibroid versus ovarian mass. If a mass lies adjacent to the ovary, it can be very hard to distinguish between a fibroid and a solid intraovarian mass such as a fibroma. Push the vaginal probe between the mass and the uterus to see whether the two can be separated. A gap between the two structures needs to be seen at all sites for a mass to be definitely considered ovarian rather than a pedunculated fibroid. Use color flow to see whether there are vessels extending from the uterus to the mass (see Fig. 31-6).
3. Endometrioma versus corpus luteum. A basically intraovarian mass with clumps of echogenic material within may represent a corpus luteum with hemorrhage, a dermoid, an endometrioma, or, much less likely, an ovarian neoplasm. Pulsed Doppler is not helpful because corpus luteum and neoplasm may both show a low-resistance pattern. A repeat examination in the next proliferative phase of the cycle in approximately 6 weeks can help to distinguish between the lesions. A corpus luteum will alter configuration, whereas a dermoid, an endometrioma, and a neoplasm will stay unchanged. At this point Doppler may be helpful because endometrioma do not have internal vascularity except in pregnancy.
4. Pulsed Doppler sampling for signs of a neoplasm. Pulsed Doppler sampling should be performed within or at the edge of a suspect ovarian mass. Sampling at other sites related to the ovary can be misleading. The arteries at the center of a malignant mass show abnormal irregular contour and pattern (abnormal angiogenesis).
5. Endovaginal scanning with a bladder containing some urine. If the bladder is not completely empty, reverberation artifacts may obscure crucial structures and problem areas may be pushed too far away from the transducer.
6. After hysterectomy. The ovaries may be very hard to find because they may fall together in the center of the pelvis or be pulled laterally.

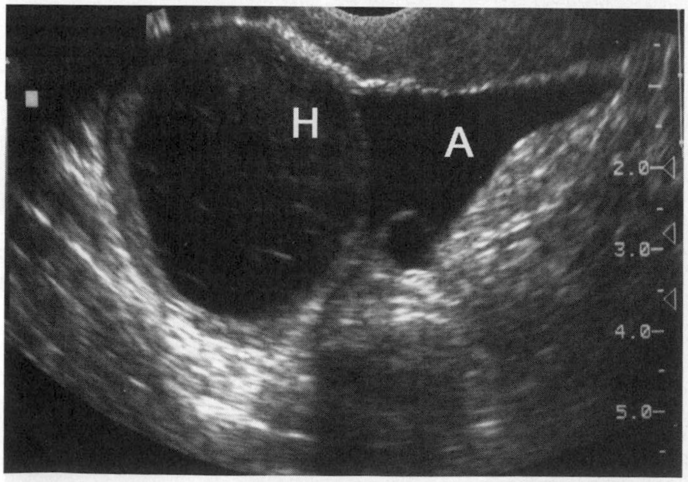

Figure 30-9. ■ *Hemorrhagic cyst. The cyst* (H) *lies within the ovary. Note the rim of ovary enclosing it, a sign of a benign mass. Small quantity of physiologic ascites* (A) *lies adjacent to the cyst. Small quantities of peritoneal fluid are often seen during the menstrual cycle particularly at the time of ovulation.*

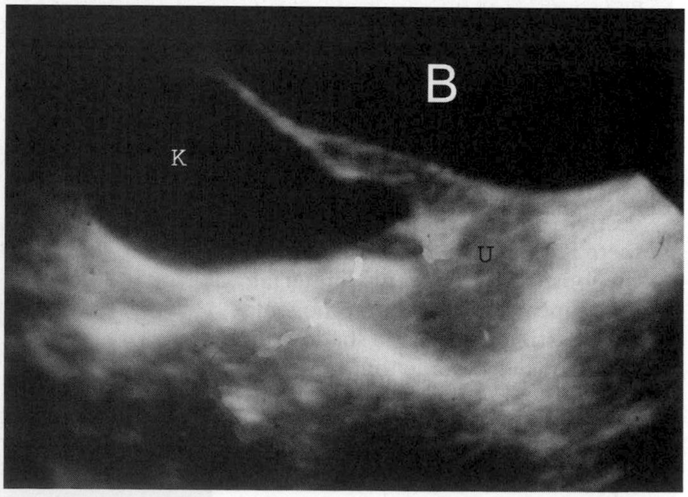

Figure 30-10. ■ *Pelvic kidney. Hydronephrotic pelvic kidney* (K) *lies adjacent to the uterus* (U) *and posterior to the bladder and mimics a pelvic cystic mass.*

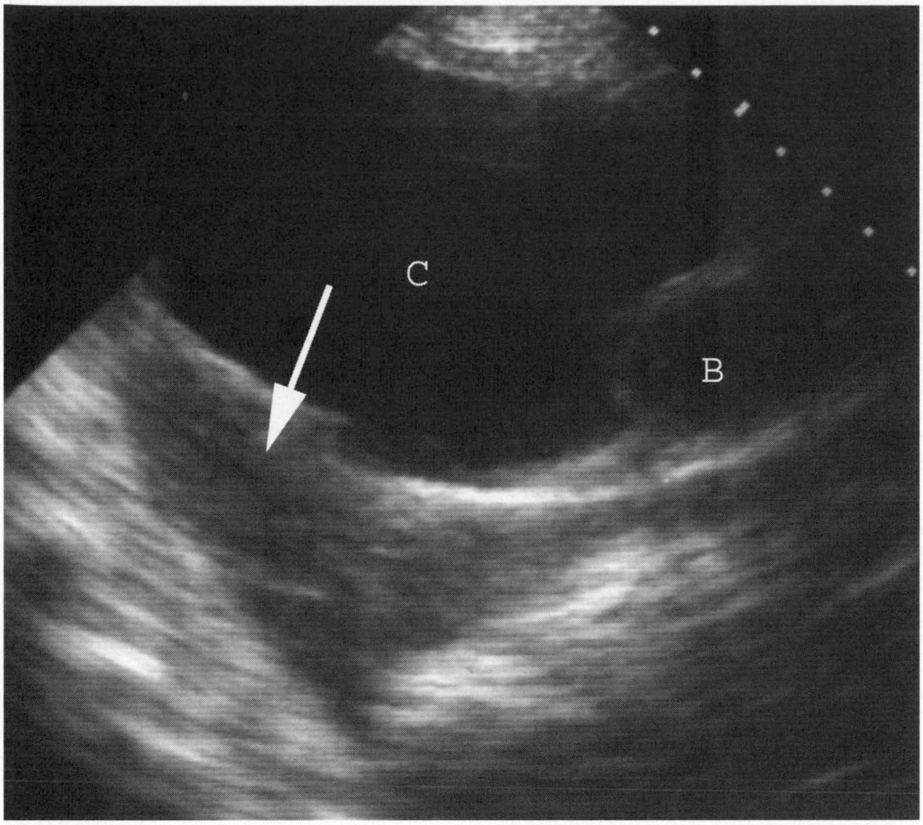

Figure 30-11. ■ *Ovarian cyst mimicking bladder. The large cystic ovarian mass* (C) *lies in the midline and compresses the tiny bladder* (B). *The cyst was initially mistaken for the bladder but did not change with voiding.*

7. Post-hysterectomy changes. A large vaginal cuff may mimic a recurrent mass.
8. Pelvic musculature can be confusing. The iliopsoas and piriform muscles may be misinterpreted as pelvic masses. A solid knowledge of pelvic anatomy is essential.
9. Fluid in the posterior cul-de-sac. Ten to fifteen milliliters of fluid is normal in women in the reproductive years (Fig. 30-9). A portion of this fluid is derived from follicular rupture.
10. Make sure the supposed pelvic mass is not a pelvic kidney (Fig. 30-10). A pelvic kidney will have a central group of sinus echoes and a reniform shape.
11. An ovarian cyst located in the midline anterior to the uterus can be mistaken for the bladder. The cyst may compress the bladder, making the patient uncomfortable when the bladder is filled (Fig. 30-11). The bladder will be seen as a small slit on the posterior-inferior aspect of such a cyst.
12. An enlarged bladder can be confused with a cyst. The patient voids incompletely and leaves a considerable amount of residual urine within the bladder. If you cannot see the bladder as well as a cyst, be cautious in diagnosing the presence of a cyst.

Where Else to Look

1. When performing a scan of a patient with a large pelvic mass of ovarian origin, the kidneys should also be examined to rule out hydronephrosis caused by pressure on the ureters.
2. If the patient is in the menopausal age group and the features of the pelvic mass suggest malignancy—large size, complex echoes, and ovarian origin—then a search for metastatic lesions, nodes, and ascites should be carried out. The most common sites of metastatic lesions from pelvic masses are the peritoneum, para-aortic nodes, and liver.
3. If you suspect that a pelvic kidney is present, examine the normal sites where the kidney should lie, and make sure that two kidneys are not present in their usual location.

SELECTED READING

Alfuhaid TR, Rosen BP, Wilson SR. Low malignant tumors of the ovary: sonographic features with clinicopathologic correlation in 41 patients. *Ultrasound Q* 2003;19:13–26.

Atri M, Nazarnia S, Bret PM, et al. Endovaginal sonographic appearance of benign ovarian masses. *Radiographics* 1994;14:747–760.

Caspi B, Appelman Z, Rabinerson D, et al. Pathognomonic echo patterns of benign cystic teratomas of the ovary: classification, incidence and accuracy rate of sonographic diagnosis. *Ultrasound Obstet Gynecol* 1996;7:275–279.

Conway C, Zalud I, Dilena M, et al. Simple cyst in the postmenopausal patient: detection and management. *J Ultrasound Med* 1988; 17:369–372.

Fried AM, Kenney CM III, Stigers, KB, et al. Benign pelvic masses: sonographic spectrum. *Radiographics* 1996;16:321–334.

Kim JS, Woo SK, Suh SJ, et al. Sonographic diagnosis of paraovarian cysts: value of detecting a separate ipsilateral ovary. *AJR Am J Roentgenol* 1995;164:1441–1444.

Hillaby K, Aslam N, Salim R, et al. The value of the detection of normal ovarian tissue (the "ovarian crescent" sign) in the differential diagnosis of adnexal masses. *Ultrasound Obstet Gynecol* 2004;23:63–67.

Jain DA. Sonographic spectrum of hemorrhagic ovarian cysts. *J Ultrasound Med* 2002;21: 879–886.

Sanders R, Parsons A. *Integrated Gynecological Ultrasound and Management.* Mosby. In press.

Sheth S, Fishman EK, Buck JL, et al. The variable sonographic appearances of ovarian teratomas: correlation with CT. *AJR Am J Roentgenol* 1998;151:331–334.

Valentin L. Pattern recognition of pelvic masses by gray-scale ultrasound imaging: the contribution of Doppler ultrasound. *Ultrasound Obstet Gynecol* 1999;14:338–347.

Woodward PJ, Kosseinzadeh K, Saenger JS. Radiologic staging of ovarian carcinoma with pathologic correlation. *Radiographics* 2004;24:225–246.

31 Midline Pelvic Mass

ROGER C. SANDERS

KEY WORDS

Adenomyosis. Common condition causing pain and heavy periods. Endometrial tissue implants in the myometrium causing uterine enlargement and a variety of sonographic changes. Can be focal or generalized.

Cuff. After hysterectomy, the blind end of the vagina is sutured and may form a fibrous mass, the cuff.

Fibroid (Myoma, Leiomyoma). A benign tumor of the smooth muscle of the uterus. Submucosal—a fibroid bordering on the endometrial cavity. Subserosal—a fibroid bordering on the peritoneal cavity. Intramural—fibroid within the wall of the uterus.

Hematometrocolpos. Metra, uterus; culpa, vagina. Condition presenting at birth or at puberty due to an imperforate hymen. Blood or other fluid accumulates in the vagina and uterus.

Hematocolpos. Obstructed vagina filled with blood. Usually found in teenagers with imperforate hymen or transverse vaginal bands shortly after the onset of menstruation.

Hematometra. Obstructed uterus filled with blood. Usually related to a cervical obstructive process such as cancer of the cervix.

Intramural. Term used to describe a lesion, such as a fibroid, that lies in the wall of the uterus.

Myoma. See Fibroid.

Pedunculated. Term used particularly for fibroids describing a mass that is connected to its site of origin by only a short pedicle.

Submucosal. Term used to describe a process, such as a fibroid, that is located adjacent to the uterine cavity within the uterus.

Subserosal. Term used to describe a lesion such as a fibroid that is on the surface of the uterus.

The Clinical Problem

Masses that appear to involve the uterus are routinely examined with ultrasound for several reasons:

1. It is difficult to assess the ovaries by clinical examination when there is a sizable uterine mass present.
2. Tracking the size of fibroids is most accurately performed with ultrasound. Very rapid growth of an apparent fibroid suggests that the mass might be a leiomyosarcoma.
3. Not all uterine masses are fibroids. Adenomyosis is a common entity enlarging the uterus that is treated in a different fashion.
4. Occasional ovarian masses in the midline are mistaken for masses of uterine origin.
5. Delineating the relationship of the myoma to the endometrial cavity is important in planning surgery.

Anatomy

See Chapter 29.

Technique

ABDOMINAL APPROACH

- Uterine masses are often so large that the entire size of the uterus and the size of individual fibroids can only be measured using the abdominal approach.
- If the ovaries are visible using the abdominal approach, measure and record their size. They may be located at too high a level to be visible with the endovaginal transducer.

VAGINAL APPROACH

- You may find that even though fibroids are large, they do not border on the endometrial cavity and are therefore not responsible for vaginal bleeding. Only the improved resolution of the vaginal probe may show this relationship if the endometrial cavity is difficult to see.
- When an intracavitary mass is suspected in the presence of fibroids, use a balloon catheter with a saline infusion study; the fibroids are solid and not easily displaced by the intracavitary fluid unless a balloon catheter is used.

Clinical

UTERINE MASSES

Solid Uterine Masses

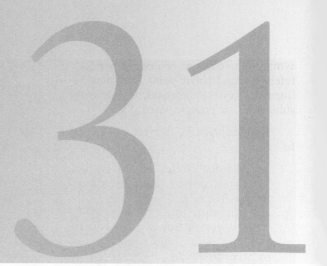

Fibroids (leiomyomas). Fibroids represent an overgrowth of uterine smooth muscle that forms a tumor. Leiomyoma is the benign form, and leiomyosarcoma is the rare malignant form. Fibroids are the most common tumors in women and are present in 40% of women aged more than 40 years. They usually grow progressively during the menstrual years but may shrink after menopause. Common symptoms are heavy, prolonged periods; infertility; and pelvic pain. They may be intracavitary, submucosal, intramural, subserosal, or pedunculated (Fig. 31-1).

Sonographically, the features are as follows:

1. An enlarged uterus, usually with a lobulated contour that may indent the bladder (Fig. 31-2). If the bladder volume is small, document the size. Frequency is a common complication of fibroids because they reduce bladder capacity.
2. Focal ovoid or circular masses within the uterus. These masses may have a similar echogenicity to the remainder of the uterus, but tissue within is organized in a whirled (circular) fashion (Fig. 31-3). Blood vessels form a rim around the fibroid, whereas with other entities they may look similar, such as in focal adenomyosis the blood vessels traverse the lesion.

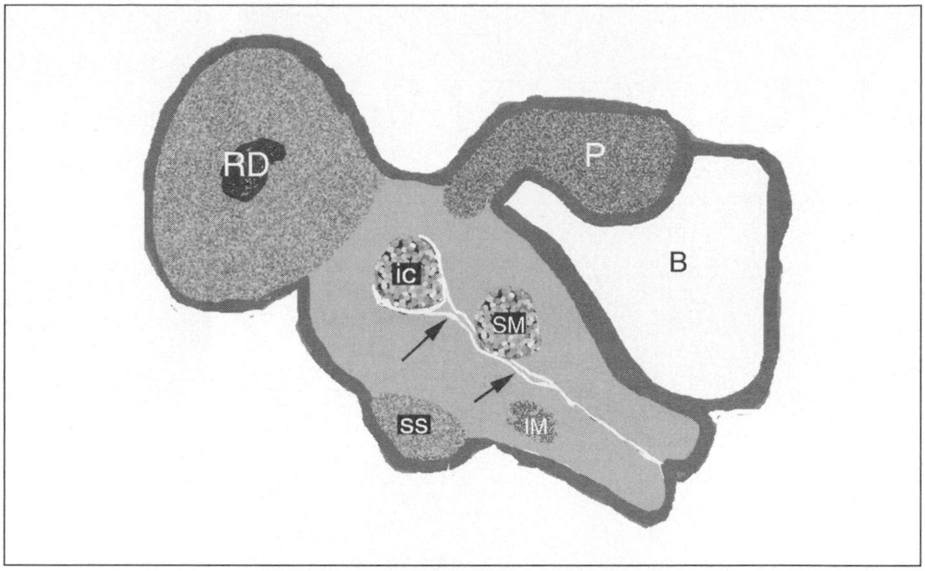

Figure 31-1. ■ *Fibroids may be located in several different sites. Subserosal fibroids* (SS) *lie on the edge of the uterus and may indent the bladder. They are almost always asymptomatic. Intramural fibroids* (IM) *lie in the center of the myometrium (the muscular component of the uterus). If they do not distort the cavity, they are usually asymptomatic. Submucosal fibroids* (SM) *lie on the edge of the endometrium. They often cause menstrual cramping and bleeding. Intracavity fibroids* (IC) *almost always cause cramping and bleeding. Pedunculated fibroids* (P) *are usually asymptomatic, but in this diagram, the fundal pedunculated fibroid has an echopenic center because it has undergone red degeneration* (RD)*. This painful condition usually occurs in pregnancy.*

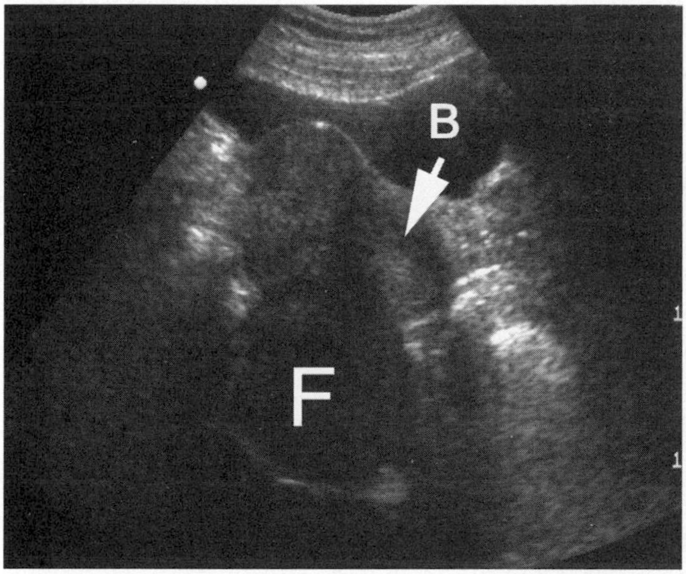

Figure 31-2. ■ *Transabdominal view of posterior pedunculated fibroid* (F)*. Note that the endometrial cavity* (arrow) *is not adjacent to the fibroid, so it is unlikely that this patient is symptomatic. The fibroid is sonolucent, yet transmission is poor and the posterior border is seen but not enhanced, indicating that the mass is not cystic but filled with homogeneous tissue. B, bladder.*

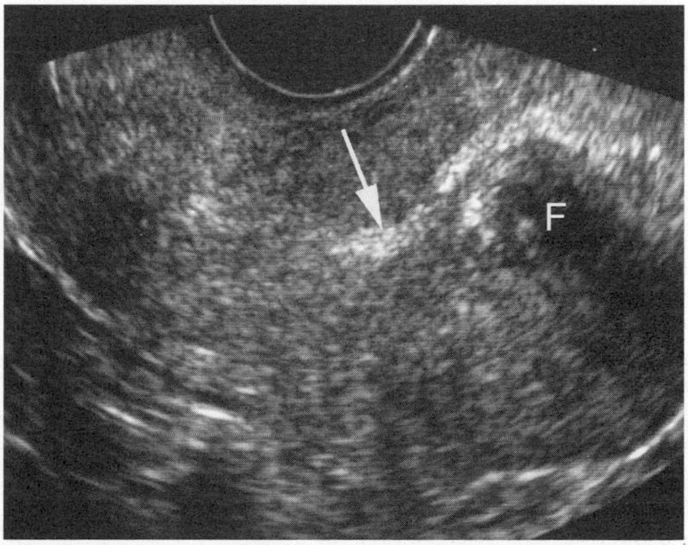

Figure 31-3. ■ *Submucosal fibroid. Posterior submucosal fibroid* (F) *indents the endometrial cavity* (arrow)*. This fibroid is likely to cause heavy periods and intermenstrual spotting.*

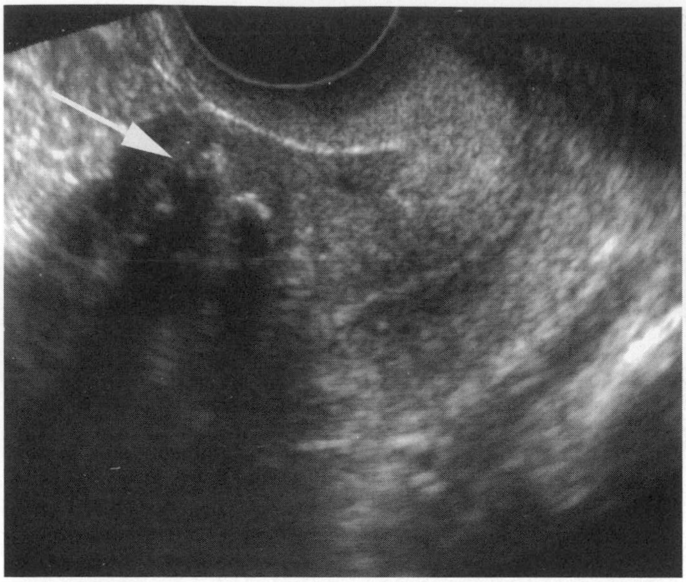

Figure 31-4. ■ *Calcified fibroid. Multiple calcified segments of a fibroid* (arrow) *are present in this fundal intramural fibroid. Note the shadowing posterior to the fibroid preventing visualization of the fundal portion of the endometrial cavity.*

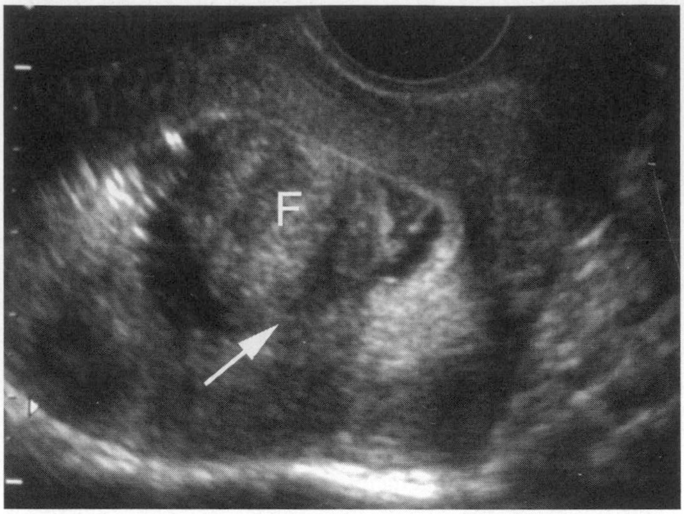

Figure 31-5. ■ *Intravital fibroid shown on saline infusion study* (arrow). *The fibroid* (F) *is mostly within the endometrial cavity, although a neck extends into the myometrium* (arrow).

3. The fibroid may be surrounded with a rim of calcification that can occasionally be so dense that the center cannot be seen with ultrasound (Fig. 31-4).
4. The relationship of the fibroid to the endometrial cavity should be defined (Figs. 31-1 and 31-3). Submucosal fibroids, which border on the endometrial cavity, often cause frequent lengthy periods with intramenstrual spotting and may cause infertility (Fig. 31-3).
5. Fibroids that lie within the cavity (intracavitary) or protrude into the cavity (Fig. 31-5) are even more likely to cause vaginal bleeding and cramping.
6. Fibroids that have a small neck and extend off the border of the uterus are termed "pedunculated" (Figs. 31-1 and 31-6). They may be hard to distinguish from adnexal masses and may twist and infarct (torsion). It should be possible to track the myometrial arteries into the pedunculated fibroid with color flow (Fig. 31-6). Pedunculated fibroids with a small neck connecting them to the main part of the uterus may otherwise be mistaken for a solid adnexal mass.
7. If a fibroid is acutely tender, "red degeneration" may have occurred (Fig. 31-1). There is usually a cystic center to the fibroid, the site of bleeding, when red degeneration has occurred.
8. Occasional fibroids contain fat and are known as lipoleiomyomas. These masses are densely echogenic and circular but without shadowing.
9. Patients with fibroids may need serial ultrasound scans at intervals. Rapid growth with an abrupt change in size suggests malignancy. Malignant change is exceedingly rare.

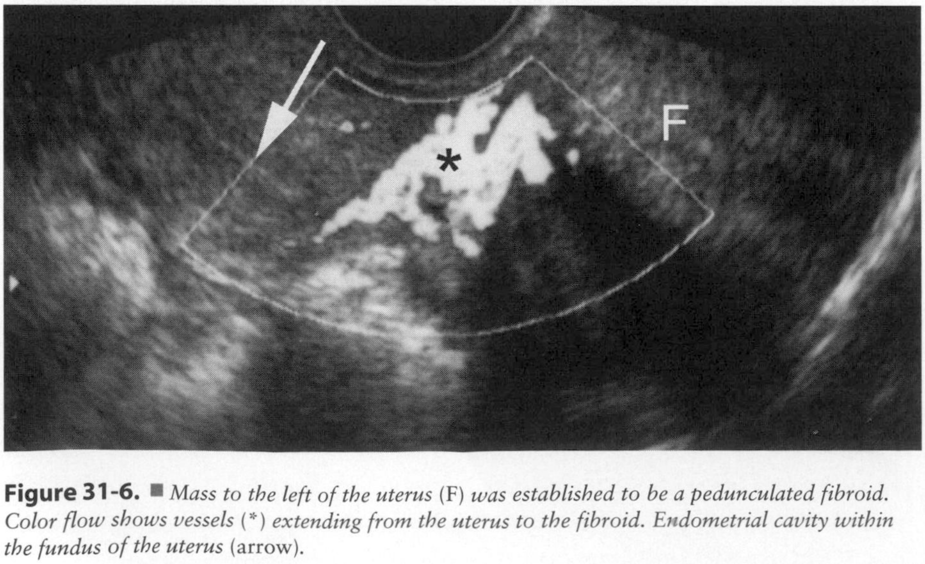

Figure 31-6. ■ *Mass to the left of the uterus* (F) *was established to be a pedunculated fibroid. Color flow shows vessels* (*) *extending from the uterus to the fibroid. Endometrial cavity within the fundus of the uterus* (arrow).

Adenomyosis

Endometrial glands invade the myometrium and respond to hormonal stimulation in the same fashion as the endometrial lining, causing cramping, heavy menstrual bleeding (menorrhagia), and uterine enlargement.

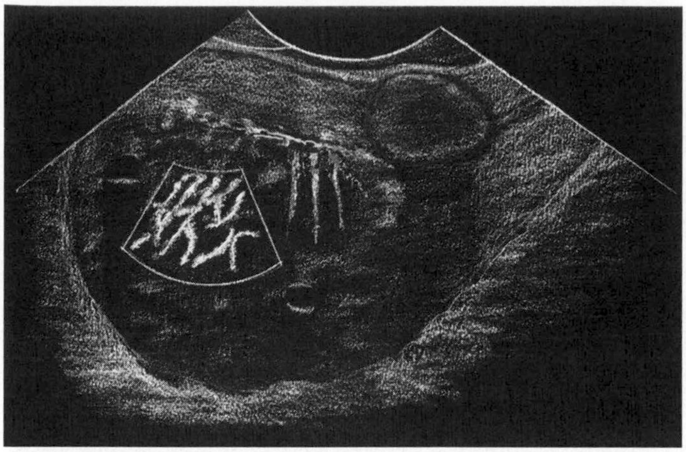

Figure 31-7. ■ *Features of adenomyosis. Vessels tracking through an area of adenomyosis in a normal fashion* (inset), *unlike fibroids where the vessels skirt the mass. The texture of the uterus is inhomogeneous typical of the process. Radiating echogenic lines coming from the endometrial cavity are a common feature. A focal mass of adenomyosis is seen anteriorly. Myometrial cysts are present.*

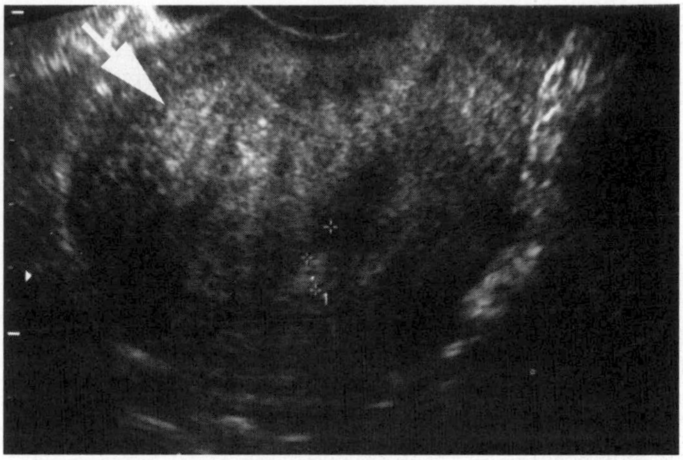

Figure 31-8. ■ *Uterus enlarged by adenomyosis. The portion of the uterus anterior to the endometrial cavity (measurement markers) is much larger than the area posterior to the cavity. There is an irregular texture within the affected area* (arrow) *with linear echogenic areas.*

The sonographic findings may be diffuse or localized (Figs. 31-7 and 31-8).

- Cysts of varying sizes may be found within the myometrium usually located close to the endometrium.
- Subtle, more or less parallel echogenic lines radiate from the endometrium into the myometrium.
- The uterus is eccentrically enlarged, usually with the anterior aspect more enlarged than the posterior.
- The myometrium has a patchy appearance, forming a "Donegal tweed"-like pattern.
- In the focal form, an ill-defined echopenic mass is found. Blood vessels traverse the lesion, unlike the findings with fibroids where blood vessels surround the mass.

Cervical cancer. The most common genital tract malignancy in women is cervical cancer. The peak age for occurrence is in the fourth decade. Often the lesion is too small to be seen with ultrasound, even if a Pap smear is suggestive or it can be seen with a speculum examination. Sonographically, the following may be seen:

1. Bulky cervix with an irregular outline, possibly extending into the vagina or peritoneum (Fig. 31-9).
2. A mass extending from the cervix to the pelvic sidewalls.
3. Obstruction of the ureters, producing hydronephrosis.
4. Invasion of the bladder, producing an irregular mass effect in the bladder wall.
5. Para-aortic node formation and metastatic lesions in the liver.

Complex Masses in the Uterus

Pyometra. A uterine cavity that contains echopenic fluid surrounded by myometrium may be caused by pyometra. Especially when significant debris or gas-forming organisms are present, echogenic areas with shadowing may occur.

Fibroids. Occasional fibroids that have degenerated have a complex appearance, with cystic areas in a predominantly solid mass.

Single "Cystic" Masses Seen within the Uterus

Hydrometrocolpos (neonatal). In hydrometrocolpos, there is distention of the vagina and uterus with fluid. This is secondary to cervical or vaginal obstruction; a common cause is an imperforate hymen. Often only the vagina is distended (hydrocolpos) and the uterus is still small; however, both the uterus and vagina may be fluid filled. The fluid contents are usually anechoic.

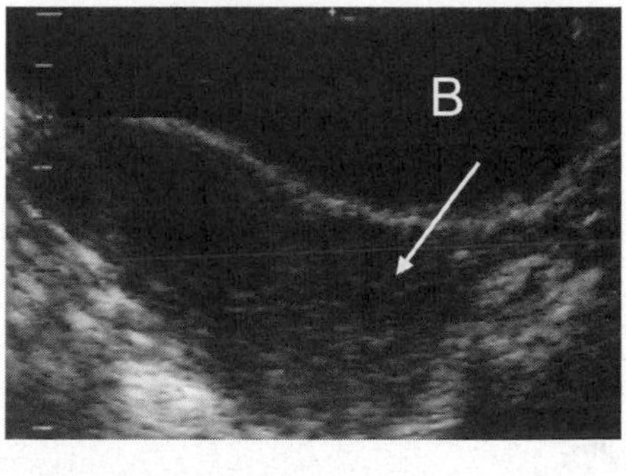

Figure 31-9. ■ *Diffuse enlargement of the cervix with subtle change in texture* (arrow) *because of carcinoma of the cervix. B, bladder.*

Hematometrocolpos (premenarche). Hematometrocolpos occurs when the vagina and possibly the uterus are distended with blood at menarche, rather than the serous fluid of hydrometrocolpos. Internal echoes within the blood are usually seen. Either the hymen is imperforate or there is a congenital septum blocking the vagina or cervix, which only becomes clinically apparent when menstruation starts. Hematometra, in which only the uterus is distended with blood, may be seen at menarche if there is a congenital occlusion of the vagina or the cervix. In older women, it may result from cervical malignancy or postradiation cervical stenosis (Fig. 31-10).

Pyometra (reproductive or postmenarche age groups). Pyometra—distention of the uterus with pus—usually occurs secondary to a cervical obstruction of drainage of the normal uterine secretions, with subsequent superinfection. The patient is febrile and very sick. Debris is seen within the fluid in the endometrial canal.

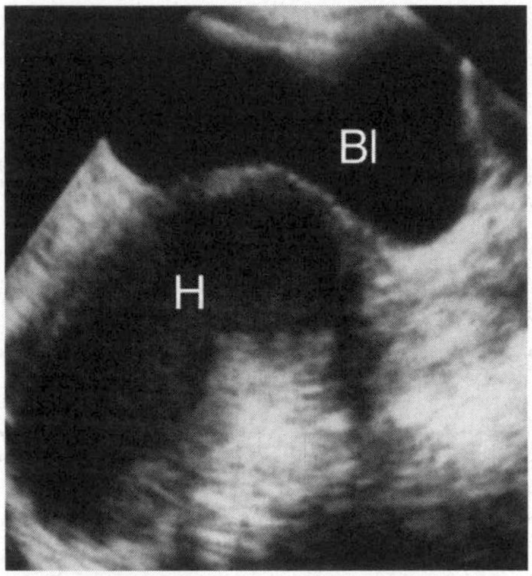

Figure 31-10. ■ *Hematometra. This patient has a small cancer of the cervix that has bled back into the uterus. Blood and fluid have slowly accumulated in the endometrial cavity* (H) *causing a hematometra. Bl, bladder.*

Fibroids. Occasional fibroids in the myometrium appear cystic and are echopenic with acoustic through transmission.

Pitfalls

1. Intracavitary masses in the secretory phase of the cycle. The endometrial cavity echoes vary between 0.2 and 0.4 cm thick in the proliferative phase of the cycle and between 0.8 and 1.3 cm thick in the secretory phase of the cycle. Small masses such as polyps or intracavitary fibroids can be concealed in the secretory phase. If possible, schedule patients with possible intracavitary masses for the proliferative phase of the cycle or repeat the study at that time.
2. On a transabdominal view, the fundus of the retroverted uterus may be difficult to delineate if the beam lies at the same angle as the uterus. When acutely retroverted, the fundus may lie adjacent to the cervix and simulate a mass. Because a retroverted uterus is globular in shape, enlargement is hard to assess. A fibroid may be mistakenly diagnosed unless endovaginal views are obtained.
3. With uterine anomalies such as bicornuate and double uterus, the second horn may be mistaken for an adjacent mass. Careful longitudinal and oblique scanning should demonstrate two endometrial cavities (see Fig. 29-16). With a double uterus, two cervices and a vagina will be present.
4. By 1 week postpartum, the uterus decreases in size to approximately one-half its size at delivery. During the next 4 to 7 weeks, the uterus gradually returns to normal size. If the history is unknown, the enlarged uterus may be misdiagnosed as fibroids or other uterine mass.
5. Calcification in a fibroid may cause shadowing that obscures the endometrial cavity (Fig. 31-4). Looking at the fibroid from a different approach using the abdominal, vaginal, or even the rectal probe may allow a decision as to the whether the fibroid is submucosal.

Where Else to Look

When performing a scan of a patient with a large pelvic mass of ovarian or uterine origin, the kidneys should also be examined to rule out hydronephrosis caused by pressure on the ureters.

SELECTED READING

Atri M, Reinhold C, Mehio AR, et al. Adenomyosis: US features with histologic correlation in an in-vitro study. *Radiology* 2000;215:783–790.

Caolli EM, Hertzberg BS, Kliewer M, et al. Refractor shadowing from pelvic masses on sonography: a useful sign of uterine leiomyomas. *AJR Am J Roentgenol* 1999; 174:97–101.

Sanders R, Parsons A. *Integrated Gynecological Ultrasound and Management*. Mosby. In press.

Serafini G, Martinoli C, Quadri P, et al. Lipomatous tumors of the uterus; ultrasonographic findings in 11 cases. *J Ultrasound Med* 1996;16:195–199.

32 Chronic Pain

ROGER C. SANDERS

KEY WORDS

Abscess. Localized collection of pus.

Adenomyosis. Endometrial glands invade the myometrium causing a painful uterus and menorrhagia.

Adnexa. The regions of the ovaries, fallopian tubes, and broad ligaments.

Anteverted. The body of the uterus is tilted forward.

Crohn's Disease. Bowel inflammation that can affect any level of the bowel from stomach to anus. Fistula is a common complication.

Cul-de-Sac. An area posterior to the uterus and anterior to the rectum where fluid often collects.

Diverticulitis. Bowel outpouchings typically found in the distal large bowel. May become infected and painful.

Dysmenorrhea. Difficult or painful menstruation.

Dyspareunia. Difficult or painful intercourse.

Endometrial Cavity, Canal. A potential space in the center of the uterus where blood or pus may collect.

Endometrium. Membrane lining of the uterine cavity.

Hydrosalpinx. Accumulation of watery fluid in the fallopian tube. The tube is blocked at the peritoneal end by adhesions and fibrosis due to a prior infection or other causes such as endometriosis.

Laparoscopy. Surgically invasive technique for viewing the pelvic anatomy in situ through a small tube using fiber-optics. The tube is inserted into the peritoneum through a small incision near the umbilicus.

Leukocyte Count. The number of circulating white blood cells. This count increases when an inflammatory process is present, as in pelvic inflammatory disease, but remains normal in ectopic pregnancy and endometriosis.

Myometrium. Smooth muscle of the uterus.

Pelvic Inflammatory Disease (PID). Infection that spreads from the uterine tubes and ovaries throughout the pelvis; commonly due to gonorrhea.

Retroverted Uterus. The long axis of the uterus points posteriorly toward the sacrum.

Salpinx. Fallopian tube.

Vulva. Region where the urethra and the vagina exit in the perineum.

Clinical

Chronic pelvic pain is common and responsible for approximately 10% of gynecologic outpatient visits. Two common causes are endometriosis and the long-term consequence of PID. Typical symptoms are pain on intercourse (dyspareunia) and dysmenorrhea (painful menstruation). Some causes such as muscular trigger pain cannot be recognized with ultrasound.

Anatomy

See Chapter 29.

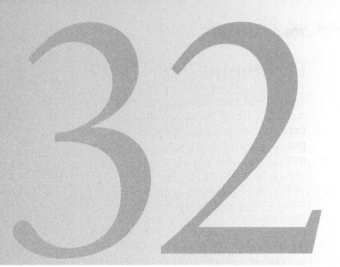

Technique

TENDERNESS

The endovaginal probe is superior to an examining finger because one can find the site of pelvic pain while pushing with the vaginal probe and see where the pain originates; for example, the pain may be arising from a neighboring portion of bowel rather than a gynecologic structure.

- Introduce the vaginal probe with care in symptomatic patients so as not to cause vaginal spasm and lack of cooperation in finding the cause of the pain.
- Carefully push with an even pressure on the pelvic structures, including the proximal fallopian tubes, asking the patient to grade the severity of the pain from 1 to 10. (A score of 10 is the worst, usually equivalent to labor pains.) Repeat the procedure several times if it is unclear where the pain is most severe so you can be sure where the pain originates. However, if it is obvious where the patient is maximally tender you do not need to repeat this painful test. Do not be unnecessarily cruel; the test only works with patient cooperation!
- If the tenderness is superior to the area that can be examined with vaginal probe, feel the abdomen for the most painful site and look with the abdominal probe.

MOVEMENT

Make sure that the uterus and ovaries move freely and slide away from neighboring structures such as the uterus, bowel, or sidewall structures. Absence of free movement suggests adhesions.

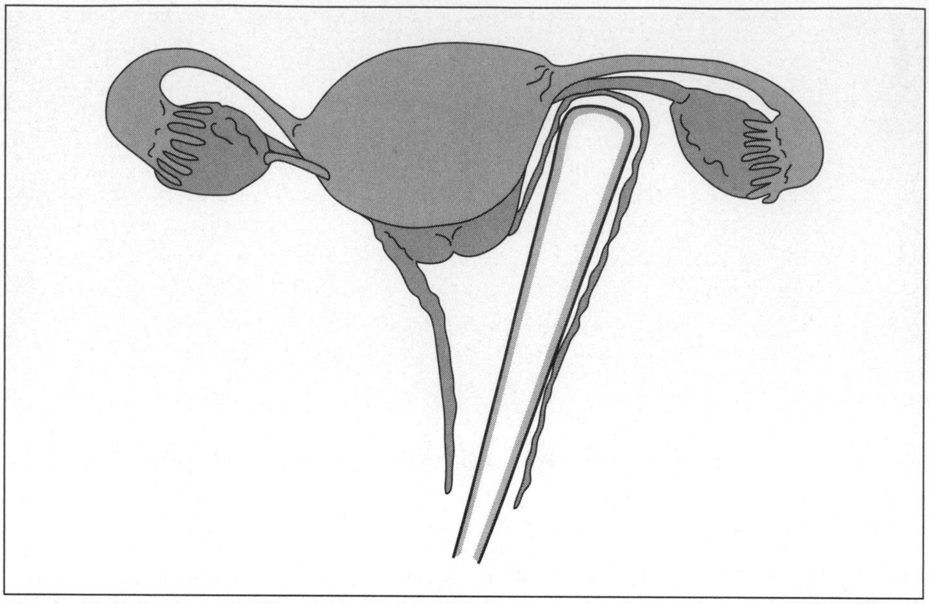

Figure 32-1. ■ *Technique and site used to assess chronic pain by pushing on the adnexa. Note that the vagina is very distensible and that the probe is alongside the uterus close to the fallopian tube origin.*

Pathology

CHRONIC PELVIC INFLAMMATORY DISEASE

Chronic pain related to an earlier infection with PID is common and usually unrecognized unless the sonographer accurately localizes the tenderness. In this situation, tenderness is maximal over the proximal fallopian tubes and to a lesser extent over the uterus (Fig. 32-1). Often cultures are negative, and the only way to confirm that the right diagnosis has been made is that the pain disappears after the administration of a course of an antibiotic such as doxycycline.

Sometimes the pain relates to a hydrosalpinx (see Fig. 29-19). There is a serpiginous or apparently septate extraovarian mass. The walls of the dilated tube are thin, but there are intermittent small nodules representing the remnants of endosalpingeal folds. Hydrosalpinges may cause pain by distending to a point where they compress other organs. Usually they are bilateral, but they may be of very different size on the two sides.

The Fallopian tubes may be enlarged and thickened due to chronic inflammation. They will be locally tender.

MASSES

Large, slowly growing uterine or adnexal masses may cause pain by compression of neighboring organs (see Chapters 30 and 31). Adenomyosis causes an enlarged tender uterus, dyspareunia, and dysmenorrhea (see Chapter 31).

INFERTILITY

Endometriosis is a common cause of pelvic pain that often causes infertility (see Chapter 29 for a detailed description). Often the typical masses seen with endometriosis are absent, and the condition can only be inferred by the presence of adhesions. Unusual sites of endometriotic implants should be sought, such as incisions on the abdominal wall, bowel, and bladder wall.

ADHESIONS

Adhesions (1) occur as a consequence of previous infection or surgery (e.g., tubal ligation); (2) may be seen with endometriosis; and (3) occur occasionally with malignancy. Adhesions may cause a chronic, nagging pelvic pain. Although the adhesions cannot be seen with ultrasound, there are several indirect signs:

1. Uterine deviation to left or right or extreme retroversion.
2. An ovary positioned in a high or low lateral position.

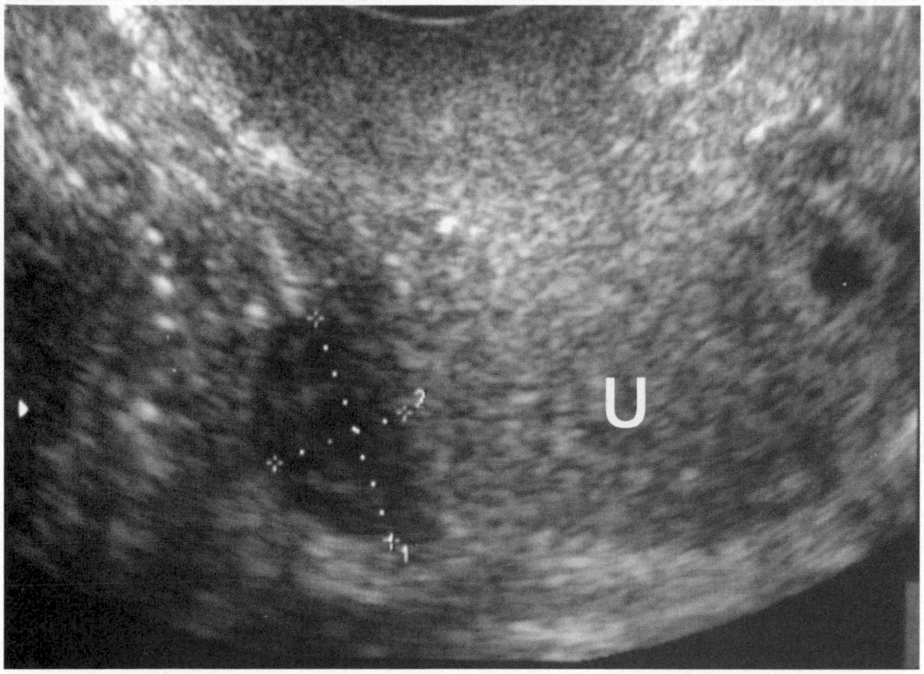

Figure 32-2. ■ *The calipers outline the right ovary, which lies adjacent to the uterus* (U) *on this transverse view. The ovary remained next to the uterus and would not move when prodded with the vaginal probe indicating adhesions.*

3. An ovary located adjacent to the uterus that cannot be moved with the vaginal probe and is locally tender. This is a very reliable sign (Fig. 32-2).
4. An ovary that feels stiff and immobile when pushed with the transducer and that remains adjacent to a loop of bowel. Normally, the ovary can be pushed away from surrounding bowel with the transducer.

OVARIAN REMNANT SYNDROME

Sometimes a remnant of one ovary remains after bilateral salpingo-oophorectomy (surgical removal of the uterus and both ovaries). The ovarian remnant produces follicles and corpora lutea; because it is surrounded by adhesions and in a confined space, cyst formation is painful and occurs at approximately monthly intervals when ovulation occurs. Make sure the patient is examined when she is symptomatic; you will be able to see the follicle or corpus luteum. Pushing on the mass will be very painful.

PELVIC CONGESTION SYNDROME

Dilated veins in the region of the ovary, particularly on the left, are found often and may occasionally be the cause of chronic pain. It is difficult to know when such varicosities are a genuine cause of symptoms and when they are coincidental. Approximately 10% of women have visibly dilated left pelvic veins, but a small minority (at most 2%) have symptoms. Local vein tenderness when compressed with the vaginal probe may be of some help in deciding if the veins have any significance. Use color flow to establish that large cystic structures in the region of the ovary are dilated veins (Fig. 32-3).

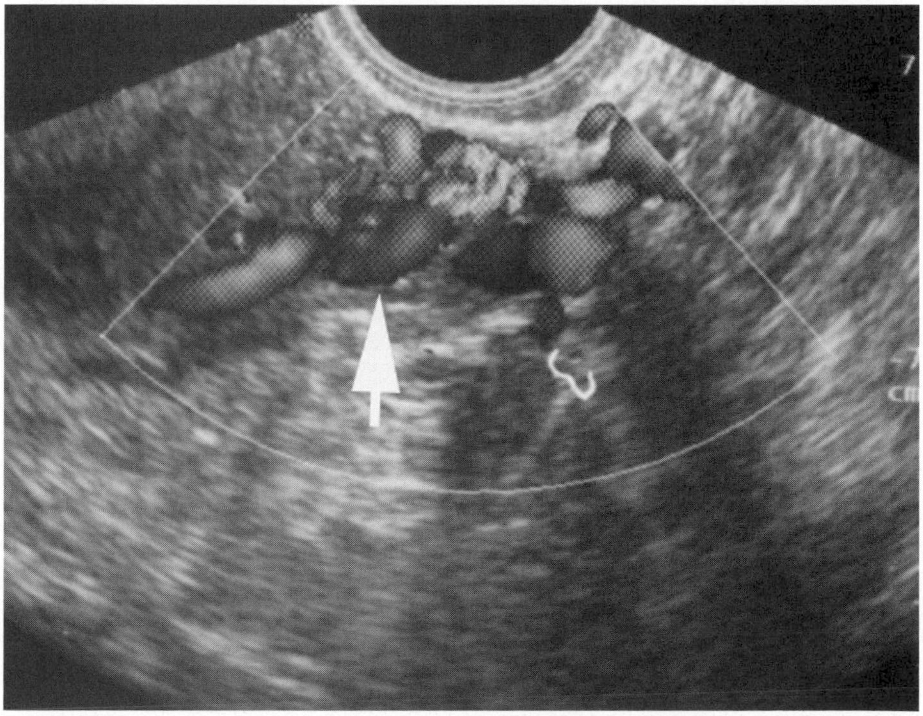

Figure 32-3. ■ *Transverse view of the left adnexa showing multiple veins in the region of the left ovary* (arrow). *Color flow shows flow in the venous structures in this case of pelvic congestion syndrome.*

DIVERTICULAR DISEASE

Painful diverticula in the sigmoid colon, which lies close to the left ovary, are often mistaken for a gynecologic process. Diverticula are common, occurring in one-third of women aged more than 45 years. The bowel wall is abnormally thickened (>2 mm) with a dome-shaped hump if a diverticular abscess is present. Small echogenic lines in the bowel wall suggest the presence of diverticula. Some contain shadowing gas. The bowel wall will be locally tender as it is pressed with the vaginal probe.

IRRITABLE COLON

This common condition leads to chronically thickened sigmoid bowel wall (>2 mm thick) presumably due to focal spasm. Vaginal pressure on the thickened bowel wall reproduces the patients' symptoms.

INTERSTITIAL CYSTITIS

Bladder wall inflammation is often mistaken for a gynecologic lesion. In this condition, the wall of the bladder is exquisitely tender, and the bladder capacity is usually small (<100 mL). (To crudely calculate bladder volume in milliliters, measure the width, length, and height of the bladder and multiply by 0.65.)

Pitfalls

1. If the patient has intermittent pain, make sure she is examined when she is having pain.
2. Some patients gain sympathy from talking about pelvic pain. If the pressure test yields inconsistent results with the site of pain varying, make sure to report this.
3. Tests for adhesions are often indeterminate. Make sure the ovary will not move and is recognizably an ovary before making this observation. The uterus is often deviated to the right or left or retroverted without adhesions being present.

Where Else to Look

1. If a hydrosalpinx is found on one side, look hard for a hydrosalpinx on the other side.
2. When a sizable mass is the cause of pain, look at the kidneys to make sure obstruction is not present.

SELECTED READING

Fleischer A, Tait D, Mayo J, et al. Sonographic features of ovarian remnants. *J Ultrasound Med* 1998;17:551–555.

Howard F, Perry P, Carter JC, et al. *Pelvic Pain: Diagnosis and Management.* Philadelphia: Lippincott Williams and Wilkins; 2000.

Park SJ, Lim JW, Ko YT, et al. Diagnosis of pelvic congestion syndrome using transabdominal and transvaginal sonography. *AJR Am J Roentgenol* 2004;182:683–688.

Patel MD, Feldstein VA, Chen DC, et al. Endometriomas: diagnostic performance of US. *Radiology* 1999;210:739–745.

Sanders R, Parsons A. *Integrated Gynecological Ultrasound and Management.* Mosby. In press.

Vaginal Bleeding with Negative Pregnancy Test

33

ROGER C. SANDERS

KEY WORDS

Adenomyosis. Endometrial tissue extends into the myometrium. Blood cysts develop with menstruation in the myometrium.

Bleeding Dyscrasia. Abnormality of the factors that control clotting and platelet function.

Breakthrough Bleeding. Erratic bleeding while taking hormones such as oral contraceptives.

Dysmenorrhea. Painful periods with excessive bleeding.

Endometrial Cavity, Canal. A potential space in the center of the uterus where blood or pus may collect.

Endometritis. Infection of the endometrial cavity.

Endometrium. Membrane lining of the uterus.

French. A measure of catheter size.

Hematometrocolpos. Metra, uterus; culpa, vagina. Condition presenting at birth or at puberty due to an imperforate hymen. Blood or other fluid accumulates in the vagina and uterus.

Hysterosonogram (Saline Infusion Study [SIS]). Procedure in which a catheter is placed in the cervical cavity and saline is infused into the endometrial cavity. Used to show intracavitary pathology.

Menorrhagia. Heavy bleeding with periods.

Metromenorrhagia. Excessive bleeding occurring with and between periods.

Proliferative. Preovulatory phase of the menstrual cycle, at which time the endometrial cavity echoes form a single thin line.

Saline Infusion Study (SIS). See Hysterosonogram.

Secretory. Postovulatory phase of the menstrual cycle, at which time the endometrial cavity echoes are thick.

Submucosal. Term used to describe a process, such as a fibroid, that is located adjacent to the endometrial cavity within the uterus.

Tamoxifen. Antiestrogenic drug used in patients with breast cancer to prevent a recurrence. It carries a small risk of endometrial neoplasm and produces a reaction in the endometrium.

The Clinical Problem

Vaginal bleeding between periods or at any time in the pre- or postmenstrual nonpregnant patient is abnormal and is an indication for a sonogram. Very heavy painful periods may indicate an endometrial process.

In a child, vaginal bleeding may be a sign of precocious puberty. Other clinical features that occur in the child with precocious puberty include large breasts (gynecomastia), excessive growth, and the development of an adult pubic hair distribution.

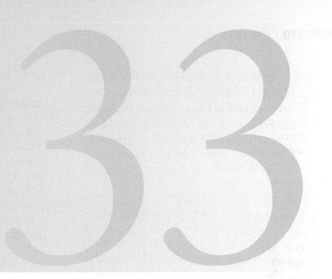

There are many possible reasons for intramenstrual bleeding. Conditions that may cause abnormal bleeding but do not distort the normal pelvic anatomy (e.g., clotting problems) cannot be detected by sonography. Sonographically visible findings include the following:

1. Retained products of conception. If the patient has been pregnant in the recent past, a retained fragment of placenta may cause persistent bleeding. This may also occur after a termination.
2. Fibroids that border on the endometrial cavity. As mentioned in Chapter 31, fibroids can occur in a number of locations. Those that border on the cavity (submucosal) and those that lie within the cavity (intracavitary) are particularly likely to cause intramenstrual bleeding.
3. Intracavitary masses. Some intracavitary lesions such as polyps form a well-defined focal mass, whereas others, such as cancer of the endometrium or endometrial hyperplasia, cause an increased thickness or focal irregularity to the endometrial cavity borders. All may cause excessively heavy periods or intermenstrual spotting.
4. Adnexal masses. Occasionally, an ovarian mass, such as a hormone-secreting ovarian neoplasm or dermoid, may cause vaginal spotting.

CHANGES WITH MENSTRUATION

The lining of the endometrial cavity is partially shed each month at menstruation, with consequent changes in cavity appearance during the course of the cycle. During the preovulatory (proliferative) phase, the endometrial cavity echo is only approximately 3 mm thick and surrounded by an echopenic halo. Shortly before ovulation, two additional linear echoes outline the echopenic area (the "three-line sign" or trilaminar appearance). The echopenic area becomes more echogenic so that in the postovulatory (secretory or luteal) phase, the cavity echo becomes brighter and thicker (see Fig. 29-7A–C). At this point, the width of the canal is between approximately 8 and 13 mm.

Ascertain the following before starting a study for vaginal bleeding:

1. What was the first day of the last period? Try to ensure that the sonogram is performed in the 13 days after the first day of the period so the endometrium is thin.
2. Are menstrual cycles regular and how long do they last?
3. How long ago did the patient stop menstruating if menopausal?
4. If the patient is postmenopausal, is she on hormone-replacement therapy (HRT)? HRT with estrogen or a combination of estrogen and progesterone thickens the endometrium. Unopposed estrogen (estrogen only) is particularly likely to thicken the endometrium. A postmenopausal endometrial cavity thickness of greater than 5 mm in an unstimulated patient is a signal for further investigation such as a saline infusion study (SIS) or endometrial sampling.
5. Is Tamoxifen being administered? Tamoxifen, a commonly administered antiestrogenic chemotherapeutic drug, is given to women who have had breast cancer. Although it reduces breast cancer recurrence, there is a slight increase in the number of endometrial neoplasms. After 6 months to 1 year, 60% of women develop secondary changes in the endometrium.

Anatomy

See Chapters 29 and 31.

Technique

TRANSVAGINAL

The endometrium can only be satisfactorily assessed with the vaginal probe. Detail is never satisfactory with the transabdominal approach.

SALINE INFUSION STUDY HYSTEROSONOGRAM

This technique is used for the further investigation of the cause of abnormal vaginal bleeding (Fig. 33-1). Informed consent is usually obtained because the procedure involves placing a catheter within the endometrial cavity, although the risks of infection and bleeding are minimal. In patients with a history of

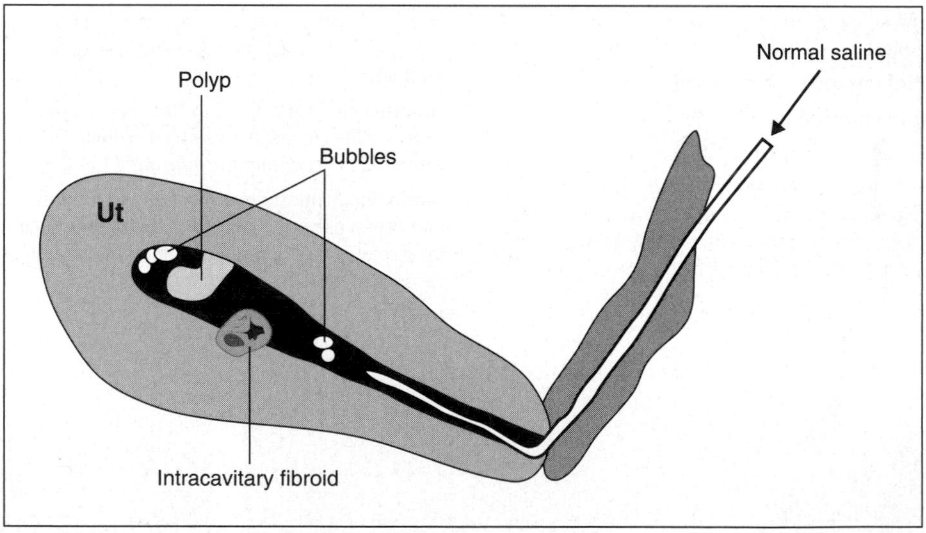

Figure 33-1. ■ *Hysterosonogram. A catheter is inserted into the endometrial cavity through which normal saline is infused. The catheter tip lies in the middle of the endometrial cavity and can be moved back or pushed forward under direct ultrasonic visualization. Normal saline causes bubbles that accumulate at the fundus if the uterus is anteverted and dissipate spontaneously if the uterus is retroverted. Polyps are typically on a stalk, mobile and echogenic, with irregular borders. Fibroids indent into the myometrium and are usually evenly echopenic with a well-defined border.*

pelvic inflammatory disease, antibiotic prophylaxis with an antibiotic such as doxycycline is given. Pain and cramping occur if a balloon catheter is inserted; if that is planned, an analgesic such as ibuprofen is given before the procedure. The procedure is performed as follows:

1. A speculum is inserted. A plastic translucent speculum with a built-in light is useful because visualization of the cervix is important.
2. The cervix is cleansed with iodine.
3. A small catheter such as a 5F Tampa catheter is inserted into the cervix using sponge forceps. If this catheter cannot be inserted or will not stay in place, a 5–7F balloon catheter is inserted. The balloon is inflated with a fluid such as normal saline to prevent air within the balloon from causing a shadow that would make visualization of uterine pathology impossible. If the balloon is difficult to insert, a technique whereby the balloon is inflated, deflated, withdrawn, pushed in again, and then reinflated may be helpful in getting the catheter in place. A tapered plastic os dilator also helps ease the passage of the catheter in some cases.

Pathology

ENDOMETRIAL CANCER

Endometrial cancer, a tumor of the uterine endometrial lining, is most common after menopause and is associated with abnormal bleeding (Fig. 33-2). Typically, there is an echogenic mass with a large (sessile) base arising from the endometrium. These cancers are highly vascular with many supplying vessels. The management is changed and prognosis is worse if the echopenic area around the endometrium in the myometrium is penetrated by the tumor. Fluid in the endometrial cavity may occasionally be an indication of an underlying endometrial neoplasm.

Benign Endometrial Hyperplasia

The endometrium becomes thickened (>8 mm thick) and echogenic. The condition can either be generalized or localized to a small segment of the endometrium. Small cysts may lie within the echogenic area in the cavity border. This condition is usually seen around the time of menopause.

Endometrial Polyp

Polyps within the endometrial cavity are common. Typically, they are round and echogenic. If the examination is performed in the secretory phase of the menstrual cycle, polyps may be concealed within the normal echogenic thickening that occurs at this phase of the cycle. Many are asymptomatic, but some present with heavy periods or intramenstrual bleeding. If there is uncertainty whether a polyp is present, a hysterosonogram is helpful. When outlined by fluid with a hysterosonogram, polyps are markedly echogenic, have an irregular border, and can be seen to move if they are on a stalk, as they often are (Fig. 33-3). Color flow usually shows a single supplying vessel to the polyp (Fig. 33-3). This finding favors a benign origin to the polyp.

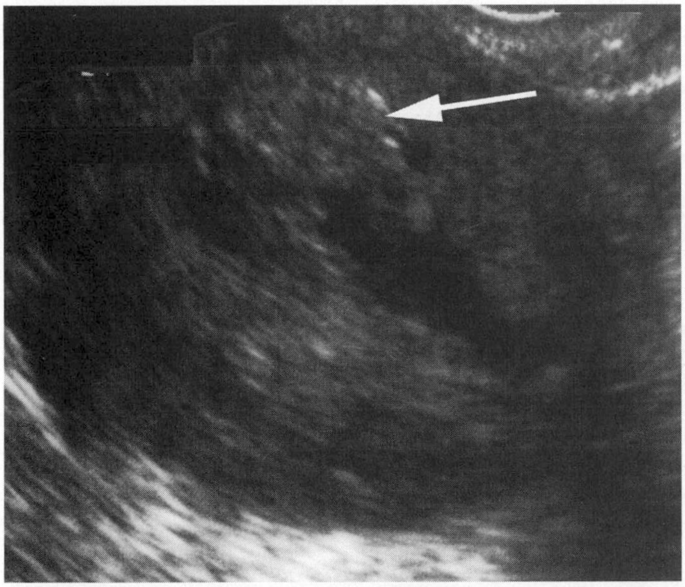

Figure 33-2. ■ *Cancer of the endometrium. Extensive intracavitary mass that was highly vascular on color flow* (arrow). *The neoplasm is arising from multiple foci and is outlined by a saline infusion study (SIS).*

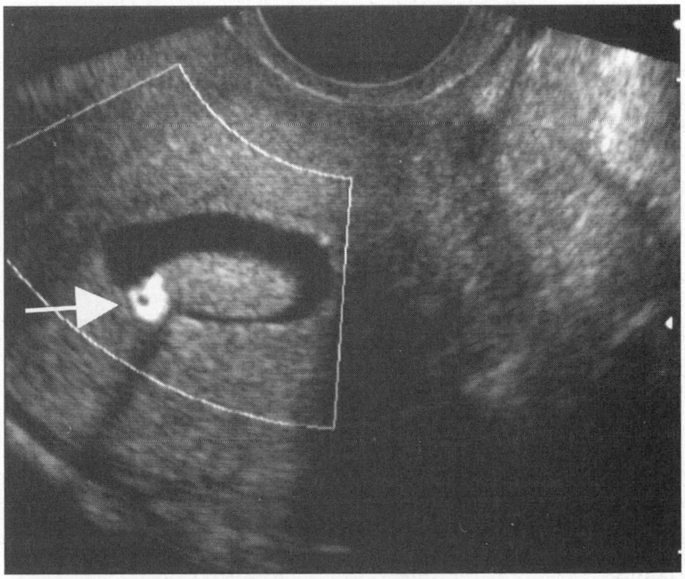

Figure 33-3. ■ *SIS showing a sessile (large-based) intracavitary polyp. Note the single supplying vessel to this benign polyp* (arrow).

Fibroids

Fibroids that abut on the endometrial cavity (submucosal) or that lie within the endometrial cavity (intracavitary) are a frequent cause of heavy periods, intramenstrual spotting, or postmenopausal bleeding. When outlined by fluid, during the performance of a hysterosonogram (SIS), they have a smooth, mildly echogenic border and less echogenic internal contents. They are immobile and can usually be seen to extend beyond the confines of the endometrial cavity (Fig. 33-4).

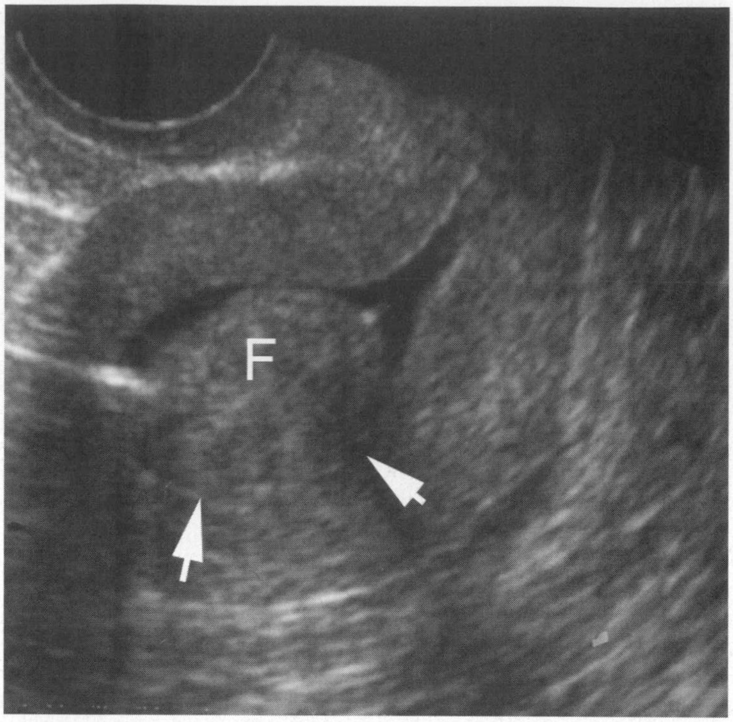

Figure 33-4. ■ *Large intracavitary fibroid* (F) *is outlined by saline on this saline infusion study* (SIS) *. Note the inhomogeneous contents, which are less echogenic than a polyp. The fibroid extends into the myometrium* (arrow).

Retained Products of Conception

This cause of endovaginal bleeding only occurs after a patient has been recently pregnant and has undergone an elective termination of pregnancy or a vaginal delivery. Endovaginal probe views will show echogenic material within the endometrial cavity, possibly with an area of acoustic shadowing related to a bony fragment (Fig. 33-5). As a rule, the retained product is a portion of the placenta and will have typical placental texture. Blood and retained products can look very similar. An SIS can help differentiate blood from retained products because retained products will adhere to the endometrium, whereas blood will float around (Fig. 33-6). Color flow Doppler is also helpful because retained placenta that is attached to the uterine wall often shows blood perfusion when examined with color flow; blood clot never lights up with color flow. If the endometrial cavity appears empty, this is helpful to the referring clinician because it means that there are no significant retained products.

Recurrence of Apparent Menstruation after an Interval of Months or Years

Menopause does not occur abruptly. A genuine period with ovulation may occur after a gap of months or years. In a patient with recurrent menstruation after a long gap the endometrium may be thick if the patient is in the secretory phase or a small cyst representing a follicle will be seen in an ovary.

Atrophic Endometrium

After the patient is menopausal, providing she is not taking HRT, the endometrium normally measures 4 mm or

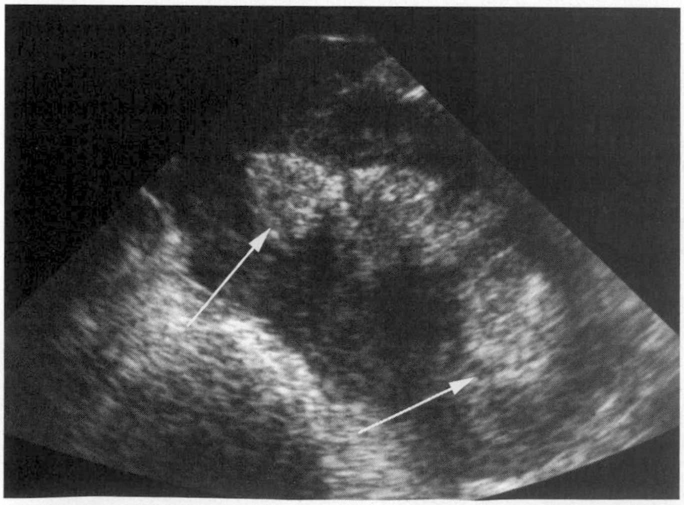

Figure 33-5. ■ *Retained products. Large amount of retained placental material within the endometrium* (arrows).

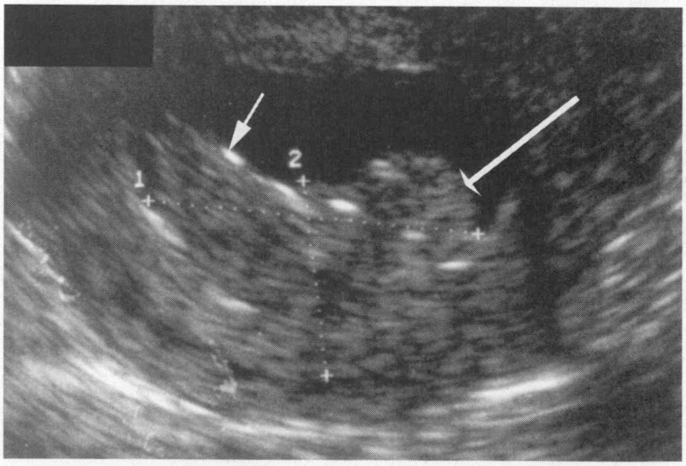

Figure 33-6. ■ *Extensive retained placental material* (arrows) *is outlined by fluid placed in the endometrial cavity in this saline infusion study (SIS).*

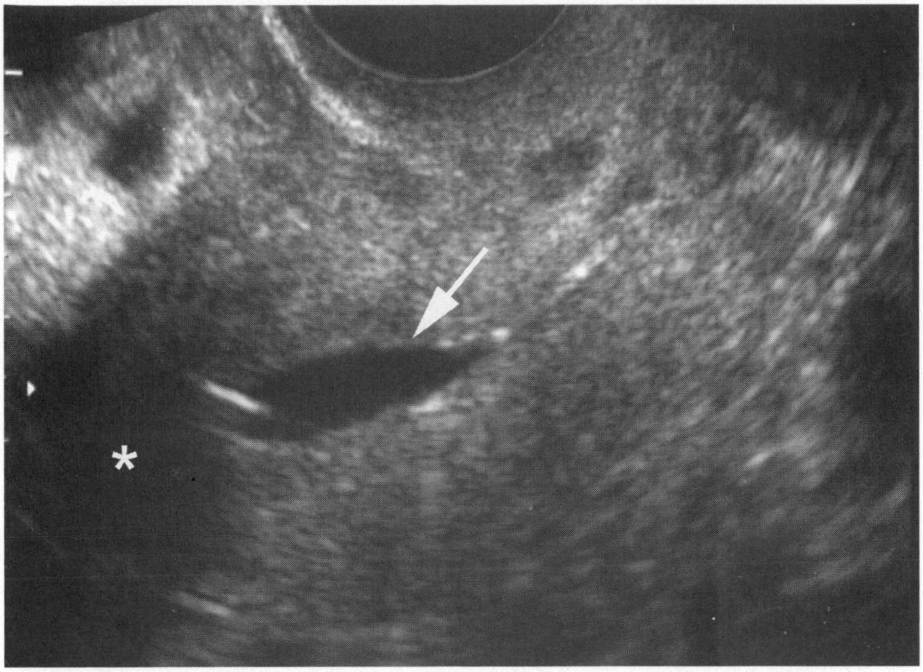

Figure 33-7. ■ *Atrophic endometrium. The endometrium is very thin* (arrow) *in this postmenopausal patient with vaginal bleeding. Note the echopenic area at the fundus* (*), *which is an artifact caused by the beam angle to uterine wall. This area can be mistaken for a fibroid.*

less. This atrophic endometrium can bleed spontaneously because it is fragile. Providing the outline of the endometrium is smooth without a focal mass (Fig. 33-7) and no blood dyscrasia is present, one can presume that postmenopausal bleeding relates to an atrophic endometrium. This is important because the patient does not need a biopsy or other invasive intervention.

Postmenopausal Hormone-Replacement Therapy

This type of therapy is much less popular than it used to be since a study showed that there was an increased risk of breast cancer with HRT and the protective effects of HRT against heart attacks had been exaggerated. Nevertheless, HRT prevents postmenopausal side effects such as hot flashes and helps to prevent osteoporosis, so it is still used by some patients. Most women take sequential estrogen and progesterone, which mimics the premenopausal appearance. In women who take estrogen alone, the endometrium can look very thick because this regimen promotes endometrial hyperplasia.

Cesarian Section Scar

Women who have had a Cesarian section performed are left with a scar. The pouch related to the scar may fill with blood at the time of menstruation; old dark blood leaks out slowly over the next few days causing intermenstrual spotting. A gaping cesarian section scar at the junction of the cervix and body of the uterus will be readily seen with the endovaginal probe (Fig. 33-8).

Tamoxifen

Tamoxifen changes are of two types:

1. Cystic and echogenic areas reminiscent of benign endometrial hyperplasia (Fig. 33-9). These changes are the result of subendometrial adenomyosis; a hysteroscopy shows a smooth surface resembling a waterbed ripple because the surface of the endometrium is uninvolved.
2. Multiple polyps, which may be very large, lie in the endometrium. These may develop into cancerous masses (Fig. 33-10).

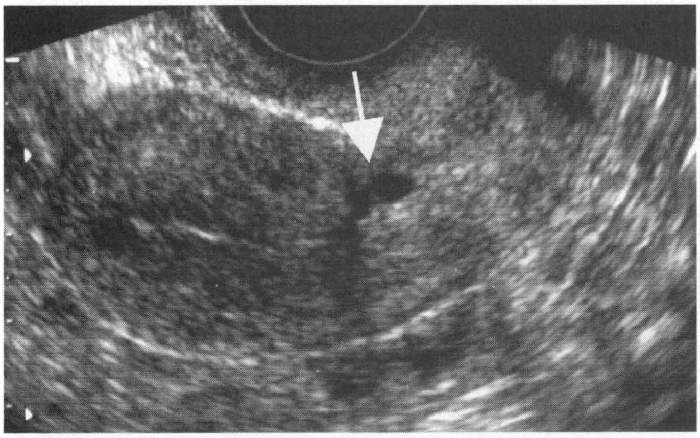

Figure 33-8. ■ *Cesarean section scar that is causing bleeding. Note the triangular cystic area* (arrow) *related to the previous cesarean section at the junction of the cervix and uterus.*

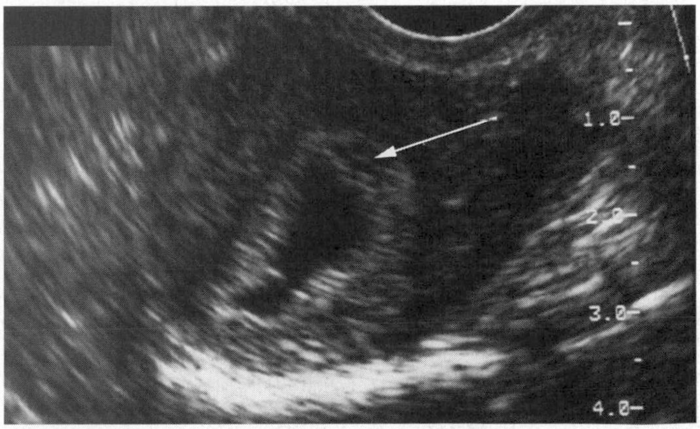

Figure 33-9. ■ *Subendometrial adenomyosis caused by Tamoxifen. The endometrium is apparently thickened, although it looked smoothly undulating at hysteroscopy; there are subendometrial cysts* (arrow).

Pitfalls

1. Intracavitary masses in the secretory phase of the cycle. The endometrial cavity echoes vary between 0.2 and 0.4 cm thick in the proliferative phase of the cycle and between 0.8 and 1.3 cm thick in the secretory phase of the cycle. Small masses such as polyps or intracavitary fibroids are often concealed in the secretory phase. If possible, schedule patients with possible intracavitary masses for the proliferative phase of the cycle or repeat the study.
2. Blood clot versus intracavitary mass. In a patient with a history of intramenstrual bleeding or heavy periods, an apparent intracavitary mass may represent a blood clot. Blood clots usually move within the cavity when an SIS is performed.
3. Endovaginal scanning with a bladder containing some urine. If the bladder is not completely empty, reverberation artifacts may obscure crucial structures and problem areas may be pushed far away from the transducer.
4. Hysterosonogram (SIS) in the secretory phase. If a hysterosonogram is performed in the secretory phase, the endometrium is fragile. The catheter can push up the endometrium so it looks like a polyp. A polyp can be suspected when none is present because the borders of the cavity are often irregular in the secretory phase.
5. Bubbles on hysterosonogram. Air can accumulate at the fundus and conceal pathology if the uterus is anteverted.

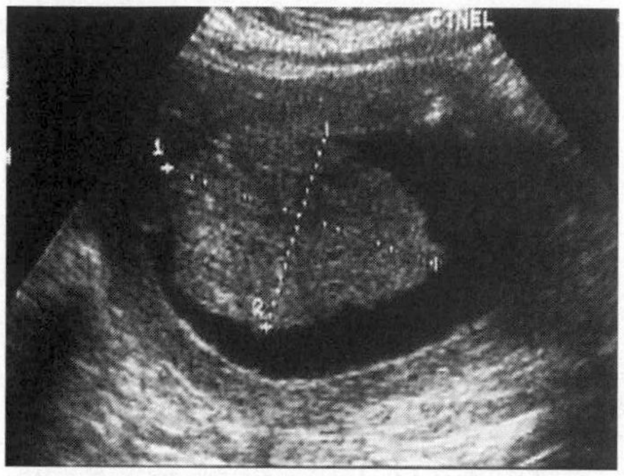

Figure 33-10. ■ *Large polypoid mass in the endometrium outlined by fluid in the endometrium. This mass was a cancerous polyp related to Tamoxifen administration.*

SELECTED READING

Atri M, Nazarnia S, Aldis A, et al. Transvaginal appearance of endometrial abnormalities. *Radiographics* 1994;14:483–492.

Berridge DL, Winter TC. Saline infusion sonohysterography: technique, indications and imaging findings. *J Ultrasound Med* 2004; 23:97–114.

Bree RL, Carlos RC. US for postmenopausal bleeding: consensus development and patient-centered outcomes. *Radiology* 2002; 222:595–598.

Fleischer AC. Color Doppler sonography of uterine disorders. *Ultrasound Q* 2003;19: 179–189.

Fong K, Kung R, Lytwyn A, et al. Endometrial evaluation with transvaginal ultrasound and hysterosonography in asymptomatic postmenopausal women with breast cancer receiving Tamoxifen. *Radiology* 2001;220: 765–773.

Lee EJ, Joo HJ, Ryu HS. Sonographic findings of uterine polypoid adenomas. *Ultrasound Q* 2004;20:1–12.

Nalaboff KM, Pellerito JS, Ben-Levi E, et al. Imaging the endometrium: disease and normal variants. *Radiographics* 2001;21: 1409–1414.

Sanders R, Parsons A. *Integrated Gynecological Ultrasound and Management.* Mosby. In press.

Intrauterine Contraceptive Devices

34

"Lost IUD"

ROGER C. SANDERS

SONOGRAM ABBREVIATIONS

IUD	Intrauterine device
IUCD	Intrauterine contraceptive device

KEY WORDS

Copper T and Copper 7 IUDs. Intrauterine devices (IUDs) containing copper that are still in use.

Lippes Loop. Obsolete but widely used serpentine-shaped IUD constructed with five parallel portions of plastic.

Levonorgestrel. Progesterone-like agent used in modern IUDs that release hormones over long periods.

Mirena Intrauterine System. T-shaped device that slowly releases levonorgestrel over a 5- to 7-year period.

Pelvic Inflammatory Disease (PID). Infection that spreads throughout the pelvis, often caused by gonorrhea. If it is secondary to an IUD, other bacteria are usually found.

Progestasert. T-shaped IUD that releases progesterone. Needs to be replaced annually.

The Clinical Problem

Intrauterine contraceptive devices (IUDs, IUCDs) are a highly effective means of contraception with relatively few systemic side effects. Although many varieties of IUDs have been used, only the most commonly used devices will be discussed here. Less than 1% of women in the United States use these devices; however, 15% to 30% of women use IUDs in Europe and Canada.

Because pelvic inflammatory disease (PID) was a common side effect in women who used IUDs, the devices fell out of favor. Modern IUDs that slowly release progesterone or a progesterone-like substance, levonorgestrel, over a number of years are making a comeback because infection is rare nowadays. Usually inserted to prevent pregnancy, IUDs may also be used to prevent dysfunctional bleeding.

The proper location of an IUD, regardless of type, is in the endometrial cavity at the uterine fundus. The remainder of the device should be above the cervix. A nylon thread, which extends from the uterus into the vagina, is attached to the proximal end of all IUDs. This string should be palpable or visible on pelvic examination. If this string cannot be identified, the patient may be referred for evaluation of a "lost IUD."

Some patients have no complaint other than a lost string. Others, however, present with cramping, pain, or abnormal bleeding. In either case, the position of the IUD must be demonstrated. If the uterus is empty, the device has been expelled or has perforated the uterus. An IUD outside the uterus is usually not seen with ultrasound because it is surrounded by gut. Although an IUD in the correct location prevents a normal pregnancy effectively, ectopic pregnancies may still occur.

Anatomy

Anatomy of the pelvic area is discussed in Chapter 29.

TYPES OF DEVICES

Lippes Loop

The Lippes loop was the most widely used IUD, and there are still some in use. In a long-axis view, the loop has two to five echogenic components, depending on whether a true long-axis IUD view has been obtained (Fig. 34-1A,B). Transversely, the device is visualized as a single line.

Dalkon Shield

Insertion of the Dalkon shield was suspended some years ago because of a large number of associated infections. There are still a few women using the device. The Dalkon shield is the smallest of the

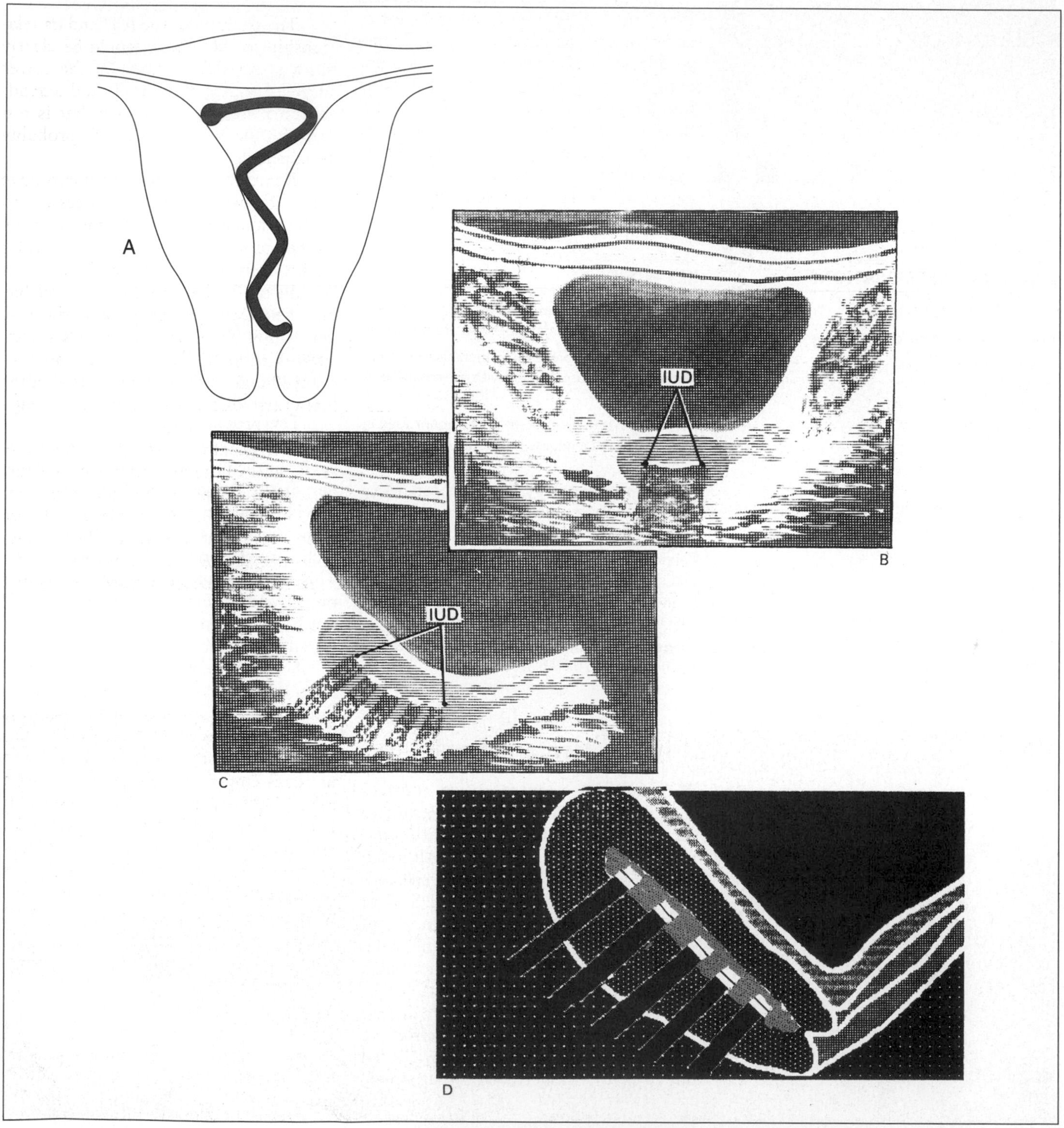

Figure 34-1. ■ *Lippes loop. A. Lippes loop in the endometrial cavity. B. Transverse view of one rung of the Lippes loop. C. Longitudinal view of five rungs of the Lippes loop. D. Lippes loop within the uterus with entrance and exit echoes.*

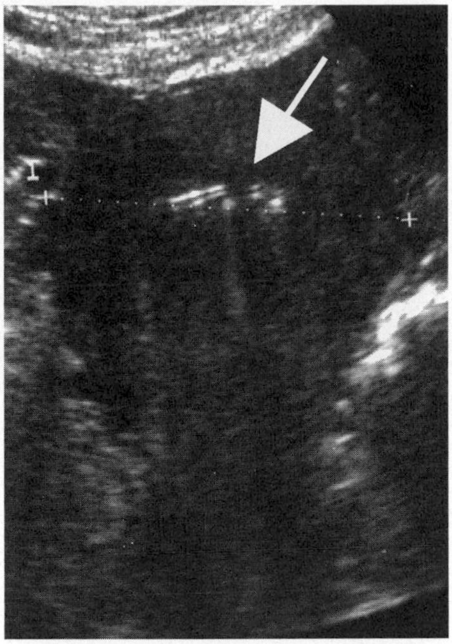

Figure 34-2. ■ *Transverse view of vertically orientated uterus showing a copper T intrauterine device (IUD)* (arrow). *Both the transverse arms and the stem can be seen. Note the entrance and exit echoes seen on the arm portion of the IUD.*

IUDs. On both longitudinal and transverse scans, it appears as two echogenic foci.

Saf-T-Coil

This unusual older IUD may still be seen occasionally. There are two spirals alongside a central stem.

Copper 7 and Copper T, Progestasert, ParaGard, and Mirena Intrauterine Devices

The Copper 7 and Copper T IUDs differ from the others in that a band of copper is wound around one end. On long-axis views, both usually appear as a line with thickening at the upper end of the bend that forms the 7 or the T and at the lower end owing to the band of copper. Transversely, the devices will appear as a dot except at the upper end, where a short line can be seen owing to the 7 or T configuration (Fig. 34-2). The Progestasert and ParaGard have an indistinguishable appearance. The Mirena IUD has a thick stem and a blurred stem echo (Fig. 34-3).

Technique

INTRAUTERINE DEVICE POSITION

The endovaginal approach has a number of advantages over a transabdominal view:

1. Providing the IUD is in the uterus, it can be seen throughout its extent, whatever the uterine position.
2. The string can be seen as a thin longitudinal echo. If it is balled up into a clump, a small echogenic mass will be found near the inferior end of the IUD (Fig. 34-3).
3. Should the IUD have perforated the myometrium, the site and amount of intramyometrial extension can be quantitated.
4. If the IUD is extrauterine, a small abscess or fluid collection may form around it and it may be visible from an endovaginal view point, even when it cannot be seen on a transabdominal sonogram.

The position of the IUD and its relationship to the uterus should be clearly shown. An IUD located in the lower uterine segment (Fig. 34-4) and extending into the vagina, or one that is too large for the uterine cavity, will probably be expelled.

Remember that not all patients have a midline uterus. It may be necessary to scan obliquely to obtain a long-axis view of the uterus. Transverse scans are useful in demonstrating that the entire device is within the endometrial cavity and has not penetrated or perforated the myometrium. There are two echoes associated with an IUD, known as the "entrance" and "exit" echoes. These subtle linear echoes are diagnostic of a foreign body (Figs. 34-1 and 34-2).

The decidual reaction in the secretory phase of the endometrial cavity may obscure an IUD. IUD echoes are more readily reproducible, are associated with shadowing, and are generally stronger than decidual echoes. If the gain is decreased, IUD echoes will still be visible.

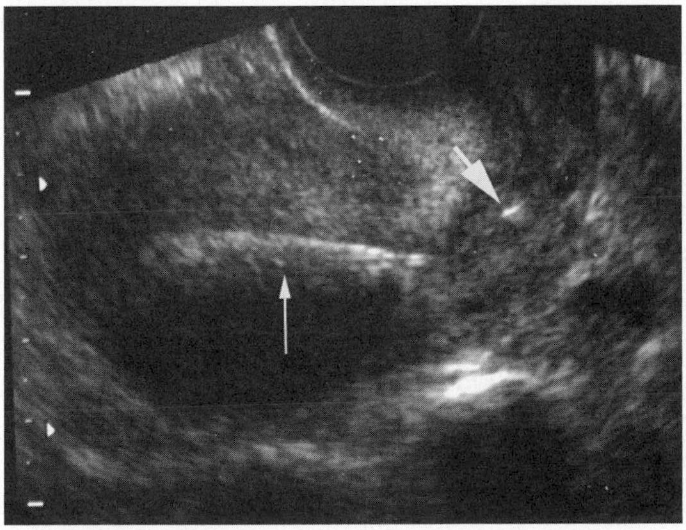

Figure 34-3. ■ *Mirena IUD. Note the relatively subtle shaft echoes with a lot of shadowing* (arrow). *The IUD string can be seen* (larger arrow). *The IUD string could not be felt.*

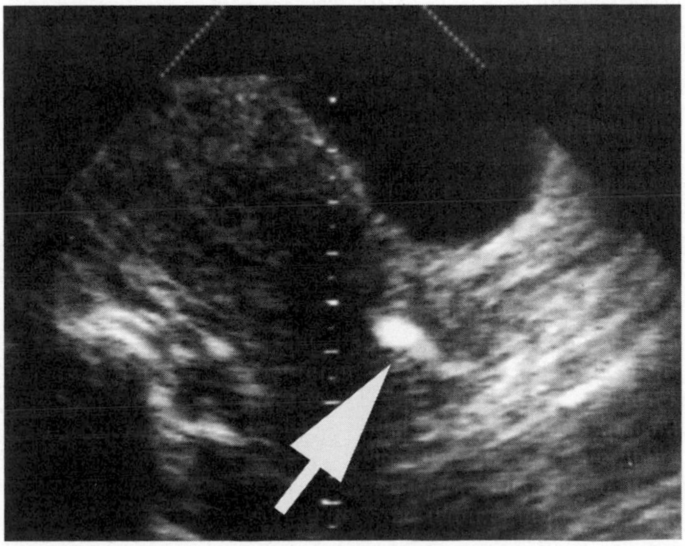

Figure 34-4. ■ *Progestasert IUD in an abnormally low position partially in the cervix. An IUD in this position will be ineffective and will fall out.*

Pathology

LOST INTRAUTERINE DEVICE

When a patient cannot feel the IUD string in the vagina, it is termed a "lost IUD." Most often the IUD is still in good position, but the string is balled up and visible in the region of the internal os (Fig. 34-3). Perforation of the uterus by an IUD may be complete or incomplete. If incomplete, a portion of the IUD may be demonstrated within the uterine wall (Fig. 34-5). If the IUD cannot be seen with ultrasound it may have fallen out or it may have perforated the uterus and be in the pelvis outside the uterus. A radiograph or computed tomography scan will show whether it is still inside the patient.

It is important to show the relationship of the IUD to the endometrial cavity. If any portion of the device is in contact with the cavity, the IUD can be withdrawn, but if the IUD is entirely in the myometrium the uterus may have to be surgically removed.

PREGNANCY

Pregnancy can occasionally occur with IUDs. This complication is almost unknown with modern IUDs that contain progesterone-like substances. When an IUD with a coexisting pregnancy is discovered, one should determine the relationship of the device to the gestational sac (i.e., superior or inferior). This relationship is important in deciding whether an IUD can be safely removed. If it is left in place, a severe infection may occur. In the later stages of pregnancy, the location of the IUD is difficult to determine because of the large volume of the uterus occupied by the fetus.

PELVIC INFLAMMATORY DISEASE

IUDs have been historically associated with a slightly increased incidence of PID. If a patient presents with pain or bleeding and the IUD is properly positioned, check the adnexal areas and the cul-de-sac for evidence of PID (as discussed in Chapter 32). Occasionally the abscess around a perforated infected IUD allows an extrauterine IUD to be seen.

Pitfalls

1. When the patient is in the secretory phase of the cycle and endometrium is thick it may be difficult to see the IUD.
2. The balled-up string in the region of the internal os may not be obvious. Magnify the image to see the subtle string components.
3. Fibroids may distort the endometrium so that the IUD appears to lie off-axis.

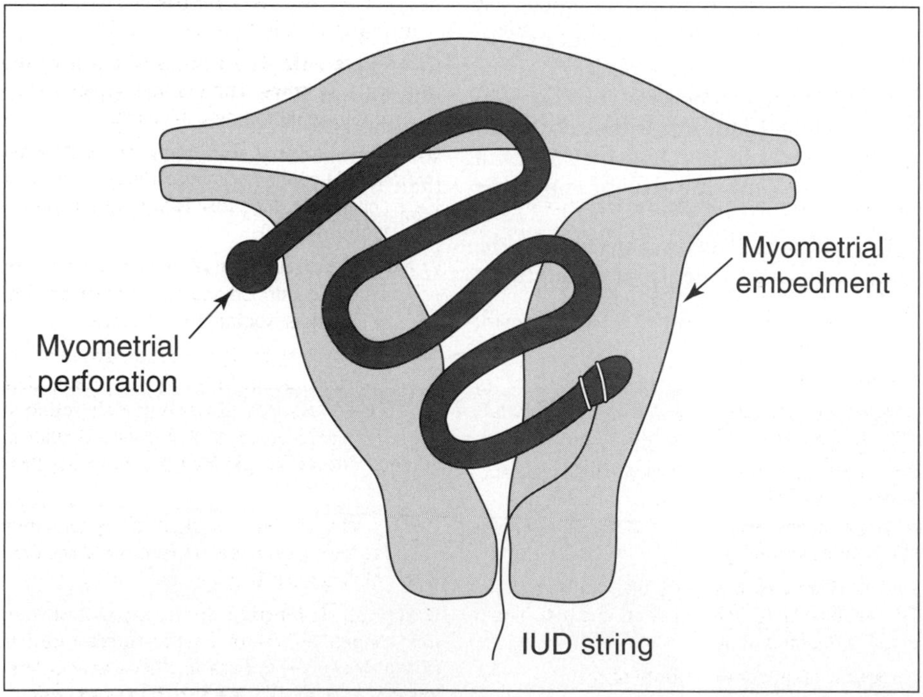

Figure 34-5. ■ *Intramyometrial IUD. Portions of the IUD are outside the cavity within the myometrium or peritoneum.*

Where Else to Look

1. If an IUD cannot be found with ultrasound despite a thorough search, and pregnancy has been ruled out, an abdominal radiograph or CAT scan will reveal the location of a migrated IUD or prove that the IUD has been expelled.
2. If the patient has pelvic pain, look in the adnexa for an ectopic pregnancy because these may occur even when the IUD is correctly positioned.

SELECTED READING

Salem S, Wilson SR. Gynecological ultrasound. In *Diagnostic Ultrasound*, 3rd ed. Rumack CR, Wilson S, Charbonneau JW, et al. eds. St. Louis: Mosby; 2005.

Sanders R, Parsons A. *Integrated Gynecological Sonography and Management.* Philadelphia: Mosby. In press.

Pediatric Abdominal Masses

35

MARILYN J. SIEGEL

KEY WORDS

Adrenal Hemorrhage. Hemorrhage into the adrenal gland is a common cause of a neonatal abdominal mass. It resolves spontaneously, often with development of calcifications.

Beckwith-Wiedemann Syndrome. Congenital malformation characterized by hemihypertrophy (overgrowth of one side of the body), enlargement of the tongue, and omphalocele (protuberance of bowel through a defect in the abdominal wall).

Choledochal Cyst. Congenital dilatation of the biliary tree. Clinical findings include jaundice, abdominal mass, and pain.

Enteric Duplication. Congenital duplication of the bowel. The involved segment does not communicate with the remainder of the bowel and presents as a fluid-filled mass.

Hemangioendothelioma. Benign tumor of the liver. Affects neonates and infants under the age of 6 months. Patients usually present with heart failure and a large liver.

Hematocolpos. Blood in a dilated vagina. Vaginal dilatation may be secondary to distal atresia, a septum, or a membrane. Patients present with a midline pelvic mass. Has been associated with uterine duplication anomalies.

Hepatoblastoma. Most common hepatic malignancy. Occurs in young children, usually under the age of 3 years.

Hepatocellular Carcinoma. Rare malignancy of the liver in older children and adolescents.

Hydronephrosis. Dilatation of the renal pelvis and calyces. Most common cause is obstruction at the level of the renal pelvis. Usually found in neonates and infants.

Infant. Individual between 1 month and 2 years of age.

Intussusception. Obstructed bowel coiled on itself. Seen in young children.

Lymphoma. Malignancy of lymphoid tissue. The non-Hodgkin form of lymphoma is most common in the abdomen. Usually involves bowel and lymph nodes, but it can involve the liver, spleen, and kidneys.

Mesenchymal Hamartoma. Rare benign liver mass. Most commonly seen in children under 2 years of age.

Meningocele. Cystic dilatation of the spinal canal at the site of a bony defect. May appear as a pelvic mass in the neonate when it protrudes anterior to the sacrum.

Mesentery. A fan-shaped fold of peritoneum that connects the small bowel and colon to the posterior abdominal wall.

Mesenteric Cyst. Cyst filled with lymph. Found in the mesentery and presents as an asymptomatic abdominal mass.

Mesoblastic Nephroma. Rare benign renal tumor occurring in neonates and young infants. Rarely metastasizes. Treated by nephrectomy.

Multicystic Dysplastic Kidney. Unilateral renal cystic disease. It develops in utero and is the result of atresia of the renal pelvis and ureter. Renal tissue is nonfunctioning.

Multilocular Cystic Nephroma. Nonhereditary, benign renal mass. Affect patients under 4 years of age. Treatment is nephrectomy.

Neonate. Infant under 1 month of age.

Nephroblastomatosis. Persistence of fetal renal tissue in the kidneys. Has been associated with Wilms tumor. Usually found in neonates and infants. Treatment is chemotherapy.

Neuroblastoma. Second most common abdominal mass after Wilms tumor. Usually arises in the adrenal gland, but it may arise in ganglia (nervous tissue) along the spine. Occurs between birth and 5 years of age. Most patients present with palpable abdominal masses.

Omentum. A fold that joins the stomach to the liver or colon. Cysts may develop in the omentum and may cause an abdominal mass.

Posterior Urethral Valves. Most common cause of urethral obstruction in male infants and children. Does not affect females.

Pyloric Stenosis. The pylorus (the exit of the stomach) is narrowed and the wall is thickened. A cause of projectile vomiting in infants.

Renal Vein Thrombosis. Usually the result of dehydration. Also seen in infants of diabetic mothers. Classic clinical findings are a flank mass and hematuria (blood in urine).

Rhabdomyosarcoma. Malignant muscle tumor that occurs in childhood and has a particular affinity for the bladder, vagina, and prostate.

Teratoma. Usually benign mass composed of elements of most tissues in the body, notably skin, hair, bone, and teeth. Most commonly found in the sacrococcygeal area in neonates and ovary in adolescent girls. Malignancy occurs in less than 10%.

Ureterocele. Dilatation of the distal ureter where it inserts into the bladder. Most often associated with a duplicated kidney.

Ureteropelvic Junction Obstruction. Most common congenital cause of renal obstruction. Results from a block of the upper end of the ureter just below the renal pelvis. Usually found in neonates.

Wilms Tumor. Most common renal malignancy in childhood. Usually affects children between 1 and 6 years of age. Associated with Beckwith-Wiedemann syndrome (mentioned previously in this section) and hemihypertrophy. Treatment is chemotherapy and surgical resection.

The Clinical Problem

The differential diagnosis of pediatric abdominal masses varies based on patient age (neonate vs. infant and older child) and the presence or absence of symptoms.

Sonography is used to confirm the presence of the mass and to suggest its size and position. Most, if not all, masses will require additional imaging studies, and the type of study can be influenced by the sonographic findings. For example, if sonography demonstrates hydronephrosis, a nuclear medicine study is performed to assess renal function, and a contrast examination of the bladder (cystogram) is obtained to determine if reflux is causing the hydronephrosis. If sonography demonstrates a benign cystic mass, further imaging is often not indicated. If sonography reveals a solid abdominal mass, however, computed tomography or magnetic resonance imaging is performed to define the extent of disease.

NEONATAL ABDOMINAL MASSES

Renal masses account for the majority (>70%) of abdominal masses in neonates and virtually all are asymptomatic. These masses come to clinical attention because they produce a palpable abdominal mass. The common renal masses are hydronephrosis and multicystic dysplastic kidney. Rarer renal masses include autosomal recessive polycystic disease, mesoblastic nephroma, renal vein thrombosis, and nephroblastomatosis.

Less often, abdominal masses in neonates arise in the adrenal glands (usually adrenal hemorrhage or neuroblastoma), the reproductive organs (ovarian cysts and hydrocolpos), liver (hemangioendothelioma), biliary tract (choledochal cyst), gastrointestinal tract (duplication and mesenteric cysts), or in the sacrococcygeal area (teratoma).

ABDOMINAL MASSES IN THE OLDER INFANT AND CHILD

In older infants (after 2 months of age) and children, most abdominal masses are of renal origin and most are detected as asymptomatic, palpable masses. Wilms tumor, which arises in the kidney, and neuroblastoma, which arises in the adrenal gland, are the most common abdominal masses. Ovarian tumors (teratomas), rhabdomyosarcoma, hepatic tumors (hepatoblastoma and hepatoma), and gastrointestinal tumors (lymphoma) may also occur in this age group. Occasionally, abdominal masses in this age group will produce symptoms. These include pyloric stenosis, intussusception, appendiceal abscess, and ovarian torsion. This chapter will first review the common asymptomatic masses in older infants and children, followed by a discussion of symptomatic masses in young infants (e.g., pyloric stenosis and intussusception). Symptomatic masses that occur in both pediatric and adult populations are discussed elsewhere in this textbook.

Technique

TRANSDUCERS

Sector-type or curved array probes are used for imaging most abdominal masses. A linear array transducer may improve visualization of bowel morphology and abnormalities in the near field. Abdominal sonograms are performed with the highest frequency transducer possible. A 5-MHz transducer usually suffices in children and thin adolescents, and a 3.5-MHz transducer may be needed in larger adolescents. A 7.5-MHz transducer is usually adequate in small infants.

SCANNING TECHNIQUES

Kidneys and adrenal glands are examined in transverse and longitudinal planes. The right kidney and adrenal gland are seen best with the patient in the supine or left lateral decubitus position, using the right hepatic lobe as an acoustic window. The left kidney and adrenal gland are imaged with the patient in the supine or the right lateral decubitus position, using the spleen as an acoustic window. Scanning the patient in the prone position may be advantageous when abundant bowel gas obscures visualization using an anterior approach. Images of the kidneys are obtained through the upper poles, midsection, and lower poles. Renal lengths are noted. Images of the urinary bladder are obtained as part of the routine renal sonogram. Always check the bladder first, and take a picture before it empties.

Although adrenal sonograms are rarely requested in adults, it is not uncommon to follow adrenal hemorrhage in neonates with ultrasound. The right adrenal is easily seen through the liver at a level just superior to the upper pole of the kidney. It lies medial to the right lobe of the liver, behind the inferior vena cava (IVC), and above the upper pole of the right kidney. The left adrenal lies lateral to the aorta, medial to the spleen and upper pole of the left kidney, and posterior to the pancreatic tail. The left adrenal gland is often best seen with the infant either supine or left side up. It helps to use a posterior approach to demonstrate the left adrenal gland. The adrenal glands can be recognized by their "V" or "Y" shape on longitudinal views and by their linear, "V,""Y," or "L" configuration on transverse views.

The liver is evaluated in both longitudinal and transverse scans with the patient in the supine position. Examining the patient in the left posterior oblique position may be helpful to evaluate the deeper posterior parts of the right lobe. Most of the liver can be imaged by a subcostal approach, although an intercostal approach with a sector transducer may be necessary for evaluating the superior parts of the liver, especially the subdiaphragmatic part of the right lobe. The use of pulsed and color flow Doppler imaging can help to differentiate blood vessels from bile ducts and can characterize vascular abnormalities. The gallbladder, spleen, and pancreas are examined as part of a routine liver sonogram.

The bowel is examined in longitudinal and transverse planes. Firm pressure is applied with a linear array transducer in order to displace normal air-filled bowel loops out of the field of view.

The peritoneal cavity is examined for ascites or tumor. The examination should include the subdiaphragmatic spaces, the space between the right kidney and liver (Morison's pouch), the paracolic gutters, and the cul-de-sac.

Pelvic sonography in children is usually performed transabdominally with a distended bladder. Adequate bladder distention can be achieved either by having the patient drink large volumes of fluid, or if the patient is not allowed oral intake, the bladder can be distended with sterile fluid through a Foley catheter. Endovaginal scanning is not used in younger children, although this approach can be useful in adolescent females when findings with the transabdominal approach are equivocal. Scans of the ovaries and uterus are obtained in both the sagittal and transverse planes. In some instances, placing the patient in a decubitus position and scanning directly over the adnexa will improve visualization of the ovaries. The use of tissue harmonics can improve organ visualization and image quality. Measurements of the ovaries and uterus are obtained in three orthogonal planes.

As the well-known adage states, "Children are not just small adults," the following tips may prove useful when scanning the pediatric patient.

SONOGRAPHER'S APPROACH TO CHILDREN

1. Start the examination in a well-lit room.
2. Do not wear a white coat.
3. Maintain steady eye contact, and concentrate on the child rather than the parents.
4. Speak with a soft voice.
5. Do not talk about sonographic findings in front of the child, although some children respond well to having their anatomy discussed. If you discuss the sonogram findings, use simple terms. For instance, "This long tube is a vessel. It has blood in it."
6. Allow the child to become familiar with the room and the system.
7. Unless contraindicated, feed small infants during the study.
8. Have the parents help hold the child. Use warm gel. Let the child put the gel on him or herself.
9. Young children may cooperate more by telling them that they are going to be on TV.
10. Show small children something dynamic on ultrasound (e.g., the beating heart) to interest them in the procedure.

IMMOBILIZATION

Infants and young children can usually be examined by having an adult, preferably a parent, restrain the shoulders and legs so that the patient falls asleep or at least lies quietly. Sandbags may help to keep infants in a desired position. Always try to distract the older patient with casual conversation about their favorite food or television show.

Older children should be shown the transducer and equipment before you perform the examination so that they will not feel threatened by the assessment. Encouraging the child to feel the transducer or switch on instrumentation to see himself or herself on TV is helpful.

When explanations, reassurance, and restraint on the examination table fail, you may try having the patient sit or lie on the parent's lap.

SEDATION

Sedation may rarely be necessary in examining uncooperative infants or children. The drugs used for sedation should be individualized for each patient and approved by the anesthesia department for each hospital.

KEEPING THE NEONATE WARM

The neonate must be kept warm. A blanket usually suffices and can also be used to restrain the patient. Small infants should be uncovered for the shortest time possible.

TRANSDUCER CONTACT

The transducer of choice should be the one with the highest frequency and the smallest footprint adequate to the task. In a neonate, this may mean using a small parts transducer. The right upper quadrant may be better visualized by angling up under the costal margin. Use warm gel to ensure good contact and patient cooperation.

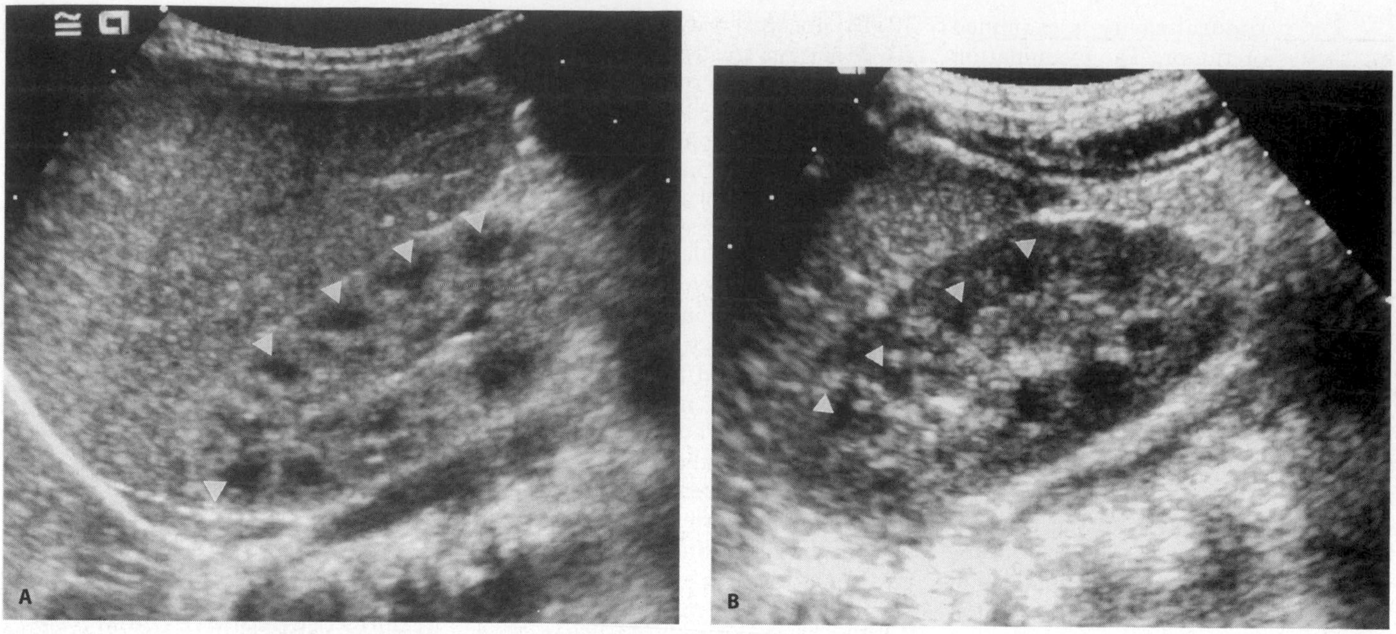

Figure 35-1. ■ *Normal renal anatomy. **A.** Neonate. Note that the echogenicity of the cortex is equal to that of the liver. The pyramids* (arrowheads) *are prominent, and there is a paucity of central renal sinus echogenicity. **B.** Older child (3 years of age). The renal cortex is hypoechoic to liver. The renal pyramids* (arrowheads) *are less prominent. There is still a paucity of central sinus echogenicity.*

Normal Anatomy

KIDNEYS

The neonatal kidney demonstrates three unique features (Fig. 35-1). The renal cortex is iso- or hyperechoic to liver or spleen. The renal pyramids are prominent, and there is a paucity of renal sinus echogenicity. The cortex usually becomes hypoechoic relative to liver or spleen by the end of the first year of life, and the pyramids become less well defined by the second or third year of life. The echogenicity of the renal pelvis increases at the end of the first decade of life. Doppler interrogation of the renal artery shows continuous forward flow in diastole, indicating low vascular resistance. Renal size is described by measurements of length (Table 35-1).

TABLE 35-1 Mean Renal Length

Age (Years)	Mean Renal Length (cm)	Standard Deviation
0 to 1 wk	4.5	0.30
1 wk to 4 mo	5.0	0.70
4 to 8 mo	6.0	0.70
8 mo to 1 y	6.0	0.60
1 to 2	6.7	0.55
2 to 3	7.0	0.55
3 to 4	7.0	0.65
4 to 5	8.0	0.50
5 to 6	8.0	0.55
6 to 7	8.0	0.70
7 to 8	8.0	0.50
8 to 9	9.0	0.90
9 to 10	9.0	0.90
10 to 11	9.0	0.80
11 to 12	10.0	0.65
12 to 13	10.5	0.90
13 to 14	10.0	0.75
14 to 15	10.0	0.60
15 to 16	11.0	0.80
16 to 17	10.0	0.90
17 to 18	10.5	0.30
18 to 19	11.0	1.15

(Adapted from Han BK, Babcock DS. Sonographic measurements and appearance of normal kidneys in children. AJR 1985;145:611.)

ADRENAL GLANDS

Normal adrenal glands are relatively large and easily seen in the neonate because the cortex is prominent. The length of each adrenal gland is between 0.9 and 3.6 cm (mean, 1.5 to 1.7 cm), and the thickness ranges between 0.2 and 0.5 cm (mean, 0.3 cm). The adrenal cortex is hypoechoic to the medulla (Fig. 35-2). Although the adrenal glands become more difficult to visualize after the first few months of life because the cortex atrophies, they often can be seen in older infants and children with the use of high-resolution sonography.

LIVER AND SPLEEN

The liver and spleen in neonates are isoechoic or hypoechoic relative to the kidneys. They become hyperechoic to the kidneys at the end of the first year of life (Fig. 35-1). The appearances of the fissures, ligaments, and vessels are similar to those seen in adults. The intrahepatic and common bile ducts should be visualized. Measurements for the common bile duct are <1 mm in neonates and infants under 1 year of age, <2 mm in infants under 2 years of age, <4 mm in children between 2 and 12 years of age, and <5 mm in adolescents.

BOWEL

With standard transabdominal scanning, the normal bowel usually has a three-layer appearance with an echogenic inner layer of mucosa and submucosa, a hypoechoic middle layer of muscle, and an echogenic outer layer of serosa and surrounding fat (with higher-frequency insonation, more bowel layers may be seen). Normal bowel wall, measured from the inner edge of the mucosa to the outer edge of the muscle, is 2- to 6-mm thick, depending on the distention. The wall thickness of distended bowel is 2 to 3 mm; the thickness of collapsed bowel ranges from 4 to 6 mm. The lumen of the bowel may contain internal echoes, representing food, air, or stool. Normal bowel wall shows little or no color flow on Doppler imaging.

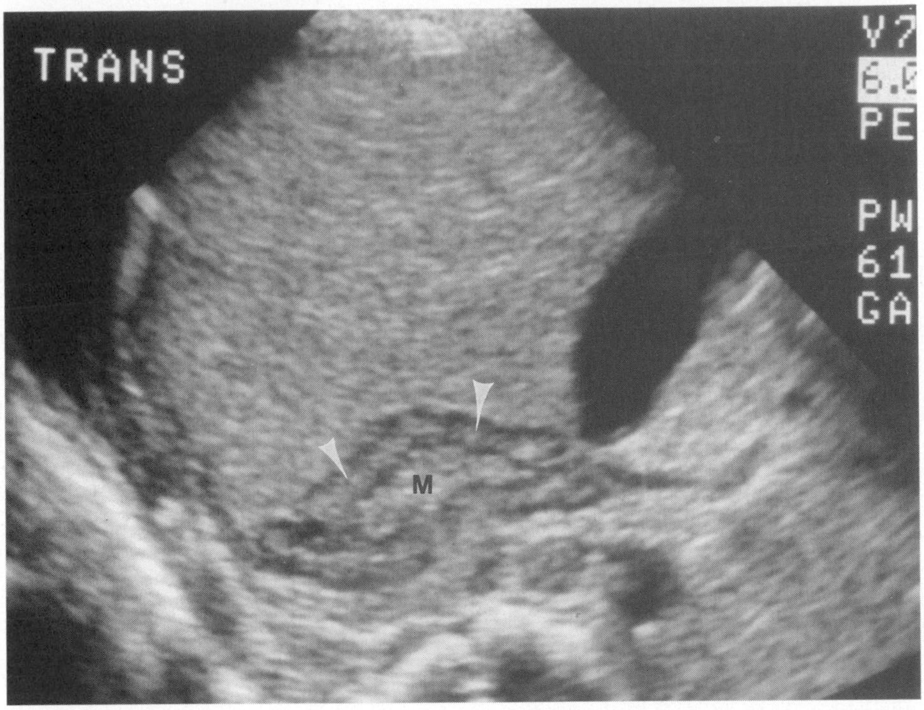

Figure 35-2. ■ *Neonatal adrenal gland. The adrenal cortex* (arrowheads) *is hypoechoic compared to medulla* (M).

OVARIES AND UTERUS

The size and appearance of the ovaries vary with age. Ovarian size is described by measurements of ovarian volume (0.52 × length × width × height) (Table 35-2). In general, mean ovarian volume in prepubertal girls under 6 years of age is less than 1.0 cm^3. Ovarian volume begins to increase after 6 years of age. Mean volumes for premenarchal girls between 6 and 13 years old range between 1.1 and 4 cm^3. In postmenarchal girls, mean ovarian volume is 9 to 10 cm^3. Normal microcystic follicles (<9 mm in diameter) are routinely seen in premenarchal girls. Normal follicles appear as hypoechoic, thin-walled cysts in the periphery of the ovary. After the onset of menses, macrocystic follicles (>1 cm in diameter) become common. These are follicles that develop in response to stimulation by follicle-stimu-

TABLE 35-2 Ovarian Volume Measurements

Age (Years)	Mean Ovarian Volume cm^3 (± 1 SD)
1 day to 1 year	1.1 (1.0)
1	1.1 (0. 7)
2	0.7 (0.4)
3	0.7 (0.2)
4	0.8 (0.4)
5	0.9 (02)
6	1.2 (0.4)
7	1.3 (0.6)
8	1.1 (0.5)
9	2.0 (0.8)
10	2.2 (0.7)
11	2.5 (1.3)
12	3.8 (1.4)
13	4.2 (2.3)
Postmenarchal	9.8 (0.6)

From: Cohen HL, Shapiro MA, Mandel FS, Shapiro ML. Normal ovaries in neonates and infants: a sonographic study of 77 patients 1 day to 24 months old. AJR 1993;160:583–586.
Cohen HL, Tice HM, Mandel FS. Ovarian volumes measured by US: bigger than we think. Radiology 1990;177:189–192
Orsini LF, Salardi S, Pilu G, Bovicelli L, Cacciari E. Pelvic organs by premenarcheal girls: real-time ultrasonography. AJR 1984;153:113–116.

lating and luteinizing hormones. One follicle becomes dominant and is destined to ovulate; the other follicles involute. The dominant follicle ranges between 17 and 30 mm in diameter.

Uterine size and shape also change with patient age. The neonatal uterus is prominent because of in utero stimulation by maternal hormones. The uterus is approximately 3.5 cm long and 1.4 cm thick. The endometrial lining is echogenic. After the neonatal period, the prepubertal uterus has a tubular shape. The fundus and cervix are equal in size. The endometrial stripe is not usually seen. The uterus is 2.5 to 4 cm long and is less than 1 cm thick. The pubertal uterus is pear-shaped; the fundus is larger than the cervix. The uterus is 5 to 8 cm long, 3 cm wide, and 1.5 cm thick. The endometrial stripe is seen and varies in thickness with the time of the menstrual cycle.

Sonographic Findings of Asymptomatic Abdominal Masses

KIDNEYS

Neonatal Renal Masses

Hydronephrosis. Renal obstruction in the newborn may be underestimated on examinations performed immediately after birth because of a normal physiologic decrease in renal function. In the neonate with an antenatal diagnosis of fetal pelviectasis or calicectasis, postnatal sonography should be performed between 4 and 7 days of age.

Ureteropelvic junction obstruction is the most common cause of congenital hydronephrosis. This is a proximal obstruction, occurring at the level of the renal pelvis and ureter. This anomaly produces dilatation of the calyces and renal pelvis; the ureter and bladder are normal (Fig. 35-3). Severe or chronic obstruction is often associated with diffuse parenchymal loss, increased parenchymal echogenicity and cortical cysts.

Distal ureteral obstruction is the next most common cause of congenital hydronephrosis, and ureterovesical junction obstruction, usually due to a stricture, and ureteral ectopia or a ureterocele associated with a duplicated collecting

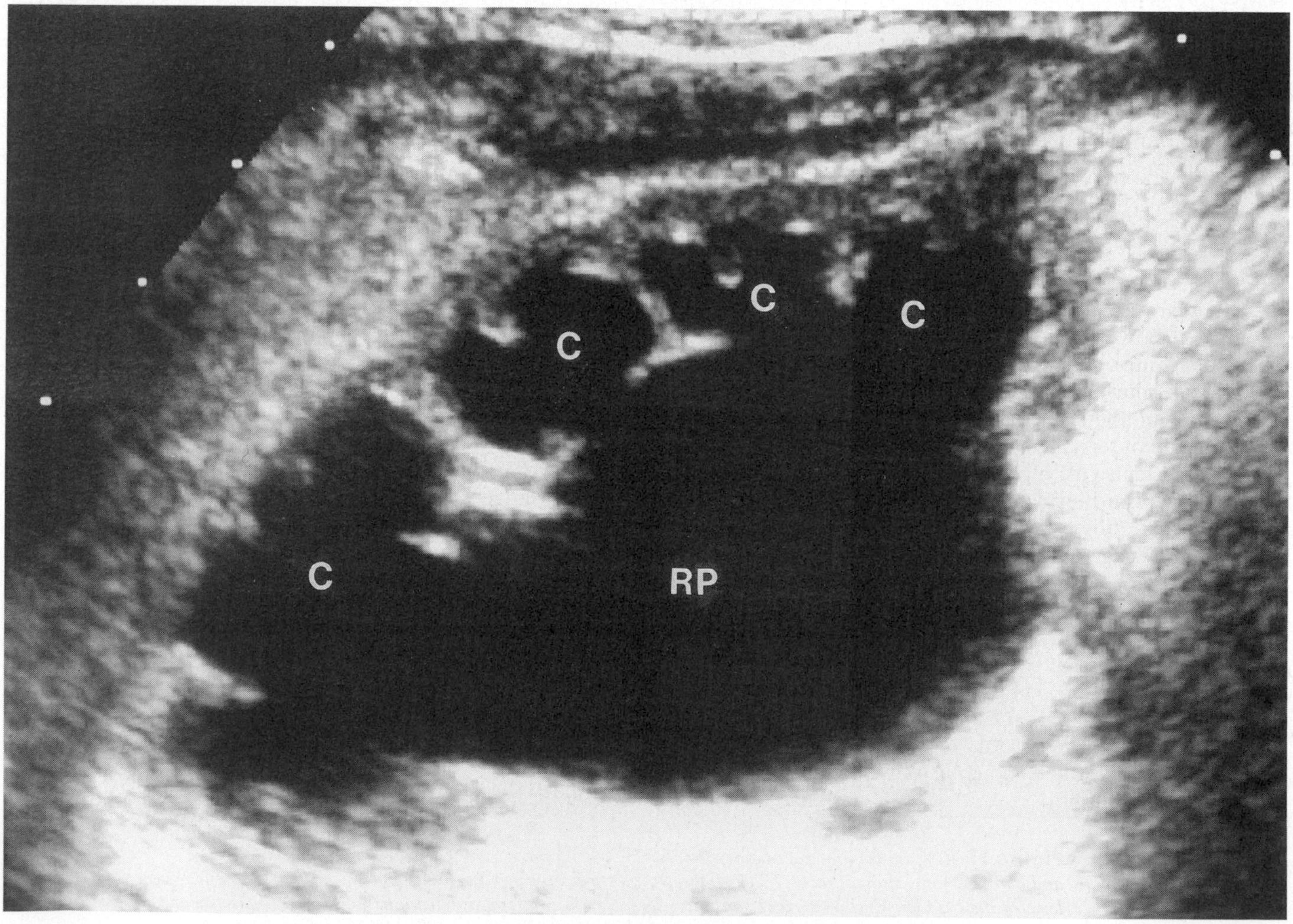

Figure 35-3. ■ *Ureteropelvic junction obstruction in a neonate. Longitudinal sonogram of the right kidney shows dilated calyces* (C) *connecting to a large renal pelvis* (RP). *A thin rim of parenchyma surrounds the dilated calyces. A distal ureter was not identified.*

system are the common causes of distal obstruction (Fig. 35-4). In patients with ureterovesical junction obstruction, the ureter is obstructed at the site where it inserts into the bladder. The ureter above the obstruction dilates to a varying degree (Fig. 35-4A,B). Reflux of urine from the bladder into the ureter may mimic an obstructed ureter. Reflux is difficult to diagnose by sonography, but the diagnosis should be suspected if there is intermittent hydronephrosis or ureteral dilatation.

In patients with ureteral ectopia or ureteroceles associated with a duplicated collecting system, the ureter draining the upper pole system is the one that is obstructed. It inserts ectopically either into the bladder neck, forming a ureterocele, or outside of the bladder in the vagina or prostate. The result is hydronephrosis of the upper pole moiety. The ectopic ureterocele appears as a round, thin-walled fluid-filled mass in the posterior aspect of the bladder (Fig. 35-4C,D). The lower pole ureter of a duplicated system inserts into its normal position, which is in the posterior-inferior part of the bladder. It may appear normal, or it may be dilated due to reflux.

Urethral obstruction is an uncommon cause of obstruction. It occurs almost exclusively in boys and is the result

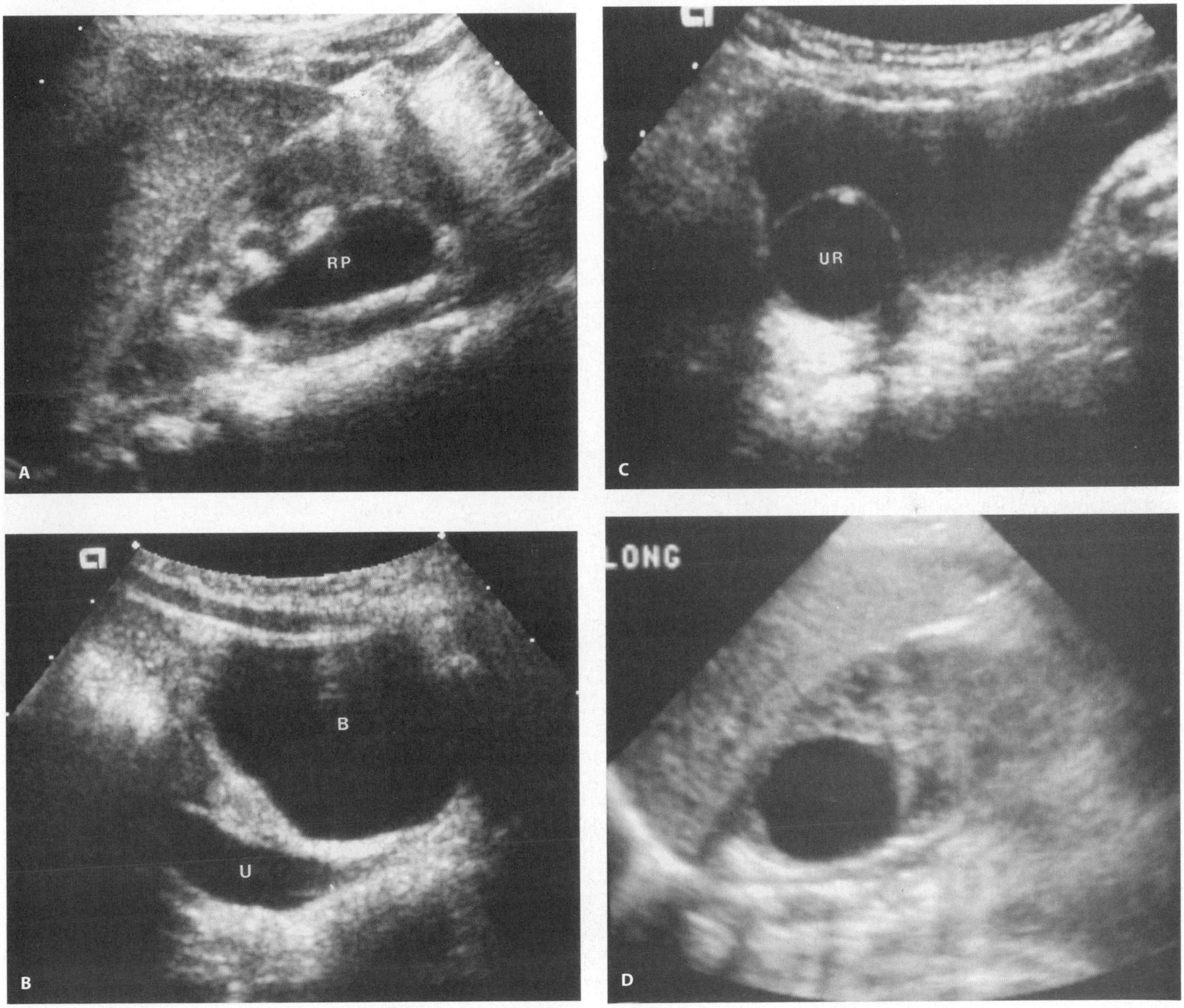

Figure 35-4. ■ *Distal ureteral obstruction. **A.** Obstruction due to stricture at junction of ureter and bladder. Longitudinal scan of right kidney shows a dilated renal pelvis* (RP). ***B.** Image at the level of the bladder* (B) *shows a dilated distal ureter* (U). ***C.** Ureteral duplication. Transverse sonogram of another patient at the level of the urinary bladder shows a urine-filled ureterocele* (UR). ***D.** A scan through the right kidney shows a dilated upper pole collecting system.*

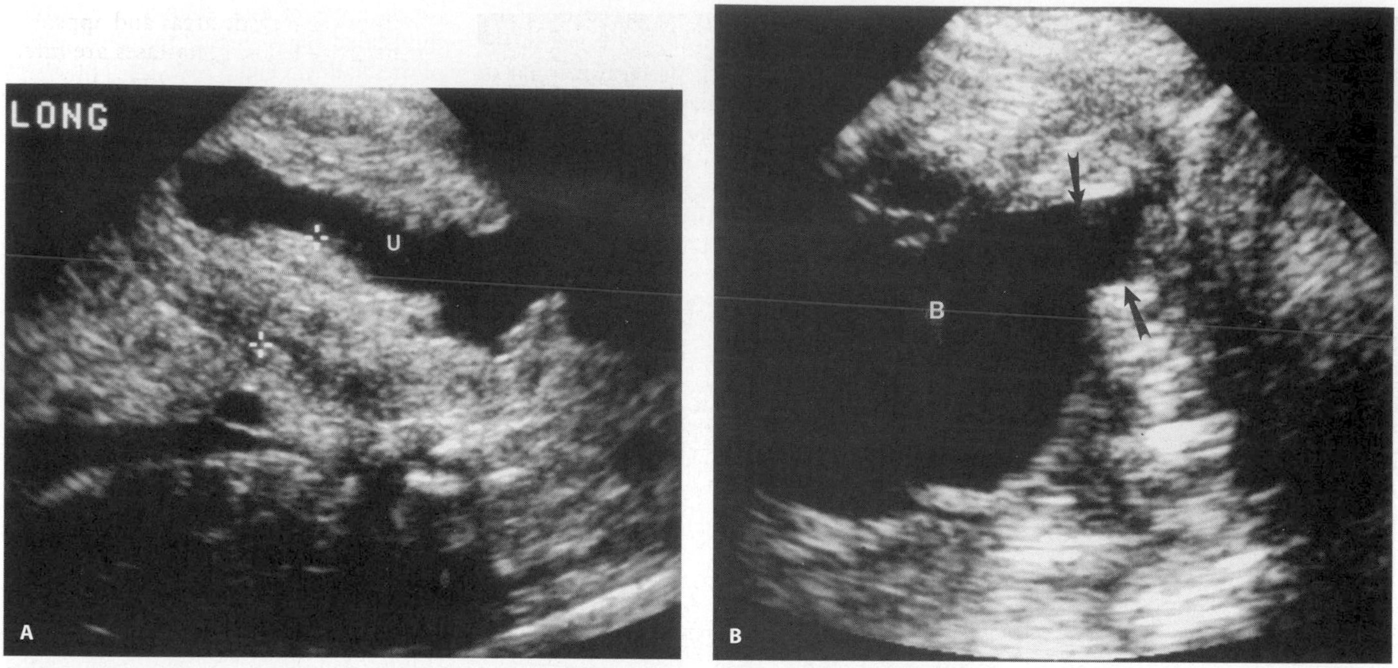

Figure 35-5. ■ *Posterior urethral valves. A. Longitudinal view of the pelvis shows a markedly thickened bladder wall (calipers), measuring 12 mm. The normal wall thickness of a distended bladder should not exceed 3 mm. Normal thickness of a partially distended bladder should not exceed 6 mm.* U, *urine within the compressed bladder lumen. B. Longitudinal view in another patient shows a urine-filled bladder and a dilated posterior urethra* (arrows).

of an obstructing valve in the posterior urethra. The resultant hydronephrosis and hydroureter are usually bilateral. The bladder wall is thick, and the posterior urethra is dilated (Fig. 35-5). The dilated posterior urethra is sometimes seen better on longitudinal scanning directly over the perineum. Severe obstruction is associated with urine ascites and subcapsular or perinephric urinomas.

Multicystic dysplastic kidney. Multicystic dysplastic kidney is the second common cause of a renal mass. It is usually unilateral. Bilateral multicystic dysplastic kidney is incompatible with survival past the newborn period. The classic features of multicystic dysplastic kidney are multiple noncommunicating cysts of varying size, which have a random distribution. No renal pelvis or renal parenchyma is identified (Fig. 35-6). Doppler waveforms are either absent and show a low systolic peak frequency and absent diastolic flow. The multicystic dysplastic kidney is large at birth but then progressively decreases in size or disappears, usually within the first year of life.

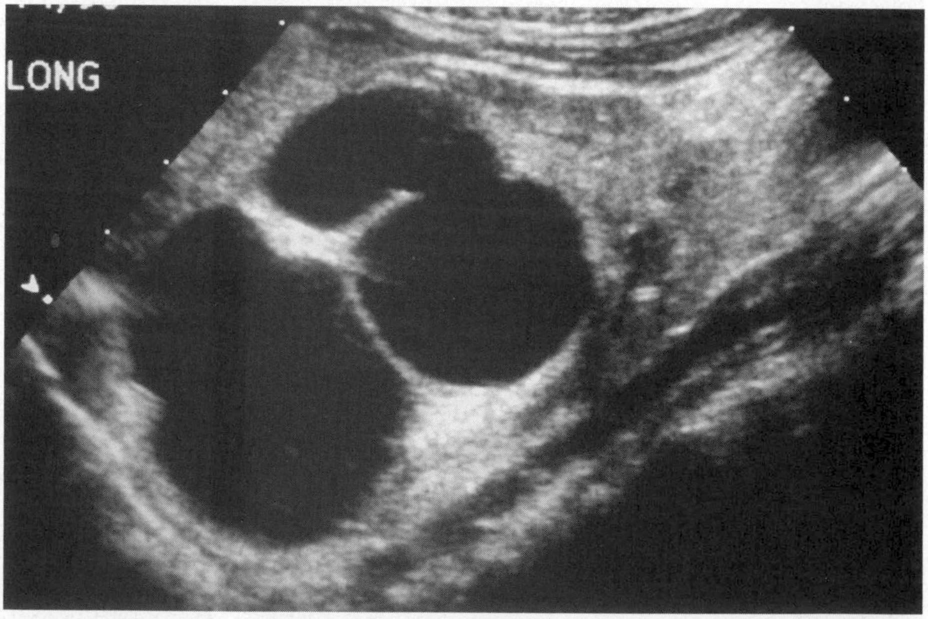

Figure 35-6. ■ *Multicystic dysplastic kidney. Longitudinal scan of the right kidney reveals multiple noncommunicating cysts of varying sizes. There is no communication between the cysts and no recognizable central renal pelvis. These findings help to differentiate the dysplastic kidney from hydronephrosis. In this case, the cysts completely involuted on a follow-up examination 1 year later.*

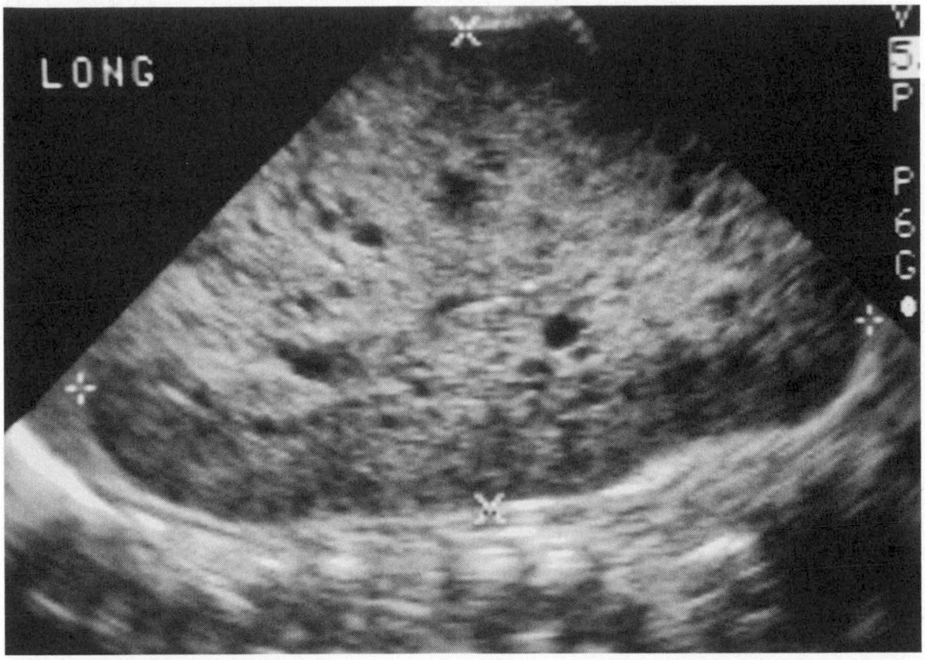

Figure 35-7. ■ *Autosomal recessive polycystic disease in a 3-month-old boy. Longitudinal scan shows an enlarged, diffusely hyperechoic right kidney (calibers). The left kidney had a similar appearance.*

Polycystic diseases. Autosomal recessive polycystic disease usually presents in the newborn. It has a spectrum of clinical findings ranging from poor renal function in the neonate to complications of hepatic fibrosis (i.e., portal hypertension and esophageal varices) in adolescents. The kidneys are markedly enlarged bilaterally and hyperechoic (Fig. 35-7). Tiny cysts may be seen in the renal parenchyma.

Autosomal dominant polycystic disease generally occurs in adults, but it can be seen in neonates and children. In the neonate, the kidneys are enlarged and echogenic. The appearance is similar to that seen in autosomal recessive polycystic disease and correlation with family history or biopsy is needed for diagnosis. Multiple discrete cysts become apparent in older children and adolescents.

Solid abdominal masses.

Mesoblastic nephroma. Mesoblastic nephroma, also known as *fetal renal hamartoma*, is a benign tumor of infancy. It replaces most or all of the kidney. The tumor is large, predominantly solid, and homogeneously echogenic. Occasional tumors have cystic areas and appear heterogeneous. Metastases are rare.

Nephroblastomatosis. This lesion is usually found in the cortex or along the columns of Bertin. It may diffusely replace the parenchyma or may appear as focal or multifocal masses. Diffuse disease presents as a peripheral rind of hypoechoic tissue (Fig. 35-8). Focal or multinodular disease presents as hypoechoic masses.

Renal vein thrombosis. Acute renal vein thrombosis produces renal enlargement and hypoechoic parenchyma, secondary to edema and hemorrhage. If there is prompt and adequate collateral vessel formation, the kidney returns to normal. If collateral formation is insufficient, the kidney atrophies and becomes hyperechoic. At any stage, thrombus may be identified in the renal vein or IVC. Color Doppler imaging may show either total absence of flow or flow around the clot. Doppler imaging of the intrarenal arteries may show absent or reversed diastolic flow.

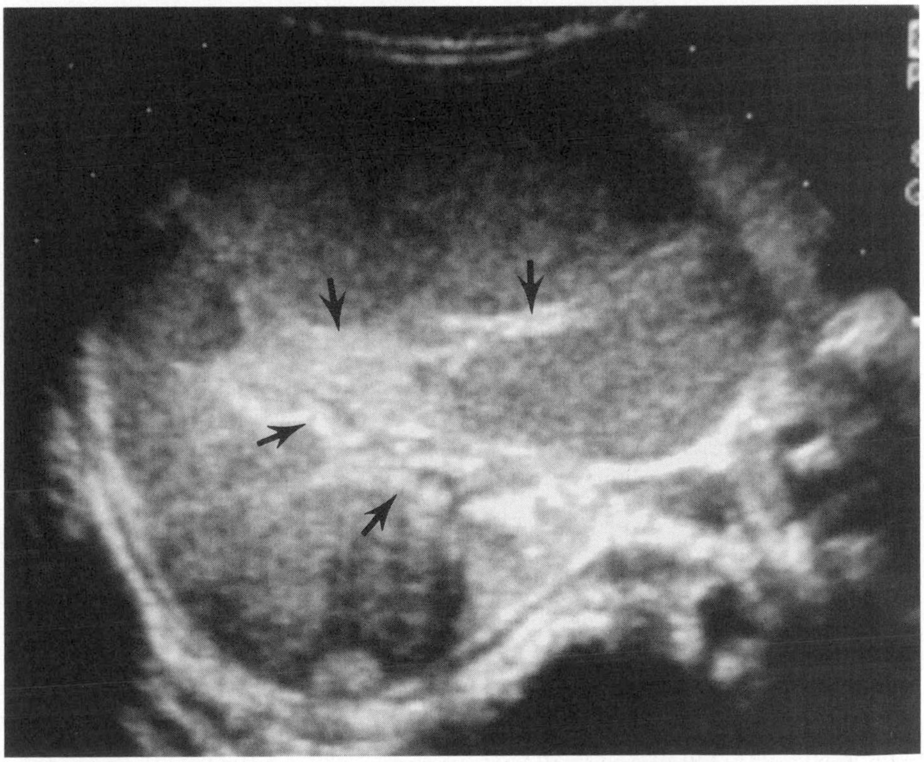

Figure 35-8. ■ *Diffuse nephroblastomatosis in a 13-month-old girl. Longitudinal scan shows an enlarged kidney with a hypoechoic rim of tumor displacing and distorting the renal sinus* (arrows).

Older Children and Adolescents

Malignant tumors.

Wilms tumor. Wilms tumor is the common malignant tumor of childhood. Mean patient age at diagnosis is 3 years. Typical sonographic findings are a large, echogenic mass with a homogeneous or heterogeneous matrix and a sharp interface between the tumor and normal parenchyma (Fig. 35-9). Calcification is present in about 10% of tumors. Mildly increased vascularity may be noted on color Doppler sonography. Tumor may spread outside of the kidney to renal vein or IVC, lymph nodes, or liver. Wilms tumor is bilateral in about 10% of cases.

Rare renal tumors. Renal cell cancer, clear cell sarcoma, and malignant rhabdoid tumor account for less than 10% of pediatric renal tumors. Mean age of patients with renal cell cancer is approximately 9 years. Malignant rhabdoid tumor affects young infants under 2 years of age, whereas clear cell sarcoma affects children between 3 and 5 years of age. The sonographic appearance of these tumors is usually similar to that of Wilms tumor, although a subcapsular or perinephric fluid collection may be noted in rhabdoid tumor. Definitive diagnosis requires tissue sampling.

Lymphoma. Renal involvement by lymphoma is more common with non-Hodgkin's lymphoma than with Hodgkin's disease. It usually appears as multiple bilateral, hypoechoic masses. The tumor is typically homogeneous. Less frequent patterns include direct renal invasion from contiguous retroperitoneal lymphoma, solitary renal mass, and diffuse infiltration.

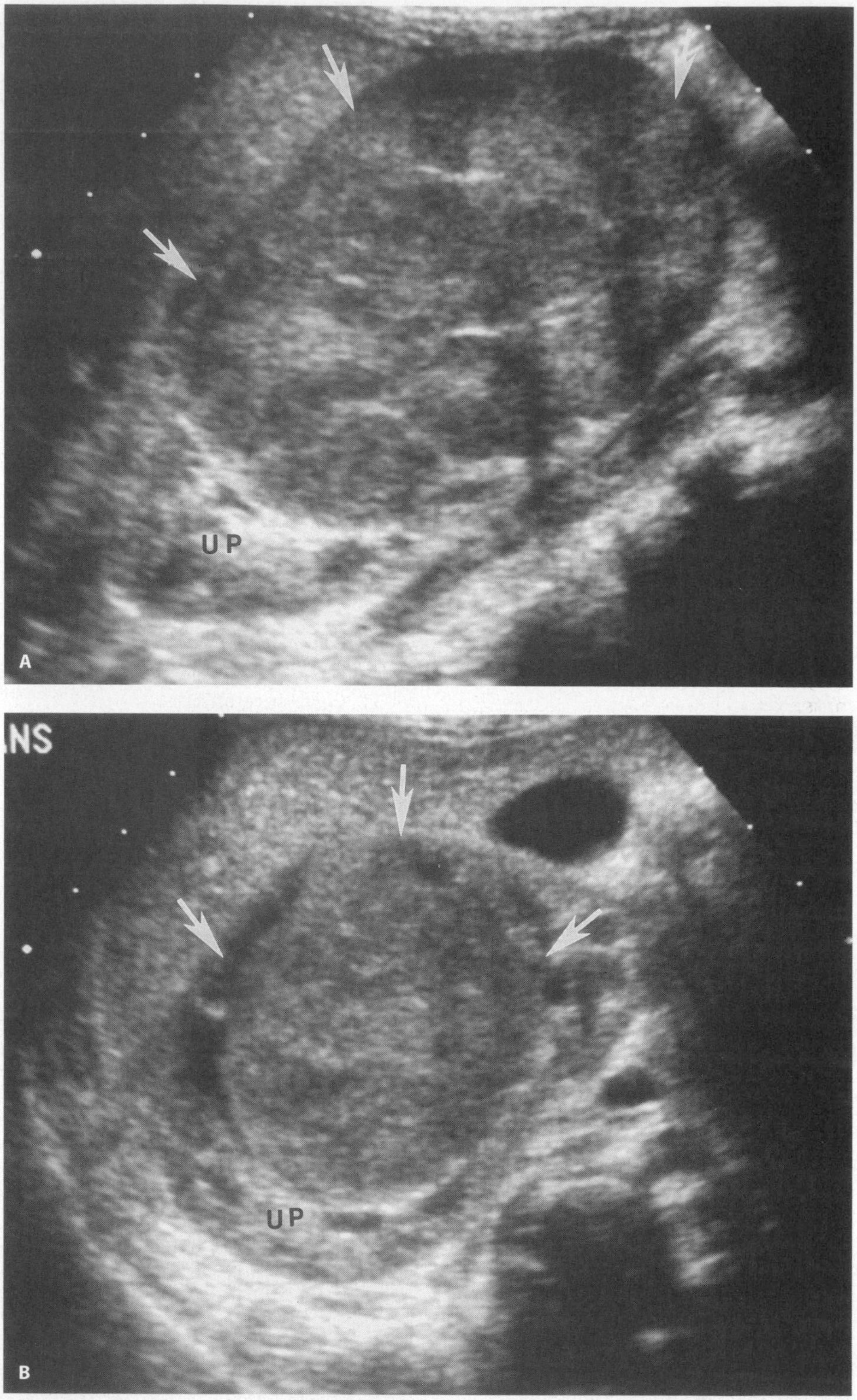

Figure 35-9. ■ *Wilms tumor. (A) Longitudinal and (B) transverse views of the right kidney show a large, slightly heterogeneous mass* (arrows) *arising from the lower pole. UP represents the normal upper pole parenchyma, which is compressed by tumor. There is a well-defined interface between the tumor and adjacent normal parenchyma.*

Benign renal masses.

Multilocular cystic nephroma. Multilocular cystic nephroma is an uncommon benign tumor. The typical sonographic appearance is that of a multicystic mass with anechoic or hypoechoic cysts separated by echogenic septa and surrounded by thick walls (Fig. 35-10). The cystic nature of this benign lesion helps to differentiate it from Wilms tumor. The characteristic multicystic appearance may not be seen, however, if the cysts are too small to be resolved or if they contain mucoid material.

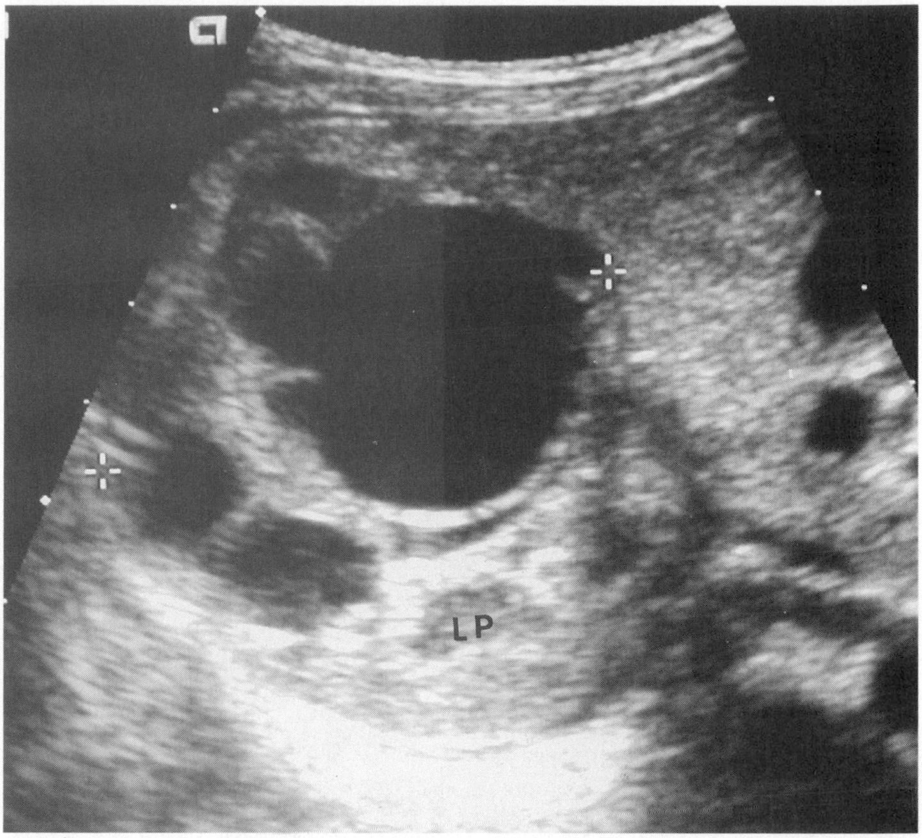

Figure 35-10. ■ *Multilocular cystic nephroma. Transverse scan of the right kidney (calipers) shows several cysts of varying sizes separated by echogenic septa. The lesion arose from the mid-pole of the kidney. Normal parenchyma of the lower pole* (LP) *is seen beneath the lesion.*

NONRENAL RETROPERITONEAL MASSES

Neonates

Adrenal hemorrhage. Adrenal hemorrhage is a common mass in neonates. The typical appearance of adrenal hemorrhage is a round or triangular suprarenal mass, replacing the entire gland. The echogenicity varies with the age of the blood. Acute hemorrhage is isoechoic or hyperechoic to the adjacent kidney. As the blood lyses, it becomes hypoechoic and eventually develops a cystic appearance (Fig. 35-11). Eventually, the adrenal gland may calcify.

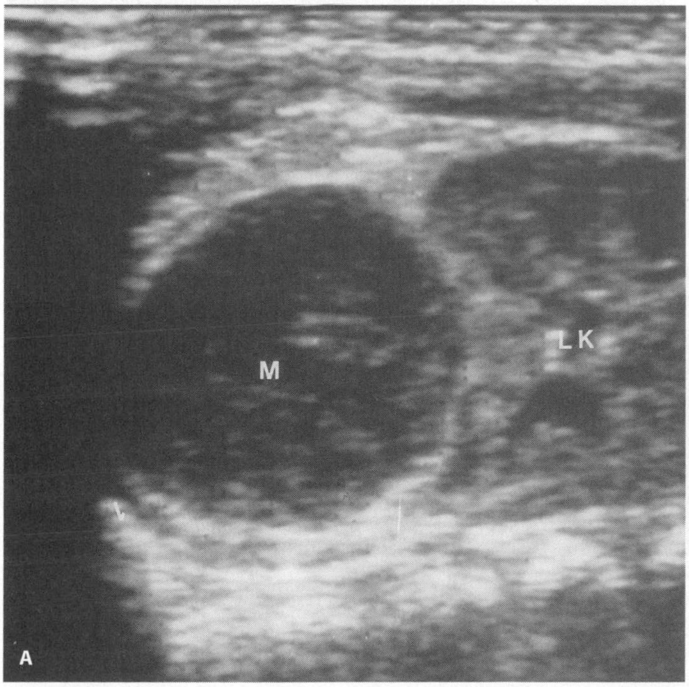

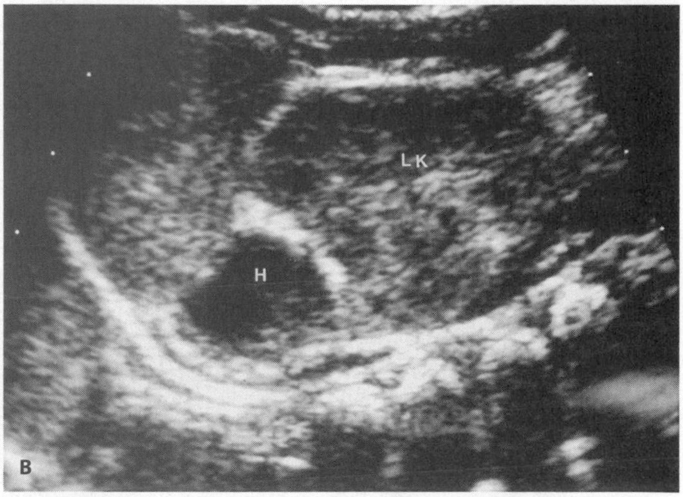

Figure 35-11. ■ *A. Adrenal hemorrhage in 2-day-old infant girl. Longitudinal scan through the left flank reveals a round mass* (M) *superior to the upper pole of the left kidney. The mass is isoechoic to kidney. B. Two weeks later, the hematoma* (H) *is hypoechoic and smaller in size.* LK, *left kidney.*

The primary diagnostic dilemma is the rare case of congenital neuroblastoma. In the neonate, neuroblastoma is a complex or predominantly cystic mass. The tumor is usually small and does not cross the midline. Neuroblastoma can be differentiated from adrenal hemorrhage if there is evidence of metastatic disease. Metastases are to the liver, skin, and bone marrow. In the absence of metastases, these two tumors can be differentiated by serial sonography. Adrenal hemorrhage decreases in size within several weeks, whereas neuroblastoma is unlikely to show an interval change in size.

Older Children

Neuroblastoma. Neuroblastoma is the most common extrarenal mass in infants and children. It is usually heterogeneous and contains hyperechoic areas related to calcification and hypoechoic areas secondary to necrosis or hemorrhage. Calcification occurs in about 85% of tumors. As noted previously, the tumor can be predominantly cystic in neonates. Tumor margins may be smooth or irregular (Fig. 35-12). Patterns of intra-abdominal extension of tumor include extension across the midline, spread to regional lymph nodes, encasement of adjacent vessels, intraspinal extension, and hepatic metastases.

Adrenal cortical neoplasms. Adrenal carcinoma and adenoma account for <5% of adrenal tumors in children. The sonographic appearance is similar to that of neuroblastoma. These tumors typically affect older children and adolescents.

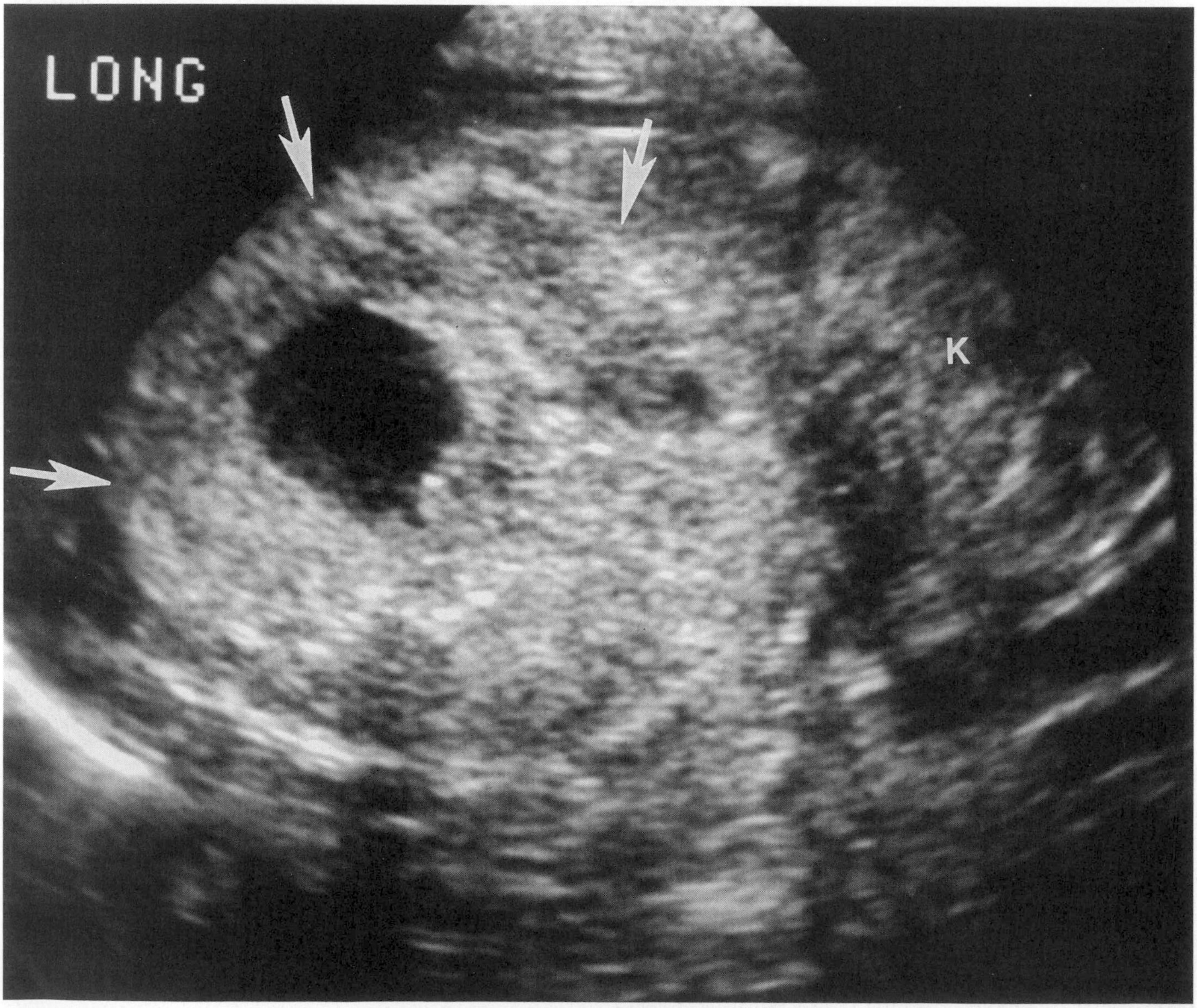

Figure 35-12. ■ *Neuroblastoma. Longitudinal sonogram through the left flank shows a large, well-circumscribed, predominantly echogenic mass* (arrows). *The hypoechoic area represents a focus of necrosis.* K, *kidney.*

HEPATIC MASSES

Neonates

Benign tumors.

Hemangioendothelioma. Hemangioendothelioma is the most common benign lesion of the liver. Histologically, it represents dilated vascular channels. This lesion may be a solitary lesion or multifocal. It is typically hypoechoic relative to normal liver, but on occasion, it may appear hyperechoic. The matrix may be homogeneous, or it may be heterogeneous related to the presence of calcification, areas of thrombus, or area of calcification (Fig. 35-13). Color Doppler imaging usually shows internal flow. Pulsed Doppler imaging may show high-frequency peak systolic frequency shifts and minimal systolic-diastolic flow variation.

Mesenchymal hamartoma. Mesenchymal hamartoma is the next most common benign tumor of the liver in neonates after hemangioendothelioma. It appears as a multicystic mass containing anechoic spaces separated by echogenic septa. If the cystic areas are small, the mass may appear relatively solid.

Malignant tumors. Although congenital hepatoblastoma has been documented in this age group, malignant hepatic tumors are rare in neonates.

Older Children

Malignant hepatic tumors.

Hepatoblastoma. Hepatoblastoma is the most common malignant tumor of childhood. This tumor may occur as a solitary mass, as a dominant mass with smaller surrounding lesions, or as multiple nodules. Tumor margins may be well defined or poorly defined. In the latter cases, secondary signs, such as

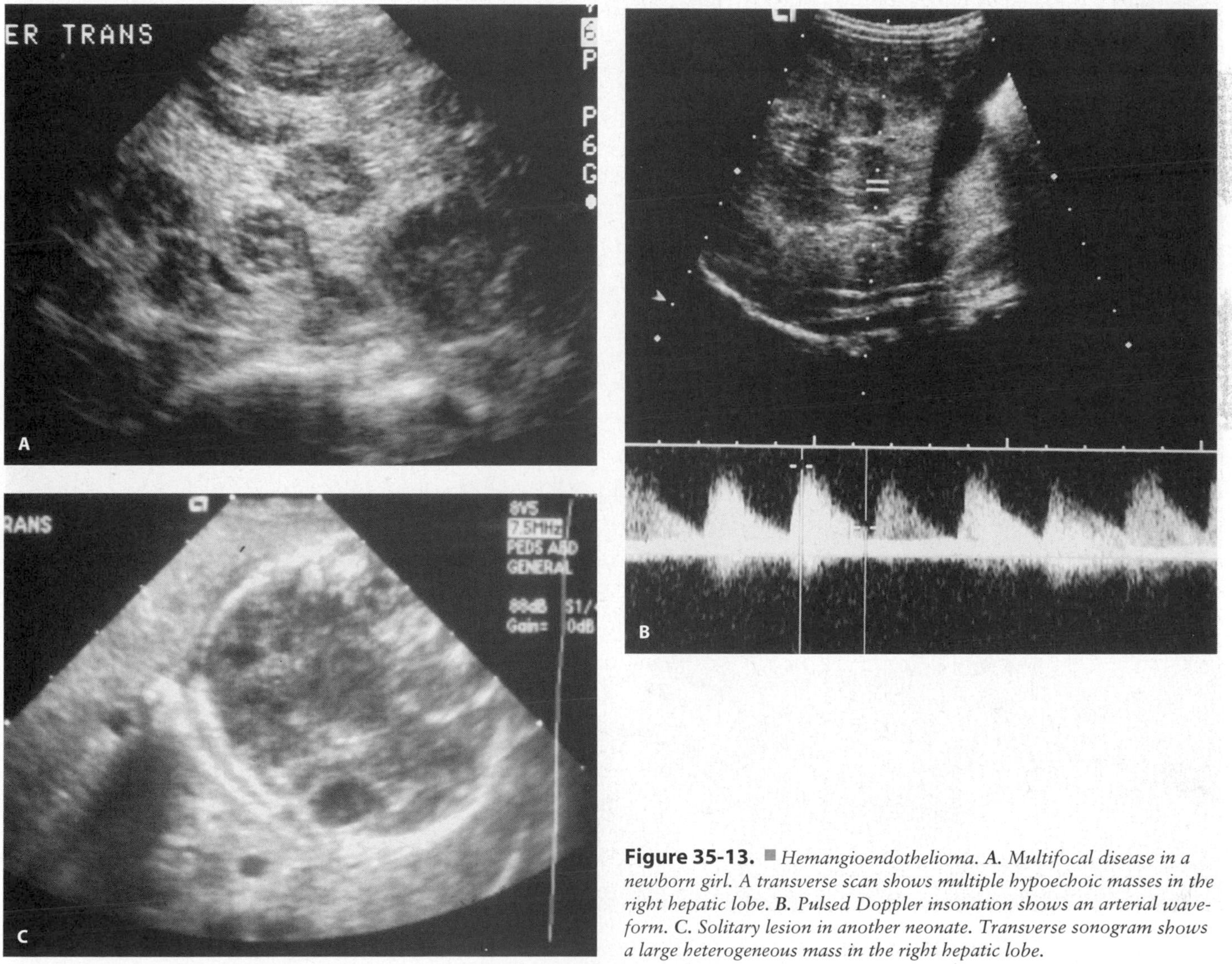

Figure 35-13. ■ *Hemangioendothelioma. A. Multifocal disease in a newborn girl. A transverse scan shows multiple hypoechoic masses in the right hepatic lobe. B. Pulsed Doppler insonation shows an arterial waveform. C. Solitary lesion in another neonate. Transverse sonogram shows a large heterogeneous mass in the right hepatic lobe.*

vessel displacement or amputation or tumor in the hepatic or portal veins can help suggest the diagnosis. Most tumors are echogenic compared with surrounding normal parenchyma. Calcifications may be present within the tumor matrix (Fig. 35-14). Most tumors are hypervascular on color flow imaging. Tumor invasion of portal or hepatic veins occurs in about 25% of cases. Tumor thrombus appears as an echogenic mass in a dilated vein. Enlarged nodes may be seen in the porta hepatis.

Hepatocellular carcinoma. The sonographic appearance is similar to that of hepatoblastoma. This tumor typically affects older children and adolescents. A definitive diagnosis requires biopsy.

Benign hepatic tumors. Cavernous hemangioma and focal nodular hyperplasia are rare benign hepatic tumors of older children and adolescents. Most hemangiomas are small, homogeneous, and hyperechoic. Focal nodular hyperplasia is a homogeneous mass that is isoechoic or hypoechoic to normal liver tissue. Doppler imaging may show a central echogenic and hypervascular scar.

BILIARY MASSES

Choledochal cysts. A choledochal cyst is a congenital anomaly of the bile ducts characterized by dilatation of the intra- or extrahepatic biliary system. The most common appearance is that of a well-defined, fluid-filled mass in the porta hepatis (Fig. 35-15). In this form, the right and left main hepatic ducts may be dilated, but the intrahepatic ducts are normal. Less common appearances include a diverticu-

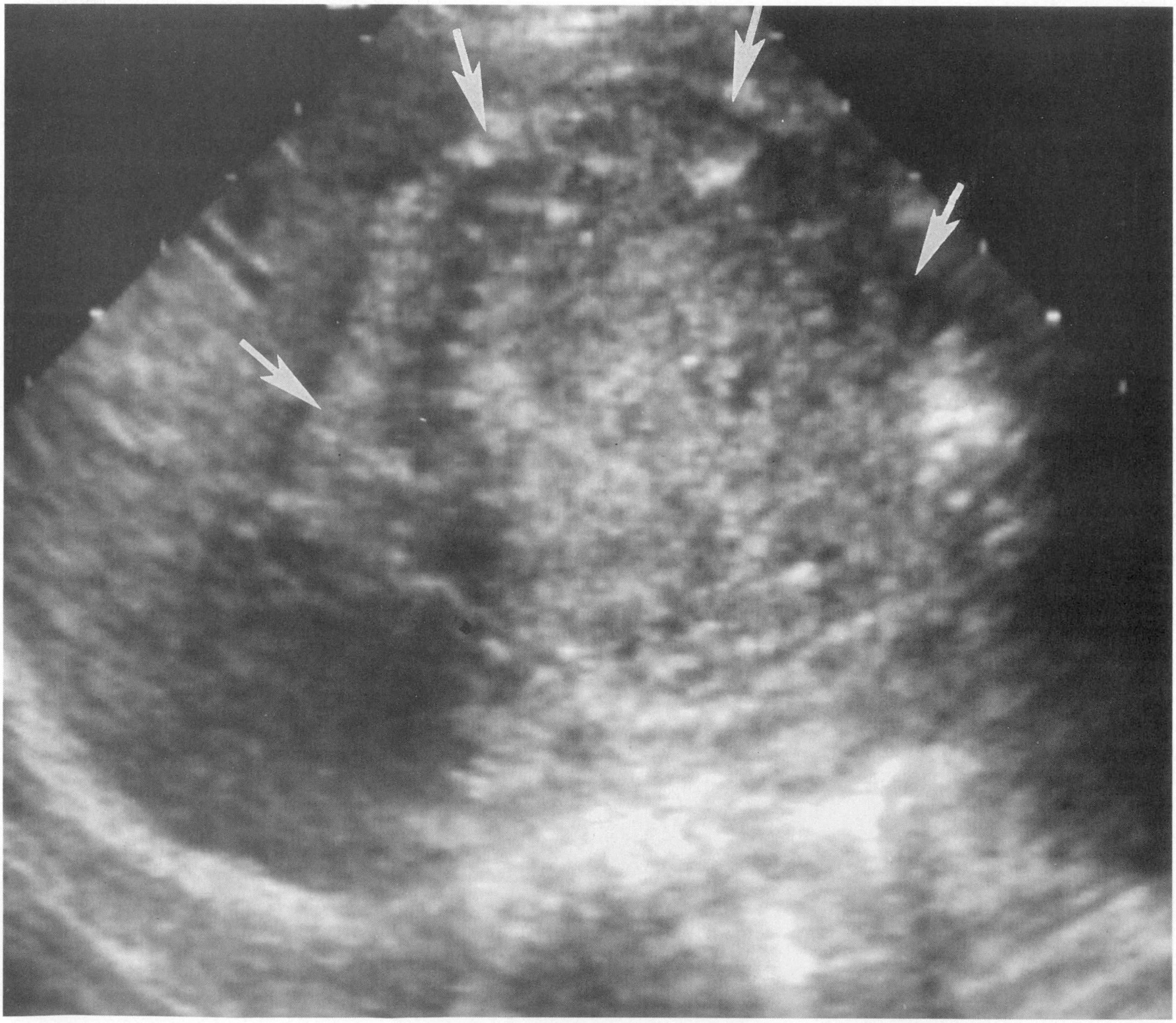

Figure 35-14. ■ *Hepatoblastoma in a 1-year-old boy. Transverse scan shows a heterogeneous mass* (arrows) *that is slightly hyperechoic to normal parenchyma. Focal areas of echogenicity within the tumor represent calcification.*

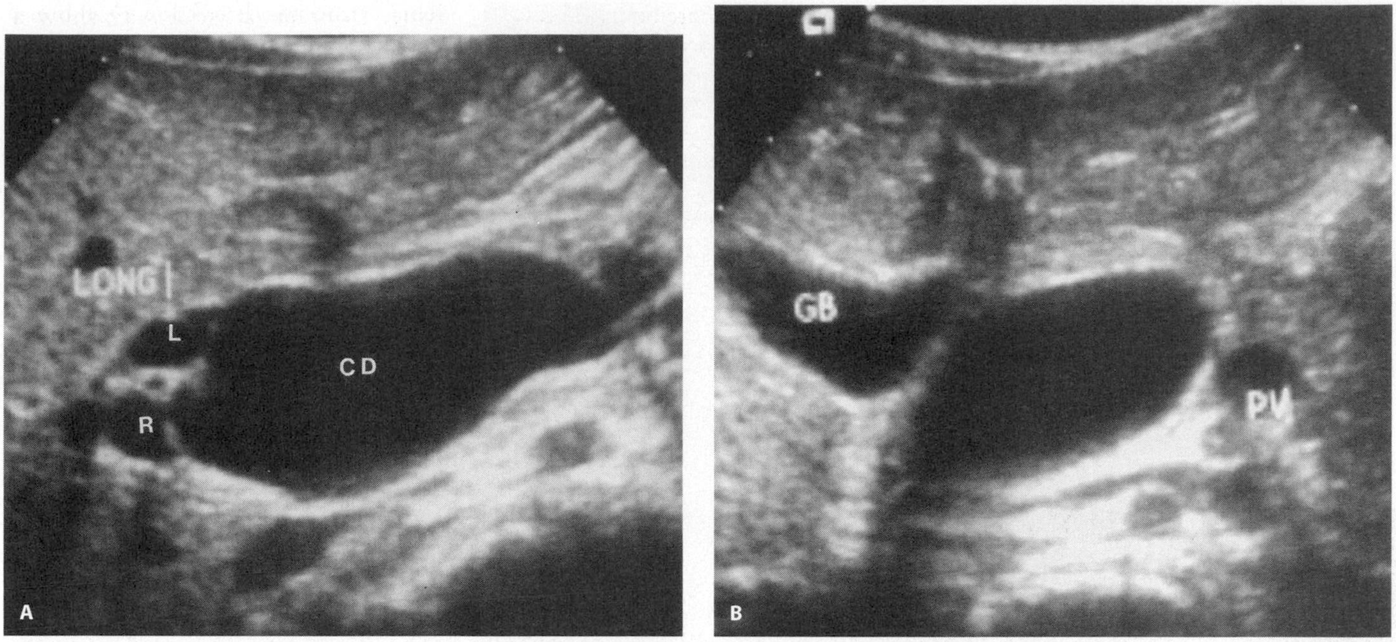

Figure 35-15. ■ *Choledochal cyst. A. Longitudinal sonogram shows dilated right* (R) *and left* (L) *hepatic ducts and a cystic mass in the porta hepatis, representing a dilated common bile duct* (CD). *B. Transverse view through the porta hepatis shows that the dilated common bile duct is separate from the gallbladder* (GB). PV, *portal vein.*

lum of the common bile duct, dilatation of the duodenal portion of the distal common bile duct, cystic dilatations of both intra- and extrahepatic ducts, and dilatation of the intrahepatic ducts.

GASTROINTESTINAL MASSES

Neonates

Enteric duplication cysts. The most common location for a duplication cyst is in the distal ileum near the ileocecal valve. Sonography usually shows an anechoic cyst with increased through transmission. An occasional cyst may contain internal echoes, representing blood or debris. The wall is smooth, and it may have a multilayered appearance similar to normal bowel. Most duplication cysts are unilocular.

Older Children

Lymphoma. Most cases of lymphoma involving the bowel in children are non-Hodgkin lymphoma, and the distal ileum is the common site of involvement. Bowel lymphoma produces circumferential hypoechoic bowel thickening (Fig. 35-16). The wall thickness exceeds 1 cm. Enlarged retroperitoneal and mesenteric lymph nodes are common.

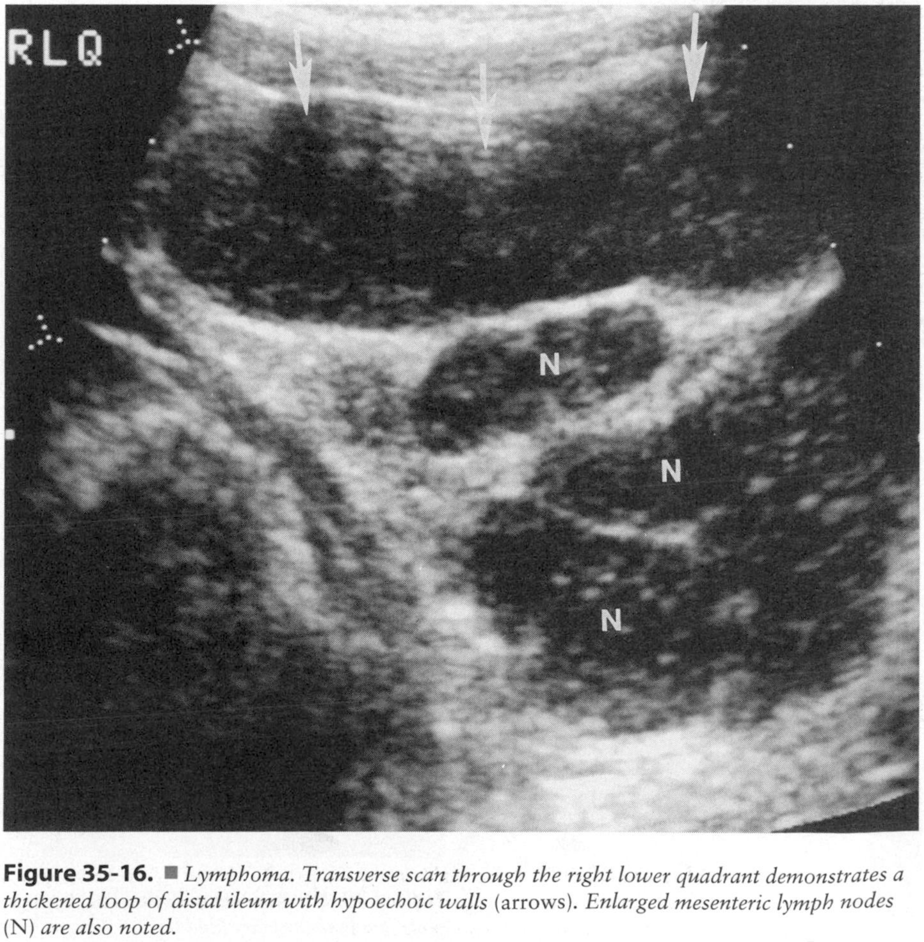

Figure 35-16. ■ *Lymphoma. Transverse scan through the right lower quadrant demonstrates a thickened loop of distal ileum with hypoechoic walls* (arrows). *Enlarged mesenteric lymph nodes* (N) *are also noted.*

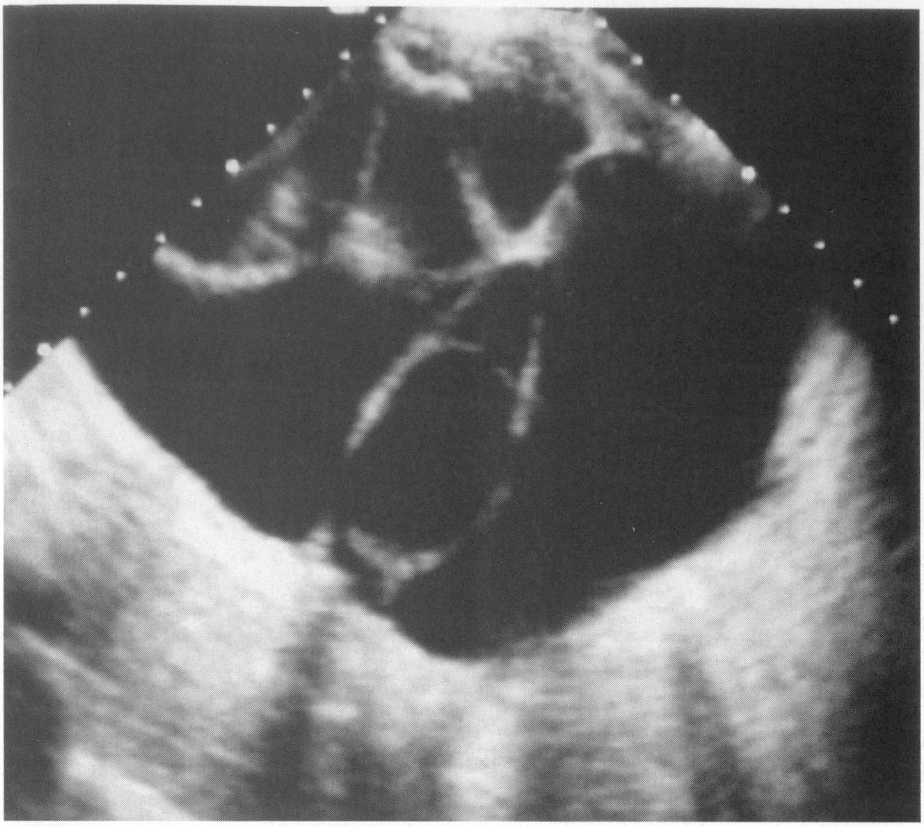

Figure 35-17. ■ *Mesenteric cyst. Longitudinal scan of the left upper quadrant shows a septated cystic mass.*

debris from the breakdown of blood products. A markedly dilated vagina can obstruct the distal ureters causing hydronephrosis. The uterine cavity may or may not be dilated (hematometra, blood in the uterine cavity).

The classic appearance of an ovarian cyst is a thin-walled mass with increased through transmission. The contents may be echo-free or they may contain low-level echoes, reflecting the presence of blood. A fluid–debris level and septations are common. Large ovarian cysts can extend into the upper abdomen and can be mistaken for a mesenteric or omental cyst.

Older Children

Ovarian and uterine masses. Cystic teratoma is the most common ovarian tumor in children and adolescents. The characteristic appearance of a benign teratoma is a predominantly cystic mass containing a highly echogenic nodular

Mesenteric/omental cyst. Mesenteric and omental cysts are usually large, thin-walled masses with internal septations (Fig. 35-17). The internal contents are usually anechoic, but they may contain internal echoes or fluid-fluid levels related to infection or hemorrhage. Mesenteric cysts occur between bowel loops. Omental cysts are usually located near the anterior abdominal wall, anterior to bowel.

PELVIC MASSES

Neonates

Ovarian and uterine masses. An obstructed, dilated vagina and ovarian cyst are the causes of most pelvic masses in girls. The obstructed vagina is usually distended by blood (referred to as *hematocolpos*). It typically appears as a tubular, echogenic midline mass between the bladder and rectum (Fig. 35-18). The echogenic contents represent cellular

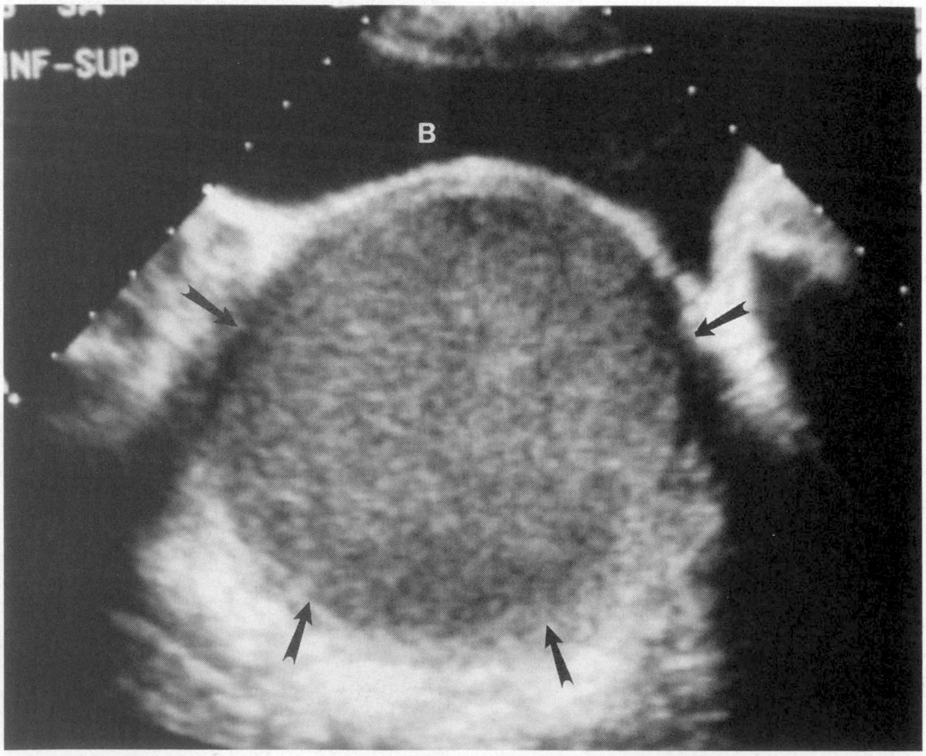

Figure 35-18. ■ *Hematocolpos. Transverse sonogram shows a markedly dilated vagina* (arrows) *posterior to the urinary bladder* (B). *The echogenic contents represent blood products.*

focus (termed a *dermoid plug*) (Fig. 35-19). The nodule may produce acoustic shadowing because it contains fat, hair, bone, or teeth. Typically, benign teratomas have thin, smooth walls. On rare occasions, benign teratomas present as purely anechoic masses. By comparison, malignant teratomas tend to have a predominance of solid components (>50%) (Fig. 35-20). Other findings of malignancy include irregular thick walls, septations and papillary projections, ascites, peritoneal implants (i.e., nodules on the peritoneal surfaces), pelvic and retroperitoneal adenopathy, and hepatic metastases.

Hematometrocolpos can present in adolescent girls after the start of menarche. The appearance is similar to that described in the neonate.

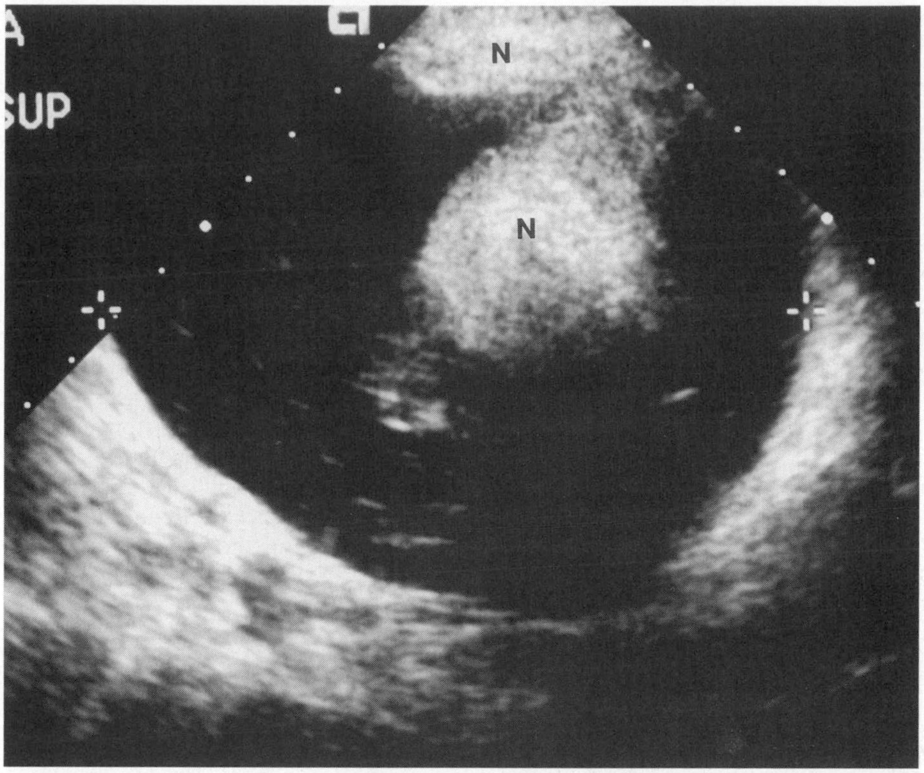

Figure 35-19. ■ *Benign cystic ovarian teratoma in a 13-year-old girl. Transverse sonogram of the right adnexa shows a predominantly cystic mass with peripheral echogenic nodules* (N).

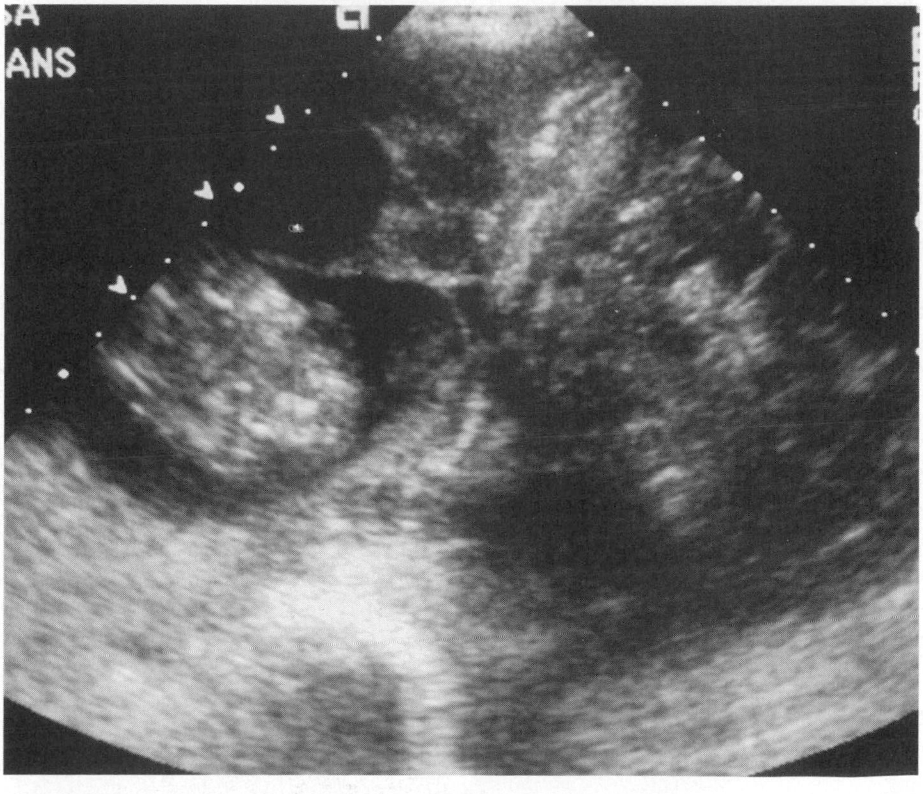

Figure 35-20. ■ *Malignant ovarian teratoma. Transverse sonogram through the lower abdomen of a 9-year-old girl shows a poorly defined, predominantly solid mass. Hypoechoic areas represent necrosis.*

Rhabdomyosarcoma. Rhabdomyosarcoma is the most common malignant tumor of the vagina, uterus, bladder, and prostate. It may appear as a discrete soft-tissue mass, or it may diffusely infiltrate the organ of origin (Fig. 35-21). Cystic areas are common. Hydronephrosis and extension into surrounding soft tissues may also be noted. Metastases are to the liver, lymph nodes, lung, and bone.

Sacrococcygeal teratoma. The sacrococcygeal teratoma arises in the presacral region and often extends into the soft tissues of the buttocks. The appearance is similar to that of the ovarian teratoma. The differential diagnosis of a cystic presacral mass includes anterior meningocele and rectal duplication.

Sonographic Findings of Symptomatic Abdominal Masses

PYLORIC STENOSIS

Patients with pyloric stenosis present at 2 to 6 weeks of age with nonbilious vomiting, which often is projectile in nature. On the longitudinal view, the thickened pyloric muscle is visualized as a mass in direct connection with the stomach (Fig. 35-22). On the transverse view, the pyloric muscle has a bull's-eye appearance, reflecting the thickened hypoechoic muscle surrounding the central echogenic mucosa. Additional findings include minimal or absent gastric emptying, exaggerated peristaltic waves that stop abruptly at the gastric antrum (distal end of the stomach), and esophageal reflux.

Measurements are made of the wall thickness. A wall thickness of greater than 3.5 mm and a pyloric length of greater than 1.7 cm indicate pyloric stenosis. Borderline muscle thickness measurements are common in premature infants with pyloric stenosis. The diagnosis in these infants is based on the thickness of the pyloric muscle, which is increased relative to the rest of the stomach and the length of the pyloric canal.

Two important pitfalls include failure to visualize the pylorus due to gastric overdistension, which causes the

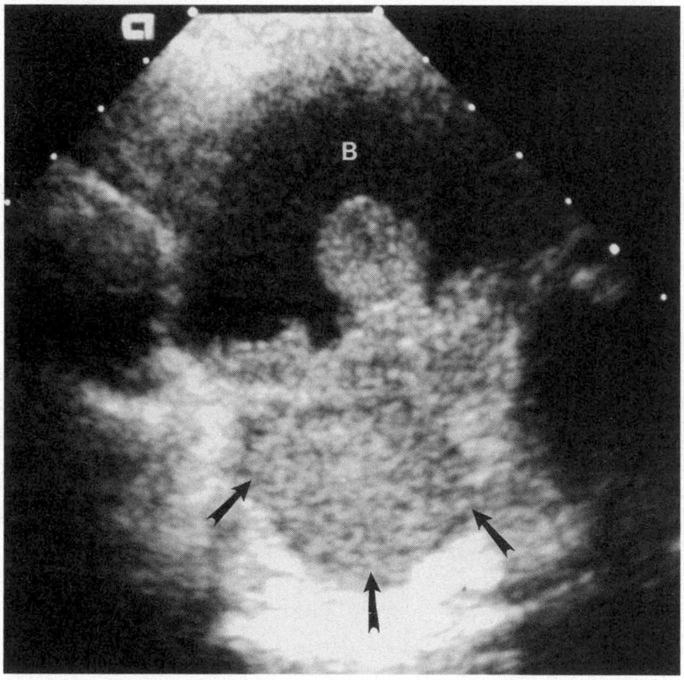

Figure 35-21. ■ *Prostate rhabdomyosarcoma in a 3-year-old boy. Transverse image shows a lobulated homogeneous mass* (arrows) *arising from the prostate and invading the bladder* (B).

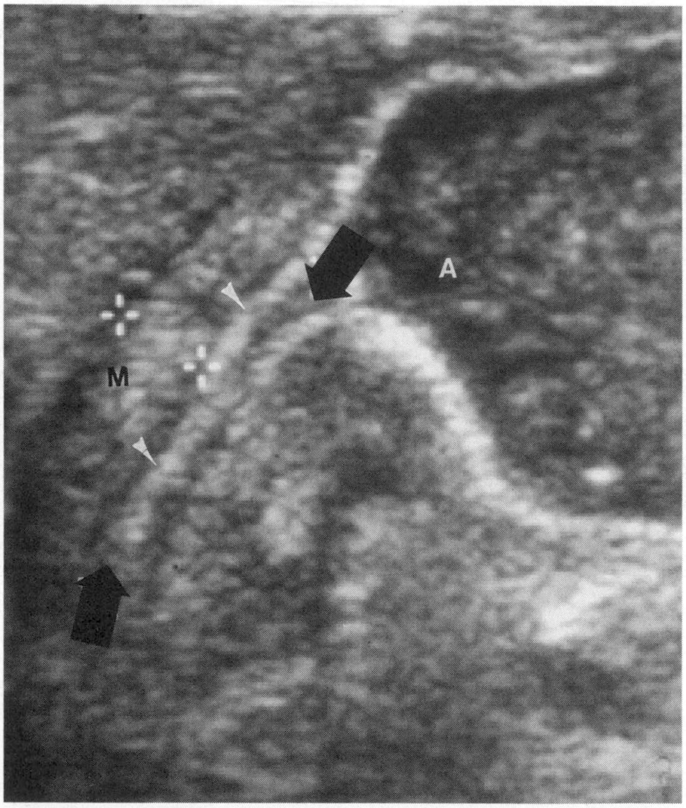

Figure 35-22. ■ *Pyloric stenosis. Long-axis sonogram with electronic calipers marking thickness of the pyloric muscle* (M) *on one side of the central echogenic mucosa* (arrowheads). Black arrows *mark the length of the pyloric canal. In this patient, the wall thickness measured 6 mm.* A, *gastric antrum.*

pylorus to be displaced posteriorly, and pseudothickening of the pyloric muscle, due to decompression of the stomach. If the antrum does not contain an adequate amount of fluid, a glucose solution or water should be given orally or through a nasogastric tube.

INTUSSUSCEPTION

Intussusception is an invagination of a segment of bowel into another segment of bowel. It affects children between 3 months and 2 years of age. In the most common form of intussusception, the distal part of the small bowel enters the cecum. The classic clinical features of intussusception are acute abdominal pain, vomiting, bloody stools, and a palpable abdominal mass. On transverse sonograms, the intussusception appears as a round, complex mass with alternating hypo- and hyperechoic layers (Fig. 35-23). On longitudinal images, the intussusception has an oval shape. The presence of blood flow in the mass suggests viable bowel, whereas the absence of blood flow suggests that gangrenous changes have occurred. Intussusception can be cured if fluid is administered rectally so that the distal small bowel is pushed out of the cecum toward the stomach. Such a procedure is often done under fluoroscopic control, but ultrasound can be used as the monitoring technique.

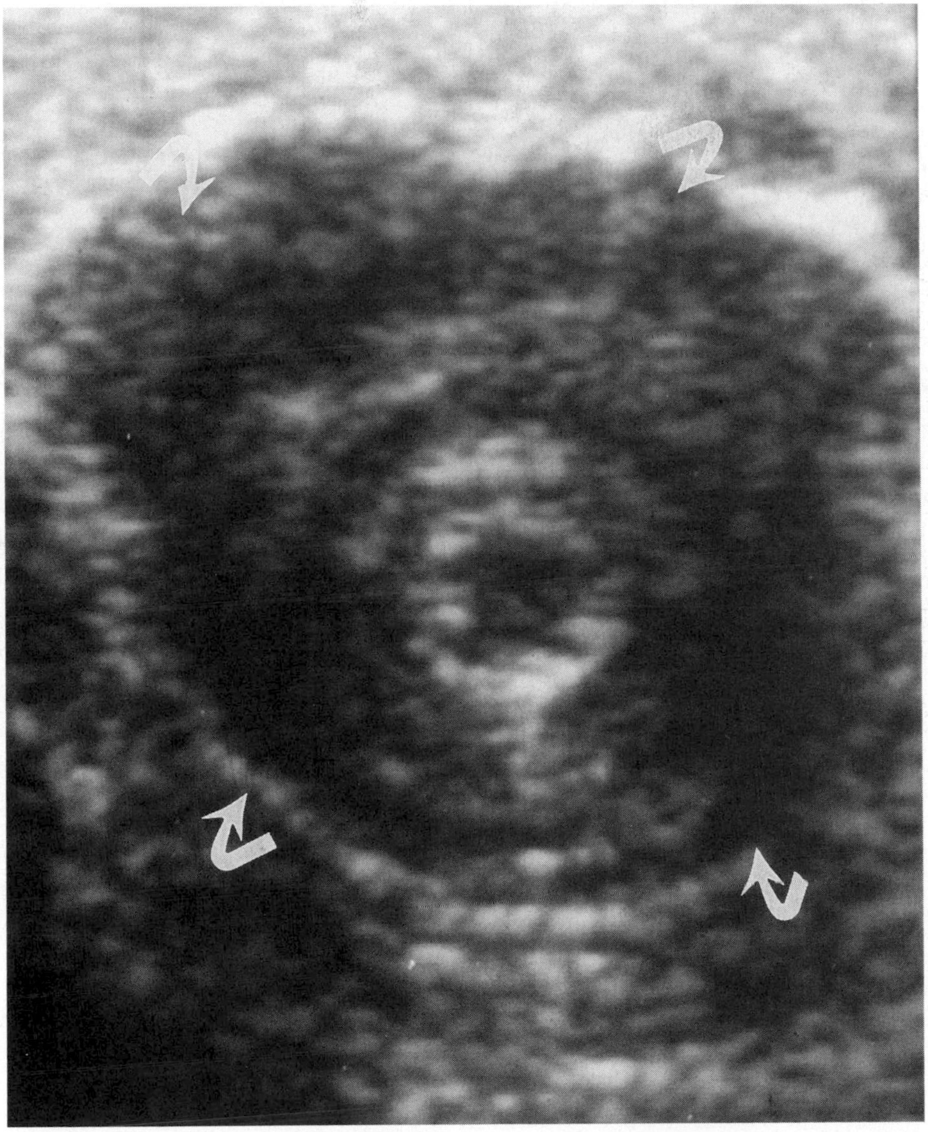

Figure 35-23. ■ *Intussusception. Transverse sonogram of the right midabdomen shows a complex mass* (curved arrows) *with multiple concentric layers of varying echogenicity.*

Diagnostic Dilemmas

1. Renal pyramids versus calyces. Renal pyramids appear hypoechoic in the neonate; do not mistake them for hydronephrosis. Pyramids do not communicate with a dilated renal pelvis, and dilated calyces do connect with the pelvis.
2. Increased renal cortical echogenicity. This is normal in the neonate; do not mistake for parenchymal disease.
3. Hydronephrosis versus multicystic dysplastic kidney. Hydronephrosis produces uniformly sized calyces and a large renal pelvis. Multicystic dysplastic kidney results in nonuniform-size cysts; there is no central renal pelvis.
4. Renal obstruction versus reflux. Both can cause dilated pelves, calyces, and ureters. Intermittent waxing or waning of the caliber of the renal collecting system or ureter should suggest reflux.
5. Adrenal hemorrhage versus tumor. Both appear as echogenic suprarenal masses. Hemorrhage will decrease in size and develop cystic areas; tumor will remain stable.
6. Solid abdominal tumors. Echogenic tumors arising in the kidney, adrenal glands, or liver are nonspecific. Correlating sonographic findings with patient age can often narrow the diagnostic possibilities. Ultimately, biopsy is required for final diagnosis.

Where Else to Look

1. If hydronephrosis is discovered, examine the pelvis to see if the cause of obstruction is visible—for example, a distal ureter or ureterocele.
2. If Wilms tumor is suspected, look for tumor in the renal vein and IVC; color flow Doppler will help. This tumor needs to be removed before the primary tumor is resected. Also

look for para-aortic area nodal enlargement, liver metastases, and tumor in the opposite kidney. These findings alter the staging.

3. If neuroblastoma is likely, look for midline spread and metastases to liver. Both of these alter staging. Also look for tumor encasement of the aorta and IVC—this may preclude immediate surgical resection.
4. If a malignant hepatic tumor is suspected, define the site of the tumor with respect to the hepatic veins because these tumors can be resected if they are confined to one lobe of the liver. Otherwise, they are treated with chemotherapy and resected later. Also examine the porta hepatis for enlarged lymph nodes. Distant spread of tumor is to lungs, brain, and skeleton.
5. If ovarian malignancy is likely, examine the pelvis and retroperitoneum for lymph nodes and look elsewhere in the abdomen for implants on the mesentery and hepatic metastases.
6. If a vaginal, bladder, or prostate mass is found, look in the abdomen for metastases in the liver or retroperitoneal lymph nodes. Also examine the kidneys for hydronephrosis.

SUGGESTED READING

Siegel MJ. Urinary tract. In: Siegel MJ, ed. *Pediatric Sonography*, 3rd ed. Philadelphia: Lippincott Williams & Wilkins; 2001:386–473.

Siegel MJ. Adrenal glands, pancreas, and other retroperitoneal structures. In: Siegel MJ, ed. *Pediatric Sonography*, 3rd ed. Philadelphia: Lippincott Williams & Wilkins; 2001:475–527.

Siegel MJ. Female pelvis. In: Siegel MJ, ed. *Pediatric Sonography*, 3rd ed. Philadelphia: Lippincott Williams & Wilkins; 2001:529–577.

States LJ, Bellah RD. Imaging of the pediatric female pelvis. *Semin Roentgenol* 1996;31:312–329.

36 Neonatal Intracranial Problems

MARILYN J. SIEGEL

KEY WORDS

Aqueductal Stenosis. Narrowing of the duct connecting the third and fourth ventricles.

Arnold-Chiari Malformation. Congenital anomaly in which the cerebellum and brainstem are pulled toward the spinal cord.

Atrium (Trigone) of the Lateral Ventricles. Site where the anterior, occipital, and temporal horns join.

Brainstem. Part of the brain connecting the forebrain and the spinal cord; consists of the midbrain, pons, and medulla oblongata.

Caudate Nucleus. Deep structure in the brain that forms the lateral borders of the frontal horns of the lateral ventricles. It lies anterior to the thalamus.

Caudothalamic Groove. The interface between the caudate nucleus and thalamus.

Cavum Septi Pellucidi. A triangular, cerebrospinal fluid-filled space that lies between the frontal horns of the lateral ventricles.

Cerebellum. Portion of the brain that lies behind the fourth ventricle and below the tentorium.

Cerebrum. The part of the brain above the tentorium; it consists of two hemispheres.

Choroid Plexus. Mass of special cells located in the cerebral ventricles that are responsible for producing cerebrospinal fluid.

Cistern. Focal enlargements of the subarachnoid space that serve as reservoirs for cerebrospinal fluid.

Corpus Callosum. Large group of nerve fibers superior to the third ventricle that connects the left and right sides of the brain.

Dandy-Walker Syndrome. Congenital anomaly characterized by a dilated fourth ventricle and small cerebellum.

Dura Mater. Fibrous membrane that surrounds the brain.

Encephalocele. Congenital anomaly in which a portion of the brain protrudes through a defect in the skull.

Encephalomalacia. An abnormal softening of the brain after infarction. Appears as cystic spaces or holes in the brain tissue.

Falx Cerebri (Interhemispheric Fissure). A portion of the dura mater that separates the two cerebral hemispheres.

Fontanelle. Space between the bones of the skull.

Germinal Matrix. Periventricular tissue that is fragile and bleeds easily.

Glomus. Bulbous area of the choroid plexus in the trigones of the lateral ventricles.

Gyri. Convolutions on the surface of the brain.

Holoprosencephaly. Abnormal brain in which there is a varying degree of ventricular and parenchymal fusion due to an in utero error in separation.

Hypoxia. Refers to decreased oxygenation of blood, typically as a result of respiratory failure.

Hydranencephaly. Congenital anomaly in which the cortex is absent. The midbrain and brainstem structures are present.

Hydrocephalus. Dilatation of the ventricles due to accumulation of cerebrospinal fluid. Usually caused by blockage of drainage pathways.

Interhemispheric Fissure. The band of dura mater that separates the two cerebral hemispheres.

Ischemia. Refers to a decrease in cerebral blood flow.

Lipoma of the Corpus Callosum. A fat-filled mass within the corpus callosum.

Massa Intermedia. Portion of the brain that bulges into the third ventricle.

Meninges. The brain coverings.

Myelomeningocele. Indicates incomplete closure of the spinal cord and surrounding vertebral column and skin. This lesion presents as a mass, usually on the lower back.

Neonate. Newborn infant.

Parenchyma. Term for tissues of the cortex.

Periventricular Halo. A normal area of increased echogenicity along the trigone of the lateral ventricles.

Periventricular Leukomalacia. An infarct or softening of the white matter surrounding the ventricles, initially seen as echogenic and later as cystic.

Porencephalic Cyst. Cystic space in the brain that develops early in gestation as a result of ischemia.

Subependyma. The area immediately beneath the floor of the lateral ventricles and above the third ventricle. Most common site of bleeding in the premature infant.

Sulcus. A groove or depression on the surface of the brain, separating the gyri.

Tentorium. Echogenic structure separating the cerebrum and the cerebellum; it is an extension of the dura mater.

Thalami. Two ovoid brain structures situated on either side of the third ventricle.

Trigone. Same as atrium of the lateral ventricles.

Ventricle. A cavity within the brain containing cerebrospinal fluid.

Ventriculomegaly. Same as hydrocephalus. Refers to enlarged ventricles.

The Clinical Problem

Cranial sonography is used in the detection and follow-up of intracranial hemorrhage (ICH), ischemia, congenital malformations, and congenital infections. Clinical signs that suggest an intracranial problem include diminished level of consciousness, lower- or upper-extremity weakness, abnormal posturing, seizures, apnea, coma, and low hematocrit. Diagnosis of these conditions is important because, although some are not treatable, they can affect outcome. This information is important for parental counseling.

Technique

Sonography of the neonatal brain is generally performed through the anterior fontanelle, which provides an excellent sonographic window for evaluation. The anterior fontanelle is available as an acoustic window through the first year of life. The fontanelle may remain open after this time period in premature infants and in those with increased intracranial pressure. High-frequency, small footprint 7.5-MHz sector or curved array transducers usually suffice to examine the brain in coronal and sagittal planes. Lower-frequency transducers (3.0 or 5.0 MHz) may be needed to improve visualization in older infants with closing fontanelles. Images are obtained in coronal and sagittal planes. In the coronal plane, the transducer is angled in a sequential manner from anterior to posterior, and symmetrical images are obtained of the cerebral hemispheres and lateral ventricles. The transducer is then turned 90 degrees for the sagittal plane. In the sagittal plane, the transducer is angled medially to laterally to examine each ventricle and hemisphere. Duplex and color flow Doppler sonography are valuable to assess vascular anatomy, cerebral blood flow, and congenital vascular anomalies.

Other important technical factors include (1) appropriate labeling, (2) adequate depth, and (3) proper gain settings. The right and left sides of the neonatal head need to be clearly labeled. The ultrasound beam's depth needs to be adjusted to allow visualization of the skull beneath the cerebellum. The gain setting needs to be adjusted to compensate for the increased ambient light levels common in most nurseries.

Cross-Sectional Sonographic Anatomy

The ventricular system and cerebrospinal fluid (CSF) spaces serve as references for identifying intracranial anatomy and selecting scan planes. The basic planes for coronal scans are the (1) frontal horns anterior to the foramen of Monro, (2) third ventricle through the foramen of Monro, (3) quadrigeminal cistern, (4) trigones of the lateral ventricles, and (5) parietal and occipital cortex.

CORONAL SECTIONS

The most anterior coronal scan is through the frontal horns of the lateral ventricles (Fig. 36-1). The frontal horns are anechoic, fluid-filled spaces with a triangular configuration. The hypoechoic corpus callosum forms the roof of the frontal horns, the cavum septi pellucidi forms the medial walls, and the echogenic heads of the caudate nucleus form the lateral walls. The hypoechoic cingulate gyrus borders the corpus callosum. The hyperechoic pericallosal sulcus separates the corpus callosum from the cingulate gyrus. The sylvian fissures appear as Y-shaped echogenic areas laterally. The relatively hypoechoic frontal and temporal lobes are also imaged at this level. Anterior cerebral arteries are

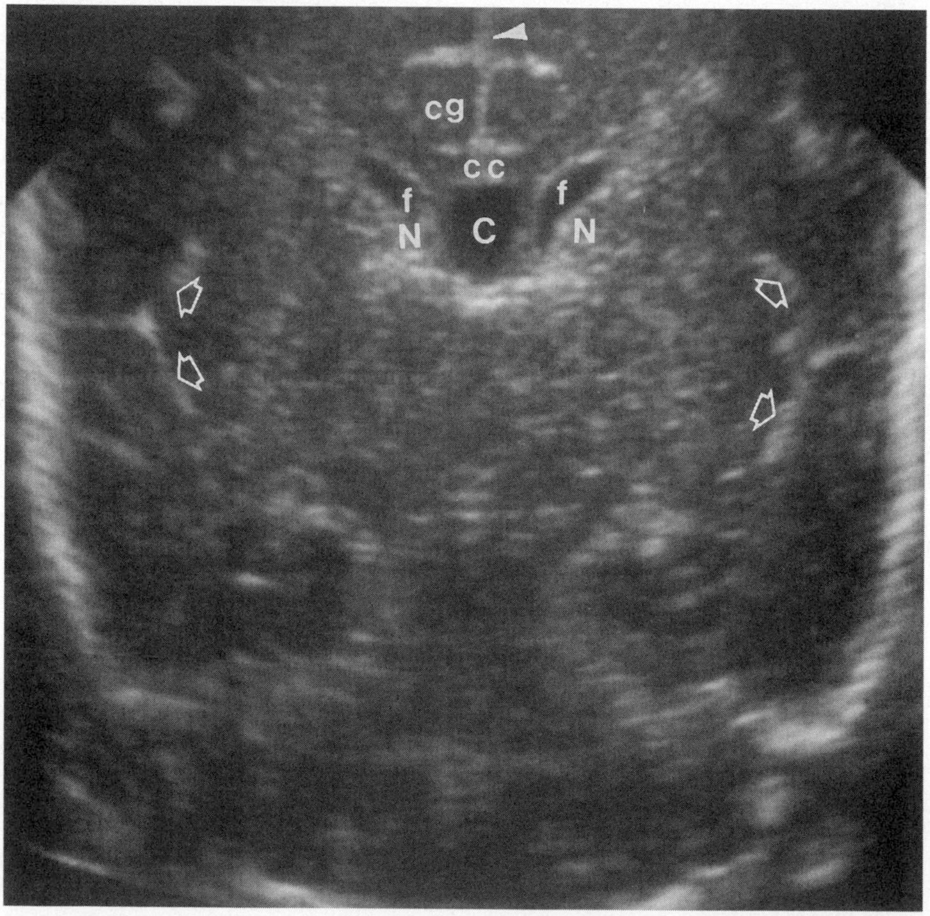

Figure 36-1. ■ *Coronal scan, frontal horns. The frontal horns* (f) *appear as triangular, fluid-filled spaces separated by the cavum septi pellucidi* (C). *The caudate nuclei* (N) *lie lateral to the frontal horns. The hypoechoic corpus callosum* (cc) *forms the roof of the cavum. The echogenic pericallosal sulcus separates the corpus callosum from the hypoechoic cingulate gyrus* (cg). *The Y-shaped sylvian fissures* (open arrows) *and anterior interhemispheric fissure* (arrowhead) *are also seen.*

visible in the sagittal fissure on color Doppler imaging.

The next scan is through the third ventricle (Fig. 36-2). Echogenic choroid plexus is visualized in the floor of both lateral ventricles and in the roof of the third ventricle just below the cavum septi pellucidi. The anechoic cavum septi pellucidi again may be seen between the lateral ventricles. The lateral ventricles are bordered by the thalami, which have an echogenicity similar to or slightly less than that of adjacent parenchyma. The normal-sized third ventricle is usually not visualized because its transverse diameter is small. When dilated, it can be recognized as a midline anechoic structure beneath the bodies of the lateral ventricles. The echogenic brainstem (i.e., the pons and medulla) and tentorium are seen inferiorly. The pericallosal artery in the interhemispheric fissure and middle cerebral artery in the sylvian fissure may be noted on color Doppler imaging.

On a more posterior scan, the echogenic, star-shaped, quadrigeminal cistern is seen superior to the cerebellum (Fig. 36-3). The cisternal echogenicity is thought to be secondary to the presence of arachnoid septations or pulsations from large vessels within the cistern. The bodies of the lateral ventricles are bordered by the thalami. The cerebellum appears as an echogenic midline structure in the posterior fossa. A small cisterna magna is sometimes seen posterior and inferior to the cerebellum. The middle cerebral and pericallosal arteries may also be observed on color Doppler imaging.

The next most posterior coronal scan is through the trigones of the ven-

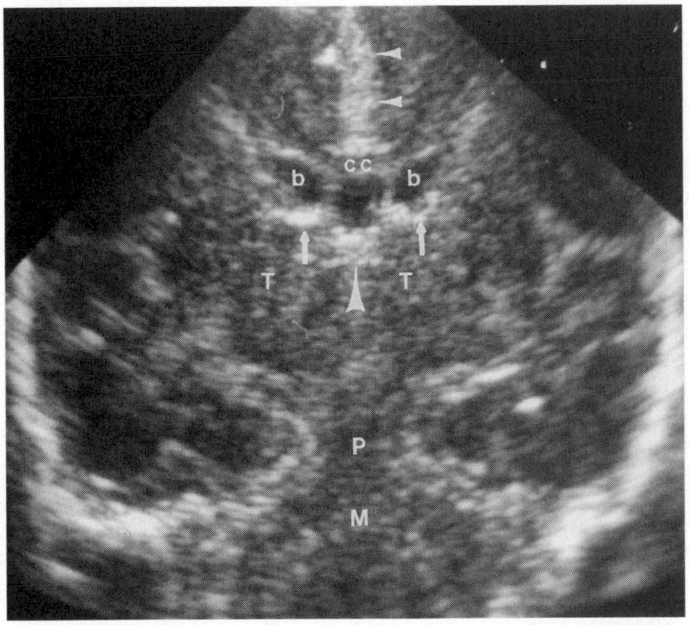

Figure 36-2. ■ *Coronal scan, third ventricle. The bodies* (b) *of the lateral ventricles and the thalami* (T) *inferior to the ventricles are imaged. The echogenic choroid plexus is seen in the floor of the lateral ventricles* (arrows) *and in the roof of the third ventricle* (arrowhead) *just below the cavum septum pellucidi. The three dots of echogenic choroid plexus indicate that this scan is through the third ventricle. The third ventricle is usually slitlike and thus often not seen in the coronal plane. The pons* (P) *and medulla* (M) *are imaged at this level, although a well-defined interface between the two structures is not usually apparent.* cc, *corpus callosum;* small arrowheads, *interhemispheric fissure.*

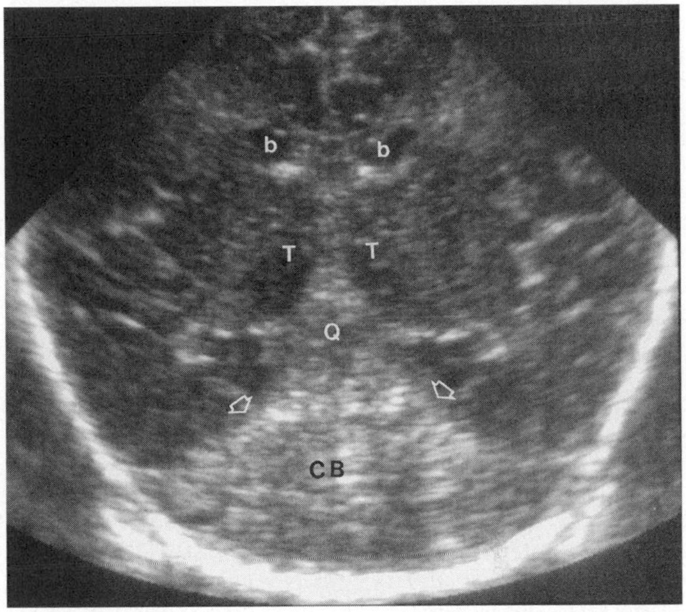

Figure 36-3. ■ *Coronal scan, quadrigeminal cistern. The quadrigeminal cistern* (Q) *appears as an echogenic, star-shaped structure just inferior to the thalami* (T). *The bodies of the lateral ventricles* (b), *cerebellum* (CB), *and tentorium* (open arrows) *are also imaged on this section.*

tricles (Fig. 36-4). The highly echogenic glomi of the choroid plexus are noted in the atria of the lateral ventricles. Prominent symmetric echogenic stripes, produced by the periventricular white matter tracts, are noted lateral to both ventricles. These echogenic stripes are referred to as a "periventricular halo" or "blush." The echogenicity of the periventricular stripes should be less than or equal to that of the choroid plexus. The top of the cerebellum is also seen.

The final scan, obtained posterior and cephalad to the trigones and cerebellum, shows the gyri and sulci of the occipital lobes and the posterior interhemispheric fissure. Again noted is the echogenicity from the periventricular white matter tracts (Fig. 36-5).

SAGITTAL SECTIONS

Sagittal images are obtained through (1) the midline, (2) the caudothalamic groove, and (3) the body of each lateral ventricle.

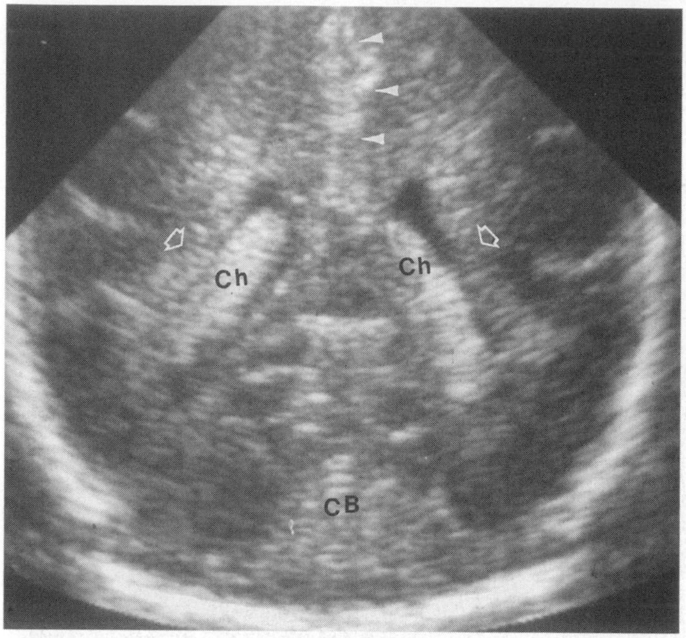

Figure 36-4. ■ *Coronal scan, trigones of lateral ventricles. The largest part of the choroid plexus* (Ch), *which is termed the* glomus, *is seen at this level. The choroid nearly totally fills the ventricles. Lateral to the trigones are the normal bands of periventricular echoes* (open arrows). *Normal periventricular echogenicity is fairly symmetric, and the echogenicity is equal to or less than that of the choroid plexus. The top of the echogenic cerebellum* (CB) *and posterior interhemispheric fissure* (arrowheads) *are also seen.*

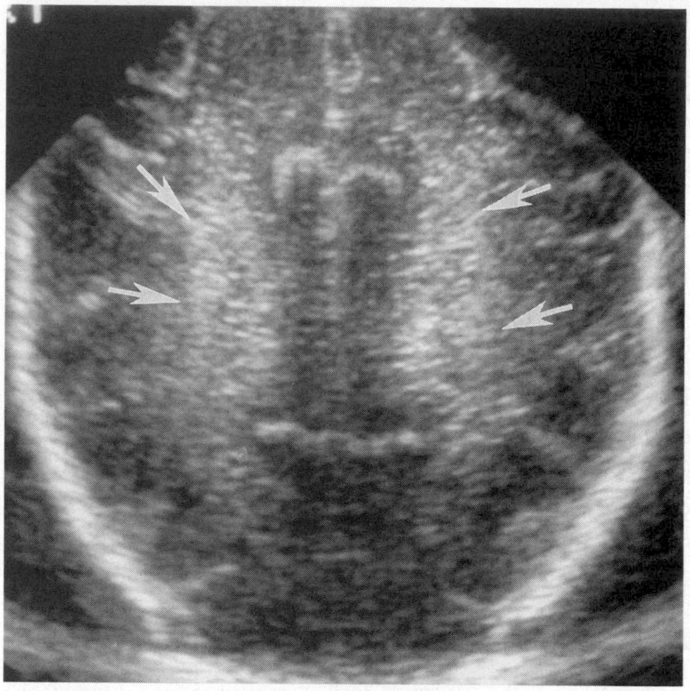

Figure 36-5. ■ *Coronal scan, periventricular white matter. Coronal scan posterior to occipital horns shows the normal periventricular white matter* (arrows). *Echogenic sulci and hypoechoic gyri are noted in the brain periphery.*

The midline image shows the cavum septi pellucidi as a comma-shaped, fluid-filled structure between the frontal horns of the lateral ventricles (Fig. 36-6). The cavum vergae is the posterior extension of the cavum septi pellucidi; it lies between the bodies of the lateral ventricles. Cephalad to the cavi septi pellucidi and vergae is the crescentic, hypoechoic corpus callosum. It is bordered superiorly by the echogenic sulcus of the corpus callosum, which contains the pericallosal arteries. Cephalad to the pericallosal sulcus is the cingulate gyrus, which is seen as a broad, curvilinear, hypoechoic band. The cingulate gyrus radiates around the lateral ventricles. Immediately below the cavum septi pellucidi is the choroid plexus in the roof of the third ventricle. The third and fourth ventricles are seen as anechoic, fluid-filled structures. Posterior to the triangular-shaped fourth ventricle is the echogenic cerebellar vermis. Anterior to the fourth ventricle is the brainstem. Inferior to the vermis is the anechoic cisterna magna.

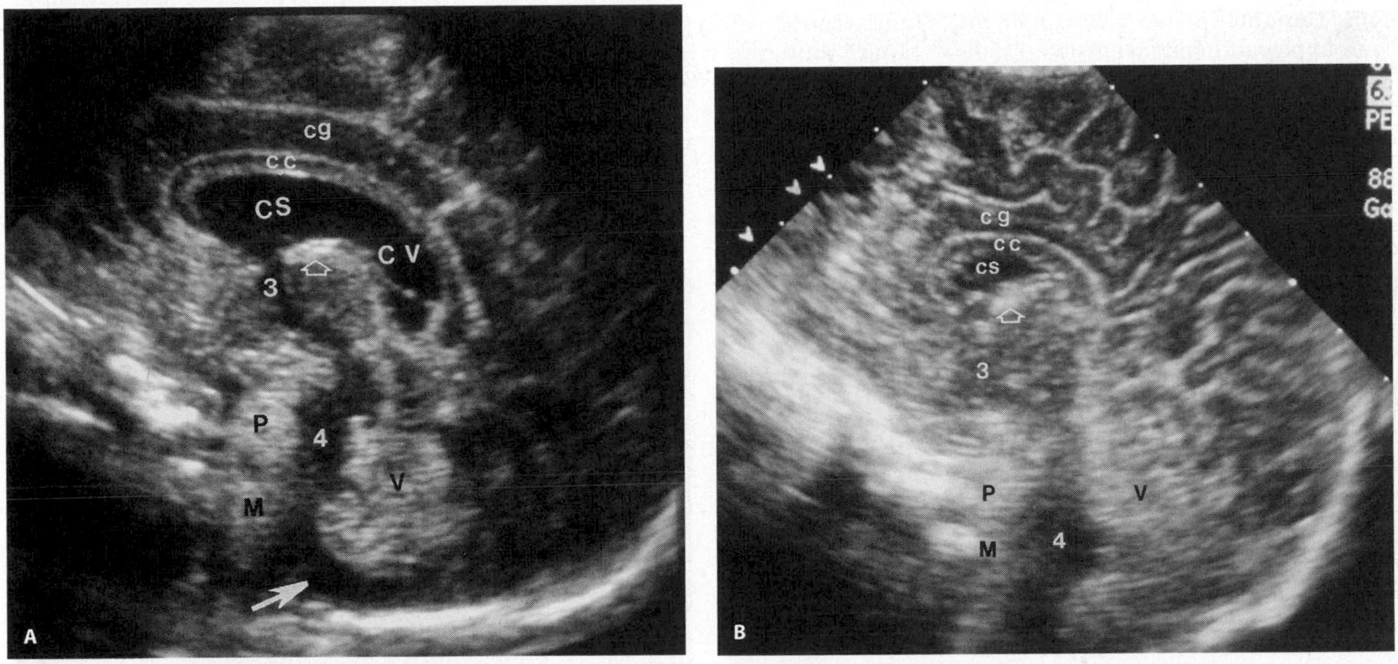

Figure 36-6. ■ *Sagittal plane, midline image. A. Immature brain. B. Mature brain. The midline cavum septi pellucidi* (CS) *and vergae* (CV) *are identified in the premature brain. Only the cavum septum pellucidum is seen in the mature brain. Gyri and sulci are more easily seen in the term infant than in the preterm infant, who has a featureless cortical surface. Note that the sulci extend to the cingulate gyrus* (cg), *never to the ventricles. Also note the hypoechoic corpus callosum* (cc) *superior to the cavum septum pellucidum and the echogenic band of choroid plexus* (open arrow) *just below the cavum. The third* (3) *and fourth* (4) *ventricles are seen in this plane. The pons* (P) *and medulla* (M) *are seen anterior to the fourth ventricle. The vermis* (V) *of the cerebellum is posterior to the fourth ventricle. Beneath the vermis is the small, fluid-filled cisterna magna* (arrow). *A cisterna magna should always be seen. Absence of the cisterna magna suggests a Chiari malformation.*

Approximately 15 degrees of lateral angulation will show the frontal horns, bodies, and occipital horns of the lateral ventricles (Fig. 36-7). The occipital horns are usually larger than the frontal horns. The important anatomic landmark on this image is the caudothalamic groove, a thin, echogenic band that lies between the caudate nuclei anteriorly and thalami posteriorly. The caudate nucleus is slightly more echogenic than the thalamus. The caudothalamic groove denotes the anterior-most extent of the choroid plexus. In premature infants, the vascular germinal matrix is located above the caudothalamic groove, which is a common site for bleeding. The glomus of the choroid plexus is seen in the lateral ventricles.

Further lateral angulation of the transducer produces an image through the frontal horns, bodies, and occipital horns of the lateral ventricles (Fig. 36-8). The transducer should be angled obliquely, with the anterior part angled medially and the posterior part laterally, to image the entire ventricle. The choroid plexus has a comma-shaped configuration as it extends from the roof of the third ventricle through the foramen of Monro into the trigones. It is most prominent in the trigones of the lateral ventricles, tapering anteriorly as it courses toward the third ventricle and tapering posteriorly as it courses toward the temporal horns. The glomus of the choroid plexus commonly has a lobulated contour. The amount of CSF within the lateral ventricles varies, ranging from a tiny anechoic collection above the choroid plexus to a larger C-shaped collection filling the ventricles. The lateral ventricles are surrounded by the caudate nuclei, thalami, and cerebral hemispheres (i.e., frontal, parietal, occipital, and temporal lobes). Posterior to the occipital horns is the echogenic periventricular halo.

A more lateral sagittal image will show the echogenic periventricular white matter tracts and the brain parenchyma. The sylvian fissure and a variable number of cerebral convolutions, which in-

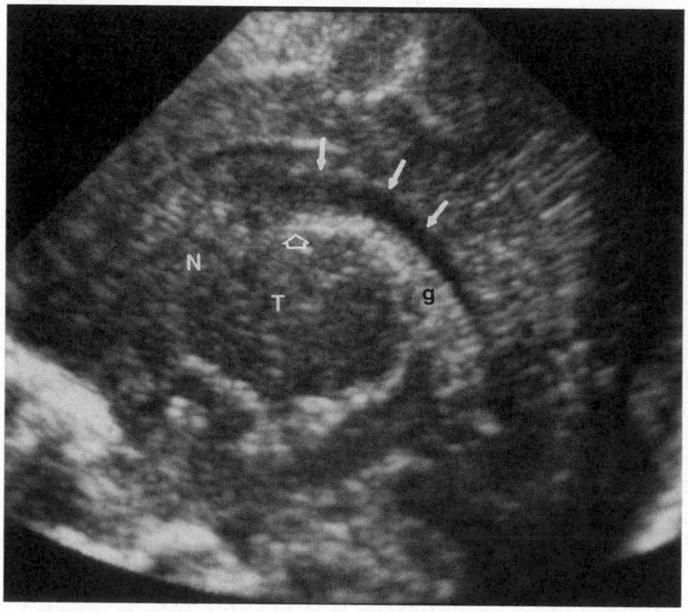

Figure 36-7. ■ *Sagittal plane, caudothalamic groove. The head of the caudate nucleus* (N) *anteriorly and thalamus* (T) *posteriorly lie inferior to the body of the lateral ventricle* (arrows). *Between these structures is the caudothalamic groove containing the anterior extent of the choroid plexus* (open arrow). *The echogenic glomus* (g) *of the choroid plexus is seen in the lateral ventricle.*

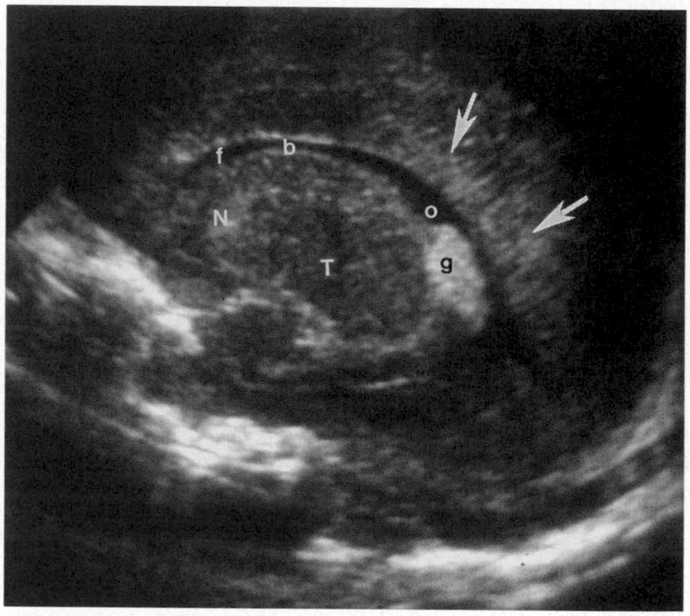

Figure 36-8. ■ *Sagittal scan, body of lateral ventricles. The frontal horn* (f), *body* (b), *and occipital horn* (o) *of the lateral ventricles are seen at this level. The echogenic glomus* (g) *of the choroid plexus is noted within the trigone of the lateral ventricle. Below the ventricle are the caudate nucleus* (N) *and the thalamus* (T). *The normal periventricular halo* (arrows) *is superoposterior to the trigones. The echogenicity of the periventricular white matter should be less than or equal to that of the choroid plexus.*

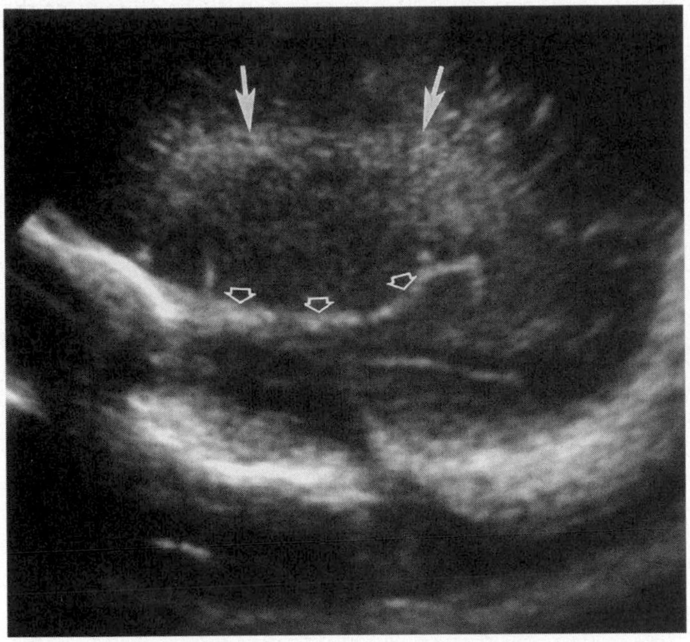

Figure 36-9. ■ *Sagittal scan, lateral to the ventricle. The normal periventricular echogenic band* (arrows) *and sylvian fissure* (open arrows) *are noted on this section.*

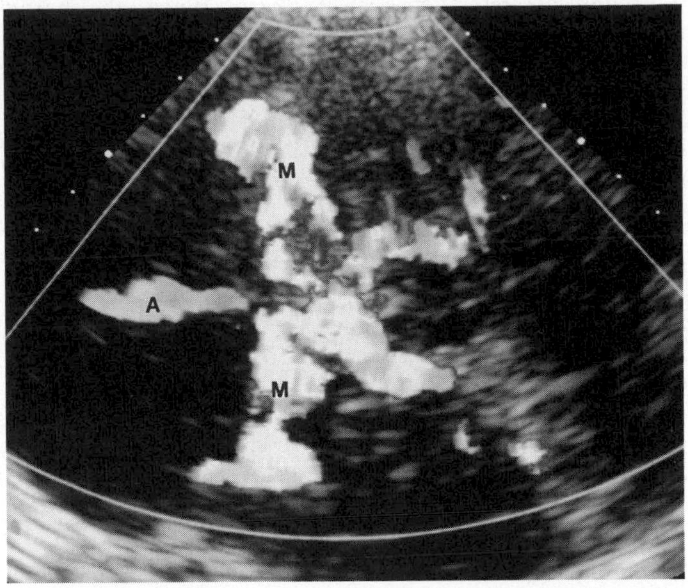

Figure 36-10. ■ *In this 10-year-old boy's axial scan through the brainstem, the middle* (M) *and anterior* (A) *cerebral arteries are identified. This image is obtained with the transducer placed in front of the ear. The part of the temporal bone anterior to the ear is thin enough to allow imaging of the brainstem to be performed even after sutural closure.*

crease with gestational age, can also be seen (Fig. 36-9).

ANATOMY IN OTHER IMAGING PLANES

The coronal and squamosal sutures, posterior fontanelle, and temporal bone can also serve as acoustic windows in the neonate. Scanning through the coronal and squamosal sutures is useful for visualizing the brain's convexities when evaluating extracerebral fluid collections. Use of the posterior fossa as an acoustic window can improve visualization of the brainstem, fourth ventricle, trigones of the ventricles, and the posterior periventricular area.

Axial scanning through the temporal bone is used for evaluating the major branches of the circle of Willis (Fig. 36-10). The transducer is placed on the lateral aspect of the head just in front of the ear and above the mandibular condyle. The ultrasound beam is directed horizontally. Axial imaging can be used after the fontanelle has closed.

ARTERIAL AND VENOUS FLOW PATTERNS

Systolic and diastolic blood flow velocities and resistive indices decrease as gestational age increases. The mean resistive index of the intracranial arteries in term infants is 0.7 with a standard deviation of 0.05. In term infants, antegrade flow is present throughout systole and diastole. In premature infants under 30 weeks' gestation, diastolic flow may be absent. ICH, brain edema, subdural effusions, periventricular leukomalacia, and hydrocephalus increase vascular resistance, which in turn reduces diastolic flow and increases the resistive index. An abnormally low resistive index has been reported in intrauterine asphyxia and growth retardation.

The larger central veins, such as the sagittal sinus and vein of Galen, show low-amplitude pulsations. The smaller intracerebral veins, such as the internal cerebral veins and terminal veins, show a monophasic continuous waveform. High-amplitude waveforms ("sawtooth" pattern) are abnormal and suggest elevated right heart pressures.

Basic Normal Anatomy

BRAIN PARENCHYMA

In premature infants, the surface of the brain is smooth because the gyri and sulci are underdeveloped. In term infants, individual gyri and sulci can be seen sonographically (Fig. 36-6).

LATERAL VENTRICLES

Asymmetry of the lateral ventricles is a common variant. More often, the left ventricle is larger than the right and the occipital horns are larger than the frontal horns. Ventricular size may also change with changes in patient positioning. When the infant is scanned in a decubitus position, the ventricle on the down side may be smaller than the ventricle on the up side.

The ventricles of the premature infant are usually larger than those of the term infant. In mature infants, the ventricles may be tiny slits, or they may appear as fluid-filled, comma-shaped structures. Slit-like ventricles also occur in infants with cerebral edema, but in this clinical setting, there are other associated findings, such as increased parenchymal echogenicity and poor definition of sulci and gyri.

On the sagittal views, the diameter of the occipital horn should not exceed 16 mm; the diameter of the body should not exceed 3 mm. The third ventricle can be measured on coronal views; it normally measures less than 2 mm in widest diameter.

CAVI SEPTI PELLUCIDI AND VERGAE

The cavum septi pellucidi is seen in the midline between the anterior horns of the lateral ventricles. The posterior part of the cavum septum pellucidi is termed the *cavum vergae*. The cavum vergae is interposed between the bodies of the lateral ventricles. The foramen of Monro marks the dividing line between these two parts of the cavum. During the sixth month of gestation, the cavum vergae normally begins to close from posterior to anterior. Closure is usually complete by 2 to 6 weeks of postnatal life. The cavum vergae is seen in very premature infants (Fig. 36-6). The cavum septum pellucidi can be seen in premature and term infants. The cavi appear as fluid-filled spaces between the lateral ventricles.

GERMINAL MATRIX

The germinal matrix is a highly vascular structure that gives rise to the nerve cells of the cerebral cortex during fetal development. It lies just above the caudothalamic groove and just beneath the ependymal lining of the ventricles. The germinal matrix begins to involute at about the third month of gestation. This involution is usually complete by 36 weeks' gestation. The clinical significance of the germinal matrix is that it is the source of bleeding in premature infants. The germinal matrix is not seen at sonography. Only the sequelae of bleeding can be recognized.

CHOROID PLEXUS

The choroid plexus is responsible for producing CSF in the ventricles. It lines the body as well as the occipital and temporal horns of each lateral ventricle. The largest part of the choroid plexus, which is known as the *glomus*, is in the trigones of the lateral ventricles (Figs. 36-7 and 36-8). At the level of the glomus, the choroid plexus tapers as it courses anteriorly to the roof of the third ventricle and posteriorly into the temporal horns of each lateral ventricle. Of note, the choroid plexus ends at the caudothalamic groove, and it never extends into the frontal or occipital horns of the lateral ventricles. Echogenicity in the floor of the ventricles anterior to the third ventricle indicates hemorrhage. Choroid plexus is also present in the roof of the fourth ventricle, although it is not usually seen on sonography.

PERIVENTRICULAR WHITE MATTER ECHOGENICITY

An echogenic band paralleling the posterior part of the lateral ventricles is a normal finding seen in virtually all neonates. This band of echogenicity is referred to as a *periventricular halo*. The degree of echogenicity should be less than or equal to that of the normal choroid plexus. The halo should have a homogeneous, brush-like appearance (Figs. 36-4, 36-5, 36-8, and 36-9). The differential of periventricular echogenicity includes cerebral hemorrhage and periventricular leukomalacia. Either of these conditions should be suspected if the periventricular halo is asymmetric or more echogenic than the choroid plexus.

CISTERNA MAGNA

The cisterna magna is a fluid-filled structure that lies inferior to the vermis and communicates with the fourth ventricle (Fig. 36-6). In the midsagittal plane, the height of the cisterna magna varies from 3 to 8 mm. Absence of the cisterna is associated with Arnold-Chiari malformation.

Intracranial Hemorrhage

GENERAL OVERVIEW: ULTRASOUND APPEARANCE OF HEMORRHAGE

The appearance of ICH changes with time. Acute hemorrhage has an echogenicity equal to or greater than that of the choroid plexus. As the blood clot lyses, it becomes hypoechoic centrally, whereas the clot's periphery is still echogenic.

BLEEDING OF THE PREMATURE NEONATE

Major risk factors for hemorrhage in the preterm neonate are gestational age of less than 32 weeks and birth weight of less than 1,500 g. The hemorrhage begins in the germinal matrix of the periventricular area. The germinal matrix contains a number of immature thin-walled vessels, which have a tendency to rupture. The portion of germinal matrix in the thalamostriate groove at the head of the caudate nucleus is the most common site for hemorrhage. Germinal matrix hemorrhage may extend into the lateral ventricles, and large germinal matrix bleeds may compress the subependymal veins leading to venous infarction and parenchymal hemorrhage.

ICH is rare beyond the first week of life. Most hemorrhages are symptomatic, but some are asymptomatic. In the latter group, routine screening sonography is performed 7 to 10 days after birth to document silent hemorrhage because this can lead to hydrocephalus.

ICH is classically divided into four grades:

Grade I, subependymal hemorrhage only

Grade II, subependymal hemorrhage with blood in nondilated ventricles

Grade III, subependymal hemorrhage with blood in dilated ventricles

Grade IV, subependymal hemorrhage, blood in dilated ventricles, and intraparenchymal blood

Isolated grade I hemorrhage has virtually no morbidity or mortality. More severe grades of hemorrhages are associated with increasing mortality and a poorer neurologic outcome. ICH may result in learning deficits, mental retardation, and developmental delays.

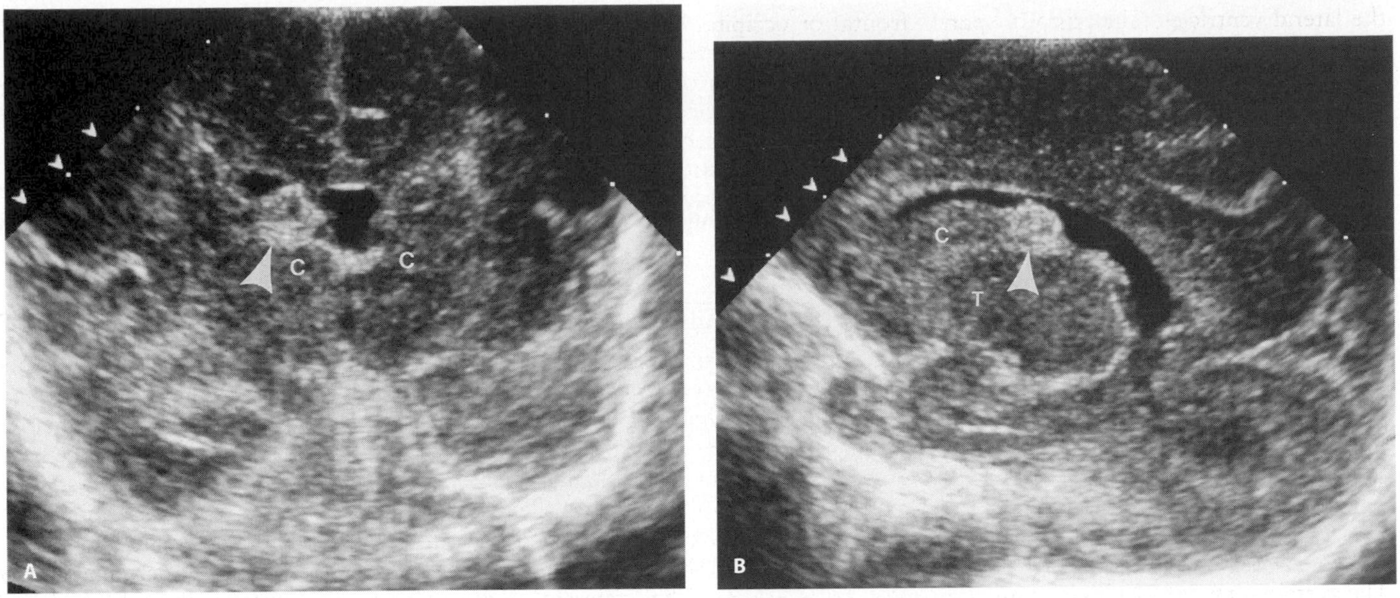

Figure 36-11. ■ *Subependymal hemorrhage. A. Coronal sonogram shows a focus of increased echogenicity* (arrowhead) *in the right subependymal area, just above the caudate nucleus. B. Right parasagittal image. The hemorrhage* (arrowhead) *appears as an echogenic mass in the caudothalamic groove.* C, *caudate nucleus;* T, *thalamus.*

Grade I Hemorrhage (Subependymal Hemorrhage)

Subependymal hemorrhage appears as a discrete focus of increased echogenicity above the caudate nucleus on coronal views and anterior to the caudothalamic groove on sagittal views (Fig. 36-11). Hemorrhage has no flow signal on color Doppler sonography. Remember that the echogenic choroid plexus in the lateral ventricle does not extend anterior to the foramen of Monro.

Over a period of days to weeks, grade I hemorrhage liquefies and evolves into a subependymal cyst (Fig. 36-12). These cysts have an echogenic wall as well as an echogenic center and bulge into the lateral ventricle. They do not communicate with the ventricle. Such cysts do not usually have long-term consequences.

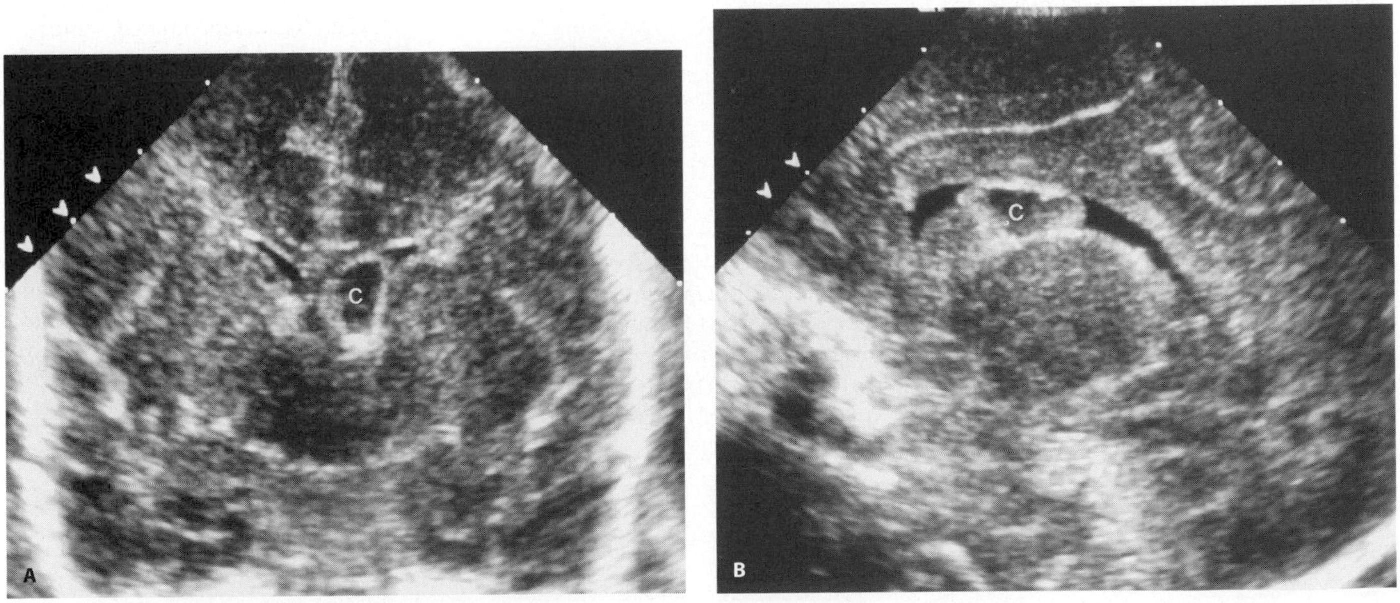

Figure 36-12. ■ *Resolving subependymal hemorrhage. A. Coronal and (B) sagittal views show a thick-walled cyst* (C) *in the subependymal area, representing a resolving hematoma.*

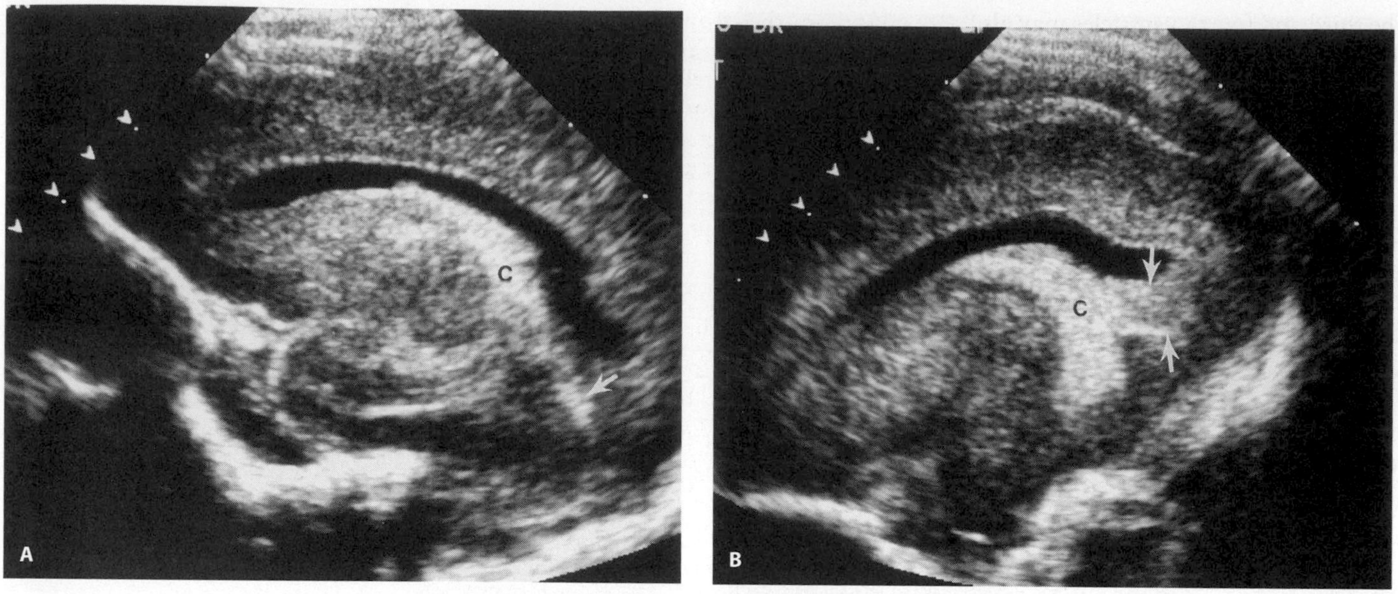

Figure 36-13. ■ *Grade II hemorrhage. A. Right parasagittal view shows faintly increased echogenicity in the occipital horn* (arrow), *which could represent blood versus volume averaging of adjacent parenchyma. B. View through the posterior fontanelle confirms clot* (arrows) *in the occipital horn.* C, *choroid plexus.*

Grade II Hemorrhage

Grade II hemorrhage results when the subependymal blood ruptures through the ventricular wall, entering the lumen. It appears as echogenic material within part or all of a nondilated ventricular system. Most often, the blood accumulates in the dependent part of the ventricle (the occipital horns). In some neonates, it can be difficult to identify small amounts of hemorrhage in a nondilated ventricle, particularly if the choroid plexus is large. In equivocal cases, scanning through the posterior fontanelle can help to determine the presence or absence of hemorrhage (Fig. 36-13). Doppler imaging may also be useful to distinguish normal vascularized choroid plexus from nonvascularized clot. As grade II hemorrhage resolves, the ventricular wall often becomes echogenic.

Grade III Hemorrhage

Grade III hemorrhage fills and also enlarges one or both lateral ventricles. Because the ventricles are dilated, grade III hemorrhage is recognized more easily than grade II hemorrhage. The blood may completely fill the lateral ventricle, appearing as an echogenic cast of the ventricle (Fig. 36-14). A blood–CSF level may be seen in the occipital horn.

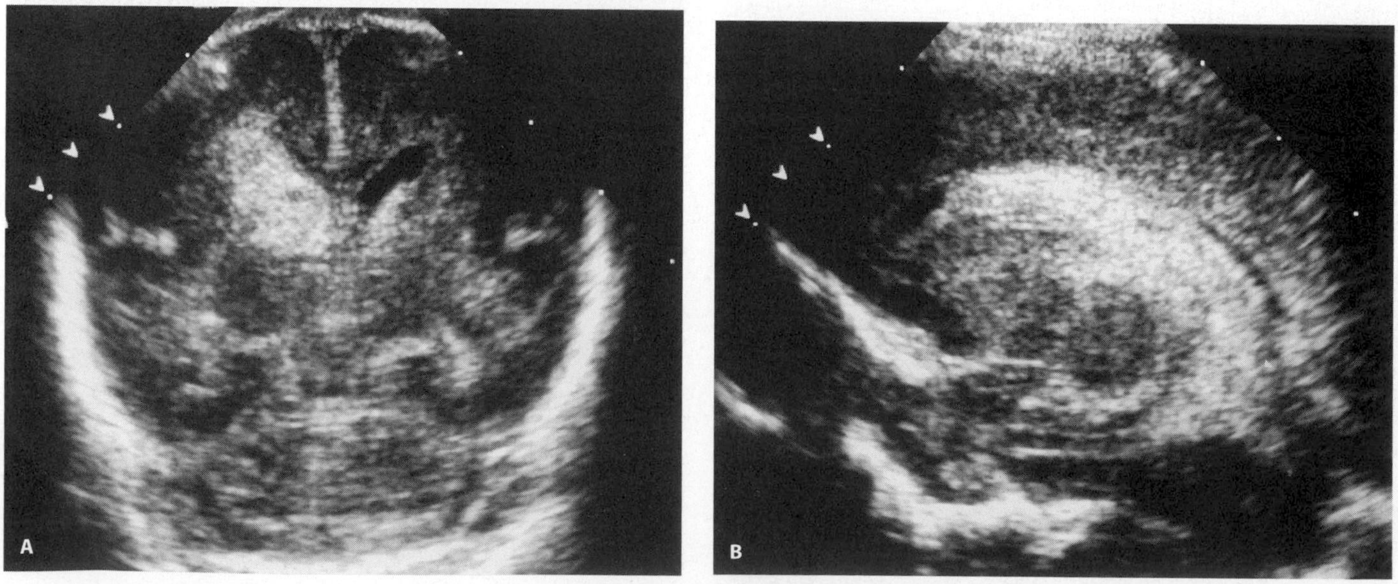

Figure 36-14. ■ *Grade III hemorrhage. A. Anterior coronal scan demonstrates a dilated, blood-filled right frontal horn. B. Sagittal scan shows blood filling virtually the entire right lateral ventricle, forming a so-called ventricular cast.*

The third and fourth ventricles may also be distended with blood. The contour of the frontal horn becomes rounded instead of tapered. As the intraventricular clot retracts, echogenic debris or floating clot fragments may be seen in the ventricles.

Grade IV Hemorrhage (Blood in the Brain Tissues)

Grade IV hemorrhage is thought to be the result of infarction and subsequent bleeding. Intraparenchymal blood is seen as an intensely echogenic focus in the brain tissues adjacent to one or both lateral ventricles (Fig. 36-15). It is most common in the frontal and parietal lobes. Shift of the midline structures to the unaffected contralateral side and ventricular dilatation are often associated findings with intraparenchymal hemorrhage. This type of hemorrhage causes brain necrosis, which results in encephalomalacia (cystic areas in the brain parenchyma).

Posthemorrhagic Hydrocephalus (Ventricular Dilatation)

Ventricular dilatation commonly results from intraventricular hemorrhage. Blood may obstruct the outflow tracts of the lateral, third, or fourth ventricles or it may obstruct the arachnoid granulations over the brain's surface. These granulations are responsible for absorbing CSF in healthy individuals. The trigones and occipital horns of the lateral ventricles dilate before the frontal horns. The lateral ventricles dilate more than the third or fourth ventricles. Most cases of hydrocephalus resolve or arrest spontaneously. A ventriculoperitoneal shunt may be required in patients with severe hydrocephalus.

Intracerebellar Hemorrhage

Intracerebellar hemorrhage is more frequent in the premature than in the full-

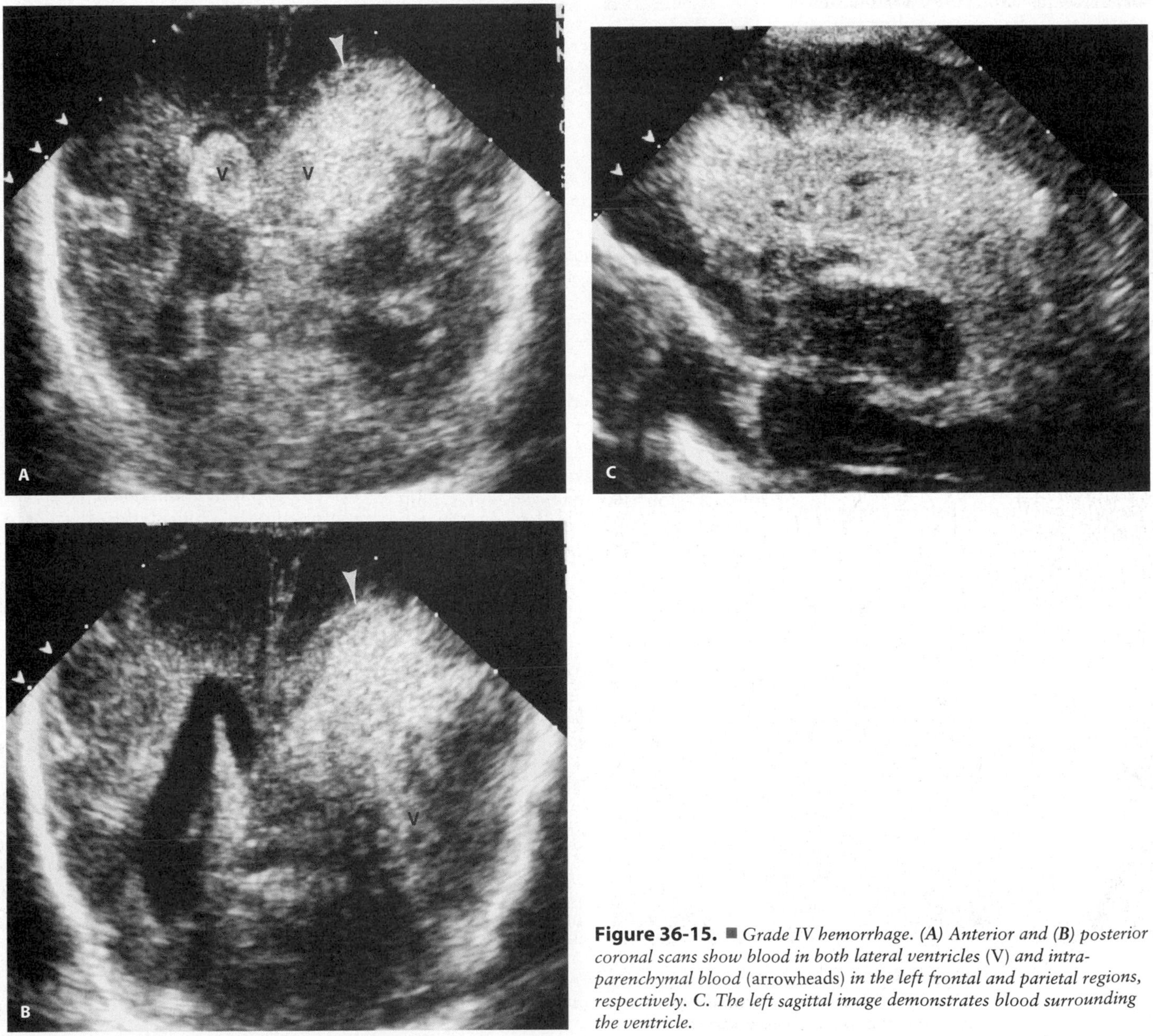

Figure 36-15. ■ *Grade IV hemorrhage. (A) Anterior and (B) posterior coronal scans show blood in both lateral ventricles* (V) *and intraparenchymal blood* (arrowheads) *in the left frontal and parietal regions, respectively. C. The left sagittal image demonstrates blood surrounding the ventricle.*

term infant. Cerebellar hemorrhage produces either ill-defined, asymmetric cerebellar echogenicity or a focal mass. The hemorrhage may resolve completely or produce an area of encephalomalacia.

BLEEDING IN THE TERM INFANT

Subarachnoid and Subdural Hemorrhages

The subarachnoid and subdural spaces are sites of hemorrhage in term infants. Grayscale sonographic features of subarachnoid and subdural hemorrhages are similar and include fluid collections over the brain's surface (Fig. 36-16), a widened interhemispheric fissure, visualization of the cortical surfaces, and mass effect with flattening of gyri, as well as displacement and compression of the ventricles. Subarachnoid, but not subdural, hemorrhages can cause widening of the sylvian fissures. A high-frequency transducer (10 MHz) will improve visualization of the periphery of the brain, as will use of a linear array transducer if the acoustic window permits.

Color flow Doppler ultrasonography is useful to separate subarachnoid and subdural fluid based on displacement of vessels. The arachnoid membrane contains superficial cortical blood vessels. Fluid in the subarachnoid space displaces the cortical vessels away from the brain surface toward the skull. These vessels and their branches can be seen crossing the subarachnoid fluid collection over the cerebral convexities. Fluid in the subdural space pushes the cortical vessels toward the surface of the brain. The subdural fluid collection contains no crossing vessels.

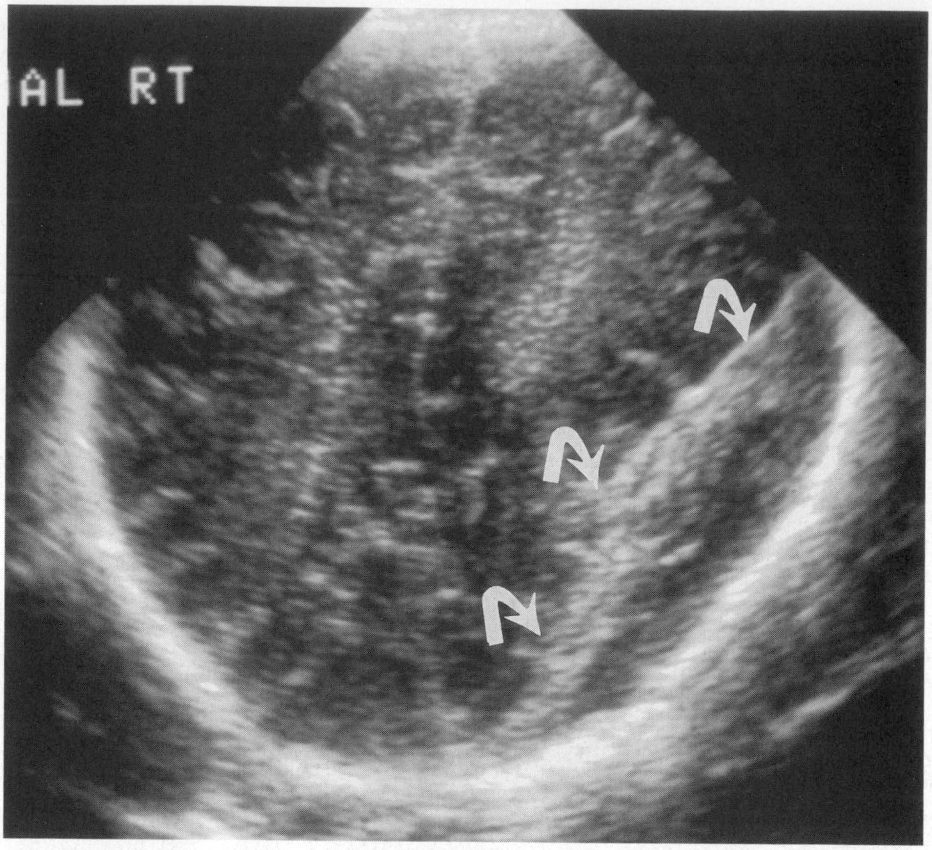

Figure 36-16. ■ *Subdural hemorrhage. Posterior coronal sonograms show an echogenic fluid collection* (arrows) *over the cortical surfaces, flattening and displacing the gyri.*

Choroid Plexus Hemorrhage

Choroid plexus hemorrhage is more frequent in term infants than in premature infants. It appears as an enlarged echogenic plexus with a lumpy contour. The diagnosis of choroid plexus hematoma can be difficult because the normal choroid plexus is echogenic and on occasion may have irregular contours. Concomitant intraventricular hemorrhage or decrease in size of the choroid plexus on serial sonograms support the diagnosis at hemorrhage.

Ischemic Brain Injury

PERIVENTRICULAR LEUKOMALACIA OF PREMATURITY

Periventricular leukomalacia is an infarction of deep white matter adjacent to the lateral ventricles. It is important to note that sonography is not very sensitive for detecting ischemic injury, and the initial examination is commonly normal. The most common sonographic finding of acute periventricular leukomalacia, occurring within a day or two of the ischemic insult, is a band of increased periventricular echogenicity (Fig. 36-17). The echogenicity exceeds that of the choroid plexus. This finding is most often bilateral and symmetric, but it may be unilateral.

The late changes are those of cystic encephalomalacia (Fig. 36-17). Cysts develop in the periventricular white matter 2 to 3 weeks after the acute insult. These cysts can be single or multiple, and they vary in size. Other findings include ventricular dilatation and interhemispheric widening due to brain atrophy.

Differential Diagnostic Considerations

The increased echogenicity accompanying periventricular leukomalacia must be differentiated from the normal periventricular halo and from parenchymal blood associated with grade IV hemorrhage. The normal periventricular halo has ill-defined borders and an echogenicity less than that of the choroid plexus, whereas periventricular leukomalacia will have better-defined borders and an echogenicity greater than that of the choroid plexus. Parenchymal hemorrhage is unilateral or asymmetric and is associated with intraventricular blood, whereas periventricular leukomalacia is

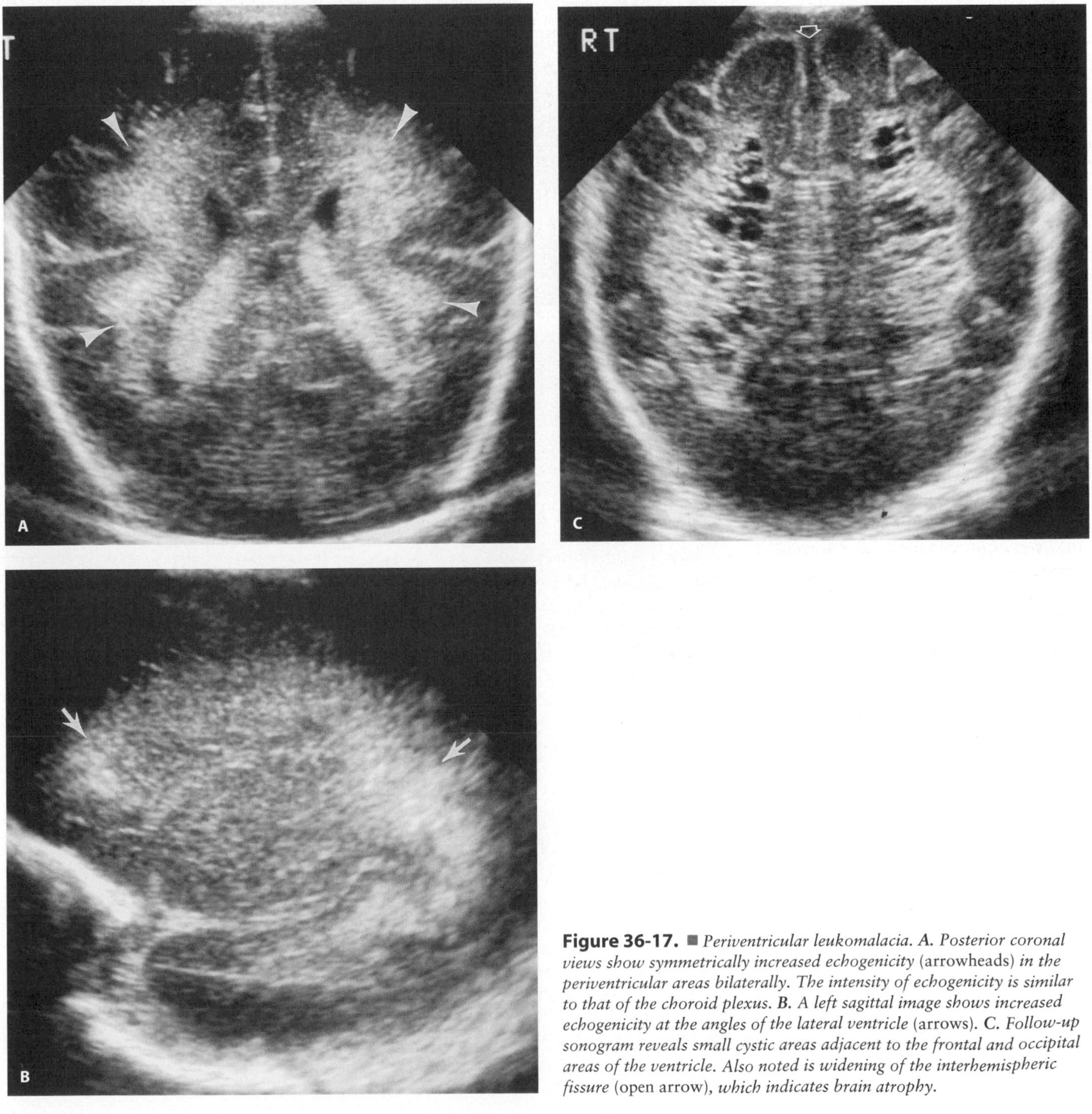

Figure 36-17. ■ *Periventricular leukomalacia. **A.** Posterior coronal views show symmetrically increased echogenicity* (arrowheads) *in the periventricular areas bilaterally. The intensity of echogenicity is similar to that of the choroid plexus. **B.** A left sagittal image shows increased echogenicity at the angles of the lateral ventricle* (arrows). ***C.** Follow-up sonogram reveals small cystic areas adjacent to the frontal and occipital areas of the ventricle. Also noted is widening of the interhemispheric fissure* (open arrow), *which indicates brain atrophy.*

most commonly symmetric and not associated with intraventricular hemorrhage.

ISCHEMIC LESIONS OF THE TERM NEONATE

Ischemic lesions in term infants have a predilection for the cerebral cortex, subcortical white matter, and basal ganglia rather than the periventricular area. In mild ischemic injury, the sonographic examination may be normal. In more severe ischemic injury, the brain parenchyma increases in echogenicity and there is poor definition of the gyral margins (Fig. 36-18). The ventricles are usually slit-like, although this finding is not specific for ischemia and can be seen in healthy term infants. The late change of ischemic injury is brain atrophy, which manifests as enlarged extra-axial spaces over the brain surface and ventricular enlargement. Other late findings include parenchymal calcifications and encephalomalacia.

Early in the course of ischemia and before the development of significant brain edema, diastolic flow may rise in an attempt to increase cerebral perfusion, leading to a low resistive index

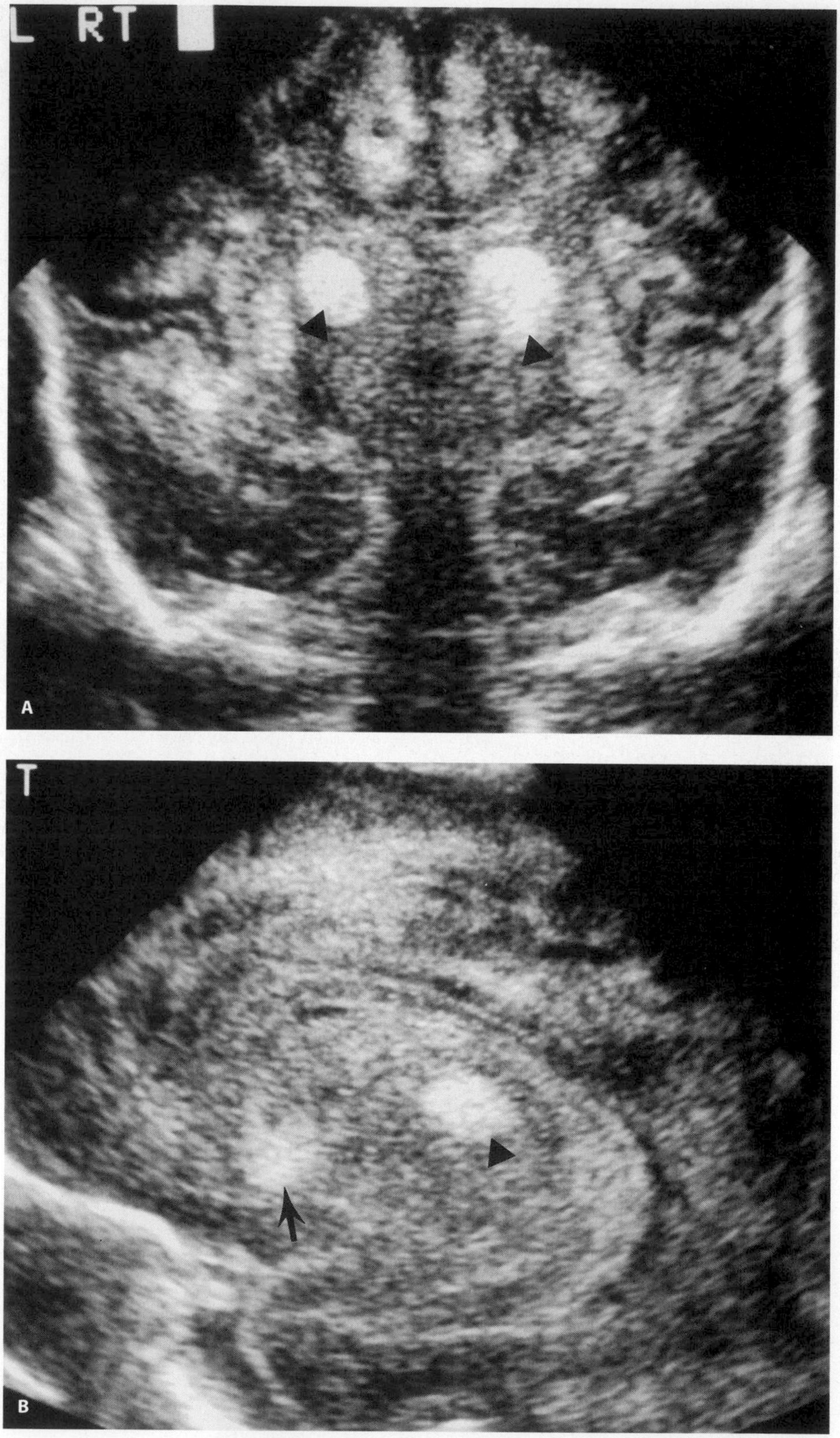

Figure 36-18. ■ *Ischemic injury in the term infant. (A) Posterior coronal and (B) left sagittal images show generalized increased echogenicity in the cortex of the brain, in the thalamus* (arrowhead) *and caudate nucleus* (arrow). *Discrete gyri cannot be identified. The ventricle is compressed by the edema and appears slit-like.*

(<0.60; normal is 0.70) (Fig. 36-19). This increase may occur in the absence of grayscale abnormalities and may be the only indication of ischemic injury. As diffuse cerebral edema develops, vascular resistance increases, which reduces diastolic flow decreases and increases the resistive index.

Congenital Malformations

Congenital brain malformations can be related to errors in vessel formation, neural tube closure, diverticulation (separation into two hemispheres), or neural tissue migration and sulcation (development of sulci). Ultrasonography can be used to diagnose and classify many of these anomalies.

ERRORS IN VESSEL FORMATIONS (VEIN OF GALEN MALFORMATION)

The vein of Galen malformation is a vascular irregularity characterized by a fistula between the cerebral arteries and the vein of Galen. Abnormal feeding vessels drain into the vein of Galen, which becomes markedly enlarged. Affected neonates present soon after birth with congestive heart failure.

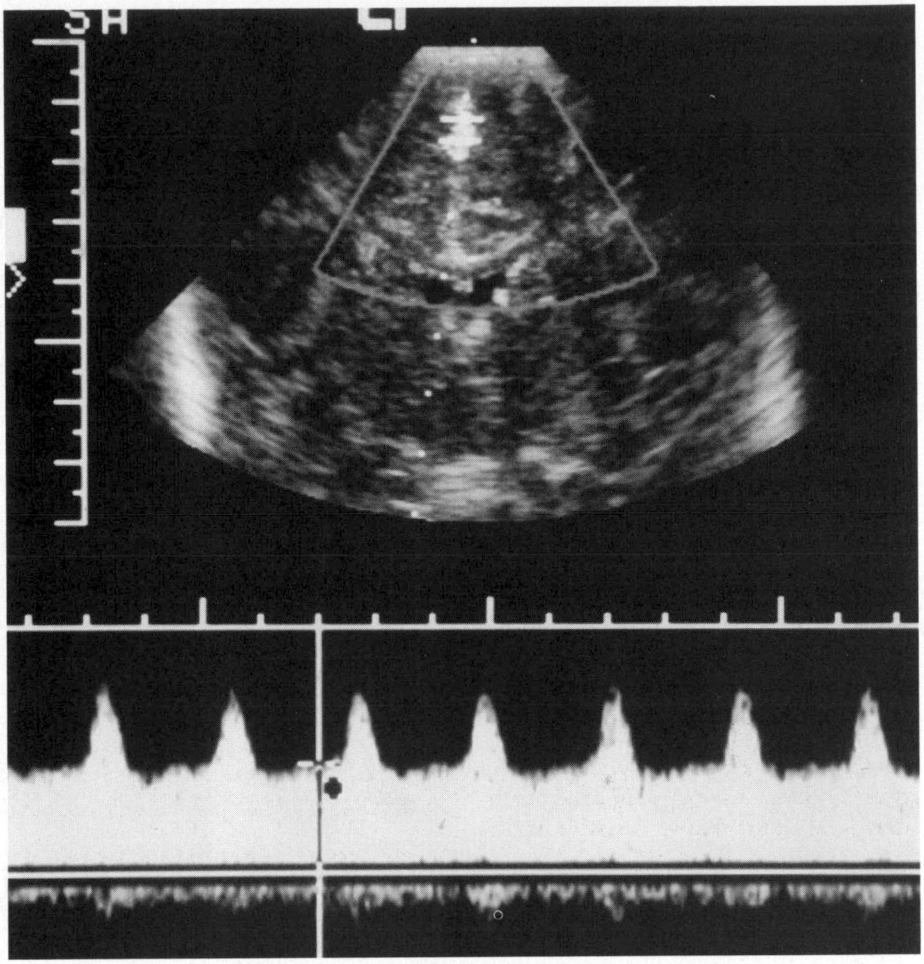

Figure 36-19. ■ *Ischemic injury. Doppler insonation of the anterior cerebral artery shows elevated diastolic flow and a slow systolic upstroke. Resistive index = 0.41.*

The vein of Galen appears as a well-circumscribed, midline cystic space posterior to the third ventricle (Fig. 36-20). It drains into a dilated straight sinus. If the vein is very large, it can compress the third ventricle resulting in hydrocephalus. Blood flow to the periphery of the brain is decreased because blood is shunted to the lower resistance vein of Galen. This decreased perfusion can result in brain atrophy and parenchymal calcifications. Doppler imaging of the dilated vein of Galen shows turbulent flow with increased diastolic and systolic flow velocities and arterialization of venous flow.

NEURAL TUBE CLOSURE DISORDERS

Encephalocele

An encephalocele is herniation of meninges or a portion of the brain through a hole in the midline of the skull. The hole is usually located in the occipital area of the skull, but it may also be lo-

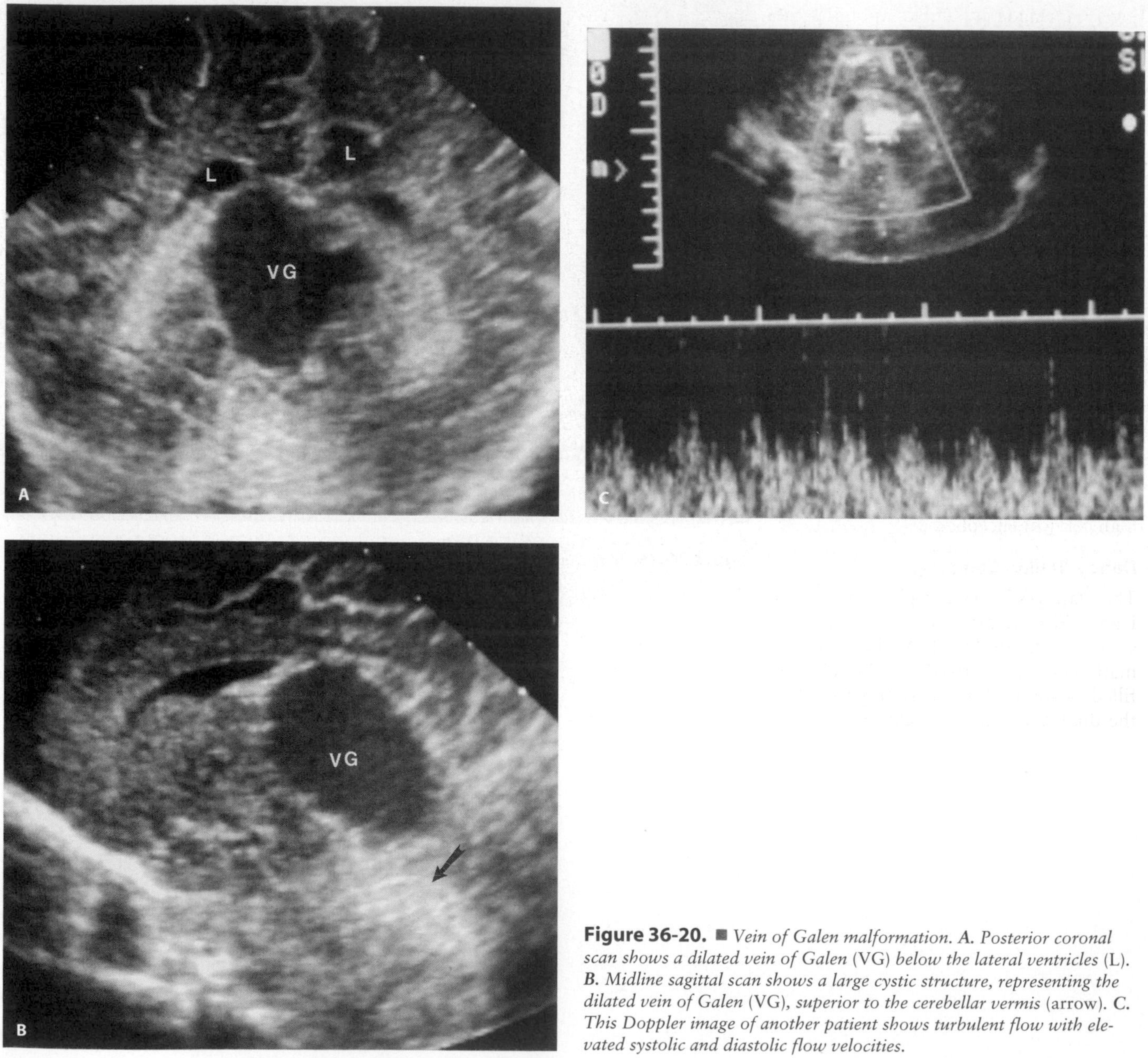

Figure 36-20. ■ *Vein of Galen malformation.* ***A.*** *Posterior coronal scan shows a dilated vein of Galen* (VG) *below the lateral ventricles* (L). ***B.*** *Midline sagittal scan shows a large cystic structure, representing the dilated vein of Galen* (VG), *superior to the cerebellar vermis* (arrow). ***C.*** *This Doppler image of another patient shows turbulent flow with elevated systolic and diastolic flow velocities.*

cated in the nasal or frontal regions. The mass is almost entirely fluid filled. Some encephaloceles may contain small amounts of echogenic brain tissue.

Arnold-Chiari Malformation

Arnold-Chiari malformation refers to three major anomalies involving the posterior fossa. Chiari II malformation is the most common type seen in neonates. It is nearly always associated with a myelomeningocele. On sonography, the posterior fossa is small, and the cerebellum is displaced inferiorly into the cervical spinal canal, obliterating the cisterna magna (Fig. 36-21). The fourth ventricle is elongated. The third and lateral ventricles are often dilated as a result of elongation and stenosis of the aqueduct draining the third ventricle. The massa intermedia in the third ventricle is large. Partial or total absence of the corpus callosum is a common associated anomaly. Scanning through the upper cervical spine can improve visualization of the low-lying cerebellum. Chiari I malformation is characterized by displacement of the cerebellar tonsils into the upper cervical spinal canal. There is no associated myelomeningocele. Chiari III malformation is herniation of the cerebellum, medulla, and fourth ventricle into a high cervical encephalocele.

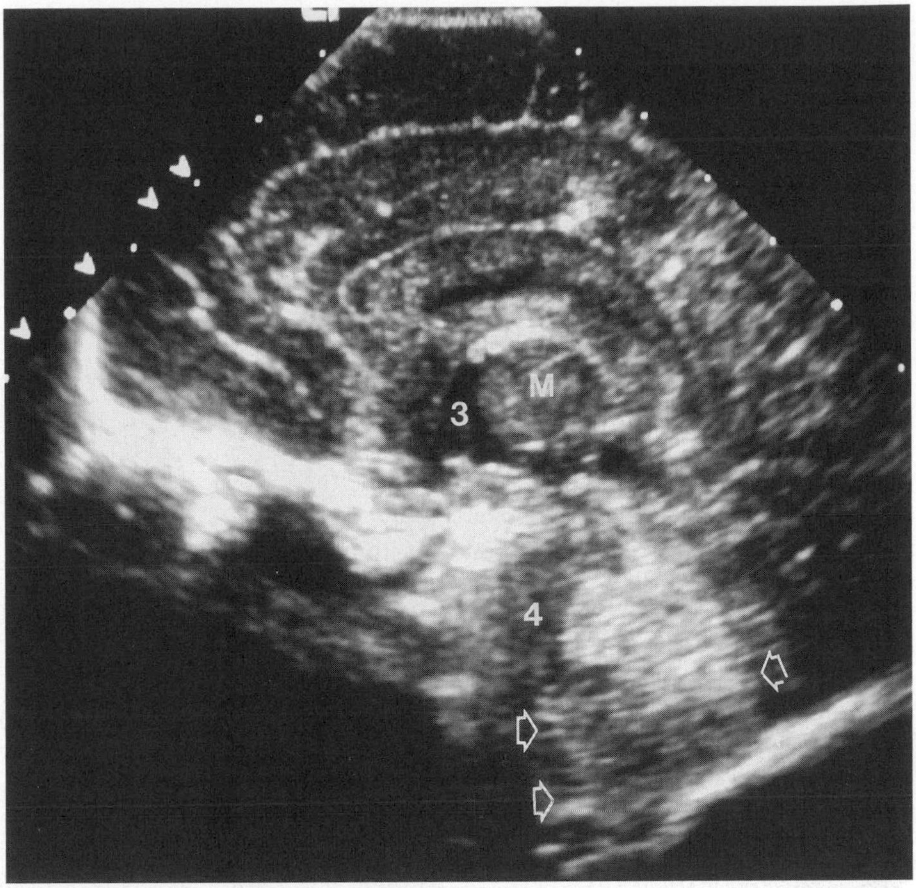

Figure 36-21. ■ *Chiari II malformation. The midline sagittal scan shows a low-lying cerebellar vermis* (open arrows), *resulting in compression of the fourth ventricle* (4) *and obliteration of the cisterna magna, which should be noted on the midline image. Also note a prominent massa intermedia* (M) *within the third ventricle* (3).

Dandy-Walker Complex

The Dandy-Walker complex consists of Dandy-Walker malformations and variants. The classic Dandy-Walker malformation is characterized by a large fluid-filled posterior fossa cyst (representing the dilated fourth ventricle), a small or absent vermis, small cerebellar hemispheres, and superior elevation of the tentorium (Fig. 36-22). Hydrocephalus is present in most cases. The Dandy-Walker variant refers to a milder abnormality of the posterior fossa. It is characterized by milder enlargement of the fourth ventricle, a hypoplastic vermis, and a near-normal-size posterior fossa. Hydrocephalus is often absent.

Dandy-Walker complex needs to be differentiated from a posterior fossa arachnoid cyst and a mega cisterna magna. An arachnoid cyst does not communicate with the fourth ventricle, although it may displace or compress the fourth ventricle, cerebellum, and brainstem. A mega cisterna magna is a normal variant (although it may be associated with aneuploidy in utero). It is associated with a normal fourth ventricle, cerebellum, and brainstem and shows no mass effect.

Agenesis of the Corpus Callosum

The corpus callosum is a midline band of tissue that bridges the two cerebral hemispheres, allowing for shared learning and memory. Agenesis may be complete or partial. The hypoechoic band of the corpus callosum is either completely absent or partially thinned or absent. The lateral ventricles are widely separated and the frontal horns are angled laterally. The occipital horns of the lateral ventricles have a parallel orientation. The third ventricle is elevated superiorly, extending between the lateral ventricles.

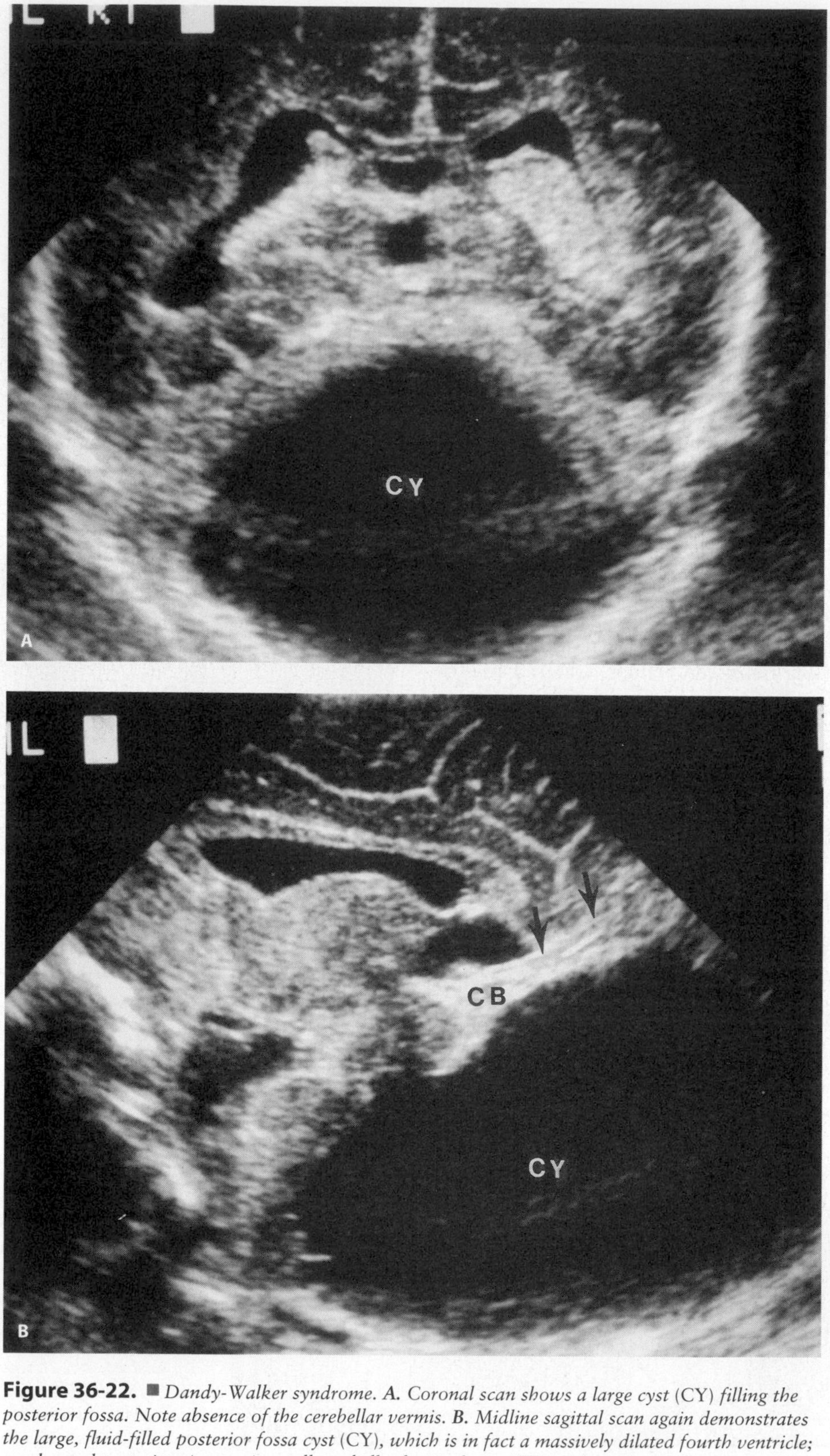

Figure 36-22. ■ *Dandy-Walker syndrome. A. Coronal scan shows a large cyst* (CY) *filling the posterior fossa. Note absence of the cerebellar vermis. B. Midline sagittal scan again demonstrates the large, fluid-filled posterior fossa cyst* (CY), *which is in fact a massively dilated fourth ventricle; an elevated tentorium* (arrows); *small cerebellar hemispheres* (CB), *and an absent vermis.*

The gyri are vertically rather than horizontally aligned (Fig. 36-23).

Lipoma of the corpus callosum is a common associated finding. This highly echogenic mass occurs in the expected location of the corpus callosum and often extends into the cerebral hemispheres.

DISORDERS OF DIVERTICULATION

Holoprosencephaly

Holoprosencephaly is a congenital malformation in which there is failure of diverticulation (separation of the brain above the tentorium into midline structures). The posterior fossa structures are normal. Three forms of holoprosencephaly have been described: alobar, semilobar, and lobar.

Alobar. Alobar holoprosencephaly is the most severe form of this condition. It is characterized by complete absence of diverticulation and is usually fatal. Affected neonates die soon after birth.

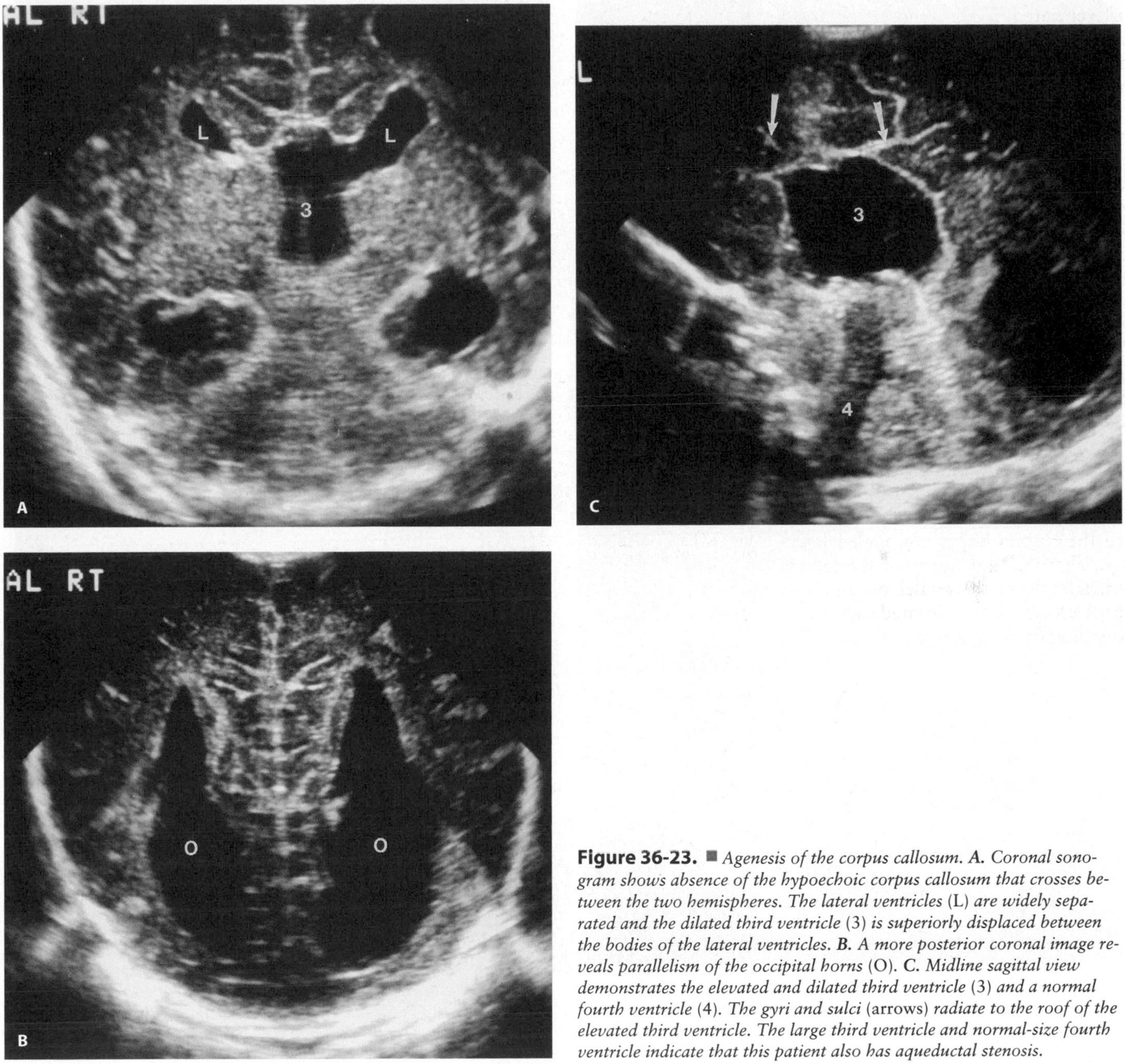

Figure 36-23. ■ *Agenesis of the corpus callosum.* ***A.*** *Coronal sonogram shows absence of the hypoechoic corpus callosum that crosses between the two hemispheres. The lateral ventricles* (L) *are widely separated and the dilated third ventricle* (3) *is superiorly displaced between the bodies of the lateral ventricles.* ***B.*** *A more posterior coronal image reveals parallelism of the occipital horns* (O). ***C.*** *Midline sagittal view demonstrates the elevated and dilated third ventricle* (3) *and a normal fourth ventricle* (4). *The gyri and sulci* (arrows) *radiate to the roof of the elevated third ventricle. The large third ventricle and normal-size fourth ventricle indicate that this patient also has aqueductal stenosis.*

This form of the anomaly has a single, horseshoe-shaped, midline ventricle that is surrounded by a thin cortical rim (Fig. 36-24). The single ventricle may dilate and herniate dorsally (referred to as a *dorsal sac*). The thalami are fused. There is no differentiation into frontal, temporal, or occipital horns. The third ventricle, corpus callosum, and interhemispheric fissures are absent.

Semilobar. Semilobar holoprosencephaly is an intermediate form of holoprosencephaly in which there is partial development of the two cerebral hemispheres. A single frontal horn and ven-

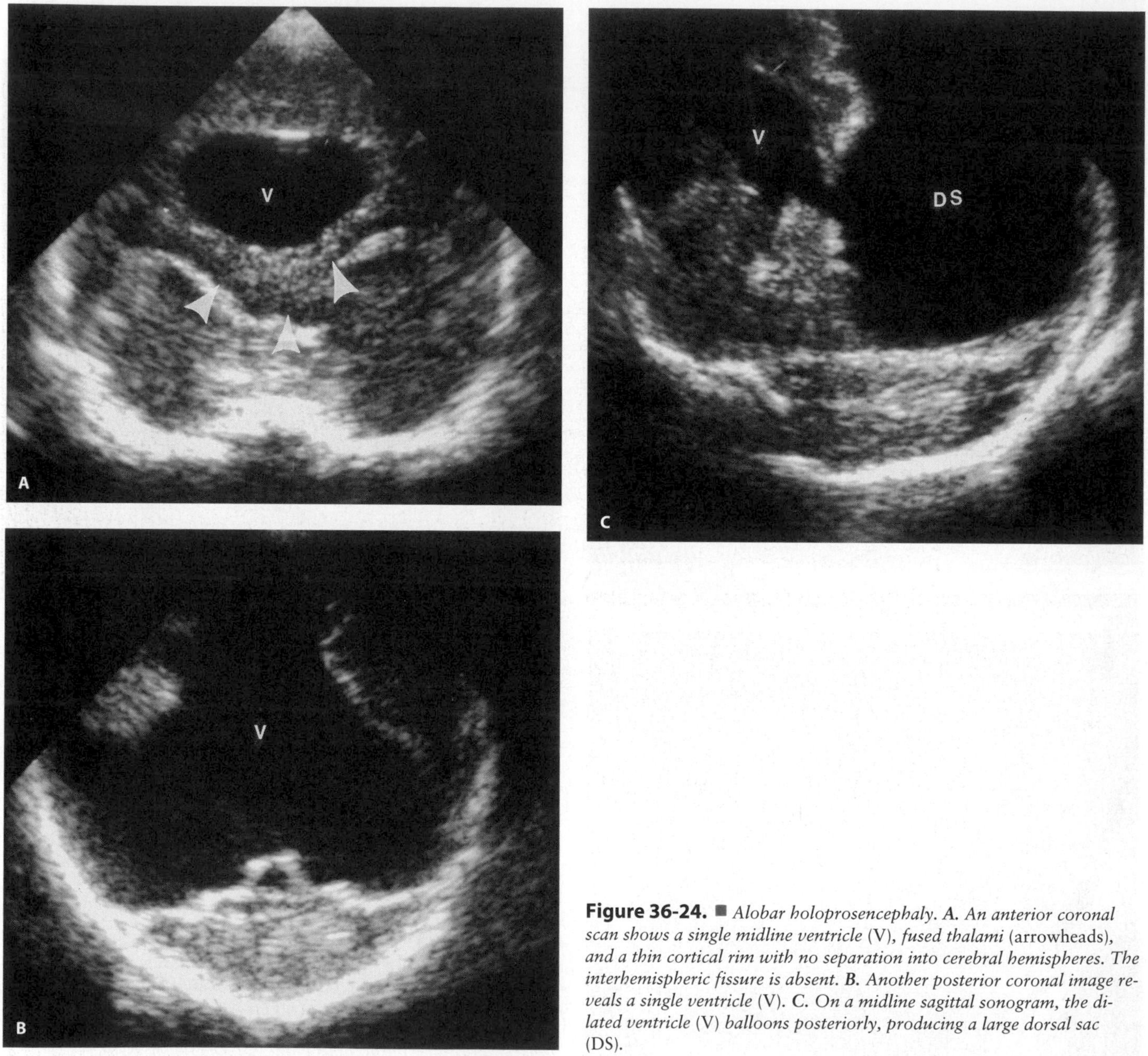

Figure 36-24. ■ *Alobar holoprosencephaly.* ***A.*** *An anterior coronal scan shows a single midline ventricle* (V), *fused thalami* (arrowheads), *and a thin cortical rim with no separation into cerebral hemispheres. The interhemispheric fissure is absent.* ***B.*** *Another posterior coronal image reveals a single ventricle* (V). ***C.*** *On a midline sagittal sonogram, the dilated ventricle* (V) *balloons posteriorly, producing a large dorsal sac* (DS).

tricular body are present, but there is some separation of the occipital and temporal horns. The thalami are partially separated (Fig. 36-25). The posterior interhemispheric fissure and the posterior part of the corpus callosum are present. The third ventricle is small or absent.

Lobar. Lobar holoprosencephaly is the mildest form of holoprosencephaly. The frontal horns are fused and have flat roofs, and the septum pellucidum is ab-

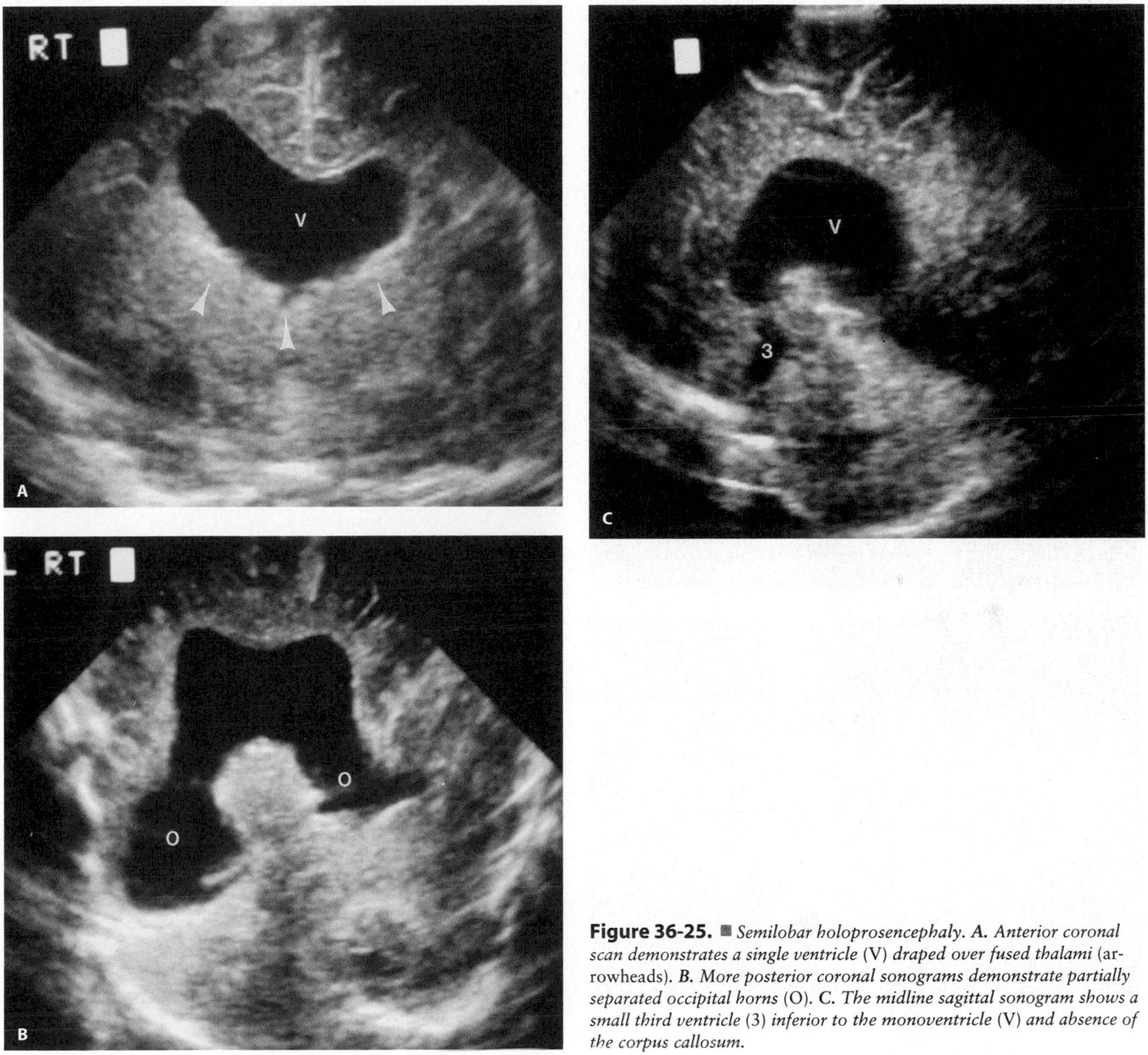

Figure 36-25. ■ *Semilobar holoprosencephaly.* ***A.*** *Anterior coronal scan demonstrates a single ventricle* (V) *draped over fused thalami* (arrowheads). ***B.*** *More posterior coronal sonograms demonstrate partially separated occipital horns* (O). ***C.*** *The midline sagittal sonogram shows a small third ventricle* (3) *inferior to the monoventricle* (V) *and absence of the corpus callosum.*

sent (Fig. 36-26). The anterior interhemispheric fissure is present but shallow. The thalami, occipital, and temporal horns of the lateral ventricles, as well as the third ventricle, are normal.

Isolated absence of the septum pellucidum can occur as a normal variant and should not be confused with lobar holoprosencephaly. The presence of a well-developed anterior interhemispheric fissure favors benign absence of the septum pellucidum, rather than holoprosencephaly. Definitive separation of the two conditions usually requires magnetic resonance imaging (MRI), however.

DISORDERS OF MIGRATION AND SULCATION

Errors in migration and sulcation (development of sulci) include lissencephaly and schizencephaly. When these malformations are severe, they can be seen by sonography. More subtle malformations require MRI for diagnosis.

Lissencephaly

Lissencephaly results in a smooth four-layered cortex instead of the normal six-layer cortex. The gyri are either absent or reduced in number. Sonographic findings include a smooth cortical surface, ventricular dilatation, widened subarachnoid spaces, and sylvian fissures.

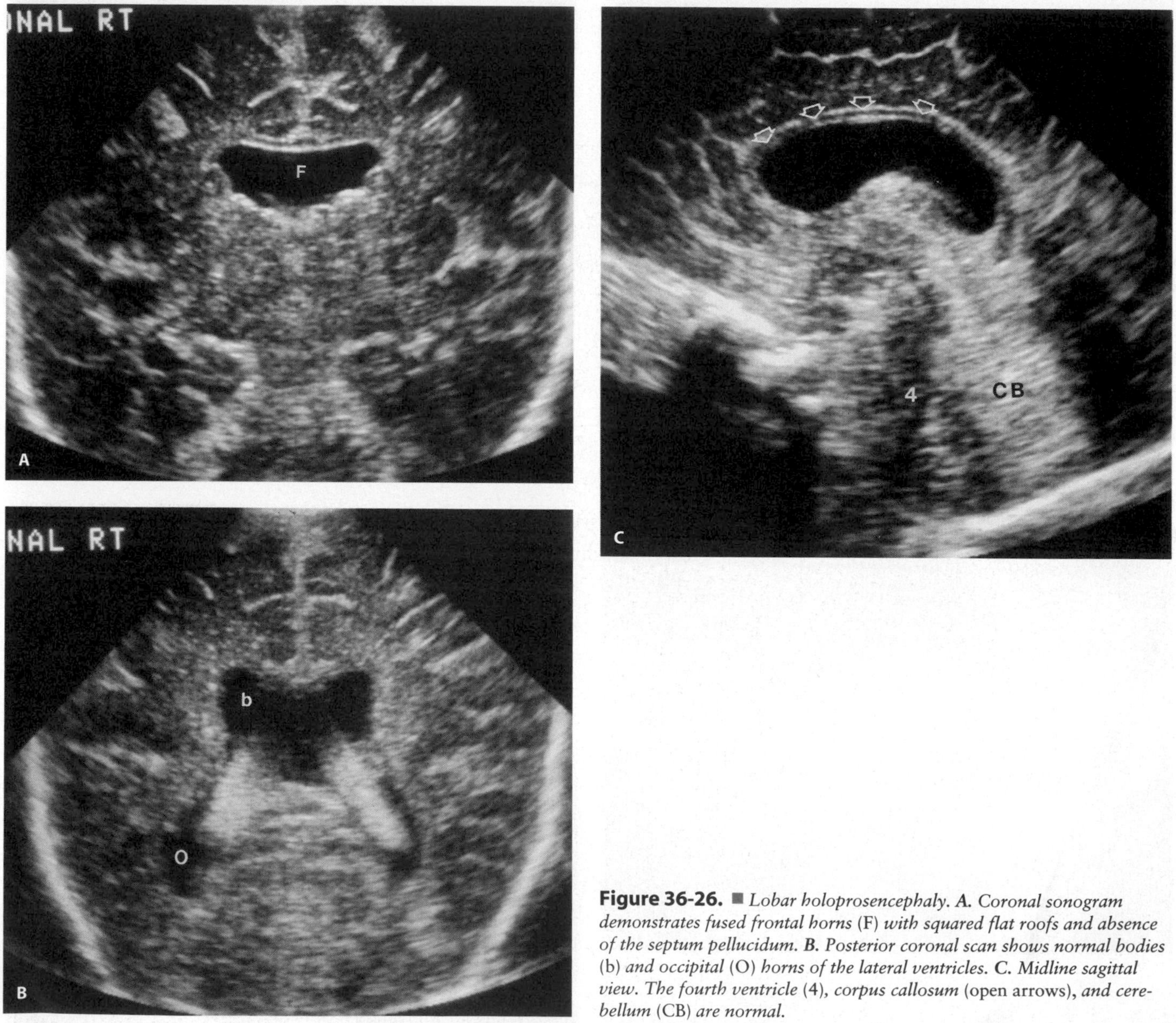

Figure 36-26. ■ *Lobar holoprosencephaly. **A.** Coronal sonogram demonstrates fused frontal horns* (F) *with squared flat roofs and absence of the septum pellucidum. **B.** Posterior coronal scan shows normal bodies* (b) *and occipital* (O) *horns of the lateral ventricles. **C.** Midline sagittal view. The fourth ventricle* (4), *corpus callosum* (open arrows), *and cerebellum* (CB) *are normal.*

Schizencephaly

Schizencephaly is characterized by irregular fluid-filled clefts that extend from the lateral ventricles to the brain's surface (Fig. 36-27). Bilateral clefts may be unilateral or bilateral and symmetric or asymmetric. They communicate with the lateral ventricles. Absence of the septum, pellucidum, and a thinned corpus callosum are other common findings.

Intracranial Infection

CONGENITAL BRAIN INFECTIONS

The common causes of infection in the fetus are cytomegalovirus, *Toxoplasma gondii*, rubella virus, and herpes simplex type 2 virus.

Parenchymal calcifications and a mineralizing vasculopathy are the characteristic findings of congenital infection. Calcifications appear as echogenic foci with or without distal acoustic shadowing. The mineralizing vasculopathy is characterized by linear, nonshadowing areas of echogenicity in the thalami and basal ganglia. The echogenic foci follow the distribution of the lenticulostriate arteries (Fig. 36-28). Other findings of fetal infection include ventricular dilatation, echogenic brain parenchyma, and

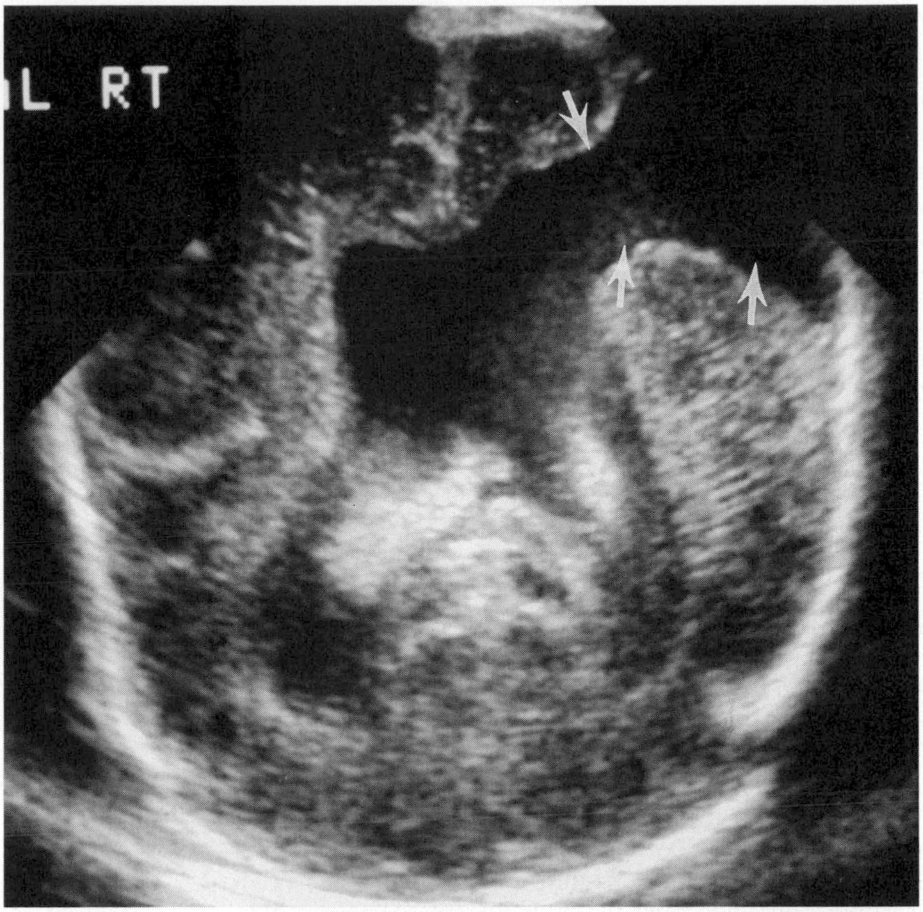

Figure 36-27. ■ *Schizencephaly. Posterior coronal sonogram shows a large, unilateral, fluid-filled cleft* (arrows) *in the left hemisphere. The cleft extends from the lateral ventricle to the brain surface.*

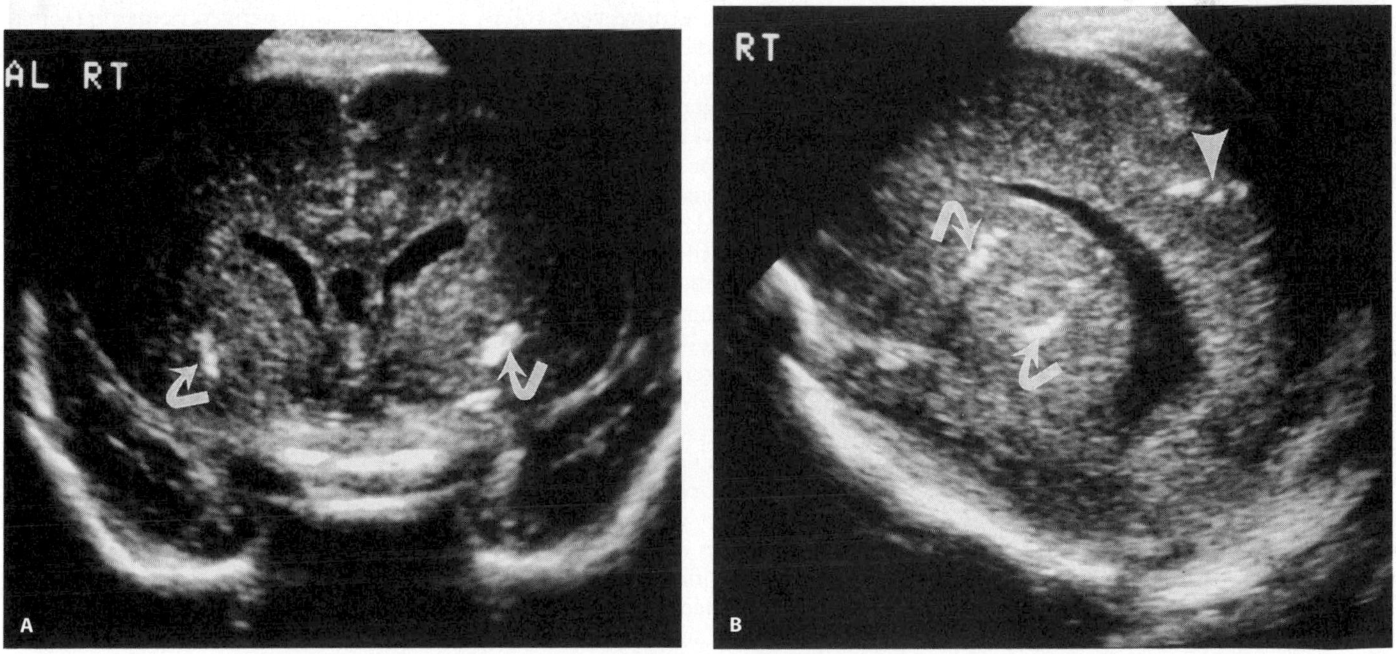

Figure 36-28. ■ *Cytomegalovirus infection. (A) Coronal and (B) sagittal images show linear, echogenic structures* (curved arrows) *within the basal ganglia, representing mineralized vessels. Also noted are clusters of punctate calcifications in the brain parenchyma* (arrowhead). *Cultures were positive for cytomegalovirus.*

encephalomalacia. Subdural effusions are relatively uncommon in intrauterine brain infections.

MENINGITIS

Sonography is often normal early in the course of meningitis. Findings in more extensive disease include fluid collections over the brain's surface and focal or diffuse areas of increased parenchymal echogenicity. Spread of infection to the ventricles causes ventricular dilatation with increased echogenicity of the ventricular walls. Echogenic fluid and debris may be noted in the lumen. Brain abscess is a complication of severe infection and causes a hypoechoic mass with thick, echogenic walls. Associated mass effect with ventricular displacement is common.

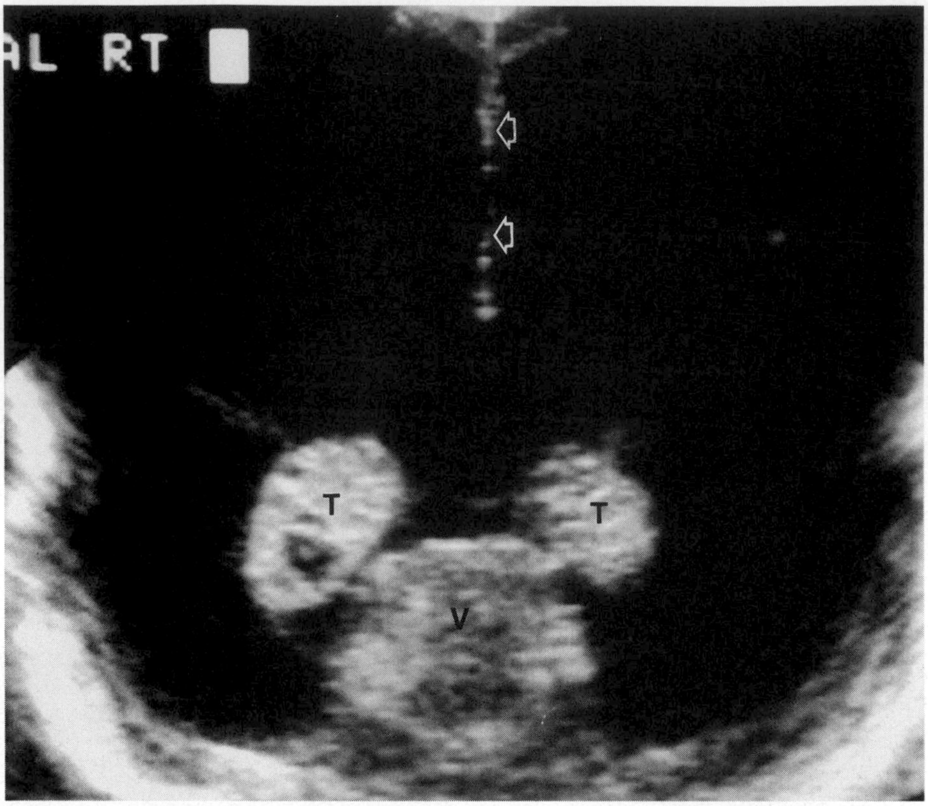

Figure 36-29. ■ *Hydranencephaly. Coronal image shows replacement of cerebral brain tissue by a large fluid-filled sac. The thalami* (T), *cerebellar vermis* (V), *and falx cerebri* (open arrows) *are normal.*

Other Brain Lesions

HYDRANENCEPHALY

Hydranencephaly is the result of in utero occlusion of both internal carotid arteries, which leads to destruction of the cerebral hemispheres. A thin-walled sac containing CSF replaces brain tissue (Fig. 36-29). The thalami and posterior fossa structures are normal. The falx is present. Identification of the falx helps differentiate this condition from the holoprosencephalies.

PORENCEPHALIC CYST

A porencephalic cyst is a cystic lesion that results from focal brain destruction early in gestation. It appears as a thin-walled anechoic cavity, usually without septations, in the cerebral hemispheres.

Pitfalls

1. Choroid plexus versus intraventricular hemorrhage. Choroid plexus is located in the nondependent part of the lateral ventricles, and hemorrhage favors the dependent part. Examining the patient in both decubitus positions can show that blood moves or forms a fluid–fluid level, whereas the choroid plexus will not change position. Moreover, a blood clot is avascular on Doppler imaging, and the choroid plexus shows flow.
2. Caudothalamic groove versus germinal matrix (subependymal) bleed. The normal caudothalamic groove is a thin echogenic line with a tapered end between the caudate nucleus and thalamus. Bleeds have a round or bulbous termination.
3. Cerebellar bleed. Cerebellar hemorrhage may be difficult to detect because the cerebellum is normally echogenic. Asymmetry of echogenicity should suggest hemorrhage.
4. Subarachnoid versus subdural fluid. Both appear as fluid collections over the brain surface. Subarachnoid fluid has crossing vessels, whereas subdural fluid does not.
5. Periventricular halo versus leukomalacia. Periventricular echogenicity is a normal finding. It is usually iso- or hypoechoic to normal choroid plexus and often has poorly defined margins. On scans through the posterior fossa, the echogenic halo becomes less evident. In patients with periventricular leukomalacia, the echogenicity is usually more intense than choroid plexus and the margins are fairly well defined. Periventricular leukomalacia persists unchanged on scans through the posterior fontanelle.

SELECTED READING

Babcock DS. Sonography of the brain in infants: role in evaluating neurologic abnormalities. *AJR Am J Roentgenol* 1995;165:417–423.

Bellah RD. Intracranial hemorrhage and ischemia in the premature infant. In: Bluth EI, Arger PH, Benson CB, et al., eds. *Ultrasound: A Practical Approach to Clinical Problems.* New York: Thieme; 1999:503–530.

Siegel MJ. Brain. In: Siegel MJ, ed. *Pediatric Sonography,* 3rd ed. Philadelphia: Lippincott Williams & Wilkins; 2002:41–121.

37 Spinal Ultrasonography

MARILYN J. SIEGEL

KEY WORDS

Cauda Equina. The nerve root fibers arising from the terminal end of the spinal cord.

Cerebrospinal Fluid. Fluid that surrounds the spinal cord to protect it from rapid movement.

Conus Medullaris. The inferior (distal) termination of the spinal cord. The normal conus tip lies above the second to third lumbar (L2 to L3) level.

Dermal Sinus. A tract that extends from the skin surface to the deeper tissues. It may end in the subcutaneous tissues, or it may extend deeper to the level of the spinal cord.

Dermoid cyst. A cystic mass that contains hair and/or skin.

Diastematomyelia. Condition in which the spinal cord is split sagittally into two hemicords by a bony, cartilaginous, or fibrous septum.

Filum terminale. A cord-like structure that extends from the conus tip to the first coccygeal (S1) segment. It is surrounded by nerve roots of the cauda equina.

Hydromyelia. Dilatation of the central canal of the spinal cord.

Lipoma. Fat-containing mass that is usually associated with dysraphism, particularly in the form of a lipomeningocele.

Lipomyelomeningocele. This lesion is similar to that of a myelomeningocele, but with the addition of a lipoma.

Meningocele. An expanded subarachnoid space.

Myelocele. A form of spinal dysraphism in which the spinal cord is open and located at the level of the skin surface posteriorly.

Myelomeningocele. This lesion is similar to a myelocele except that it lies above the skin surface. There is no fluid-filled sac surrounding nerve fibers.

Neural Placode. The open spinal cord that protrudes onto the skin surface posteriorly.

Pilonidal Sinus. Deep hair-containing tract in the skin that overlies the sacrum and coccyx.

Spina Bifida. Refers to incomplete closure of the spine's bony elements.

Spinal Dysraphism. Refers to a group of spinal anomalies, all of which have bony spina bifida and incomplete closure of the spinal canal, overlying soft tissues, and skin. The spinal canal contents may protrude posteriorly onto the skin.

Subarachnoid Space. Fluid-filled space that surrounds the cord and is lined by meninges. The outer meningeal layer, closest to the bony spine, is the dura mater. The inner layer, closest to the cord, contains the pia mater and the arachnoid. The subarachnoid space extends to about the second to fourth coccygeal (S2 to S4) level.

Syringomyelia. Fluid-filled space within the cord. Usually located outside of the central canal.

Tethered Cord. Abnormal low position of the spinal cord's distal end in the spinal canal. The cord normally ends around L2 or L3.

The Clinical Problem

Sonography is an excellent method for evaluating the spinal canal and cord in neonates and young infants. The incompletely ossified midline posterior arches of the vertebral column provide an acoustic window that allows transmission of the ultrasound beam. The most common clinical indication for spinal sonography is a midline cutaneous lesion on the lower back, which has a high association with spinal dysraphism. Such lesions include skin dimples, hemangiomas, sinus tracts, hyperpigmented plaques, and hairy patches. Sonography is also performed in newborns with bony defects of the spine noted on plain radiographs (e.g., sacral absence) and/or the VATER syndrome (*v*ertebral anomalies, *a*nal atresia, *t*racheo*e*sophageal fistula, *r*enal and radial anomalies). Both of these conditions also have an increased frequency of dysraphism. Finally, sonography is performed in neonates with lower-extremity weakness or paralysis to detect cord compression or tethering and in newborns with suspected birth-related spinal cord injury to detect cord or nerve root lesions. Early detection of spinal lesions through the use of sonography may help treatment planning and decrease long-term morbidity.

High-resolution sonography can reliably show the spinal canal and its contents, and thus demonstrate the presence or absence of disease. If sonography is normal, no further imaging is necessary. If sonography shows spinal malformations, further imaging can be done with computed tomography or magnetic resonance imaging.

Sonographic Technique

Ultrasound of the spine is a reliable method of screening for spinal cord anomalies in infants <6 months of age. After 6 months of age, the acoustic window begins to close as a result of normal ossification of the posterior spinal elements. Subsequently, acoustic shadowing by the ossified spine makes evaluating intraspinal contents difficult.

Spinal sonography is performed with 7- to 15-MHz linear- or curved-array transducers. Scans are obtained with the neonate or infant in the prone position and with the legs flexed to create a relative kyphosis. This position produces splaying of the spinous processes, which improves acoustic access to the spinal canal. Scans are obtained with the transducer positioned in the midline over the unossified spinous processes. In infants with partially ossified posterior spinal elements and smaller acoustic windows, paramedian scans with the transducer positioned lateral and parallel to the spinous processes may improve visualization of spinal anatomy. Images are obtained in both longitudinal and transverse planes from the craniocervical junction to the cauda equina. A split-screen function or the newer extended field of view technology can help in demonstrating the relationship of pathology to normal structures. The level of the spine should be labeled on the image.

Normal Anatomy

On longitudinal scans, the spinal cord is a hypoechoic tubular structure with echogenic anterior and posterior walls and an echogenic central complex, which represents the central canal. The spinal cord is bordered posteriorly by the hypoechoic cartilaginous spinous processes, the echogenic posterior dura mater, and the anechoic posterior subarachnoid space. The cord is bordered anteriorly by the anechoic anterior subarachnoid space and echogenic vertebral bodies. The cord gradually tapers at the level of the first or second lumbar vertebral body to form the conus medullaris. The conus medullaris is continuous with the fibrous filum terminale, which extends into the distal sacral canal. The filum terminale is an echogenic structure, which is surrounded by echogenic nerve roots (cauda equina). It inserts on the dorsal aspect of the first sacral segment (S1) (Fig. 37-1). Differentiation of the filum from adjacent nerve roots of the cauda equina is sometimes not possible by sonography. The subarachnoid space extends to about the second to fourth coccygeal (S2 to S4) level.

On transverse images, the spinal cord appears as a hypoechoic, round or oval structure with a central echogenic complex. Paired echogenic anterior and posterior nerve roots border the conus in the subarachnoid space. Transverse scans further caudad show the echogenic

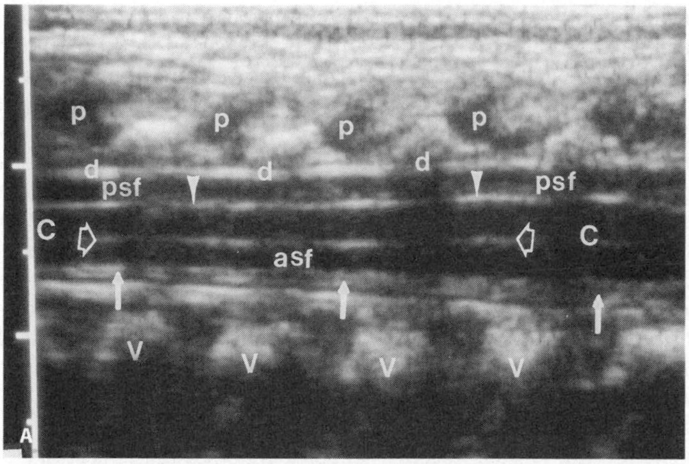

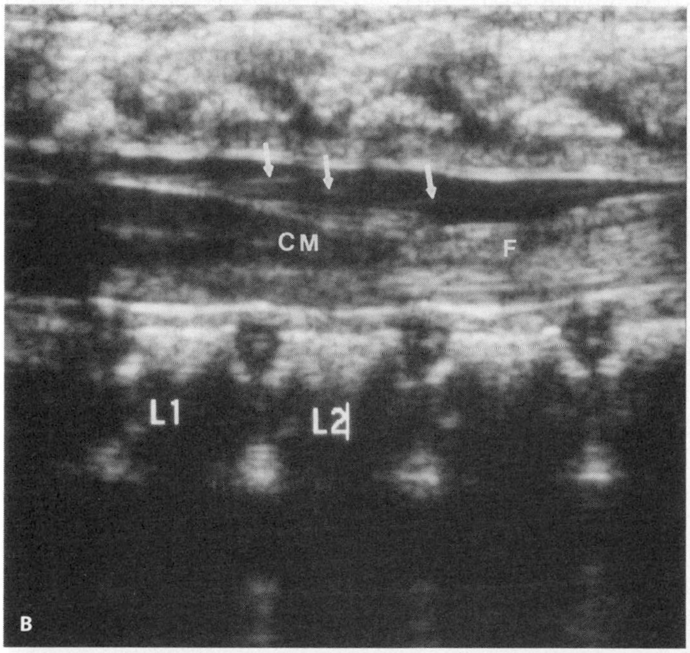

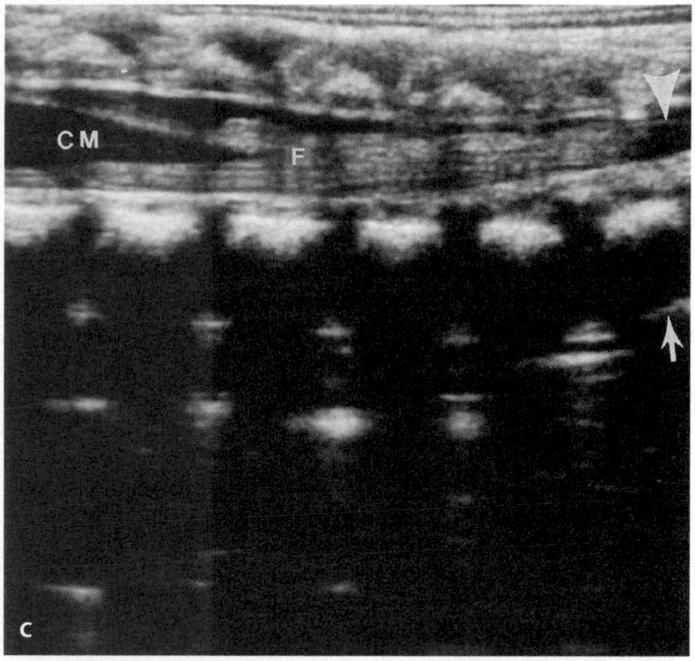

Figure 37-1. ■ *Normal longitudinal anatomy of the spinal cord.* ***A.*** *Longitudinal scan through the lower thoracic and upper lumbar region shows the hypoechoic cartilaginous spinous processes* (p), *echogenic posterior dura mater* (d), *hypoechoic fluid in the posterior subarachnoid space* (psf), *posterior surface of the spinal cord* (arrowheads), *hypoechoic cord* (C) *with central echogenic complex* (open arrows), *anterior surface of the cord* (arrows), *hypoechoic fluid in the anterior subarachnoid space* (asf), *and echogenic vertebral bodies* (v). ***B.*** *Longitudinal scan through the distal cord shows the smoothly tapering conus medullaris* (CM), *nerve roots* (arrows), *and the filum terminale* (F). L1, *first lumbar vertebral body;* L2, *second lumbar vertebral body.* ***C.*** *Longitudinal scan in another neonate shows a normal tapered conus medullaris* (CM) *and the most distal part* (arrowhead) *of the filum terminale* (F). *The filum terminale extends to the level of the S1 vertebral body* (arrow). ***D.*** *Longitudinal extended field of view image shows the conus medullaris* (CM) *and the entire extent of the filum terminale* (F).

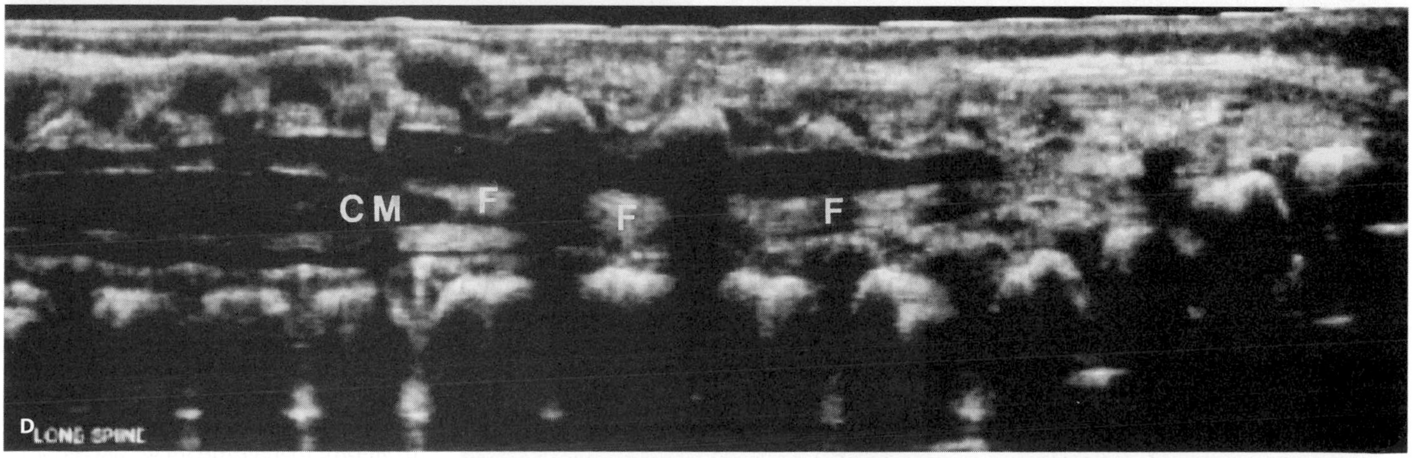

Subacute or chronic hemorrhage is hypo- or anechoic.

On occasion, the dura mater may be lacerated during a lumbar puncture, resulting in cerebrospinal fluid leakage and resultant compression of the subarachnoid space, spinal cord, and/or nerve roots. Typically, the fluid resolves within a few days.

Diagnostic Dilemmas

1. A transient dilated central canal versus hydromyelia. The spinal canal can show transient dilatation in the first week of life. Clinical findings are absent. Hydromyelia (central canal dilatation) is associated with pathologic conditions, does not resolve, and may produce symptoms.
2. Ventriculus terminalis versus syringomyelia. The former resolves and causes no symptoms, whereas the latter is usually associated with pathologic conditions and produces symptoms.
3. Simple meningocele versus myelocele or myelomeningocele. The simple meningocele contains no neural tissue. In the other two conditions, a portion of the spinal cord and its membranes protrude outside the spinal canal.

Where Else to Look

1. If spinal cord tethering is discovered, examine the spinal canal and lower back to see if the cause of tethering is visible.
2. If the cord has a blunted end, look for other signs of caudal regression syndrome, such as renal abnormalities.

SELECTED READING

Barkovitch AJ. Congenital anomalies of the spine. In: Barkovitch AJ, ed. *Pediatric Neuroimaging*, 3rd ed. Philadelphia: Lippincott Williams & Wilkins; 2000:621–684.

Coley BD. Spine. In: Siegel MJ, ed. *Pediatric Sonography*, 3rd ed. Philadelphia; Lippincott Williams & Wilkins; 2002.

Kriss VM, Desai NS. Occult spinal dysraphism in neonates: assessment of high-risk cutaneous stigmata on sonography. *AJR Am J Roentgenol* 1998;171:1687–1692.

Unsinn KM, Geley T, Freund MC, et al. US of the spinal cord in newborns: spectrum of normal findings, variants, congenital anomalies, and acquired diseases. *Radiographics* 2000;20:923–938.

Developmental Dysplasia of the Infant Hip

LYNDAL MACPHERSON

38

KEY WORDS

Acetabular Dysplasia. Abnormal development of the acetabulum tissue.

Acetabular Labrum (Limbus Cartilage). Cartilaginous ring surrounding the periphery of the acetabulum that aids in stabilizing the femoral head within the acetabulum.

Acetabulum. Cup-shaped bony structure formed by the ilium, ischium, and pubis that articulates with the femoral head.

Clicky Hip. As the hip joint is dislocated and reduced, a "click" is heard as the femoral head passes over the posterior labrum of the acetabulum.

Congenital Hip Dislocation. Displacement of the hip joint existing from or before birth. The term is interchangeable with developmental dysplasic hip.

Developmental Dysplastic Hip. Displacement of the hip joint caused by the femoral head moving out of the socket, or the socket not having formed properly. The term is interchangeable with *congenital hip dislocation*, although *developmental dysplasic hip* is more commonly used at the present time.

Dislocatable Hip. The femoral head displaces from the acetabulum during certain stress maneuvers of the leg but returns to its normal position spontaneously once the pressure is released.

Fovea. Indentation (pit) on the femoral head, which provides attachment for the ligamentum teres.

Gluteus Medius Muscle. This muscle originates from the ilium and inserts at the greater trochanter. It stabilizes the hip.

Greater Trochanter. Bony process arising from the superolateral portion of the proximal femoral shaft.

Ilium. Bone that forms the superior portion of the acetabulum.

Intertrochanteric Crest. Prominent ridge between the greater and lesser trochanters on the posterior portion of the proximal femoral shaft.

Ischium. Forms the inferoposterior portion of the acetabulum.

Lesser Trochanter. Bony process located at the posteromedial portion of the proximal femoral shaft.

Ligamentum Teres. Ligament that extends from the edges of the fovea on the femoral head to the edges of the acetabular notch; it contains a branch of the obturator artery.

Ossific Nucleus or Ossification Center. Bony formation appearing as early as 4 weeks of age in the center of the femoral head.

Pavlik Harness. Corrective harness that supports the hips in flexion and abduction without force.

Pubis. Bone that forms the inferoanterior portion of the acetabulum.

Subluxation. Incomplete displacement of the femoral head from the acetabulum during certain stress maneuvers of the leg.

Triradiate Cartilage. Cartilaginous connection between the ilium, ischium, and pubis of the acetabulum.

The Clinical Problem

Ultrasound is widely used for assessing developmental dysplasia of the neonatal hip because it effectively depicts the soft tissue and cartilaginous structures and has the advantage that dynamic movement of the hip joint can be examined. Alternative imaging techniques include:

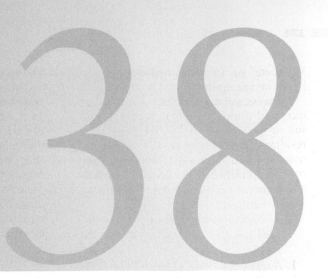

- Radiography: The traditional diagnostic modality used for developmental hip dysplasia. It is not reliable in neonates, as the hip is still a cartilaginous structure that has not yet ossified.
- Arthrography: Demonstrates hip anatomy; it is rarely used because it is invasive and sedation or a general anesthetic are needed.
- Computed tomography: Is helpful in infants confined to a cast; it is not routinely used in diagnosing congenital hip dislocation because it is nondynamic, results in gonadal radiation exposure, and requires sedation.
- Magnetic resonance imaging: Provides exquisite anatomic detail of the soft tissue, cartilage, and bony structures with no radiation expo-

sure, but requires sedation, has a long scanning time, is expensive, and is not dynamic.

Ultrasound is the first tool used because:

1. One can differentiate the cartilage components of the acetabulum and femoral head from other soft-tissue structures.
2. The relationship of the femoral head position to the acetabulum can be seen.
3. A dynamic study of the hip position including the application of stress maneuvers to assess joint laxity can be performed.
4. Fluid in the joint space can be assessed.
5. No ionizing radiation is used.
6. No contrast media is required.
7. It is inexpensive.
8. No sedation is required.
9. The infant hip is easily accessible, and comparable follow-up studies can be performed even when corrective devices such as traction, a cast, or a Pavlik harness are in place.

The cause of developmental hip dysplasia unknown, but:

1. Females are affected substantially more frequently than males (5:1). This gender difference is thought to be due to the maternal hormonal effect of estrogen, which increases muscle laxity (helping with childbirth). This effect is reduced by male hormones.
2. The left hip (60%) is more often involved than the right hip (20%) or both hips (20%).
3. Developmental hip dysplasia is more common in breech presentations; this is thought to be due to extension of the fetal knees and hyperflexion of the fetal hip while the fetus is in the breech position.
4. Developmental hip dysplasia is more common when there has been oligohydramnios.
5. Hip dysplasia is more common in children with a family history of developmental dysplasia of the hip (e.g., a parent or sibling).
6. Firstborns are affected more often.
7. Neuromuscular abnormalities (e.g., spina bifida and arthrogryposis), congenital torticollis, skull-molding deformities, and certain congenital foot deformities have a higher incidence of developmental hip dysplasia.
8. Caucasians, certain Native American tribes, Scandinavians, and people from some regions of Japan appear to have a higher incidence of congenital dislocation of the hip as compared to people of African or Asian descent.

Clinical Examination Technique

The clinical examination remains the principal screening tool for detecting developmental hip dysplasia and is most valuable when performed with experienced hands on a passive infant. The clinical examination usually consists of the Ortolani and Barlow maneuvers.

1. The examiner holds the infant's thigh and positions his or her middle finger over the greater trochanter.
   a. The Ortolani test is performed by abducting and lifting the thigh to bring the femoral head into the acetabulum. The examiner will sense reduction by a palpable "click" if the hip was in fact, dislocated.
   b. The Barlow test is performed by adducting the hip with gentle downward pressure. Dislocation is felt by the examiner as the femoral head slips out of the acetabulum over the posterior labrum. The diagnosis can be confirmed with the Ortolani test.

Certain ancillary signs may be seen with congenital hip dislocation, although they are not conclusive:

1. Asymmetric skin folds, both gluteal and thigh
2. Limited abduction of less than 45 to 60 degrees often noticed during a diaper change
3. Poor movement of the affected limb
4. Limb maintaining a position of outward rotation
5. Shortening of the femur

Early diagnosis and treatment of congenital hip dislocation is essential for proper hip joint development. The most favorable time for sonographic screening evaluation appears to be 6 weeks of age, for the following reasons:

1. Newborns may have minimal subluxation, which corrects itself without intervention by 4 weeks of age.
2. Orthopaedic surgeons like to begin treatment by 2 months of age.
3. Some dysplasia may not occur until after the newborn period.

An ultrasound examination of both hips will be requested in the following circumstances:

1. When the clinical examination is indeterminate
2. To confirm a clinical impression of dislocation or "clicky hip" and to quantitate severity
3. As follow-up to show proper migration of the femoral head with treatment

Anatomy

ACETABULUM

- The newborn pelvic girdle is made up of two coxal bones, each with three components: the ilium, pubis, and ischium. The ilium is the superior component, the pubis is located in the inferoanterior position, and the ischium is inferior and posterior. The triradiate cartilage is a useful landmark that connects the ilium, ischium, and pubis (Figs. 38-1 and 38-2). Sonographically, this cartilage appears hypoechoic and allows penetration of the sound beam. The triradiate cartilage becomes ossified in adulthood and fuses with the ilium, ischium, and pubis to form the acetabulum. Sonographically, these bony segments appear echogenic and cast an acoustic shadow.
- The acetabulum is a cup-shaped structure that articulates with the femoral head as a ball-and-socket joint. The articular surface in the acetabulum is horseshoe shaped and smaller than the articular surface of the femur.
- The acetabular labrum, sometimes called the *limbus cartilage*, is a cartilaginous ring that surrounds the periphery of the acetabulum and forms an extension of the acetabular roof. The labrum is rounded off at the superior and posterior positions of the acetabulum. It narrows the acetabulum and increases its depth, thus supporting and stabilizing the femoral head within the acetabulum. The labrum is best seen in the coronal view as a triangular structure adjacent to the ilium and superolateral to the femoral head. The acetabular labrum is composed of hyaline cartilage with a fibrocartilaginous tip; sonographically, it appears mainly hypoechoic except for the echogenic fibrocartilaginous tip.
- The superior portions of the femur—the femoral head, femoral neck, and greater and lesser trochanters—are cartilaginous in the neonate and can be well visualized by ultrasound.
  1. The femoral head appears as a hypoechoic circle with smooth borders containing fine-stippled echoes spread evenly throughout. The fovea (pit) of the femoral head provides attachment for the ligamentum teres.

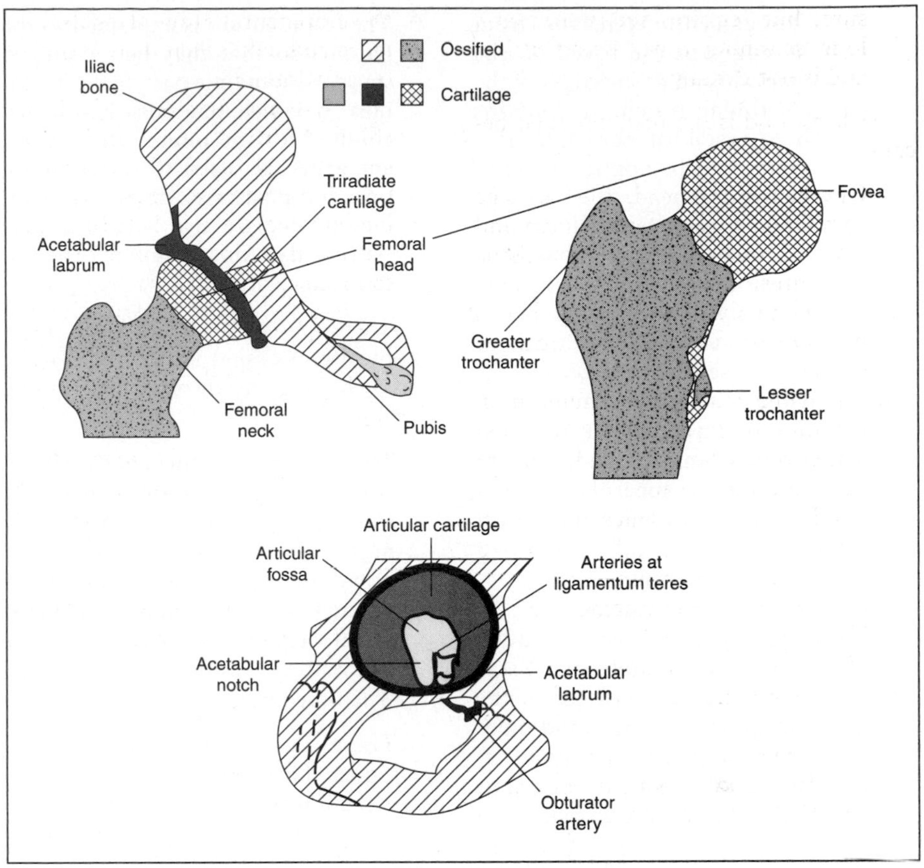

Figure 38-1. ■ *Anatomic drawing of the acetabulum and femur.*

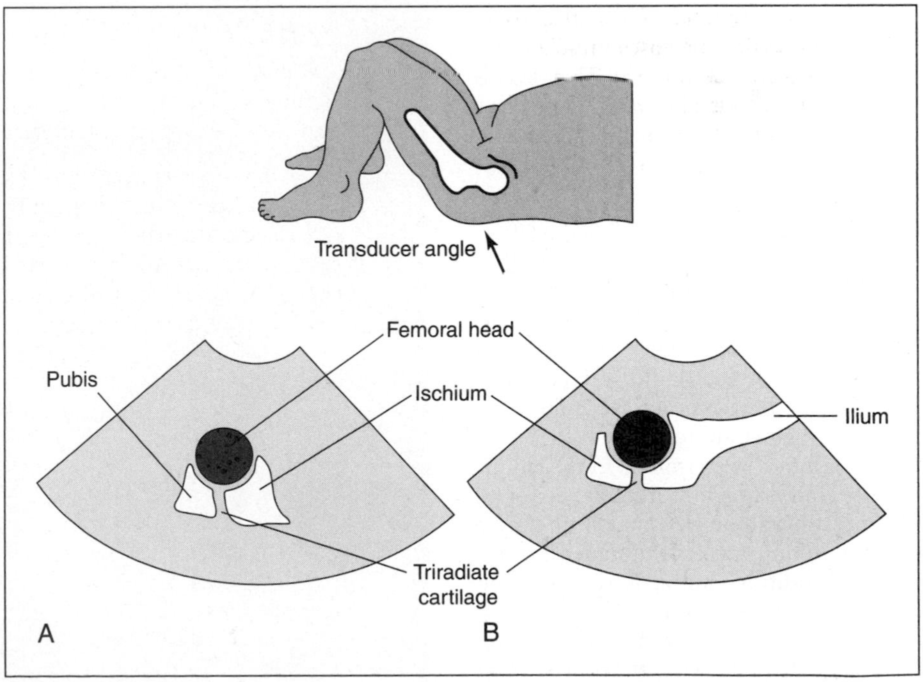

Figure 38-2. ■ *Sketch of an infant showing the transverse (**A**) and coronal (**B**) approach.*

2. The ligamentum teres runs from the edges of the fovea on the femoral head to the edges of the acetabular notch. It contains the branch of the obturator artery, which supplies blood to the femoral head.
3. The echogenic femoral neck angles medially, superiorly, and anteriorly as it tapers toward the femoral head.
4. The greater and lesser trochanters are seen as echogenic areas at the base of the femoral neck protruding from the proximal femoral shaft. The greater trochanter is superolateral, and the lesser trochanter projects off the posteromedial portion of the proximal femoral shaft.
5. The intertrochanteric crest of the femur is the area found between the greater and lesser trochanters at the base of the neck on the posterior portion of the proximal femoral shaft.
6. The femoral shaft is ossified at birth, appearing echogenic and casting an acoustic shadow.
7. The ossific nucleus is a bony formation that appears in the center of the femoral head. It is seen as early as 4 weeks after birth but normally develops between 3 and 8 months, and it appears as an echogenic focus that gradually increases in size with age. If large enough, the ossific nucleus may cast an acoustic shadow.

Technique

1. The ultrasonic features of both hips should be compared using a 5- to 10-MHz real-time linear array transducer. Sector and curved transducers are less desirable because they distort anatomy.
2. The infant is examined in the supine or lateral position. Ideally, a second person/parent helps to immobilize the infant; a cradle designed for lateral position can be used to help immobilize the infant.
3. It is essential that the infant is relaxed for the examination so that the stress and nonstress measurements can be accurately interpreted. The examination is explained to the parents so that they better understand the dynamic part of the examination, which may cause a little discomfort for the infant. Still images are generally used to differentiate pre- and poststress views; however, digital clips are also helpful in presenting dynamic results to the orthopaedic surgeon.

There are two techniques for sonographically assessing the hip: the static Graf technique and the dynamic Harcke technique.

- The Graf technique consists of a coronal image taken from the lateral aspect of the hip. It was previously performed with the femur extended; however, more recently, the usual practice is for the femur to be flexed at 90 degrees consistent with any follow-up examinations required when the infant is in a harness.

There are two types of measuring techniques. Lines and angles are used to assess the hip as follows:

Line 1 is aligned with the ilium, extending through the head of the femur.

Line 2 is drawn from the ilium along the labrum giving the α angle.

Line 3 extends from the bony edge of the acetabulum at the triradiate cartilage to the lowest point of the ilium giving the β angle, which is shown in Figure 38-3.

By measuring α and β, the depth of the acetabulum and the position of the labrum can be determined. The smaller the α angle, and the larger the β angle, the more likely dysplasia is to occur.

The position of the femoral head, labrum, and acetabulum may also be subjectively evaluated.

Another widely used measuring technique is the femoral head coverage method, which calculates the percentage of acetabular coverage around the femoral head. These measurements are simply done by measuring the height of the femoral head and the height of acetabular coverage

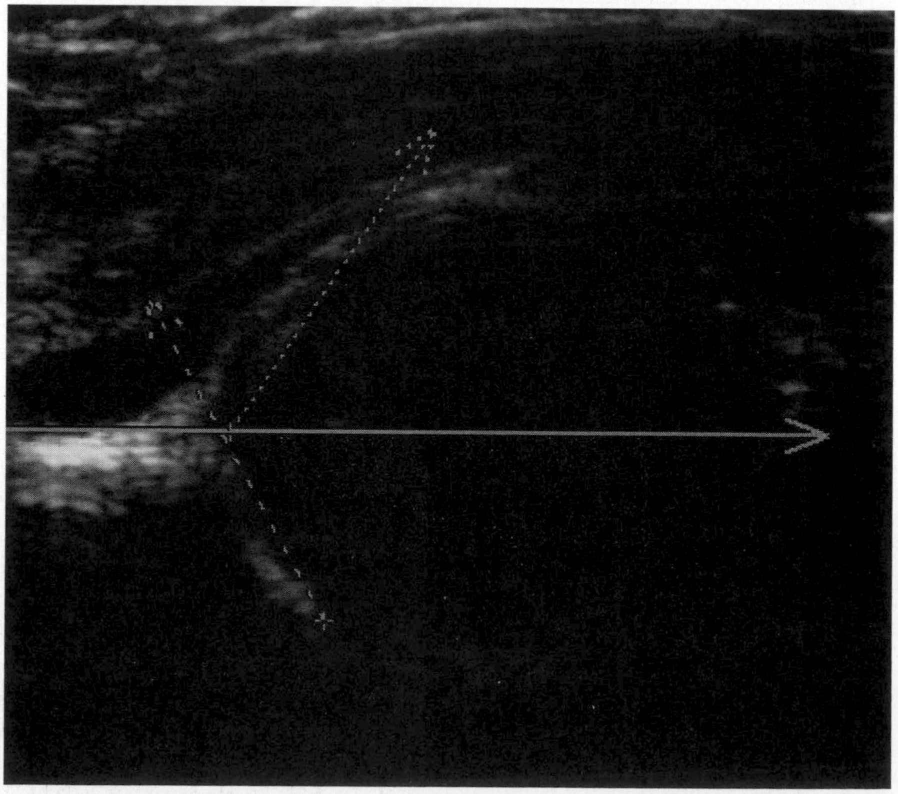

Figure 38-3. ■ *Image showing a normal coronal view measuring alpha and beta angles.*

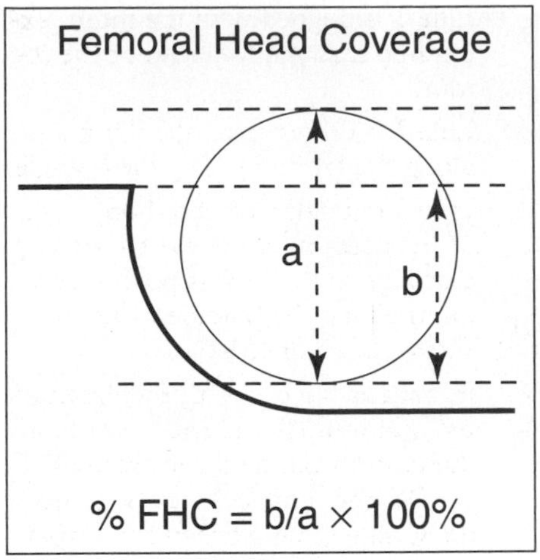

Figure 38-4. ■ *Diagram showing a normal transverse view with a vertical line through the femoral head at ischial and triradiate cartilage borders.*

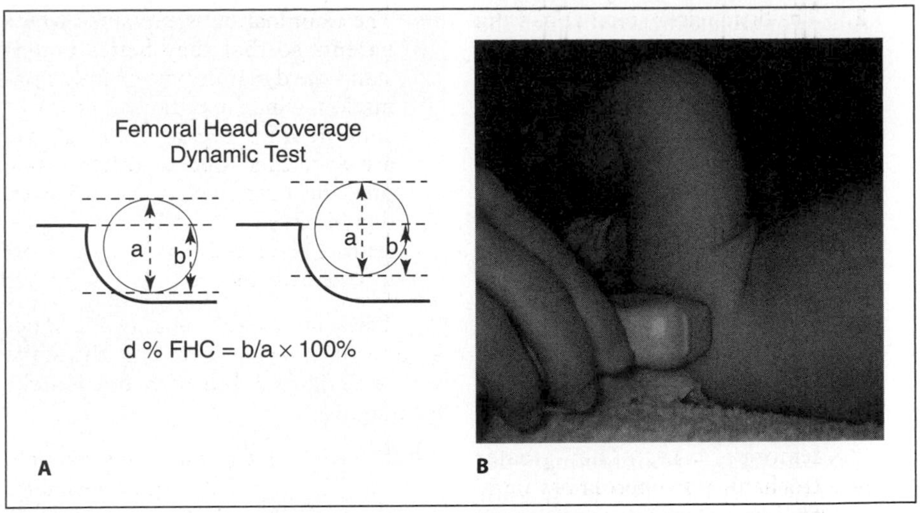

Figure 38-5. ■ *A. Left: Diagram showing a normal coronal view with a horizontal line through the femoral head from the ilium. Right: Coronal view showing dislocation. The horizontal line passes through the upper third of the femoral head. **B.** An infant positioned for the coronal flexion view.*

within the femoral head (Fig. 38-4). This number is then given as a percentage of coverage for both pre- and poststress views (Fig. 38-5).

- The Harcke technique uses a dynamic multiplanar examination making use of clinical techniques, that is, the Ortolani and Barlow maneuvers to assess the hip. Begin by imaging the hip in the transverse neutral position. The hip is then flexed to 90 degrees and imaged both coronally and in the transverse plane. Gentle posterior pressure is applied while the hip is flexed at 90 degrees as it is adducted and abducted. At the same time, the position of the femoral head and its relationship to the acetabulum and any abnormal motion should be noted.
- Both hips are always scanned for comparison. A typical protocol for hip ultrasound is:
  1. Coronal flexion views
     —two images without stress
     —two images with stress
  2. Transverse flexion
     —one image without stress
     —one image with stress
- In cases of dislocation:
  1. Transverse neutral—one image without stress
  2. Posterior lip—one image without stress

CORONAL VIEW

The coronal view is taken in the midacetabular plane and is crucial for assessing acetabular development.

1. Coronal flexion. Place the transducer over the lateral aspect of the infant's hip in a coronal plane (Fig. 38-5B). The femur is flexed at 90 degrees. The echogenic ilium should be seen parallel to the face of the transducer and superior to the femoral head (Fig. 38-6). Adjust the transducer's angle to align the largest diameter of the femoral head with the deepest portion of the acetabulum.

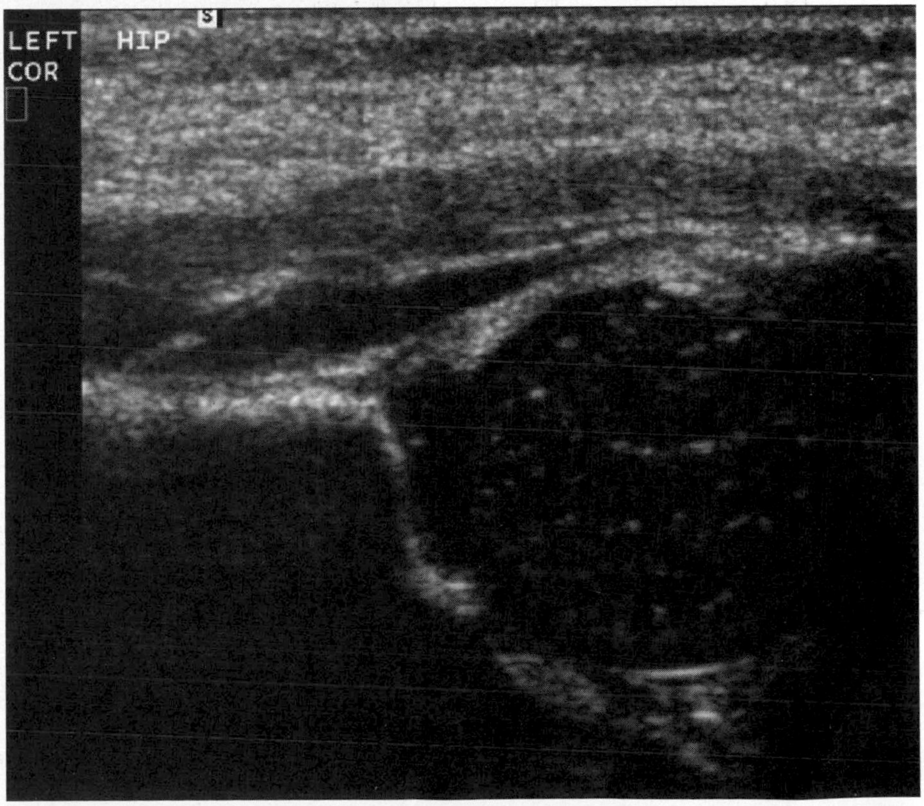

Figure 38-6. ■ *Normal hip seen on a coronal view.*

A horizontal line drawn through the femoral head contiguous with the ilium demonstrates the depth of the acetabulum. The triradiate cartilage is seen at the base of the acetabulum (Fig. 38-2). The acetabular labrum is seen adjacent to the ilium and superolateral to the femoral head. The gluteus medius muscle of the hip joint can also be visualized superolateral to the femoral head and lateral to the ilium. Measurements are taken using Graf or percentage coverage techniques to quantify the femoral head position (Fig. 38-7).

2. Flexion-stress. Maintaining the transducer in the same plane with the echogenic line of the ilium, a small amount of pressure is applied posteriorly to the hip while adducting and maintaining 90-degree flexion. This refers to the stress view and corresponds to the Barlow test used to clinically assess a hip for possible subluxation. The same measurements used in the coronal flexion view can be used here to quantify the femoral head position within the acetabulum after stress is applied, which will help differentiate laxity within the hip joint.

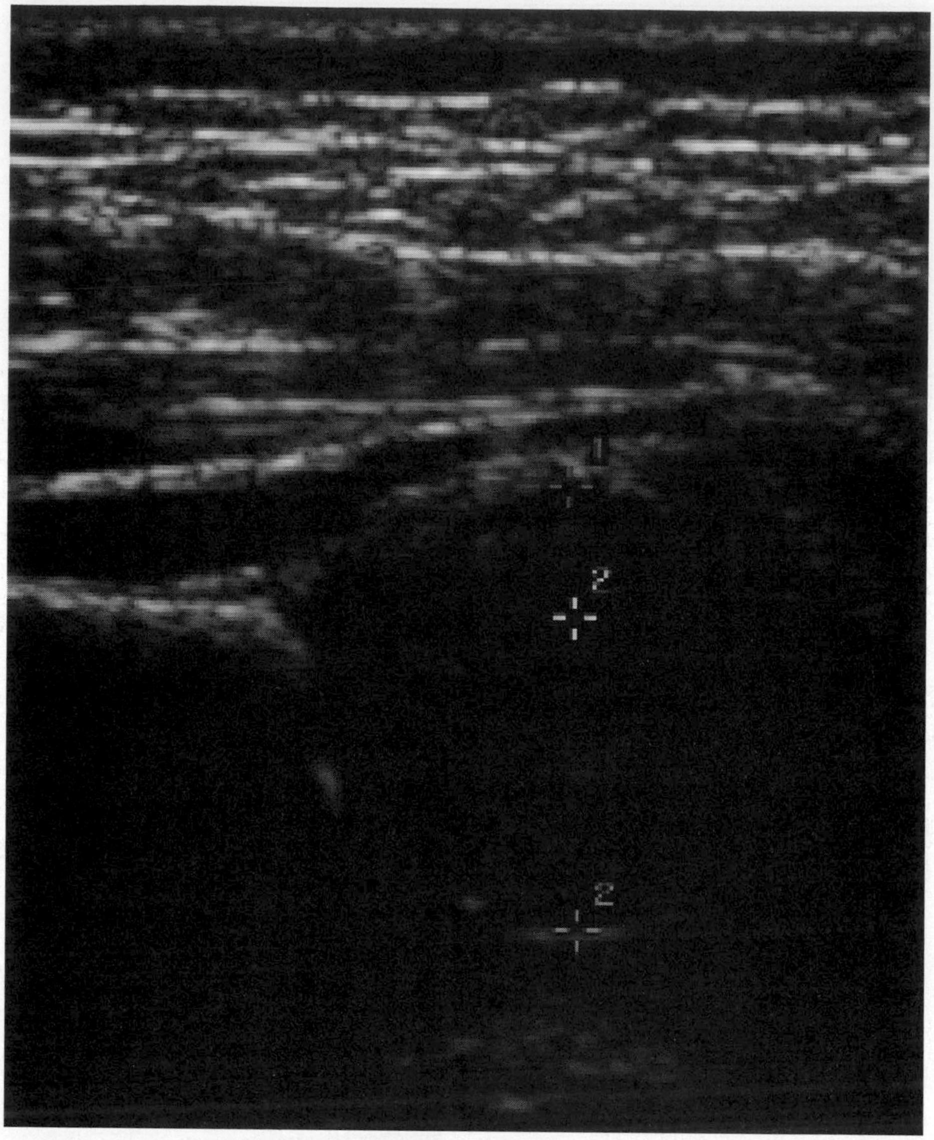

Figure 38-7. ■ *Measurements using the percentage coverage technique to assess femoral head coverage by the acetabulum.*

Figures 38-8 and 38-9 demonstrate mild dysplasia of the acetabulum. Note the echogenic center or ossification center of the femoral head in Figure 38-9. Figure 38-10 shows slightly more severe dysplasia of the acetabulum compared to Figure 38-8. Figure 38-11 shows a femoral head severely displaced from the acetabulum, with no formation of the acetabulum.

3. Posterior lip. Maintaining the transducer in the same plane as the coronal flexion position, flex the infant's hip and knee 90 degrees to bring the femoral shaft perpendicular to the table top. Slide the transducer posteriorly to visualize the posterior portion of the triradiate cartilage. The ilium and ischium border the triradiate cartilage and will have a linear appearance. With the transducer fixed in this plane, gently stress the leg (similar to the Barlow test of the

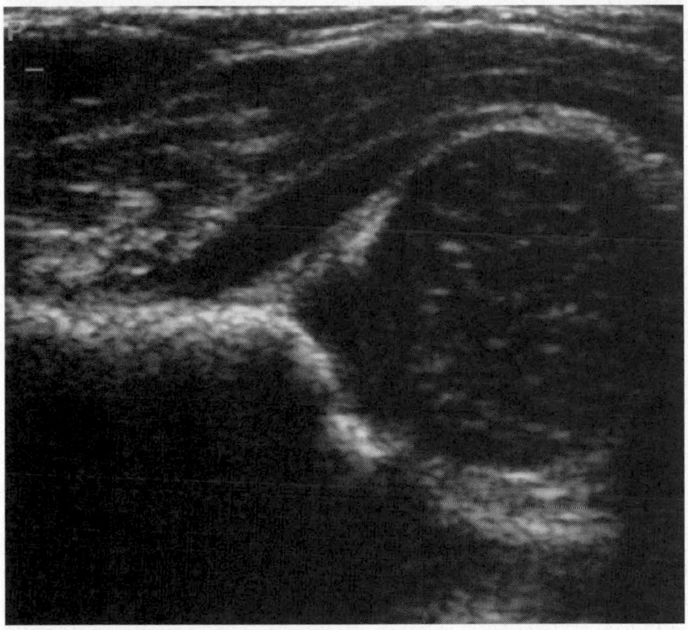

Figure 38-8. ■ *Mild acetabular dysplasia seen on a coronal view.*

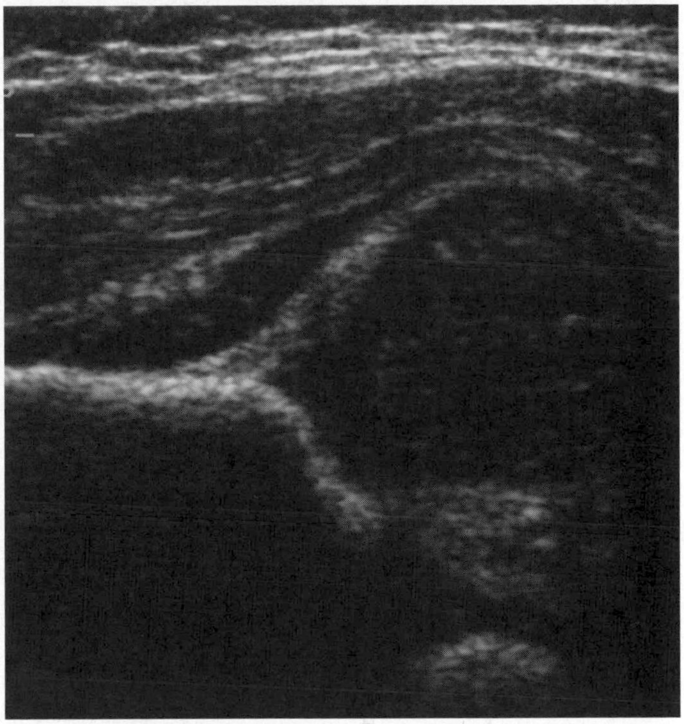

Figure 38-10. ■ *Even more severe acetabular dysplasia on a coronal view.*

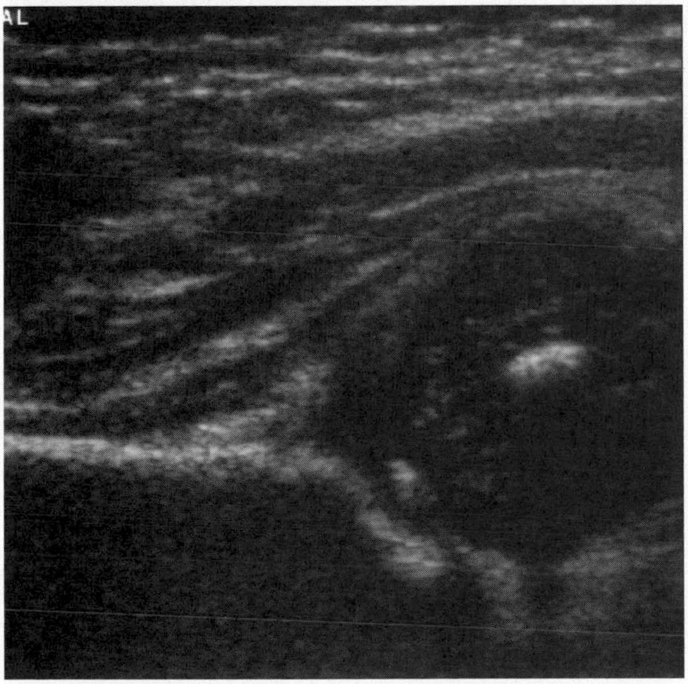

Figure 38-9. ■ *Slightly more severe acetabular dysplasia on a coronal view. Note the echogenic center of ossification within the femoral head.*

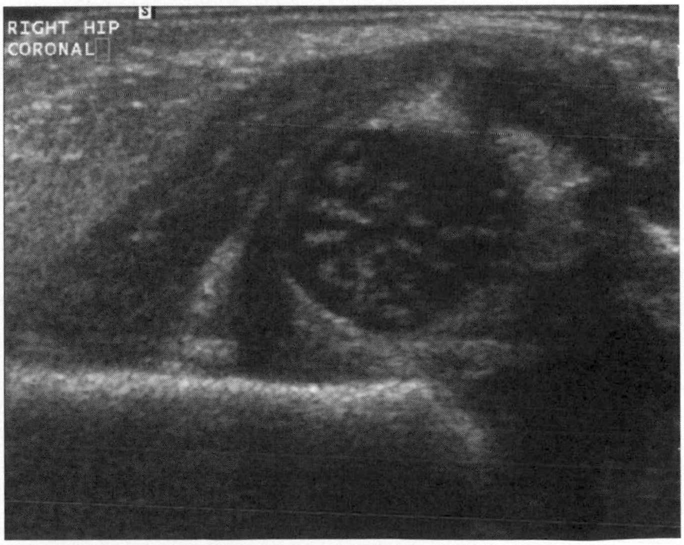

Figure 38-11. ■ *Very severe acetabular dysplasia with no formation of the acetabulum and proximal displacement of the femoral head.*

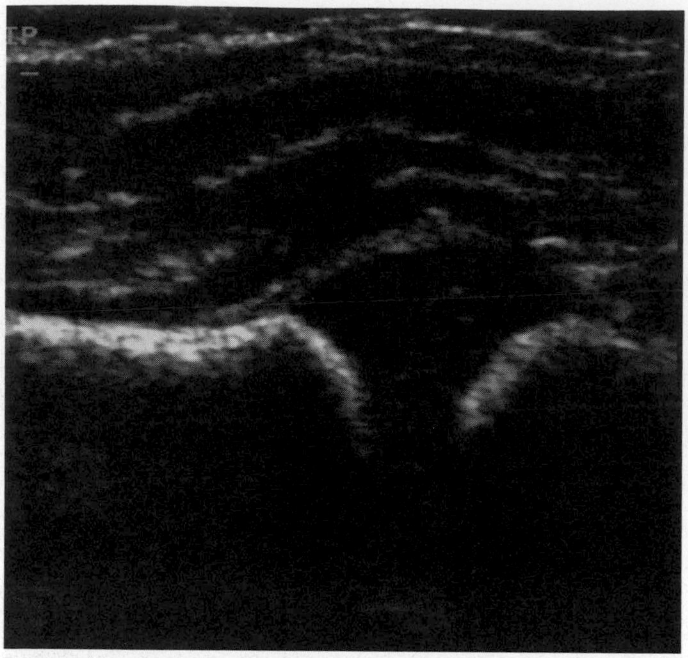

Figure 38-12. ■ *Posterior lip view of a normal hip.*

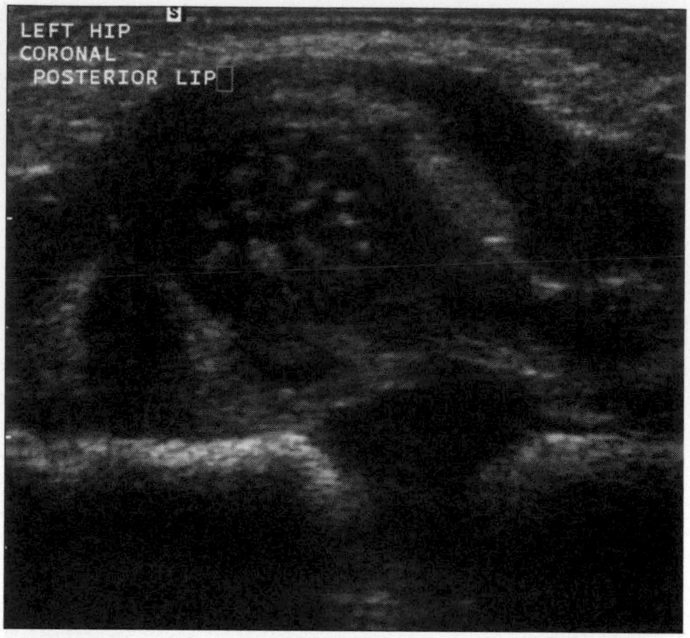

Figure 38-13. ■ *Posterior lip view with severe dislocation of the femoral head.*

clinical examination). If the femoral head is visualized to any degree in this plane, there is posterior displacement. The amount of displacement varies from minimal subluxation to total dislocation, depending on how much of the femoral head is seen over the posterior portion of the acetabulum. Figure 38-12 demonstrates the posterior lip view of a normal hip. Figure 38-13 demonstrates the posterior lip view with severe dislocation of the femoral head.

TRANSVERSE VIEW

1. Transverse flexion. Rotating the transducer 90 degrees from the coronal flexion view—that is, transverse to the infant's body—flex the infant's hip and knee 90 degrees to bring the femoral shaft perpendicular to the table top (Fig. 38-14). The femoral shaft will now be more anterior to the femoral head, demonstrating the metaphysis and shaft of the femur. While viewing the femoral head under real time, gently

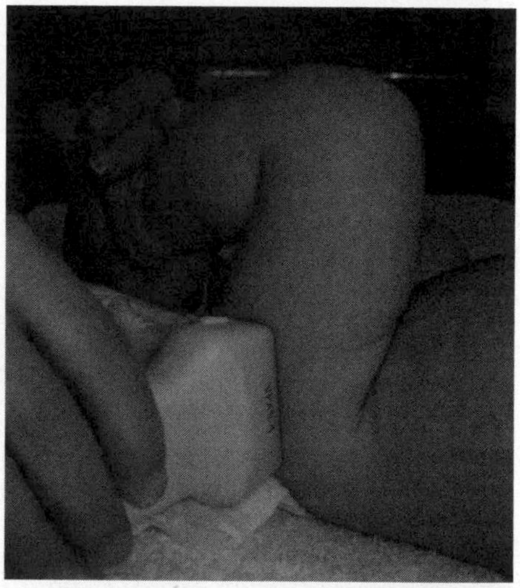

Figure 38-14. ■ *An infant positioned for a transverse flexion view.*

push the femur posteriorly while adducting the hip (Barlow test of the clinical examination) to provoke dislocation. If the hip dislocates, reduction of the dislocated hip can be assessed by gently pulling and abducting the femur (Ortolani test of the clinical examination). Stability of the femoral head can be evaluated by gently moving the hip from maximum abduction, which stabilizes the hip, to maximum adduction, which stresses the hip.

In the transverse-flexion view, the echogenic femoral shaft and metaphysis lie adjacent to the femoral head, and the echogenic acetabulum surrounds the femoral head posteriorly to produce a U-shaped configuration, as in Figure 38-15. If the hip is dislocated, this U configuration cannot be obtained but appears more V shaped (Figs. 38-16 and 38-17).

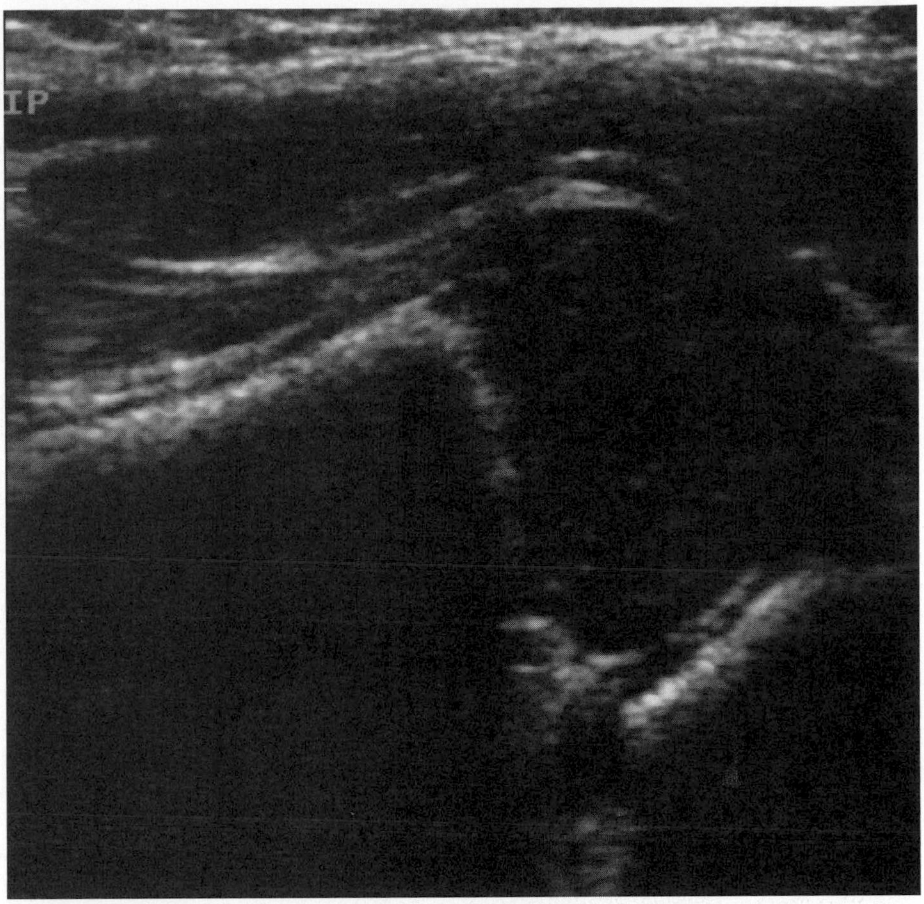

Figure 38-15. ■ *Sonogram of normal hip in transverse flexion view.*

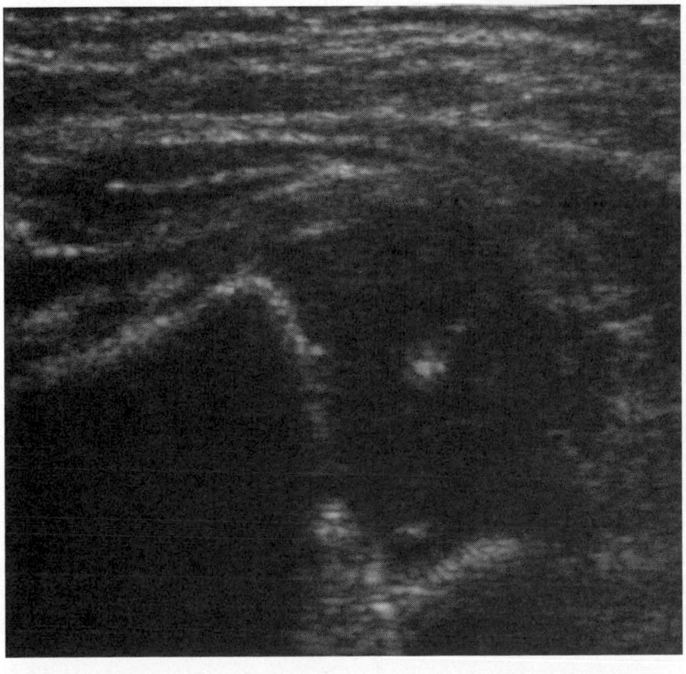

Figure 38-16. ■ *Mild dislocation of the femoral head and the V-shaped appearance of the acetabulum seen on a transverse flexion view.*

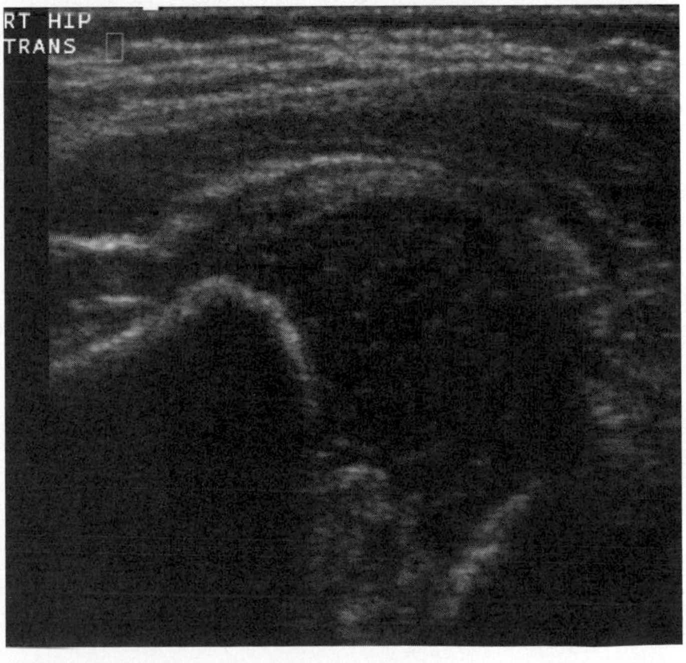

Figure 38-17. ■ *Severe dislocation of the femoral head on a transverse flexion view.*

2. Neutral position. Place the transducer on the infant's lateral thigh transversely as mentioned previously with the femur extended (Fig. 38-18). Slide the transducer cephalad along the femoral shaft until it widens at the intertrochanteric crest. The femoral head can be visualized slightly cephalad. Using slight changes in beam angulation, find the largest diameter of the femoral head as it relates to the acetabulum. The femoral head should sit firmly on the ischial and pubic portions of the acetabulum and concentrically over the triradiate cartilage (Figs. 38-19 and 38-2). A vertical line drawn through the femoral head at the junction of the ischium and triradiate cartilage should dissect it into two equal portions (Figure 38-20).

Pathology

DISLOCATION

Dislocation of the neonatal hip is present when the femoral head is completely dis-

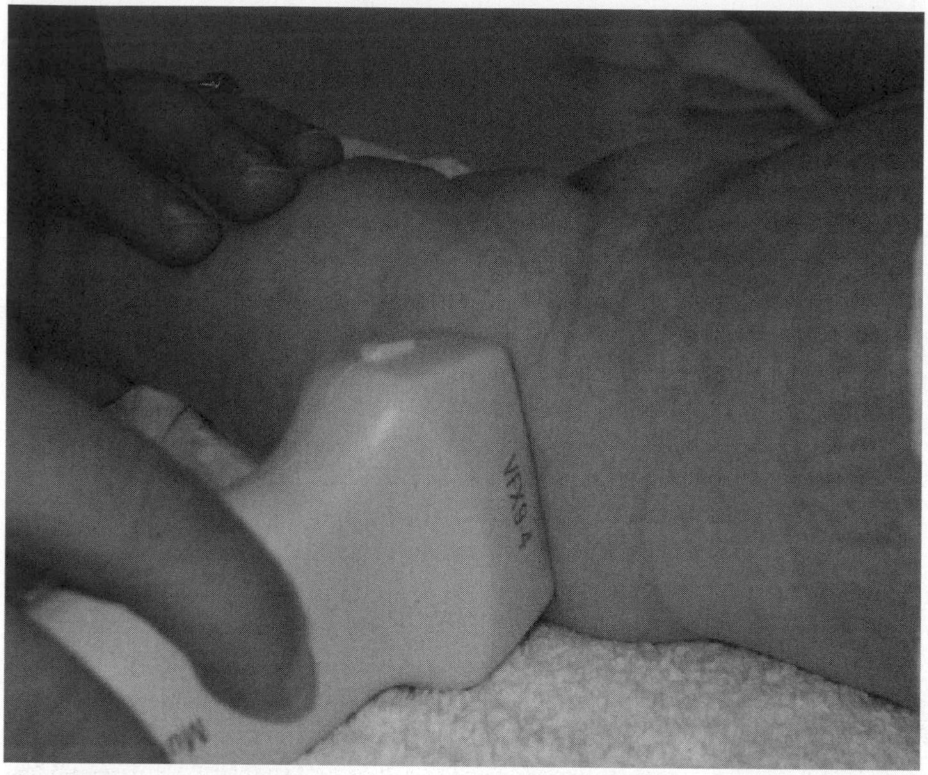

Figure 38-18. ■ *Photo showing the position of the probe and infant for a transverse neutral image of the hip.*

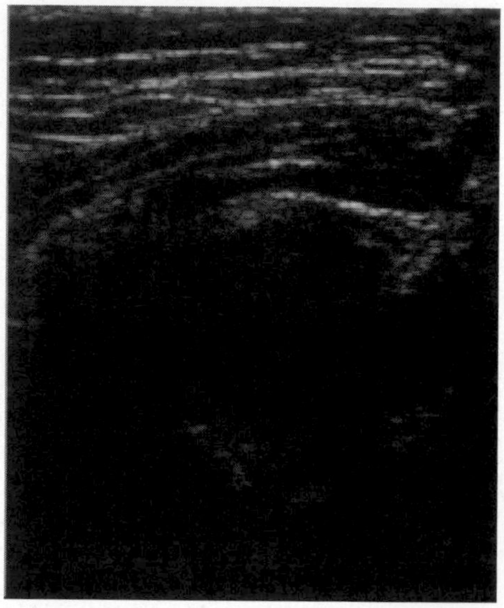

Figure 38-19. ■ *Sonogram showing the normal position of the femoral head over the triradiate cartilage.*

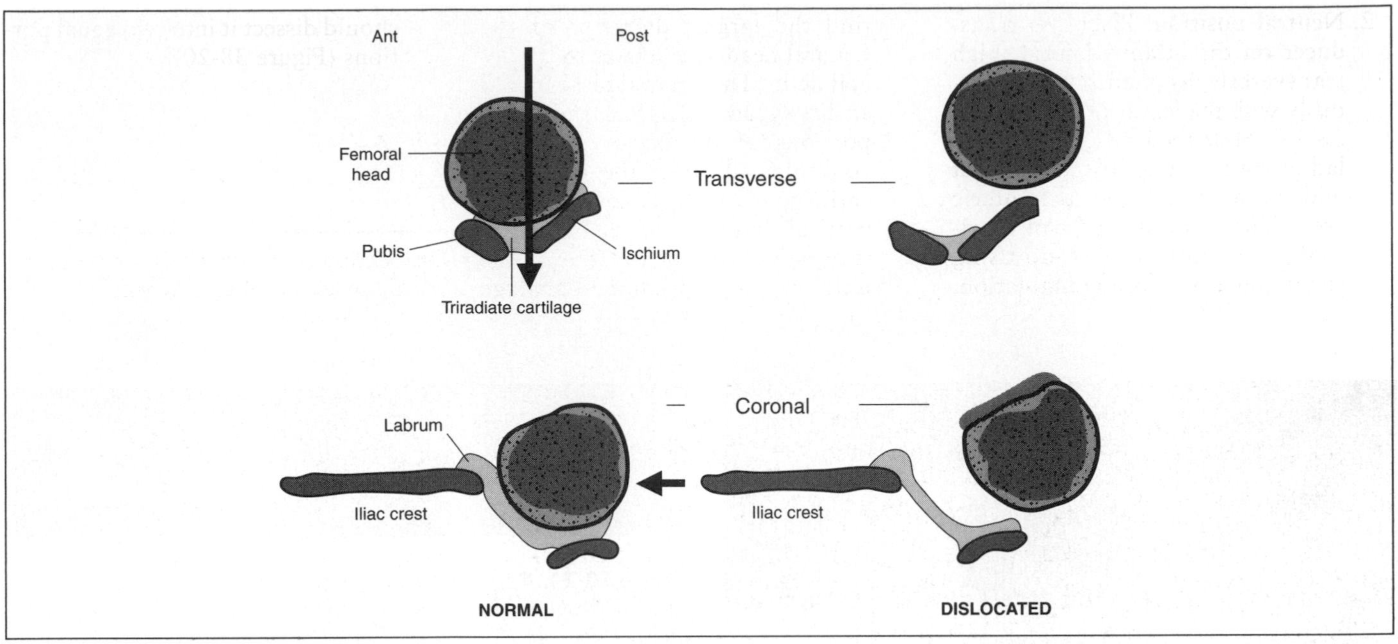

Figure 38-20. ■ *Top left: Normal transverse view with a vertical line through the femoral head at ischial and triradiate cartilage borders. Bottom left: Normal coronal view with a horizontal line through the femoral head from ilium. Upper right: Transverse view showing dislocation. Bottom right: Coronal view showing dislocation.*

placed from the acetabulum. The femoral head most commonly dislocates laterally and superiorly over the posterior acetabular rim onto the iliac wing (Fig. 38-21). Sonographically, there is a loss of normal anatomic landmarks and an empty acetabulum.

Superior dislocation often results in the bony femoral shaft obscuring the acetabulum and triradiate cartilage. On the coronal view, the femoral head will rest against the bony ilium rather than inferior to it.

When dislocation occurs, it is important to visualize the acetabular labrum and show its relationship to the femoral head. If the labrum becomes inverted (Fig. 38-22), it will obstruct the femoral head from relocating into the ac-

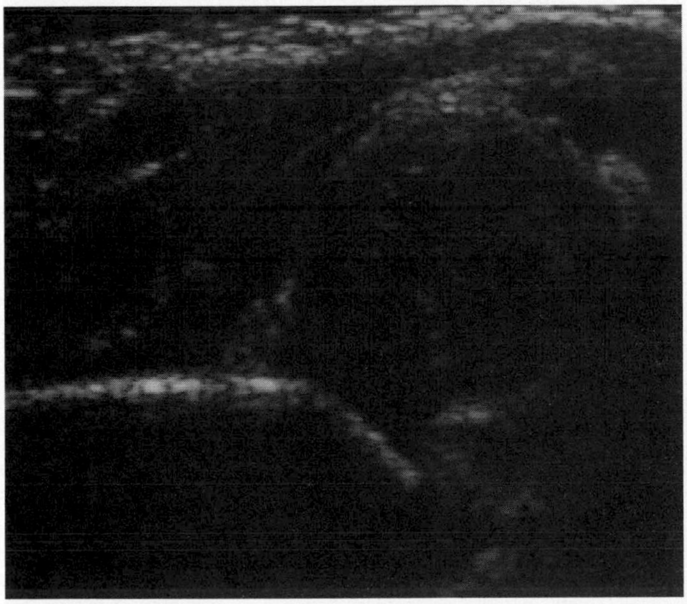

Figure 38-21. ■ *Dislocation of the femoral head.*

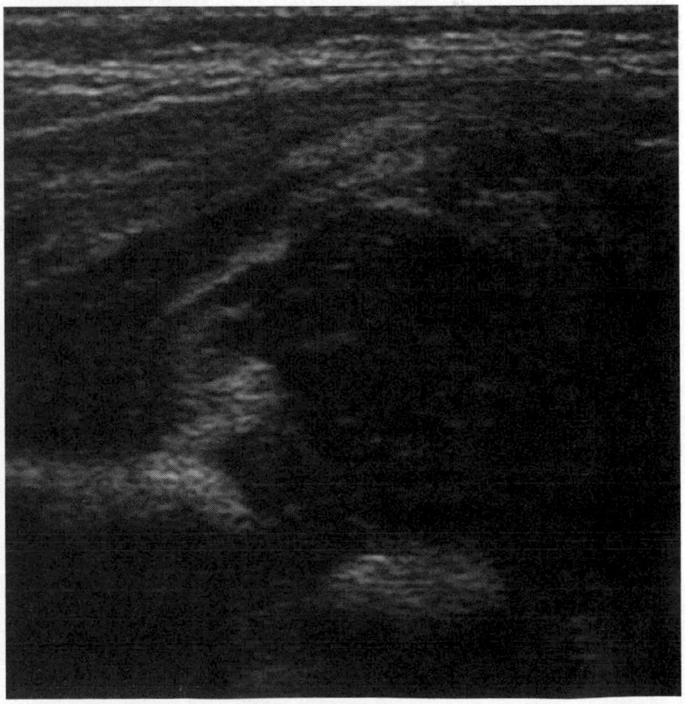

Figure 38-22. ■ *An inverted labrum obstructing the femoral head.*

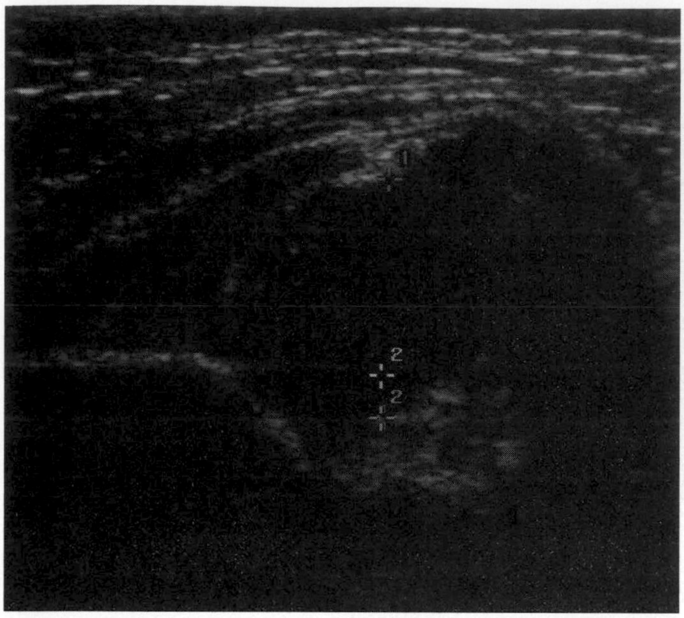

Figure 38-23. ■ *Coronal view during the stress maneuver showing poor acetabular coverage.*

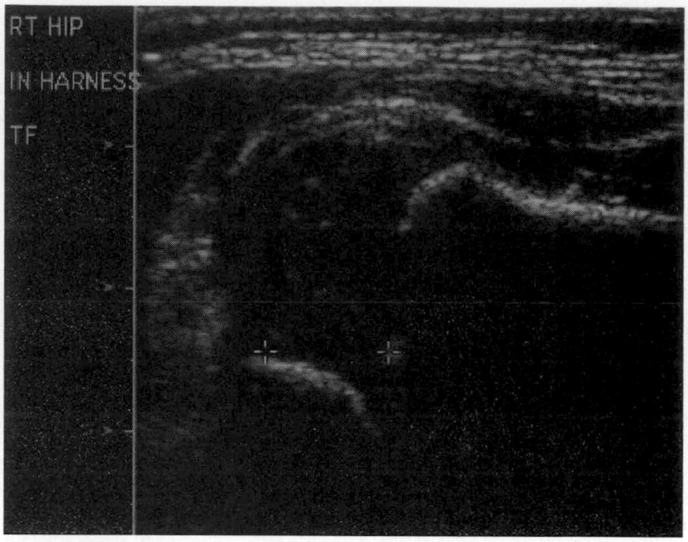

Figure 38-24. ■ *Same infant as shown in Figure 38-23. The transverse flexion view during the stress maneuver confirming poor acetabular coverage.*

etabulum, and surgical correction may be the only management option. Figure 38-16 shows a dislocated femoral head with very little acetabular development.

DISLOCATABLE HIP

The hip is said to be dislocatable when the femoral head is properly positioned within the acetabulum, but during the flexion-stress maneuver it completely displaces from the acetabulum. Once the pressure is released, the femoral head returns to its normal position within the acetabulum (Figs. 38-23 and 38-24).

SUBLUXATION

Subluxation occurs when the femoral head incompletely displaces from the acetabulum during the flexion-stress maneuver (Fig. 38-25). This is best seen on the transverse view.

Normal newborn hips may show signs of minimal subluxation during the stress maneuver, which resolves within the first month of life without intervention.

Using the percentage coverage method, disorders of the infant hip can be graded in increasing severity.

1. Joint laxity. The femoral head has a small amount of movement on the dynamic test. The femoral head coverage ranges from 33% to 50% with stress.

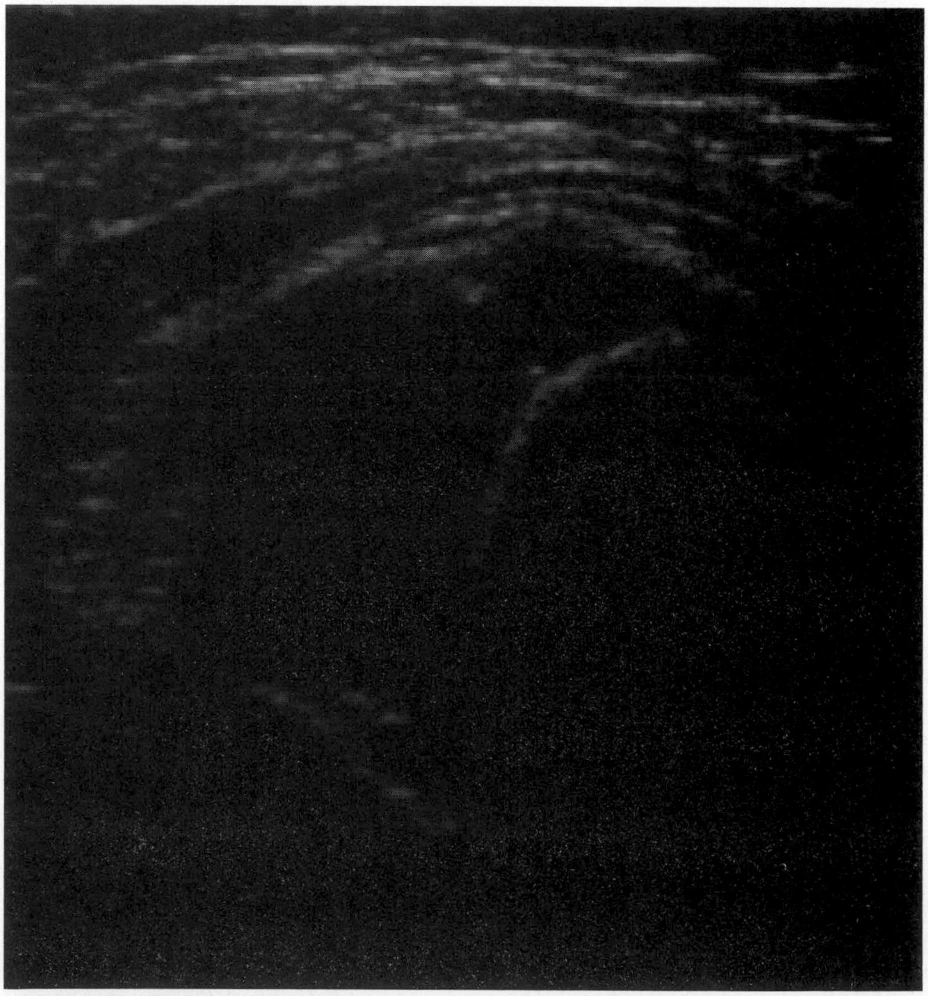

Figure 38-25. ■ *Incomplete displacement (subluxation) of the femoral head from the acetabulum during the flexion-stress maneuver.*

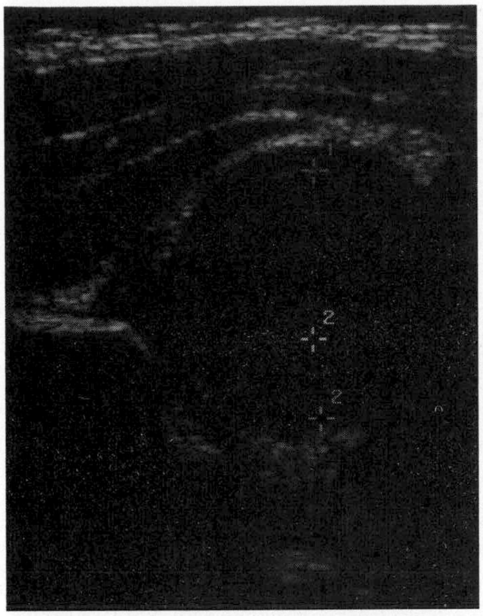

Figure 38-26. ■ *This hip is graded as subluxable.*

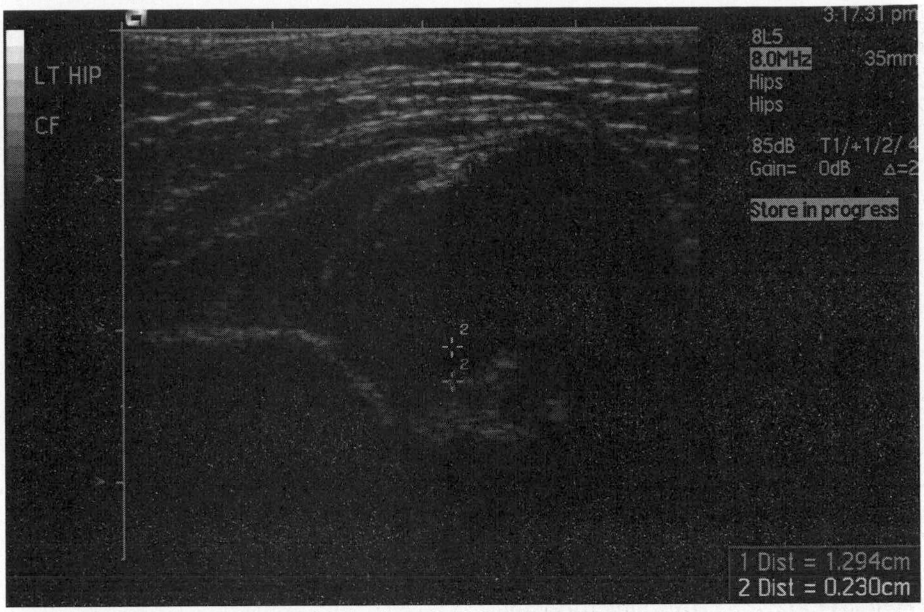

Figure 38-27. ■ *Infant hip showing a percentage coverage of 18%.*

2. Subluxable. The femoral head has a greater degree of movement within the acetabulum. Femoral head coverage is less than 33% with stress (Figs. 38-26 and 38-27).
3. Dislocatable. The femoral head is reduced but may be manually dislocated.
4. Dislocation. The head is outside the acetabulum.
   a. Fixed: cannot be manually reduced
   b. Reducible: may be reduced

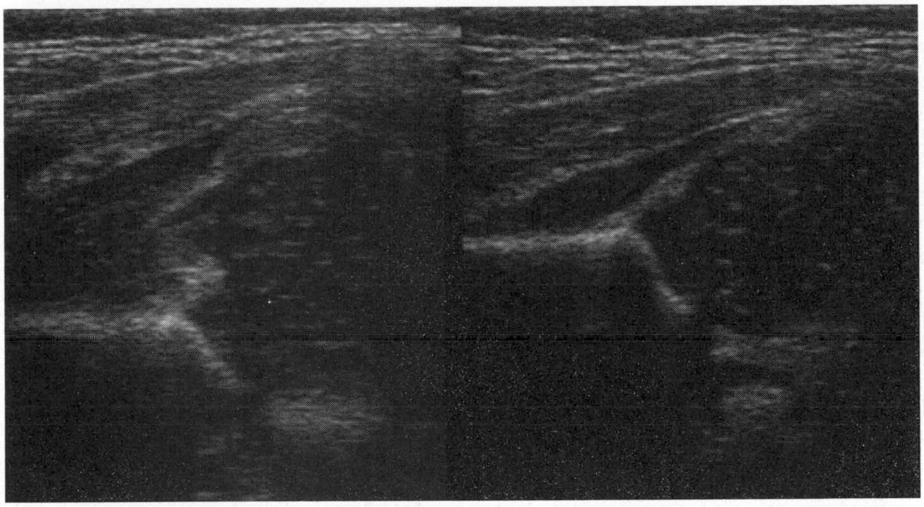

Figure 38-28. ■ *Shallow development of the acetabulum with inverted labrum on the left. The infant's other hip demonstrates normal development.*

ACETABULAR DYSPLASIA

The bony development of the acetabular roof can be assessed sonographically by determining what portion of the femoral head is covered by the ilium on the coronal view. Acetabular dysplasia should be considered when the ilium covers significantly less than one half of the femoral head. Dysplasia occurs secondary to the abnormal position of the femoral head within the acetabulum.

The normal acetabulum is deep with a concave contour and a sharp superolateral margin. The labrum will appear narrow and triangular as it covers the femoral head. An abnormal acetabulum becomes more shallow and flattened, losing its sharp superolateral margin. The labrum also becomes deformed and displaces cranially. With dysplasia, the labrum often becomes fibrotic, causing the hyaline cartilage to become thickened and more echogenic (Fig. 38-28).

Pitfalls

1. Ossific nucleus. Acoustic shadowing produced by the ossific nucleus may be mistaken for the triradiate cartilage or may make the medial acetabulum and triradiate cartilage difficult to identify on the transverse view. The transducer must be angled above or below the ossific nucleus to see the triradiate cartilage medially and avoid false interpretation.
2. Ossification of the femoral head and acetabulum. Acoustic shadowing produced by the bony femoral head and acetabulum prohibits visualization of the hip by ultrasound. Ossification of the femoral head and acetabulum occurs at different ages. Radiographic evaluation may replace ultrasound once ossification has occurred.
3. Neonates confined to a corrective device such as a cast, traction, or

Pavlik harness. A lateral window large enough to accommodate the transducer may be cut from the cast to allow an ultrasonic examination. The window should be cut no larger than necessary and needs to be replaced as quickly and securely as possible after the ultrasound examination. When a lateral approach is not possible, an anterior ultrasound examination can be performed through the perineal opening.

4. Improper alignment of the normal anatomic landmarks. False-positive results can occur from improper alignment of the femoral head with the acetabulum and triradiate cartilage. Accurate angulation of the sound beam must be attained. When performing a coronal view, the transducer may be placed either too anteriorly or posteriorly so that the ilium becomes concave or convex. This incorrect placement means the ultrasound beam is not going through the center of the acetabulum; therefore, assessment is not accurate. The transducer should be moved slightly anterior or posterior until the ilium is parallel to the transducer face.

Acknowledgments

The authors acknowledge Associate Professor Albert Lam, Radiologist at Westmead Children's Hospital, Sydney, Australia, and Cain Brockley, Senior Sonographer at the Melbourne Children's Hospital, Australia.

SELECTED READING

Boal DKB, Schwentker EP. Assessment of congenital hip dislocation with real-time ultrasound: a pictorial essay. *Clin Imag* 1991; 15:77–90.

Graf R. *Guide to Sonography of the Infant Hip*. New York: Thieme Medical Publishers; 1987.

Harcke HT. Screening newborns for developmental dysplasia of the hip: the role of sonography. *AJR Am J Roentgenol* 1994; 162:395–397.

Harcke HT, Grissom LE. Infant hip sonography: current concepts. *Semin Ultrasound CT MR* 1994;15:256–263, 1994.

Joseph KN, Meyer S. Discrepancies in ultrasonography of the infant hip. *J Pediatr Orthop* 1996;5:273–278. Part B.

Keller MS, Chawla HS, Weiss AA. Real-time sonography of infant hip dislocation. *Radiographics* 1986;6:447–456.

Morrissey RT. *Lovell and Winter's Pediatric Orthopaedics*, vol. 2, 3rd ed. Philadelphia: J. B. Lippincott Company; 1990.

Nimityongskul P, Hudgens RA, Anderson LD, et al. Ultrasonography on the management of developmental dysplasia of the hip (DDH). *J Pediatr Orthop* 1995;15:741–746.

Novick GS. Sonography in pediatric hip disorders. *Radiol Clin N Am* 1988;26:29–53.

Sochart DH, Paton RW. Role of ultrasound assessment and harness treatment in the management of developmental dysplasia of the hip. *Ann R Coll Surg Engl* 1996;78:505–508.

South Australian Orthopaedic Registrars' Notebook. Available online at http://som.flinders.edu.au/FUSA/ORTHOWEB/notebook/paediatrics/hip.html. Accessed April 13, 2006.

First Trimester Bleeding

39

ROGER C. SANDERS

KEY WORDS

Abortion. Termination of pregnancy prior to 26 weeks; various types of abortion are discussed in the text.

Amniotic Membrane. Thin membrane sometimes visible in the first trimester sac. Not visible after 12 to 16 weeks because it lies adjacent to the chorionic membrane.

Anembryonic. Gestation without development of a fetal pole (blighted ovum).

Bleeding Dyscrasia. An abnormality of the factors that control clotting and platelet function.

Blighted Ovum. See *Anembryonic*.

Chorionic Membrane. Membrane that surrounds the amniotic cavity and lies within the gestational sac. Normally lies adjacent to the amniotic membrane after 12 to 16 weeks.

Decidual Cast (Reaction). If a pregnancy is located outside the endometrial cavity, hormonal stimulants cause the endometrium to thicken.

Dilatation and Curettage (D & C). Dilatation of the cervical canal and surgical removal of the uterine contents.

Double Decidual Sign. If a pregnancy is intrauterine and not ectopic, thick decidual tissue surrounds the gestational sac and HCG causes a second decidual thickening in the endometrium, resulting in a double layer of decidua surrounding a normal gestational sac.

Embryo. Term used to describe the developing fetus before 10 weeks when organogenesis is incomplete.

Endometrium. Membrane lining the cavity of the uterus.

Estrogen. Hormone secreted by the ovary and, in pregnancy, by the placenta.

Extracelomic Space. The area between the chorion and amnion.

Fetal Pole. See *Embryo*.

Gestational Sac. Sac-like structure that is normally within the uterus and that houses the early developing pregnancy.

Human Chorionic Gonadotropin (HCG) (Beta Subunit). Hormone that rises to very high levels in pregnancy. Assessed with a radioimmunoassay test, which is very sensitive and accurate when performed on a blood sample (serum). Pregnancy testing is almost as accurate with urine samples for HCG.

Hydatidiform Mole. Benign neoplasm thought to develop from the placenta of a missed abortion. High levels of HCG are produced by the tumor.

Last Menstrual Period. The first day of the last menses before conception. It is 40 weeks to the delivery date from the last menstrual period, but pregnancy only lasts 38 weeks after conception.

Macerated Fetus. The degenerative changes and eventual disintegration of a fetus retained in the uterus after fetal death.

Missed Abortion. A fetus that has died prior to approximately 13 weeks. Only macerated remnants may be seen.

Progesterone. Hormone produced by the corpus luteum in the second half of the menstrual cycle that modifies the endometrium in preparation for implantation of a fertilized ovum.

Septic. Pertaining to the presence of pathogenic bacteria and their products in blood or tissue; the patient becomes ill.

Spontaneous Abortion. An unplanned abortion (miscarriage) of the fetus and gestational sac before 23 weeks' gestation. After 23 weeks, the spontaneous loss of pregnancy is termed *premature delivery*.

Triploidy. Chromosomal anomaly that often causes early pregnancy failure.

Trophoblast. Tissue that supports the developing pregnancy, for example, the gestational sac.

Vitelline Duct. A tube connecting the yolk sac and embryo visible only before 10 weeks.

Yolk Sac. Circular structure seen between 4 and 10 weeks that supplies nutrition to the fetal pole. It lies within the extracelomic space between the amnion and the chorion.

The Clinical Problem

Vaginal bleeding in the first trimester is common and very worrisome to the patient. A sonogram can greatly soothe maternal fears by showing a normal, live fetus. Obstetric disorders that may cause abnormal bleeding in the first trimester include threatened abortion, early embryonic demise, spontaneous abortion, ectopic pregnancy, and trophoblastic neoplastic conditions such as hydatidiform mole and choriocarcinoma.

Second and third trimester bleeding problems such as placenta previa and abruptio placentae are discussed in Chapter 42. This section focuses on spontaneous abortions. Ectopic pregnancy, which can also cause vaginal bleeding in the first trimester, is described in Chapter 40.

The majority of spontaneous abortions occur between the 5th and 12th weeks of pregnancy; a patient may therefore consult her physician for abnormal bleeding without suspecting that she is pregnant. A pregnancy test is usually performed; occasional false-negative results may occur with an early pregnancy when a urine pregnancy test is used. Urine tests are, however, often waived in favor of blood tests, which are increasingly available and completely reliable. The physician may then send the patient for a sonogram to determine the viability and location of the pregnancy. Follow-up with a combination of serum beta subunit (blood) pregnancy estimations and ultrasound studies is continued until it is evident whether the fetus is normal and viable or in an abnormal location or dead.

Seven different types of spontaneous abortion can be distinguished sonographically:

1. Threatened abortion: a viable fetus with vaginal bleeding.
2. Incomplete abortion: partial evacuation of the fetus and placenta.
3. Complete abortion: no retained products.
4. Missed abortion: retained dead fetus and placenta.
5. Blighted ovum: anembryonic pregnancy.
6. Inevitable abortion: abortion in progress.
7. Septic abortion: infected dead fetus or retained products.

Differentiation between a blighted ovum and an early pregnancy can be difficult to determine transabdominally; endovaginal ultrasonic analysis allows much earlier diagnosis of viable pregnancy at about 5 1/2 weeks and is essential in early diagnosis. It does not harm the pregnancy.

Hydatidiform mole is a condition in which the pregnancy develops abnormally into a form of neoplasm. The uterus is filled with grape-like structures (vesicles). This condition causes bleeding, vomiting, and an enlarged uterine size for dates. The HCG titer is very high. Dilatation and curettage (D & C) is performed because the condition may develop into a neoplasm that spreads to other portions of the body.

Anatomy

GESTATIONAL SAC

The uterus enlarges in relation to the length of pregnancy. A gestational sac is visible as a well-defined circle of echoes in the fundus of the uterus. The sac may be seen as early as 4 weeks' gestational age using the endovaginal approach (Fig. 39-1), and by 6 weeks, it can be demonstrated reliably on a transabdominal scan. At first, the sac appears echo-free because echoes from the fetal pole and yolk sac are too small to see.

The embryo is usually first visible at about 5 1/2 weeks. A yolk sac is visible before the fetal pole can be seen (Fig. 39-2).

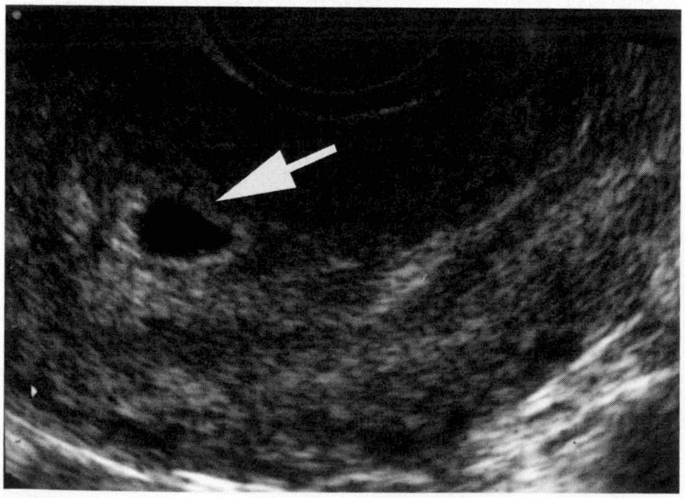

Figure 39-1. ■ *Early gestational sac at about 4 1/2 weeks* (arrow). *Note that the sac is largely enclosed within the decidual reaction and is eccentrically located. There is secondary thickening of the endometrial lining.*

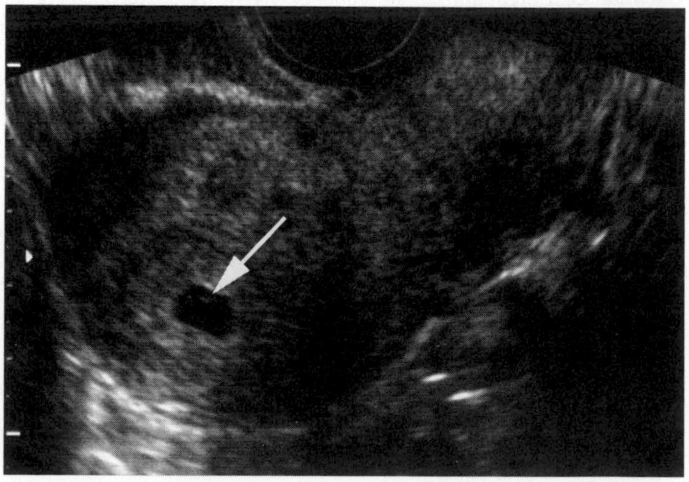

Figure 39-2. ■ *Early gestational sac at about 5 weeks. A yolk sac* (arrow) *can be seen within this small gestational sac.*

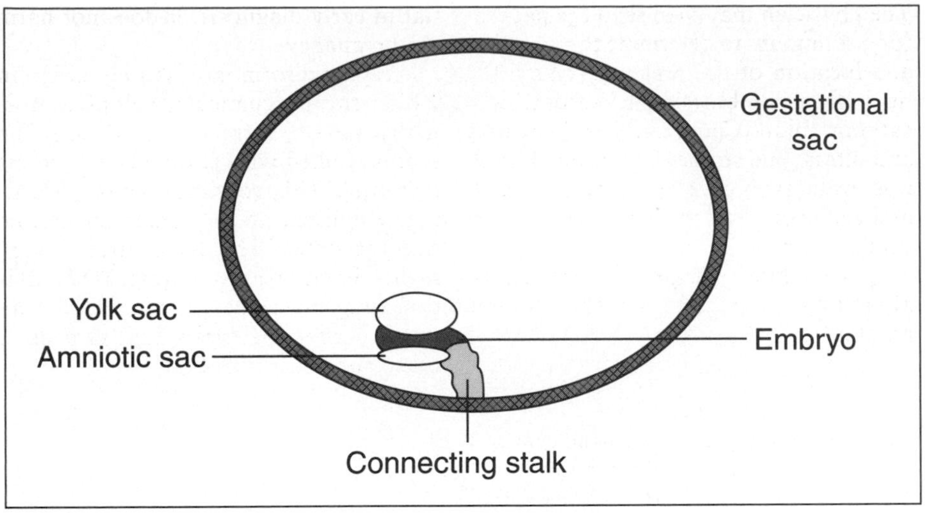

Figure 39-3. ■ *When the fetal pole is first seen, it lies between two small cysts: the yolk sac and the amniotic sac. Fetal heart motion can be seen at this 4 1/2- to 5-week stage.*

The fetal pole (embryo) may lie between two small sacs, the yolk sac and the amniotic sac, at this very early stage (Figs. 39-3 and 39-4). The amniotic sac expands thereafter, but it is difficult to see. An additional linear structure, the vitelline duct, may be seen (Fig. 39-4).

By 8 weeks, the sac should occupy approximately one half of the uterine volume, and by 10 weeks, the entire uterine cavity should be encompassed (see Appendix 3). The gestational sac is encompassed by a ring of echoes (the decidual reaction), which should be well defined and of uniform thickness except at the site where the placenta will develop. At this implantation site, the ring is single and slightly thickened. Elsewhere, it is double layered, although the second layer is sometimes subtle (Fig. 39-5). The inner layer is composed of the chorion and the decidua capsularis. The outer layer is the decidua vera; together, they are considered the double decidual sac (see Fig. 40-3) seen around true intrauterine gestations.

A sonolucent extra gestational sac space ("implantation bleed") (Fig. 39-5) is a relatively common feature of normal pregnancy between the 6th and 10th weeks. Sometimes, an apparent implantation bleed contains venous flow on color flow Doppler.

YOLK SAC

The yolk sac can be seen slightly earlier than the fetal pole, at about 4 1/2 weeks

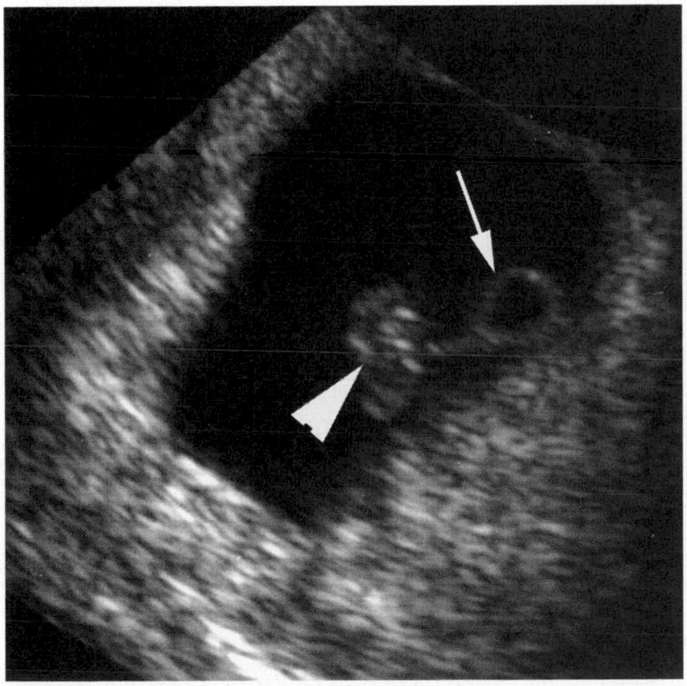

Figure 39-4. ■ *A yolk sac* (arrow) *and fetal pole* (arrowhead) *can be seen. The line connecting the two structures is the vitelline duct.*

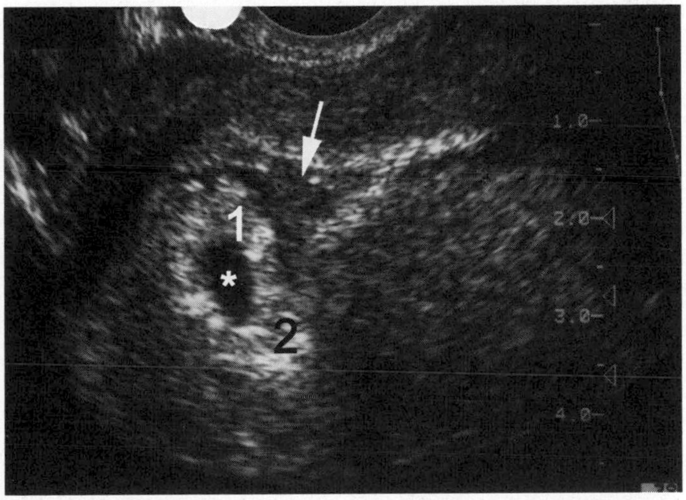

Figure 39-5. ■ *The gestational sac* (*) *can be seen surrounded by the gestational sac chorionic tissue* (1). *The decidual reaction of the endometrium forms a second outline* (2) *around part of the gestational sac outline. Surrounded by endometrial decidual reaction but outside the gestational sac is a triangular echopenic area* (arrow) *thought to represent an implantation bleed.*

transvaginally and 5 1/2 weeks transabdominally. It disappears by 10 weeks (Figs. 39-2, 39-3, 39-4, and 39-6).

AMNIOTIC MEMBRANE

The tiny crescentic line that constitutes the amniotic membrane can be seen within the gestational sac in the first trimester with high-quality ultrasound systems (Fig. 39-7). It encloses the amniotic cavity. The yolk sac lies in the extracelomic cavity outside the amniotic membrane. At about 4 weeks, the amniotic sac is about the same size as the yolk sac. Both lie within the chorion. A second membrane, the vitelline duct, may be seen leading to the yolk sac (Fig. 39-4).

FETAL POLE (EMBRYO)

By 5 to 6 weeks with transvaginal ultrasound, and by 7 weeks transabdominally, the fetus should be seen within the uterus as a small collection of echoes known as an *embryo*, or less correctly, as a *fetal pole* (Figs. 39-3, 39-4, and 39-6).

Measuring maximum fetal length (crown-rump length [CRL]) is a very accurate method of dating between 5 and 12 weeks (Figs. 39-6 and 39-7) (see Appendix 4).

Almost as soon as the fetus is visible, the fetal head and body can be made out, and facial structures can be seen. A mass may be seen at the cord insertion site, which is related to midgut herniation. This mass represents the normal gut rotation occurring outside the fetal trunk; it is a normal variant present about half

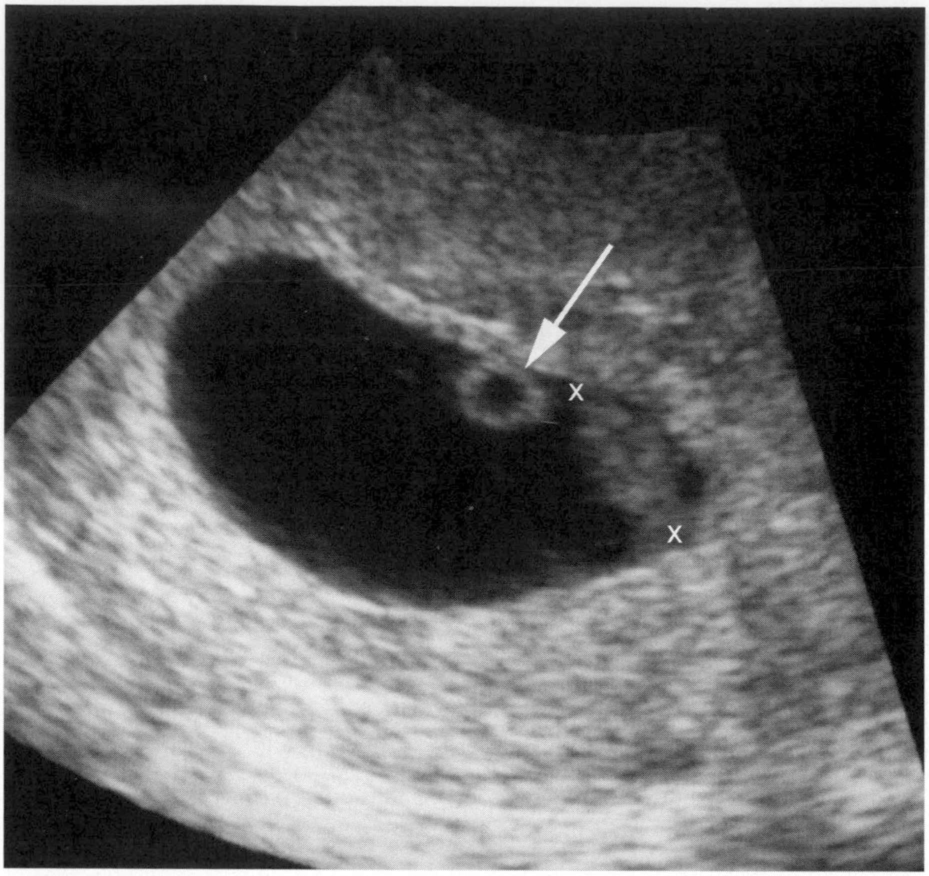

Figure 39-6. ■ *A tiny fetal pole is seen (between Xs). The measured CRL gives a very accurate gestational age. The yolk sac is visible* (arrow).

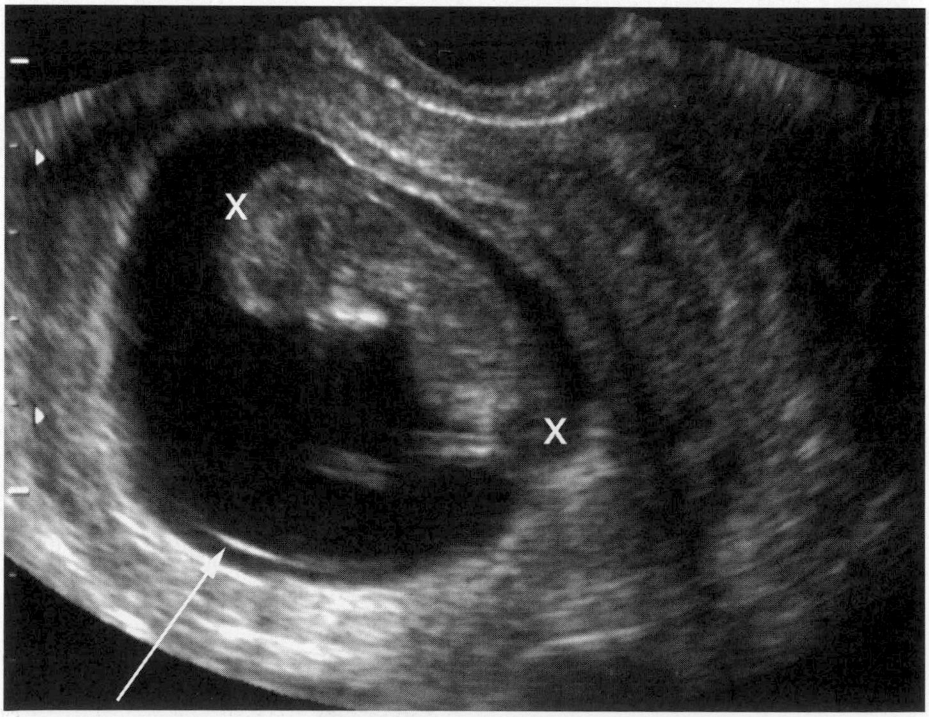

Figure 39-7. ■ *The measurement calipers show the sites where the CRL measurements are obtained in a 9-week pregnancy. Note the unfused amniotic membrane* (arrow).

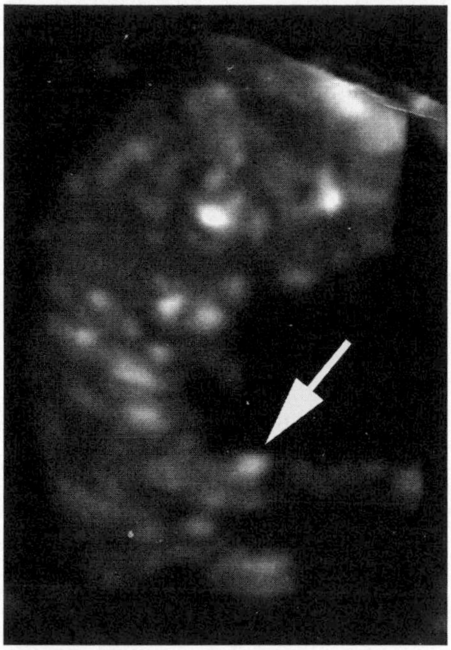

Figure 39-8. ■ *Three-dimensional view of a 9-week-old fetus showing some gut rotation* (arrow) *outside the fetal abdomen. The cord is much thinner beyond the site of gut rotation.*

the time between 6 and 10 weeks (Fig. 39-8).

Fetal heart motion is visible with good equipment almost as soon as the fetal pole is seen. It is always seen when the fetal pole is 5 mm long or greater.

The fetal heart is seen as a tiny fluttering structure within the fetal body. It beats at about double the maternal rate if the fetus is normal. If the fetus is sick, the rate will be slow or irregular. The fetal pulse rate increases during the first trimester (see Appendix 25).

Technique

ENDOVAGINAL TECHNIQUE

The endovaginal technique is a preferable method for examining the first trimester pregnancy. It is particularly helpful in the following circumstances:

1. When it is uncertain whether there is a fetus or whether it is alive
2. When the patient has an empty bladder
3. To look for bleeds in or around the sac
4. If ectopic pregnancy is a possibility

MEASURING GESTATIONAL SACS

The gestational sac measurement is an average of the width, length, and anteroposterior dimensions of the sac (Fig. 39-9). Measurements for width are taken at the transverse view demonstrating the widest portion of the sac, and measurements for the length are taken on the longest sagittal view. It is important to obtain the anteroposterior diameter from a sagittal image as well because the angle of the uterus can be taken into account. Sac shape can change owing to extrinsic factors such as fibroids or bladder distention; all three dimensions should be measured on-screen within a few minutes of each other so that all of the measurements relate to each other. Measure at the fluid–sac interface; do not include the decidua in your measurements.

MEASURING CRL

The dominant feature in a very early embryo is the pulsating heart in the center of a small lump of tissue—the crown and rump are the same size and virtually indistinguishable. At this stage, it is easy to obtain an accurate measurement of the whole embryo.

Later, the cranium is seen as a separate entity from the fetal body. A crown-rump measurement is taken at the longest axis, which may require patience because of fetal movement and varying axis (Figs. 39-6 and 39-7). It is worth taking a few measurements to determine whether the longest axis has been recorded; however, it is not appropriate to average the shorter measurements—this decreases your accuracy. If your machine averages the shorter measurements automatically, go into the OB program and remove the CRLs that are too short. The CRL is still the dating method of choice until the intracranial anatomy is clear enough (at about 12 weeks) to begin measuring the biparietal diameter.

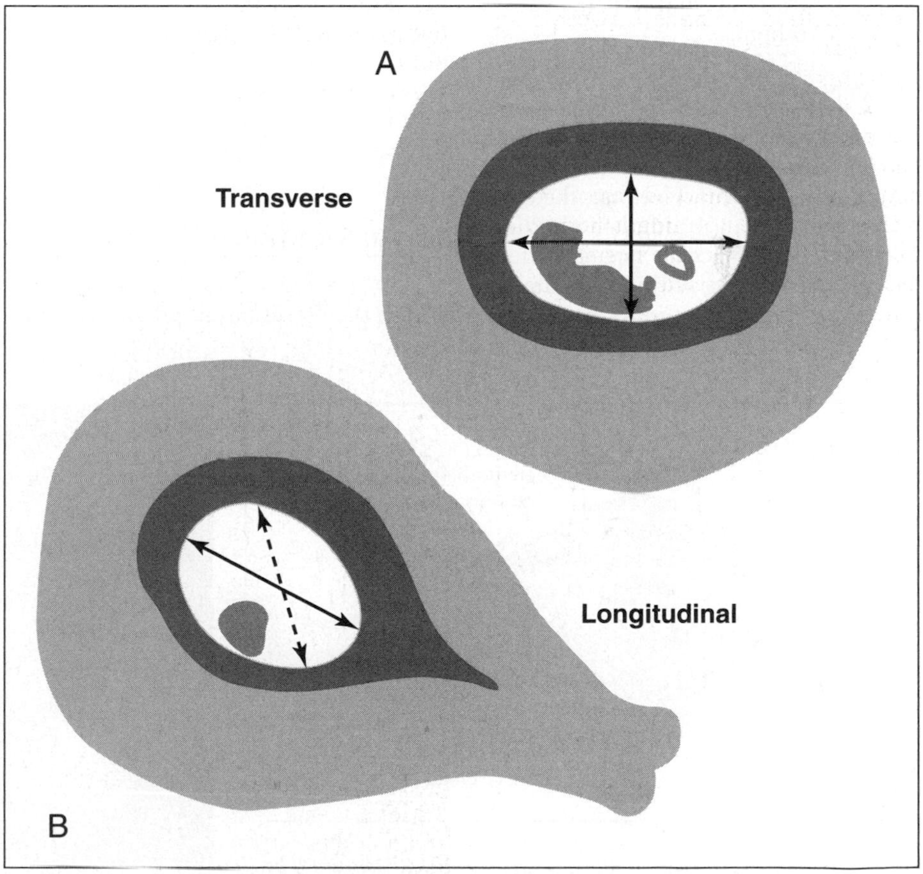

Figure 39-9. ■ *Longitudinal and transverse views of the uterus showing the views to measure a gestational sac. The width, length, and height diameters are obtained. The measurement is averaged. Take the longest length, rather than an oblique shorter measurement as shown in the longitudinal diagram in dots.*

DOPPLER AND COLOR FLOW

Avoid using color flow and Doppler at this stage of pregnancy as much as possible; the dose is high and potentially harmful, and there are few clinical uses.

Pathology

THREATENED ABORTION

Threatened abortion may not be visible sonographically. This diagnosis is made whenever vaginal bleeding occurs within the first 20 weeks of pregnancy with a closed cervix. The sonogram should demonstrate a pregnancy corresponding to the patient's dates. A bleed in or around the gestational sac may be seen (Fig. 39-10).

Most such pregnancies will proceed to term, but because of the threat of abortion and increased risk of bleeding later in pregnancy, serial sonograms during the pregnancy may be requested.

A low fetal cardiac rate (less than 100 bpm) suggests impending fetal death. Death is inevitable if the rate is less than 90 bpm.

INCOMPLETE ABORTION

If a threatened abortion progresses, and if some of the products of conception are passed as tissue with bleeding, the clinical diagnosis is an incomplete abortion. Portions of the placenta and some fetal parts may remain within the uterus, however, resulting in continued bleeding. Sonographically, the uterus appears enlarged. With incomplete abortion, the sonographer may note an empty, ill-defined gestational sac within the uterus or a sac with internal echoes that are not clearly fetal. Occasionally, no sac at all can be identified, but large clumps of echoes in the center of the uterus may be seen. These echoes may represent parts of the fetus, placenta, or blood. This sonographic confirmation of diagnosis is useful because D & C may be necessary to complete the process of abortion. If the uterus appears normal by ultrasound, D & C is unnecessary.

COMPLETE ABORTION

With complete abortion, all products of conception pass. Sonographically, the uterus appears enlarged, but a gestational sac or fetus cannot be identified. A line of central echoes—a prominent thickening of the central cavity interface—within the uterus representing a decidual reaction may be present, however. The uterus may remain enlarged for up to 2 weeks after the abortion. After the initial passage of clots, bleeding is minimal, and the patient usually does not require any further treatment.

The sonographer's role is to confirm that the uterus is empty. Echoes within the cavity may represent blood rather than retained products of conception.

MISSED ABORTION

When the fetus dies but is retained within the uterus, a missed abortion has occurred. Sonographically, the uterus is often too small for the expected dates. Most frequently, missed abortions occur between 6 and 14 weeks of gestation. In an early missed abortion, the gestational sac contains the fetal pole, which shows no heart motion.

A diagnosis of a missed abortion can be made if a fetus measures 5 mm or more but if no fetal heart motion is seen. If the fetal pole is less than 5 mm and if no fetal heart motion is seen, it is wise to rescan in a few days to confirm fetal death.

The fetal pole may assume an abnormal shape. With later missed abortions, the placenta may become large, resembling a hydatidiform mole; these changes are termed *hydropic changes*.

INTRASAC AND PERISAC BLEEDS

Bleeds in or around the sac (Fig. 39-10) are common. Bleeds are seen (1) as a group of echoes within the amniotic sac adjacent to the fetus, (2) as low-level echoes in the space between the amniotic and chorionic membranes (extracelomic space), (3) as a group of echoes in a crescentic shape in a subchorionic location, or (4) between the gestational sac and the decidual reaction (Fig. 39-11). In any location, as long as fetal heart motion is seen, management of the bleed should include a follow-up sonogram in 1 or 2 weeks.

Fetal survival is much more common (92%) than death if fetal heart motion is seen.

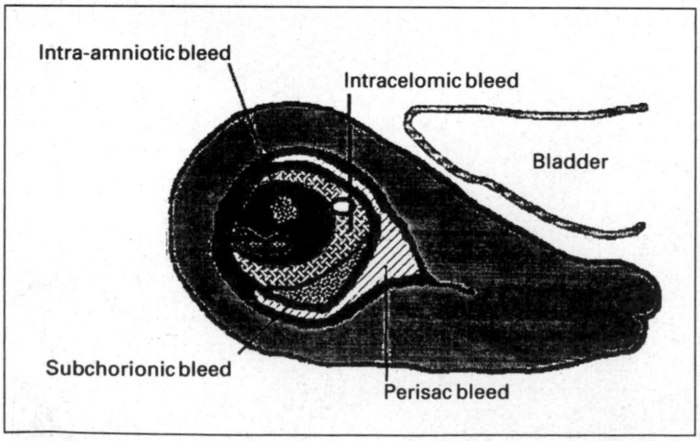

Figure 39-10. ■ *Bleeding with threatened abortion may occur (1) between the gestational sac and the endometrial cavity, (2) in a subchorionic location, (3) within the chorionic sac, and (4) within the amniotic sac.*

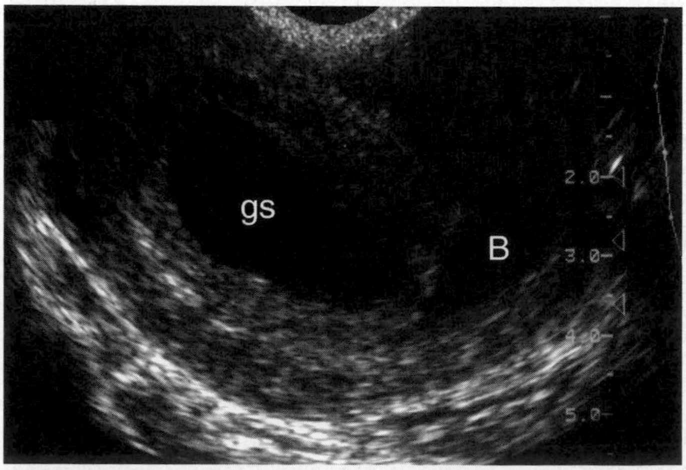

Figure 39-11. ■ *Large empty gestational sac* (gs) *related to a blighted ovum. Average sac measurements measured 22 mm. At this size, a fetal pole should be visible. An extra gestational sac bleed* (B) *can be seen alongside the gestational sac.*

BLIGHTED OVUM

The definition of a blighted ovum is an anembryonic pregnancy. This means that the sac develops but the embryo does not. Clinically, the patient usually has slight vaginal bleeding. The pregnancy test may be positive although no embryo is present because there is continued production of HCG by the trophoblasts in the sac. Although a blighted ovum will eventually abort, the physician may intervene with D & C before that occurs.

The main sonographic finding is a trophoblastic ring within the uterus. This ring may look like a gestational sac, although the borders are usually less regular and are ill defined. No fetal pole is seen within the sac (Fig. 39-11).

Using the endovaginal probe, a fetal pole should be seen when the gestational sac diameter is 17 mm or more. A yolk sac should be seen when the gestational sac has a mean diameter greater than 8 mm. Be cautious about using these measurements in the diagnosis of blighted ovum if there is a possibility of monoamniotic monochorionic twins.

There may be a fluid–fluid level due to blood within the gestational sac; this is definitive evidence of fetal death.

The absence of a fetal pole is inconclusive evidence of blighted ovum if the gestational sac is small, because early normal gestational sacs with a diameter of less than 8 mm also appear to be without a fetal pole. To solve this dilemma, the patient may be asked to return in a week or two for a repeat sonogram. Serial serum beta subunit pregnancy tests may be performed. Unduly large or small sacs for gestational age with absence of embryo and yolk sac are both seen with blighted ovum. The trophoblastic reaction around the gestational sac is often irregular or thin.

INEVITABLE ABORTION

Pregnancies suffering an inevitable abortion are usually clinically obvious. The patient consults her physician because she is experiencing some bleeding. The physician examines her and discovers that her cervix is dilating and that pregnancy is doomed to be aborted. Sonographically, the area of the cervix may appear to be widened and fluid filled owing to blood and dilatation. A sonolucent space around the sac may be present where the sac has dissected away from the uterine wall. A fluid–fluid level may be present within the aborting sac. The gestational sac may lie at the level of the cervix and may be in the process of being aborted (Fig. 39-12).

SEPTIC ABORTION

In septic abortion, there are infected products of conception in the uterus, perhaps as a result of a surgical abortion with a nonsterile device. Alternatively, infection may occur in retained products after a spontaneous or induced abortion. Sonographically, the uterus is enlarged, and there are increased endometrial echoes. If the infection is caused by gas-forming organisms, areas of shadowing may be produced. Shadowing may also be caused by retained bony fragments after an attempted abortion.

HYDATIDIFORM MOLE

Vaginal bleeding, excessive vomiting (hyperemesis gravidarum), and high blood pressure suggest the presence of a mole. The uterus will be filled with echoes interspersed with a few echopenic areas (Fig. 39-13).

Large echo-free spaces may occur within a mole, and the process may be confused with a missed abortion or a fibroid; however, the HCG titers will be markedly elevated. Large cysts may be seen in the ovaries. These theca lutein cysts represent follicles greatly stimulated by increased HCG.

INVASIVE MOLE

Some hydatidiform moles recur after the performance of a curettage and invade the muscle of the uterus. Residual molar tissue is highly vascular and lights up using color flow. Without color flow, remaining invasive tissue may be overlooked.

CHORIOCARCINOMA

Molar tissue has the potential to develop into an aggressive malignancy known as

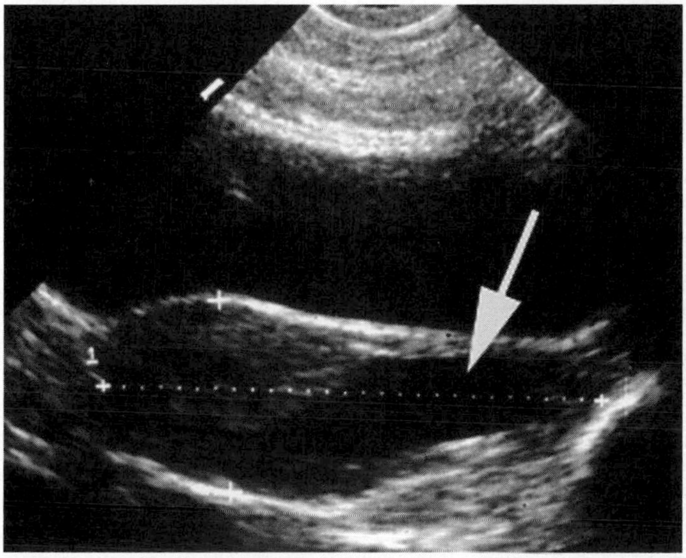

Figure 39-12. ■ *Aborting sac. A fluid collection with a subtle border* (arrow) *can be seen within the cervix, which represented an aborting sac.*

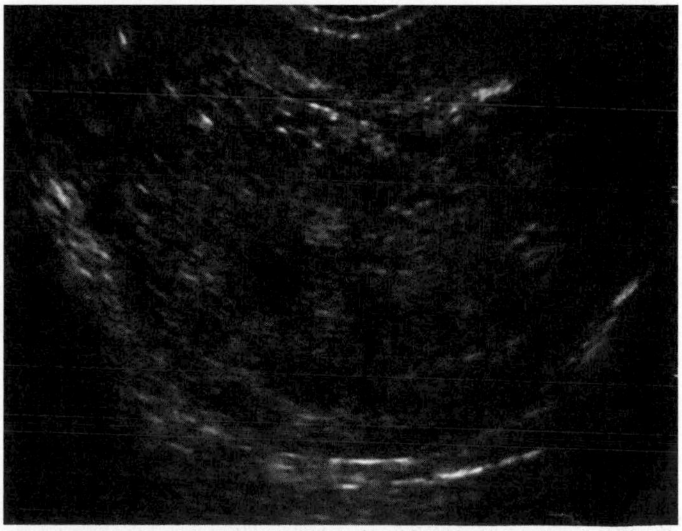

Figure 39-13. ■ *Hydatidiform mole. The uterus is filled with echogenic material with some less-echogenic areas within, presumably representing bleeding because the mass is very vascular. Much flow was seen with color flow.*

a *choriocarcinoma*. When seen in the uterus, this tumor has cystic centers with echogenic borders. Although easily treatable, it metastasizes early. When a patient with a positive pregnancy test is seen with a very high HCG, and if masses with an irregular appearance are present within the uterus, the liver should be examined for metastatic lesions, which are generally echopenic.

PARTIAL MOLE

When an apparent mole and a fetus are present together, it is possible (1) that there are twins and that one twin has become a mole or (2) that there is a "partial mole." A chromosomal anomaly, triploidy, causes placental changes that resemble a mole. The fetus is anomalous and almost always dies. Sometimes, the fetus is hydropic (see Chapter 45).

Pitfalls

1. Changes in sac shape may be caused by external compression due to an overdistended bladder or bowel or to fibroids in the uterine wall (Fig. 39-14). Myometrial contractions may distort the sac shape in the first trimester.
2. If the sac is located to one or the other side of the uterus with a relatively thin adjacent myometrium, consider the following possibilities: (1) cornual or interstitial pregnancy (see Chapter 40); (2) fibroid displacing the sac (see Fig. 39-14); (3) septate or bicornuate uterus (see Fig. 40-10); or (4) normal variant. Rescanning with a different degree of bladder filling may show a normal appearance.
3. Other entities may mimic the complex echo pattern seen in a molar pregnancy (e.g., degenerating fibroid, missed abortion, and necrotic placenta).
4. A sonolucent space around a portion of the gestational sac may be seen between the 6th and 8th weeks of pregnancy as a normal variant. Subtle venous flow is usually visible within the area.
5. A cervical pregnancy and an impending abortion appear similar. If the pregnancy is aborting, the sonographic findings will change rapidly, and the patient will be bleeding.
6. Underdistention and overdistention of the bladder may prevent gestational sac visualization. The bladder should rise approximately 1 to 2 cm above the uterine fundus for satisfactory transabdominal evaluation.
7. Although a gestational sac size of greater than 17 mm with no evidence of fetal pole or yolk sac using an endovaginal probe suggests blighted ovum, monozygotic twins may still be present. The gestation is earlier than the sac makes it appear; rescan later if twins are suspected.

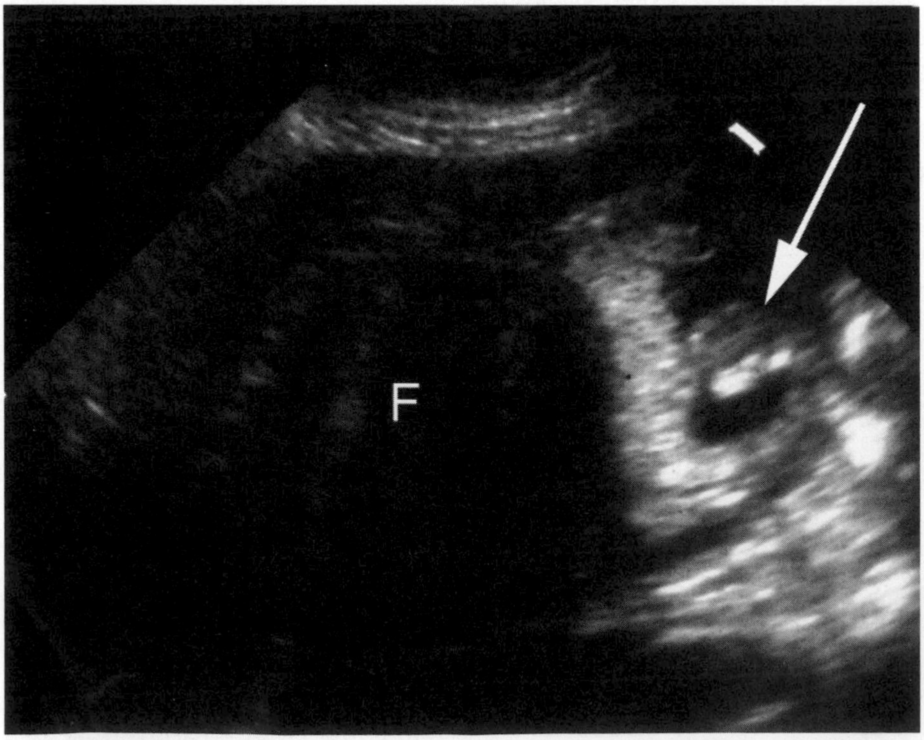

Figure 39-14. ■ *A fibroid* (F) *markedly displaces the gestational sac to the left. The wall of the sac appears thin due to the distorted position, and one could worry about an interstitial pregnancy.*

Where Else to Look

HYDATIDIFORM MOLE

If a mole-like appearance is seen in the uterus (Fig. 39-13):

1. Look hard for evidence of an intrauterine fetus. Missed abortion with a macerated fetus can look like a mole.
2. Look for a theca lutein cyst, which is seen with 40% of moles.
3. Look for liver metastases, which are commonly seen with choriocarcinoma.

SELECTED READING

Condous G, Okaro E, Bourne T. The conservative management of early pregnancy complications: a review of the literature. *Ultrasound Obstet Gynecol* 2003;22:420–430.

Oh JS, Wright G, Coulam C. Gestational sac diameter in very early pregnancy as a predictor of fetal outcome. *Ultrasound Obstet Gynecol* 2002;20:206–209.

Jauniaux E. Ultrasound diagnosis and follow-up of gestational trophoblastic disease. *Ultrasound Obstet Gynecol* 1998;11:367–377.

Johns J, Hyett J, Jauniaux E. Obstetric outcome after threatened miscarriage with and without a hematoma on ultrasound. *Obstet Gynecol* 2003;102:383–387.

Laboda LA, Esroff JA, Benacerraf BR. First trimester bradycardia: a sign of impending fetal loss. *J Ultrasound Med* 1988;8:561–563.

Nyberg D, Filly R. Predicting pregnancy failure in "empty" gestational sacs. *Ultrasound Obstet Gynecol* 2003;21:9–12.

Sohaey R, Woodward P, Zwiebel WJ. First-trimester ultrasound: the essentials. *Semin Ultrasound CT MR* 1996;17:2–14.

Wagner BJ, Woodward PJ, Dickey GE. From the archives of the AFIP: gestational trophoblastic disease; radiologic-pathologic correlation. *Radiographics* 1996;16:131–148.

Acute Pelvic Pain

40

ROGER C. SANDERS

KEY WORDS

Abdominal Pregnancy. A pregnancy that occurs outside the fallopian tube or uterus and therefore expands without causing bleeding. Occasionally, abdominal pregnancies go to term.

Abscess. Localized collection of pus.

Adnexal Ring. Extraovarian adnexal mass with thick echogenic border; this finding is suspicious for ectopic pregnancy.

Adnexa. The regions of the ovaries, fallopian tubes, and broad ligaments.

Amenorrhea. Absence of menstruation. Can be primary if menstruation never occurs or secondary if menstruation occurred in the past.

Anteverted. The body of the uterus is tilted forward.

Beta Subunit. Portion of human chorionic gonadotropin (HCG) measured to determine pregnancy status.

Cervical Pregnancy. Ectopic pregnancy located in the cervix. It is a dangerous site because there is heavy bleeding when the pregnancy is lost.

Cornual Pregnancy. Ectopic pregnancy located at the origin of the fallopian tubes from the endometrial cavity.

Corpus Luteum. Small cyst or complex mass that develops within the ovary in the second half of the menstrual cycle and secretes progesterone.

Crohn's Disease. Bowel inflammation that can affect any level of the bowel from stomach to anus. Fistula is a common complication.

Cul-de-sac. An area posterior to the uterus and anterior to the rectum where fluid often collects.

Dysmenorrhea. Painful menstruation.

Dyspareunia. Painful intercourse.

Ectopic Pregnancy. Pregnancy that is located in a site other than within the fundus of the uterine cavity.

Endometrial Cavity, Canal. A potential space in the center of the uterus where blood or pus may collect.

Endometritis. Infection of the endometrial cavity.

Endometrium. Membrane lining the interior of the uterus.

Follicle (Graafian Follicle). An intraovarian saclike structure in which the ovum matures prior to rupture at ovulation. The follicle is visualized as an ovoid cavity with fluid.

Hematocrit. The percentage of red blood cells in a given volume of blood.

Hydrosalpinx. Accumulation of watery fluid in the fallopian tube. The tube can be blocked at the peritoneal end by adhesions and fibrosis due to a previous infection.

Laparoscopy. A surgical procedure in which a tube is introduced into a small incision made, as a rule, adjacent to the umbilicus. Carbon dioxide is placed within the maternal abdomen. This allows visualization of pelvic structures through a small, movable tube.

Leukocyte Count. The number of circulating white blood cells. This count increases when an inflammatory process is present, as in pelvic inflammatory disease (PID), but remains normal in ectopic pregnancy and endometriosis.

Methotrexate. Chemotherapeutic drug that can eliminate an ectopic pregnancy, leaving no scarring. It is now used as the first approach with unruptured ectopic pregnancies.

Myometrium. Smooth muscle of the uterus.

Pelvic Inflammatory Disease (PID). Infection that spreads from the uterine tubes and ovaries throughout the pelvis; commonly due to gonorrhea.

Peritonitis. Inflammation of the peritoneum, which is the serous membrane lining the abdominal cavity.

Purulent. Containing pus.

Pyosalpinx. Accumulation of pus in the fallopian tube.

Retroverted Uterus. The long axis of the uterus points posteriorly toward the sacrum.

Salpinx. Fallopian tube.

Tubo-ovarian Abscess (TOA). An abscess involving the ovary and the fallopian tube.

Vulva. Region where the urethra and the vagina exit in the perineum.

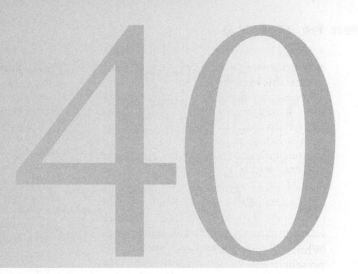

The Clinical Problem

One of the most common indications for a pelvic sonogram is pelvic pain. The differential diagnosis is narrowed by the duration of the pain. If the pain is acute and severe, obstetric disorders should be considered if the patient is of childbearing age. In most parts of the world, rapid, reliable pregnancy tests are available. Because serum pregnancy tests are so reliable, referral to the ultrasound unit should ideally wait until pregnancy test results are performed.

The most common cause of pelvic pain with a positive pregnancy test is ectopic pregnancy. This is a common diagnosis, now occurring in as many as 1 in 200 pregnancies. Pregnancies occurring outside the uterine cavity are termed *ectopic pregnancies.*

Ectopic pregnancies are most frequent in the following types of patients:

1. Patients with a history of pelvic inflammatory disease (PID)
2. Patients with a previous or current intrauterine device
3. Patients undergoing infertility treatment
4. Patients with a history of previous tubal surgery

After successful nonsurgical treatment of an infection, thickened and scarred fallopian tubes may remain. Although these injured tubes may not prevent the passage of sperm for fertilizing ova, the scarring may retard the return of a fertilized zygote to the uterine cavity. The zygote may begin to develop and grow in the fallopian tube, and eventually pain will result due to distention and rupture of the fallopian tube.

Ectopic pregnancy may occur at various sites, including the abdominal cavity, the fallopian tube, the cornu of the uterus, and the cervix (Fig. 40-1). Pregnancies in the interstitial portion of the fallopian tube are the most difficult to diagnose because they lie within the uterine myometrium. If misdiagnosed, they will progress to a more advanced stage than distal tubal ectopics before causing symptoms.

The clinical symptoms and tests that suggest an ectopic pregnancy are as follows:

1. Acute pelvic pain (before or after rupture)
2. Vaginal bleeding (before or after rupture)
3. Amenorrhea (consistent with pregnancy)
4. Adnexal mass (before or after rupture)
5. Positive pregnancy test
6. Cervical tenderness (usually after rupture)
7. A drop in hematocrit (usually after rupture)
8. Shock (after rupture)

A feared complication of ectopic pregnancy is rupture of the ectopic sac. Rupture usually occurs at or before the 8th week of gestation. A ruptured ectopic pregnancy is an urgent surgical emergency. The diagnosis usually cannot be made on clinical grounds alone; pelvic sonography is helpful in making a more specific diagnosis. Free fluid (blood) in the peritoneal cavity suggests ruptured ectopic pregnancy. Unruptured ectopic pregnancy is much less of an emergency and is often treated conservatively with methotrexate. Sonography in a patient with the clinical features of ectopic pregnancy often demonstrates an intrauterine pregnancy, thus precluding surgical intervention.

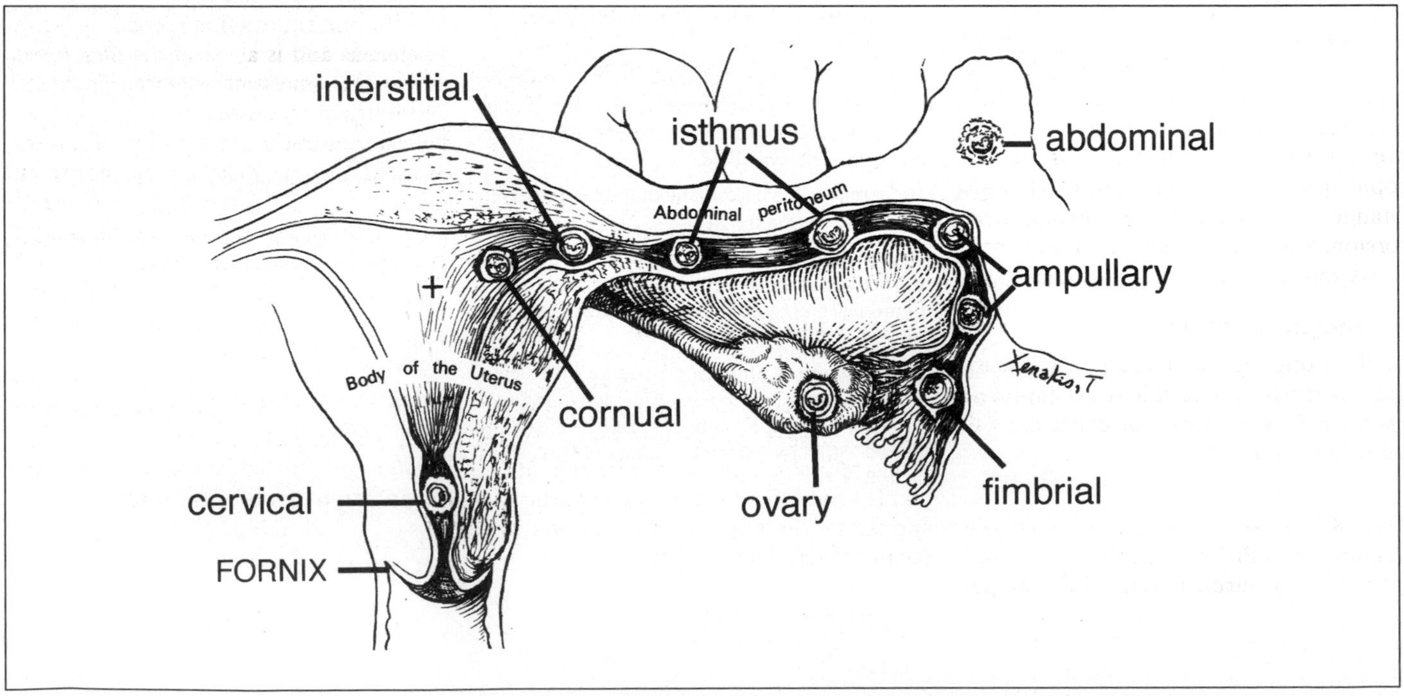

Figure 40-1. ■ *Possible sites for ectopic pregnancy. Note that the type of ectopic pregnancy is named after its site. The fornix is the structure in which the vaginal probe is normally placed. The fornices are very distensible so the vaginal probe transducer can be adjacent to the ectopic pregnancy site.*

Although unruptured ectopic pregnancies may be medically treated with methotrexate administration, the diagnosis is still one that requires an immediate call to the referring doctor.

Abdominal pregnancy outside the tube and uterus is rare. Although abdominal pregnancies can be carried to term, they are most often removed when diagnosed because they have a poor outcome and are associated with many complications.

Quantitation of the beta subunit helps in the diagnosis of ectopic pregnancy. In a normal pregnancy, the level should double every other day. Once it reaches a level of about 1,500 IU (depending on the test used), a normal gestational sac will be seen within the uterus. Falling levels may be due to complete or incomplete spontaneous abortion rather than dead ectopic pregnancy. The pregnancy test may remain positive for as long as 2 months after an abortion or after an ectopic pregnancy has been removed.

TORSION OR RUPTURE OF CORPUS LUTEUM CYST

Rupture or bleeding of any pelvic mass in a pregnant patient causes acute pelvic pain similar to that seen in rupture of an ectopic pregnancy. Torsion (twisting of a cyst on a pedicle), hemorrhage, and rupture are the three complications that cause pain in cysts. Hemorrhage often results from torsion. The sonographic findings of corpus luteum cyst rupture are confusingly similar to those of ectopic pregnancy, but more specific changes are seen with hemorrhage and torsion, especially if there has been a previous sonogram showing a simple cyst.

Nonpregnant Patient

In the nonpregnant patient with acute pain of recent onset, PID and a ruptured or twisted ovarian cyst or ovary are the most likely diagnoses.

PID

Patients with PID are usually febrile and often have a purulent vaginal discharge. An adnexal mass may be felt on clinical examination, and the patient may have pain associated with movement of the cervix. Physical examination is often so painful that a thorough search cannot be completed. In these cases, a pelvic sonogram is needed as a supplemental examination, and at times, it may replace the physical examination completely.

Acute or chronic PID is most commonly caused by gonorrhea or chlamydia. Pyogenic (*Escherichia coli*) and tuberculous infections are other, more unusual causes. There is an association with the use of older intrauterine contraceptive devices. Although PID due to gonorrhea and chlamydia spreads along the mucous membranes and travels from the vulva to the adnexa, the main site of localization is the fallopian tube. If left untreated, the course of tubal infection progresses as follows:

1. Endometritis
2. Acute salpingitis with cul-de-sac pus
3. Chronic salpingitis
4. Pyosalpinx: A blockage of the peritoneal (fimbriated) end of the tube with an accumulation of pus (see Fig. 40-14)
5. Tubo-ovarian abscesses (TOAs): Pus surrounded by tubal and ovarian tissue
6. Pelvic abscess: Abscesses outside of the tube in the region of the ovary or cul-de-sac
7. Hydrosalpinx: The pus from a pyosalpinx resorbs and over months or years becomes sterile, watery fluid (see Fig. 29-19).

The purulent contents of a TOA may escape the confines of the tube and ovary area and cause peritonitis or multiple pelvic abscesses.

The pelvic sonogram helps determine the extent of the disease, including the presence and size of adnexal masses. If large echo-free areas compatible with pus are present, surgical drainage rather than antibiotic therapy may be appropriate. If antibiotic therapy is given, the response to therapy can be followed by means of serial sonograms.

CYSTIC MASSES

Rupture or bleeding of any pelvic mass causes acute pelvic pain similar to that seen in rupture of an ectopic pregnancy. Torsion (twisting of a cyst on a pedicle), hemorrhage, and rupture are the three complications that cause pain in cysts. Hemorrhage often results from torsion.

Anatomy

See Chapter 29, Infertility.

Approximately 95%of ectopic pregnancies occur in the fallopian tubes; it is increasingly easy to visualize the tubes with endovaginal sonography. There are four subdivisions: (1) the mouth of the fallopian tube as it enters into the endometrial cavity is termed the *cornu*; (2) the short "interstitial" portion, which is intramural and surrounded by the wall of the uterus; (3) the long tubal segment termed the *isthmus*; and (4) the ampulla, which opens into the abdominal cavity and receives the ovulated egg into the tube at the fimbria (Fig. 40-1). The normal tube is about 10 cm long.

Technique

See Chapter 29, Infertility.

Use the endovaginal probe. It is not dangerous and is an essential diagnostic tool in this emergency clinical situation. Endovaginal views are usually obtained first because the patient is often instructed to take nothing by mouth in preparation for surgery. If nothing is seen in or outside of the uterus on endovaginal views and if the pregnancy test is positive, then perform transabdominal views for ectopic pregnancies that lie high in the abdomen.

The endovaginal transducer is also routinely used with patients who have acute pelvic pain, either as a first approach or after an apparently normal transabdominal real-time study.

Pathology

ECTOPIC PREGNANCY

The ultrasonic features of ectopic pregnancy are as follows:

1. A gestational sac in the adnexa containing a fetal pole with heart motion and a yolk sac is a diagnostic finding (Fig. 40-2). This used to be a rare finding, but is not uncommon when an endovaginal transducer is used.

   Endovaginal visualization of the fetus is possible as early as 4 weeks and 3 days after menstruation. A yolk sac has such a distinct shape that a diagnosis of ectopic pregnancy can also be made when only a yolk sac is seen in an adnexal sac. Fetal heart motion may be seen with high-quality equipment when the fetal pole itself is barely seen and when the gestational sac is very small (Fig. 40-2).
2. Uterine enlargement or a decidual reaction in the endometrium without a gestational sac. The uterus enlarges when an ectopic pregnancy is present. A cystic structure resembling a gestational sac may be seen within the uterus. This decidual reaction has a single outline, whereas an early gestational sac has a double decidual reaction (Fig. 40-3). Echogenic fluid due to blood often occurs within the pseudogestational sac (Fig. 40-4).

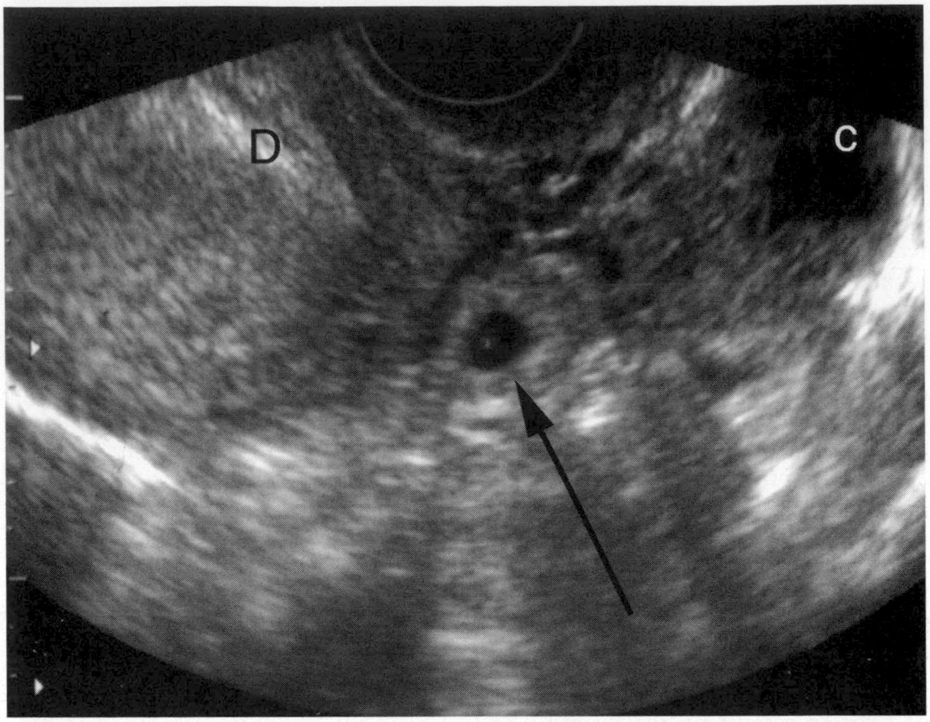

Figure 40-2. ■ *Ectopic pregnancy with yolk sac and cardiac motion at 5 weeks. The arrow points to the ectopic pregnancy. A gestational sac is present between the uterus and the left ovary. Although the fetal pole is very small, cardiac motion was observed within the gestational sac. Note the prominent decidual reaction* (D) *in the uterus. There is a corpus luteum cyst within the left ovary* (C), *which has a thick echogenic border around it and could be mistaken for a gestational sac, except that it lies within the ovary.*

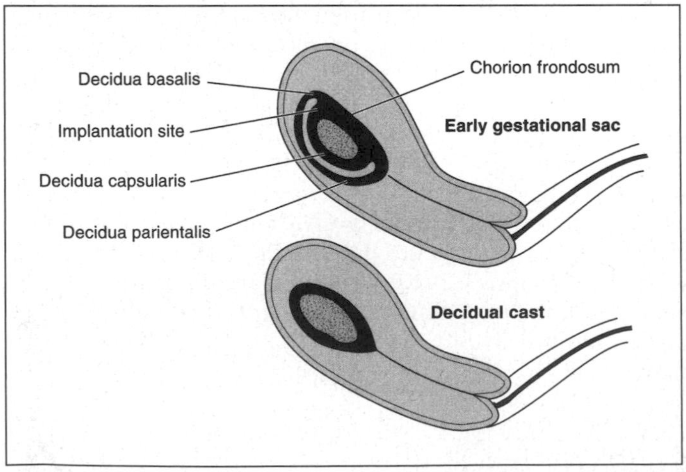

Figure 40-3. ■ *Decidual reaction compared with early gestational sac. Note the double outline to the normal pregnancy, which is eccentrically located to the endometrial cavity. The decidual cast (pseudosac) contains low-level echoes due to blood.*

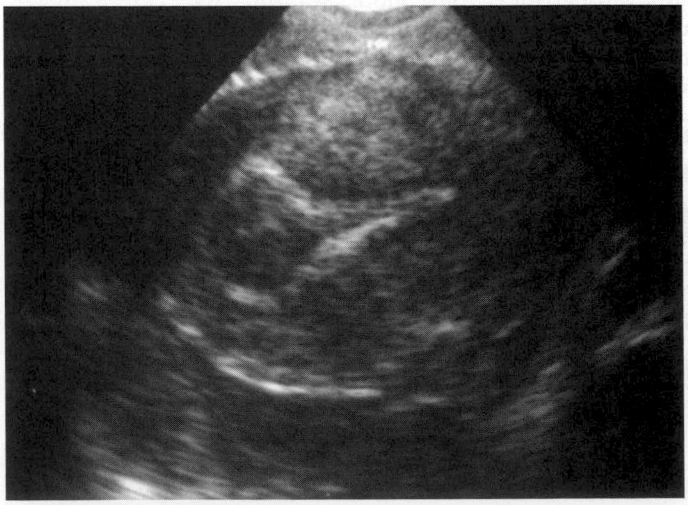

Figure 40-4. ■ *Pseudogestational sac within in the uterus. Note the single wall and the echogenic fluid within the "sac" representing blood. The endometrial cavity echoes extend around the pseudosac.*

The endometrial cavity echoes may also be exceptionally thick due to a decidual reaction without a pseudosac (Fig. 40-5).

3. An adnexal mass, which may be echo filled or hypoechoic (Fig. 40-6). The use of color flow Doppler may be helpful because a low-resistance pattern in the center of a nonspecific extraovarian mass is typical of an ectopic pregnancy; however, this pattern is also seen in association with corpus luteum cysts.
4. Free fluid in the pelvis. When the ectopic pregnancy grows to a size too large for the fallopian tube, it may rupture and induce severe bleeding. Usually, the blood escapes into the peritoneal cavity (see Figs. 40-7 and 40-8) rather than the endometrial cavity.
5. Intra-abdominal blood. If there are many adhesions, free intraperitoneal fluid will not pool in the cul-de-sac but will be seen in the subhepatic space or the paracolic gutters. Those areas should be examined whenever pelvic findings are negative and when ectopic pregnancy is suspected (Fig. 40-8).

The presence of free fluid suggests a ruptured ectopic pregnancy, especially if internal echoes are visible within the free fluid. This represents a dangerous situation, and an

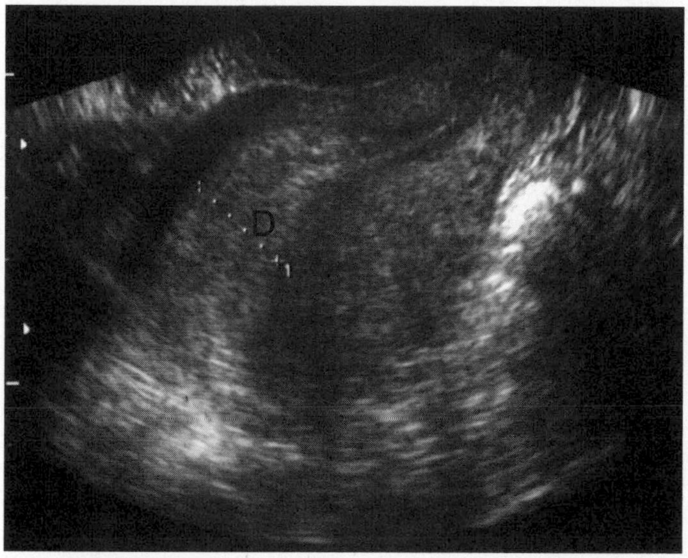

Figure 40-5. ■ *Decidual reaction in another ectopic pregnancy* (D). *The endometrial cavity echoes (being measured) are about three times as thick as is usual in the secretory phase of the endometrial cycle.*

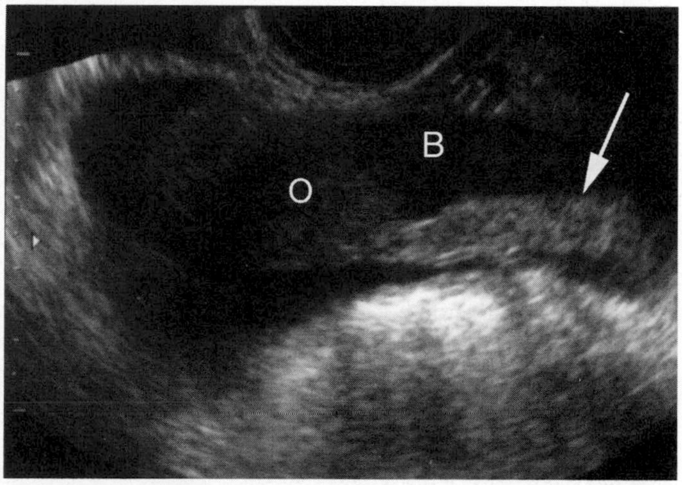

Figure 40-7. ■ *Fluid that is recognizably blood* (B) *because there is an even echogenic texture, due to a ruptured ectopic pregnancy, outlines the ovary* (O) *and the right tube* (arrow). *The ectopic pregnancy was not seen, but the combination of adnexal tenderness, sonographic appearance, and increased beta subunit level made the diagnosis. Because there was a hemoperitoneum, the patient was taken immediately to surgery, where a ruptured ectopic was found.*

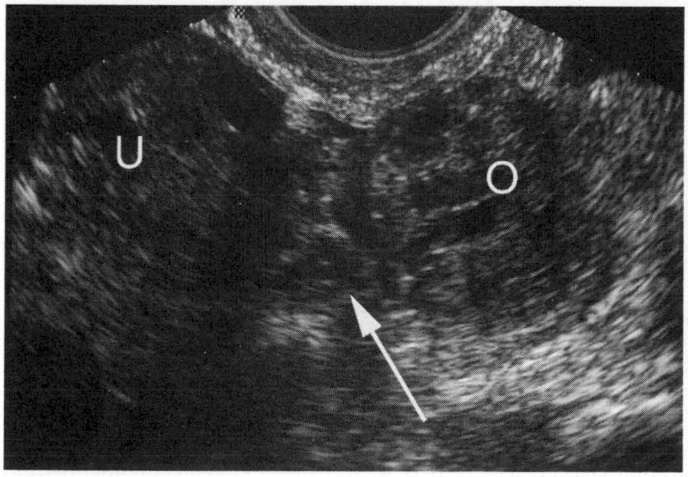

Figure 40-6. ■ *Mass* (arrow) *representing blood clot is seen between the uterus* (U) *and the left ovary* (O). *An ectopic pregnancy with some blood around it was found at surgery.*

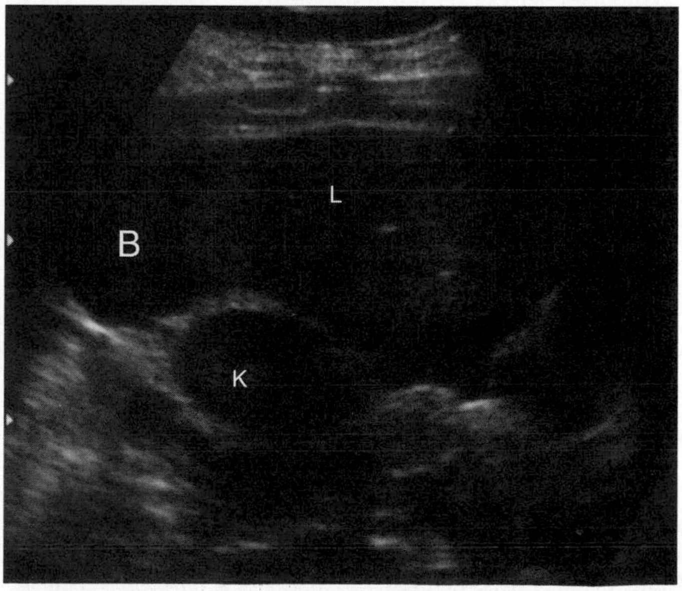

Figure 40-8. ■ *Blood* (B) *in the upper abdomen surrounding the liver* (L) *and anterior to the kidney* (K) *due to a ruptured ectopic pregnancy.*

immediate call should be made to the referring physician.

6. Empty uterus with a positive pregnancy test. If the pregnancy test is positive, but nothing is seen in the pelvis, an ectopic pregnancy is possible. A more likely diagnosis is early pregnancy (before the gestational sac can be seen) or complete spontaneous abortion (if the patient has vaginal bleeding). An ectopic pregnancy becomes almost certain on endovaginal examination if:
   a. There is no intrauterine pregnancy
   b. The patient has had no vaginal bleeding
   c. The beta subunit is more than 1,500 IU.
7. Periuterine blood. If bleeding has occurred, there is a loss of uterine outline due to hematoma. Blood may surround the uterus, giving a "pseudouterus" effect. The presence of blood may not be obvious because the complex mass can look like the uterus.

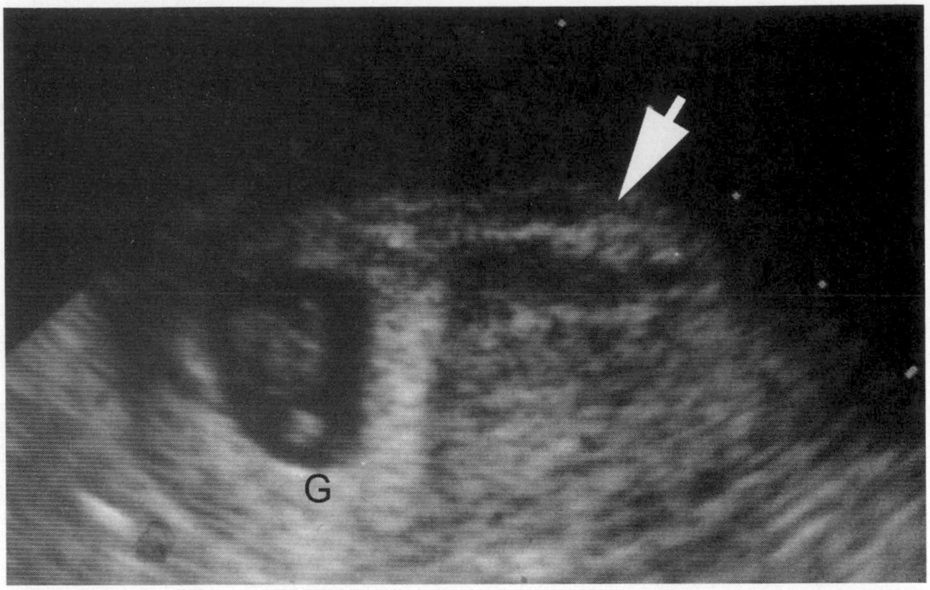

Figure 40-9. ■ *Interstitial pregnancy. The ectopic gestational sac* (G) *lies within the uterine outline. The interstitial line* (arrow) *leads to, but does not enclose, the sac.*

INTERSTITIAL PREGNANCY

When the fertilized egg implants in the intrauterine portion of the tube (intramural), it is termed an *interstitial pregnancy* (Fig. 40-1). Interstitial pregnancies are difficult to diagnose because the gestational sac appears to be within the uterus, although there is a relative absence of surrounding myometrium. An interstitial pregnancy usually presents at a later date than an ectopic pregnancy (8 to 10 weeks) with catastrophic bleeding. The pregnancy may look as if it is in the edge of the myometrium or may lie very close to the uterus (Fig. 40-9). The endometrial cavity line (interstitial line) leads but does not enclose the abnormally placed sac.

This is a very confusing location because a normal gestational sac may not lie in the center at the fundus of the uterus. In addition to a variant of normal, there are two other common causes of lateral gestational sac location:

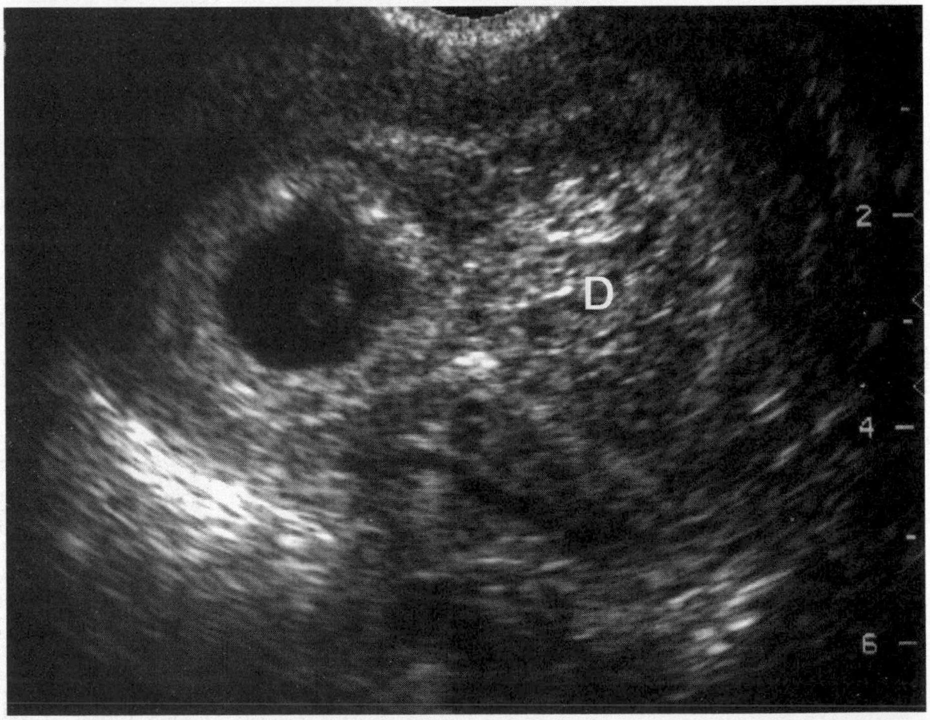

Figure 40-10. ■ *Bicornuate pregnancy (transverse view). The gestational sac is located to the right, and there is a sizable decidual reaction* (D) *in the left horn.*

1. Fibroids at the fundus. The gestational sac is displaced to one side by a fibroid. The texture of the fibroid is usually distorted and easily distinguished from the normal uterus.
2. Bicornuate or subseptate uterus (Fig. 40-10). The pregnancy develops in one horn and is, therefore, eccentrically located. A second well-defined decidual reaction should also be seen on the other side of the uterus.

If neither of these previously mentioned entities are present and if the gestational sac is eccentrically located, reexamine with a different degree of bladder filling. The sac may then appear in the midline. Managing gestational sacs in this location is not easy because so many turn out to be normal variants, yet there is a serious risk of rupture. On re-examination at another time, the gestational sac may adopt a normal location. If the myometrium is very thin (less than 3 mm) over the lateral side of the gestational sac, the diagnosis becomes more likely, but even then, a later examination may be normal.

CERVICAL PREGNANCY

Another rare ectopic location where a pregnancy can implant is the cervix (Fig. 40-11). The gestational sac will be in a low position with little or no myometrium surrounding its inferior aspect. Cervical pregnancies present at a later date than ectopic pregnancies (8 to 10 weeks), often with severe bleeding. An oral dose or an intra-amniotic injection of methotrexate under ultrasound visualization is used to treat this condition.

ABDOMINAL PREGNANCY

Abdominal pregnancy is rare. The pregnancy develops outside the tubes within the peritoneal cavity. These pregnancies may grow to a large size, since they are not surrounded by the fallopian tube and can present at term with unsuccessful labor. Three sonographic findings suggest an abdominal pregnancy (Fig. 40-12):

1. The fetus, placenta, and amniotic fluid are outside the uterus. The uterus may lie between the bladder and the pregnancy; the endometrial cavity in the uterus is the giveaway finding. Less commonly, the uterus may lie posterior to the pregnancy, in which case the diagnosis is often missed.
2. The surrounding membrane around an abdominal pregnancy will be very thin because there is no myometrium.
3. The pregnancy lies close to the abdominal wall.

Abdominal pregnancies often fail before term. During the surgical removal of an abdominal pregnancy, the placenta may be left in place because it is too dangerous to remove. If it is attached to the intestines, it slowly regresses over the ensuing months under the influence of the chemotherapeutic agent methotrexate.

CORPUS LUTEUM PROBLEMS IN PREGNANCY

1. Hemorrhage. Corpus luteum cysts may become filled with blood and form a painful mass, which can be mistaken for an ectopic pregnancy. The corpus luteum will lie within the ovary, whereas an ectopic pregnancy lies outside the ovary. A search for the normal ovary should enable one to differentiate between ectopic pregnancy and a corpus luteum with hemorrhage.
2. Rupture of corpus luteum. The sonographic features of a ruptured corpus luteum include the following:
   a. An adnexal mass with an irregular shape
   b. Cul-de-sac fluid
   c. Evidence of bleeding with development of a relatively echogenic mass of blood (hard to separate from the uterus)

The ovary will lie in the center of this mass. This pattern may be indistin-

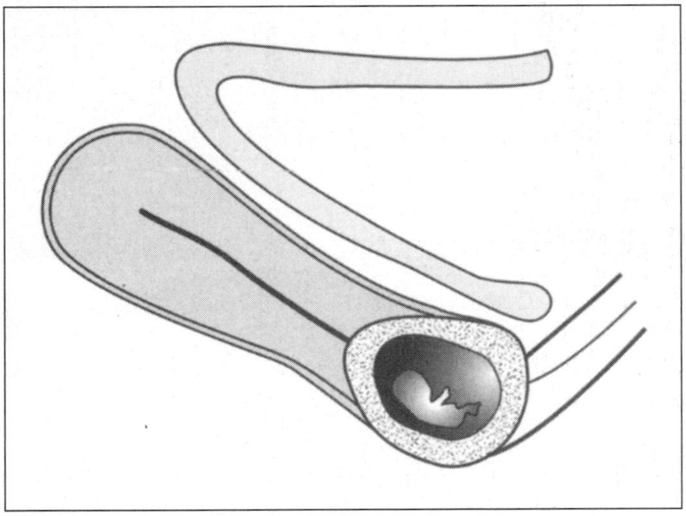

Figure 40-11. ■ *Cervical pregnancy. The gestational sac lies within the cervix. An impending abortion could have a similar appearance but would be at this site for a very short time, and the cervix would likely be open.*

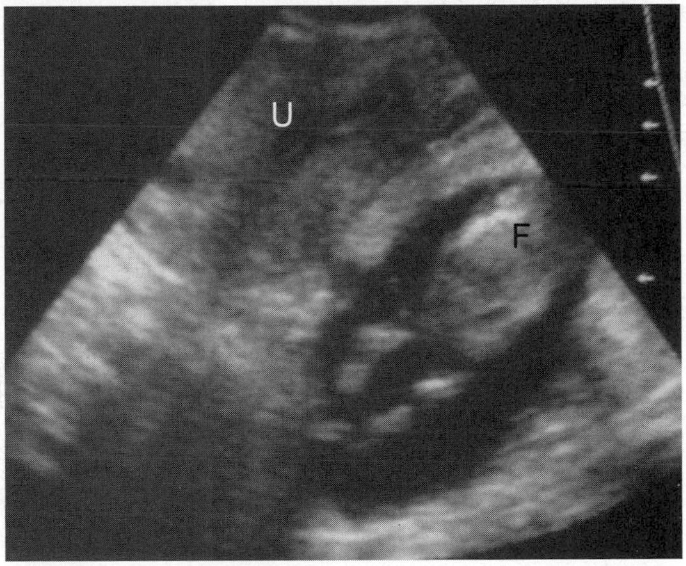

Figure 40-12. ■ *Abdominal pregnancy. The uterus* (U) *lies anterior to the pregnancy. A fetus* (f) *can be seen outside the uterus in the cul-de-sac.*

guishable from ruptured ectopic pregnancy. In both, a low-resistance Doppler pattern is seen within the mass.

ACUTE PID

In a patient with PID, the sonogram is difficult to perform because the uterus and adnexa are so tender when the vaginal probe is inserted. The tenderness is maximal over the uterus and tubal region.

1. Uterus. On some occasions, there is fluid within the endometrial cavity (endometritis) (Fig. 40-13).
2. Cul-de-sac. Fluid often develops in the cul-de-sac. Such fluid almost always contains echoes and perhaps a fluid–fluid level when examined with the vaginal probe.
3. Adnexa. Bilateral cystic or complex masses located lateral, posterior, or superior to the uterus may be seen. These masses represent pyosalpinx or a closely related entity, TOA.

On endovaginal examination, the typical appearance of a pyosalpinx is a smooth-walled curving tubular structure with a club shape (Fig. 40-14). The walls of the dilated tubes may be thickened and irregular if the acute infection has been present for awhile. The tubal contents may contain internal echoes. Unilateral pyosalpinx is uncommon because most infections relate to venereal diseases such as gonorrhea or chlamydia. Local inflammatory disease such as Crohn's disease or diverticulosis may cause a unilateral pyosalpinx. Although the ovaries may be surrounded by infected material, they are practically never directly involved with PID.

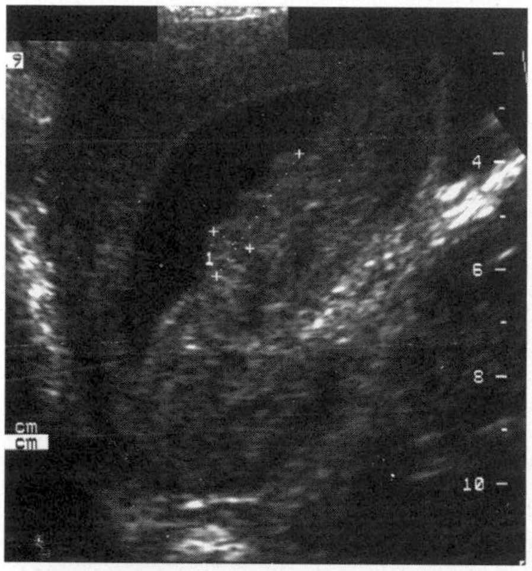

Figure 40-13. ■ *Enlarged uterus in a patient who has recently been pregnant and now has pus within the endometrial cavity. Note the debris within the endometrial cavity* (measurement markers).

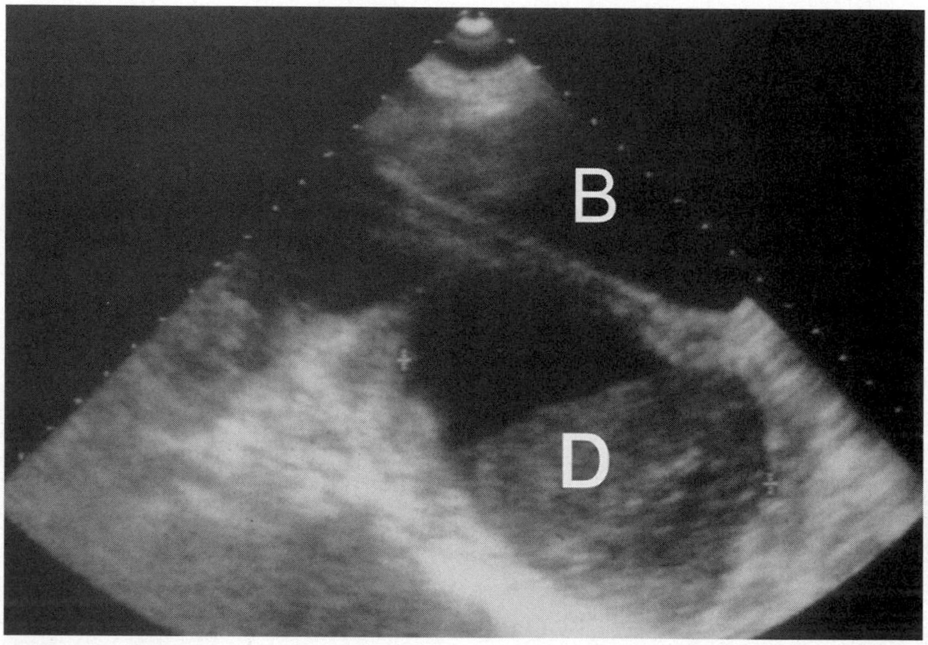

Figure 40-14. ■ *Pyosalpinx. The dilated club-shaped fallopian tube has thickened walls and contains echogenic pus* (D). *B, bladder.*

HEMORRHAGIC CYSTS

Hemorrhagic cysts are blood-filled cysts containing echoes that may form a fluid–fluid level (Fig. 40-15) or a clump-like pattern due to clot. Severe pain develops when the bleeding into the cyst takes place. Bleeding into a cyst sometimes occurs at the time of ovulation with the formation of the corpus luteum. In some women, large hemorrhagic cysts, in association with ovulation, occur repeatedly. In other women, bleeding into a cyst occurs when a pre-existing cyst, either a follicular cyst or a cystadenoma, twists and torts. In both situations, a cystic mass is seen in the ovary that contains either (1) a fluid–fluid level; (2) a crescent-shaped mass of low-level echogenicity; (3) clumps of echogenic material; (4) diffuse, even, echogenic material; or (5) diffuse low-level echoes.

TORTED OVARY OR CYST

If the ovary twists on its mesenteric attachment, much pain develops. Some blood will usually be seen in the region of the ovary, and the ovary will be very tender and enlarged on endovaginal examination. Color flow analysis of the blood supply to the ovary in torsion has been confusing because there is a double arterial supply. If no flow can be demonstrated while flow to the other ovary can be seen, torsion is probable. Evidence of normal flow does not rule out torsion, however, since blood supply from the ovarian artery can continue while the uterine artery supply is occluded, or vice versa.

Cysts in the ovary may be associated with torsion. The cyst is very tender with the endovaginal probe and often contains a fluid–fluid level. A thick rim may surround the ovary.

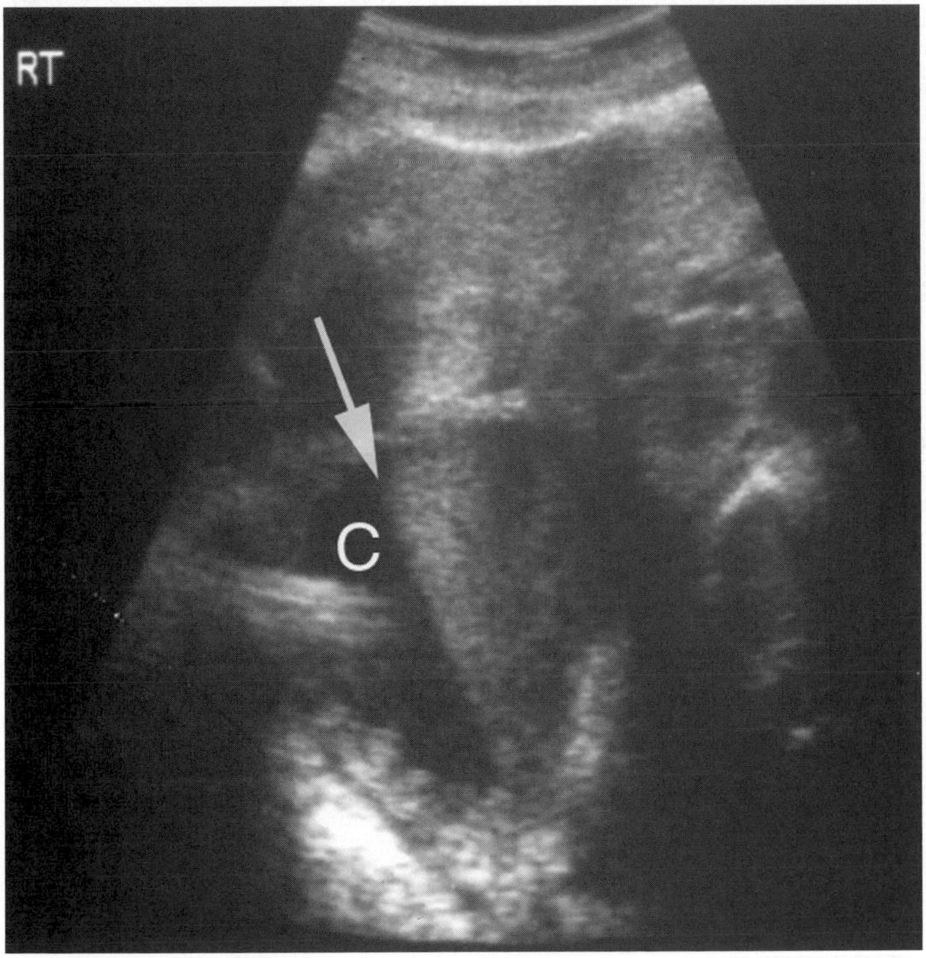

Figure 40-15. ■ *Endovaginal view of a bleed into a cyst* (C). *The cyst contains a fluid–fluid level* (arrow), *which appears at a more or less vertical axis in the usual way endovaginal views are displayed, although it is actually horizontal.*

RUPTURED CYST

Common features of a ruptured cyst include the following:

1. An adnexal mass with an irregular shape
2. Cul-de-sac fluid
3. Evidence of bleeding with development of a relatively echogenic mass of blood (hard to separate from the uterus), as in ruptured ectopic pregnancy

Pitfalls

1. A cervical pregnancy and an impending abortion appear similar. If the pregnancy is aborting, the sonographic findings will change rapidly, and the patient will be bleeding.
2. Pelvic adhesions in pregnancy. Check in the upper abdomen if nothing is seen in the pelvis. If many adhesions are present in the pelvis, free fluid may only be seen in the lateral paracolic "gutters" or in the subhepatic space.
3. Abdominal pregnancies. Abdominal pregnancies are easily missed unless the empty uterus is recognized lying between the bladder and the pregnancy. Always look for myometrium surrounding the amniotic fluid and placenta in any pregnancy.
4. Decidual reaction versus gestational sac. Many decidual casts have been mistaken for intrauterine pregnancies. The clue to the diagnosis of decidual reaction with a pseudosac is the absence of the double outline that is normally seen in an early intrauterine gestational sac.
5. Cornual ectopic versus eccentrically located normal pregnancy. It is hard to distinguish these two entities because the normal gestational sac may be eccentrically located. A fibroid may displace the sac to one side. With a bicornuate uterus, there will be an eccentric gestational sac position, but a second decidual reaction will be seen.
6. Color flow Doppler. Low-resistance Doppler flow can be found both with a corpus luteum with hemor-

rhage and with ectopic pregnancy. This finding is only helpful if the normal ovary has been located, if a separate mass is seen, and if flow is found within the mass.

Where Else to Look

1. Empty uterus with positive pregnancy test. If the uterus appears normal but the pregnancy test is positive, look in the cul-de-sac and the adnexa for evidence of ectopic pregnancy. If there is nothing to see, the possibilities are (1) early pregnancy, (2) complete spontaneous abortion. or (3) ectopic pregnancy. Profuse vaginal bleeding favors complete spontaneous abortion.
2. Look for nongynecological causes of pain.
   a. Appendicitis. Some retrocecal cases of appendicitis lie low in the pelvis and can mimic an adnexal cause of acute pain. Sonographic appearances are described in Chapter 15. Some cases of appendicitis are best seen with the vaginal probe.
   b. Renal colic. Pain referred into the adnexa can originate from a ureteric stone (see Chapter 20). The endovaginal probe is a good way to see renal calculi impacted at the ureterovesical junction. Calculi have been seen with the endovaginal probe that were not visible from the standard abdominal approach.
   c. Gut lesions. Gut problems located in the true pelvis can present with adnexal pain. Crohn's disease is particularly likely to involve the adnexa and can create fistulous connections to the fallopian tube. The typical appearances are described in Chapter 15.

SELECTED READING

Ackerman TH, Levi CS, Dashefsky SM, et al. Interstitial line: sonographic findings in interstitial (cornual) ectopic pregnancy. *Radiology* 1993;189:83–87.

Atri M, Leduc C, Gillett P, et al. Role of endovaginal sonography in the diagnosis and management of ectopic pregnancy. *Radiographics* 1996;16:755–774.

Chiang G, Levine D, Swire M, et al. The intradecidual sign: is it reliable for diagnosis of early intrauterine pregnancy? *AJR Am J Roentgenol* 2004;183:725–731.

Dialani V, Levine D. Ectopic pregnancy: a review. *Ultrasound Q* 2004;20:105–117.

Ignacio EA, Hill MC. Ultrasound of the acute female pelvis. *Ultrasound Q* 2003;19:86–98.

Sanders RC, Parsons A. *Integrated Sonography and Management in Gynecology*. Elsevier. In press.

Timor-Tritsch E, Lerner JP, Montaguedo A, et al. Transvaginal sonographic markers of tubal inflammatory disease. *Ultrasound Obstet Gynecol* 1998;12:56–66.

Wachsberg RH. Ectopic pregnancy: recent developments and changing concepts. *Ultrasound Q* 2003;14:247–257.

Uncertain Dates

Elective Cesarean Section, "Late Registrant"

ROGER C. SANDERS
NANCY SMITH MINER

41

KEY WORDS

Amniocentesis. Procedure involving the insertion of a small needle into the amniotic cavity to obtain fluid for cytogenic or biochemical analysis.

Brachycephaly. Short, wide fetal head—a third-trimester normal variant.

Breech Presentation. The fetal head is situated at the fundus of the uterus (see Fig. 41-21).

Cephalic Presentation. The fetal head is the presenting part in the cervical area; also known as a *vertex presentation* (see Fig. 41-21).

DeLee's Test. The first time the fetal heart can be heard with the fetal stethoscope, usually at about 16 weeks' gestation.

Dolichocephaly. Long, flattened fetal head—a normal variant.

Ductus Venosus. Fetal vein that connects the umbilical vein to the inferior vena cava and runs at an oblique axis through the liver.

Face Presentation. The fetal face is the presenting part. This suboptimal position is more likely in a fetus that is lying on its back.

Gestational Age. As used with ultrasound studies, this term refers to the pregnancy age since the first day of the last menstrual period.

Gravid. Pregnant.

High-Risk Pregnancy (HRP). Pregnancy at high risk for an abnormal outcome. Typical examples of high-risk pregnancies are those that involve (1) maternal disease (e.g., kidney or heart disease), (2) maternal drug ingestion (e.g., alcohol or cigarettes), (3) a previous pregnancy with a small fetus, and (4) a family history of congenital malformations.

Hydrocephalus. Enlargement of the cerebral ventricles; can be associated with spina bifida.

Late Registration. A pregnant woman who first attends the obstetric clinic when she is 20 or more weeks pregnant is termed a *late registrant.* At this stage of pregnancy, clinical dating is difficult because several important dating landmarks have passed (e.g., quickening and the DeLee's test).

Menstrual Age. Age of the pregnancy calculated from the last menstrual period.

Microcephaly. Unduly small skull and brain. Associated with mental deficiency.

Para. Term used to describe how many pregnancies a woman has undergone and their outcome. The first number represents the total number of pregnancies. The second number represents the number of abortions. The third number indicates the total number of premature births. The fourth number shows the number of full-term pregnancies. For example, para 4112 represents four pregnancies, one abortion, one premature birth, and two full-term deliveries.

Quickening. The time when the mother first feels the baby move—about 16 to 18 weeks.

Shoulder Presentation. The fetal shoulder is the presenting part (see Fig. 41-21).

Transverse Lie. A fetus that is lying transversely so that the head and trunk are at approximately the same level (see Fig. 41-21).

Umbilical Vein and Arteries. Vessels within the cord. There are two arteries and one vein.

Ventricular Outflow Tracts. Term used for a view showing the chambers of the heart and the aorta and a second view showing the pulmonary artery as it leaves the main chambers of the heart.

Vertex Presentation. The fetal head is the presenting part. This is the usual presentation; it can be face first or brow first (see Fig. 41-21).

The Clinical Problem

UNCERTAIN DATES

Pregnant women are often referred to ultrasound to confirm gestational age. One of the common reasons for referral is uncertainty about when the mother became pregnant. The mother (1) may be uncertain whether her last menstrual period was a genuine period, (2) may have a history of infrequent periods, or (3) may be a late registrant, first attending the clinic after dating landmarks (such as the DeLee's test, quickening, and findings on the first trimester physical examination) have already passed. A sonogram is also usually recommended to confirm the maternal dates when a woman has had a previous cesarean section. Another cesarean section is often performed with any subsequent pregnancy, and in such patients, the gestational age must be accurately determined so that a cesarean section will not be performed too early, possibly resulting in a child with immature lungs.

Many patients undergo a sonogram between 11 and 14 weeks. Dating is most accurate at this time, twins can be diagnosed and, in addition, the test for nuchal thickening (Chapter 45) can be performed. In any event, dating by ultrasound should take place before 28 weeks, because at a later stage in pregnancy the biparietal diameter may vary within a 4-week range of possible dates.

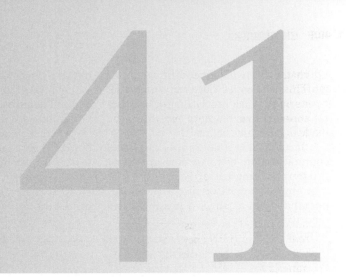

Often the first, or an additional sonogram, is performed between 16 and 20 weeks so that the timely diagnosis of fetal anomalies or placenta previa can be made.

If an earlier sonogram is available, continue to date by those measurements. If dating is being performed for the first time after 28 weeks, be sure to issue a report that gives a range of possible dates (and weights) for a given measurement. Reporting by computer saves a lot of time because a date and a range of possible dates can be generated effortlessly without the tedium and possible inaccuracy associated with gathering the information from tables (see Appendices 6, 7, 8, 10, 11).

Fetal Presentation

It can be difficult for the clinician to tell which part of the baby is going to be delivered first. Most babies are delivered head first (cephalic or vertex presentation). Others are delivered foot or bottom first (breech presentation). The latter is a much more dangerous mode of delivery and generally requires cesarean section. Other dangerous fetal positions are shoulder presentation and transverse lie. The sonographer should therefore make a point of mentioning the fetal position if a preliminary report is being issued.

If the fetus is lying on its back with the head presenting, this is known as a *dorsoposterior fetal position*. There is a greater chance that a fetus in this position will be difficult to deliver because the face is the presenting part.

The sonographer's preliminary report on an obstetric sonogram should include (1) fetal position, (2) number of fetuses, (3) placental position, (4) measurements of the biparietal diameter, femoral length, and abdominal and head circumference (after 16 weeks), and (5) whether evidence of fetal movement or fetal heart movement was observed. It is wise to document images that correspond with those suggested by ACR/AIUM/ACOG guidelines (see Appendix 32).

Anatomy

The anatomy described in this chapter is limited to that required for a basic obstetric ultrasound examination. In a basic exam, a series of transverse views of the fetus are obtained (Fig. 41-1).

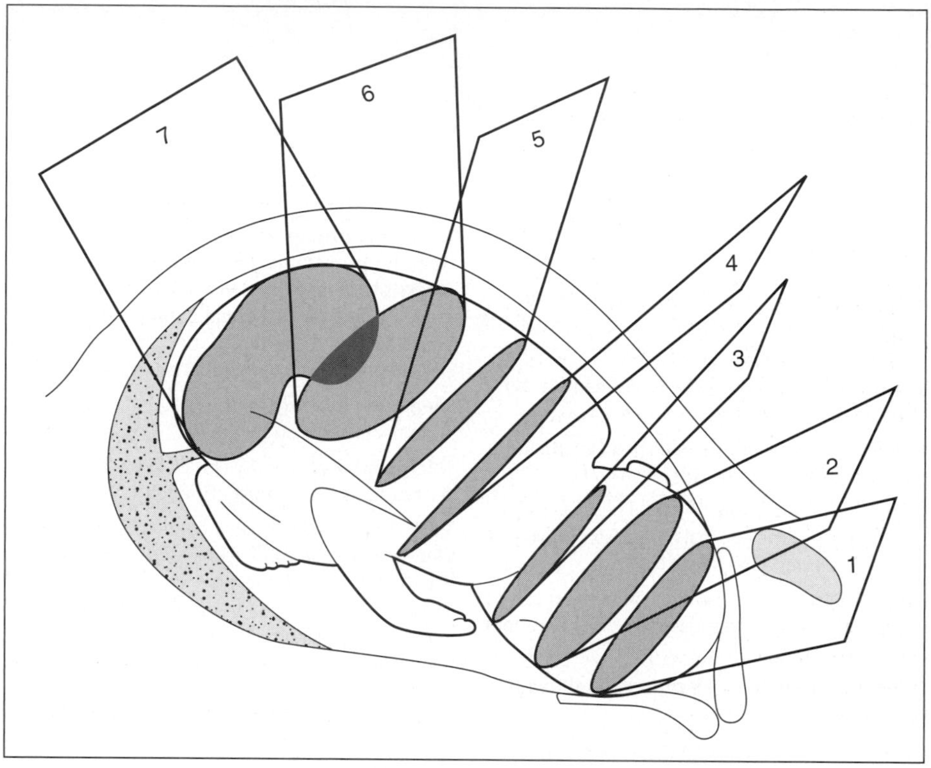

Figure 41-1. ■ *View of the fetus showing the levels at which the transverse images of the fetus are obtained to satisfy the ACR/AIUM/ACOG guidelines. Level 1 is obtained at the level of the lateral ventricles; level 2 at the level of the biparietal diameter; level 3 at the level of the cerebellum; level 4 at the level of the fetal heart; level 5 at the trunk circumference level; level 6 at the level of the fetal kidneys; and level 7 is obtained at the level of the lumbar spine and bladder.*

FETAL HEAD

Cross-sectional anatomy of the fetal head should be defined at varying levels, starting at the level of the lateral ventricles (Fig. 41-2) and moving inferiorly

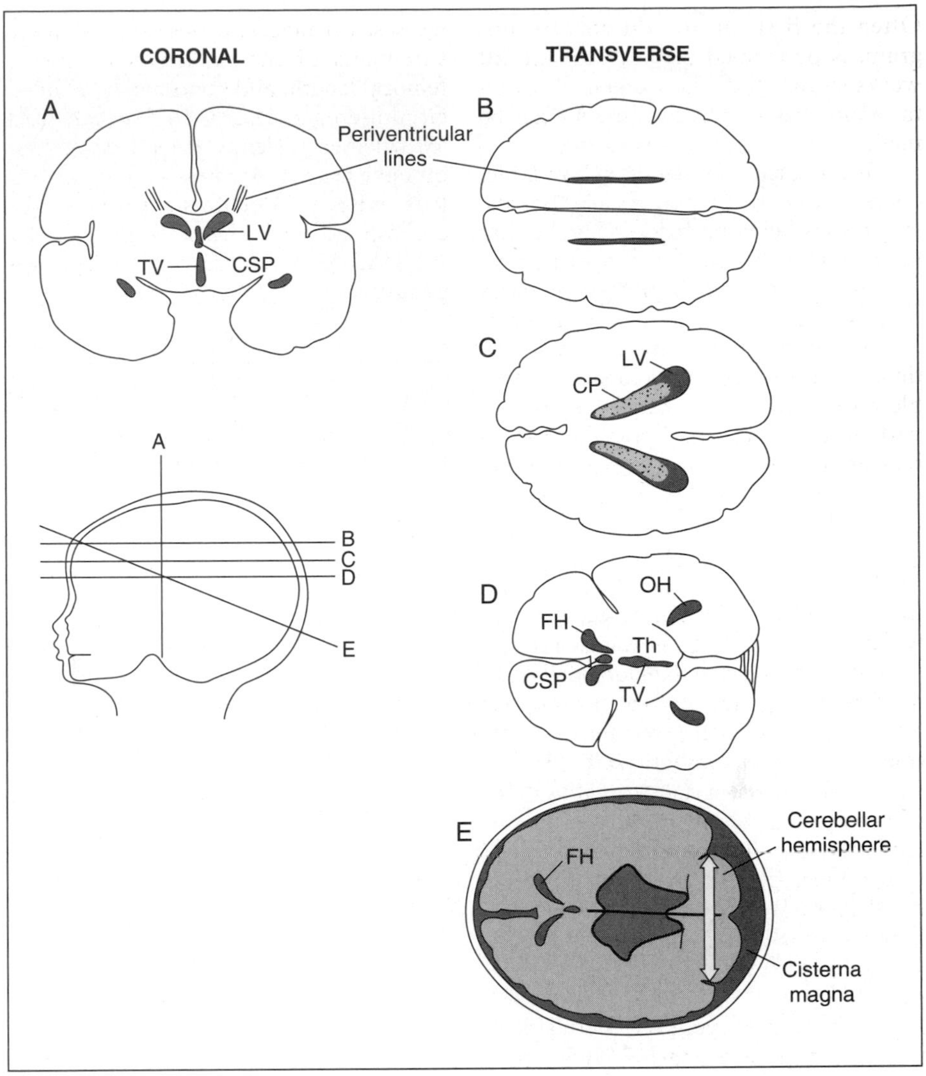

Figure 41-2. ■ *Series of normal transverse sections and coronal sections. On the coronal view (**A**), note the lateral ventricles* (LV) *and the cavum septum pellucidum* (CSP) *between them. The third ventricle* (TV) *is immediately inferior. The transverse (**B**) shows the periventricular line that can be seen on the coronal view. These periventricular lines were at one time mistaken for the lateral ventricles. They actually represent a series of blood vessels that lie superior to the lateral ventricles. Section (**C**) is taken at the level of the lateral ventricles* (LV). *The choroid plexus* (CP) *can be seen within the lateral ventricles. Section (**D**) is taken at the level normally used for the biparietal diameter. One can see the cavum septum pellucidum* (CSP), *the frontal horns* (FH), *and the occipital horns* (OH). *The thalamus* (Th) *surrounds the third ventricle* (TV). *Section (**E**), which is more oblique, is a section through the cerebellum and the front horns* (FH). *This is the section used to measure skin thickness, cerebellar width, and cisterna magna size. (Reprinted with permission by D Nyberg.)*

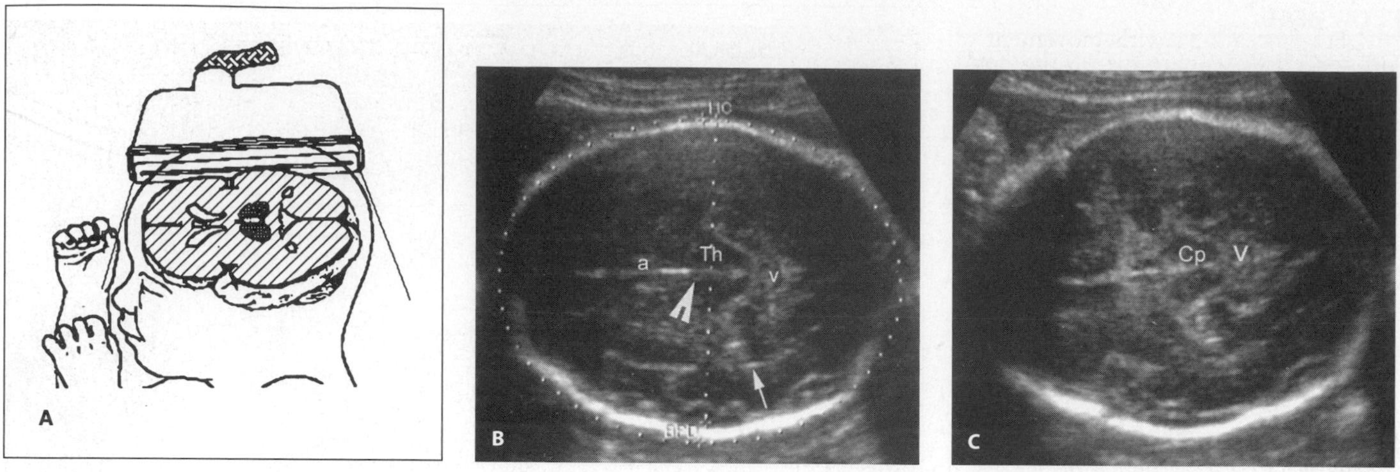

Figure 41-3. ■ *A. Diagram showing the axial approach to obtaining views of the thalami (level D on the inset of Fig. 41-2). **B.** Sonographic appearances of a normal BPD and head circumference view. The thalamus* (Th) *should have a diamond shape, and the third ventricle* (arrowhead) *should be seen between them. The cavum septum pellucidum* (a) *is visible. Too much of the cerebellar vermis* (v) *should not be visible in an acceptable head circumference view. The occipitofrontal diameter is obtained at this level. The biparietal diameter should be taken from the near-side echoes to the inner aspect of the far-side echo (central line of dots). The head circumference measurement is taken around the outside of the skull echoes (dotted line around the outside of the skull)* (arrow indicates sylvian fissure). *Image **(C)** is taken at the level of the cerebral peduncles* (Cp). *The vermis of the cerebellum is shown* (v). *This level may give an erroneously small biparietal diameter measurement because it is inferior to the thalamus.*

(Figs. 41-3 and 41-4). Structures that should be routinely identified are the thalamus (Fig. 41-3), the lateral ventricles (Figs. 41-2 and 41-3B), the third ventricle (Fig. 41-3B), the cavum septi pellucidi (Fig. 41-3B), the sylvian fissures (Fig. 41-3B), the cerebellar hemispheres (Fig. 41-4), the vermis of the cerebellum (Fig. 41-3A,B), and the cisterna magna (Fig. 41-4).

Abnormalities in the posterior fossa structures or enlargement of the ventricles raise suspicion of spinal abnormalities.

FETAL CHEST

On either side of the heart, one can see the fetal lungs, which are evenly echogenic but have a slightly different texture from the liver. The diaphragm can be seen as an interface between the liver and the lung (Fig. 41-5).

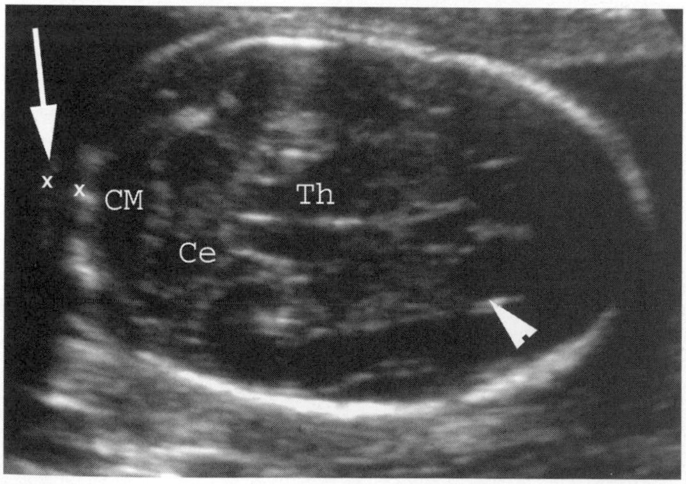

Figure 41-4. ■ *Axial view of the cerebellum* (Ce) *at 20 weeks. The cisterna magna* (CM) *can be seen between the cerebellum and occiput. The arrow points to the measurement markers, which are used for measuring nuchal thickening. This view is critical in excluding spina bifida. In almost all instances of spina bifida, the cerebellum will become banana shaped, and the cisterna magna will not be seen. The arrowhead points to the lateral ventricles. Th, thalamus.*

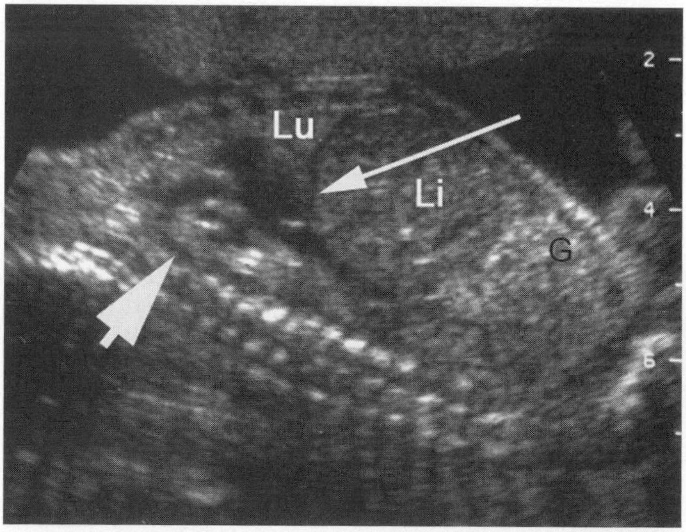

Figure 41-5. ■ *Sagittal view of a supine fetus showing the diaphragm* (thin arrow) *and the heart. The aortic arch* (thick arrow) *is well demonstrated. Note the slight difference in texture of the liver* (Li) *below the diaphragm and the lungs* (Lu) *above the diaphragm. G, gut.*

Fetal breathing with movement of the diaphragm is commonly present after approximately 24 weeks. The ribs cast acoustic shadows across the chest.

FETAL HEART

On a transverse section through the chest, a normal heart will occupy about one third of the chest, predominantly on the left side. The four chambers of the fetal heart should be routinely identified on a four-chamber view (Fig. 41-6).

The right and left ventricular outflow tract views (see Fig. 47-3) are useful additional views. If normal four-chamber and outflow tract views of the heart are obtained, most cardiac malformations can be excluded. A brief look to see whether the rhythm is regular and if the rate is normal is desirable.

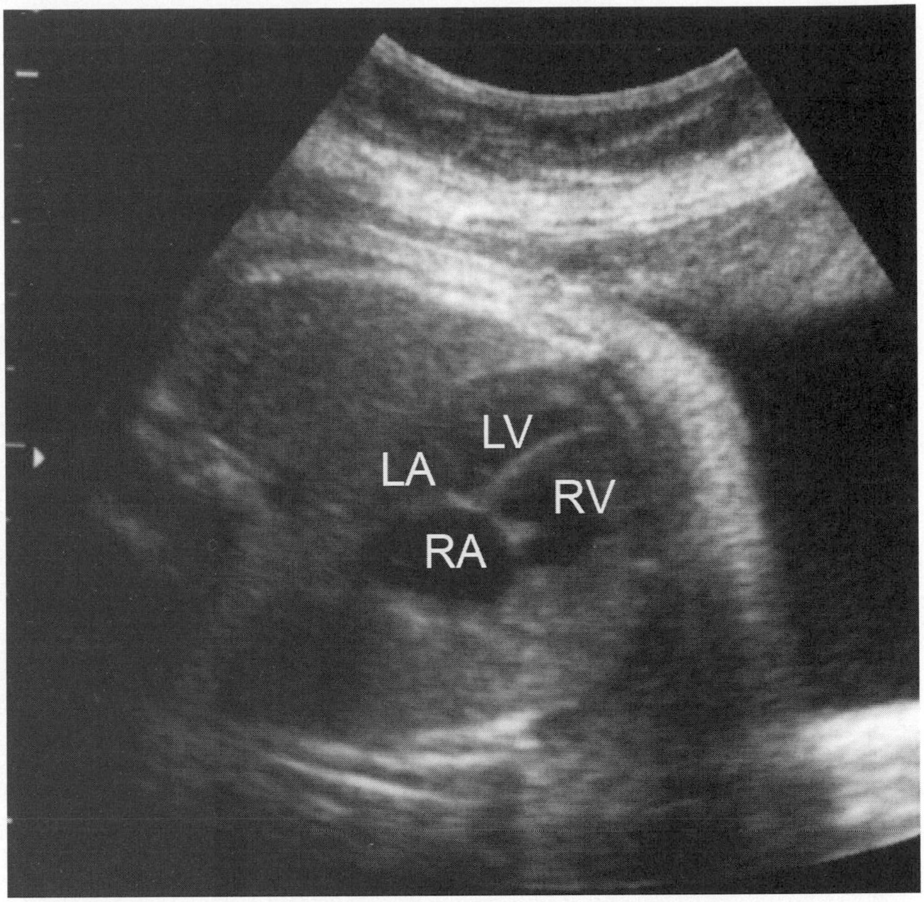

Figure 41-6. ■ *Four-chamber view of the fetal heart. The right* (RV) *and left ventricle* (LV) *and the right* (RA) *and left atria* (LA) *are labeled. As long as the situs is normal, the heart is on the left side of the fetus, and the left ventricle points left. This is the normal degree of obliquity of the heart as it relates to the spine.*

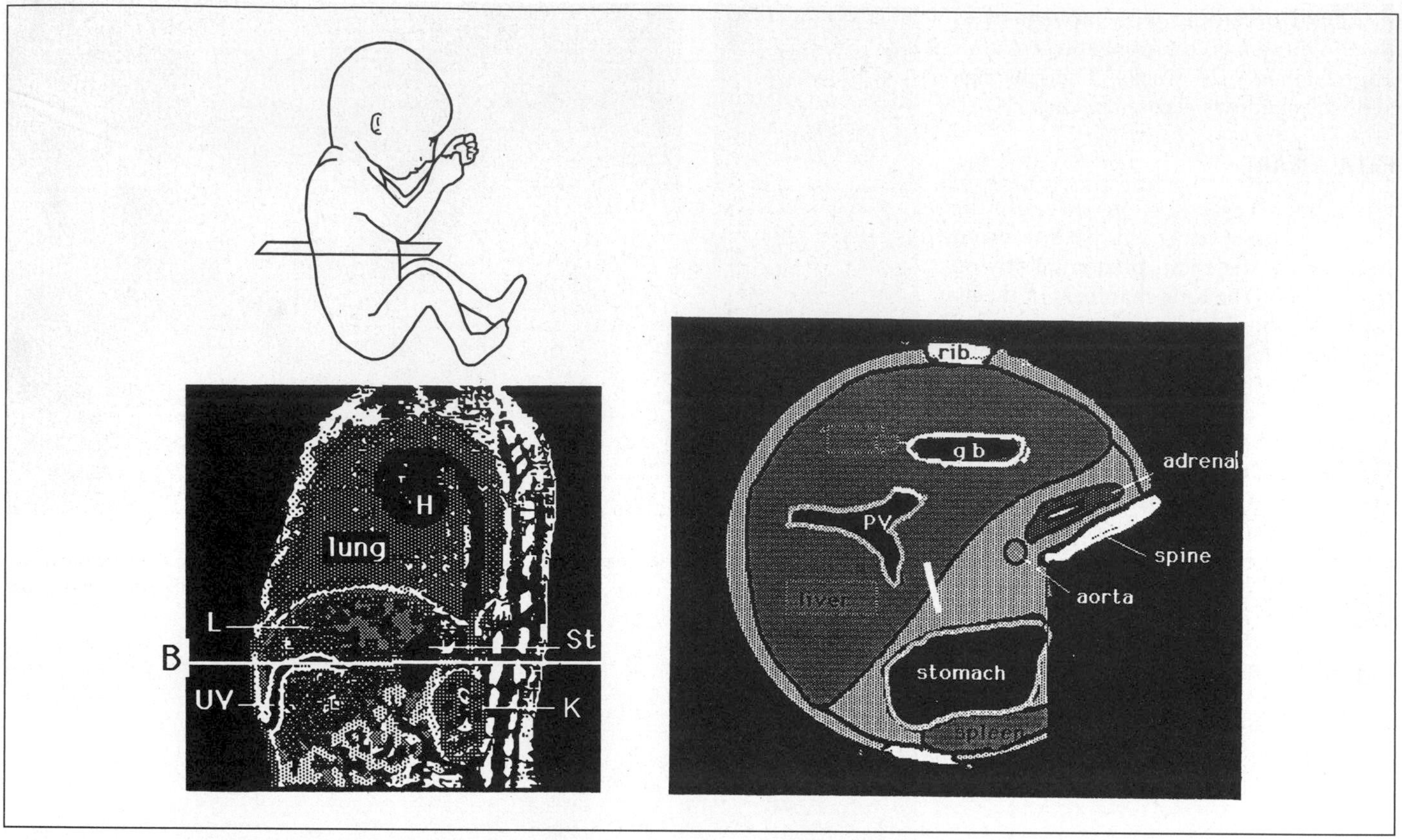

Figure 41-7. ■ *Longitudinal section of the fetus through the chest and abdomen (left). A transverse section taken through the liver shows the aorta, stomach, and portal vein. The inset diagram* (top) *shows the level at which the trunk circumference is obtained. Trunk circumference view* (right) *shows the gallbladder* (gb), *the portal vein* (pv), *the adrenal gland, the aorta, stomach, and symmetrically placed ribs if the view is of good quality. Shadowing behind the spine obliterates part of the abdominal outline.*

FETAL ABDOMEN, LIVER, GALLBLADDER, AND SPLEEN

On a high transverse section of the fetal abdomen, the liver, umbilical and left portal veins, stomach, aorta, adrenal glands, and spine should be visible (Figs. 41-7 and 41-8).

The gallbladder can often be seen within the liver contour and may be confused with the umbilical vein. A fetal liver has the same homogeneous appearance as an adult liver. The liver edge can usually be delineated adjacent to fetal bowel (Fig. 41-5).

The spleen may be visible on the side of the abdomen opposite the liver (see Fig. 41-11). The pancreas is hard to distinguish from the liver; the vascular anatomy is often the best clue to finding the fetal pancreas.

KIDNEY AND BLADDER

On lower transverse sections, the fetal kidneys can be seen (Fig. 41-9). They are

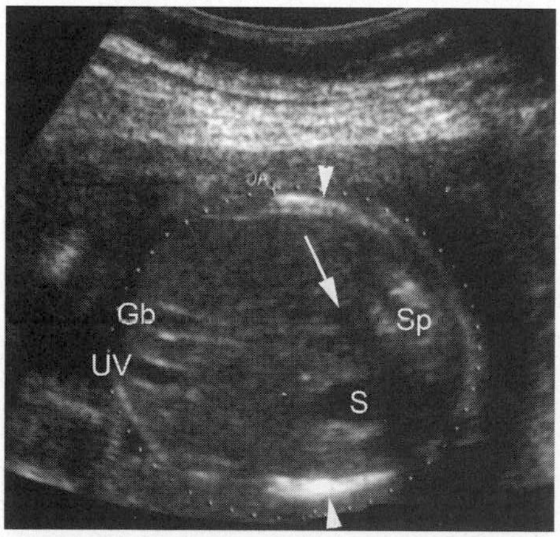

Figure 41-8. ■ *Transverse view of the fetal abdomen. S, stomach; Sp, spine; UV, umbilical vein. The arrow points to the aorta. GB, gallbladder. Both ribs are symmetrical* (arrowhead), *an indication that the abdominal circumference is not oblique. The dotted line outlines the normal measurement site for the abdominal circumference.*

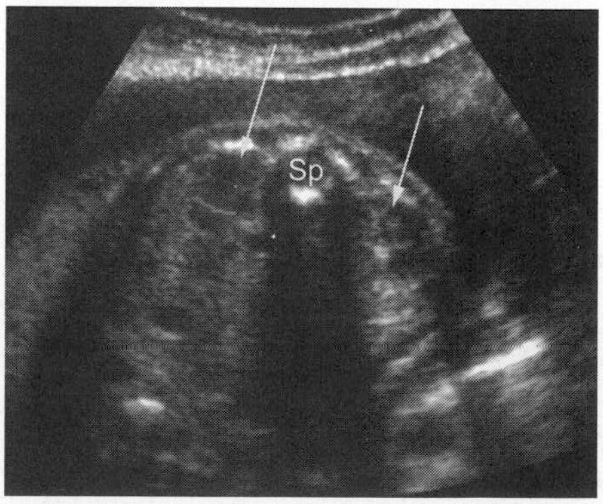

Figure 41-9. ■ *Transverse view of the kidneys* (arrows) *showing their position alongside the spine* (Sp).

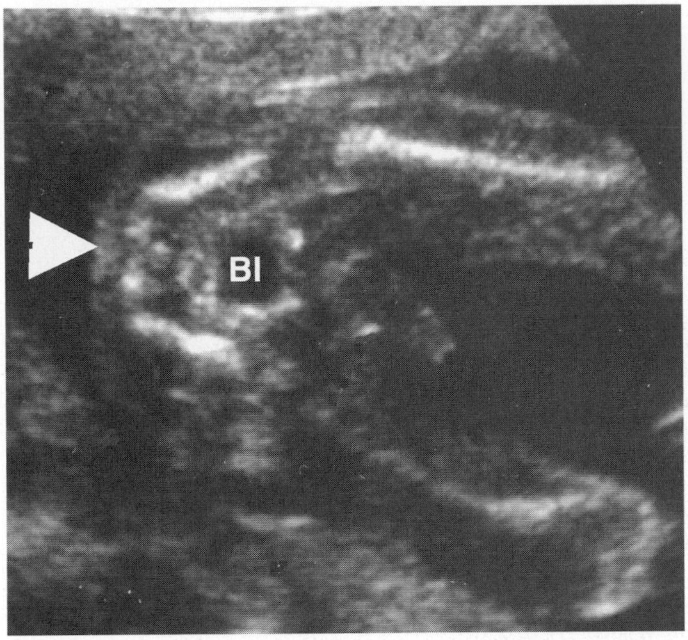

Figure 41-10. ■ *Transverse view of the bladder* (Bl). *The lumbar spine* (arrowhead) *can be seen posterior to the bladder. Spina bifida is often located at this level and seen well on this view. The femurs are also visible.*

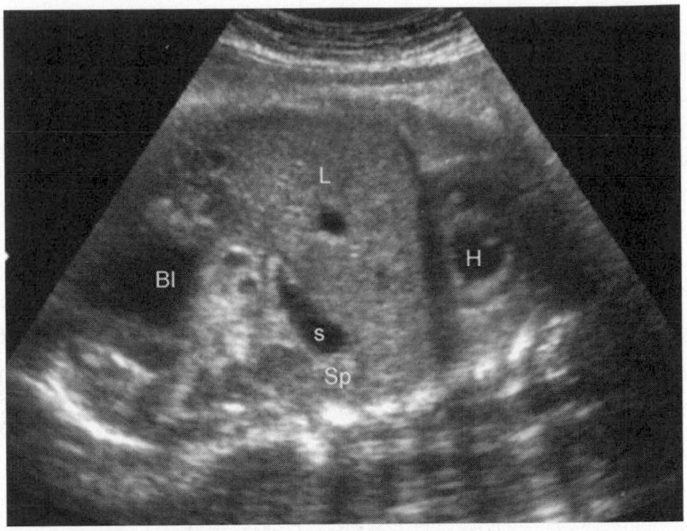

Figure 41-11. ■ *Coronal view of the fetal abdomen showing the fetal bladder* (Bl), *the stomach* (S), *the liver* (L), *the spleen* (Sp) *and, above the diaphragm, the heart* (H).

paraspinous and have a configuration similar to that of adult kidneys. A small degree of dilatation of the central sinus echoes is permissible as a normal variant. The dilatation is accepted as a normal variant if it is less than 5 mm and probably normal if it is between 5 and 10 mm.

At a still lower section, the fetal bladder should be recognizable (Fig. 41-10); it empties and fills over the course of about an hour and is rarely completely empty.

While small bowel is echogenic, large bowel contains meconium, which can look echopenic or echogenic in the third trimester. A fetal long-axis section that demonstrates the bladder, stomach, and heart is desirable (Fig. 41-11).

GENITALIA

From as early as 13 weeks on, the penis and scrotum can be seen (Fig. 41-12). The testicles normally descend into the scrotum at 28 weeks. Females can be recognized by seeing the echogenic labia with a linear echo from the vagina in between (Fig. 41-13).

Most patients are anxious to know the fetal sex. We inform the parents of the fetal gender but say that there is a chance that we are wrong (even if we are certain).

The gender of the fetus can be important information from an obstetric point of view; there may be sex-linked chromosomal anomalies or a need to determine the type of twin. The fetal sex is often important to the parents, and not only from a planning point of view. Studies have shown that parents who see their baby on ultrasound undergo a sort of prenatal bonding experience, which can result in greater compliance with prenatal care. Problems that interfere with gender identification, such as swollen labia from maternal hormones or difficult fetal lie, should be carefully explained to the parents to temper their expectations.

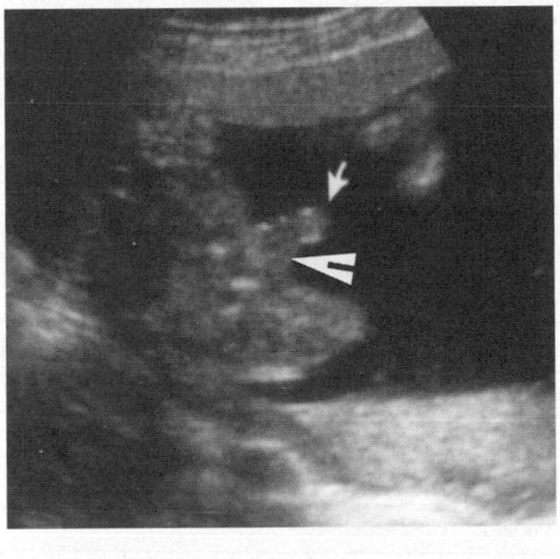

Figure 41-12. ■ *Transverse view of the male fetal genitalia. The arrowhead points to the testicles, and the arrow points to the penis.*

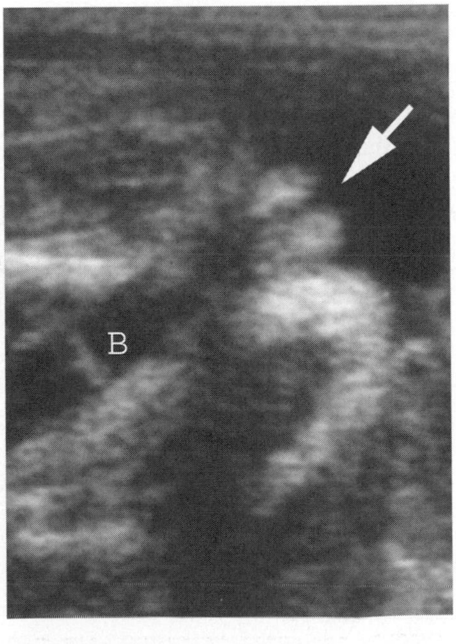

Figure 41-13. ■ *Female genitalia. The labia can be well seen* (arrow). B, *bladder.*

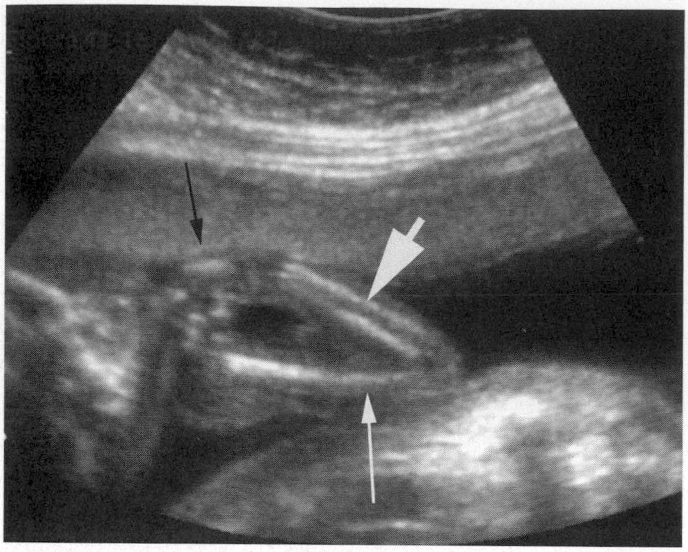

Figure 41-14. ■ *View of the left arm and hand. The single bone of the upper arm (the humerus) can be seen* (thin arrow). *Two parallel bones in the lower arm (the radius and ulna) are visible* (thick arrow). *The small black arrow points to the hand.*

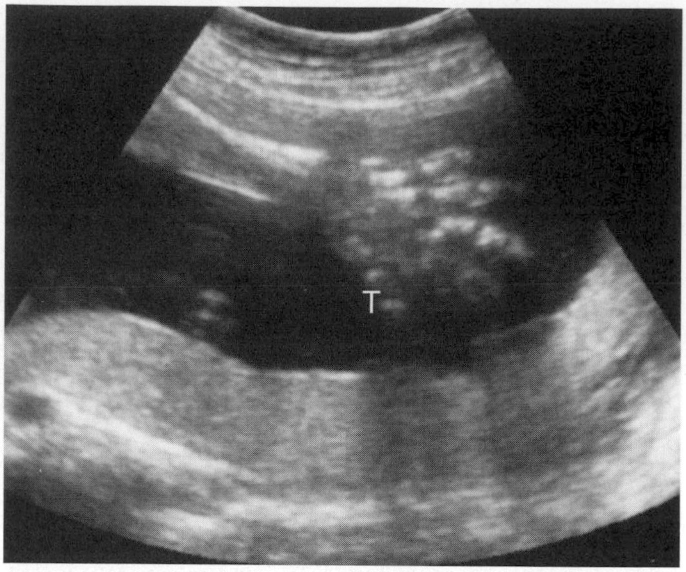

Figure 41-15. ■ *View of the fetal hand showing the four fingers and the thumb* (T).

BONES

The upper arm and thigh (femur), which contain single bones, generate only a single linear echo, whereas the distal limbs generate two parallel linear echoes. Bones are seen as echogenic lines with acoustic shadowing (Fig. 41-14).

Individual digits can be counted reliably from about 16 weeks' gestational age (Fig. 41-15), earlier in ideal patients. Soft tissues can be seen around the bones, and some epiphyses can be seen. Cartilaginous structures such as the femoral head are visible (Fig. 41-16). Visualization of the ossified distal femoral epiphysis, the proximal humeral epiphysis, and the proximal tibial epiphysis is used to aid dating (see Fig. 41-17 and Appendix 20). New guidelines from a combined group representing the AIUM, ACR, and ACOG (see Appendix 32) require documentation of the presence of all limbs.

FETAL SPINE

Although a comprehensive examination is not required by the ACR/AIUM/ACOG guidelines, it is imperative to take a good look at the spine. To rule out spina bifida, serial transverse views must be obtained of the entire spine. On a transverse view of the fetal spine, three echogenic structures that form a complete ring can be seen (Fig. 41-10). These are the posterior elements and the poste-

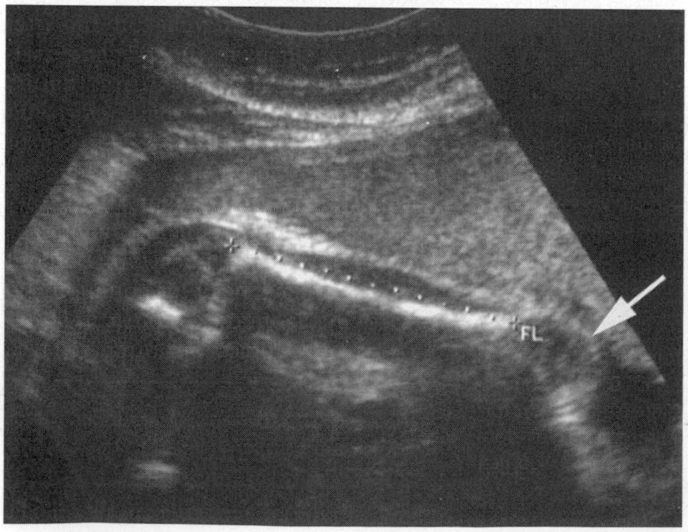

Figure 41-16. ■ *View of the femur and knee. The longest length is being measured. The cartilaginous femoral head can be seen* (arrow).

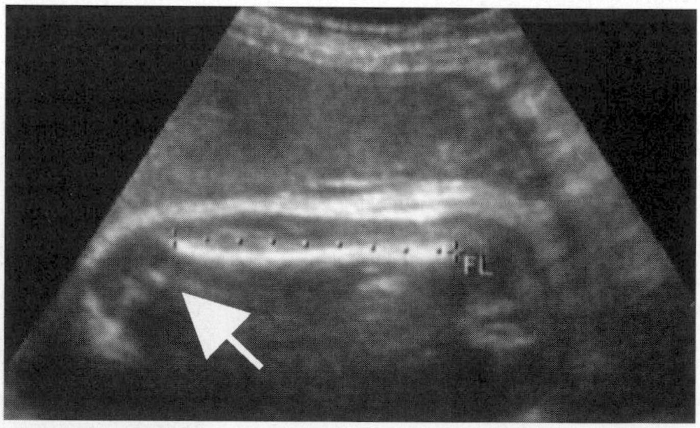

Figure 41-17. ■ *View of femoral length* (FL) *showing the femoral epiphysis* (arrow). *The femoral epiphysis is seen from 32 weeks' gestational age and thereafter.*

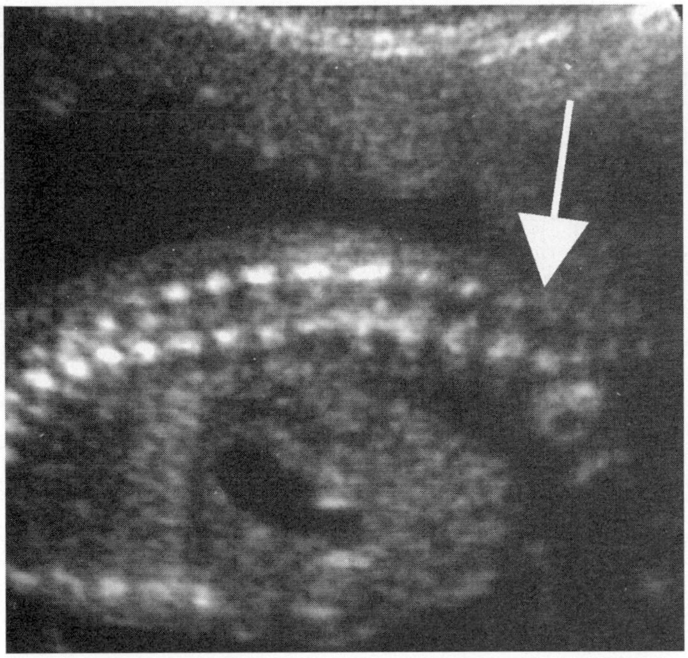

Figure 41-18. ■ *Sagittal view of the lumbar spine showing two ossification centers. Note the posterior angulation of the sacral portion of the spine* (arrow). *This is an important view to exclude spina bifida.*

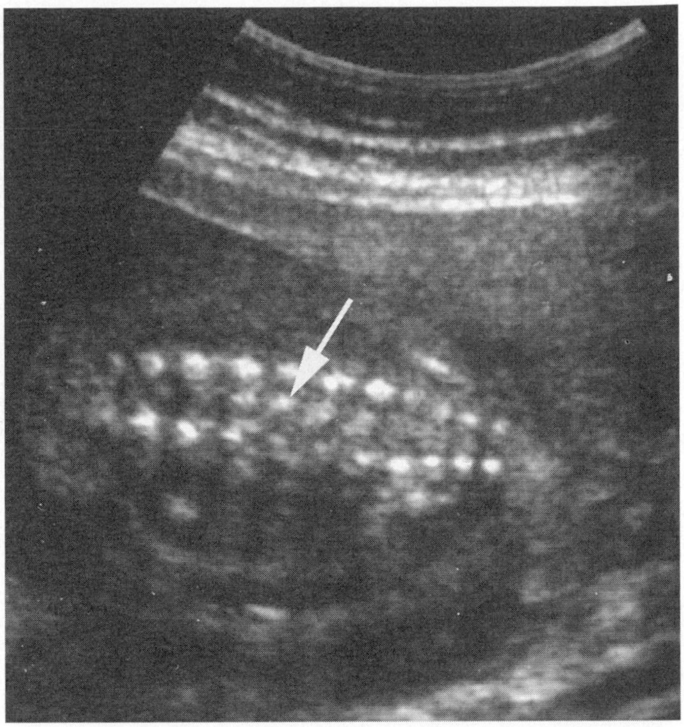

Figure 41-19. ■ *Coronal view of the lumbar spine. The posterior element pedicle ossification centers can be seen throughout the visible length of the spine. The spinal processes* (arrow) *are also seen over a short distance.*

rior ossification center of the vertebrae (Figs. 41-9 and 41-10). On long-axis views (Fig. 41-18), two of the three ossification centers, the posterior ossification center of the vertebrae, and the posterior elements are seen.

On a coronal view, both posterior elements can be seen by 12 weeks (Fig. 41-19). The posterior elements are partly composed of the pedicles and partly of the lamina. The bony ring formed by these ossification centers contains the spinal canal. The spinal cord may be seen within the spinal canal (see Fig. 45-13B) and can be traced to about the level of L2. It is more echopenic than the other contents of the spinal canal. The normal spine has a gentle curve forward in the thoracic area and a posterior bend in the sacral region on the longitudinal view. The fetal spine widens slightly in the cervical and lumbar areas (Fig. 41-20).

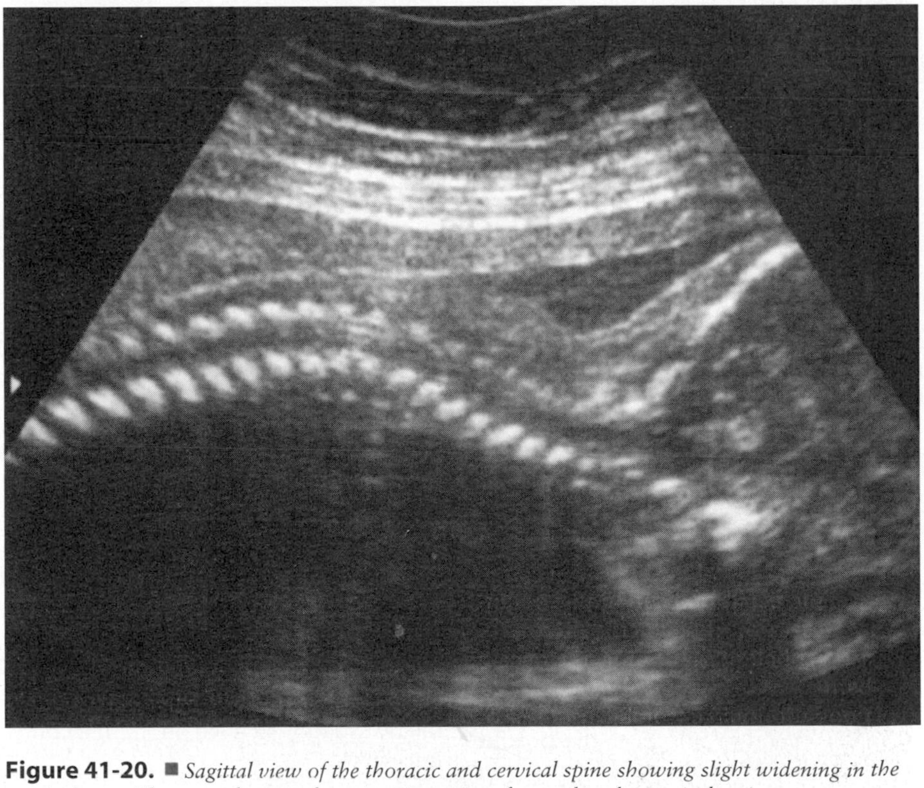

Figure 41-20. ■ *Sagittal view of the thoracic and cervical spine showing slight widening in the cervical area. The normal upper thoracic spine curves forward in the cervical region.*

AMNIOTIC FLUID

The amount of amniotic fluid varies with the gestational age, so no single measurement can be used throughout pregnancy. The amniotic fluid index is a crude method of quantifying amniotic fluid. The uterine cavity is divided into quadrants, and the vertical depth of the largest fluid pocket is measured. Values between 10 and 20 are considered normal; the normal values vary with gestational age, however (see Appendix 24 and Chapter 46). There should be a large amount of fluid in the second trimester and a steadily lessening amount in the third trimester, so not much is present at term.

If the only fluid present is a pocket of less than 2 cm, this is abnormal at any stage of pregnancy. A pocket of more than 8 cm indicates polyhydramnios.

PLACENTA

The placenta is discussed in Chapter 42. The placental position can be well seen from about 13 weeks on. The placenta may lie adjacent to the cervix in the second trimester. The placental position changes as the pregnancy proceeds, and most such pregnancies are normal. Nevertheless, provided the bladder is empty, follow-up of a placenta that covers the cervix is desirable because a few such cases will end up with a placenta previa.

Technique

BONDING

A sonogram is a powerful experience for a pregnant woman and should, if possible, be shared with the father. The mother and the father appreciate, often for the first time, that a little person lies within. Once it is determined that the fetus is sonographically normal, the maternal feelings induced by the sonogram should be reinforced by showing the mother the heart, limbs, genitalia, and other structures. If an abortion is planned, we do not recommend that the patient view the fetal anatomy unless the patient insists. If an anomaly is found, we do not show the mother the details of the abnormality until we are as clear as possible about the diagnosis and have contacted the referring physician.

Giving the Patient a Picture

Most patients request a picture of the fetus. We believe the psychological benefit in giving them an image of the profile, the genitalia, or the hand far outweighs any legal hazard. Allowing the patient to watch in real time as the sonogram is being performed enhances the bonding process.

Videotaping

Many patients request that a videotape of the obstetric sonogram be made. Some institutions do not permit videotaping because they fear that the videotape will be used as evidence were there to be a malpractice suit. Our practice is to perform a standard obstetric study first. If the sonogram is normal, the doctor videotapes selected areas at the end of the study. If the sonogram is abnormal and if termination or still birth is a possibility, we do not provide a videotape because we feel that repeated viewing of the tape may exacerbate the grieving process. Three-dimensional images of the normal fetus enhance the bonding process.

ENDOVAGINAL APPROACH

A complete fetal survey can be performed by means of the vaginal probe with a pregnancy that is less than 15 weeks; this is particularly helpful in obese patients. We prefer to use the endovaginal approach as a primary imaging technique in fetuses that are less than 14 weeks in age and whenever we have a question about the cervix or fetal anatomy that lies close to the cervix.

Although such exams are increasingly commonplace, they are sometimes unexpectedly invasive for the patient, and she may be ill at ease. It is appropriate (if sometimes inconvenient) to have a female in the room, at least during insertion of the probe.

Gel is placed on the transducer, then a sterile condom is placed over it and fastened on with a rubber band. Further instructions for ensuring sterile technique are discussed in Chapter 55.

The patient should be instructed to empty her bladder before she gets on the table. Because so much manipulation of the transducer is necessary to see all of the anatomy, these exams are much more easily accomplished on a gynecological table. If such a table is not available, it is usually necessary to build up the patient's hips with pillows or towels; this creates enough space to angle the transducer up or down as needed. The patient's knees are also dropped to allow movement from side to side, visualizing the adnexae. To demonstrate the cervix, the transducer is pulled out until it comes into view.

TRANSDUCER CHOICE

Most current systems provide a curved linear array as the primary tool for obstetrical work. Multiple frequencies and focal zones are available on most systems with standard transducers. A large field of view can usually be seen. Linear arrays that allow one to place two images alongside each other may be helpful for obstetric work. A composite long view of the fetus can be created. Three-dimensional imaging is helpful if you cannot see a fetal structure (such as the face) with the standard approach.

PATIENT PREPARATION

It is not necessary to have the bladder full before starting an obstetrical ultrasound study. A scan taken on a patient with a full bladder may make you suspect a placenta previa when none is present. Some urine in the bladder may be helpful if the pregnancy is under 20 weeks. The patient's bladder should be empty before an endovaginal exam.

ROUTINE APPROACH

The following is the suggested routine when examining women with an apparently normal pregnancy. Bear in mind, however, that when a sonogenic view of the spine rolls by, or if the fetus waves at you—affording a lovely view of five normal fingers and a photo-op for mom—freeze it and photograph it. You may not get another chance. Conversely, don't waste time sticking to a routine if the fetus refuses to cooperate. Come back later.

1. Sweep first. A quick scan through the uterus to check for gross pathology and fetal viability allows you to set the tone for how much to share the exam with the patient and family.
2. Lower uterine segment. Do it early, before the bladder fills, potentially distorting the cervical length or its relationship to the placental margin. Include the presenting fetal part.
3. Long-axis and transverse views of the spine, if the fetus is in a convenient position. This localizes the fetus for the axial views to follow.
4. The head (it may not be as easy to view later in the exam).
5. Transverse views of the chest to show a four-chamber view.
6. The trunk circumference view, making sure to include the stomach.
7. Transverse and long views of the kidneys.
8. Views of the cord insertion.
9. Bladder views (long view to include the stomach, heart, and diaphragm).

10. Femur views and evidence that all four extremities are present.
11. A sweep through the entire fetus and an informal biophysical profile.
12. Views of the placental site and amniotic fluid volume.

Fetal Lie

Demonstrate the fetal position by taking a view that shows the fetal head and the maternal bladder if there is a vertex (head first) position. The term *cephalic presentation* may be preferable because it doesn't imply whether the face or the back of the head is coming first. If the fetus is foot or bottom first (breech) or in an oblique position, take a view that shows the lower uterine segment and the presenting fetal structures (Fig. 41-21). It helps the obstetrician to know if the legs in a breech presentation are extended or flexed.

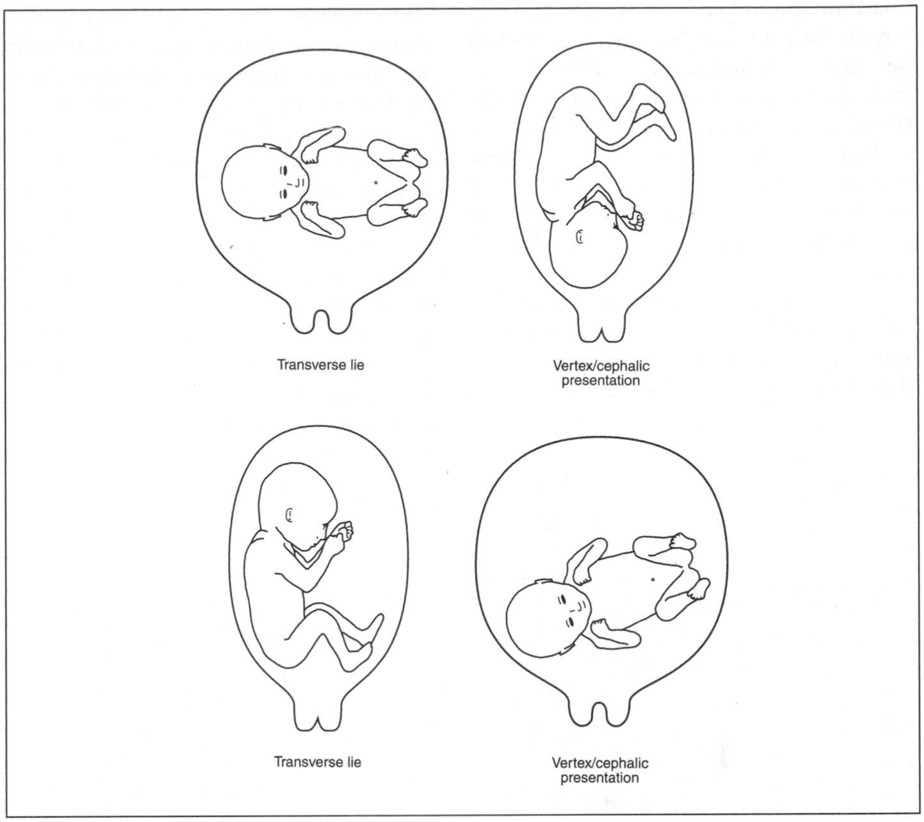

Figure 41-21. ■ *Diagram of different fetal positions. A fetus in the breech position can have its legs extended or flexed. This information is helpful to the referring obstetrician. To determine the situs of the fetal organs, use the following rule: If the fetal head is down and the fetal back is to the left, the left side of the fetus (stomach, heart) is down. Conversely, if the fetal head is up (breech) and the fetal back is to the mother's right, the right side of the fetus is up. If the fetal head is up, and if the fetal back is to the left, the left side is up.*

Lower Uterine Segment

Views of the lower uterine segment in the midline are helpful. If the maternal bladder is empty, the relationship of a low-lying placenta to the cervix can be shown and the presence of a placenta previa can be established.

A postvoid view of the normal cervix and vagina should be obtained. The normal cervical length is 3.5 cm or more. Translabial or endovaginal views of the cervix are often performed because they give a superior view of the placenta/cervix relationship and show whether cervical incompetence is present (Fig. 41-22) (see Chapter 42).

Spine

Localize the spine next. Many views such as those of the kidneys and the trunk circumference require knowledge of how the spine lies for orientation.

1. It may be impossible to get the entire spine on a single cut if the fetus is curled. Dual or "long" linear array views may be used for the long axis.

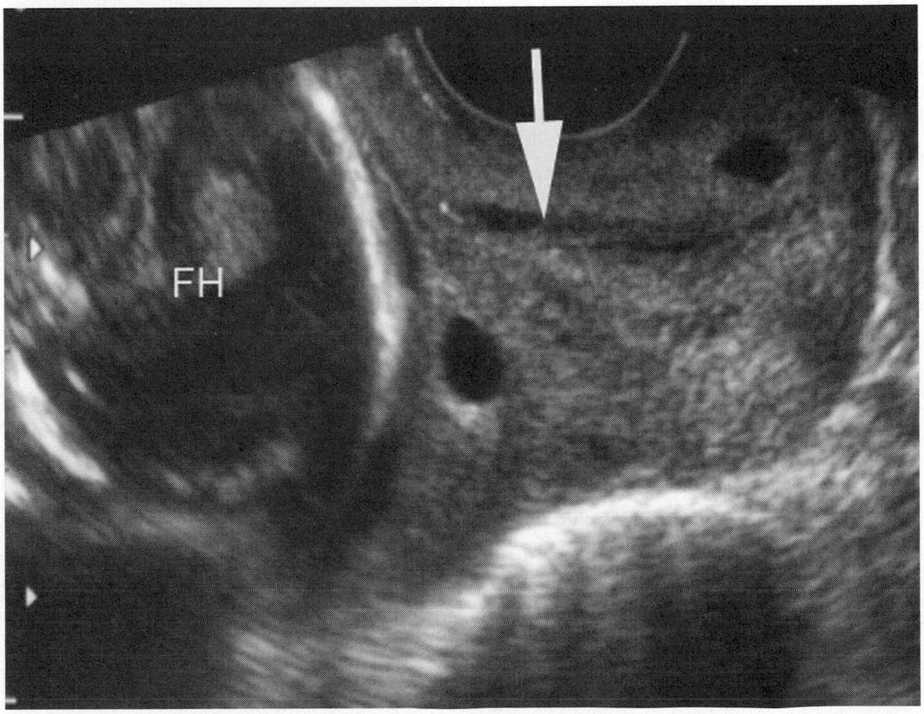

Figure 41-22. ■ *Normal endovaginal view of the cervix. The fetal head* (FH) *lies adjacent to the cervix (a normal finding). The arrow points to the cervical canal. This cervix is closed and is normal, about 3.5 cm long. The two cystic areas in the cervix are coincidental nabothians cysts of no clinical importance. Internal detail of the brain is well shown.*

2. The iliac crests may conceal the sacrum. Views from a more dorsal approach are needed for this area. Inclusion of the iliac crests on the transverse view is evidence that the scan was obtained in the lumbosacral region.
3. If possible, get prone long-axis views of the fetus that show the skin covering over the spine; this is a good way to show subtle myelomeningoceles (see Fig. 45-18). The skin over the lumbar spine must be shown from a sagittal posterior aspect for this approach to be useful. This image must be pursued if an abnormal cerebellum suggests spinal pathology.
4. Transverse views showing the relationships of the posterior elements to the vertebral body should be obtained at several sites in the lumbosacral area and at several sites in the abdomen and chest. Show some other anatomy, such as the iliac crest or kidneys, so the level can be recognized later (Figs. 41-9 and 41-10).
5. Coronal views obtained in a long axis, from the side of the fetus, are an excellent way of showing widening of the spinal canal (Fig. 41-19). This view is especially valuable if the fetus is in a supine position. Check to make sure there is an equal amount of soft tissue on either side of the spine to ensure that you are in the best plane.

Four-Chamber View

Once the spine is localized, turn the transducer 90 degrees at the level of the heart and record an image documenting four chambers and the interventricular septum (Fig. 41-6). The septum between the atria doesn't always look intact on still images because the foramen ovale is flipping in and out of the left atrium; watch this in real time. The cine loop option is very helpful in finding the optimal image on this view.

Truncal Views

Once the spine has been plotted out, it is easy to take transverse views at the level of the stomach, kidneys, bladder (see Figs. 41-9 and 41-10), heart, and trunk circumference (Figs. 41-6 and 41-8).

If the stomach is not seen, come back and try later. Some fluid should be visualized in a normal fetal stomach during the course of an exam. When the kidney view is taken, try to slide the transducer to a position where the spine's shadow does not obscure the second kidney. Turn the transducer at right angles and take a longitudinal view that shows the diaphragm, stomach, and bladder, if possible, on a single view (Fig. 41-5).

Gut extending through the fetal anterior abdominal wall, a normal finding until about 11 weeks, can confuse the long-axis image in the first trimester (Chapter 39). In early pregnancy, the fetal anatomy is poorly seen. One should measure the longest length on a view that shows the fetal heart. Don't include the yolk sac in the measurement. Very small fetuses may lie adjacent to the yolk sac. Always do more than one measurement to find the longest one, and use the system's electronic calipers.

Limbs

Once the proximal femur is found below the iliac crest, rotate the transducer so the rest of the bone is lined up. Use the same technique for other bones. In a dating series, all that is required are images that show there are four extremities. If possible, demonstrate both feet and hands.

Always start from a known landmark in the trunk and work outward through the femur or humerus. The lower leg can easily be mistaken for the forearm.

Amniotic Fluid

Document the largest pocket of amniotic fluid by taking two views of it at right angles. Look for evidence of internal echoes or septa within the amniotic fluid. Views across the short axis of the fetus and the fluid pocket in true transverse and longitudinal planes show the fluid amount. Oblique views may be misleading. A view that shows all four limbs extending into the amniotic fluid is useful evidence that all four limbs exist and that the fluid quantity is normal or increased.

Placenta

Document the placental site, size, and texture by taking views at right angles that show its maximal extent. A long-axis view of the lower segment of the uterus and cervix shows placental maturation and placental relationship to the cervix.

If the placenta appears to obscure the cervix, repeat this view with an empty bladder. If it is still unclear whether the placenta relates to the cervix, examine the area with the endovaginal probe (see Chapter 42).

Cord

Take a short-axis view of the cord that shows whether there are two or three vessels (Fig. 41-23). If the cord is very

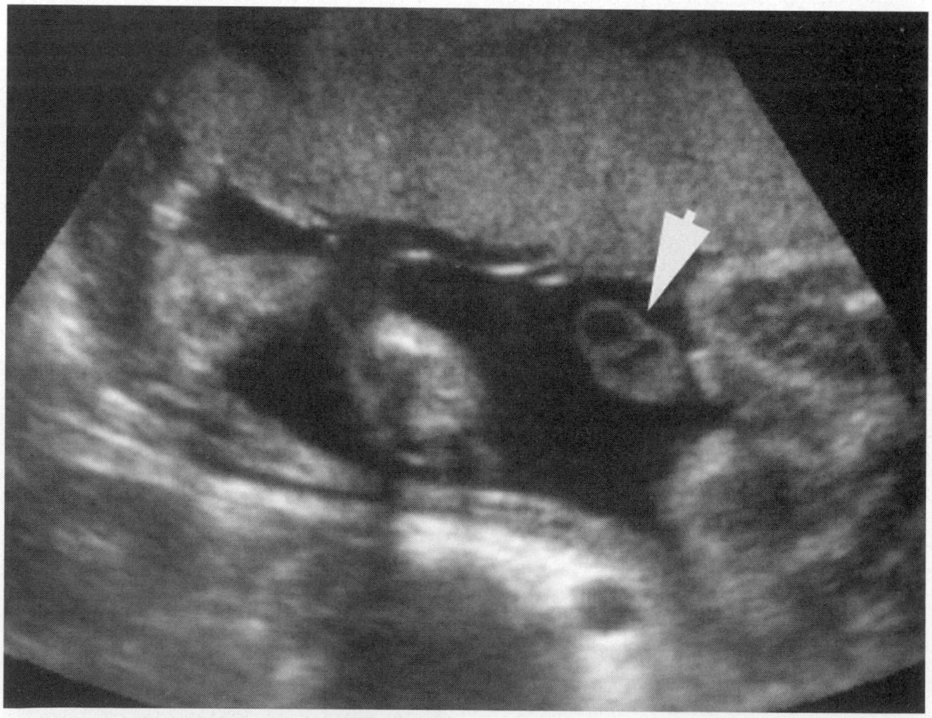

Figure 41-23. ■ *Three-vessel cord. A transverse section of the cord* (arrow) *shows three vessels—a large vein and two smaller arteries.*

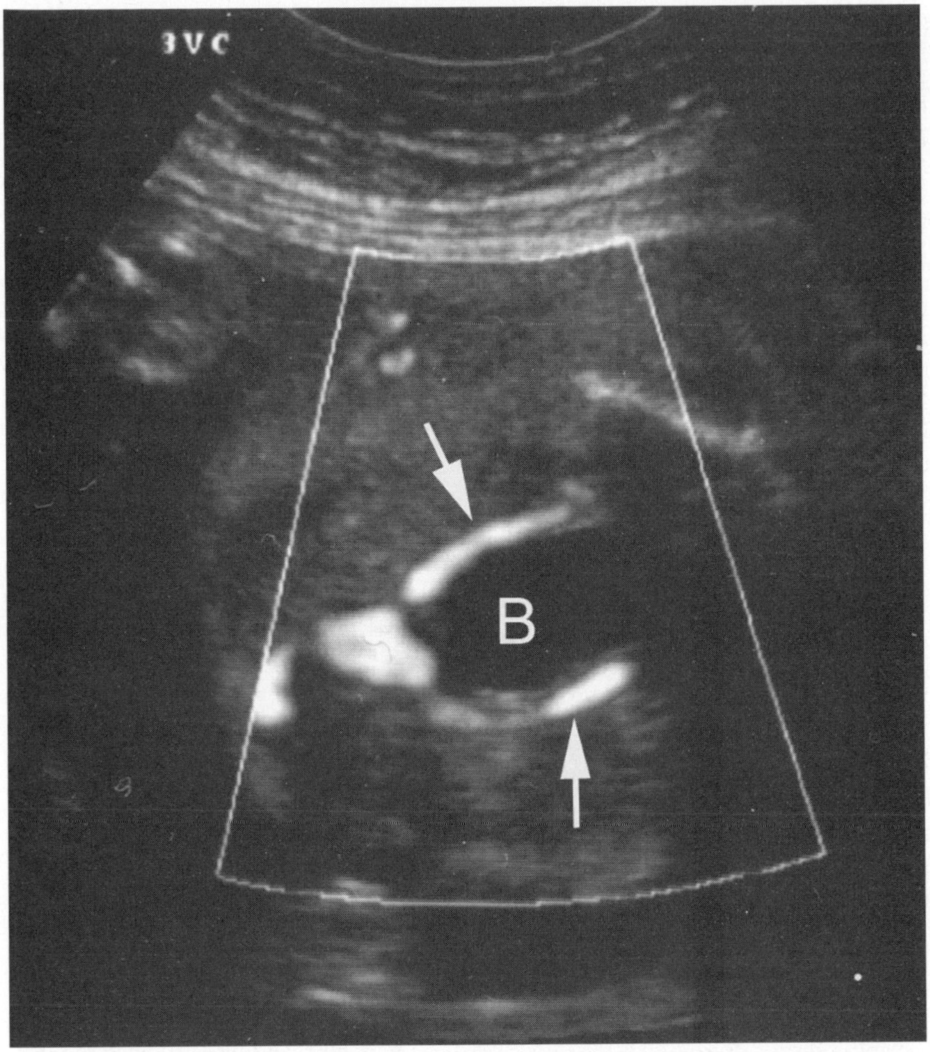

Figure 41-24. ■ *Color flow view of the cord insertion and bladder area showing the two umbilical artery branches on either side* (arrows) *of the bladder* (B), *proving that a three-vessel cord exists and that there is no mass extending out of the cord insertion, such as an omphalocele.*

twisted, it may be difficult to decide whether there are one or two arteries present. Look with color flow for pulsating arteries on either side of the bladder within the fetus (Fig. 41-24). If the cord is uncoiled, take an image. A noncoiled cord is a nonspecific indicator that the fetus is at increased risk for perinatal morbidity and mortality. If amniocentesis is being performed, show the cord's entrance site into the placenta. Take a view of the cord insertion.

MEASUREMENTS TO PERFORM

Critical obstetric management decisions hinge on accurate measurements, so be certain that the system is properly calibrated.

Crown-Rump Length

In a dating examination performed in the first trimester, the crown-rump length is the optimal method of establishing fetal age (see Fig. 39-7). This measurement is performed using a real-time system by finding the longest axis of the fetus. This value can be obtained between approximately 5 and 12 weeks quite easily (see Appendices 4 and 5).

Biparietal Diameter

For dating after 12 weeks, the biparietal diameter is used (Fig. 41-3) (see Appendix 8). Find the cervical spine as it enters the head at its widest point. Place the transducer at right angles to this axis and adjust the angulation of the transducer so that it is at a right angle to the midline echo. Take images at the level of the thalami (Fig. 41-3), which are recognizable as hypoechoic, blunted, diamond-shaped structures in the center of the brain. Structures visible at the desirable level include the thalamus, the third ventricle, and the cavum septi pellucidi (Fig. 41-3). Do not take a biparietal measurement at the level of the two lines parallel to the midline, which were formerly thought to represent the lateral ventricles and which have now been shown to represent venous structures. Make sure to obtain the ovoid shape that is desirable. Measurements are made from the outer side of the near skull to the inner side of the distal skull echoes.

Accuracy with this technique is ±1 week prior to 20 weeks and ±10 days until about 28 weeks. Beyond this point, accuracy diminishes to ±2 to 4 weeks, as do all other measurement dating parameters; therefore, dating by sonographic measurement data is undesirable after about 28 weeks.

A ratio of the biparietal diameter to the longest distance from the front of the head to the back of the head (occipitofrontal diameter) is useful in the diagnosis of dolichocephaly. This normal variant—a long, flattened fetal head in the third trimester—produces erroneous biparietal diameters. The normal ratio is 0.74 ± 0.08 (see Appendix 9).

An unduly wide head (brachycephaly) is less frequently seen and is also usually of little significance.

Head Circumference

The head circumference is obtained from a good biparietal image that shows the thalamus, third ventricle, and falx and does not show the cerebellum (Fig. 41-3) (see Appendix 7). If the cerebellar hemispheres are visible, the section is too steeply angled (Fig. 41-4). If the fetal head is deep in the pelvis or if the face is looking in the direction of the transducer, it may be difficult or impossible to obtain a head circumference, although a biparietal diameter is usually possible.

Changing the maternal position may allow visualization. Use of the endovaginal probe approach is helpful with a vertex presentation.

Measure around the perimeter of the skull, including the bone but not fetal hair and scalp. Use the electronic ellipse or trackball if possible; always move the posterior caliper from the inside of the cranium to the outside before taking circumference measurements. If the system only allows for diameter measurements, measure the diameter from outside to outside and then move to a right-angle position and repeat the measurement. Average the two measurements and use this with the formula IID.

Femoral Length

The femoral length is an additional method of estimating gestational age (Figs. 41-16 and 41-17). Overall, it is a slightly more accurate predictor of age than the biparietal diameter. Tables of normal values are available (see Appendix 10). The lateral and medial aspects of the femur have different appearances. The lateral aspect is straight, whereas the medial aspect is curved. If a femur length is obtained from the medial surface, the femur may be thought to be bowed.

To ensure that one has the longest femoral length, measurements should be taken along an axis that show both the round, echopenic, cartilaginous femoral head, and the femoral condyles (Fig. 41-25). A portion of the femoral condyle may be ossified as the distal femoral epiphysis (Fig. 41-17). Angle to show the entire femoral shaft. It is easy to underestimate length, so take more than one measurement. Measure the straight lateral surface rather than the bowed medial surface. Noting the date of the first appearance of condyles can be used as a dating technique (see Appendix 20). The distal femoral epiphyses are visible after 32 weeks (Fig. 41-17). The proximal tibial epiphysis becomes visible at around 35 weeks and can also be used for dating purposes.

The proximal humeral epiphysis appears so late that its appearance has a good correlation with fetal lung maturity.

Abdominal Circumferences (or Diameter)

The abdominal circumference (Fig. 41-8) is usually used for detecting intrauterine growth retardation (IUGR) (see Chapter 43), as well as for dating the fetus (see Appendices 11 through 14).

For further details, see Chapter 43.

Femoral Length/Abdominal Circumference Ratio

The femoral length/abdominal circumference ratio is 22 and is constant from 22 weeks on. It may be of help in the diagnosis of fetuses with the long, lean type of IUGR.

Dating with Other Measurements

There are tables that allow one to obtain the gestational age from the size of numerous other body parts, such as the orbits, foot, and clavicle. These measurements are useful if only a small segment of the fetus can be seen or if much of the fetus is abnormal (see Appendices 2 and 16–19).

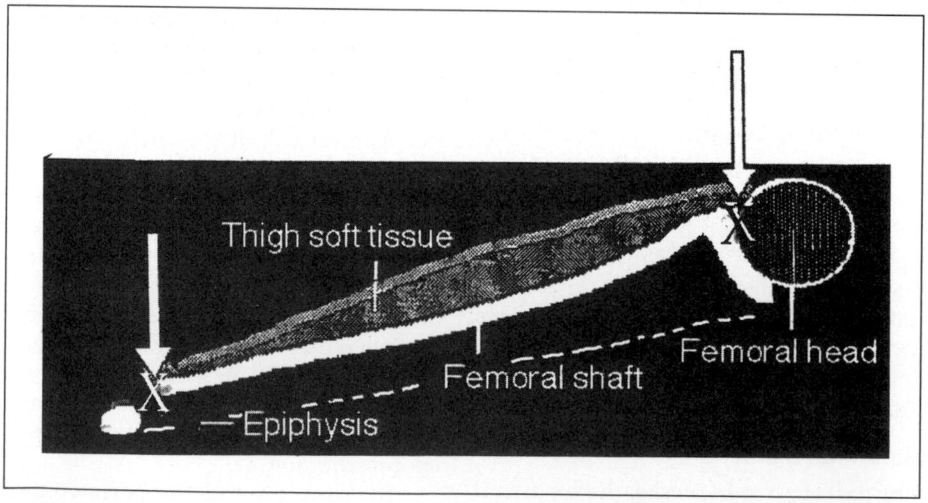

Figure 41-25. ■ *View of the femur. The femoral length is measured along the shaft from X to X* (arrows). *The cartilaginous femoral head can be poorly seen. The hook at the proximal end of the femur is now considered to represent the undersurface of the femoral head rather than the greater trochanter. Note the epiphysis at the distal end of the femur* (white dot). *This structure first appears at 32 weeks. The soft tissue on the underside of the femur is dotted in. It is normally shadowed out by the femoral bone.*

CEREBELLAR VIEW (POSTERIOR FOSSA)

An inferiorly angled view to show the cerebellar hemispheres (useful in excluding spina bifida) will also, if obtained at 18 weeks, show the skin thickening around the neck that is seen in Down syndrome (Fig. 41-4). Now required by the guidelines, this is an essential screening view. Be sure to include the shape of the cerebellar lobes, and try to demonstrate the cisterna magna. The transcerebellar diameter can be used as a dating technique. The diameter in millimeters corresponds to the gestational age throughout the first 20 weeks of pregnancy. This image is easy to obtain once the transducer is positioned for a biparietal diameter by angling the posterior aspect of the transducer inferiorly on the fetal head. The cisterna magna should be photographed on this view. It should not measure more than 9 mm wide.

Pitfalls

1. An inaccurate biparietal diameter is obtained if:
   a. The biparietal diameter is not taken at the level of the thalamus and cavum septi pellucidi
   b. The head is round (brachycephalic) or flattened (dolichocephalic) rather than ovoid
   c. The head measurement is taken at a point where the distance between one side of the skull and the midline is not the same as the other side and is asymmetrical
   d. The measurement is first obtained in the third trimester when there is a wide variation of dates for any given measurement
   e. The measurement is taken inferior to the thalamus at the level of the cerebellar peduncles and cerebellar hemispheres (Fig. 41-3C).
2. The crown-rump length is inaccurate if:
   a. It is obtained after 12 weeks
   b. No persistent effort is made to find the longest length by varying the transducer axis
   c. The yolk sac is included in the length measurement.
3. The femoral length may be erroneous if:

a. It is really the humerus that is being measured
b. The femur is scanned at an oblique axis
c. The measurement is faulty because the calipers were put at the wrong site
d. Too much gain is used or abnormal ossification occurs at the distal end of the femur.

4. The head circumference will be underestimated if:
   a. Too steep an axis is used so that the cerebellum is prominent
   b. The measurement line does not follow the external borders of the head outline.
5. The biparietal diameter in the third trimester is less than caliper measurements at birth because of the measurement site used and because the assumed speed of sound is slightly slower than it really is—1,540 m/sec versus 1,610 m/sec.
6. Failure to check the calibration system may lead to incorrect measurements. Wrong measurements can have serious clinical and legal consequences. Fortunately, modern digital systems rarely vary.
7. By not using the calipers on screen that were incorporated into the system, it is easy to mismeasure the image by 1 cm.
8. Using the wrong nomogram for the measurement technique employed will yield erroneous dates. The technique used in creating the measurement tables for dating must be used. For example, different biparietal diameter measurement sites, such as outer table to outer table of the skull, have been used in some older tables.

Where Else to Look

1. If the biparietal diameter and femoral length do not indicate the same fetal age, perform the measurements suggested for IUGR (see Chapter 43).
2. If the biparietal diameter is less than expected, consider the possibility of microcephalus by looking at the head circumference/abdominal circumference ratio. Check the intraorbital distance and look for ventriculomegaly.
3. If the biparietal diameter is more than expected, make sure that hydrocephalus is not present (see Chapter 45) and look for evidence of IUGR (see Chapter 43).
4. If the femoral length is too short, consider the possibility of dwarfism (see Chapter 45).
   a. Check the length of the humerus, tibia, fibula, radius, and ulna.
   b. Count the number of digits, and look at the hand and feet position.
   c. Look at the ratio of abdomen to chest size; it should be greater than 0.87.
   d. Examine the head and spine for the appearances described in Chapter 45.
5. If the femur is too long or too short, check the size of the parents to see whether they are short or tall.
6. If the abdominal circumference is unusually large relative to other measurements later in pregnancy, consider diabetes mellitus. Look for scalp edema and skin thickening, and ask the patient whether she is diabetic or if there is a family history of diabetes.
7. If no fetal movement or fetal breathing is seen, do a biophysical profile (see Chapter 46).
8. If the fetal head is unduly large relative to other measurements and dates and there is no hydrocephalus, perform views of the orbits, hands, and feet. There may be a chromosomal anomaly present. Hand, foot, and face problems are common with chromosomal anomalies. Check the maternal and paternal head size. Familial large head is common.
9. If the measurement data are less than expected, perform a biophysical profile and use the protocol suggested for IUGR (see Chapters 43 and 46).

SELECTED READING

Bowerman RA, DiPietro MA. Erroneous sonographic identification of fetal lateral ventricles: relationship to the echogenic periventricular "blush." *AJNR Am J Neuroradiol* 1987;8:661–664.

Callen PW, ed. *Ultrasonography in Obstetrics and Gynecology*, 4th ed. Philadelphia: Saunders; 2000.

Gardberg M, Tuppurainen M. Dorsoposterior fetal position near term—a sonographic finding worth noting? *Acta Obstet Gynecol Scan* 1995;74:402–403.

Hearn-Stebbins B. Normal fetal growth assessment: a review of literature and current practice. *J Diagn Med Sonogr* 1995;11:176–187.

Shepard M, Filly RA. A standardized plane for biparietal diameter measurement. *J Ultrasound Med* 1982;1:145–150.

42

Second and Third Trimester Bleeding

ROGER C. SANDERS

KEY WORDS

Abruptio Placentae (Accidental Hemorrhage; Abruption). Bleeding that occurs when the placenta separates from the uterine wall. A serious condition that threatens the life of the fetus and the mother. It is usually seen by the sonographer only when it is relatively mild; other cases go straight to the operating room.

Amnion, Amniotic Sac Membrane. The membrane that lines the fluid cavity (amniotic cavity) within the uterus in pregnancy. The membrane is not normally seen sonographically after the first trimester, except when the separation between two amniotic sacs is visualized in a multiple pregnancy.

Cervix. Most inferior segment of the uterus. It is more than 3.5 cm long during a normal pregnancy but decreases (effaces) in length during labor (Fig. 42-1).

Cesarean Section (C-section). Operation performed to deliver a fetus. An incision is made transversely in the lower anterior wall of the uterus. In a "classic" cesarean section, the incision is made vertically at the fundus of the uterus.

Chorionic Plate. Term used to describe the interface between the amniotic fluid and the placenta.

Circumvallate Placenta. A rim develops around the placental edge. This condition is thought to be associated with bleeding at delivery.

Effaced. The cervix becomes shortened toward the end of labor. When it is very thinned out and when there is a lot of fluid within the internal os, it is known as *effaced*.

Infarct of the Placenta. Loss of tissue blood supply due to arterial occlusion.

Low-Lying Placenta. The inferior edge of the placenta is close to but does not cover the inner aspect of the cervical os. Of no clinical significance.

Marginal Placenta Previa. The edge of the placenta is at the margin of the internal os.

Migration. Term used to describe the apparent shift in position of the placenta from the cervical to the fundal area that often occurs during the course of pregnancy.

Myometrium. The muscle that forms the wall of the uterus.

Oligohydramnios. Too little amniotic fluid for a given pregnancy stage.

Os. Term used to describe the upper (internal) and lower (external) entrances to the cervical canal (Fig. 42-1).

Partial Placenta Previa. The internal os is just covered by the placenta.

Placenta Creta. The placenta burrows into the myometrium, causing an unduly firm attachment that bleeds at delivery because it does not separate normally.

- **Acreta.** Entering the surface of the placenta.
- **Increta.** Involving much of the center of the placenta.
- **Percreta.** Has extended through the placenta to the structures beyond the placenta such as the bladder wall.

Placenta Previa (Total). The placenta completely covers the internal os.

Polyhydramnios. Too much amniotic fluid for a given pregnancy stage.

Ripening. As the cervix softens and the internal and external os dilate close to the end of pregnancy, the cervix is said to be ripening.

Succenturiate Lobe. Anomaly in which the placenta is divided into two segments that are connected by blood vessels. The second lobe may be so small that it is overlooked sonographically. This anomaly occurs in less than 1% of pregnancies.

Vasa Previa. The umbilical cord vessels as they enter the placenta are the presenting part of the internal os.

Velamentous Insertion. The cord bifurcates before reaching the placenta and lies within a membrane. Especially common in twins.

The Clinical Problem

Vaginal bleeding in the second or third trimester is an ominous clinical sign. Although such bleeding may be due to unimportant conditions such as cervical erosions or vaginal varices, it may signify placenta previa or abruptio placenta.

PLACENTA PREVIA

In placenta previa, the placenta covers the internal os of the cervix and bleeds because the placenta has separated from the myometrium. When the placenta covers the cervix (total placenta previa), cesarean section is necessary because vaginal delivery would endanger the fetus. With lesser degrees of placenta previa, vaginal delivery may be attempted. Ultrasound is the best noninvasive method of establishing a diagnosis of placenta previa.

ABRUPTIO PLACENTAE (ABRUPTION)

Although placental abruption is about as common in clinical practice as placenta previa, ultrasonic examinations may not be performed because many patients with abruptio placentae are taken straight to the operating room as a clinical emergency. The primary event is a bleed between the placenta and the uterine wall, but blood also frequently enters the amniotic cavity, where it can be visualized sonographically. Abruption may be present yet not visualized sonographically.

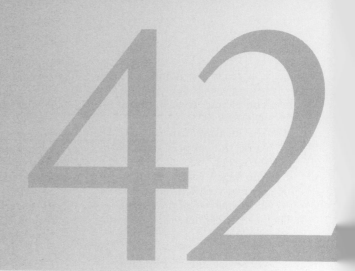

Anatomy

PLACENTA

In the second trimester, the placenta is evenly echogenic with a smooth, well-defined border marginated by the chorionic plate. An irregular border and textural changes often occur in the third trimester (see section under Placental Maturation in Chapter 43, Small for Dates).

Echopenic areas in the placenta in a subchorionic location are a normal finding. Venous lakes, which are echo-free areas, may show flow with real time. Alternatively, echopenic areas may represent deposits of a material known as Wharton's jelly, of no pathologic significance.

VAGINA AND CERVIX

The vagina can be seen transabdominally as an echogenic line with echo-free walls. It ends at the cervix. The internal os, external os, and cervical canal can be seen within the cervix (Fig. 42-1).

These structures are best examined with the endovaginal probe but may often be well seen using the translabial approach. Occasionally, they can be seen adequately on a postvoid transabdominal view.

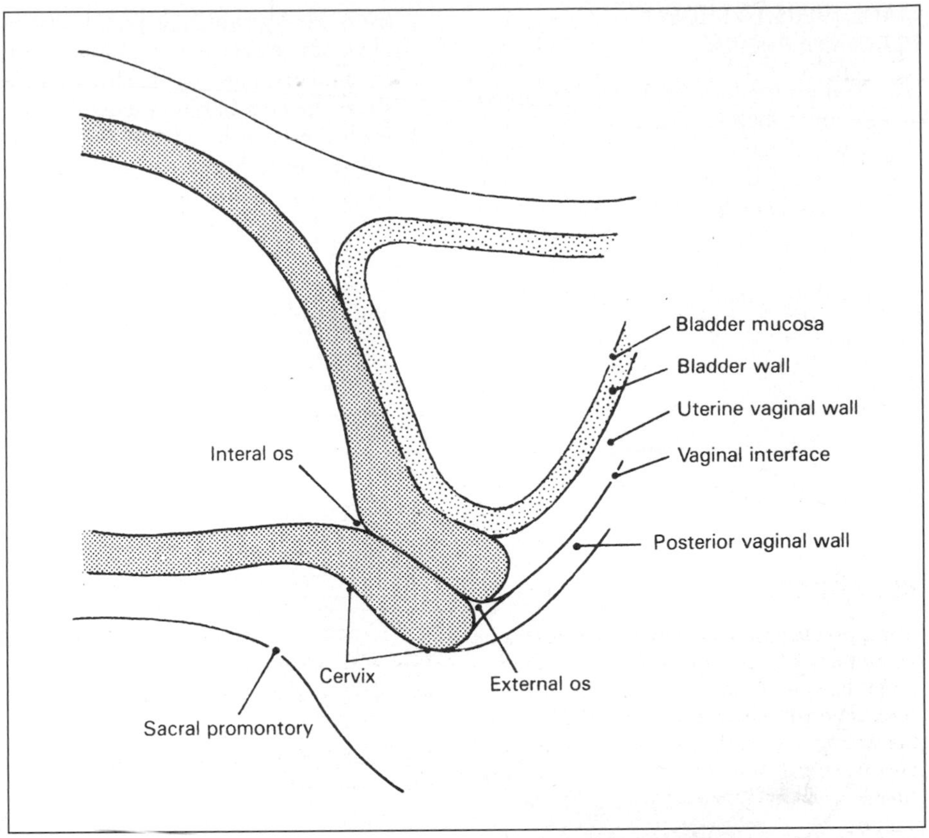

Figure 42-1. ■ *Diagram showing the cervix and surrounding structures.*

CORD

The cord normally comprises three vessels—two small arteries and one large vein. About 2% of the time, there are only two vessels with one of the arteries missing. There is an increased incidence of fetal abnormalities when there are only two vessels.

AMNIOTIC FLUID

Amniotic fluid is produced by the mother until between 15 and 18 weeks. After that time period, it is produced by the fetus. The fetus swallows the fluid, absorbs it, and excretes it through the kidneys. If the fetus cannot swallow, polyhydramnios develops. If the fetus cannot urinate, oligohydramnios occurs. There is a steady reduction in amniotic volume as the pregnancy proceeds. Fluid volume is maximal between 20 and 30 weeks. In the third trimester, small particles known as *vernix* can be seen in the normal amniotic fluid.

Technique

FILLED BLADDER AND UTERUS

Fluid in the bladder makes the cervix appear longer than it really is and creates a spurious appearance suggesting placenta previa. Avoid it if you can. Before approximately 13 to 14 weeks, the fetal examination is best performed using the endovaginal approach, which requires an empty bladder. Between 16 and 20 weeks, it may be helpful to examine pregnant women with some urine in the maternal bladder. Beyond 20 weeks, the fetus lies at a sufficiently high level that urine in the bladder is unnecessary. At this time, any fetal structure lying close to the cervix that is poorly seen with a transabdominal approach can be examined with the vaginal probe.

If the placenta extends into the lower uterine segment, examine the vagina and cervix when the patient's bladder is empty because there may be a placenta previa. Only with the bladder empty can you be sure the cervix is not artificially lengthened when the anterior and posterior uterine walls are squashed together by the distended bladder. The axis of the vagina and cervix may not be longitudinal, and oblique sections may be required to show this critical relationship. If the placenta appears to lie adjacent to the cervix, scan transversely at right angles to see whether the placenta is centrally located or whether it lies to one side of the cervix and lower uterine segment. This relationship is easy to determine if the fetus is breech, but more difficult with a cephalic (vertex) presentation.

MANEUVERS TO SHOW PLACENTA PREVIA

1. Make sure that the patient's bladder is empty before trying any of the following maneuvers. When the bladder is filled, the anterior wall of the uterus may be compressed against the placenta, giving a false impression of placenta previa (Fig. 42-2). If the fetal head is more than 2 cm from the sacrum, the possibility of placenta previa exists, and certain maneuvers can be performed to show the area behind the fetal head.
2. Push the transducer into the maternal abdomen just superior to the pubic symphysis, and while scanning, arch it longitudinally toward the patient's feet.
3. Have a physician move and hold the fetal head out of the pelvis with an abdominal (rather than a vaginal) approach and scan the lower uterine segment.

   These techniques have, for the most part, been replaced by the transvaginal and transperineal (translabial) approaches.
4. Transperineal (translabial). Place a covered curved linear array probe (5 MHz) against the labia and optimize settings so that the bladder can be

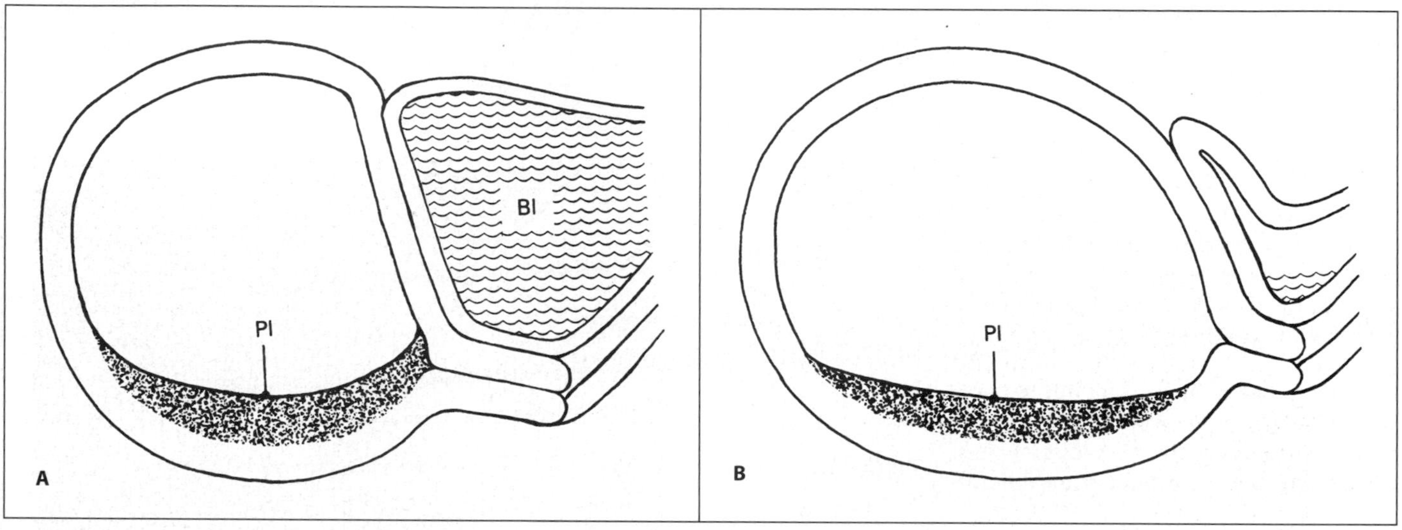

Figure 42-2. ■ *Overdistended bladder and placenta previa.* ***A.*** *An overdistended bladder may compress the anterior wall of the uterus against the posterior wall, causing an appearance resembling a placenta previa.* ***B.*** *With the bladder empty, the true length of the cervix is seen: the placenta ends above the cervix.*

seen (Fig. 42-3). The vagina will be seen as an apparently vertically placed echopenic area and the cervix will be visualized at right angles at the lower end of the vagina. The fetal head or fetal parts will be seen posterior to the bladder, which should be almost empty. The cervix will be somewhere between 2.9 and 5 cm long and should be closed. If there is a V-shaped opening at the fetal end of the cervix, this indicates cervical incompetence (Fig. 42-3B). The cervix is an active structure and may be closed at times and open at others. To provoke it to open, press gently but firmly on the maternal abdomen at the fundus to increase pressure at the internal os, the proximal end of the cervix. Occasionally, the entire cervix is then filled with fluid and the membranes balloon out of the external os. This is an emergency situation, and an obstetrician needs to be called immediately.

Gas in the rectum sometimes obscures the external os when using a transperineal approach, so the entire cervical length cannot be mea-

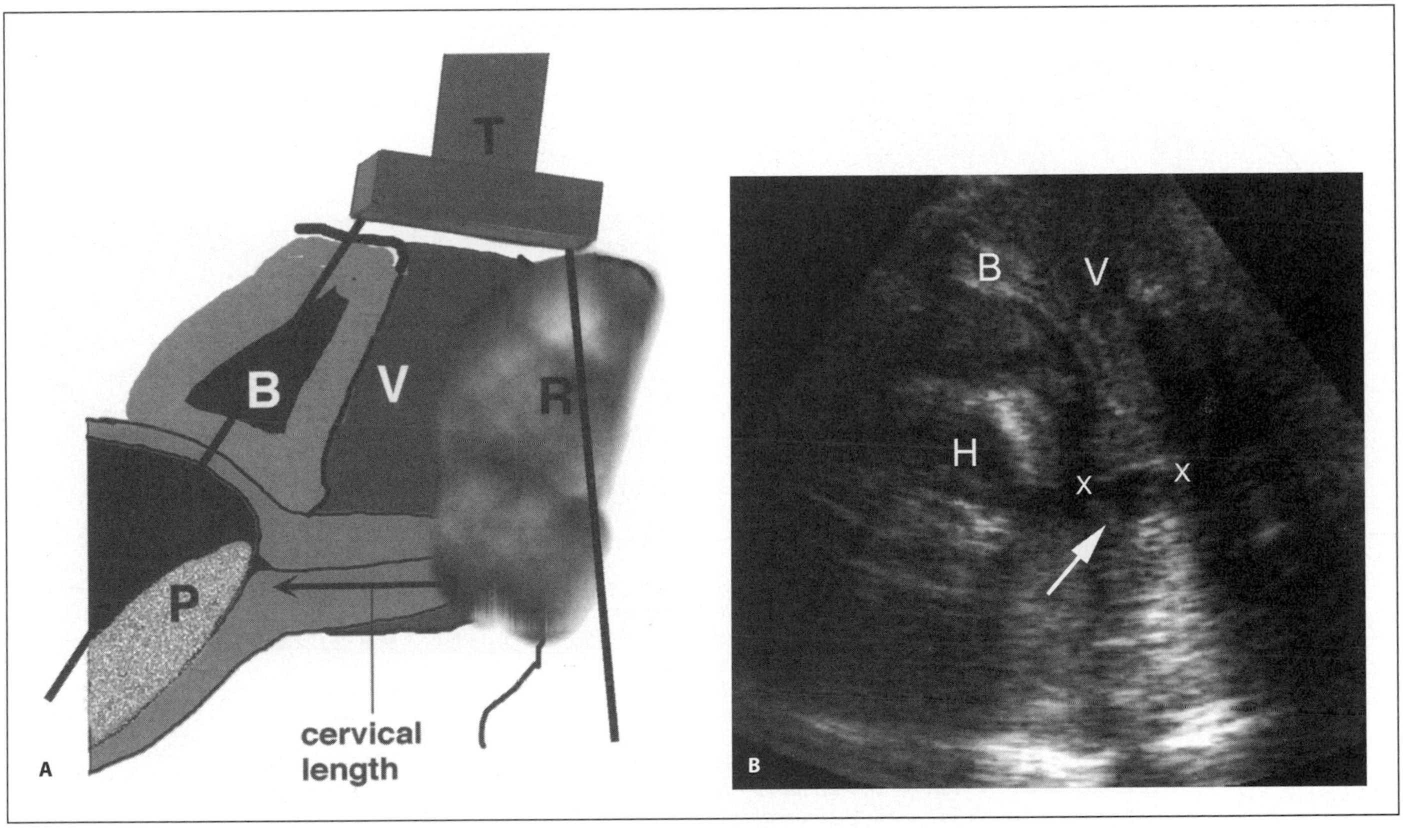

Figure 42-3. ■ *A. Diagram of translabial view of the cervix displayed in the way it is seen on the monitor. The transducer* (T) *is placed against the labia while the patient is supine or in the left lateral position with her legs flexed and wide apart. The transducer is covered with gel and plastic wrap to prevent infection. The vagina* (V) *is an echopenic vertical structure leading directly down to the cervix. The bladder lies superiorly, as does the fetus. The cervix is almost always "horizontal" to the vagina, although it may be oblique or even angulated toward the bladder* (B). *The rectum* (R) *may interfere with the image and may prevent the inferior end of the cervix from being seen. In this case, the entire placental length cannot be examined, and the external os cannot be seen. If rectal gas interferes, an endovaginal probe view will be required. In this example, the placenta* (P) *covers the cervix and is a marginal previa.* ***(B)*** *Transperineal or translabial view. The probe is placed on the labia so the vagina* (V), *although horizontal, appears to run at a vertical axis down to the cervix, which is normally at right angles to the vagina (between Xs). The bladder* (B) *is almost empty. Fetal parts* (H) *can be seen superior to the cervix. The cervix is very short and partly open in this case of incompetent cervix.*

sured. The patient may then be placed in the left-side-down decubitus position. If this maneuver fails, an endovaginal examination of the cervix shows the entire cervical length.

5. Endovaginal. The endovaginal probe is cautiously introduced, viewing the cervix as one puts it in place. After only a short distance, the cervix will be seen (Fig. 42-4). Because the cervix is usually at right angles to the vagina, the procedure is not dangerous, providing that the cervix is watched as the probe is introduced. In addition to allowing a beautiful look at the entire cervix, one can gently probe for cervical firmness with the endovaginal probe. If it is soft, the cervix is ripening and becoming effaced. Again, press on the fundus to provoke dilatation of the internal os.

Using either technique, the relationship of the placenta to the internal os will be seen well.

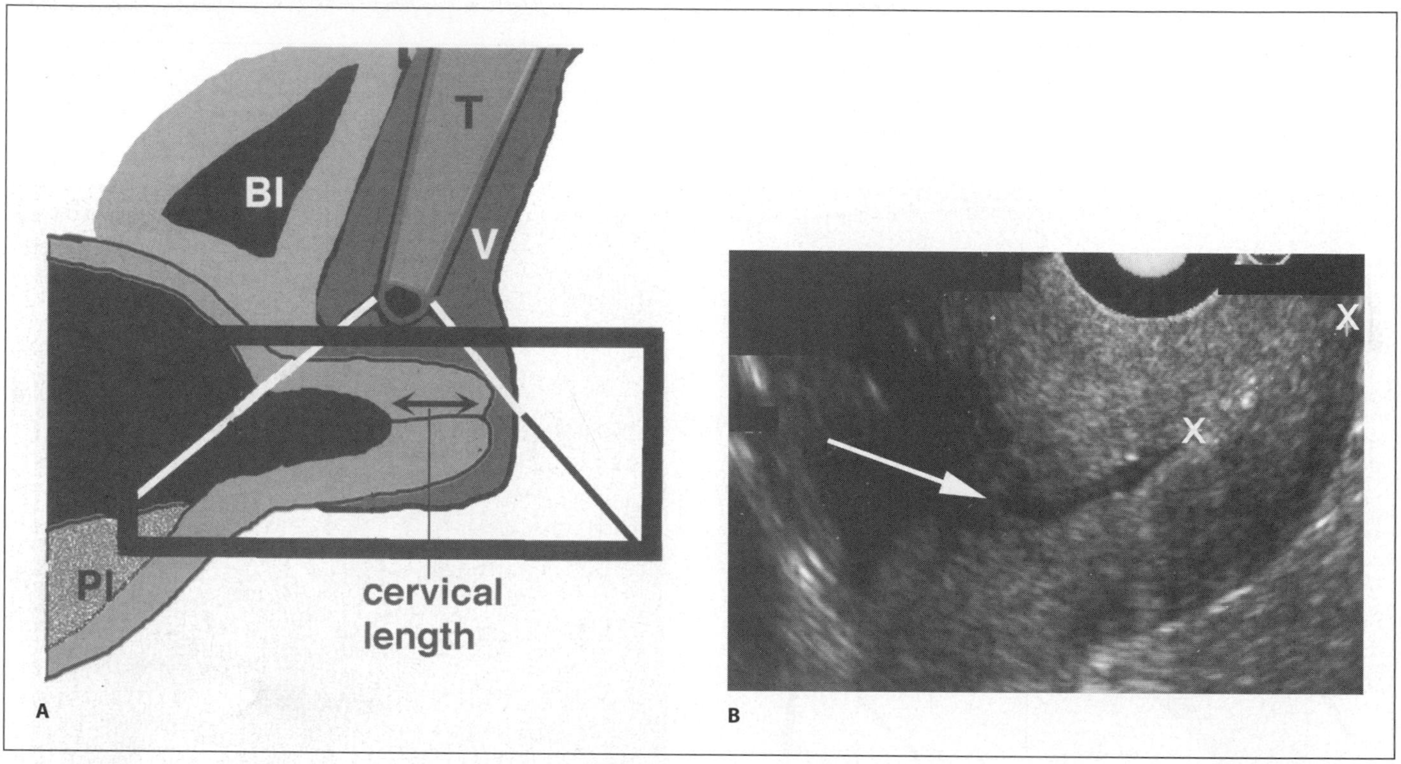

Figure 42-4. ■ *A. Endovaginal view of the cervix. Note that the vaginal probe* (T) *is located directly adjacent to the cervix. Cervical incompetence is present. Cervical length can be accurately measured, and the cervix is gently prodded with end of the transducer to see if it is soft. When the cervix is partially effaced, as in this case, the remaining cervical length is measured* (arrow). *The placenta* (Pl) *is low lying but is not a placenta previa. The box shows the area seen on the monitor. B. Endovaginal view of the cervix. The probe is adjacent to the cervix, which is at right angles to the probe. This cervix is showing funneling due to cervical incompetence* (arrow). *Only the closed portion of the cervix is measured (between Xs) when assessing cervical length.*

Pathology

PLACENTA PREVIA

Placenta previa is present whenever the placenta can be shown to lie adjacent to the internal cervical os. There are three low placental positions (Fig. 42-5):

1. Low-lying when the placenta is close to the os but not overlying it. This is not a placenta previa.
2. Marginal or partial when the placenta extends to or just covers the internal os but does not cross it (Figs. 42-6 and 42-7).

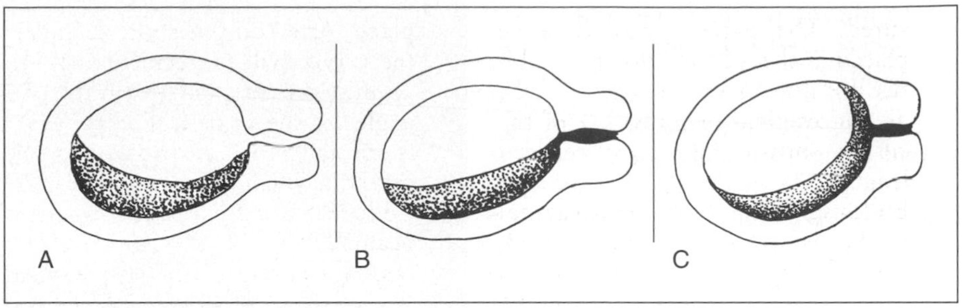

Figure 42-5. ■ *The types of placenta previa. A. Low-lying: abutting on the internal os but not covering it. B. Partial or marginal: extending to the internal os. C. Total: completely covering the internal os.*

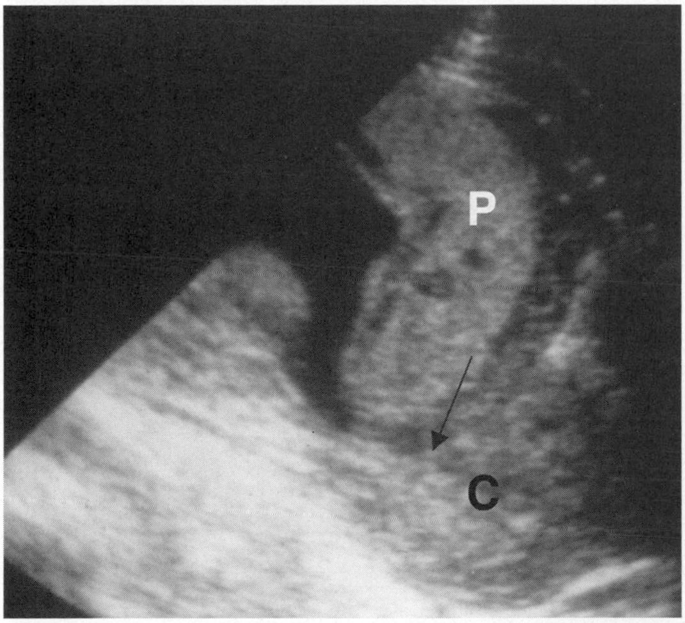

Figure 42-6. ■ *Transabdominal view of marginal placenta previa. The bladder is empty, and fortunately, the fetus was in a breech position so the cervix was well seen. The placenta* (P) *just covers the internal os of the cervix* (arrow). C, *cervix.*

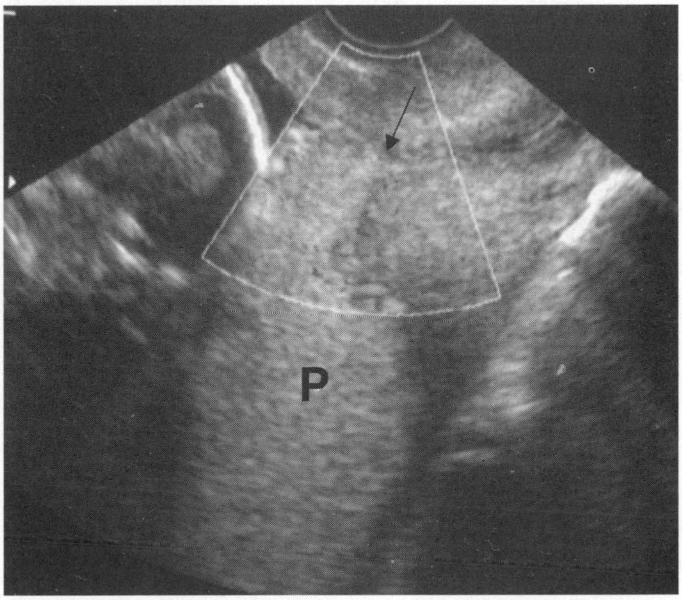

Figure 42-7. ■ *Endovaginal view of partial placenta previa at 23 weeks. The placenta* (P) *extends about 2 cm beyond the internal os* (arrow). *It is unlikely that this mild degree of placenta previa will persist to term.*

3. Complete or total when it completely overlies the internal os (Fig. 42-8).

An apparent placenta previa in the second trimester usually ceases to be a placenta previa in the third trimester. Possible explanations include the following:

1. Overdistention of the fetal bladder (Figs. 42-2 and 42-9A,B).

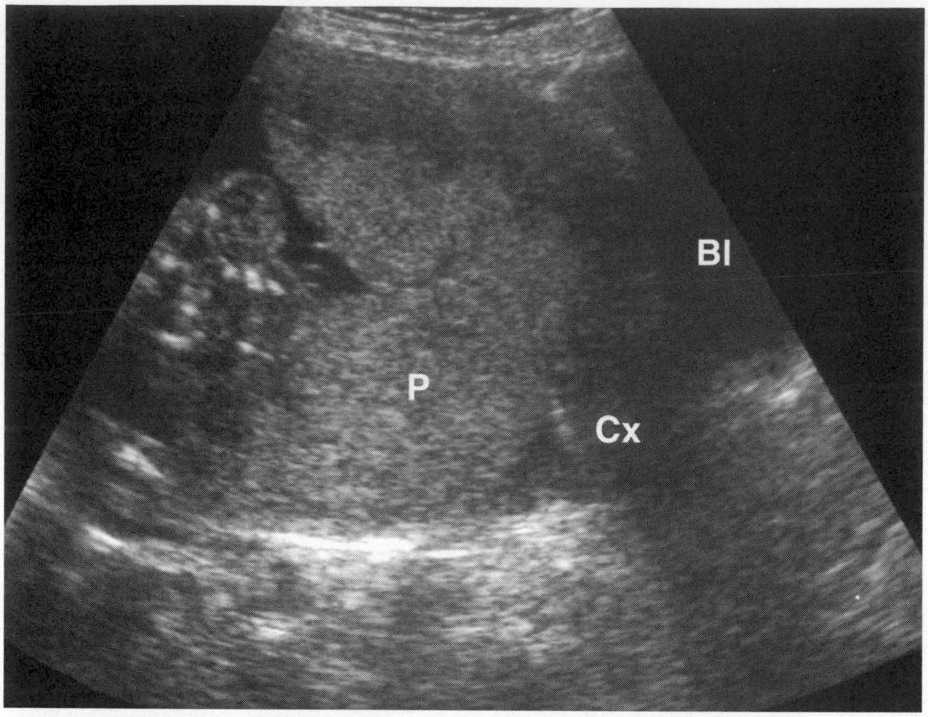

Figure 42-8. ■ *Abdominal view of total placenta previa. Although there is a small amount of urine in the bladder* (Bl) *(not ideal), the placenta* (P) *is a complete previa extending anterior and posterior to the cervix* (Cx). *Delivery by cesarean section is inevitable.*

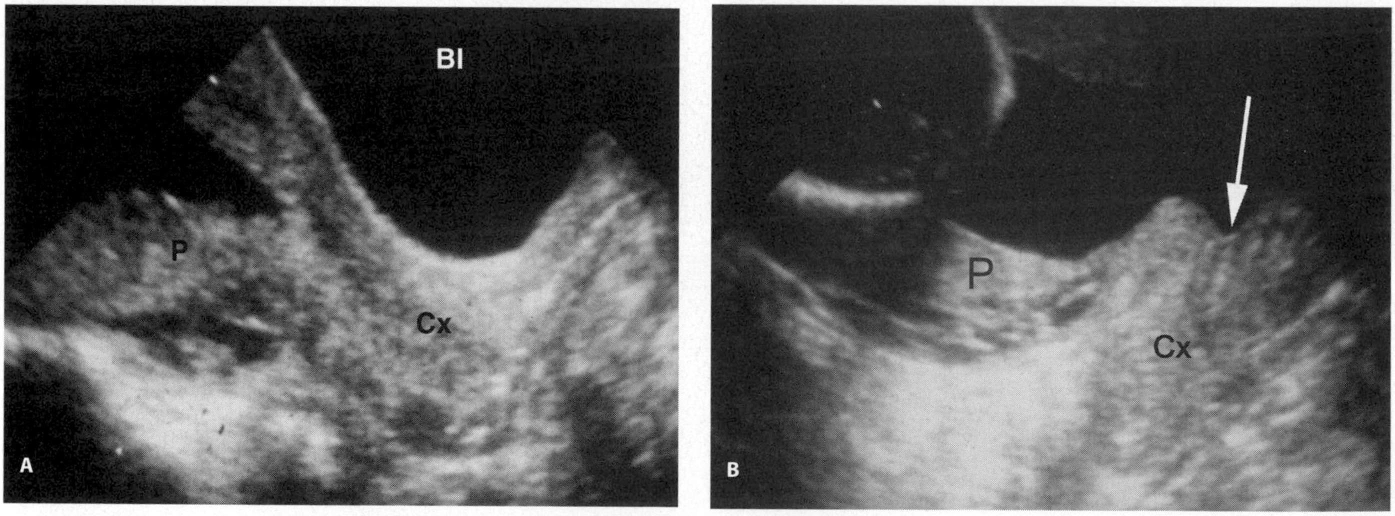

Figure 42-9. ■ *A. Apparent placenta previa* (P) *with full bladder* (Bl). *The cervix* (Cx) *is spuriously lengthened by the overdistension of the bladder.* ***B.*** *Same case with empty bladder. The axis of the cervix* (Cx) *has changed; it is now vertical. The inferior end of the placenta* (P) *lies well above the internal os* (arrow) *of the cervix.*

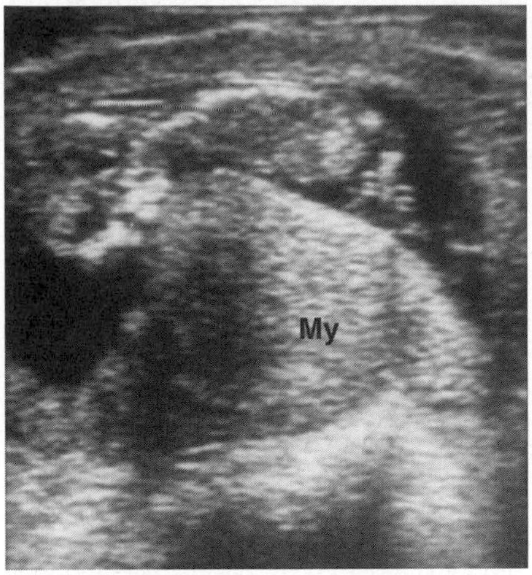

Figure 42-10. ■ *A huge myometrial contraction* (My) *involves much of the posterior aspect of the uterus including a portion of the cervix mimicking a placenta previa. Thirty minutes later, the contraction had disappeared.*

2. Myometrial contractions giving the impression of a placenta previa (Fig. 42-10).
3. A placenta that lies adjacent to the cervix but is not attached to the placental wall at that site.
4. Placental atrophy. It is thought that the placenta atrophies at sites where there is poor blood supply, such as in the cervical region.

In our practice, serial ultrasonic examinations are obtained when placenta previa is discovered, with the hope that the placenta will change position during the course of pregnancy. At term, it frequently lies at the fundus, whereas previously it was close to the cervix (Fig. 42-11). In asymptomatic patients, the placenta often covers the cervical os early in the second trimester.

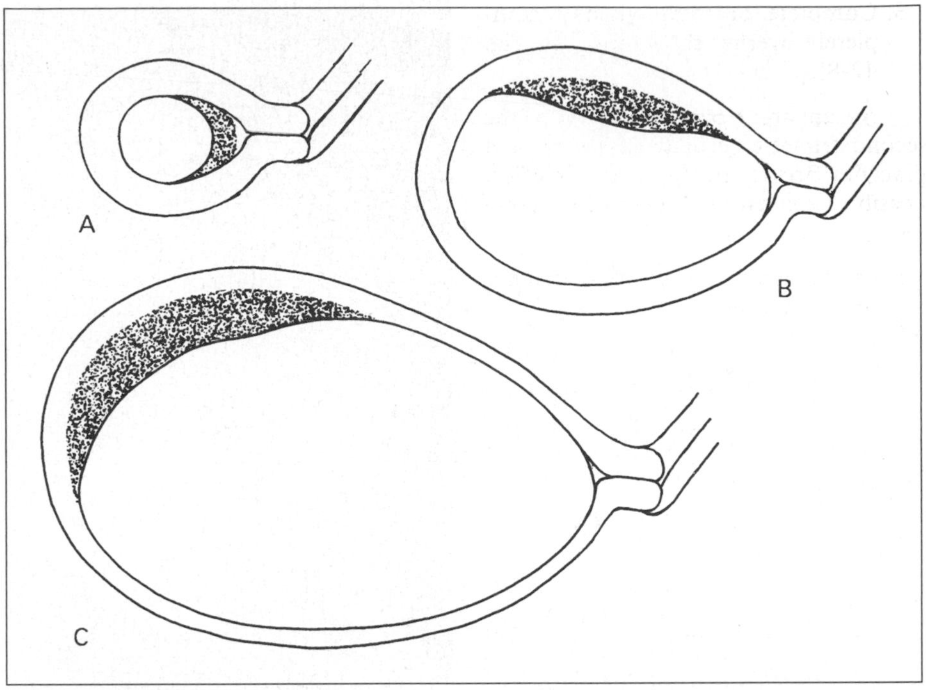

Figure 42-11. ■ *Placental "migration."* **A.** *Early in pregnancy, the placenta overlies the internal os.* **B.** *With selective growth of the lower uterine segment, the placenta moves to an anterior site.* C. *Late in pregnancy, the placenta typically lies at the fundus of the uterus.*

VASCULAR CONNECTIONS BETWEEN A SUCCENTURIATE LOBE AND THE PLACENTA

Occasionally, the placenta is split into two segments (Fig. 42-12). The smaller satellite segment is called a *succenturiate lobe*. If a succenturiate lobe is found near the cervix, and if the main portion of the placenta is located on the other side of the cervix, it is possible that the vessels that communicate between the two por-

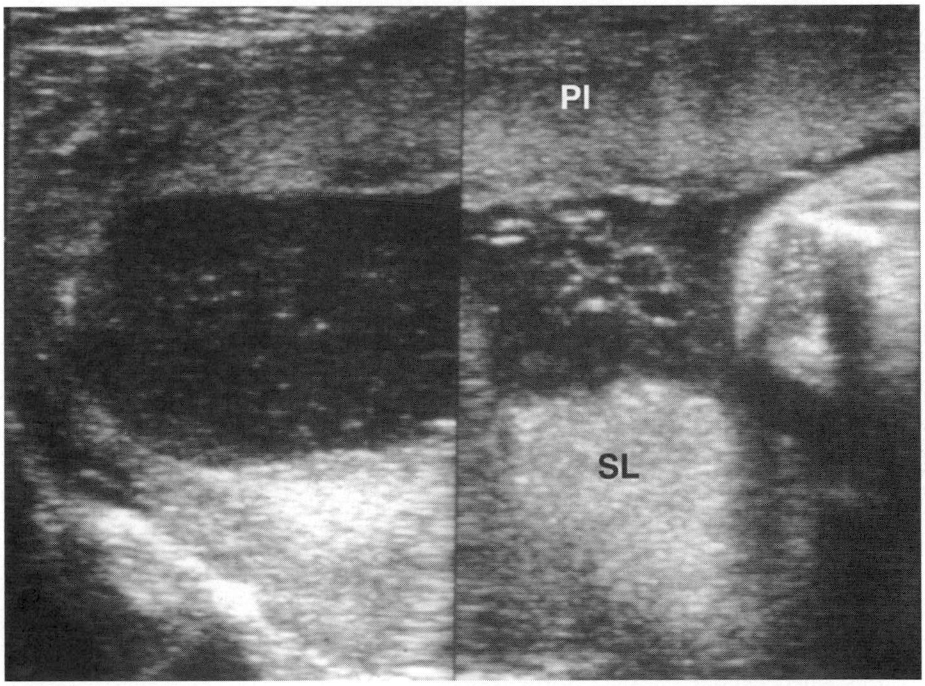

Figure 42-12. ■ *Transverse view of uterus with a succenturiate lobe. The main segment of the placenta* (P) *can be seen anteriorly, but another large segment of placenta* (Sl) *lies on the posterior aspect of the uterus. This type of placenta is potentially hazardous. The vessel connecting the smaller subsidiary part of the placenta to the main segment may cross the cervix. Both segments of the placenta need to be identified after delivery.*

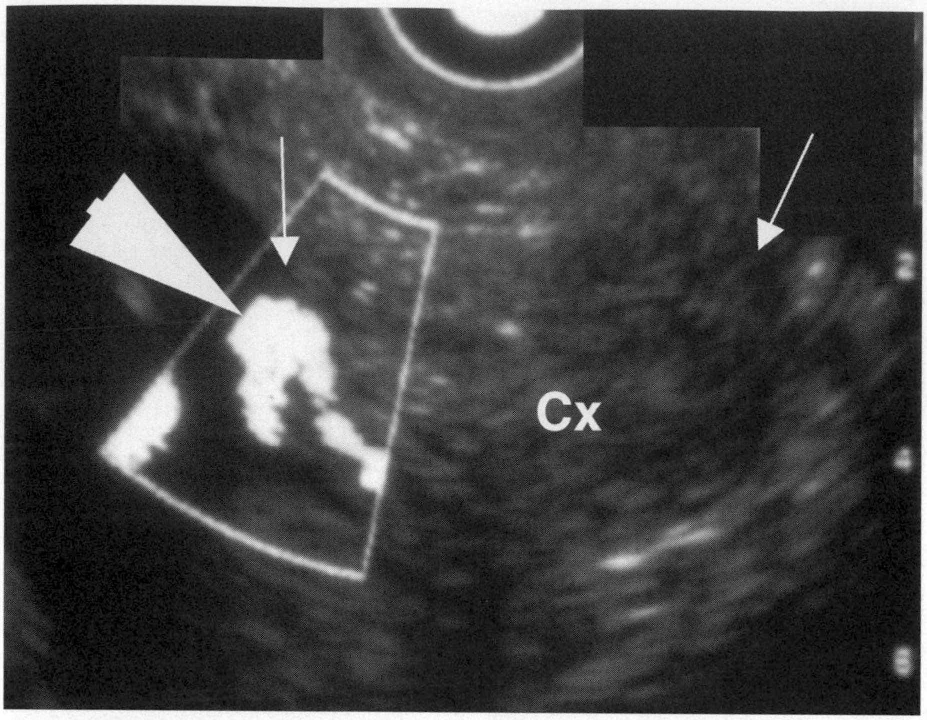

Figure 42-13. ■ *Color flow view of cervix showing vessels* (arrowhead) *adjacent to the cervix* (Cx) *due to velamentous insertion of the cord. Arrows show the internal and external os.*

tions of the placenta run across the internal os (Fig. 42-13). If the fetus breaks these vessels as it delivers, the blood loss could be disastrous.The only way to discover this very unusual finding is to look at the cervical region with color flow. Prominent vessels will be seen running across the cervix.

VASA PREVIA

If the placenta is located in a low position and if the cord insertion into the placenta is at the placenta's rim, there is a possibility of vasa previa. With a velamentous insertion, the three vessels that make up the cord become separated and lie in a membrane as they reach the placenta. If this membrane lies across the cervix, it can act in the same way as a placenta previa and can cause even more serious blood loss.

A velamentous insertion can only be easily recognized with color flow; look for this whenever the placenta is low lying and if vaginal bleeding occurs. Velamentous insertions occur much more commonly with twin pregnancies than with singleton pregnancies.

INCOMPETENT CERVIX

A cervix that starts to dilate prematurely in the absence of labor contractions is known as an *incompetent cervix* (Figs. 42-3B and 42-4). The mucous plug that fills the cervix can be lost at the time that this dilatation takes place, which causes a brief episode of vaginal bleeding.

Whenever a patient presents with vaginal bleeding in the second or third trimester, cautiously examine the cervix with the vaginal probe. The probe can be inserted about 2 cm to see whether there is any evidence of cervical incompetence. There will be a V-shaped indentation at the internal os if incompetence is present.

If cervical incompetence is not seen, the vaginal probe can be moved onto the cervix to look for placenta previa, vasa previa, or crossing vessels. Cautiously apply pressure to the cervix with the vaginal probe to see whether it has softened. Put pressure on the maternal abdomen to see whether the internal os opens. If there is evidence of fluid in the cervical canal, these maneuvers are not performed. Be especially vigilant if there is evidence of fluid throughout the canal with "ballooning" membranes prolapsing out of the external os into the vagina.

CORD PROLAPSE

Prolapse of the umbilical cord into the endocervical canal occurs at delivery in 0.5% of cases. There is a high chance of fetal loss secondary to cord compression if the cord is in this location. This rare problem occurs most often with polyhydramnios, a nonvertex presentation, and multiple gestations. If the cord is found with color flow to be the presenting structure at term or if the patient is in labor, then the obstetrician should be called.

ABRUPTIO PLACENTAE (ACCIDENTAL HEMORRHAGE)

Bleeding from the placenta in a number of different sites is known as *abruptio placentae*. The condition has several sonographic manifestations (Fig. 42-14).

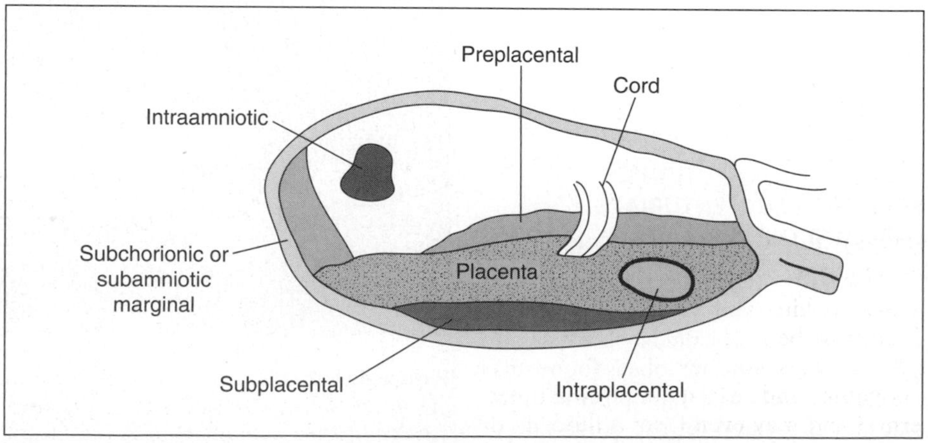

Figure 42-14. ■ *The various sites of abruptio placenta:* (1) *Blood between the placenta and myometrium (subplacental).* (2) *Blood within the amniotic fluid (intra-amniotic).* (3) *Blood between the amniotic sac membrane and chorionic membrane (subchorionic or subamniotic). The blood is usually adjacent to the placenta. If it is in a preplacental location, the cord may be compressed.* (4) *Intraplacental blood.*

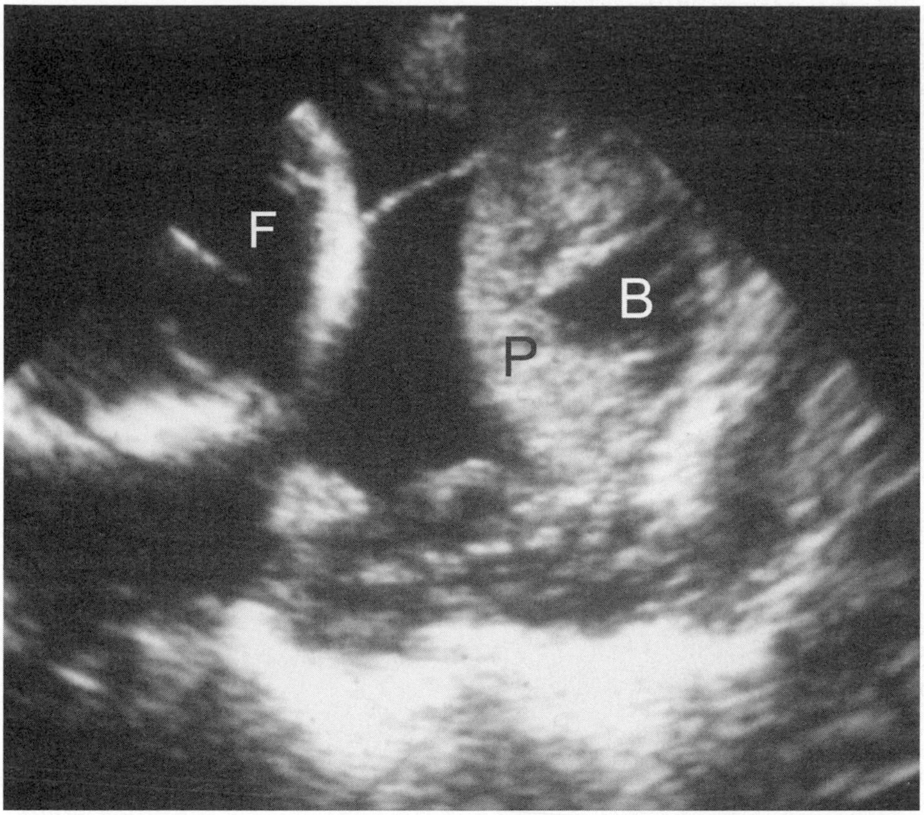

Figure 42-15. ■ *Abruptio placenta. A bleed is present* (B) *and lies posterior to a portion of the placenta* (P). *The fetal head* (F) *can be seen superior to the placenta.*

A Gap between the Myometrium and the Placenta

The collection of blood between the myometrium and the placenta may be completely sonolucent, or it may contain low-level internal echoes due to the blood (Fig. 42-15). The border of the placenta will be displaced away from the myometrium. The textures of the blood clot and of the placenta can be similar—this type has the worst prognosis. Using color flow helps in showing that myometrium is present rather than clot because vessels will be seen.

Echoes within the Amniotic Fluid due to Blood

Echoes within the amniotic fluid due to blood may be focal and may present in small clumps or they may be evenly echogenic and extensive, resembling vernix, and may even form a fluid–fluid level.

Bleeding in a Subchorionic or Subamniotic Location

The blood within the subchorionic or subamniotic space may be relatively similar in texture to that of the placenta, but it will eventually become sonolucent (Fig. 42-16).

Subchorionic blood in front of the placenta is considered particularly dangerous because it may compress the cord. The amniotic or chorionic sac membrane is displaced away from the placenta in a marginal location (Figs. 42-14 and 42-16), which is the most common form of abruptio. In most instances, the collection develops at the edge of the placenta (a marginal bleed).

With normal gain settings, the only sign of this type of abruption may be a membrane within the amniotic fluid adjacent to one end of the placenta. If gain is increased, the blood within this area becomes more echogenic than neighboring amniotic fluid because it has a more proteinaceous composition. The prognosis with this type of bleed is good.

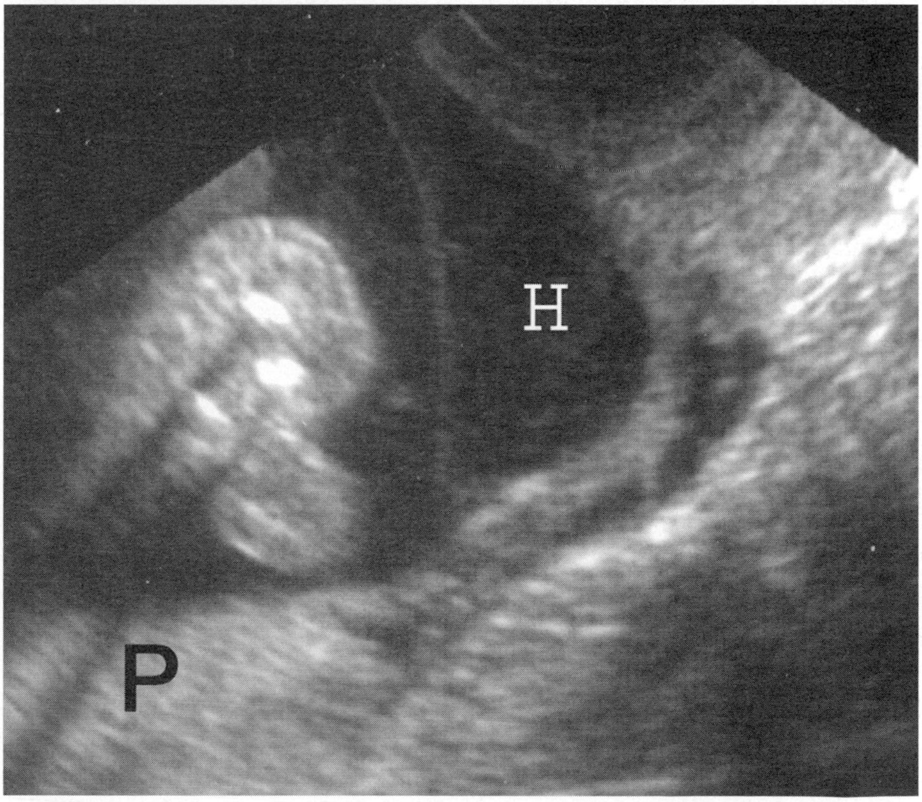

Figure 42-16. ■ *Subchorionic bleed adjacent to the placenta* (P). *This bleed* (H) *has a similar appearance to amniotic fluid but is enclosed by a membrane and contains echoes. Increasing gain would cause obvious echoes in the blood but not in the amniotic fluid.*

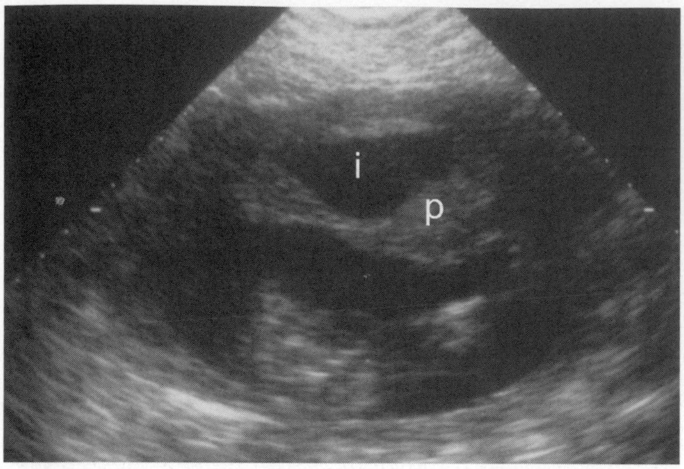

Figure 42-17. ■ *Placental infarct. This placental infarct* (i) *was tender. It is located close to the placental base pate and is more or less triangular. Some infarcts are more echogenic.* P, *placenta.*

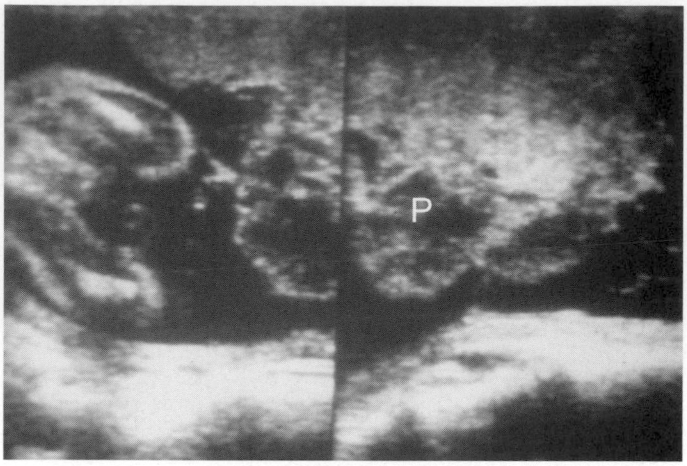

Figure 42-18. ■ *Chorioangioma. Large vascular mass* (P) *arising from the placenta. In this case, there was no evidence of hydrops in the fetus.*

Intraplacental Bleed

An echopenic or echogenic area within the placenta can represent an intraplacental bleed or infarct (Figs. 42-14 and 42-17). Areas of infarction, although initially echopenic, may eventually calcify. Intraplacental bleeds or infarcts may be locally tender, allowing distinction from Wharton's jelly deposition.

Flow will be seen in real time in an echopenic area due to vascular lakes, although the flow is usually too slow to be detected with Doppler.

CHORIOANGIOMA

A benign tumor arising from the amniotic surface of the placenta, chorioangioma is highly vascular (Fig. 42-18). Profuse blood flow can be seen within it. Chorioangiomas are quite common and are almost always of no consequence.

On extremely rare occasions, so much blood goes to the mass that the fetus becomes anemic and shows evidence of hydrops. Chorioangioma of a size greater than 5 to 6 cm needs careful follow-up (Fig. 42-18).

INTRA-AMNIOTIC MEMBRANES

Membranes within the amniotic cavity may have a number of possible causes (Fig. 42-19).

1. Abruptio (previously mentioned).
2. Amniotic sheets (Fig. 42-20). These membranes, which do not enclose a space, are double and have a small circular echopenic area in the portion adjacent to the amniotic cavity.

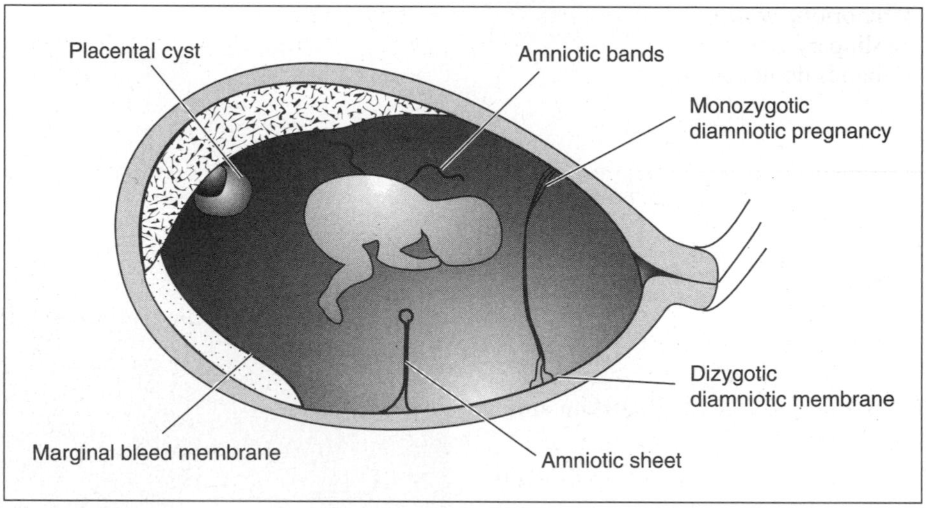

Figure 42-19. ■ *Five types of membranes are seen in the amniotic fluid:* (1) *Membranes related to subamniotic blood. Increasing the gain shows low-level echoes within the enclosed space.* (2) *Amniotic sheets. There is a double membrane with a cystic area at the tip.* (3) *Amniotic bands adhering to the fetus. These are rare.* (4) *Placental cysts.* (5) *Amniotic sac membranes related to a twin pregnancy that has resorbed.*

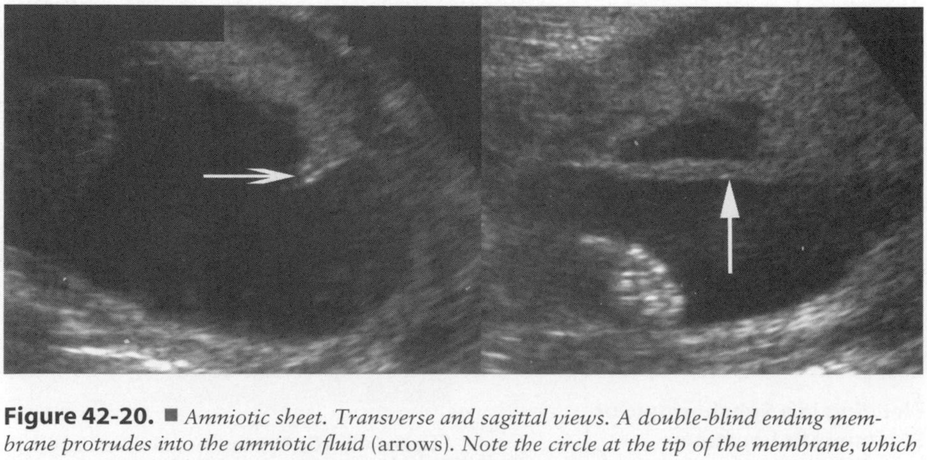

Figure 42-20. ■ *Amniotic sheet. Transverse and sagittal views. A double-blind ending membrane protrudes into the amniotic fluid* (arrows). *Note the circle at the tip of the membrane, which represents a vessel* (left arrow). *This membrane is thought to be a synechia within the amniotic fluid coated with amniotic and chorionic membranes.*

Vascular flow can often be seen at the tip of the amniotic sheet where it widens. This area is thought to represent a site where the amnion and chorion surround subamniotic adhesions (synechiae) present before the pregnancy occurred.

3. Amniotic sac membrane. In a proportion of twin pregnancies, one twin dies. The sac membrane enclosing amniotic fluid may persist when the fetus has disappeared or resorbed.
4. Amniotic bands. The amniotic membranes can break and curl up in amniotic fluid so the chorionic membrane is exposed to the amniotic fluid and the fetus. Portions of fetal limbs may be truncated if amniotic bands are present, perhaps because the fetus becomes attached to the chorion, which is not smooth and slippery like the amnion. Amniotic bands do not enclose amniotic fluid.
5. "Unfused" amnion. The extracelomic fluid between the amnion and chorion disappears by about 14 weeks. Occasionally, resorption of this fluid is delayed, which is of little clinical consequence. After amniocentesis, blood may enter the extracelomic space between the amnion and chorion. If this takes place, premature delivery may occur. Echogenic fluid will be seen between the amnion and chorion, representing blood.
6. Placental cysts. Cysts consisting of fluid and debris may form on the amniotic surface of the placenta; they relate to a preplacental hemorrhage. The cysts have no pathologic significance, but the membrane around the cyst may be confused with an amniotic band or other structures.

PLACENTA PERCRETA

If the placenta implants onto a previous cesarean section incision, placental tissue may invade the myometrium at the cesarean section site (Fig. 42-21). The invasion may be slight (acreta), into the myometrium (increta), or through the muscle wall (percreta). This is a rare but very dangerous condition with a high mortality rate. At the time of delivery, a large bleed occurs as the placenta and myometrium attempt to separate. The sonographer can detect placenta percreta by concentrating on a previous cesarean section site and seeing the absence of myometrium. Many prominent arterial vessels will be seen flowing at right angles to the placental interface with the myometrium. Vessels will be seen on the inner bladder wall surface if a placenta increta is present.

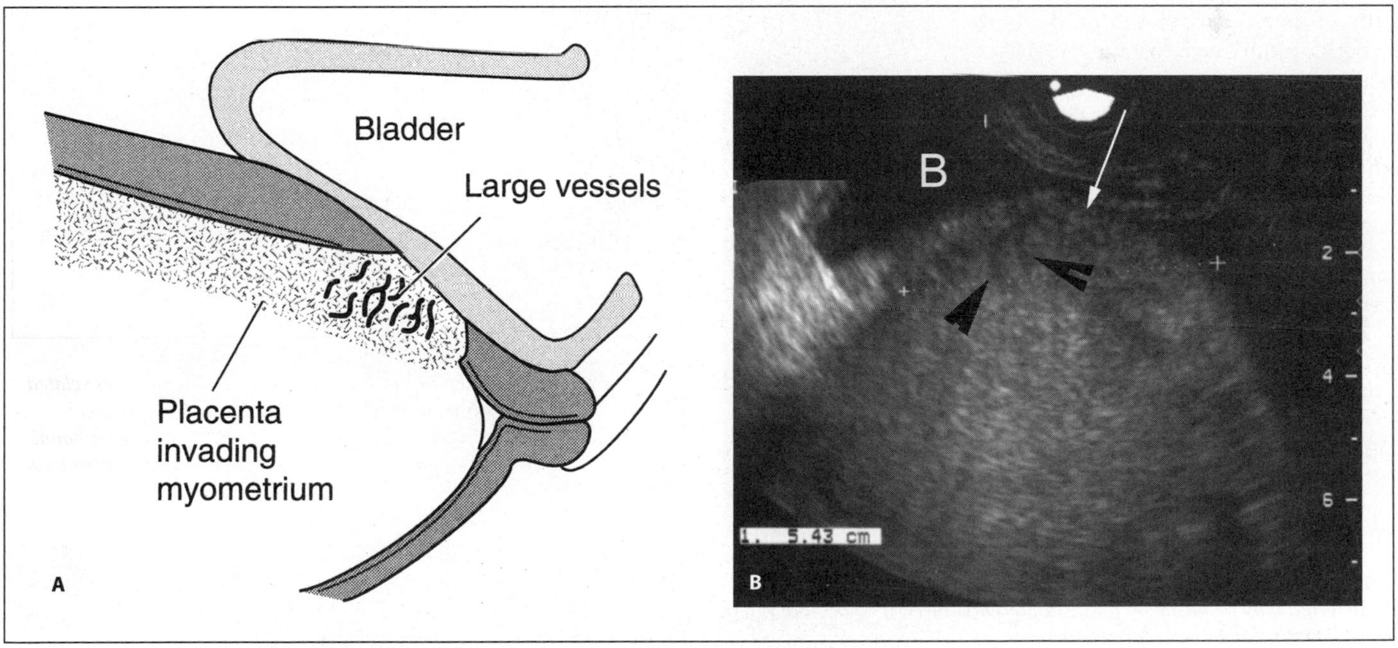

Figure 42-21. ■ *A. Placenta percreta. At the cesarean section incision site, the placenta invades the myometrium and bladder wall. Large vertically aligned vessels can be seen within the placental invasion site. They may extend into the bladder.* ***B.*** *Placenta percreta. Endovaginal view. The placenta previa is entering the myometrium adjacent to the bladder. Note the small vertically aligned vessels at the percreta site* (black arrowheads), *which do not run parallel with the myometrium (as in a normal placenta). The myometrium is thin or absent at the site of the placenta percreta.*

Pitfalls

1. Placental and uterine vessels. Sometimes, the blood vessels that supply the placenta are large and form spaces in the myometrium adjacent to the placenta (Fig. 42-22), which may be mistaken for abruptio placentae. Real-time visualization will document venous flow in these sinuses.
2. Overdistended bladder. An overdistended bladder may create an appearance that suggests a placenta previa because the anterior wall of the uterus is compressed against the posterior wall (Fig. 42-2). Postvoid films resolve this false-positive finding.
3. Myometrium. Mistaking the myometrium (uterine wall) for abruptio is possible. The normal sonolucent space around the placenta should be symmetrical at all sites, although this space is particularly obvious at the fundus of the uterus. An increase in gain will cause echoes in this area and not in adjacent amniotic fluid. Flow will be seen in uterine vessels with color flow Doppler.
4. Myometrial contraction. A myometrial contraction can temporarily displace the placenta and simulate a placenta previa when the contraction occurs in the lower uterine segment (Fig. 42-10). If the placenta appears to be visible at two separate sites, rescan after 30 minutes. One of the possible placentas will usually turn out to be a myometrial contraction. These are painless contractions of the uterine wall with no pathologic significance.
5. Succenturiate lobe. A succenturiate lobe is a rare placental variant occurring in approximately 1% of pregnancies (Fig. 42-12). The placenta is split into two parts. If the second part is small and located adjacent to the cervix, sonographic detection may be difficult.
6. Subchorionic echopenic areas. Sonolucent areas may be seen adjacent to the chorionic plate or within the placenta. These areas represent either fibrin deposition or large placental vessels and are of no pathologic significance (Fig. 42-23).
7. Thinned myometrium at cesarean section site. The myometrium can be markedly thinned at the cesarean section site. Although this condition is worth commenting on in a report, it is rarely of clinical significance. The myometrium can be so thin at the time of cesarean section that the fetus is visible within.
8. A circumvallate placenta. The placenta can burrow into the my-

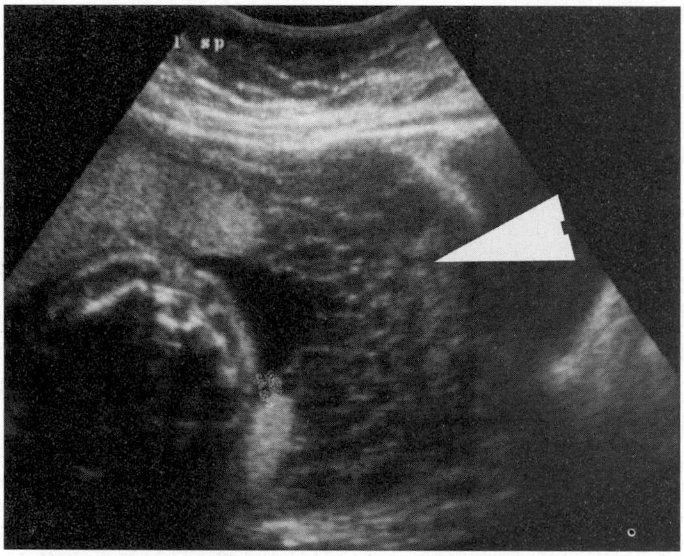

Figure 42-22. ■ *Large normal blood vessels* (arrowhead) *supplying the placenta may be mistaken for a subplacental bleed if color flow is not used to confirm their vascular origin.*

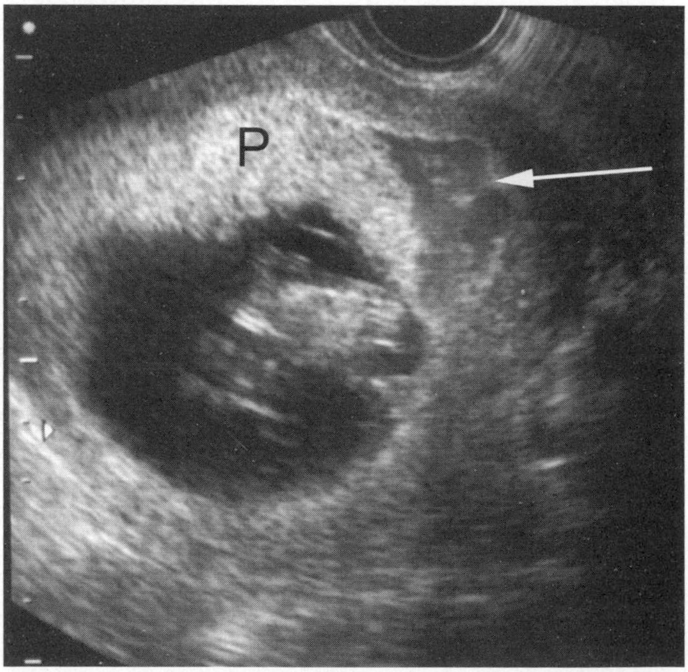

Figure 42-23. ■ *Venous lake. The sonolucent area on the uterine border of the placenta* (arrow) *showed subtle venous flow on real-time and is a venous lake. The flow may be so slow that it is difficult to detect on color flow.* P, *placenta.*

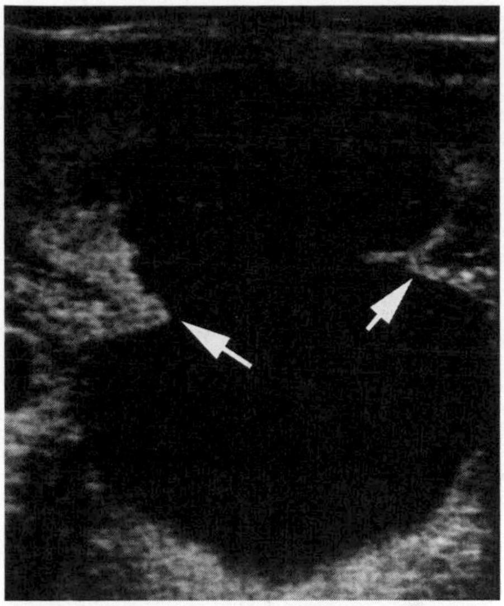

Figure 42-24. ■ *Circumvallate placenta. There is a raised rim* (arrows) *around the edge of an anterior placenta. This appearance is characteristic of circumvallate placenta.*

ometrium. An echogenic rim forms around the placenta's border (Fig. 42-24). This circumvallate appearance is worth noting. The placenta is more difficult to deliver if this abnormality is present.

9. Low lateral placenta mimicking a placenta previa. If the placenta lies lateral to the cervix but in the region of the lower segment, casual scanning may give the impression of a placenta previa. Make sure that a section is taken through the cervix and lower uterine segment simultaneously to be confident that a placenta previa is present.
10. Intra-amniotic bleed versus fetal mass. Maternal blood can collect in the amniotic fluid and create a mass that may look as if it arises from the fetus. It will change appearance if reexamined in a few days. If the maternal abdomen is jogged, the blood clot will move separately from the fetus.
11. Placental lakes. Echopenic areas within the placenta known as *vascular lakes* are common. Real time will show vascular flow in these areas (Fig. 42-23).
12. Nuchal cord. In about 20% of second and third trimester pregnancies, the cord is wrapped around the fetal neck. As a rule, this is an unimportant normal variant, but if the cord is wrapped around twice or if the cord appears to be straightened and under tension, the obstetrician should be informed because fetal death could occur at the time of delivery.
13. Unusual axes to the cervical canal. When the cervix is examined, either with a translabial or endovaginal approach, the cervical canal is usually at a horizontal axis to the probe (Fig. 42-25A). On some occasions, the axis of the cervical canal is oblique to the vagina (Fig. 42-25B). A rare variant occurs when the uterus is retroverted and the cervix flips anteriorly (Fig. 42-25C). This type of cervix can be difficult to see because it is displaced anterosuperiorly. When the uterus is retroverted with an anteverted and retroflexed cervix, there is a danger of uterine incarceration. In this condition, as the uterus expands, it compresses the bladder and eventually causes urinary retention.

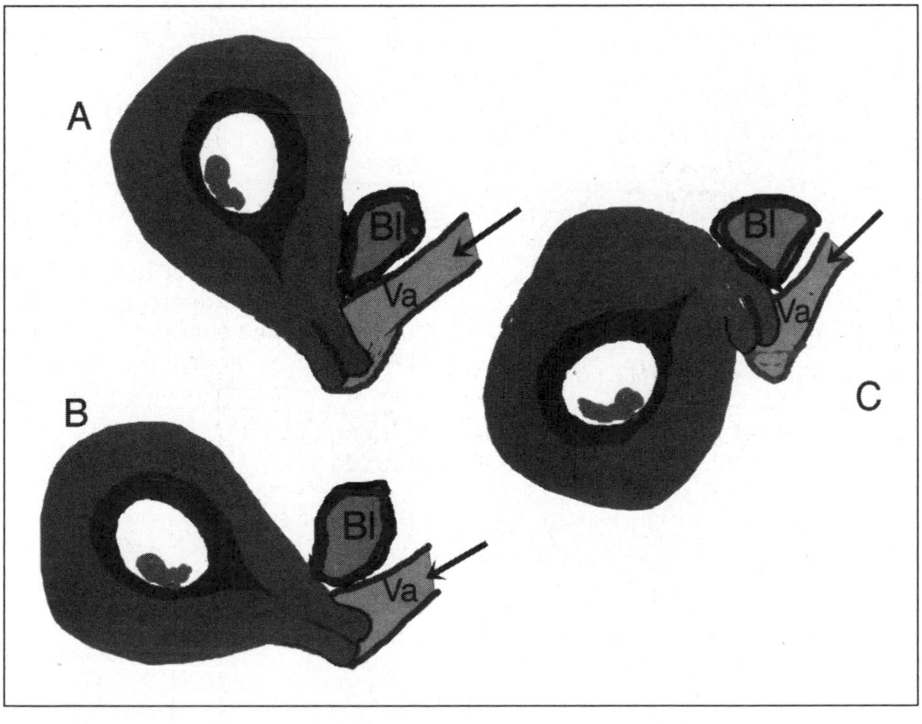

Figure 42-25. ■ *A. This is the normal position for the cervix. The black arrow indicates the transducer or beam axis. B. The cervix is at an oblique axis to the transducer. C. The cervix is anteverted but retroflexed. Note that most of the cervix is not readily seen through the vagina because it is more anteriorly located than usual. This type of cervix may be missed completely using the vaginal probe.*

SELECTED READING

Callen PW, ed. *Ultrasonography in Obstetrics and Gynecology*, 4th ed. Philadelphia: Saunders; 2002.

Clerici G, Burnelli L, Lauro V, et al. Prenatal diagnosis of vasa previa presenting as a amniotic band. "A not so innocent amniotic band." *Ultrasound Obstet Gynecol* 1996; 7:61–63.

Comstock CH, Love JJ, Brosnteen RA, et al. Sonographic detection of placenta acreta in the second and third trimesters of pregnancy. *Am J Obstet Gynecol* 2004;190: 1135–1140.

Farine D, Fox HE, Jakobson S, et al. Vaginal ultrasound for diagnosis of placenta previa. *Am J Obstet Gynecol* 1988;159:566–569.

Harris RD, Cho C, Wells WA. Sonography of the placenta with emphasis on pathological correlation. *Semin Ultrasound CT MR* 1996;17:66–89.

Heinonen S, Ryynanen M, Kirkinen P, et al. Perinatal diagnostic evaluation of velamentous umbilical cord insertion: clinical, Doppler and ultrasonic findings. *Obstet Gynecol* 1996;87:112–117.

Huntington DK, Sanders RC. Ultrasound of the placenta and membranes. *Ultrasound Q* 1994;12:45–64.

McCarthy J, Thurmond AS, Jones MK, et al. Circumvallate placenta: sonographic diagnosis. *J Ultrasound Med* 1995;14:21–26.

43

Small for Dates

ROGER C. SANDERS

KEY WORDS

Eclampsia. High blood pressure with urinary protein loss occurring in pregnancy. In its most severe form, it is associated with epileptic seizure. It is a very serious condition that causes intrauterine growth restriction and often leads to fetal death.

Hyaline Membrane Disease (Respiratory Distress Syndrome). Respiratory condition occurring in the neonate as a consequence of delivery when the fetal lungs are still immature.

Intrauterine Growth Restriction (Intrauterine Growth Retardation; IUGR). A fetus is suffering from IUGR when it is below the 10th percentile for weight at a given gestational age or weighs less than 2,500 grams at 36 weeks' gestational age.

Oligohydramnios. Too little amniotic fluid. No fluid or only small pockets of fluid are present.

Pre-eclamptic Toxemia. High blood pressure and proteinuria that precedes eclampsia.

Premature Rupture of Membranes (PROM). Leakage of fluid from the amniotic cavity occurring before the patient goes into labor. Most often results in premature delivery.

Trimester. Pregnancy is divided into three periods of 13 weeks each, known as *trimesters*. Obstetric problems are conveniently related to a given trimester.

The Clinical Problem

Three possibilities should be considered when a fetus is small for dates.

1. The mother's dates are wrong, and the fetus is actually younger than indicated by her dates.
2. Palpation is misleading because of obesity or unusual uterine lie.
3. A small uterus with oligohydramnios is present owing to:
   a. Premature rupture of membranes (PROM)
   b. Intrauterine growth restriction (IUGR) with a small fetus and placenta and diminished amniotic fluid
   c. Fetal renal anomaly (see Chapter 45) with diminished fluid

PREMATURE RUPTURE OF MEMBRANES

The rupture of membranes (a "show") early in pregnancy is an obstetric management problem. If the fetus is too small to survive outside the uterus, no efforts are made to salvage it. If the fetus is large enough to survive, the mother is put on bed rest and treated with antibiotics to stop infection of the uterine contents. Ultrasound is valuable in the following ways:

1. Showing how large the fetus is
2. Giving an idea of the mother's true dates
   a. Excluding a fetal anomaly associated with polyhydramnios that might have caused PROM
   b. Showing how much amniotic fluid is still present

This is an obstetric emergency study.

IUGR

In IUGR, insufficient nutrition is supplied to the fetus. Fetuses are at risk if the mother is chronically ill (e.g., chronic heart disease), takes drugs (e.g., alcohol or cigarettes), does not eat well, is under 17 or over 35, or has had previous pregnancies in which there was poor fetal growth.

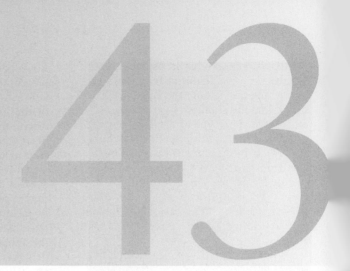

IUGR can exhibit an asymmetric, a symmetric, or a femur-sparing pattern. In asymmetric IUGR, the fetal trunk is small, but the skull is more or less normal in size. This type of IUGR is thought to be associated with placental problems that result in defective transfer of nutrients from the mother to the fetus. When the onset of fetal nutritional insufficiency is abrupt, the fetal brain is relatively spared, but the liver is severely affected, leading to an asymmetric growth pattern.

In symmetric IUGR, the entire fetus is smaller than normal. This type of IUGR is thought to relate to a continued insult such as chronic maternal illness or drug intake.

In the femur-sparing type of IUGR, all measurements apart from the femur length are small. The femur-sparing type of IUGR is relatively common. So far, no specific clinical features have been recognized.

Diagnosis of symmetric IUGR requires accurate dating at an early stage. Most obstetricians feel that a routine biparietal diameter measurement at 17 to 20 weeks' gestation is desirable in mothers who are at risk for IUGR so that accurate dates are known. A sonogram between 11 and 14 weeks is an even more accurate way of establishing the gestational age. Nuchal thickening can also be assessed (see Chapter 45).

IUGR is usually diagnosed by ultrasound when growth is less than expected in the third trimester. Establishing the diagnosis is crucial due to increased risk of difficult delivery and risk of stunted stature and intellect at a later age if the condition is not detected and remedied in utero. The fetal condition may be improved by maternal bed rest and, if applicable, having the mother quit cigarette smoking. The ultrasonic diagnosis depends on comparing the sizes of different structures in the fetal body, such as the overall size of the abdomen with the head size, and correlating these measurements with those expected according to standard obstetrical ultrasound measurements for a given obstetric date (see Appendices 11, 12, and 13). If a fetus is first examined in the late second or third trimester, and if the trunk is too small or if the femur is too long for other measurements, think of IUGR.

Anatomy

For the standard approach to the fetal anatomy, see Chapter 41.

Technique

See the techniques described in Chapter 41.

Pathology

RENAL ANOMALIES

Eliminate the possibility of a renal anomaly by finding the kidneys and looking for the fetal bladder (see Chapter 45). If a normal-size bladder is present, the possibility of agenesis (absence) of the kidneys can be eliminated. The bladder normally fills and partially empties over the course of about an hour. Slower rates of filling are associated with IUGR.

PROM

In evaluating PROM, the obstetrician needs to know the following:

1. How much amniotic fluid there is
2. Whether there is a fetal anomaly that might cause polyhydramnios and thus induce PROM
3. The gestational age and size of the fetus

If there is uncertainty as to whether PROM has occurred, the cervix should be examined (see Chapter 42). Place a sterile condom on the endovaginal probe and gently examine the cervix. If it looks short (less than 2.5 cm) and the internal os is open (see Figs. 42-3 and 42-4), it is likely that there has been PROM. If it looks normal, compress the fundus and re-examine the cervix—the internal os may open up. Gently compress the cervix with the vaginal probe to see if it is softer than normal.

IUGR

Measurements

IUGR is diagnosed by obtaining the following measurements:

Biparietal Diameter. Normal growth charts of the biparietal diameter according to week of pregnancy are available. If the mother has accurate dates or if she has been dated by an earlier biparietal diameter measurement before 26 weeks, a diagnosis of IUGR can be made if a subsequent sonogram shows unduly small growth for the stage of pregnancy (see Appendix 8 and Chapter 41).

Trunk Circumference. The trunk or abdominal circumference is measured at the level of the portal sinus and the liver (see Figs. 43-1 and 41-8). Adequate abdominal circumference measurements can be made using a small footprint transducer if the fetal trunk is not too large for the field of view, although a curved linear array system is more appropriate.

Make sure that the trunk is more or less round at the point of measurement and that the umbilical vein, aorta, adrenal gland, stomach, and spine are visible. If the kidneys are present, the section is too low or angled improperly.

To measure a trunk circumference, either find the circumference with the caliper-based system built into the ultrasound machine, or measure the trunk diameter. The two approaches are comparable in accuracy. Two trunk diameters (D) at right angles are measured, and their averages are calculated to yield an average trunk diameter (see Appendix 11). The circumference can be derived from the diameter by using the formula: transverse trunk diameter + anteroposterior diameter × 1.67 ($\pi/2$). Weight can then be estimated from the combination of the biparietal diameter and the trunk circumference and using Appendix 12 to make the calculation.

Other tables use the combination of head size, femur length, and abdominal circumference to compute weight (see Appendix 12). The abdominal circumference also represents another method of dating the fetus (see Appendix 6).

Head Circumference. The measurement of the head circumference is valuable because the head-to-trunk ratio will allow the diagnosis of asymmetric IUGR. The head circumference should be obtained at a level that shows the thalami, the cavum septum pellucidum, the intrahemispheric fissure, and the third ventricle, for calculating a biparietal diameter. Dating tables based on the head circumference are available (see Appendix 7).

Head/Trunk Circumference Ratio. Finding the head/trunk circumference ratio and comparing it with normal tables (see Appendix 14) allows the recognition of asymmetric IUGR when the liver is unusually small (Fig. 43-1) even if dates are unknown, providing intracranial structures appear normal.

If there is an abnormal head/trunk circumference ratio with the head unduly large, consider the possibility that the fetus has hydrocephalus, which will give similar measurement findings. A low head/trunk circumference ratio suggests the possibility of microcephalus or a large fetal trunk with macrosomia.

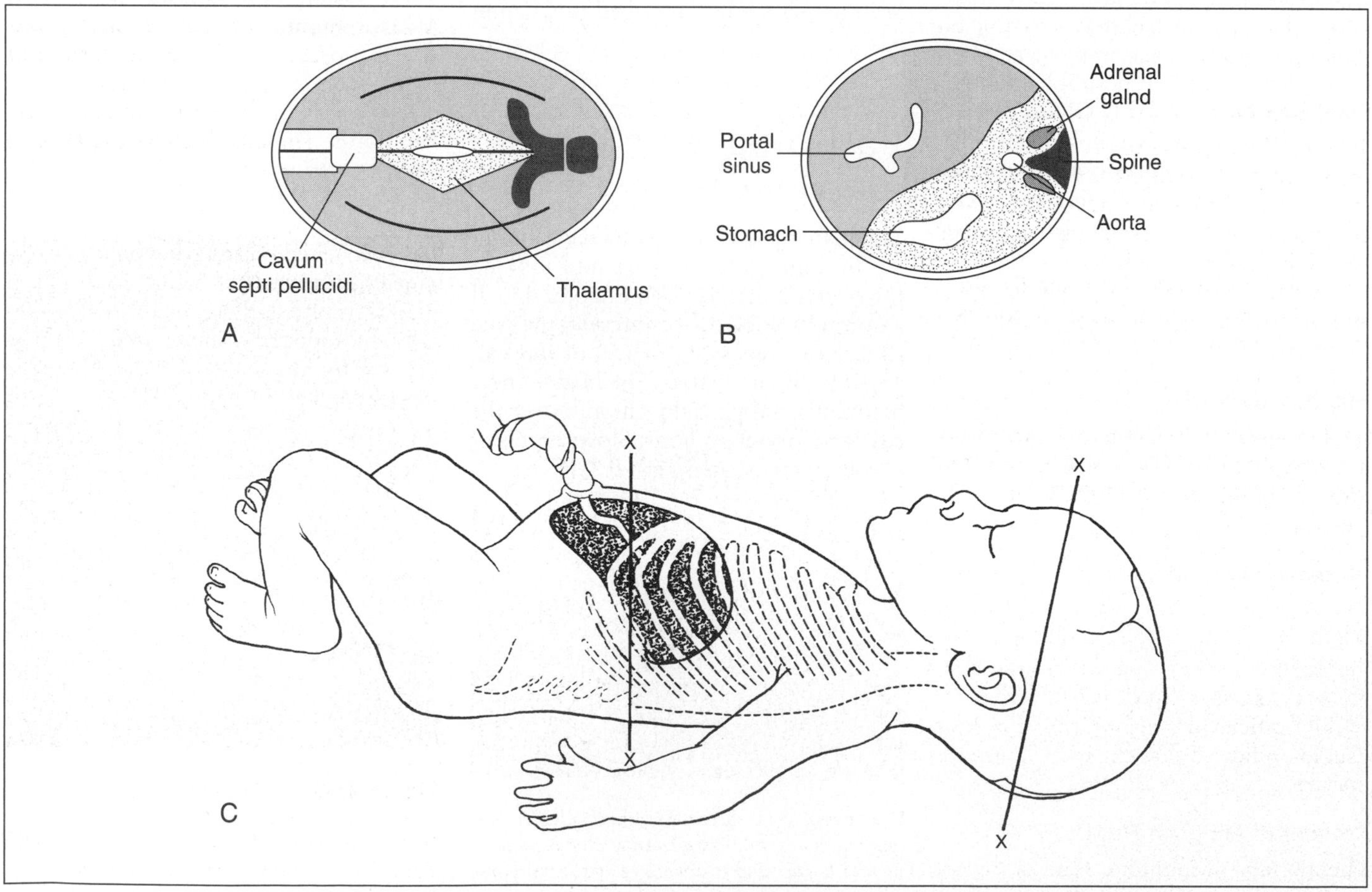

Figure 43-1. ■ *Trunk circumference measurement. **A.** The appropriate head circumference for comparison is made through the thalamus and falx cerebri. **B.** The trunk circumference or trunk diameter is obtained at a level that passes through the stomach and liver. The section should show the umbilical vein, or portal sinus, aorta, stomach, and spine. **C.** Diagram showing level at which trunk circumference and head circumference should be measured.*

Femoral Length. The femoral length measurement is described in Chapter 41 (see Fig. 41-17). It is valuable in diagnosing IUGR because it represents another method of determining whether adequate fetal growth has occurred (see Appendix 10). The femur is often spared by IUGR when the head and trunk are small.

Femoral Length/Biparietal Diameter Ratio. The femoral length/biparietal diameter ratio may reveal one type of IUGR in which the fetus is long but skinny. The femoral length/biparietal diameter ratio should be 0.79 ± 0.06.

Cerebellar Width. The cerebellar width in millimeters is equivalent to the age in weeks up to 20 weeks, and standards for dating exist beyond 20 weeks (see Appendix 26). This measurement is less affected by excessive growth or IUGR than other measurements such as the abdominal circumference or head measurements. If a patient presents with no early sonogram or accurate last menstrual period, measurement of the cerebellar width may be valuable.

Fetal Anatomy

The fetal anatomy should be examined in considerable detail, because approximately 10% of IUGR cases are due to a congenital fetal anomaly (see Chapter 45). The kidneys and bladder should be examined in detail to exclude renal anomalies causing oligohydramnios (see Chapter 45).

Biophysical Profile

If a fetus is found to have IUGR, perform a biophysical profile (see Chapter 46) and an umbilical artery Doppler study (see Chapter 46).

Placental Maturation

The placenta is likely to be small with IUGR. Signs of premature placental aging (early calcification deposition) before 36 weeks suggest IUGR (Fig. 43-2).

Calcification within the placenta usually indicates that the fetal lungs are mature.

Amount of Amniotic Fluid

The amount of amniotic fluid is low in most cases of IUGR (oligohydramnios). Reduced amounts of amniotic fluid are normally seen in the third trimester. Measurements of the largest pocket that is less than 2 cm in size is one method of quantifying oligohydramnios with IUGR, but if the fluid has diminished to this tiny quantity, the situation is grave. Recognizing lesser amounts of oligohydramnios requires experience and comparison with gestational age.

The amniotic fluid index is a measure of amniotic fluid volume. Calculating the index allows one to follow changes in the amniotic fluid volume. The uterine contents are divided into four regions. The greatest depth of amniotic fluid is measured in each quadrant. The four measurements are then totaled and compared with the values in a standard graph (see Chapter 46 and Appendix 24).

Pitfalls

1. IUGR versus hydrocephalus. Remember that an abnormal head-to-trunk ratio may occur not only with IUGR, but also with hydrocephalus. Examine the ventricles carefully if you find an abnormally high head-to-trunk ratio.
2. Inaccurate trunk circumference. The trunk circumference will be inaccurate if:
   a. Too much umbilical vein is visible
   b. The kidneys are visible (Fig. 43-3)
   c. The view is oblique, showing ribs on only one side
   d. Too much compression by the transducer has flattened the trunk shape so it is ovoid
   e. The circumference is not measured along the outside border of the abdominal image
   f. The measured outline does not correspond to the real outline (Fig. 43-4). Place the tracing at the edge of the trunk outline. (Some machines have calipers that wander from the trunk outline. If you have such a cumbersome system, use the averaged diameter approach.)
   g. The fetus is prone, so the umbilical vein cannot be found. Results are still reasonably satisfactory if the kidneys and chest are not on the view.
3. An ideal trunk circumference may not be obtained because the fetus is

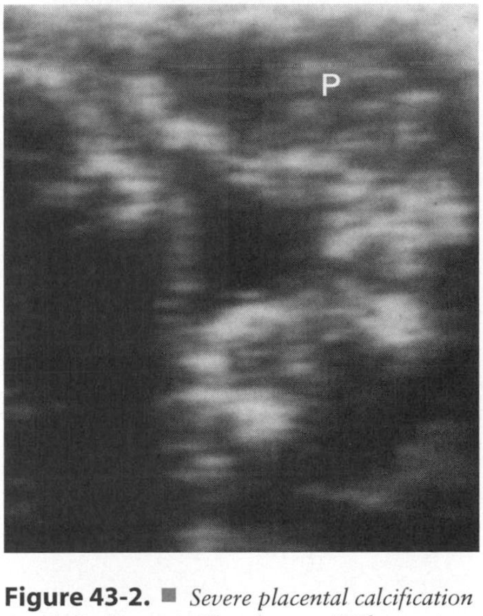

Figure 43-2. ■ *Severe placental calcification (grade 3 placenta). The placenta* (P) *has an irregular border and many echogenic areas representing calcification.*

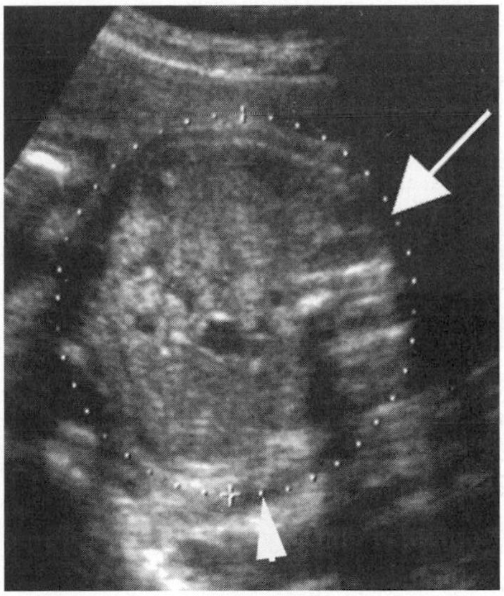

Figure 43-3. ■ *Suboptimal abdominal circumference. The kidneys* (arrow) *are included in the view. The umbilical vein is not seen well. The calipers include some nonfetal tissue* (arrowhead).

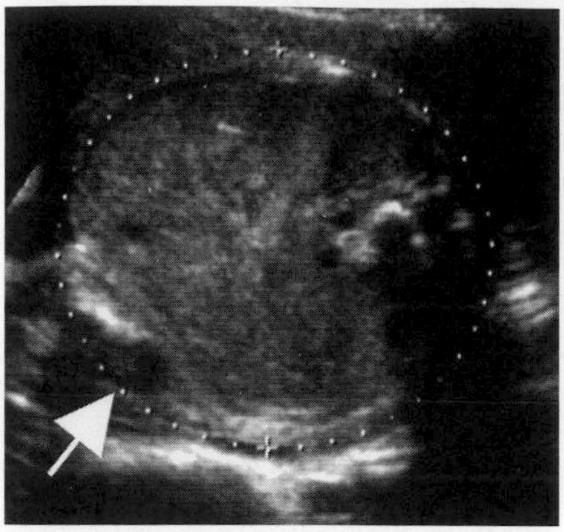

Figure 43-4. ■ *Suboptimal abdominal circumference. The abdomen is not ovoid, and a portion of amniotic fluid is included in the circumference. This may be the best one can do if the fetus is in an awkward position.*

squashed by a twin or is lying in an unusual position (Fig. 43-4). If you cannot obtain an ideal abdominal circumference however hard you try, make a note of the problem in your provisional report.

Where Else to Look

1. If IUGR is present, make a particular effort to look for signs of a chromosomal anomaly.
2. If apparent symmetric IUGR occurs at 30 weeks or more, check whether the parents are small or of Asian origin. The small fetal size may be normal if the parents are also small.

SELECTED READING

Callen PW, ed. *Ultrasonography in Obstetrics and Gynecology*, 4th ed. Philadelphia: Saunders; 2000.

Doubilet PM, Benson CB. Sonographic evaluation of intrauterine growth retardation. *AJR Am J Roentgenol* 1995;164:709–717.

Nyberg D, McGahan JP, Pretorius D, et al. Diagnostic imaging of fetal anomalies. Philadelphia: Lippincott Williams and Wilkins; 2003.

Gardosi J. Ethnic differences in fetal growth. *Ultrasound Obstet Gynecol* 1995;6:73–74.

Large for Dates

ROGER C. SANDERS

44

KEY WORDS

Acardiac Acephalic Twin. One twin is malformed. No heart is present, and circulation is pumped from the second twin. Either partial or complete absence of the head with cystic hygroma.

Conjoined (Siamese) Twins. Twins that are joined at some point in their bodies.

Corpus Luteum Cyst. A cyst developing as a response to human chorionic gonadotropin (HCG) in the first few weeks of pregnancy. Such cysts usually disappear by 14 to 16 weeks after the last menstrual period.

Cytomegalic Inclusion Disease (CMV). Viral disease characterized in utero by fetal ascites, intrauterine growth restriction, intrafetal calcification, and cardiac anomalies. The placenta is often enlarged.

Dizygotic Dichorionic. Twin pregnancies in which there are two nonidentical fetuses and two placentas.

Erythroblastosis Fetalis (Rh Incompatibility). A form of fetal anemia in which the fetal red cells are destroyed by contact with a maternal antibody produced in response to a previous fetus. Severe fetal heart failure results.

Fifth Disease. See Parvovirus.

Fraternal Twins. Dizygotic dichorionic nonidentical twins (Fig. 44-1).

Gestational Diabetes. A form of diabetes mellitus that manifests itself only in pregnancy. Discovered by performing a glucose tolerance test and associated with large babies.

Hydrops Fetalis. The fetal abdomen contains ascites, and the skin is thickened by excess fluid. This condition has a variety of causes, of which the most well known is Rh (rhesus) incompatibility. Other causes are associated with what is known as *nonimmune hydrops* (see Chapter 45).

Locking Twins. Because the twins are not separated by an amniotic sac membrane, they become entangled and are consequently difficult to deliver.

Macrosomia. Exceptionally large infant with fat deposition in the subcutaneous tissues; seen in fetuses of diabetic mothers.

Monochorionic Diamniotic. Identical twins in two amniotic cavities.

Monochorionic Monoamniotic. Identical twins in a single cavity.

Monozygotic Monochorionic. Twin pregnancies in which the fetuses are identical; usually an amniotic sac membrane divides the two amniotic cavities, but it may be absent.

Multiple Pregnancy. More than a singleton fetus (e.g., twins, triplets, or quadruplets).

Myometrial Contraction. Localized slow, asymptomatic contraction of the uterine wall. Re-examination after 20 to 30 minutes will show it to have disappeared.

Nonimmune Hydrops. Hydrops not related to underlying immunologic problems. There are many different causes. A cardiac origin is the most common.

Parvovirus. Viral disease characterized by severe fetal anemia. It may result in hydrops. It usually occurs in child care providers.

Polyhydramnios. Excessive amniotic fluid. Defined as more than 2 L at term.

Rubella. Viral disease occurring in utero with a number of associated fetal anomalies including congenital heart disease.

"Stuck" Twin. Massive polyhydramnios around one twin and severe oligohydramnios around the second. There is a shared placental circulation and one twin gets most of the blood supply. It is usually a fatal condition unless some of the amniotic fluid is withdrawn or if the connection between the twins' vascular supply in the placenta is surgically interrupted.

Toxoplasmosis. Parasitic disease affecting the fetus in utero, often resulting in intracranial calcification.

Twin-to-Twin Transfusion Syndrome. When monozygotic twins share a placenta, most of the blood from the placenta may be appropriated by one fetus at the expense of the other. One twin becomes excessively large, and the other is unduly small.

VACTERL. Combination of findings seen mostly in diabetics. There are *v*ertebral, *a*nal, *c*ongenital heart, *t*racheo*e*sophageal, *r*enal, and *l*imb findings.

The Clinical Problem

If the pregnancy appears clinically more advanced than predicted by dates, the sonographer should consider several detectable causes. Most commonly, the mother is wrong about her dates. Other possible causes of a uterus that is too large for dates include (1) polyhydramnios, (2) multiple pregnancy, (3) a large fetus, (4) a mass in addition to the uterus, and (5) a large placenta.

HYDRAMNIOS (POLYHYDRAMNIOS)

In polyhydramnios, there is excess amniotic fluid; consequently, the limbs stand out, separated by large, echo-free areas devoid of any fetal structures. Detailed sonographic visualization of the fetal gastrointestinal tract and the skeletal and central nervous systems is required because anomalies in these areas are associated with polyhydramnios (see Chapter 45). Other causes of polyhydramnios include maternal diabetes mellitus, multiple pregnancy, and hydrops. Isolated mild-to-moderate polyhydramnios at 20 to 30 weeks is common (about 3%) and often precedes macrosomia.

TWINS

It is important to establish whether there is a multiple pregnancy in a uterus that appears large for dates. Twins are at risk for a number of problems during pregnancy and have to be followed with serial sonograms to see that growth is adequate, that death has not occurred, and that one twin is not growing at the expense of the other. Careful sonographic examination of multiple pregnancy is necessary because the fetuses often adopt an unusual fetal lie. Additional fetuses, as in quintuplets, may be missed if careful scanning is not performed.

MACROSOMIA

Unduly large fetuses (over 4,000 g at birth) pose management dilemmas for the obstetrician because they are difficult for the mother to deliver. They are often the fetuses of diabetic or obese mothers. Weight estimation is important here because the obstetrician must decide whether to perform a cesarean section and must be alert to the delivery problems that occur with the fetuses of diabetic mothers.

MASS AND FETUS

Additional masses may give the impression that the uterus is larger than it really is, as with fibroids or ovarian cysts. Such problems are particularly important if an abortion is being considered because the clinician may incorrectly estimate the dates as being beyond the legal limits for abortion. Because fibroids cause a number of problems during pregnancy, such as spontaneous abortion and difficulty in delivery, size estimation and location of fibroids are important.

HYDATIDIFORM MOLE

Hydatidiform mole causes uterine enlargement in the first and early second trimester. This condition is described in detail in Chapter 39.

Anatomy

The following are important concepts to keep in mind regarding twins:

- Amnionicity—the number of sacs
- Chorionicity—the number of placentas
- Monozygotic—single zygote that divides to form identical twins
- Dizygotic—two zygotes that form fraternal twins

AMNIONICITY

Each sac is surrounded by an amniotic membrane, and each placenta gives rise to a chorionic membrane. In a dichorionic pregnancy—that is, one with two placentas—it is possible to see four "leaves" of the membranes that separate the fetuses (possible but, unfortunately, unlikely). Because these layers are difficult to separate, a subjective evaluation of the thickness is done; if only the amnions are present, the membrane is quite thin and may be difficult to see. No measurement of amniotic membrane thickness is used because the apparent thickness varies depending on the membrane angle to the ultrasonic beam. It is thickest at right angles to the beam. When there are two sacs and two placentas (diamniotic dichorionic), placental tissue often grows into the gap between the two amniotic cavities, creating the "twin peak," or lambda sign (Fig. 44-1A–C).

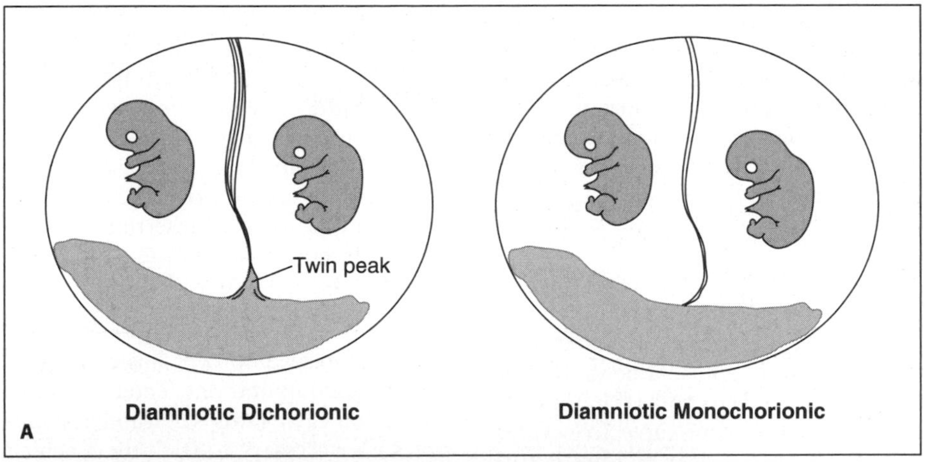

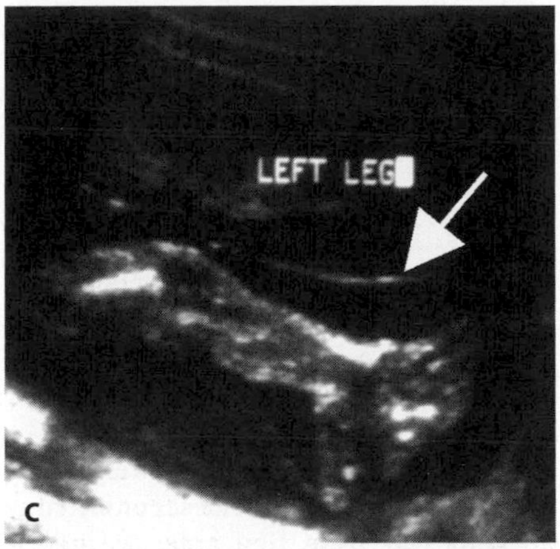

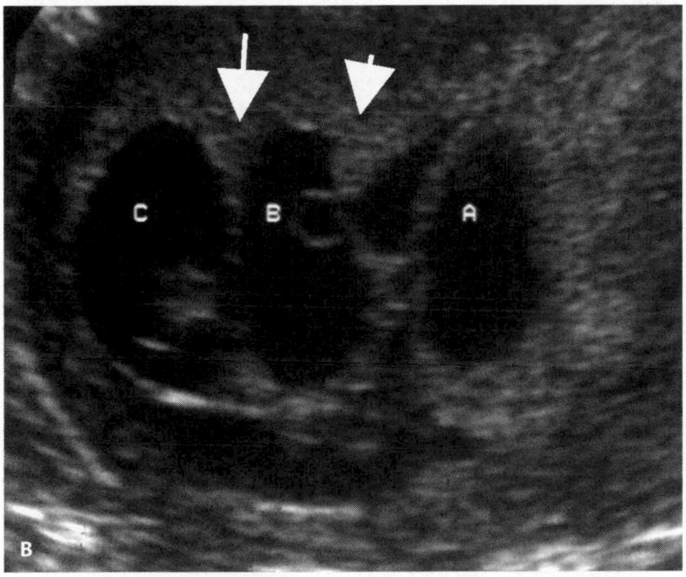

Figure 44-1. ■ *A. Diagram showing the two types of diamniotic pregnancy. In a dichorionic diamniotic pregnancy, four separate components make up the intervening membrane between the two cavities. There are separate chorionic and amniotic membranes from each pregnancy. In a dichorionic diamniotic pregnancy, the placenta grows into the gap between the two amniotic cavities forming the twin peak sign. The presence of the twin peak sign is strong evidence in favor of a diamniotic dichorionic pregnancy. In a monochorionic pregnancy, only two amniotic membranes make up the intervening membrane, so the membrane is thinner and has only two components. No twin peak sign will be seen in a monochorionic diamniotic pregnancy.* ***B.*** *Diamniotic dichorionic triplets. The twin peak or lambda sign is seen adjacent to the placenta* (arrows). *Note that the membrane looks thick elsewhere.* ***C.*** *Thin membrane with absent lambda sign in monochorionic diamniotic pregnancy. Note the thin membrane with only two components* (arrow).

CHORIONICITY

The most common type of twins are dichorionic diamniotic (about two thirds). In a monochorionic diamniotic pregnancy, there is a shared placenta, but there are two separate cord insertions, with each fetus in its own sac. In monochorionic monoamniotic pregnancies, there is a single common sac with no sac membrane visible (Fig. 44-2).

In dichorionic pregnancies, there may be adjacent placentas or two separate placentas. It can be difficult or impossible to tell a fused from an adjacent placenta, but it is important to try and make this distinction (Fig. 44-3).

Technique

When a patient is large for dates owing to a multiple gestation, the scanning routine changes. The first rule of finding twins is: look for the third. Woe be to the sonographer who gets caught up in the excitement of discovering twins and neglects to hook that femur up to trunk number three.

COUNTING AND ASSIGNING POSITION

The first order of business is to do a sweep through the uterus and count heads. Establish that each fetus has a beating heart, because there is a higher incidence of fetal death in multiple gestations. Next, assign a number or letter to each head, traditionally starting with the first to present—but not necessarily the lowest head. If both twins, for example, are cephalic, and twin A on the right is clearly lower, it still must be labeled as "A, right side," because on the subsequent exam, it may be breech. With twins, this is easy; with more than two, follow the membranes and placentas and draw a map to assign the letters, so anyone can perform the follow-up work, and be sure to give the right set of measurements to each fetus.

When and how you tell the parents during this process depends on the rules of your department (some obstetricians like to break any unusual news, but that can be impossible to pull off in these circumstances) and your subjective evaluation of how the patient and her partner will take it. It's a nice touch to be sure the father is seated first.

DETERMINING AMNIONICITY AND CHORIONICITY

Usually, multiple gestation patients are clinically large for dates early enough that it is not too crowded, and it is relatively easy to count placentas and look for membranes. Monochorionic membranes can be so hard to see that a higher frequency may help; don't just give up if you don't find the membrane easily, because a monochorionic monoamniotic pregnancy is a worrisome diagnosis. Use a high magnification and look for the twin peak sign (Fig. 44-1A,B) and at least three membranes to diagnose diamniotic dichorionic twins. Try squeezing the uterus up and down gently with the transducer while you watch the membrane to see if you can get the leaves to separate. Cine loop may be helpful in documenting temporarily splayed membranes. Look for cord insertions to help match placentas with fetuses.

KEEPING MEASUREMENTS STRAIGHT

Because most equipment has computer-generated computations, enter measurements for each fetus separately; sometimes it's necessary to trick the machine into thinking you are working on a different patient by erasing the mother's name, then re-entering "Nancy Smith—B" for the next one.

Before every measurement, start at the proper head and follow the spine to your destination. Healthy twins interact a lot in utero; arms and legs become surprisingly entangled.

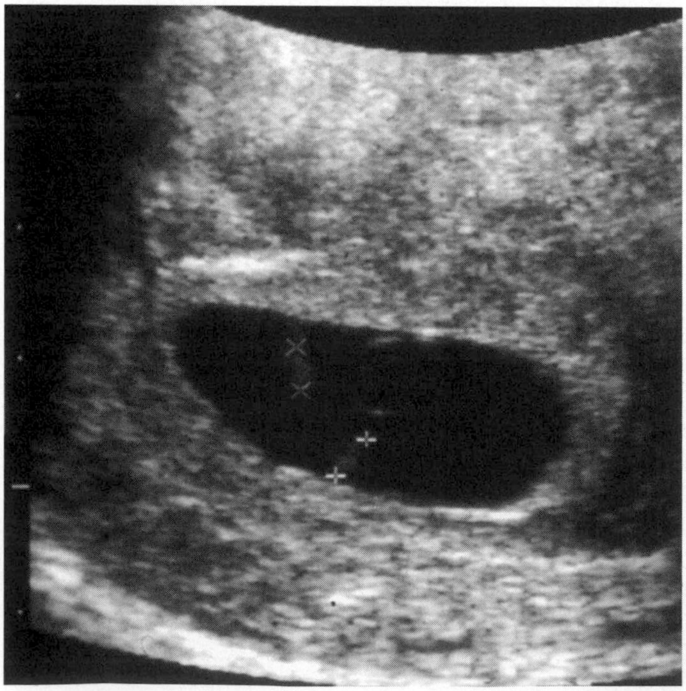

Figure 44-2. ■ *Monochorionic monoamniotic pregnancy. Although two small embryos are present, there is no intrasac membrane.*

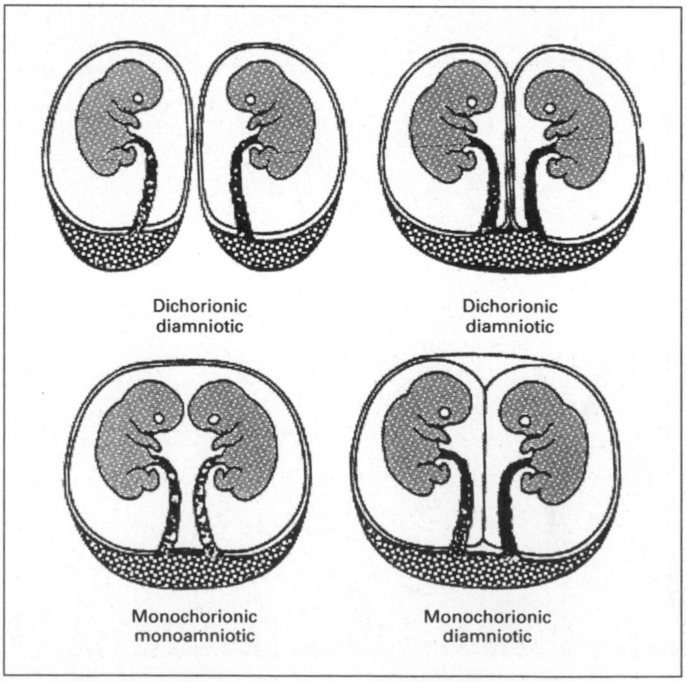

Figure 44-3. ■ *Diagram showing the different types of twins. Dichorionic diamniotic twins may have separate or adjacent placentas.*

GENDER DETERMINATION

Establishing the fetal sex becomes important clinically in twins. If two genders are present, it proves that they are dizygotic and rules out monochorionicity even if no membrane is found. Fetuses of the same sex, with one placenta, thin membranes, and no lambda sign, are monochorionic diamniotic; if amniocentesis is necessary, the greatest care should be taken ensure there is a sample from each sac (see Chapter 54). If they are the same sex with no membranes (monoamniotic monochorionic), they are at risk for various problems, such as entangled cords and acardiac acephalic twins.

SPECIAL VIEWS

Although measurements are taken separately, some views should show the fetuses together. A view with both heads is definitive proof of twins. A split screen with a good abdominal circumference from each baby shows comparable growth at a glance and can document the position of both fetuses. How is baby B relative to baby A or C? Don't forget to label whose part is presenting on the cervical evaluation views. These composite views are especially important when pathology is present and if the growth of one or more fetus is affected.

Pathology

LARGE FETUS (MACROSOMIA)

Exceptionally large fetuses cause discrepancies between estimated dates and examination findings. Sometimes, these fetuses are normally large infants. In many cases, the mother has mild diabetes mellitus, and the fetus is macrosomic. Polyhydramnios is commonly seen with macrosomia and often develops before the fetus enlarges.

When a large fetus is found, the following procedures are in order:

1. Measure the biparietal diameter.
2. Measure the trunk circumference. The normal head-to-trunk ratios are inappropriate in such babies, but the fetal weight can still be estimated. If the weight estimate is above the 90th percentile, the fetus is considered "macrosomic." If all measurements are normal, but the abdominal circumference is above the 90th percentile, this finding is very suspicious for macrosomia, although the overall weight is still less than the 90th percentile.
3. Search for evidence of scalp or trunk skin thickening; the skin is thickened to a width of greater than 5 mm. This thickening is a common finding in infants of diabetic mothers and is due to subcutaneous fat deposition. The fetal cheeks are especially prominent (Fig. 44-4).
4. Examine the placenta. In diabetic mothers, the placenta is often increased in size.
5. The fetal liver is often enlarged, and there may be thickening of the cardiac intraventricular septum.
6. Fetal anomalies related to the genitourinary tract, central nervous system, and cardiovascular system are more common in diabetic pregnancies than in others. Make sure that these areas are examined in detail. This constellation of anomalies is known as the VACTERL syndrome (*v*ertebral, *a*nal, *c*ardiovascular, *t*racheo*e*sophageal, *r*enal, and *l*imb).

MULTIPLE PREGNANCY

As mentioned in the Technique section, it is essential to determine whether there is a monochorionic or dichorionic pregnancy and whether an intersac membrane exists, because complications such as stuck twin and twin-to-twin transfusion only occur if there is a monochorionic pregnancy.

The membrane is absent in about 10% of monochorionic pregnancies.

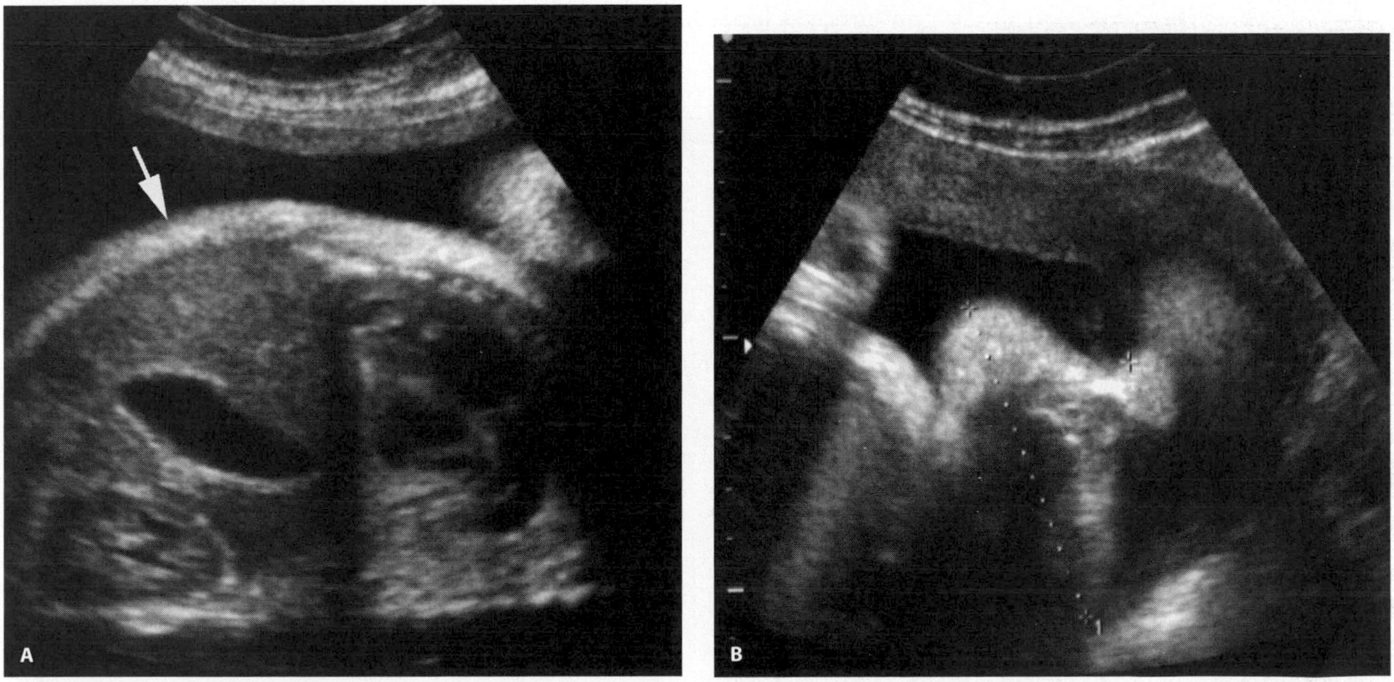

Figure 44-4. ■ *A. Macrosomic fetus with skin thickening around the fetal abdomen* (arrow). *There was moderate polyhydramnios. B. Large cheeks due to macrosomia (see measurement markers).*

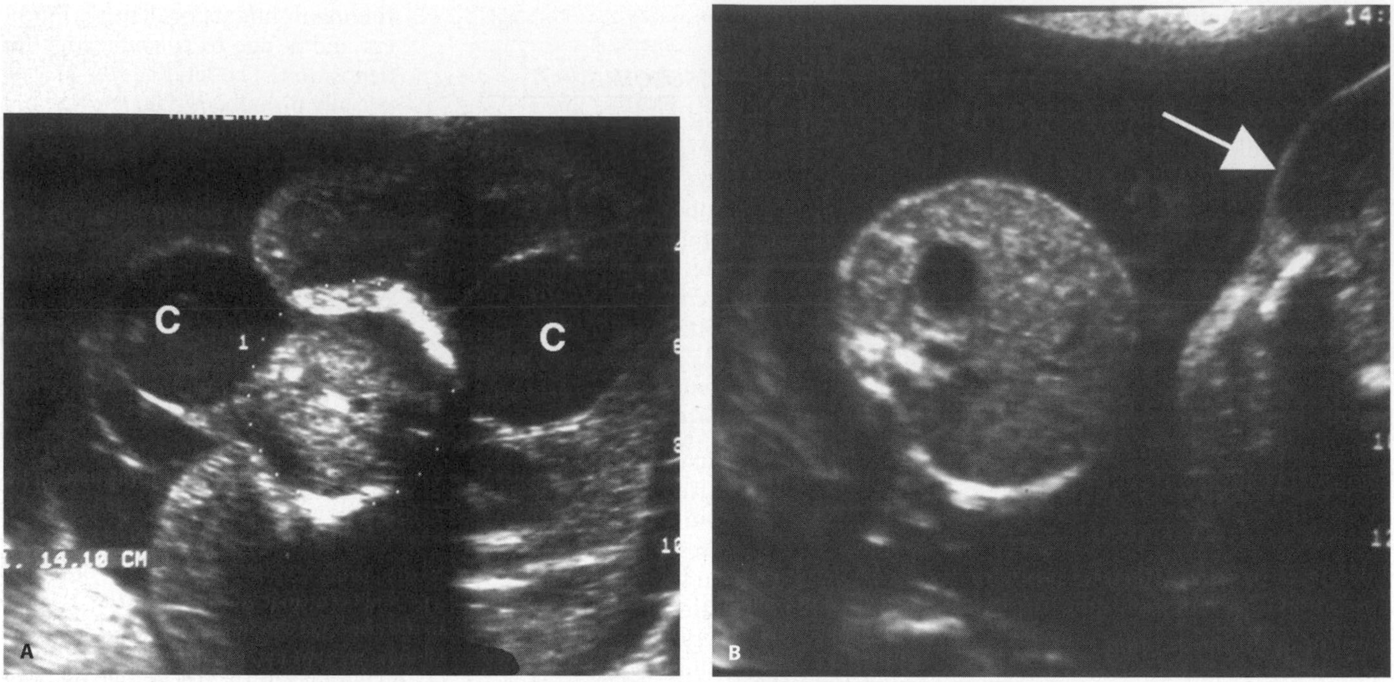

Figure 44-5. ■ *Transverse view of the abdomen (outlined by ellipse measurement) in a twin acardiac fetus. There is massive skin thickening. Within the thickened skin are large cystic spaces filled with lymph known as* cystic hygroma (C). *(Reprinted with permission from Saunders RC, ed.* Structural Fetal Abnormalities: The Total Picture, *2nd ed. New York: Mosby-Year Book Publishers, 2002.)*

Absence of the membrane is associated with various abnormalities (e.g., conjoined twins, locking twins, polyhydramnios, asymmetric growth, and tangled cords).

Cord Problems

If there appears to be only one amniotic cavity, try to follow each cord and see whether they are entangled. The two cords will be twisted around each other and may have as many as twelve twists.

Acardiac Acephalic Twins

An unusual variant of a twin pregnancy with no amniotic membrane present is an acardiac acephalic monster. A twin is seen with no heart, yet it may show movement. There is massive skin thickening of the trunk with large cystic spaces known as *cystic hygroma*. The legs are spared. The head may be absent or partially present (Fig. 44-5).

Conjoined Twins

Conjoined and locking twins should be ruled out by noting position changes. The body components of both fetuses move together if they are conjoined. If conjoined twins are found, make sure that there are two heads, two trunks, and eight limbs (Fig. 44-6).

Death

Make sure all fetuses are alive—there is an increased incidence of fetal death in multiple pregnancy.

Twin-to-Twin Transfusion Syndrome

Identical twins share a common placental circulation. One twin may grow at the expense of the other (twin-to-twin transfusion syndrome), receiving some of the blood that should have reached the second. One twin becomes plethoric

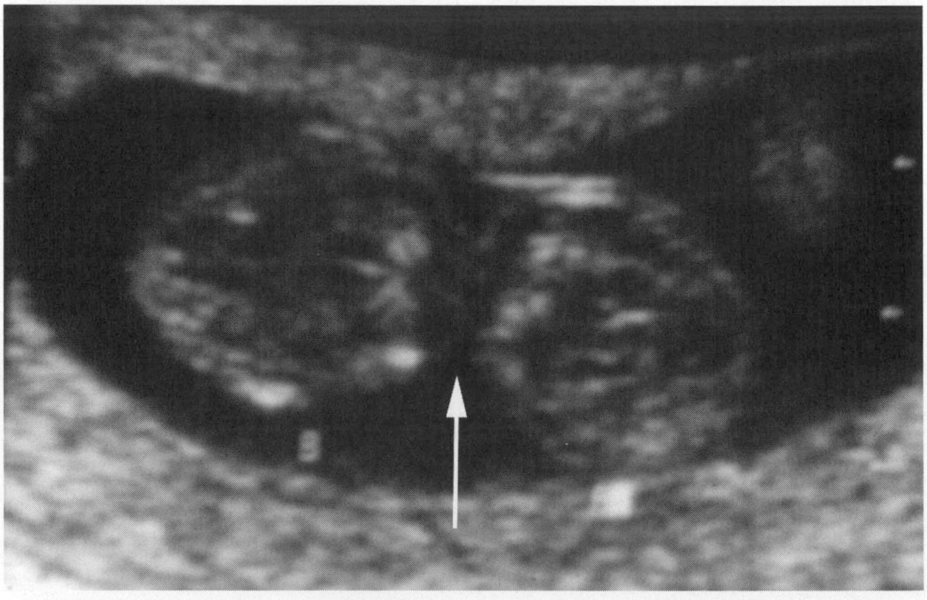

Figure 44-6. ■ *Conjoined twins. Two fetal heads lie adjacent to each other joined by skin. There was no change in the position of the two fetal heads as the fetuses moved around.*

(too much blood), and the second twin becomes anemic. Polyhydramnios may be present.

If one twin is bigger than the other and if the twin-to-twin transfusion syndrome seems possible, look for ascites in the larger twin, which is an early indication of heart failure (Fig. 44-7). The other, smaller twin will have features of IUGR (see Chapter 43). IUGR of one twin also occurs with greater frequency than in singletons in the absence of twin-to-twin transfusion syndrome and may be seen in dizygotic pregnancies.

If the twin-to-twin transfusion syndrome is severe, there will also be pleural and pericardial effusions, as well as skin thickening in the larger twin (Fig. 44-7). Look for IUGR or asymmetric growth. On follow-up examinations, measure the biparietal diameter, trunk circumference, and head/abdomen ratio on both twins every time. These measurements may be difficult to obtain because multiple pregnancies often result in an unusual fetal lie. Examine the placenta in detail. The cord from the smaller twin often enters at one end of the placenta or in a velamentous fashion (see Chapter 42). The segment of the placenta supplying the smaller fetus may be thinner and smaller than the portion related to the larger fetus. A large superficial blood artery visible on color flow may connect the two circulations allowing the larger fetus to take most of the blood circulation.

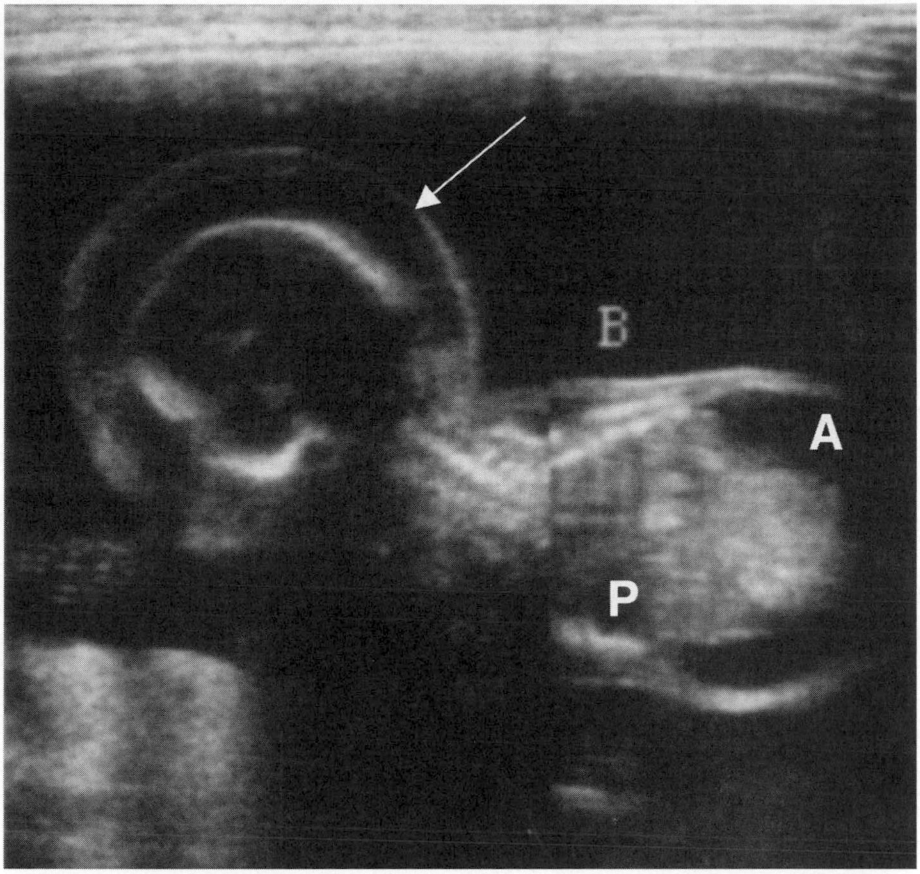

Figure 44-7. ■ *Fetal hydrops. There is severe skin thickening* (arrow). *Fetal ascites is present* (A), *and there is a small pleural effusion* (P). *In this case, this hydrops was due to severe twin–twin transfusion syndrome, but the appearances are the same with the many other causes of fetal hydrops (see Chapter 45).*

Stuck Twin

The "stuck twin" syndrome is usually fatal unless recognized by ultrasound (Fig. 44-8). There is severe polyhydramnios around one twin and oligohydramnios around the second twin. It may be difficult to see the membrane around the stuck twin. The stuck twin will not move and may appear to be adhering to the anterior or lateral aspect of the uterus. Magnified views will show the membrane alongside the fetus. Aspirating large amounts of fluid from the polyhydramniotic sac may allow survival of the stuck twin. Fluid may then return within the sac that previously showed severe oligohydramnios. In most instances, this syndrome is related to the twin-to-twin transfusion syndrome.

FETAL HYDROPS

A large-for-dates fetus may be the first indication of fetal hydrops with polyhydramnios (Fig. 44-7). Until a few years ago, this condition was almost always due to Rh incompatibility (erythroblastosis fetalis). Hydrops due to Rh incompatibility is known as *immune hydrops*. This condition is now uncommon and is considered further in Chapter 45. Today, hydrops is more commonly due to certain congenital fetal anomalies and infections, in which case it is known as *nonimmune hydrops*. Nonimmune hydrops has diagnostic sonographic findings.

The presence of any two of the following features allows a diagnosis of hydrops:

1. Fetal edema. The fetus may show evidence of scalp and skin edema as a double outline around the fetal parts (Fig. 44-7).
2. Placental enlargement. The placenta is often markedly enlarged with fetal hydrops and has an abnormal, homogeneous, echogenic texture. A large placenta is most likely to occur with Rh incompatibility, placental tumors, and fetal cardiac problems.
3. Polyhydramnios. Polyhydramnios is usually present and is responsible for the enlarged uterus.
4. Ascites. Fluid can be seen surrounding the bowel or liver and outlining the greater omentum, which is seen as a membrane.
5. Pleural effusion. Fluid outlines the lungs and diaphragm.
6. Pericardial effusion. Fluid surrounds the heart.

Underlying Causes

Nonimmune hydrops is a consequence of a number of different conditions, some of which can be detected ultrasonically.

Placental Tumors. Placental tumors siphon off the blood destined for the fetus, and the fetus becomes anemic. A mass is seen adjacent to the placenta or within it (see Fig. 42-18). Almost all placental tumors are chorioangiomas. These tumors are very vascular and show visible real-time flow or flow on Doppler. Fetal ascites is a sign that the fetus is in danger and has heart failure due to anemia.

Cardiac and Chest Anomalies and Fetal Tumors. Cardiac and chest anomalies and fetal tumors are considered in Chapters 45 and 47. All may cause hydrops.

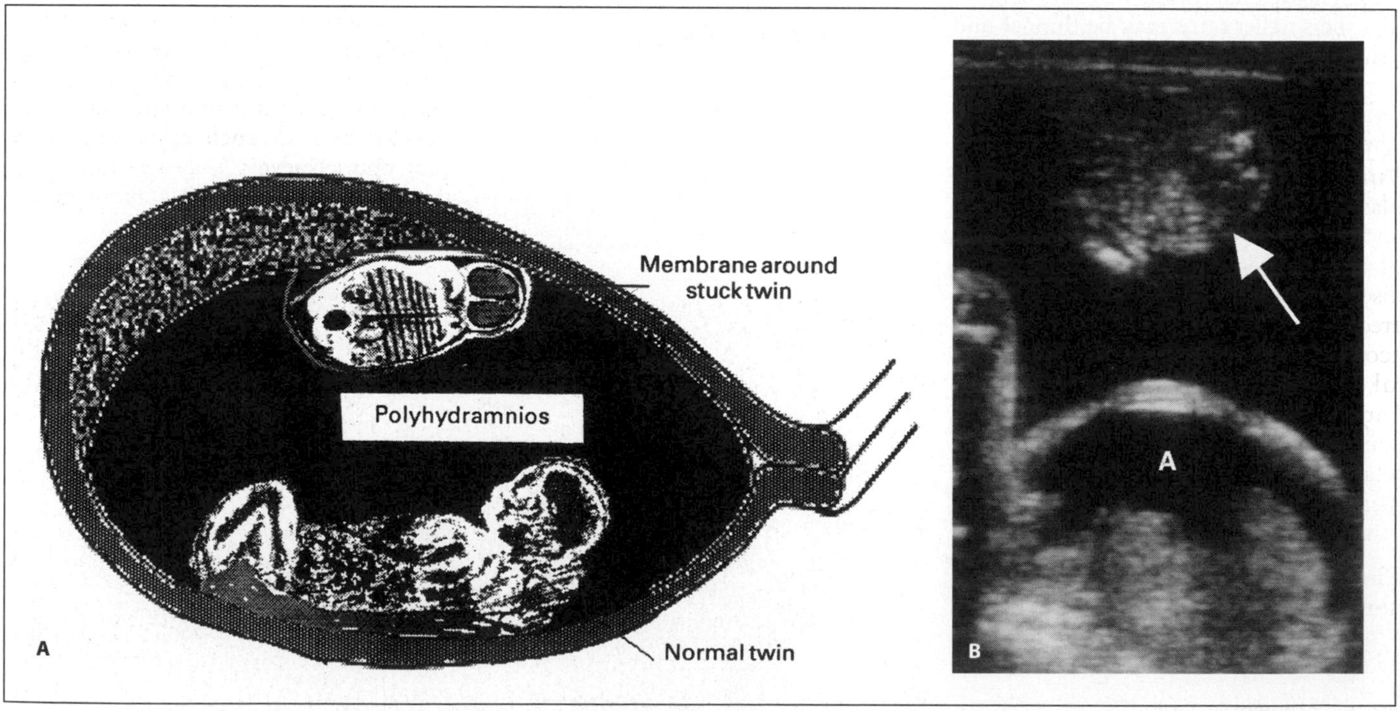

Figure 44-8. ■ *A. Stuck twin. There is polyhydramnios surrounding the plethoric and normal-appearing twin. The smaller fetus is apparently attached to the anterior abdominal wall. The amniotic membrane can just be seen around the "stuck" twin. B. Stuck twin and twin-to-twin transfusion syndrome. Diamniotic monochorionic twins are present. One fetus* (arrow) *is much smaller than the other and remained on the anterior aspect of the uterus throughout the study. The amniotic membrane is "shrink-wrapped" around this fetus and is not visible. The larger fetus has hydrops with fetal ascites* (A) *within the fetal abdomen. There is polyhydramnios around the larger fetus.*

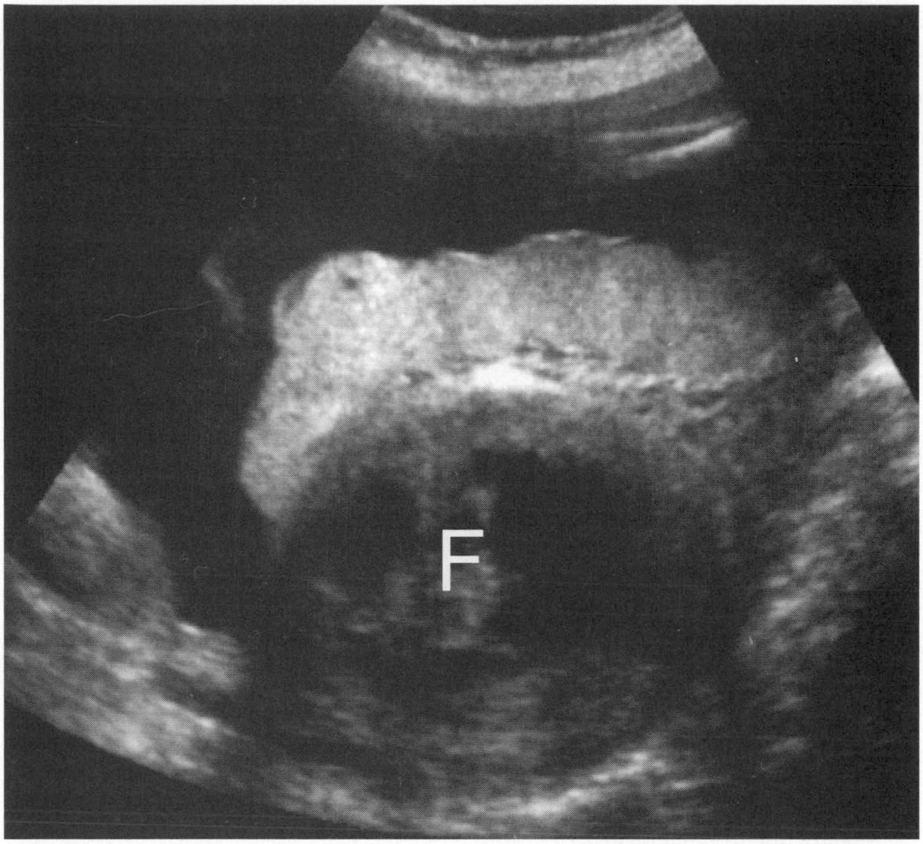

Figure 44-9. ■ *Fibroid with pregnancy. A large fibroid is seen on the posterior wall of the uterus* (F), *which enlarges the uterus so the pregnancy felt bigger than expected for the gestational age. This fibroid is just above the cervix and has cystic changes within it.*

Viral Diseases. Diseases such as toxoplasmosis, cytomegalic inclusion disease, and fifth disease (parvovirus) are causes of fetal hydrops. Cytomegalic inclusion disease and toxoplasmosis may be associated with intracranial calcification and acoustic shadowing within the brain. Fetal hepatosplenomegaly is common. Large placentas may be seen with these conditions. Parvovirus infection causes fetal anemia and thus hydrops. Treatment with intracord blood transfusion is possible.

Chromosomal Anomalies. Some chromosomal anomalies are associated with hydrops (see Chapter 45). Discovery of hydrops is followed by:

1. Chromosomal analysis
2. Fetal echocardiogram
3. Tests for toxoplasmosis and cytomegalic inclusion disease

ADDITIONAL MASSES

The uterus may appear large for dates because of a mass. Either an ovarian cyst or mass or a uterine mass may be present in addition to pregnancy.

Fibroids

Fibroids (leiomyomas) are a common cause of apparent uterine enlargement. Fibroids may be confused with the placenta because they have a somewhat similar acoustic texture, but the texture of a fibroid is usually more disorganized and tends to bulge beyond the outline of the uterus. The uterine outline is distorted by a fibroid, but not by a myometrial contraction or placental process (Fig. 44-9). Fibroids located in the lower uterine segment near the cervix are clinically important because they can interfere with delivery. As fibroids are followed through pregnancy, they may change in texture, becoming less echogenic because of cystic degeneration. Most fibroids become difficult to find in the third trimester but are visible again after delivery. Bleeding into a fibroid (red degeneration) is rare. A fibroid undergoing red degeneration is very tender and larger than on a previous study.

Ovarian Cysts

Physiologic ovarian cysts, known as *corpus luteum cysts*, are common in pregnancy. In the first few weeks of pregnancy, the increased amount of human chorionic gonadotropin stimulates the development of such cysts. Although they may achieve a large size (up to 10 cm) (Fig. 44-10), they involute sponta-

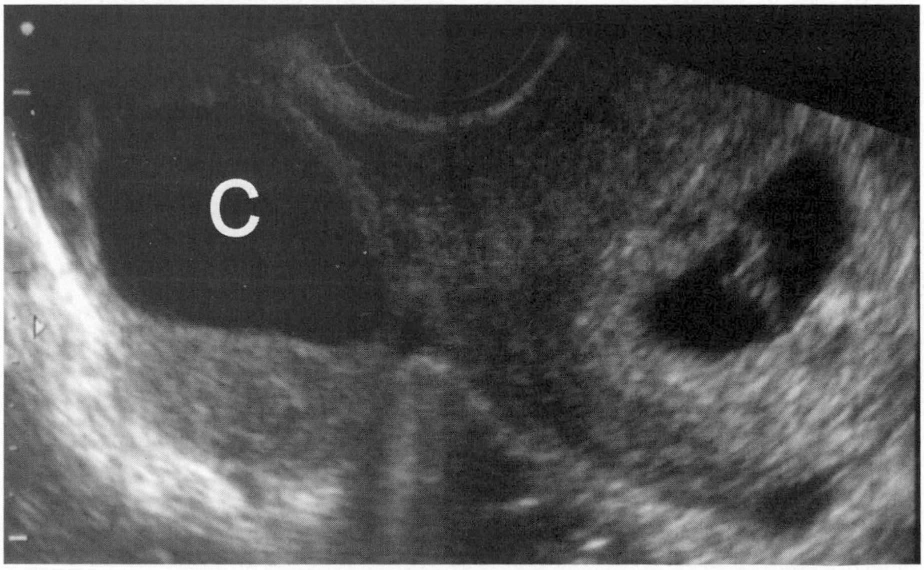

Figure 44-10. ■ *Corpus luteum cyst with pregnancy. A 5-cm cyst* (C) *was seen with an almost 8-week pregnancy. By 15 weeks, it had disappeared.*

neously as pregnancy continues and usually disappear by 16 weeks. These cysts are echo-free, apart from an occasional septum, unless bleeding has occurred within them.

Other types of cysts may occur in the ovaries, notably dermoids and serous cystadenomas. These cysts often contain internal structures such as calcifications or septa and do not decrease in size on follow-up sonograms. Cysts arising from the kidney or liver may appear on palpation to be associated with the uterus.

Occasionally, a cyst or ovary may twist on itself. The cyst or ovary is locally tender and may contain internal echoes due to hemorrhage. There may be blood around the cyst.

Abscess Formation

Abscess formation due to a ruptured appendix or pelvic inflammatory disease may occur at the same time as pregnancy. An abscess has a complicated internal texture, as described in Chapter 16, and is usually locally tender.

Pitfalls

1. Fibroids versus myometrial contraction. Uterine contractions occur throughout pregnancy but are most common in the first half and are known as *myometrial contractions* (Fig. 44-11). They last for up to half an hour and may simulate a fibroid or placenta while in progress, although the internal texture is more even than that of a fibroid and different from placenta. To differentiate a myometrial contraction from a fibroid, re-examine the patient after approximately half an hour, or document a change in shape and size at the end of the exam. Most machines document the time onscreen.
2. Cysts versus bladder. Cysts located anterior to the uterus have been mistaken for the bladder. The normal bladder should have a typical shape. Ovarian cysts are generally spherical. Asking the patient to void or fill the bladder will make the distinction apparent.
3. Overlooking a triplet or twin. A thorough search of the entire uterine cavity is the only way to avoid this disaster.
4. Pseudoascites. When the fetus appears to have ascites in a nondependent area, think of pseudoascites. In this condition, the sonolucent space is related to the paraspinous muscles and not to fluid.
5. Fetal ascites versus polyhydramnios. If the fetus has massive fetal ascites mainly due to renal obstruction, the vast amount of fluid in the abdomen may be mistaken for polyhydramnios, because fetal renal ascites is associated with very severe oligohydramnios. Close inspection will show that the fetal bowel is floating in the ascites.
6. Succenturiate lobe. Although there are two apparent placentas, there still can be a monochorionic diamniotic pregnancy if one of the apparent two placentas is actually a succenturiate lobe. Unless the twin peak sign is present or if the fetuses are of different gender, continue to look for complications of twin pregnancies such as twin–twin transfusion syndrome and stuck twin syndrome.

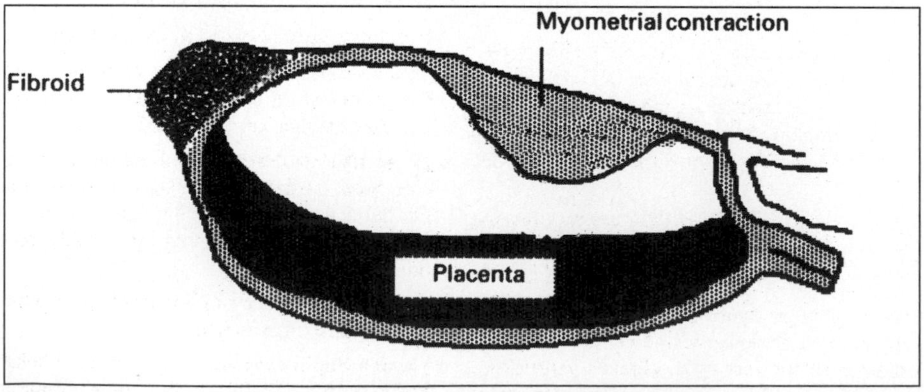

Figure 44-11. ■ *Fibroid versus myometrial contraction. The fibroid distorts the outline of the uterus. The myometrial contraction has uterine texture, is smoothly contoured, and expands toward the fetus.*

Where Else to Look

1. Cystic masses should be followed sonographically because most, but not all, will go away. Those that do not disappear, or even grow, may be surgically removed.
2. Polyhydramnios necessitates a detailed anomaly search and extra growth parameters, such as limb lengths.

SELECTED READING

Abramowicz JS, Sherer DM, Woods JR Jr. Ultrasonographic measurement of cheek-to-cheek diameter in fetal growth disturbances. *Am J Obstet Gynecol* 1993;169:405–408.

Benson CB, Doubilet PM. Ultrasound of multiple gestations. *Semin Roentgenol* 1991;26:50–62.

Bethune M, Bell R. Evaluation of the measurement of the fetal fat layer, intraventricular septum and abdominal circumference percentile in the prediction of macrosomia in pregnancies affected by gestational diabetes. *Ultrasound Obstet Gynecol* 2003;22:586–590.

Callen PW, ed. *Ultrasonography in Obstetrics and Gynecology*, 4th ed. Philadelphia: Saunders; 2002.

Elliott JP, Urig MA, Clewell WH. Aggressive therapeutic amniocentesis for treatment of twin-twin transfusion syndrome. *Obstet Gynecol* 1991;77:537–540.

Finberg HJ. The "twin peak" sign: reliable evidence of dichorionic twinning. *J Ultrasound Med* 1992;11:571–577.

Monteagudo A, Timor-Tritsch IE, Sharma S. Early and simple determination of chorionic and amniotic type in multifetal gestations in the first fourteen weeks by high-frequency transvaginal ultrasonography. *Am J Obstet Gynecol* 1994;170:824–829.

Sanders RC, ed. *Structural Fetal Abnormalities: The Total Picture*, 2nd ed. St. Louis: Mosby-Year Book; 2001.

Tan TYT, Sepulveda W. Acardiac twin: a systematic review of minimally invasive treatment modalities. *Ultrasound Obstet Gynecol* 2003;22:409–419.

Possible Fetal Anomalies

45

ROGER C. SANDERS

KEY WORDS

Acetylcholinesterase. An enzyme found in the amniotic fluid when a neural crest anomaly is present. It may be found in trace amounts if an abdominal wall defect, such as omphalocele, is present.

Achondrogenesis. A lethal type of dwarfism similar to thanatophoric dwarfism.

Achondroplasia. A type of dwarfism characterized by a bulging forehead and short limbs.

Alpha-Fetoprotein (AFP). An enzyme found in maternal blood and amniotic fluid that is elevated in the presence of neural crest anomalies, some gastrointestinal anomalies, fetal death, twins, wrong estimation of dates, fetal masses such as sacrococcygeal teratoma and cystic hygroma, and maternal liver problems. Low levels of AFP are associated with Down syndrome.

Amniotic Band Syndrome. Bands within the amniotic fluid adhere to the fetus and amputate portions of limbs. In its most severe form, it causes the limb/body wall complex.

Anal Atresia. Intestinal obstruction at the anal level due to failure to form the rectum; usually without sonographic features.

Anencephaly. Most common fetal intracranial anomaly. The base of the brain and face are the only features present in the head; the cranium is absent.

Anhydramnios. No amniotic fluid.

Arnold-Chiari Malformation (Type II). Low position of the cerebellum in the upper cervical spinal canal due to cord tethering. Associated with "lemon" skull shape, banana-shaped cerebellum, and hydrocephalus.

Banana Sign. Change in the shape of the cerebellum (it becomes curved) that occurs in the presence of spina bifida.

Cisterna Magna. Fluid-filled space at the back of the head that lies between the cerebellum and the skull. Absent if there is cord tethering as with spina bifida.

Cleft Palate. Congenital gap in the midface that variably involves the palate, maxilla, and lip.

Cloaca. Fluid-filled bag into which the ureters, rectum, and vagina enter; seen with certain developmental anomalies.

Closed Neural Defects. Neural defects in which the spinal cord and brain are not in contact with the amniotic fluid and thus are not associated with an elevated alpha-fetoprotein level.

Clubfoot. The foot is abnormally angled in relation to the leg. This abnormal foot position may be a sign of chromosomal anomaly.

Cyclops. A single eye is present. Associated with holoprosencephaly.

Cyllosoma (Limb/Body Wall Complex). Lethal abnormality thought to be due to amniotic bands. Features are gastroschisis, spina bifida, kyphoscoliosis, and absent limbs.

Cystic Adenomatoid Malformation. Anomaly in which a part of the lung is replaced by cysts.

Cystic Hygroma. Large fluid-containing sac filled with lymph, usually located in the region of the neck. May be part of a generalized fatal condition—lymphangiectasia—or a benign focal process. Associated with Turner's and Down syndrome.

Cytomegalic Inclusion Disease (CMV). Fetal viral disease sometimes resulting in intracranial calcification, microcephaly, and mental deficiency.

Dandy-Walker Syndrome. Brain anomaly with a dilated fourth ventricle and possible secondary dilation of the rest of the brain's ventricles. A small vermis of the cerebellum is the cardinal feature.

Diaphragmatic Hernia. A portion of one diaphragm is missing and the bowel or liver lies in the chest.

Diastematomyelia. Bony spur in the center of the spinal canal, splitting the cord.

Double Bubble Sign. Sign of duodenal atresia in which two circular, fluid-filled structures, representing the stomach and duodenum, are seen in the upper abdomen.

Down Syndrome (Mongolism). Syndrome seen more often in the fetuses of women who are over 35 years old; recognizable at amniotic fluid analysis or chorionic villus sampling by the presence of an abnormal chromosome. Sonographic features are usually present and include congenital heart disease and duodenal atresia.

Duodenal Atresia. Intestinal obstruction at a duodenal level with subsequent distention of the duodenum and stomach by fluid. Associated with polyhydramnios and Down syndrome.

Duplication Cyst. Congenital anomaly. A portion of the gastrointestinal tract, usually the stomach, is reduplicated. If a cystic mass can be seen with ultrasound, there is generally not a patent connection between the gut and the cyst.

Dysplasia. See *Multicystic (Dysplastic) Kidney.*

Ectopia Cordis. The heart lies partially outside and anterior to the chest. Associated with omphalocele and the pentalogy of Cantrell.

Encephalocele. Herniation of the brain's coverings through a defect in the skull. Brain tissue may be contained within the herniation, although most of the sac's contents are usually cerebrospinal fluid.

Exencephaly. Variant of anencephaly in which some cortical brain remains.

Finnish Nephropathy. A cause of renal failure and increased AFP. The kidneys are often normal but may be large and echogenic.

Gastroschisis. Condition similar to omphalocele except that no membrane covers the herniated material. Gut floats freely in the amniotic fluid. The wall defect is in the right lower part of the abdomen.

Holoprosencephaly. Intracranial anomaly. A horseshoe-shaped ventricle replaces the two lateral ventricles. Either fatal or causes severe mental retardation. Associated with trisomy 13 and facial defects such as cleft lip, palate, and hypotelorism and, in extreme cases, cyclopia and proboscis.

Holt-Oram Syndrome. Congenital syndrome consisting of a combination of heart disease and absence of a digit or the radius in the arm.

Hydranencephaly. Absence of the cortical brain. Portions of the midbrain and brainstem are present. Not compatible with life.

Hydrocephalus. Marked enlargement of the cerebral ventricles. Implies ventricular obstruction. A better term is *ventriculomegaly* or *ventricular enlargement*.

Hydronephrosis. An obstructed kidney with a dilated collecting system.

Hydrops Fetalis. Two or more of the following findings: fetal ascites, pleural effusion, pericardial effusion, skin thickening, and placentomegaly. This condition has a variety of causes, of which the most well known is rhesus incompatibility (Rh disease). Other causes are grouped as nonimmune hydrops.

Hypoplastic Left Heart Syndrome. Congenital abnormality in which the aorta and left side of the heart are too small. This condition is often fatal after birth, even with surgery.

Hypotelorism. Condition in which the orbits are too close together.

Ileal Atresia. Intestinal obstruction at a midgut level. Filling of small bowel loops with fluid; associated with polyhydramnios.

Infantile Polycystic Kidney (Autosomal Recessive Polycystic Kidney Disease). A congenital condition in which large kidneys are filled with tiny cysts.

Iniencephaly. Defect consisting of an encephalocele that involves the posterior aspects of the skull and the cervical vertebrae; some vertebrae may be missing.

Karyotype. Process of performing chromosomal analysis on a fetus.

Kleeblattschädel Deformity (Cloverleaf Skull). Skull deformity in which there is a large bony bulge off the superior aspect of the head.

Kyphoscoliosis. Spine that is bent sideways and unduly flexed.

Lamina. Lateral bridge of bone covering the posterior spinal canal.

Lemon Sign. Deformity of the skull in which it assumes a shape similar to a lemon. The frontal areas become flattened. This type of anomaly is seen when spina bifida is present.

Limb/Body Wall Syndrome. See *Cyllosoma*.

Lymphangioma. See *Cystic Hygroma*.

Meckel's Syndrome (Meckel-Gruber Syndrome). A lethal syndrome consisting of infantile polycystic kidney, encephalocele, and extra digits (polydactyly).

Meconium. Contents of the fetal bowel.

Meconium Peritonitis. Bowel rupture in utero, which leads to meconium spillage with consequent calcification. There is usually bowel obstruction.

Megacystis Microcolon Syndrome. Rare anomaly with huge bladder, dilated ureters and calyces, and minute large bowel. Only the bladder is visible with ultrasound. Most patients are female, and there is often polyhydramnios.

Meningocele. Spinal bone defect with cerebrospinal fluid pouch.

Microcephaly. Unduly small skull and brain; associated with mental deficiency.

Micrognathia. Small or absent jaw. A feature of a number of rare syndromes.

Multicystic (Dysplastic) Kidney. Developmental abnormality of the kidney in which the normal renal parenchyma is totally replaced by cysts of varying sizes. If bilateral, it is not compatible with survival.

Myelocele. Spinal bone defect with spinal cord protrusion but no cerebrospinal fluid pouch.

Myelomeningocele. Bone defect associated with tethering and distortion of the spinal cord and a fluid-containing cavity at the level of the abnormality.

Mutation. Spontaneous change in the chromosomal makeup of a cell.

Neural Crest Anomaly. A brain/spinal defect in which there is no skin covering on the spine or brain, and therefore contact between some portion of the central nervous system and the amniotic fluid occurs. This combination gives rise to a raised alpha-fetoprotein level. Anencephaly, encephalocele, and spina bifida are examples of neural crest anomalies.

Omphalocele. Herniation of some of the gut, including the liver, out of the abdomen through an umbilical opening (see *Gastroschisis*). A membrane covers the herniated contents. Associated with other congenital anomalies.

Osteogenesis Imperfecta. Congenital anomaly in which bone fractures occur.

Pentalogy of Cantrell. Combination of partial diaphragmatic absence, ectopia cordis, omphalocele, sternal abnormality, and pericardial deficiency.

Phocomelia. Most of the arms or legs are absent so that flippers originate from the trunk. Used to be seen following thalidomide administration.

Posterior Urethral Valves. Valves situated in the posterior urethra cause partial or complete obstruction of the bladder, ureters, and kidneys. Occurs only in males.

Potter's Syndrome. Fetus with bilateral renal abnormalities, which may consist of absent kidneys, bilateral hydronephrosis, bilateral multicystic dysplastic kidneys, or infantile polycystic kidney. Anhydramnios accompanies this syndrome. The consequences of absent amniotic fluid—unusual face, deformed limbs, and hypoplastic lungs—will be seen at birth. Most such fetuses are stillborn.

Proboscis. Instead of a nose, this soft tissue tubular structure may be seen above the eyes in holoprosencephaly.

Prune Belly (Eagle-Barrett) Syndrome (Agenesis of the Abdominal Muscles). Congenital condition in which there are weakened or absent abdominal wall muscles, markedly distended ureters with tiny or hydronephrotic kidneys, and a large bladder.

Pulmonary Hypoplasia. Condition associated with oligohydramnios and extrinsic pressure on the chest, due to fluid or masses, in which the lungs never function adequately after birth.

Rachischisis. The bone and soft tissues that cover the posterior aspects of the spinal canal are unfused so the spinal cord is exposed.

Reflux (Vesicourethral). In the normal fetus, the ureter enters the bladder through a long tunnel that allows urine to pass into the bladder but not to go back to the kidney. If this tunnel is wide and short, urine can pass in either direction. Reversal of urine flow back to the kidney is known as *reflux*.

Rhesus (Rh) Incompatibility (Erythroblastosis Fetalis). The fetal blood possesses a different Rh group from the maternal blood. When maternal blood cells leak into the fetal circulation, they interact, forming antibodies. In the next pregnancy, there is hemolysis, and the fetus is left anemic with hydrops.

Rockerbottom Foot. Abnormal foot with very prominent heel. May be an indication of a chromosomal anomaly.

Rubella. Viral disease that is associated with a number of fetal anomalies, including congenital heart disease, when occurring in utero.

Sequestration. Anomaly in which a segment of the lung does not connect with the trachea and has its own blood supply. Sometimes, the abnormal segment of the lung develops below the diaphragm.

Spina Bifida. Bony spinal defect over the spinal canal. Nearly always accompanied by some form of myelomeningocele, sometimes with hydrocephalus.

Teratoma. Tumor composed of multiple different tissues that may arise anywhere in the body, but usually in the sacrum.

Tethering. The lower end of the cord normally ascends from the sacrum to level L2 in utero. With anomalies such as spina bifida and lipoma, it does not ascend, but it terminates at a lower level, for example, L5.

Thanatophoric Dwarf. Form of dwarfism that affects not only the limbs but also the chest, which is too small. Invariably fatal.

TORCH. Group of congenital infectious diseases with similar features: *t*oxoplasmosis, *r*ubella, *cy*tomegalic inclusion disease, and *h*erpes.

Toxoplasmosis. Parasitic disease affecting the fetus in utero and causing intracranial calcification.

Tracheoesophageal Fistula. Obstruction of the esophagus usually associated with a fistula to the trachea. Sometimes, there is also a connection to the stomach through the trachea. In the most severe form, no fluid reaches the stomach.

Triploidy. There are one and one half times as many chromosomes as there should be. Causes fetal death and a large, abnormal placenta that may look like a mole.

Triradiate. The fingers in thanatophoric dwarfism are separated and short, forming a triradiate shape.

Trisomy. Abnormal chromosomes are present; three are present where a specific pair should be (hence, trisomy). The most common types are 13, 18, and 21.

Turner's Syndrome. One sex chromosome is absent. Associated with cystic hygroma, a webbed neck, and mental deficiency.

Vein of Galen Aneurysm. A large arteriovenous fistula seen as a sizable cyst in the posterior aspect of the brain, above the tentorium.

Ventriculomegaly. Enlargement of the intracranial ventricles, not necessarily associated with obstruction.

The Clinical Problem

Fetal anomalies as small as an extra digit or an abnormal little finger can be discovered by an accomplished sonographer. To distinguish normal from pathologic, all sonographers should have a detailed knowledge of normal fetal anatomy.

Anomalies should, if possible, be discovered before the fetus is 23 to 24 weeks old. If the fetus has a condition not compatible with normal life, therapeutic abortion may be elected; in many states, it cannot be legally performed after 6 months' gestational age. A practical limit of 23 weeks is often used because a fetus may be viable beyond this age.

Discovery of an anomaly at a later stage of pregnancy is of practical importance because the optimal fashion and time of delivery can be arranged, and the patient can, if necessary, be transferred to a hospital that has neonatal care and pediatric surgical facilities. Fetuses with anomalies that may rupture at the time of delivery (such as an encephalocele) may be best delivered by cesarean section. If the fetal prognosis is very poor, those with a fluid-distended abdomen or head may be decompressed under ultrasound control before delivery in order to avoid a needless cesarean section.

Some clues to the presence of a fetal anomaly are discussed in the following sections.

ELEVATED ALPHA-FETOPROTEIN LEVELS

Elevated alpha-fetoprotein (AFP) levels are associated with a number of anomalies, among which are:

1. Neural crest problems: anencephaly, spina bifida, and encephalocele
2. Abdominal wall problems: omphalocele and gastroschisis

For a detailed list, see the Pathology section later in this chapter.

AFP can be measured in the mother's blood (serum AFP; evaluates AFP produced by both mother and fetus) and in the amniotic fluid at amniocentesis (evaluates only AFP produced by the fetus). Levels increase with gestational age. Acetylcholinesterase, found in the amniotic fluid, is increased only with anomalies.

FAMILY HISTORY

Most hereditary anomalies are dominant, in which case there is a one in two chance of recurrence, or recessive, when the chance of recurrence is one in four. There is usually a family history of an affected sibling, parent, or cousin, but the condition can be seen for the first time if a spontaneous mutation occurs. Examples of genetic conditions are adult polycystic kidney (dominant), infantile polycystic kidney (recessive), and osteogenesis imperfecta (dominant and recessive types). The mother is usually referred for an ultrasound study because her family history is suspicious. On other occasions, the family history is elicited only when an anomaly is seen and the patient is questioned.

MATERNAL AGE

The risk of chromosomal anomalies increases as the mother ages. Amniocentesis for Down syndrome is suggested for pregnant women aged 35 or older. The risk of other chromosomal defects is also increased (Table 45-1).

TRIPLE SCREEN

Maternal blood screening for AFP, estriol, and human chorionic gonadotropin (HCG) is widely used between 16 and 22 weeks. Down syndrome and trisomy 18 result in changes in the level of these three substances in the mother's blood and reflect changes in the fetus. Levels of estriol and HCG are elevated and AFP levels are depressed with Down syndrome, whereas with trisomy 18, the level of all three substances is decreased from the normal maternal blood screening level. An additional substance, inhibin A, is now also being measured by some laboratories. Increased AFP is suspicious for a neural crest anomaly or an abdominal wall defect, as stated earlier.

Thickening of the membrane at the back of the fetal neck is now widely used at 11 to 13 weeks as a marker for chromosomal abnormalities and congenital heart disease (see Fig. 45-61A,B). Elevation of beta-HCG and depression of plasma protein-A are two substances that can be measured at this gestational age and, with nuchal translucency thickening, detect about 85% of Down syndrome cases.

TERATOGENIC DRUGS

Many drugs are said to have been responsible for fetal anomalies. Appendix 23 provides a list of drugs with a confirmed risk. The most important in practice is the relationship between antiepileptic drugs and facial/spinal deformities. A dangerous nonprescription drug that causes intrauterine growth retardation is nicotine.

TABLE 45-1 Incidence of Down Syndrome and Chromosomal Abnormalities According to Maternal Age

Maternal Age	Down Syndrome	Chromosomal Abnormalities
20	1/1,923	1/526
21	1/1,695	1/526
22	1/1,538	1/500
23	1/1,408	1/500
24	1/1,299	1/476
25	1/1,205	1/476
26	1/1,124	1/476
27	1/1,053	1/455
28	1/990	1/453
29	1/935	1/417
30	1/885	1/384
31	1/826	1/384
32	1/725	1/322
33	1/592	1/285
34	1/465	1/243
35	1/365	1/178
36	1/287	1/149
37	1/225	1/123
38	1/177	1/105
39	1/139	1/80
40	1/109	1/63
41	1/85	1/48
42	1/67	1/39
43	1/53	1/31
44	1/41	1/24
45	1/32	1/18
46	1/25	1/15
47	1/20	1/11
48	1/16	1/8
49	1/12	1/7

POLYHYDRAMNIOS

Polyhydramnios is a clue to the presence of fetal anomalies that interfere with the intake and absorption of amniotic fluid. For a detailed list of the causes, see the Pathology section later in this chapter.

SMALL FOR DATES WITH OLIGOHYDRAMNIOS

Look for a genitourinary problem when the fetus is small for dates and there is oligohydramnios. Very severe intrauterine growth retardation with oligohydramnios occurring before 28 weeks has a strong chance of being related to a chromosomal anomaly.

LACK OF FETAL MOBILITY

Fetal activity is often absent or slowed with anomalies. Take a very good look around if the fetus is unduly still.

Anatomy

The relevant anatomy is described in Chapter 41.

Technique

See Chapter 41 for appropriate technique in routine scanning of pregnant women. Additional areas that need examining when an anomaly search is being performed are the following.

THE HANDS

The hands are usually mildly flexed, with all fingers and thumbs aligned. They should flex and extend frequently (Fig. 45-1). After 15 to 16 weeks, the number of fetal digits (fingers and toes) can be counted.

To find the hands, start scanning at the trunk. Find the humerus, and continue out to the radius and ulna until you see the hands. When you have found the knuckles, angle the transducer slightly until you can see all fingers and the thumb simultaneously (Fig. 45-1A,B). If the fetus is moving, snap an image of the hands as they fly by, or use cine loop. Obtain a view that shows four or five digits simultaneously and see if any digit is out of alignment.

If the fourth finger is overlapped by the third and fifth finger, a chromosomal anomaly may be present. Unusual thumb positions may be a clue to a chromosomal anomaly or a particular type of dwarfism (e.g., Hitchhiker's thumb in diastrophic dwarfism). Count the number of digits, especially when investigating syndromes in which extra digits are present (e.g., Meckel's syndrome) or in which a digit is missing (e.g., Holt-Oram syndrome). A small, incurved fifth finger (clinodactyly) with a short middle phalanx is seen with Down syndrome.

THE FEET

A side-on view of the feet shows the leg and the foot at the same time. The foot is normally at a right angle to the distal leg. As a rule, only one long bone is seen in the distal leg. A plantar view showing the feet and toes is helpful for counting toes and making sure the toes are in the right position.

Showing the feet and legs simultaneously is difficult. Inspect the toes like you inspect the fingers, for number, alignment, and position. Find the feet by tracing the hips to the femur to the fibula and tibia. It is not difficult to obtain a view that shows the bones of the foot and the toes. The trick is to line up the lower leg and foot together so you can

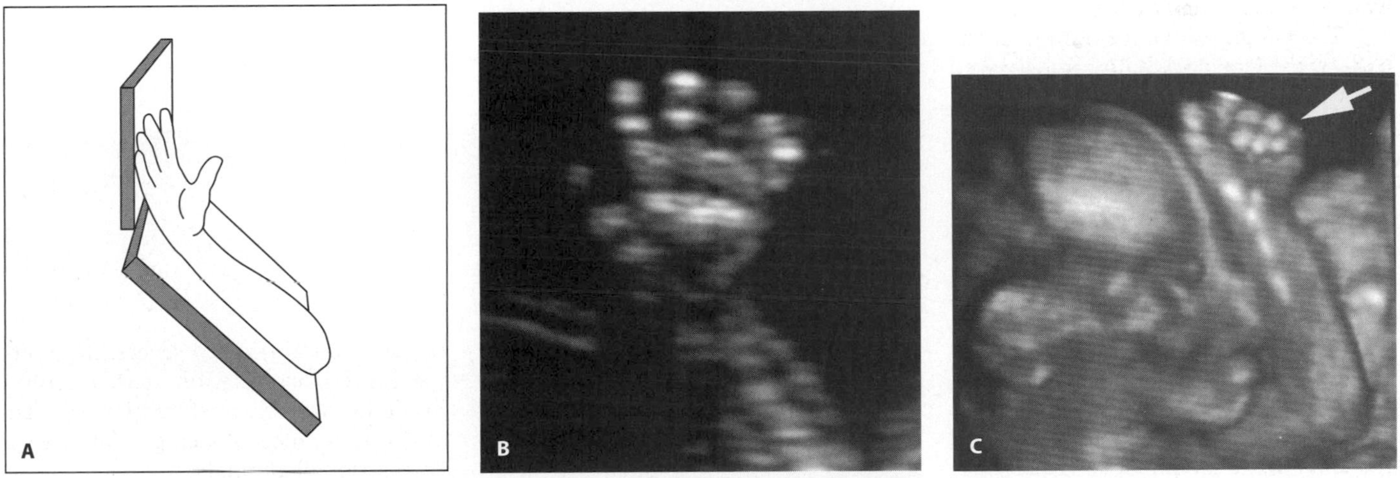

Figure 45-1. ■ *A. View showing the angle at which the hand and arm should be imaged to show the lower arm and hand position. B. Sonogram of a hand showing five digits and the palm of the hand obtained with this angulation. C. Three-dimensional view showing the face and the hand* (arrow). *Four fingers and the thumb are seen.*

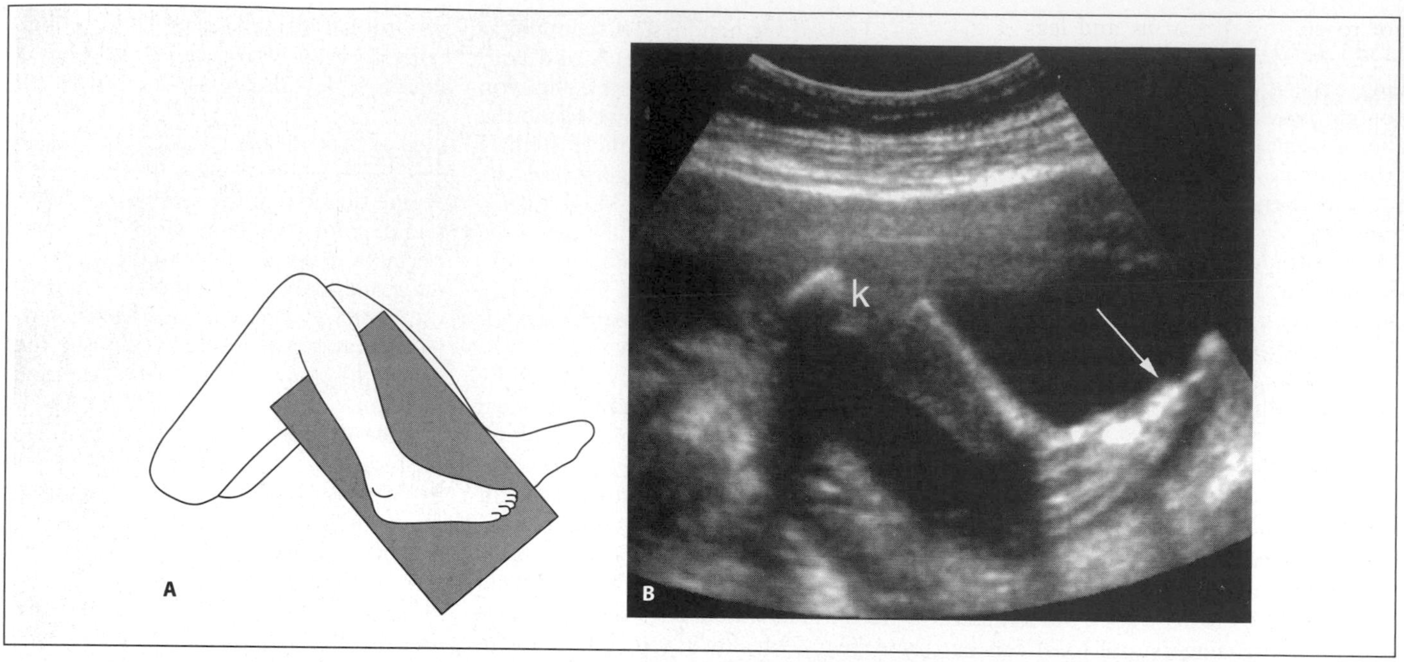

Figure 45-2. ■ *A. View diagramming the angle at which the foot and leg should be imaged to show the relative position of the leg and foot to exclude clubfoot. B. Sonogram showing the normal foot and lower leg. K, knee. Note that only one bone (the tibia) is seen in the distal leg.*

determine whether there is an abnormal angle (Fig. 45-2A,2B). This requires patience and subtle angulation of the transducer.

The angle between the foot and the lower leg should not be too large or too small. Acute or extended angulation of the foot is a feature of clubfoot. In addition, the foot is inverted so that the long axis of the foot and both long bones can be seen at the same time. Strange foot positions are often seen with chromosomal anomalies (Fig. 45-3). A gap between the big toe and the remaining toes suggests Down syndrome.

THE LIMBS

In addition to the femur (see Chapter 42), the tibia and fibula, radius and ulna, as well as the humerus, should all be imaged and measured in an anomaly search. Be systematic about the measurements of long bones. Start with the femur or the humerus, and work out to the tibia and fibula or radius and ulna so as

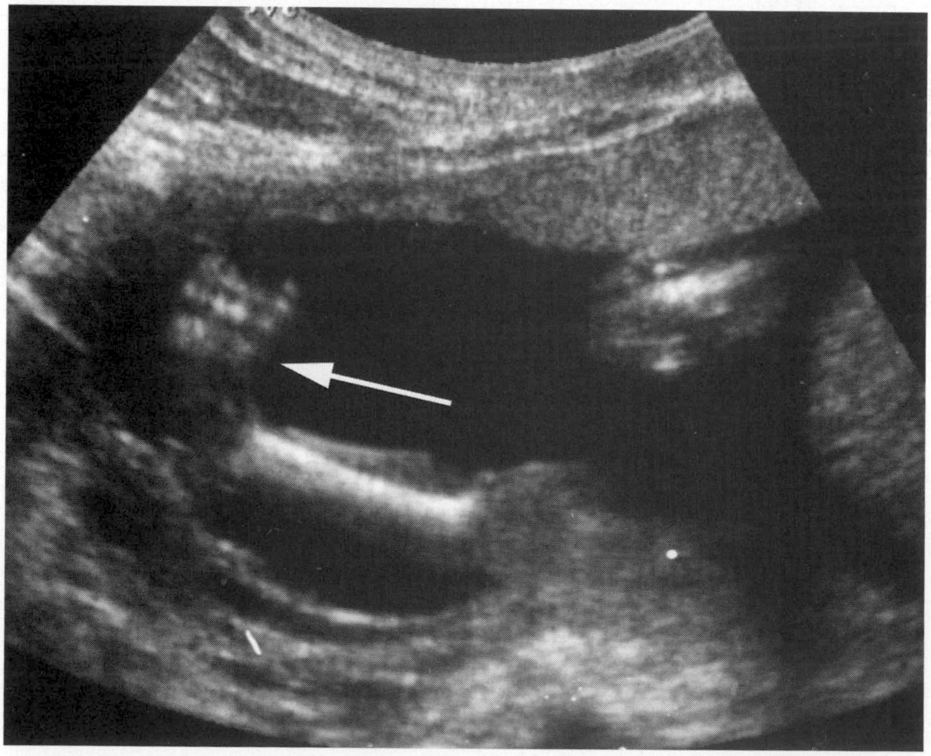

Figure 45-3. ■ *The most common form of clubfoot is shown. Note the unusual angulation of the foot and that a portion of both bones in the distal leg can be seen.*

not to confuse the arms and legs (Fig. 45-4). In distal limbs, photograph one long bone after the other, and label as you go. Bowing is a clue to some anomalies. Absent limbs are seen in some syndromes (e.g., limb/body wall complex).

If the femur length is short by more than two standard deviations, all long bones should be measured. Normal length tables for all bones are available (see Appendix 2).

Grossly short (less than the fifth percentile), barely visible long bones are associated with polyhydramnios. Unduly short or large limbs may indicate fetal anomalies. If a long bone such as the humerus or femur is short and if the condition is symmetrical and localized, however, there may be familial focal limb shortening.

To diagnose specific lethal defects described later in this chapter, look at the following:

1. Chest/abdomen ratio
2. Amount of soft tissue around the limbs
3. Amount of ossification of the spine
4. Shape of the head

Look for angulation and fractures in the long bones if the bones appear poorly ossified. With less-marked limb shortening, check for asymmetry, epiphyseal changes, bowing, increased digit number, or angulation with a fracture.

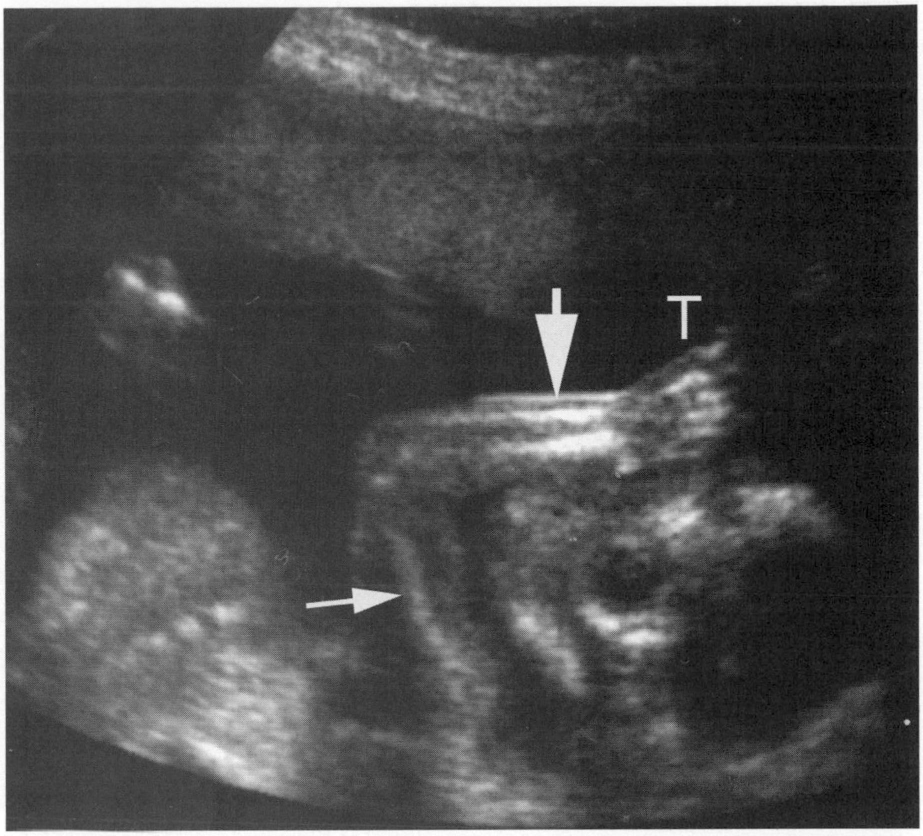

Figure 45-4. ■ *View of a flexed arm showing the humerus, radius, ulna, and the hand. The radius* (large arrow) *is the long bone closest to the thumb* (T). *The small arrow points to the humerus.*

THE BRAIN

In addition to visualizing the cerebellum, take note of the cisterna magna, which is a cystic space between the occipital bone and the cerebellum. The cisterna magna should be no more than 10 mm in diameter (see Fig. 41-4) as measured on a cerebellar view. In Dandy-Walker syndrome, the cisterna magna will be larger than 10 mm, whereas in spina bifida, the cisterna magna will usually not be seen. The entire cerebellum may not be visualized in cases of severe spina bifida because the cerebellum partially lies in the upper spine. The cavum septum pellucidum is absent in holoprosencephaly and related conditions.

The lateral ventricular width should be measured at the atrium (Fig. 45-5A). Its normal width is 10 mm or less. Demonstrate that the cisterna magna, cavum septi pellucidi, and atrium of the lateral ventricle are normal. If all are present and normal, this is a quick screening technique that shows that the brain as a whole is normal. The side of the brain closest to the transducer is often obscured by reverberation artefact in the axial position. An oblique transabdominal view sometimes shows the "up" ventricle (Fig. 45-5B). Endovaginal views are very helpful if the fetus is in a vertex position (as it usually is) in showing the hidden ventricle (Fig. 45-5C) and also permit the sonographer to get the sagittal view that excludes agenesis of the corpus callosum (discussed later in this chapter) (Fig. 45-5D).

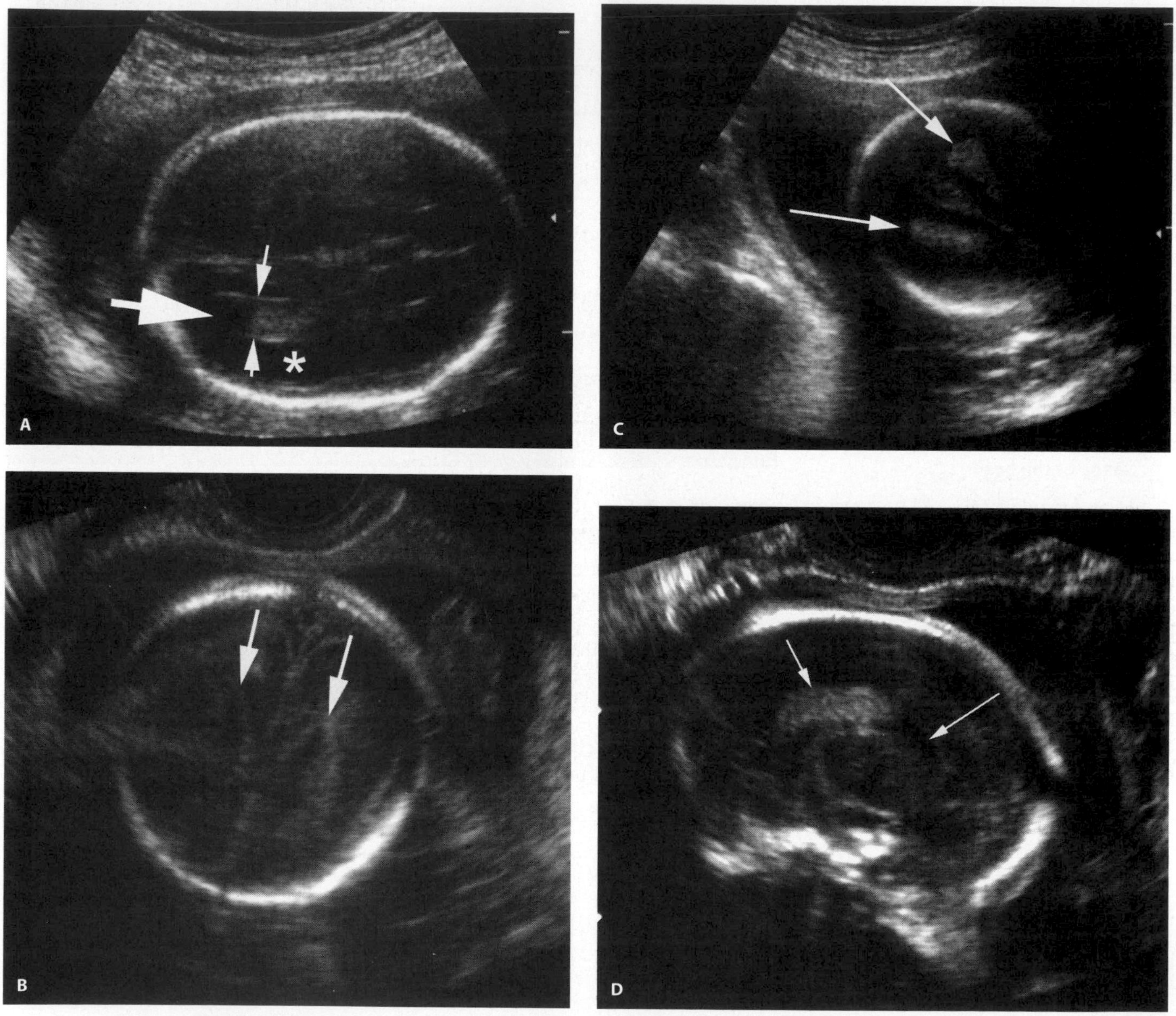

Figure 45-5. ■ *A. Standard axial view of the lateral ventricle* (large arrow) *showing the atrial location where measurements of lateral ventricular width are made* (small arrows). *Do not mistake the echopenic area lateral to the lateral ventricle* (*) *for an enlarged lateral ventricle. Note that the lateral ventricle on the transducer side of the head cannot be seen due to a reverberation artefact from the skull. B. Endovaginal view of the brain showing both lateral ventricles to be normal* (arrows). *C. Angled transabdominal coronal view of the lateral ventricles showing that both lateral ventricles* (arrows) *are normal in size. Coming from an oblique axis sometimes allows the near lateral ventricle to be seen. D. Sagittal endovaginal view of brain at 18 weeks showing the choroid and lateral ventricle* (arrows). *This view is often difficult to obtain from an abdominal approach and is important in excluding agenesis of the corpus callosum. In a third trimester pregnancy, it shows the corpus callosum and the horizontal (normal) or vertical (seen in agenesis of the corpus callosum) axis of the gyri well.*

THE ORBIT

To find the orbit, obtain the standard axial view, as for the biparietal diameter, and then change to a right-angle axis. Continually change the axis until you have determined where the orbits appear largest and where the intraorbital distance is greatest (Fig. 45-6A,B).

A small intraorbital distance is associated with cranial problems, particularly holoprosencephaly. Measuring the orbits represents another method of estimating gestational age (Fig. 45-7; see Appendices 17 and 18).

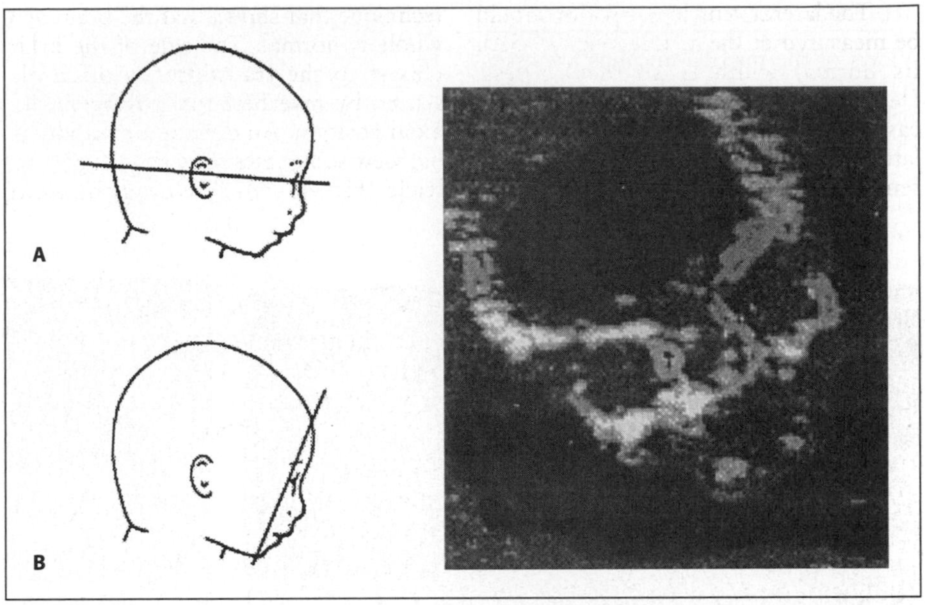

Figure 45-6. ■ *Diagram and images showing position used to show the orbits. Technique A is more likely to be accurate than technique B because it is harder to be off axis.*

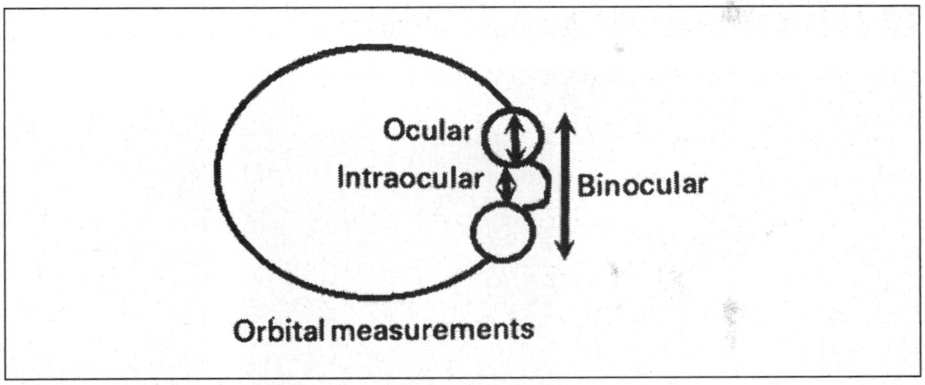

Figure 45-7. ■ *Sites for taking the orbital measurements.*

THE FACE

Views of the maxilla and lips are essential to exclude cleft palate. Angle inferiorly to display the maxilla, the lips, and the mandible (Figs. 45-8 and 45-9).

To see a gap in the upper lip and maxilla beneath the nose, as in cleft lip and palate, obtain a transverse view through the face and orbits, and then shift anteriorly to the maxilla and upper lip, which lie just beneath the nose (Fig. 45-9).

Three-dimensional views are very helpful in seeing the full extent of cleft deformities.

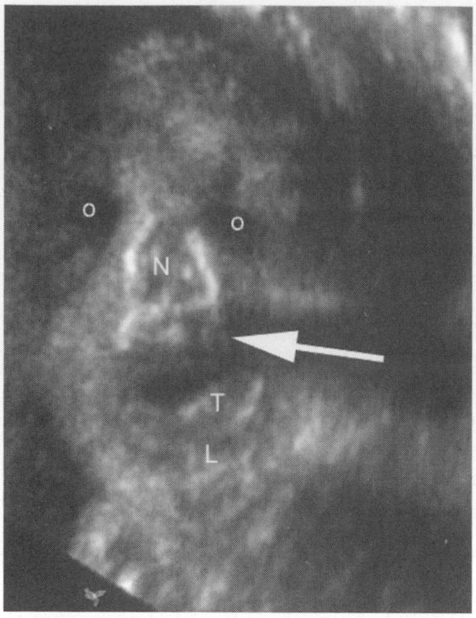

Figure 45-8. ■ *Coronal view of the face showing the orbits* (o), *nose* (N), *and mouth. Note the teeth buds superior to the mouth* (arrow). *The tongue* (T) *lies just above the lower lip* (L).

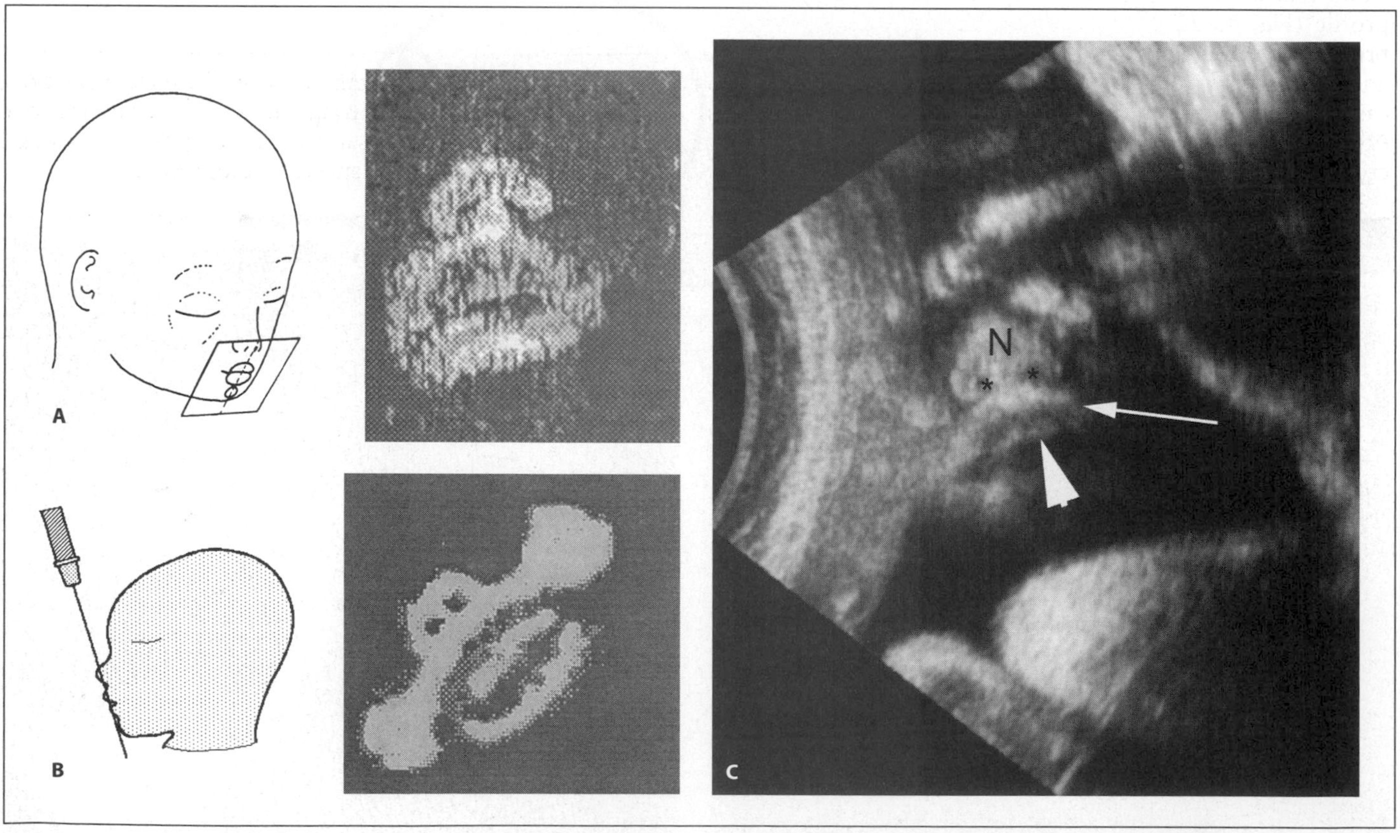

Figure 45-9. ■ *A,B. Diagrams demonstrating transducer angulation to show the face. To ideally show the lips, image the nose and lips only. C. The image shows the frenula* (small arrow), *the upper lip* (arrowhead), *and the nostrils* (*). N, *nose.*

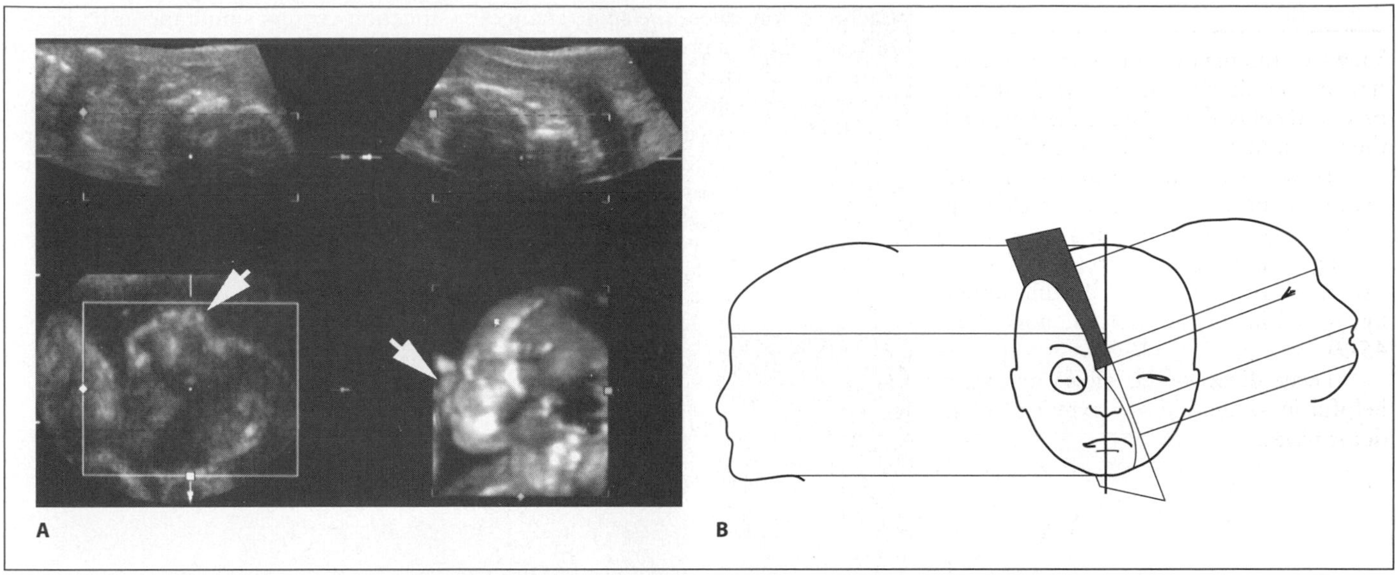

Figure 45-10. ■ *A. Profile view showing the nose* (arrows). *A profile could not be obtained using the standard approach, but 3D views showed that the chin and nose were normal.* ***B.*** *Diagram showing the technique used to obtain a straight view of the profile (on the left). The oblique view (on the right) will show the orbits and a small chin.*

THE PROFILE

Place the transducer at right angles to the views that show the maxilla to see the profile (Fig. 45-10A). Ensure that the profile view does not include the orbits and includes the chin (Fig. 45-10B). It is easy to take a profile view that is slightly oblique and create a diagnosis of micrognathia. Three-dimensional views are very helpful in obtaining profile views when they cannot be obtained in a standard fashion (Fig. 45-10A).

THE EARS

Make an attempt to show the position of the ears in relation to the cervical spine on a single view (Fig. 45-11). A low position of the ears is seen with anomalies, but deciding whether the ears are too low is very difficult. Abnormally small or misshapen ears suggest a chromosomal anomaly.

THE NOSE

When taking views of the maxilla, take a view through the nose to ensure that two nostrils are present (Fig. 45-12). A single nostril suggests holoprosencephaly.

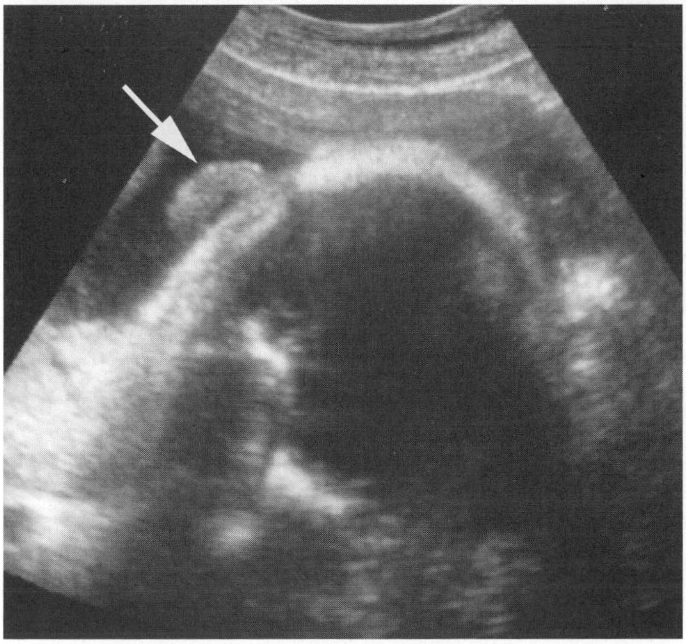

Figure 45-11. ■ *Side-on view of the ear* (arrow). *The normal fetal position of the ear is lower than in the adult.*

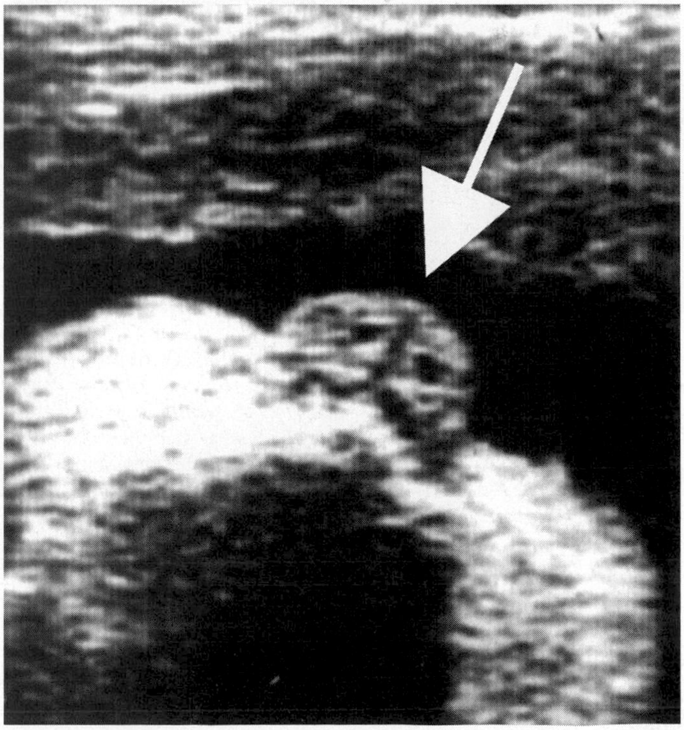

Figure 45-12. ■ *View of the nostrils* (arrow) *and the cheeks.*

THE SPINE

Take transverse views at many levels at right angles to the long axis view of the spine to show the relationship of the posterior elements to the vertebral bodies and to exclude spina bifida (Fig. 45-13A). This is especially difficult in the lumbosacral region where the spine changes direction. Obtain a prone sagittal view of the distal spine that will show the skin posterior to the spine (Fig. 45-13B).

Obtaining this view will bring out a subtle meningocele and is also helpful in showing the cord termination. The coronal view, which shows both posterior ossification centers simultaneously, is also valuable (Fig. 45-13C) and will help to exclude diastematomyelia. Obtain a view that shows the thoracic and cervical spine, although abnormalities in this region are much more unusual (Fig. 45-13D).

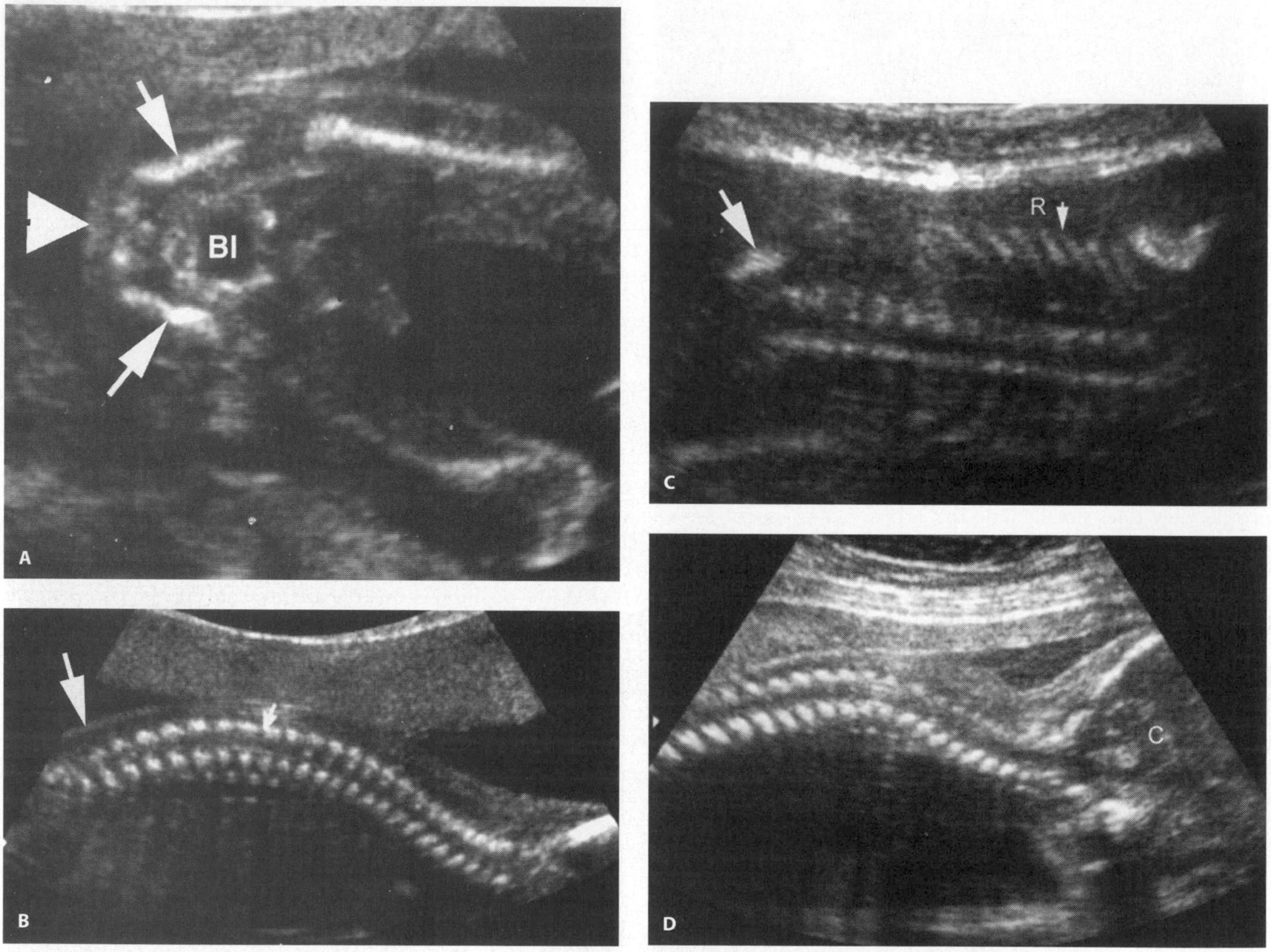

Figure 45-13. ■ *A. Transverse view of the lumbar spine* (arrowhead) *at the level of the iliac crests* (arrows). *The three bony components of the spine seen on transverse views are visible* (arrowhead). *This view is essential to exclude spina bifida most common at this level.* Bl, *bladder.* ***B.*** *Sagittal view of the lumbar spine. This view is very sensitive for the detection of spina bifida and vertebral abnormalities. Note the posterior angulation of the sacral segment of the vertebra* (large arrow). *This angulation helps to detect the level of spinal abnormalities. The skin over the spine can be well seen. If a neural tube defect were present, there would be a depression at the defect, or the cyst of a meningocele would be visible disrupting the skin line. A more accurate way to determine the level of vertebral anomalies is to count down from the level of the lowest rib. The termination of the spinal cord is visible at L2 within the spinal canal* (small arrow). ***C.*** *Coronal view of the spine. This is a valuable view if you cannot obtain the standard sagittal and transverse views. One iliac crest is shown* (arrow). *The ribs are visible* (R). ***D.*** *Sagittal view of the cervical spine showing the normal cervical curve below the cranium* (C).

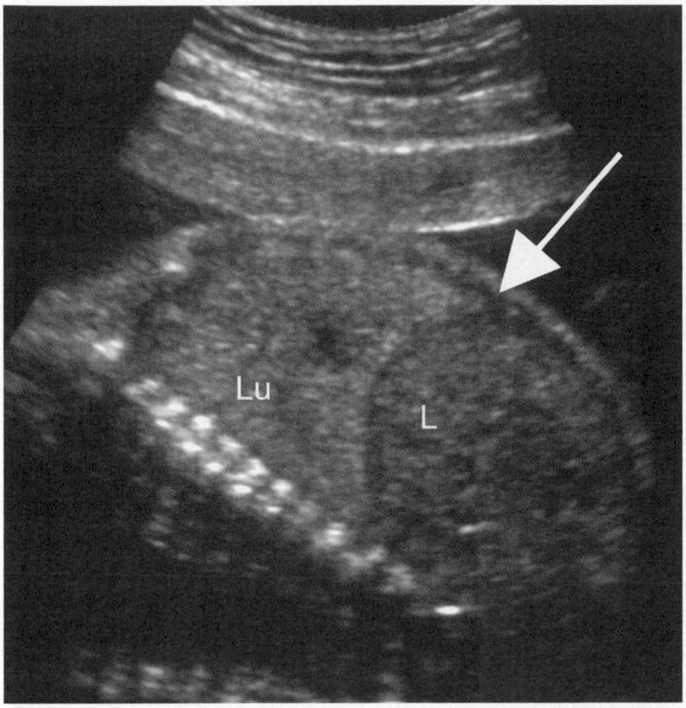

Figure 45-14. ■ *Sagittal view showing the lung* (Lu), *liver* (L), *and the diaphragm* (arrow).

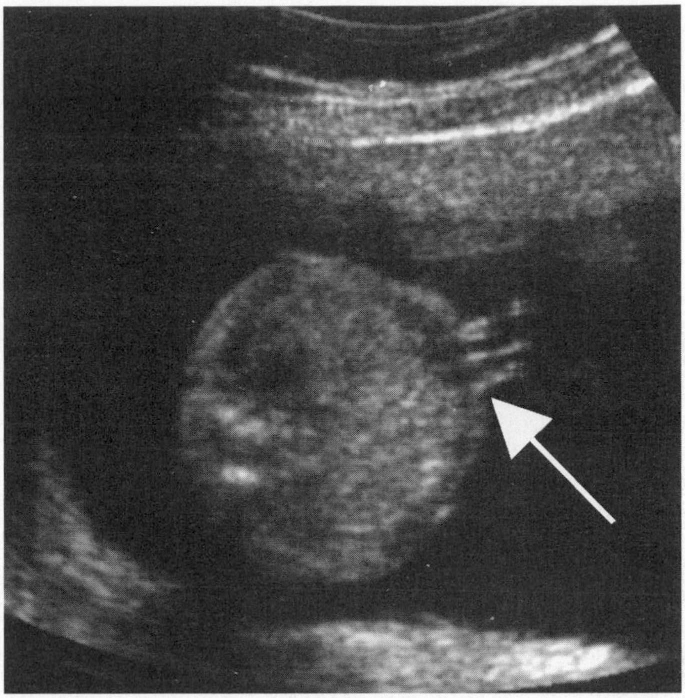

Figure 45-15. ■ *Cord insertion. Normal cord insertion* (arrow) *with three vessels.*

THE DIAPHRAGM

Find the diaphragm bilaterally to exclude diaphragmatic hernia. When the fetus is breathing, visualization of the diaphragm on longitudinal views is easier (Fig. 45-14).

THE CORD INSERTION

Make sure the cord inserts into the abdominal wall normally (Fig. 45-15). Small omphaloceles might be overlooked, and this view gives you an opportunity to count the three vessels in the cord. If only one artery is present, an anomaly is more likely.

THE NECK

Look at the cervical spine area of the neck to exclude small cystic hygromas and to check for small encephaloceles. Examine the thyroid size for goiter (Fig. 45-16) (see Appendix 27).

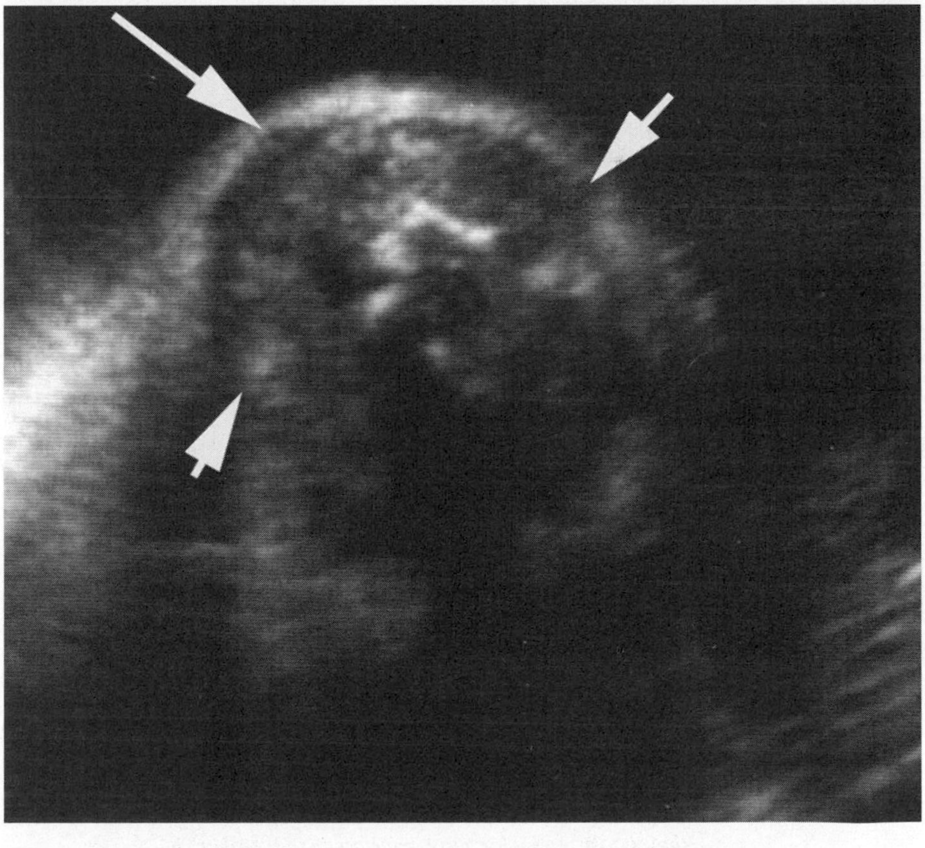

Figure 45-16. ■ *Transverse view of the fetal neck showing the thyroid* (small arrows).

THE LIVER AND SPLEEN

Try to visualize the liver length at right angles to the diaphragm. There are normal size standards (see Appendix 19). Also make an effort to see the spleen lateral to the stomach (Fig. 45-17). There are also normal standards for spleen size when its length is measured on a coronal view.

MASS ARISING FROM THE HEAD OR NECK

Most masses arising from the head or neck are cystic. First establish whether the mass arises from the head or neck by carefully showing landmarks such as the jaw and shoulder. If a cystic mass arises from the head, whether anterior or posterior, look for a bony defect in the skull, which is seen with encephalocele. Check for brain tissue within the mass and secondary intracranial ventricular dilation.

If the cystic mass arises in the neck, see whether it is bilateral and in a posterolateral location, as this favors cystic hygroma. Septations are seen in most cystic hygroma, and skin thickening with hydropic changes is common. If the cystic mass is posterior, look for spinal defects as with iniencephaly or a low encephalocele; also look for secondary hydrocephalus.

MASS ARISING FROM THE TRUNK

If the mass is anterior, determine whether it is cord or bowel loops. The cord will show flow on Doppler and will light up with color flow. Slightly dilated bowel loops can look like cord. If the mass is enclosed in a membrane as seen in omphalocele, see whether there is liver or gut within the mass.

If the mass is posterior, check to see whether the spine is intact and look at the head for evidence of Arnold-Chiari malformation. Also see whether the bladder and kidneys are obstructed and look for evidence of hydrops.

When investigating omphalocele, define the extent of the defect on transverse and longitudinal views. Also take a view that shows the cord insertion, the omphalocele, and the spine simultaneously, if possible.

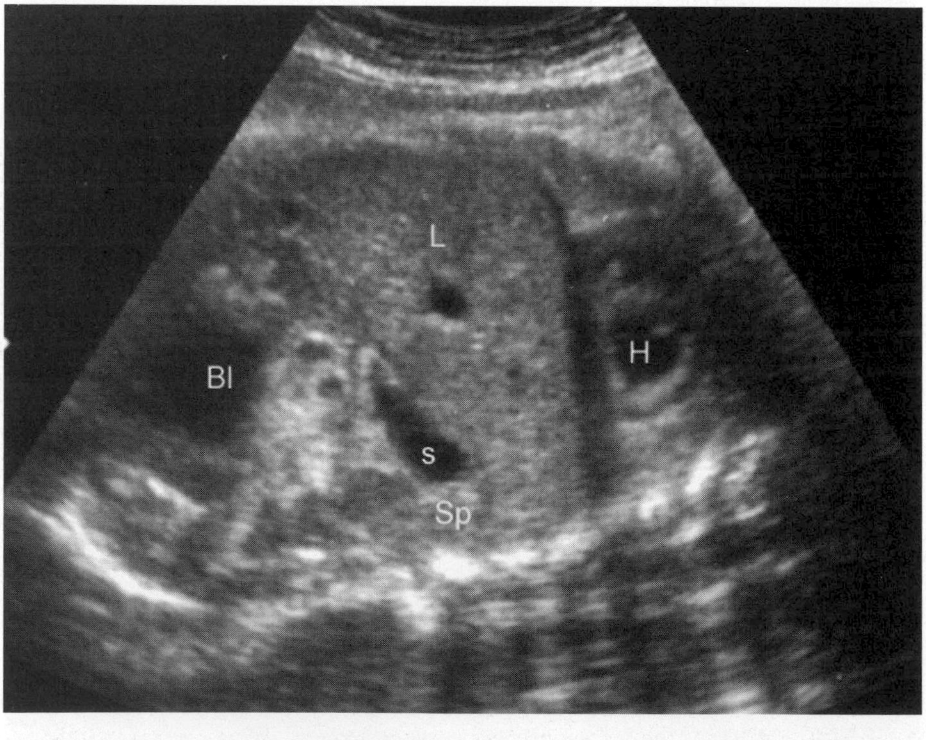

Figure 45-17. ■ *Coronal view of the fetal trunk showing the liver* (L) *and spleen* (Sp). *The stomach* (S), *bladder* (Bl), *and the heart* (H) *are also labeled.*

Pathology

Most fetal anomalies are unsuspected prior to the sonogram. If there is a family history or a risk factor such as maternal drug intake, then the examination is much simplified because a specific anomaly can be sought. Three important nonspecific clues channel the way the fetus is examined because they are associated with defined groups of anomalies.

1. Polyhydramnios. The following anomalies are associated with polyhydramnios.
   a. Gut anomalies
      Duodenal atresia
      Omphalocele
      Gastroschisis
      Diaphragmatic hernia
      Esophageal atresia and tracheoesophageal fistula
      Small bowel atresia
   b. Swallowing problems
      Cleft palate
      Tracheoesophageal fistula
      Small lower jaw (micrognathia)
   c. Central nervous system anomalies (if the swallowing center is impaired)
      Anencephaly
      Hydrocephalus
      Encephalocele
   d. Neck problems
      Goiter
      Cystic hygroma
      Cervical teratoma
   e. Short-limbed dwarfism with small chest (presumably compressing the esophagus)
      Thanatophoric dwarfism
      Achondrogenesis
      Osteogenesis imperfecta

f. Lung problems (with esophageal compression)
   Cystic adenomatoid malformation
   Isolated pleural effusion
g. Nonimmune or immune hydrops
h. Renal problems with renal enlargement compressing gut as with ureteropelvic junction obstruction (UPJ)
i. Sacrococcygeal teratoma

2. Oligohydramnios. Too little urine output causes less amniotic fluid or no amniotic fluid at all.
   a. Renal anomalies
      Bilateral renal agenesis
      Infantile polycystic kidney (autosomal recessive polycystic kidney disease)
      Bilateral dysplastic kidney
      Posterior urethral valves (PUV)
      Prune belly syndrome
   b. Others
      Limb/body wall syndrome (amniotic bands)
      Some spina bifida
      Some cranial problems
   c. IUGR
3. Increased AFP.
   a. Open neural crest defects
      Spina bifida variants
      Encephalocele
      Anencephaly
      Iniencephaly
   b. Abdominal wall defects
      Omphalocele
      Gastroschisis
      Limb/body wall syndrome (amniotic bands)
   c. Tumorous lesions
      Cystic hygroma
      Sacrococcygeal teratoma
   d. Renal problems (rarely)
      Renal agenesis
      PUV
      Hydronephrosis
      Finnish nephropathy
   e. Placental problems (e.g., triploidy)
   f. Rudimentary or dead twin

Most fetal anomalies, however, are unexpectedly discovered during a sonographic study. This section is therefore organized by the presenting sonographic finding, in the following order:

Cyst in the abdomen
Cysts and masses in the chest
Cyst in the head
Head and brain malformations
Mass arising from the head or neck
Limb shortening
Blood tests or maternal age suspicious for Down syndrome
Mass arising from the trunk
Stomach not seen
Hydrops
Skin thickening
Bilateral large echogenic kidneys
Absent or small kidneys
Masses in the region of the kidneys

CYST IN THE ABDOMEN

Three normal cystic structures lie in the abdomen: the stomach in the left upper quadrant, the gallbladder, and the bladder. Abnormal cystic processes occur in three locations between the diaphragm and the genitalia: those related to the kidney, those related to the gastrointestinal tract, and intraperitoneal and pelvic cystic processes.

Kidney (Renal) Cystic Processes

Cystic structures of renal origin normally occur in a paraspinal location. Provided the kidneys are present, gastrointestinal processes do not extend to contact the spine or into the paraspinal area. Establish whether one or more cysts are present and whether the cysts interconnect and connect with the renal pelvis. (The cysts in a dysplastic multicystic kidney may not connect, will vary in size, and are laterally placed.) If kidney parenchyma can be seen around the suspect lesion, the process is most likely related to hydronephrosis.

Look for a dilated ureter or ureters. Check the bladder to see whether it is enlarged. Note whether the kidney process is bilateral. Horseshoe and pelvic kidneys may lie at a low level in front of the spine in the midline. If these anomalies are present, no kidneys will be seen in the normal location. Dysplastic changes are more common in pelvic kidneys.

Renal Obstruction

Some renal cysts are related to obstruction, either unilateral or bilateral hydronephrosis. These conditions can be detected and explored sonographically. Renal pelvicaliceal distention suggestive of hydronephrosis has been subclassified depending on whether there is calyceal as well as pelvic distention.

Type 0: No pelvic distention
Type 1: Pelvic distention only
Type 2: Pelvic and calyceal distention
Type 3: Pelvicaliceal distention with parenchymal narrowing

Technique

1. Measurements of renal pelvic dilation are made in an anteroposterior direction at the level of the renal pelvis (Fig. 45-18).

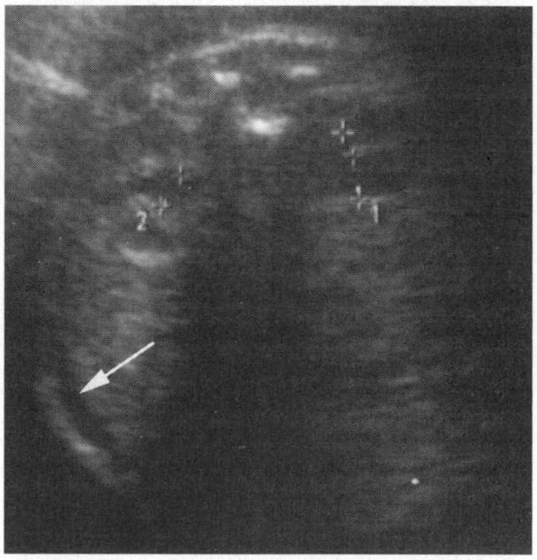

Figure 45-18. ■ *Mild renal pelvic dilation. Measurements are made in an anterior-posterior direction (see markers). Measurements of 4 mm or more are a low-grade indicator of Down syndrome. Measurements of less than 7 mm are of no long-term clinical significance, and those of 7 mm or more may indicate later hydronephrosis.*

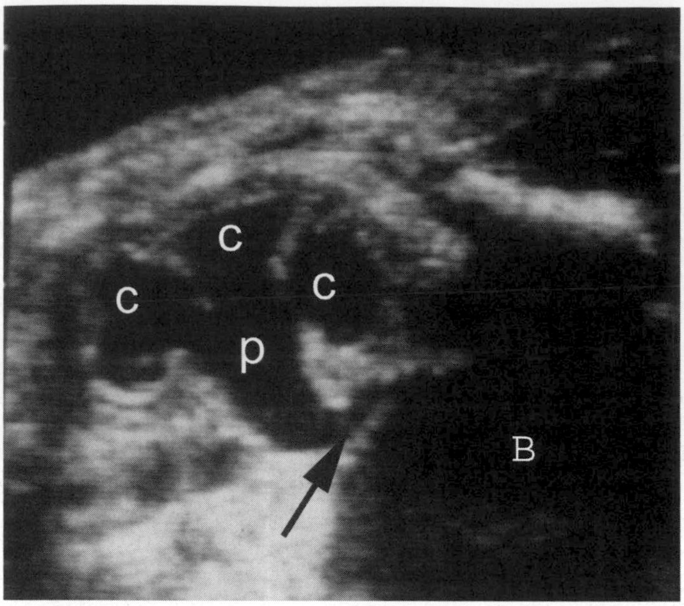

Figure 45-19. ■ *Hydronephrotic kidney with dilated ureter* (arrow) *leading to an enlarged bladder* (B). *Dilated calyces* (c) *are seen adjacent to an enlarged renal pelvis* (p).

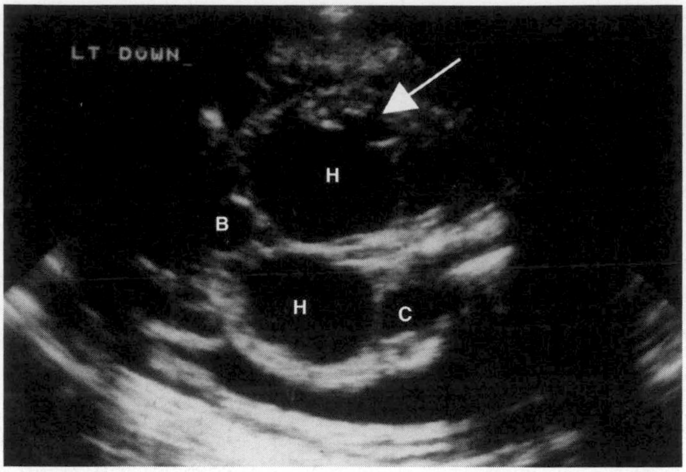

Figure 45-20. ■ *UPJ. Both kidneys are obstructed at the ureteropelvic junction; the renal pelves are very large, and there is secondary calyceal dilation* (C). *The renal pelves were so large that there was secondary polyhydramnios, which disappeared when the renal pelves were drained.*

2. A longitudinal coronal view angled so that the bladder is also seen shows the full extent of the pelvicaliceal system well. This view may show the ureter passing toward the bladder (Fig. 45-19). The ureter can be confused with the fetal psoas muscle and the iliac artery; color flow can help with this. Also, try to demonstrate the ureter emerging from the renal pelvis.
3. Watch the dilated renal pelvis for several minutes. If the renal pelvic size varies over the course of the examination, reflux should be considered. Alternatively, the renal pelvic dilation may be a response to fetal bladder dilation and may disappear when the fetus voids. Re-examine the renal pelvis after the fetus voids, if possible.
4. Examine the renal parenchyma. If it is markedly echogenic, dysplasia should be suspected. The earliest definitive sign of renal dysplasia is the presence of tiny peripherally placed cysts that enlarge as the condition becomes more severe.

UPJ

1. If the renal pelvis is large and rounded, the diagnosis is likely to be UPJ (Fig. 45-20). Generalized calyceal distention is seen with a large renal pelvis having a rounded shape.
2. Echogenic parenchyma due to dysplasia is very uncommon with UPJ.
3. Sometimes, the renal pelvis is very large with or without calyceal distention; it may appear to be a cyst in the midabdomen (Fig. 45-20)
4. Both renal pelves may have a UPJ configuration. As a rule, the degree of renal pelvic dilation is asymmetrical, and one renal pelvis is larger than the other. If the hydronephrosis is bilateral and severe, there may be decreased amniotic fluid (oligohydramnios).
5. Alternatively, with severe unilateral or bilateral renal pelvic enlargement (Fig. 45-20), there can be polyhydramnios. Gut compression by the dilated renal pelves causes the polyhydramnios.

Unilateral Hydronephrosis. There will be a normal amount of amniotic fluid with unilateral hydronephrosis.

1. UPJ. Generalized calyceal distention is seen with a large renal pelvis with a rounded shape. This condition is common (Fig. 45-20). There can be polyhydramnios, thought to be due to gut compression by the dilated renal pelvis.
2. Hydronephrosis due to ureterocele. A tortuous dilated ureter can be traced from the renal pelvis to the bladder. The dilated ureter can be so redundant with multiple dilated loops that it looks like many centrally placed cysts and seems to be of gut origin. A small spherical membrane, the wall of the ureterocele, may be seen within the bladder (Fig. 45-21). If a ureterocele is very large,

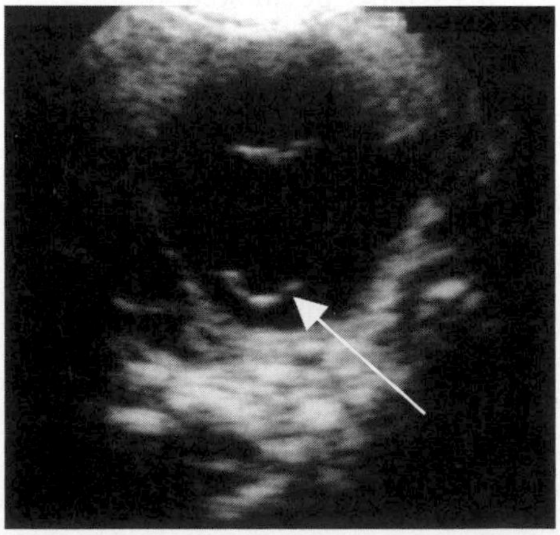

Figure 45-21. ■ *View of the bladder showing curvilinear membranes* (arrow) *within the bladder representing two of the borders of the circular ureterocele.*

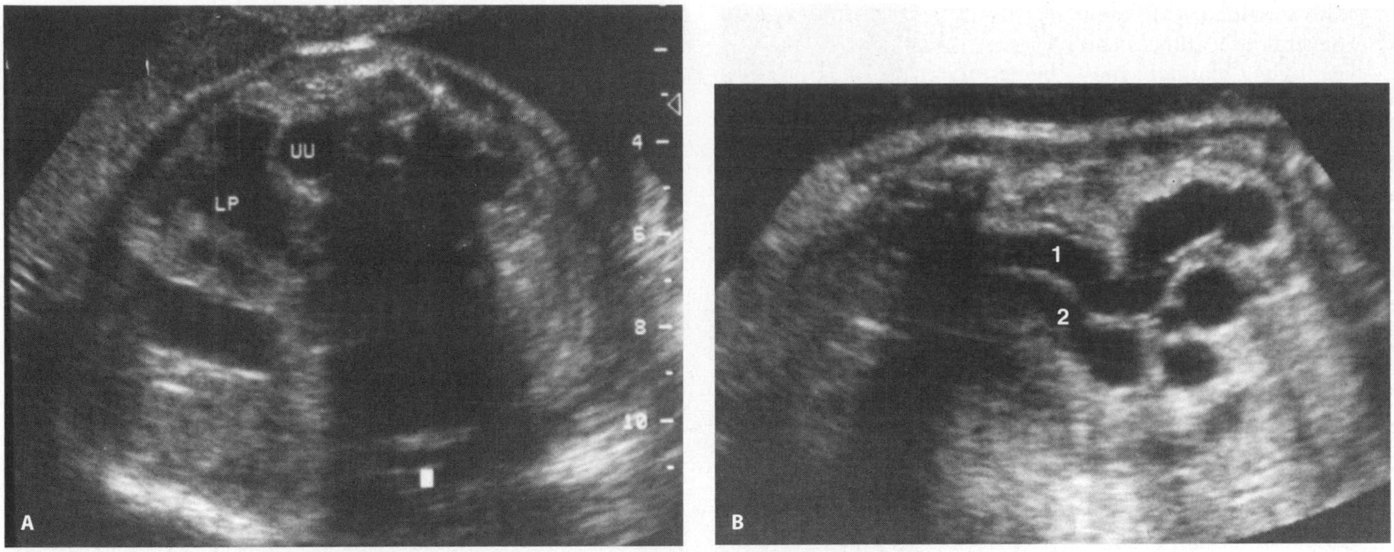

Figure 45-22. ■ *A. Transverse view of duplication. The view was obtained at the lower pole. The dilated lower collection system is visible* (LP). *The dilated ureter* (UU) *from the upper pole collecting system lies alongside. B. Sagittal view of duplication with hydronephrotic collecting systems showing both dilated ureters* (1 and 2). *(Reprinted with permission from Sanders RC, ed.* Structural Fetal Abnormalities: The Total Picture, *2nd ed. New York: Mosby-Year Book Publishers, 2002.)*

it can obstruct the ureter draining the other kidney. Many ureteroceles are found in kidneys with double collecting systems (Fig. 45-22A,B). The ureterocele may be draining only the upper half of the kidney, and the lower half of the kidney may not be hydronephrotic if it is a double collecting system. Alternatively, the lower pole may be dilated related to reflux or lower pole ureteropelvic junction obstruction. With the similar entity ectopic ureteric insertion, the dilated urethra inserts low and can be traced to a site at the inferolateral aspect of the bladder. Both ureterocele and ectopic ureter can occur in single kidneys.

Vesico Ureteric Reflux. Reflux is a condition in which some urine returns from the bladder to the kidney when the fetus voids. The one-way valve at the junction between the ureter and the bladder may not be fully formed in utero; this valve may leak so some urine flows back to the kidney from the bladder when the bladder contracts. Ultrasonic signs are (1) dilated pelvicaliceal system, (2) dilated ureter that shows much peristalsis, and (3) distention of the renal pelvis as the bladder empties. Often, the bladder is large but thin walled because it never empties well. This condition is much more common in males than females in utero and is the reverse of the situation in small children, when reflux is much more common in girls than in boys. Usually, reflux seen in utero resolves over the course of the pregnancy or in the first few months of life.

Bilateral Hydronephrosis. If the hydronephrosis severely compromises renal function, there will be decreased amniotic fluid (oligohydramnios).

1. Bilateral UPJ. Renal function is rarely impaired, but with severe obstruction, the dilated kidney compresses intestines, and polyhydramnios may result (Fig. 45-20). Oligohydramnios is rare. The degree of hydronephrosis is usually asymmetrical. The renal pelves are large in comparison with the calyces.
2. PUV. Valves in the posterior urethra of males may obstruct the urethra. An obstruction in the posterior urethra causes the bladder to dilate. Oligohydramnios is usual. The bladder has a V-shaped area known as a "keyhole" arising from its inferior end—the dilated posterior urethra (Fig. 45-23). The kidneys often

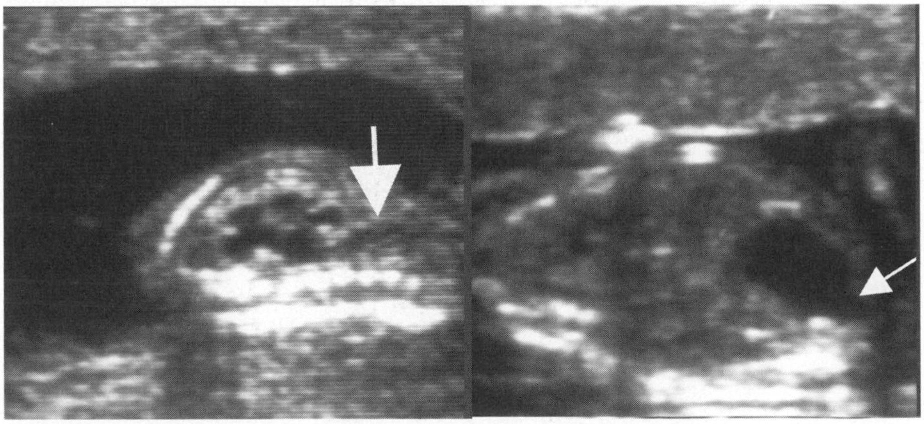

Figure 45-23. ■ *PUV. Mild case with dilated collecting system and ureter* (large arrow) *without dysphasia. A dilated posterior urethra* (small arrow) *drains a mildly dilated bladder (double linear array view).*

show evidence of renal dysplasia. Several appearances can be seen:

a. The bladder may be enormously distended without the kidneys showing hydronephrosis (Fig. 45-24). The kidneys are often densely echogenic because they are dysplastic. Confusion with a large pelvic cyst can occur. This form of PUV is always fatal. There will be no amniotic fluid if this form is seen after 18 weeks because complete urethral obstruction is present.
b. The bladder may be quite large with both kidneys hydronephrotic. Dilated tortuous ureters are seen (Fig. 45-23).
c. Severe fetal ascites can be seen without the skin thickening, pleural effusions, or placentomegaly of hydrops. The bladder, ureters, and kidneys are distended. This variant of PUV is thought to result in the prune belly anomaly (Eagle-Barrett syndrome).

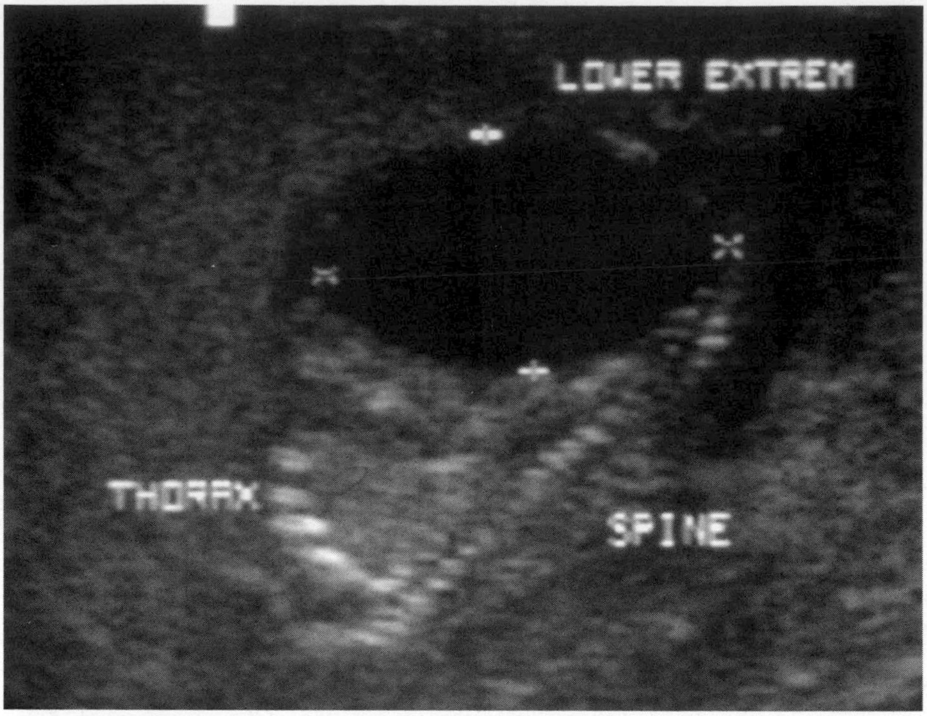

Figure 45-24. ■ *PUV. The bladder is greatly distended (see measurement markers). There is no amniotic fluid (anhydramnios). This form of PUV is lethal.*

Fetuses with PUV may be considered for in utero drainage. Before a procedure is performed, the diagnosis must be well established and the following problems must be excluded:

a. Chromosomal abnormality. Before a drainage procedure is used, karyotyping is performed because there is an association with chromosomal abnormalities, particularly trisomy 21.
b. Dysplasia. The fetal kidneys are inspected carefully to ensure that dysplasia is not present. If the kidneys are echogenic with peripherally placed cysts, one can be sure that dysplasia is present. Often, the kidneys are echogenic but no cysts can be seen, so a diagnosis of dysplasia can be suspected but not definitively made (to be discussed later in this chapter).
c. Amniotic fluid. Most groups only perform drainage procedures when amniotic fluid is still present but is decreasing in amount.

The fetal bladder is punctured under ultrasound control, and a double pigtail catheter is pushed through a wide metal catheter so that one pigtail end lies in the bladder and the other lies in the amniotic fluid. A special introducer with a pigtail catheter and a pusher on a single needle is used. This technique is difficult and should only be performed in specialized units.

3. Ureterovesical junction obstruction. In this rare condition, both ureters are dilated, and there may be pelvicaliceal dilation. The bladder may be small or normal in size because the partial obstruction is at the level of the insertions of the ureters into the bladder.
4. Idiopathic megaureter. The ureters are dilated, and there may be some dilation of the renal pelvis. There is no urethral obstruction. The distal portions of the ureters do not function normally. It is hard to distinguish this condition from reflux, which may also occur in utero. Watch for changes in size of the kidneys and ureters after fetal voiding.

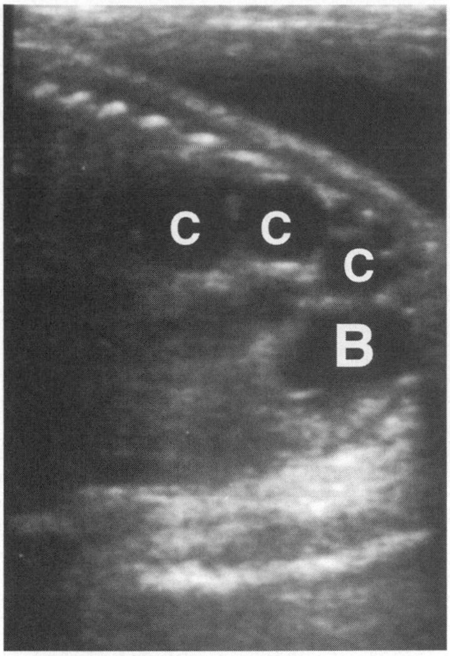

Figure 45-25. ■ *Pelvic multicystic kidney. Pelvic kidneys become obstructed more often than normally placed kidneys. A previously obstructed pelvic kidney is now dysplastic. Note the large separate cysts* (C) *alongside the bladder* (B).

Multicystic Dysplastic Kidney. If renal obstruction occurs early in pregnancy, before approximately 15 weeks, permanent damage to the kidneys (dysplasia) may occur (Figs. 45-25 and 45-26). When dysplastic changes are present the kidneys become more echogenic and develop parenchymal cysts. The cysts vary in size and do not generally communicate. If the cysts are large, the condition is known as *multicystic kidney* rather than *dysplasia*. If dysplasia is generalized with visible cysts, the kidneys do not function. Dysplasia may result from ureteropelvic, distal urethral, or ureteric obstruction; both kidneys are involved if the urethra is obstructed, and fetuses with this condition do not usually survive.

Gastrointestinal Cystic Processes

With the exception of duplication, proximal gastrointestinal processes associated with gut obstruction cause polyhydramnios. Distal gut atresias such as anal or colonic atresia are not associated with polyhydramnios.

If the obstruction is below the level of the stomach, there will be several cyst-like structures that are really dilated loops of small bowel (Fig. 45-27).

Small Bowel Atresia. The most common cause of obstruction is gut atresia, when a loop of bowel does not form or atrophies due to inadequate blood supply.

1. Obstruction occurs either in the jejunum, when both the stomach and small bowel are dilated, or in the ileum, when the stomach is usually not enlarged. Both processes cause polyhydramnios. Multiple fluid-filled tubular structures are seen in the abdomen (Fig. 45-27). Occasionally, peristalsis may be visible.
2. Malrotation with an unusual axis to the stomach and duodenum may be seen. Sometimes, the obstruction is due to volvulus; a single, very distended loop of bowel will be seen with other, less-dilated loops.
3. Distal gut atresias such as anal or colonic atresia are not associated with polyhydramnios.

Dilated large bowel is occasionally seen with these abnormalities. Usually, intestinal appearances are normal because the colon does very little in utero.

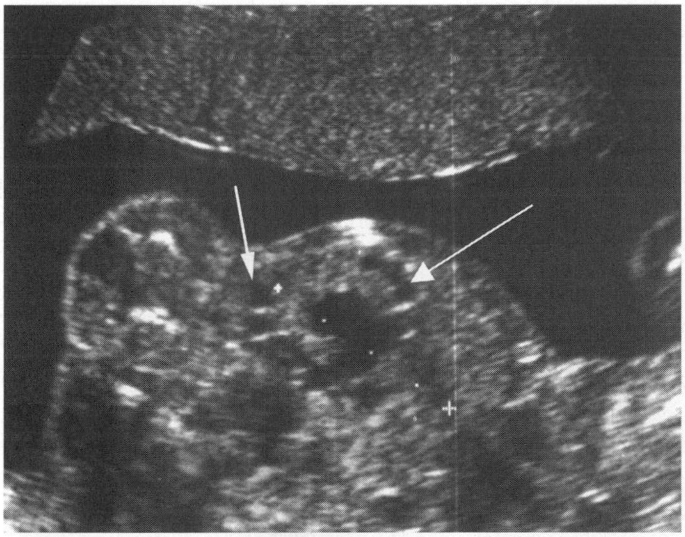

Figure 45-26. ■ *Early multicystic kidney due to PUV. Numerous cysts are seen around the edge of the kidney* (arrows). *This is the location where the cysts associated with renal dysplasia (multicystic kidney) are seen first.*

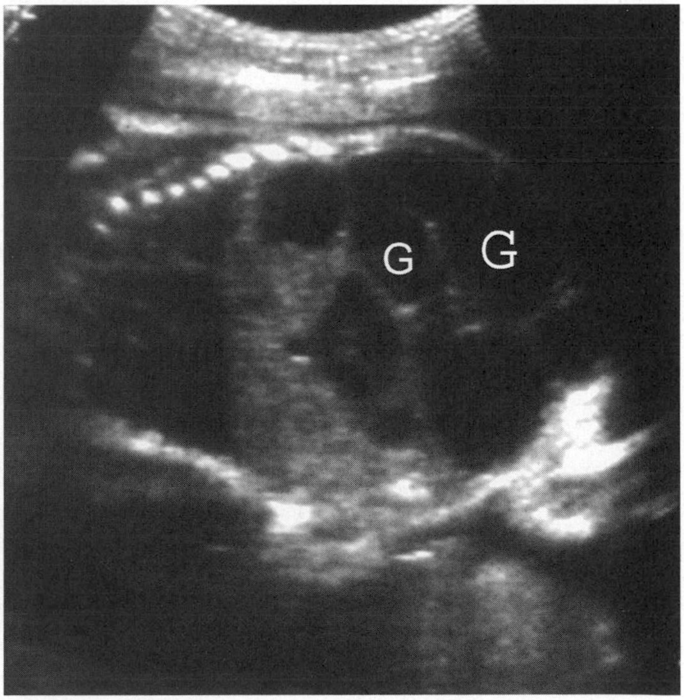

Figure 45-27. ■ *Small bowel atresia. There are a number of dilated loops of fluid-filled small bowel* (G) *due to an ileal atresia. There was polyhydramnios because this was a small-bowel obstruction.*

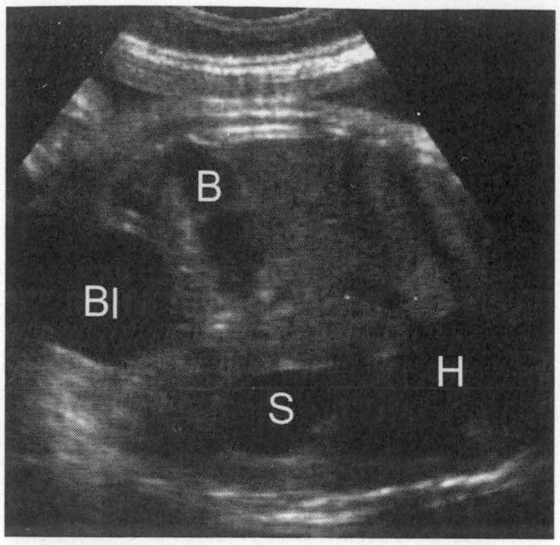

Figure 45-28. ■ *Third trimester normal colon. In the third trimester, the bowel can be fluid filled and relatively large* (B). *This is a normal variant appearance.* Bl, *bladder;* S, *stomach;* H, *heart.*

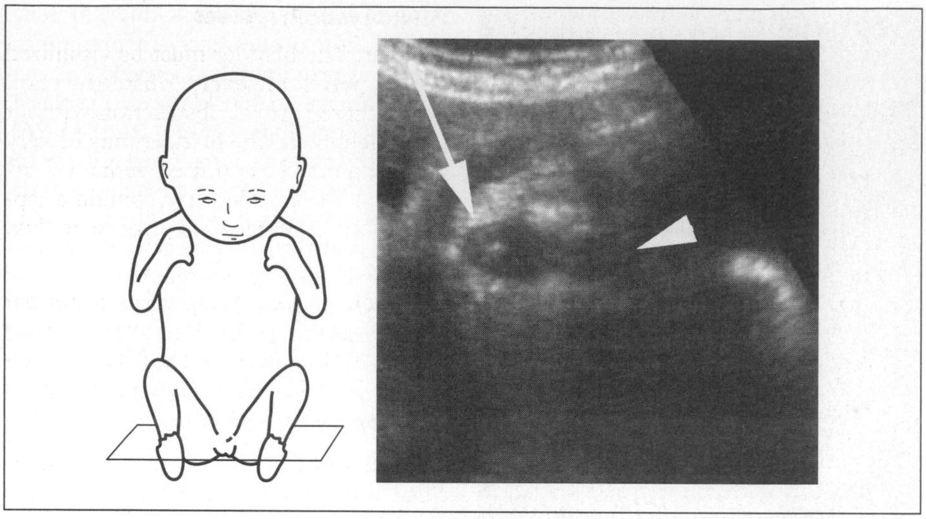

Figure 45-29. ■ *View of the anus in a female patient (arrowhead shows genitalia). The anal orifice is a small echogenic area* (arrow) *surrounded by echopenic anal muscles.*

In the third trimester, normal colon may be fluid filled and up to 28 mm in diameter normally (Fig. 45-28). An echogenic spot seen on a transverse view that includes the genitalia is normally present and represents the anus (Fig. 45-29). It is absent with anal atresia (imperforate anus).

Duodenal Atresia. Two large sonolucent spaces (the double bubble sign) are visible within the upper abdomen in duodenal atresia.

1. Demonstrate the connection between the distended fluid-filled stomach and the duodenum, which form the two spaces (Fig. 45-30).
2. Between 30% and 50% of duodenal atresia cases are associated with Down syndrome and cardiac anomalies.
3. Severe polyhydramnios is always present.
4. With duodenal atresia, obstruction may not develop until as late as 24 weeks, so an 18-week sonogram may appear normal.

Intraperitoneal Cystic Processes

This category includes cystic processes that lie outside the kidney and the gut in the midabdomen at a distance from the spine.

Meconium Cyst and Peritonitis. Spillage of fetal intestinal contents (the meconium) results in calcification, usually in a ring-like shape, in the fetal abdomen.

1. This condition may be associated with bowel obstruction.
2. Initially, a cyst with irregular echogenic walls is seen (Fig. 45-31). Over time, the cyst often disappears, and calcification develops at the cyst site.
3. Linear groups of calcification, typically superior to the liver, are considered to represent the remnants of similar episodes that were not seen with ultrasound. Extraintestinal calcifications not associated with gut dilation have no long-term clinical significance.

Mesenteric Cyst and Duplication. Mesenteric cysts and duplication are extremely rare echo-free cysts. They are indistinguishable from an ovarian cyst, except they may occur in males.

Choledochal Cyst. Choledochal cysts are bile filled and occur only adjacent to the liver. A dilated bile duct may be seen entering the cyst. The gallbladder should be seen as well as the cyst. These are also very rare.

Ovarian Cysts. In the late second and third trimester, the mother's hormones affect the fetus, occasionally causing the formation of breasts in male and female fetuses (gynecomastia). In the female fetus, the hormones affect the ovary and cause ovarian cyst formation. A cyst may be round and echo-free, or it may contain echoes that are due to bleeding fol-

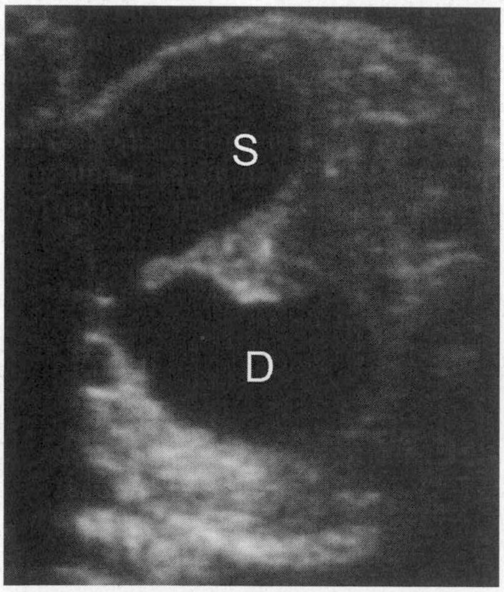

Figure 45-30. ■ *Duodenal atresia. Both the stomach* (S) *and duodenum* (D) *are dilated and are connected. There was polyhydramnios. No small or large bowel loops contain air or fluid.*

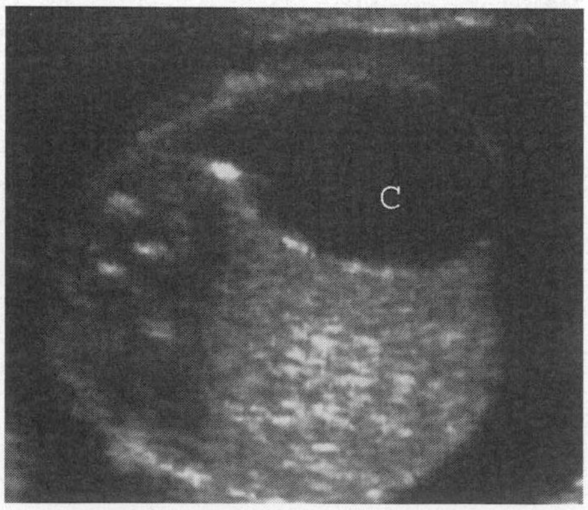

Figure 45-31. ■ *Meconium cyst. The meconium cyst* (C) *has a faint rim of calcification around it, typical of meconium cysts. The cyst often contains some echogenic debris.*

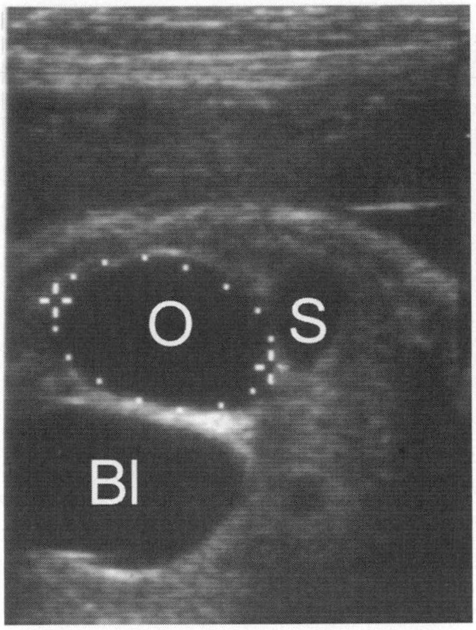

Figure 45-32. ■ *Ovarian cyst. The cyst* (O) *lies adjacent to the stomach* (S). *It is common for ovarian cysts in utero to lie in the upper abdomen adjacent to the liver. The bladder* (Bl) *is seen in addition to the cyst.*

lowing twisting (torsion) (Fig. 45-32). Echoes may be seen throughout the cyst, or they may form a curved area to one side thought to represent retracting clot. The cysts lie in the anterior part of the abdomen but are often close to the liver rather than in the pelvis.

Pelvic Cystic Processes

Bladder. The bladder must be visualized in the pelvis on every obstetric scan. When there is renal obstruction without hydronephrosis, the bladder may be very large and may be confused with an ovarian cyst. The bladder may contain a septum when a ureterocele is present (Fig. 45-21).

The bladder may be large as a normal variant. Examine the fetus over a 2-hour period to see whether the bladder contracts. The bladder normally empties partially within an hour.

Rectum and Colon. Normal meconium-filled large bowel can appear cystic in the third trimester (Fig. 45-28). The rectum may be mistaken for a cyst.

Hydrometrocolpos. In the female fetus, a cystic structure posterior to the bladder extending out of the pelvis is likely to be an obstructed vagina due to an imperforate hymen (Fig. 45-33). The uterus is not usually dilated or seen. The bladder and kidneys may also be obstructed. A cloaca, a combined bladder and vagina, may be present.

Megacystis Microcolon Syndrome. If the bladder is overdistended but there is polyhydramnios, consider the megacystis microcolon syndrome. The ureters and kidneys may or may not be dilated. The bowel is small, malformed, and obstructed, but not seen as such, and there is a normal or excessive amount of amniotic fluid. The fetus is almost always female with this very rare syndrome.

CYSTS AND MASSES IN THE CHEST

Pleural Effusion. Pleural effusions can be recognized surrounding the lungs at the level of the heart or above it (Fig. 45-34). They may be unilateral or bilateral. Although pleural effusions are usually associated with the changes of hydrops, they may be an isolated finding. Isolated pleural effusions are usually composed of lymph. As a rule, they are small and do not push the diaphragm down (diaphragmatic eversion) or displace the heart. Small pleural effusions often disappear over the course of the pregnancy. Large pleural effusions with these findings may cause secondary hydrops. Catheter drainage in utero has been advocated for this type of effusion. Some perinatologists have performed needle aspiration shortly before birth for large effusions. Aspiration after birth is usually rapidly curative.

Cystadenomatoid Malformation of the Lung

1. In the type 1 and 2 forms of cystadenomatoid malformation of the lung (CCAM), there are multiple cysts with echogenic areas in between.

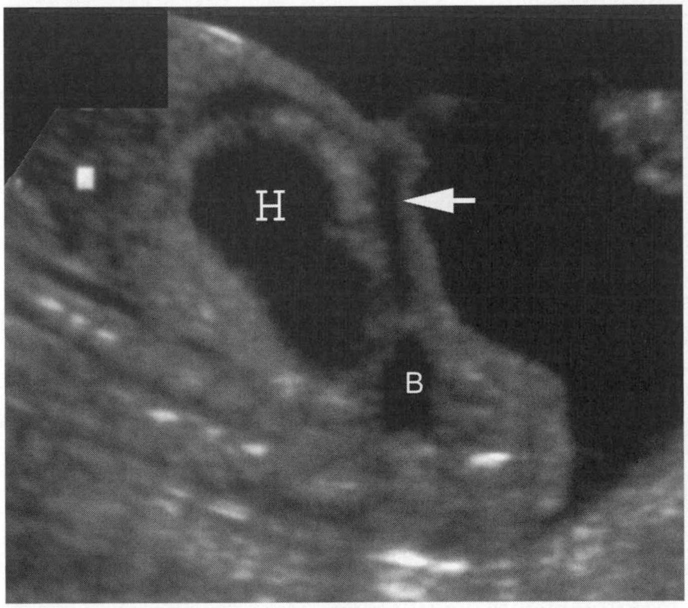

Figure 45-33. ■ *Hydrometrocolpos, dilated uterus, and vagina* (H) *on sagittal view. The bladder* (B) *lies anterior to the dilated hydrometrocolpos. (Reprinted with permission form Sanders RC, ed.* Structural Fetal Abnormalities: The Total Picture, *2nd ed. New York: Mosby-Year Book Publishers, 2002.)*

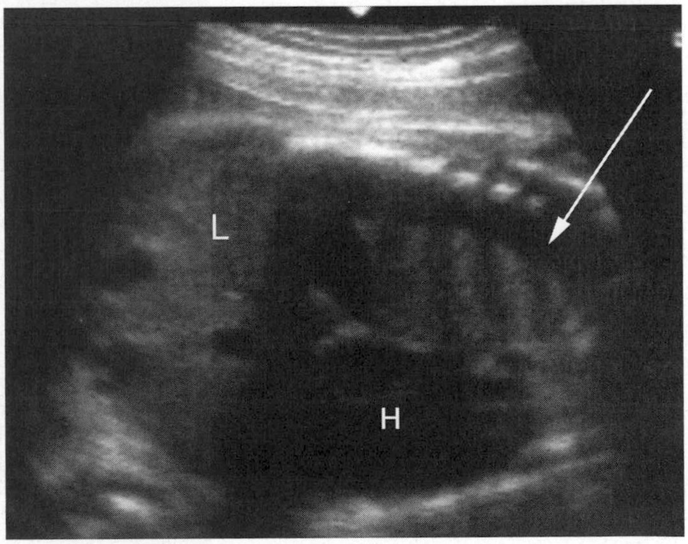

Figure 45-34. ■ *Pleural effusion. A moderately large pleural effusion* (arrow) *surrounds the lung.* H, *heart;* L, *liver.*

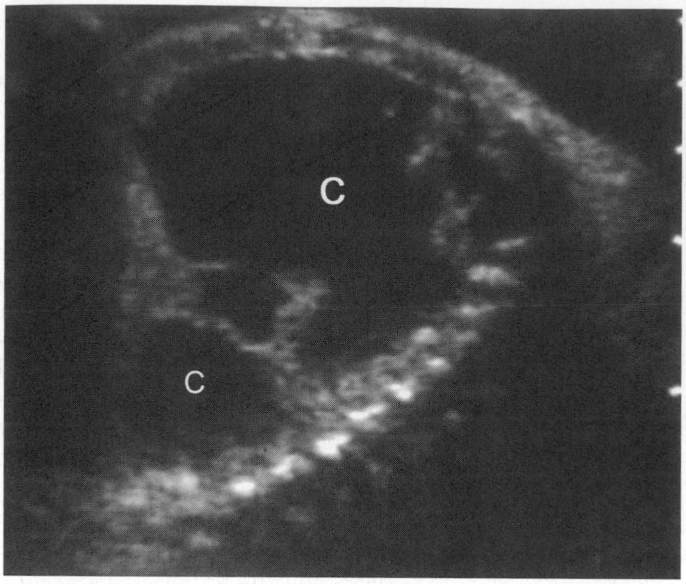

Figure 45-35. ■ *Type 1 CCAM. Multiple large cysts* (C) *occupy the right side of the chest on this sagittal view.*

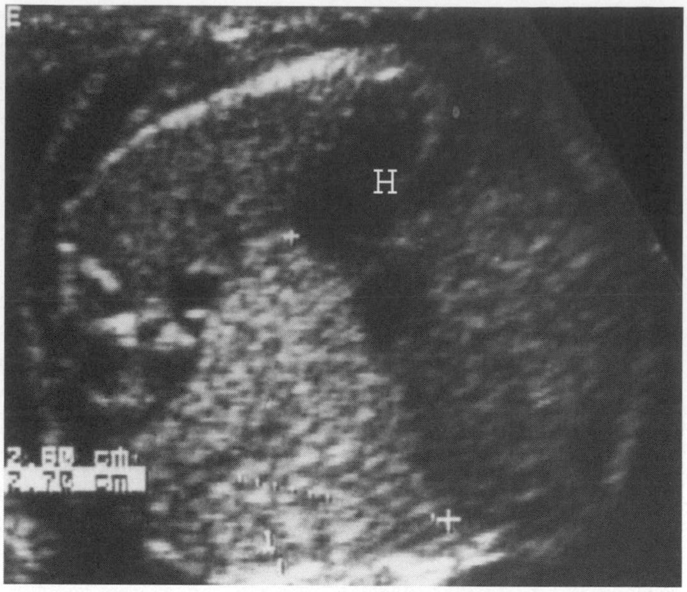

Figure 45-36. ■ *Type 3 CCAM. The outlines of the echogenic CCAM are being measured. The heart* (H) *is compressed and distorted by the CCAM. The appearance of this mass is very similar to extralobar sequestration of the lung except that the supplying artery comes from the pulmonary hilum rather than from below the diaphragm.*

The heart is displaced, and the entire chest or a portion of the chest appears filled with cysts. The cysts are large in type 1 (Fig. 45-35) and are smaller, but visible, in type 2.

2. In the type 3 form, cysts are present but too small to be seen as cysts. There is an echogenic area in the lung (Fig. 45-36).
3. Polyhydramnios and nonimmune hydrops are often present with any of the three types. Hydrops usually results in stillbirth. In utero drainage of large cysts has been helpful. In utero surgical removal of the abnormal portion of lung in type 3 abnormality has successfully cured this otherwise fatal situation.
4. All three types may regress in utero, and the lung may be normal at birth.
5. Sequestration can look the same as a type 3 CCAM; however, a large supplying artery coming from below the diaphragm may be visible on color flow.

Left-Side Diaphragmatic Hernia. Left-side diaphragmatic hernia is a difficult condition to recognize because the small bowel in the chest resembles lung.

1. The stomach is not seen in the abdomen but lies alongside the heart in the chest; the heart is shifted to the right (Fig. 45-37). No left hemidiaphragm is visible.

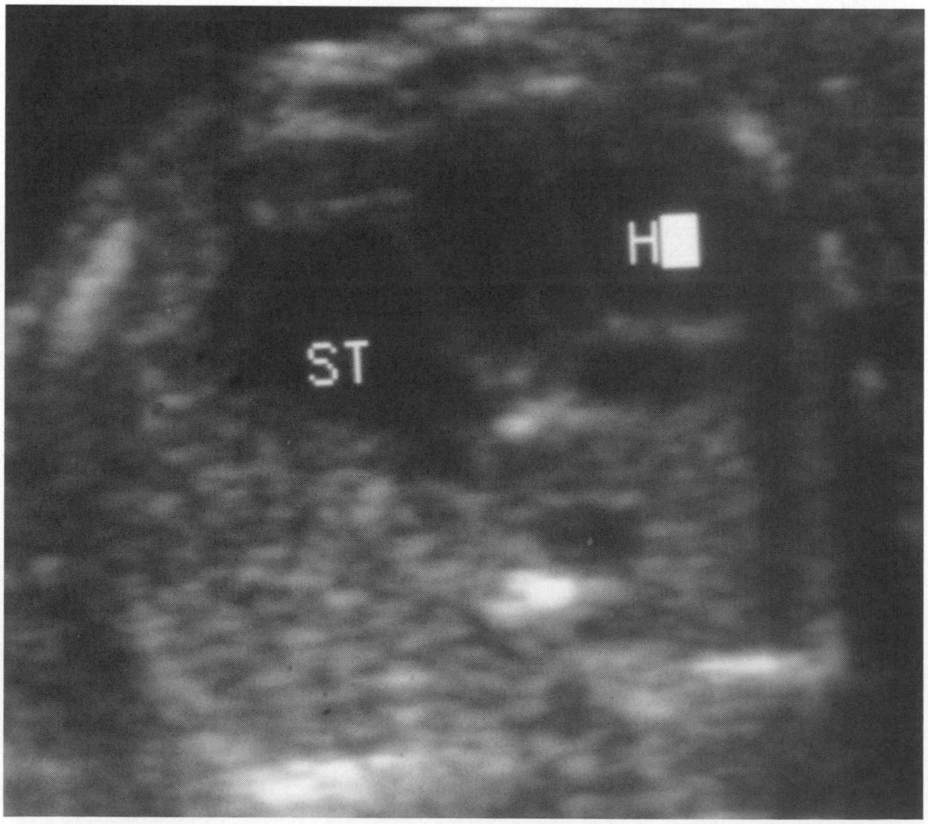

Figure 45-37. ■ *Diaphragmatic hernia. Both the heart* (H) *and the stomach* (ST) *can be seen on the same transverse section. The heart has a distorted shape because it is compressed by the stomach and small bowel that lie in the chest.*

2. The left lung's texture will be slightly different from that of the right lung. Because there are multiple loops of small bowel in the chest, fluid-filled loops may be seen, but empty gut and lung can look amazingly similar.
3. The liver will be displaced to the left and often lies partially in the chest. The presence of the liver in the chest makes in utero surgery very difficult and almost always unsuccessful. Sonographic clues to the presence of the liver in the chest are the distortion and posterior position of the liver vessels and the position of the stomach in the chest.

Right-Side Diaphragmatic Hernia. A right-side diaphragmatic hernia is even more difficult to diagnose because the herniated liver looks so similar to the lung.

1. The stomach will not be seen or will be deviated to the right.
2. The apparent lung on the right will have visible portal veins within that can be tracked to the liver with color flow.
3. The heart will be displaced to the left.
4. Right-side hernia is much less common than left-side hernia. Both types of hernias are associated with other anomalies such as hemivertebrae and hydronephrosis.

Bronchogenic and Neuroenteric Cysts. Bronchogenic and neuroenteric cysts are rare. A single cyst is seen in the posterior midline portion of the lung near the spine. As a rule, these cysts are echo-free. They are associated with vertebral anomalies.

CYST IN THE HEAD

Technique

1. Most cystic lesions in the head represent dilation of two or more ventricles, so it is first necessary to identify the ventricles and the choroid plexus. Lateral ventricles can be recognized by the presence of the choroid plexus, even when it is very distorted.
2. Reverberations from the skull obscure the ventricle closest to the transducer on axial views; apparent asymmetrical dilation of the down-sided ventricle is often a technical artefact because the superficial ventricle cannot be well seen.
   a. Try to scan the head from a coronal axis when side-to-side comparisons are made.
   b. It is usually possible to see the hidden lateral ventricle if the probe is placed in a good position to see the down ventricle on an axial view and then angled inferiorly (Fig. 45-5B–D).
   c. If the fetus is in a cephalic presentation, try an endovaginal probe to visualize the ventricular system in a fashion similar to neonatal head imaging (see Chapter 37).
3. Bananas and lemons. Be sure your images show the entire shape of the skull and the posterior fossa; both are abnormally shaped in the Arnold-Chiari malformation (see discussion later and Fig. 45-41).

The Lateral Ventricles

1. Normal lateral ventricular size. The lateral ventricles and choroid plexus do not change size during the second and third trimesters. At any stage of pregnancy beyond 12 weeks, the lateral ventricular width toward the

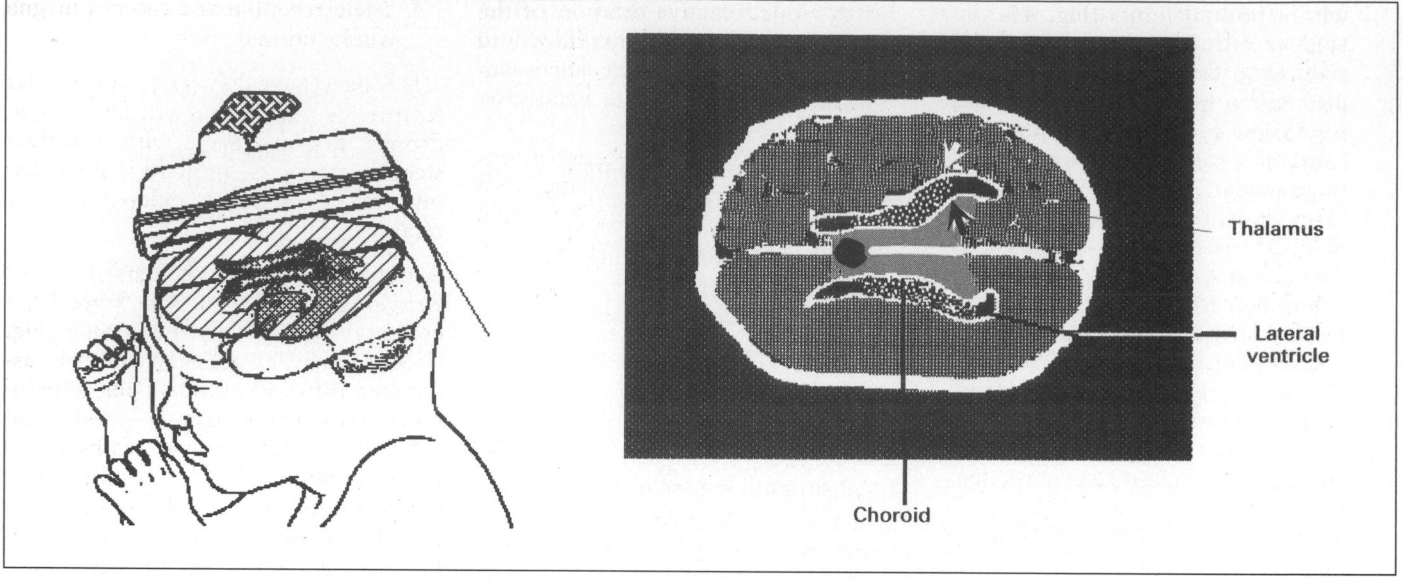

Figure 45-38. ■ *Axial view showing the way the lateral ventricles are imaged. The normal choroids should fill the lateral ventricle. The lateral ventricle width, measured at the atria, should be less than 10 mm.*

posterior aspect of the ventricle (atrium) should be no more than 10 mm, and the choroid plexus should fill most of the ventricle (Figs. 45-38 and 45-39).

2. Mild ventriculomegaly. There should be a gap of no greater than 3 mm between the choroid plexuses and the walls of the lateral ventricles. The choroid plexuses are compressed in hydrocephalus. Noting the discrepancy between the choroid plexus and ventricle sizes allows a diagnosis of mild ventriculomegaly when the ventricular size is still

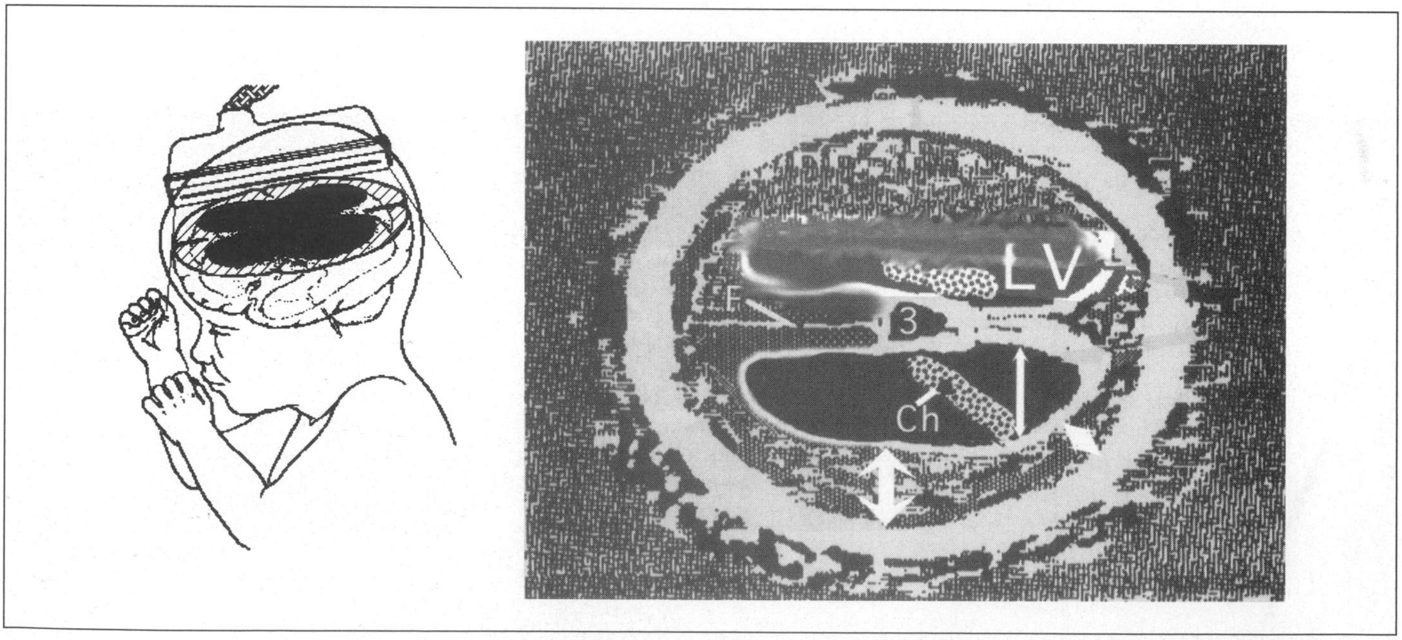

Figure 45-39. ■ *The usual type of hydrocephalus. Much of the skull is filled with two large structures obstructed by the lateral ventricles. The* cortical mantle thickness *is the term used to describe the width of the remaining brain. Details of the dilated lateral ventricle on the side of the brain near the transducer are usually poor due to the reverberations. Note the choroid plexus within the dilated ventricle, assuming an angle of greater than 75 degrees (dangling choroid). The arrow is placed at the site in the atrium of the lateral ventricle, just behind the choroids, where measurements of lateral ventricular width are made.*

within normal limits (Fig. 45-39). (The ventriculohemispheric ratio of midline-to-lateral ventricular wall distance to hemispheric distance is no longer considered helpful because the normal ratio changes over the course of pregnancy.)

3. Hanging choroid sign. The choroid plexuses are gravity dependent. In the normal ventricle, they are angled at less than 25 degrees from vertical. In hydrocephalus, the angle is greater, and the choroid plexuses "dangle" (Fig. 45-39). An angle of 75 degrees or more is pathologic, even if the choroid plexuses are in contact with the lateral ventricular wall.
4. Mantle thickness. It is important to obtain a good view of the amount of cortex (the "mantle") around the ventricle, because the mantle's width has some relationship to whether the fetus will have diminished mental capacity. Measure the mantle; measuring the thickest and thinnest points may be helpful in follow-up (Fig. 45-39).
5. Establishing the level of obstruction. If hydrocephalus is present and if the lateral ventricles are symmetrical, try to visualize the third and fourth ventricles to establish the level of obstruction. Selective dilation of the lateral ventricle without third and fourth ventricle involvement is unusual and suggests brain atrophy or holoprosencephaly.
6. Look elsewhere. Most cases of ventricular dilation are associated with an anomaly elsewhere. The spine, orbits, face, feet, and hands may be affected.

Hydrocephalus

If the fourth ventricle is not dilated, consider the following possibilities:

Aqueductal Stenosis. A relatively common form of ventriculomegaly known as *aqueduct stenosis* results from narrowing of the aqueduct of Sylvius, which connects the third and fourth ventricles (Fig. 45-40). The sonographic features are as follows:

1. Symmetrical dilation of both lateral ventricles with intact intrahemispheric fissure. The degree of dilation is usually relatively mild with considerable preserved brain mantle.
2. Dilated third ventricle without dilation of the fourth ventricle.
3. Dilated aqueduct. This structure may be seen as a small tube extending toward the tentorium on a sagittal midline view.
4. The cerebellum and cisterna magna will be normal.

Mild ventriculomegaly with similar features is associated with Down syndrome. The prognosis with aqueduct stenosis diagnosed in utero is poor; the outcome for almost all children is severe retardation or death.

Arnold-Chiari Malformation. The Arnold-Chiari malformation (type II), a common type of hydrocephalus (Fig. 45-41), is usually, but not necessarily, associated with spina bifida. Long-term intellectual capacity can be good, even when the cortical mantle width is very nar-row. With spina bifida, the spinal cord ends at a lower level than L2 owing to tethering, so a portion of the cerebellum often lies below the skull and is compressed as it is pulled through the cisterna magna. The sonographic features are as follows:

1. Dilation of the lateral ventricles—usually asymmetrical and often severe
2. Dilation of the third ventricle and aqueduct
3. "Banana" shape to the cerebellum instead of the usual bilateral "apple" shape. The cerebellum may not be seen if it is in the upper cervical spine.

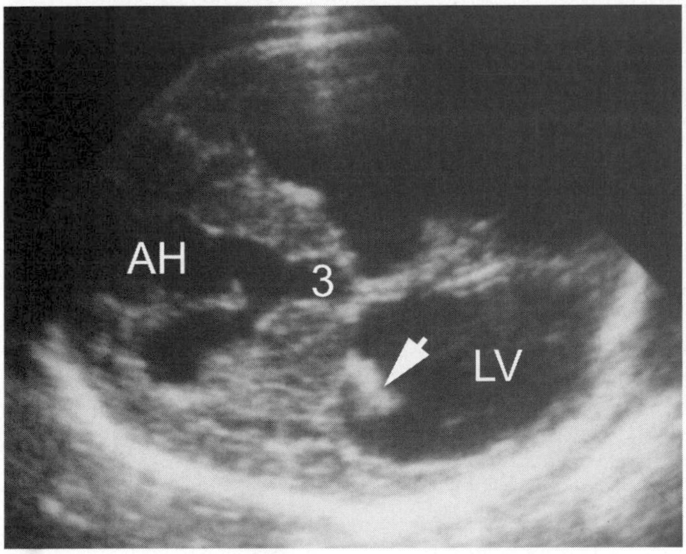

Figure 45-40. ■ *Aqueduct stenosis. The lateral and third ventricles* (3) *are dilated but not the fourth ventricle. The anterior horn* (AH) *and occipital horn* (LV) *of the lateral ventricle are both dilated. Note the dangling choroid* (arrow). *The lateral ventricle on the side closest to the transducer cannot be seen well due to reverberation artefact. It is also dilated.*

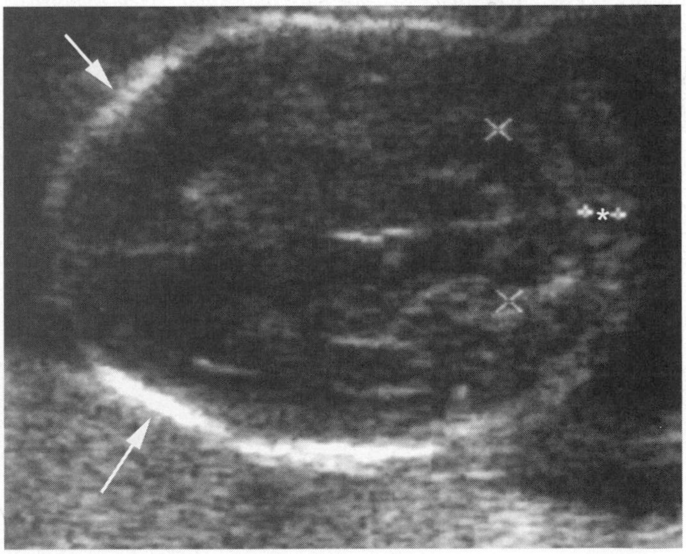

Figure 45-41. ■ *Arnold-Chiari type II malformation. Although the lateral ventricles are not dilated, other features of Arnold-Chiari malformation are seen. The cerebellum (between markers) is banana shaped. The anterior part of the skull* (arrows) *slopes, giving it a lemon shape. The cisterna magna is extremely small* (*). *These early findings secondary to spina bifida may be seen when the spinal changes are absent.*

4. There is usually a "lemon" shape to the skull with a narrower anterior portion
5. Overall small cranial size. In general, small head size associated with ventricular dilation suggests atrophy, but in a case of Arnold-Chiari malformation, considerable ventriculomegaly can be present, although the overall head size is smaller than expected.

Hydranencephaly. Hydranencephaly is an uncommon anomaly and is lethal (Fig. 45-42). It is due to an infarct of the brain's cortex.

The sonographic features are as follows:

1. No cortical mantle; a membrane surrounding the fluid where the cortex should be (the dura) can be mistaken for brain tissue.
2. No midline intrahemispheric septum and falx

In hydranencephaly, the brainstem is visible, as are cerebral peduncles and variable amounts of the thalamus and midbrain. There is no third or fourth ventricular dilation. The brainstem structures protrude into the fluid that replaces the brain in a characteristic fashion (Fig. 45-42).

Holoprosencephaly. Holoprosencephaly is a malformation with a dismal prognosis—death if the case is severe, mental retardation if it is mild (Figs. 45-43 and

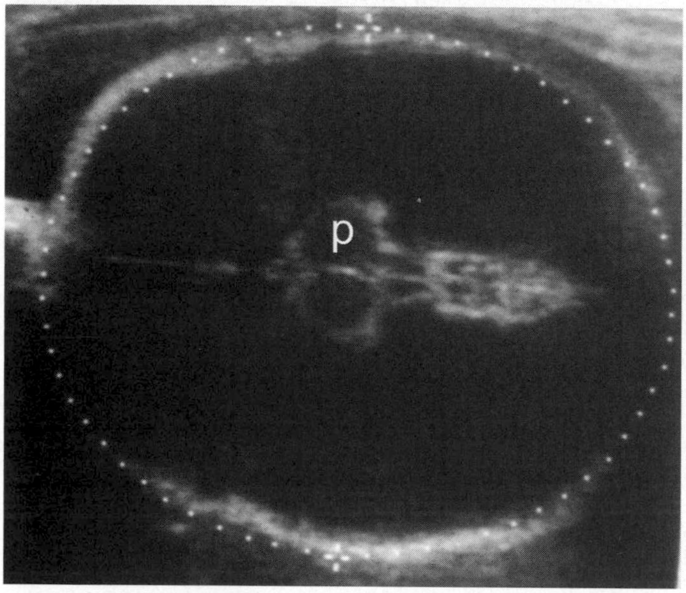

Figure 45-42. ■ *Hydranencephaly. Most of the brain tissue is absent. Only the brainstem structures such as the cerebral peduncles* (p) *remain. Sometimes, the falx persists, but it is often absent. (Reprinted with permission form Sanders RC, ed.* Structural Fetal Abnormalities: The Total Picture, *2nd ed. New York: Mosby-Year Book Publishers, 2002.)*

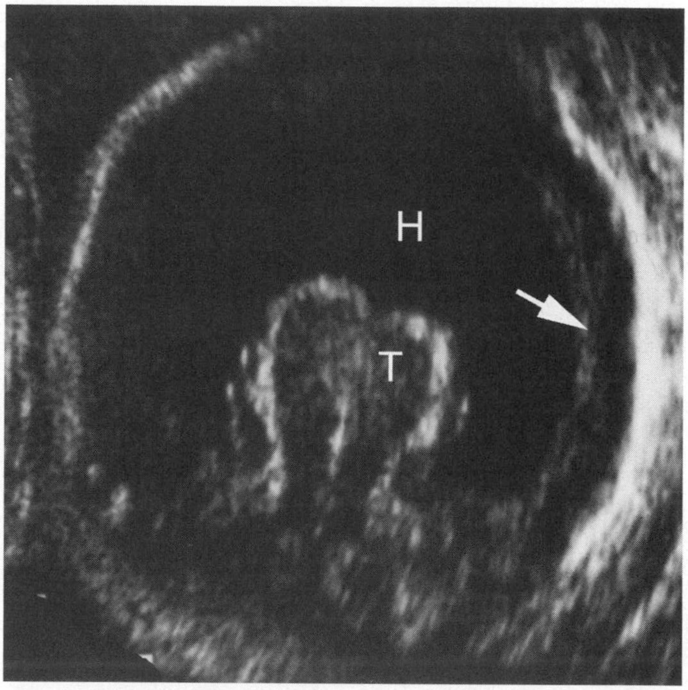

Figure 45-43. ■ *Alobar holoprosencephaly. Coronal view (best shows the horseshoe shape, although it does not show the dorsal cyst or hippocampal ridge). There is a single horseshoe-shaped ventricle* (H) *with a small cortical mantle* (arrow). *The thalami* (T) *are fused with no complete septum or third ventricle between them.*

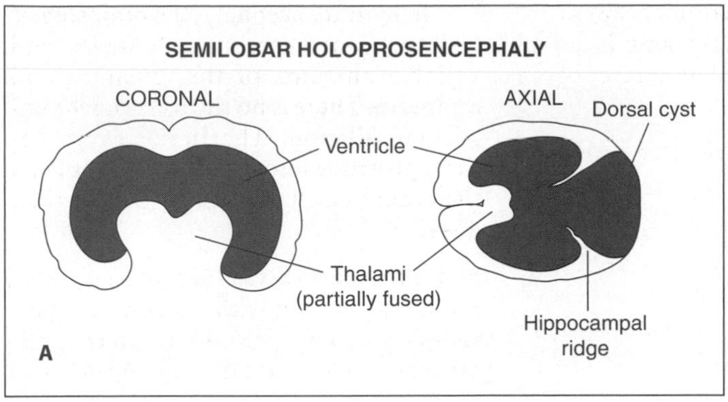

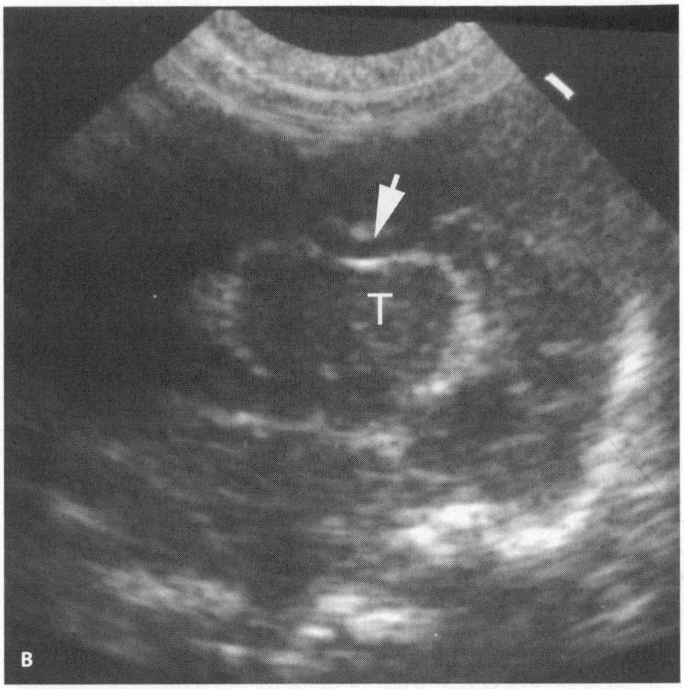

Figure 45-44. ■ *A. Diagram showing the components of semilobar holoprosencephaly. Notice the dorsal cyst separated from the main portion of the single ventricle by the hippocampal ridge. B. Lobar holoprosencephaly. In this mild version, the ventricles are not dilated, but there is a single horseshoe-shaped ventricle* (arrow), *and the thalami are fused* (T) *with no third ventricle. Coronal view.*

45-44). There is a strong association with trisomy 13. The sonographic features are characteristic:

1. A single horseshoe-shaped ventricle that may be so large that there is virtually no mantle (alobar) (Fig. 45-43), a variably sized and asymmetrical horseshoe-shaped ventricle (lobar) (Fig. 45-44), or a common ventricle that is fused only posteriorly (semilobar).
2. Fused thalami with no third ventricle visible.
3. A ridge along the lateral border of the ventricle known as the *hippocampal ridge*.
4. A bulge along the posterior aspect of the common ventricle, known as the *dorsal cyst* or *sac*, is seen in the alobar form. Whereas cortical mantle may be seen lining the anterior portion of the skull, none may be seen posteriorly.
5. Absence of corpus callosum and cavum septum pellucidi.
6. Often unusually close together orbits (hypotelorism) or only a single orbit (cyclops) (see Appendices 17 and 18).
7. Often, a central cleft palate or cleft lip (see Fig. 45-75).
8. Often no nose, which is replaced by a proboscis lying above the eyes. If the nose is present, a single nostril may be seen.
9. Other anomalies such as clubfoot or omphalocele are often seen—also IUGR, because trisomy 13 is a common association.
10. In the milder form, which can be subtle, the only finding is the absence of the septum pellucidum and the cavum septum pellucidum.

Dandy-Walker Cyst. Dandy-Walker cyst is due to a cerebellar abnormality (Fig. 45-45A,B). Mental deficiency is common in survivors. Chromosomal anomalies may be associated. The sonographic features are as follows:

1. Cystic enlargement of the fourth ventricle. The cisterna magna is enlarged above a 10-mm distance. The hypoplastic cerebellum and vermis are separated by a fluid-filled tubular structure that may be small or large and extends from the fourth ventricle to the cisterna magna.
2. Dilation of the third ventricle and aqueduct may be present.

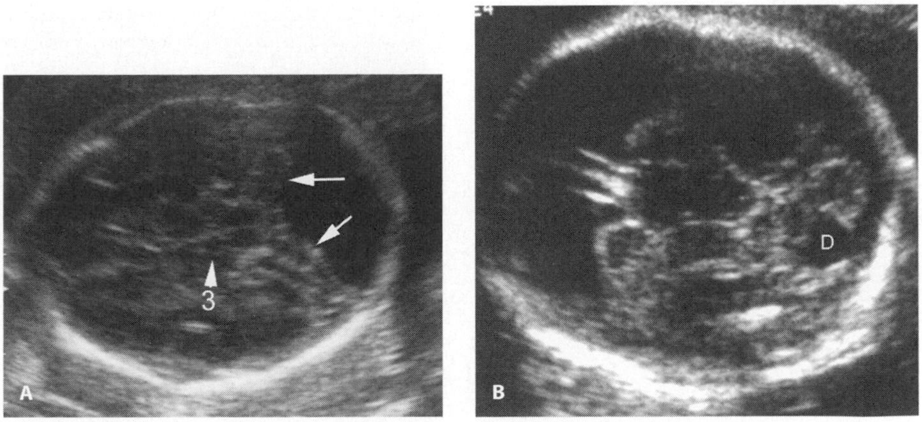

Figure 45-45. ■ *A. Dandy-Walker cyst. In this mild case of Dandy-Walker syndrome, the lateral ventricles are not dilated; however, the third ventricle* (3) *is slightly enlarged. The vermis* (arrows) *of the cerebellum are small and the cisterna magna is much enlarged. B. Another example of mild Dandy-Walker syndrome. The Dandy-Walker cyst* (D) *is much smaller, but the vermis are again decreased in size.*

3. Dilation of the lateral ventricles to a variable degree.
4. The cerebellar lobes, particularly the vermis, are split apart, smaller than usual, and are abnormal in shape.
5. Agenesis of the corpus callosum is an important and difficult-to-diagnose association. If agenesis (see Fig. 45-50) is present, the chance of mental retardation is much increased. Agenesis of the corpus callosum is described later in this chapter.

Vein of Galen Aneurysm. A large arteriovenous malformation, a vein of Galen aneurysm, causes high-output congestive failure (Fig. 45-46A,B).

The lesion is rare and is usually fatal at birth, despite surgery. The sonographic features are as follows:

1. Posterior midline pulsatile structure connected to a central tubular vascular space extending posteriorly from above the thalamus to a vein called the *straight sinus* superior to the cerebellum.
2. Pulsatile flow on Doppler with arterial and venous components within the vein.
3. Numerous collateral arteries supplying the vein will be seen. Attempt to define the number and location of the supplying vessels with color flow.
4. Possible compression of the aqueduct by the cyst may cause secondary ventriculomegaly.
5. Enlarged heart and vessels supplying the brain (e.g., the carotid artery).
6. Fetal ascites and pleural effusion are possible secondary consequences.

Porencephalic Cyst and Intracranial Hemorrhage. Porencephalic cysts are a sequel to an intraparenchymal bleed. A cystic area forms that communicates with the ventricle.

1. The ventricle bulges at the site of a porencephalic cyst.
2. Echogenic clot may be seen in the porencephalic cyst, the brain, or the dilated ventricle.

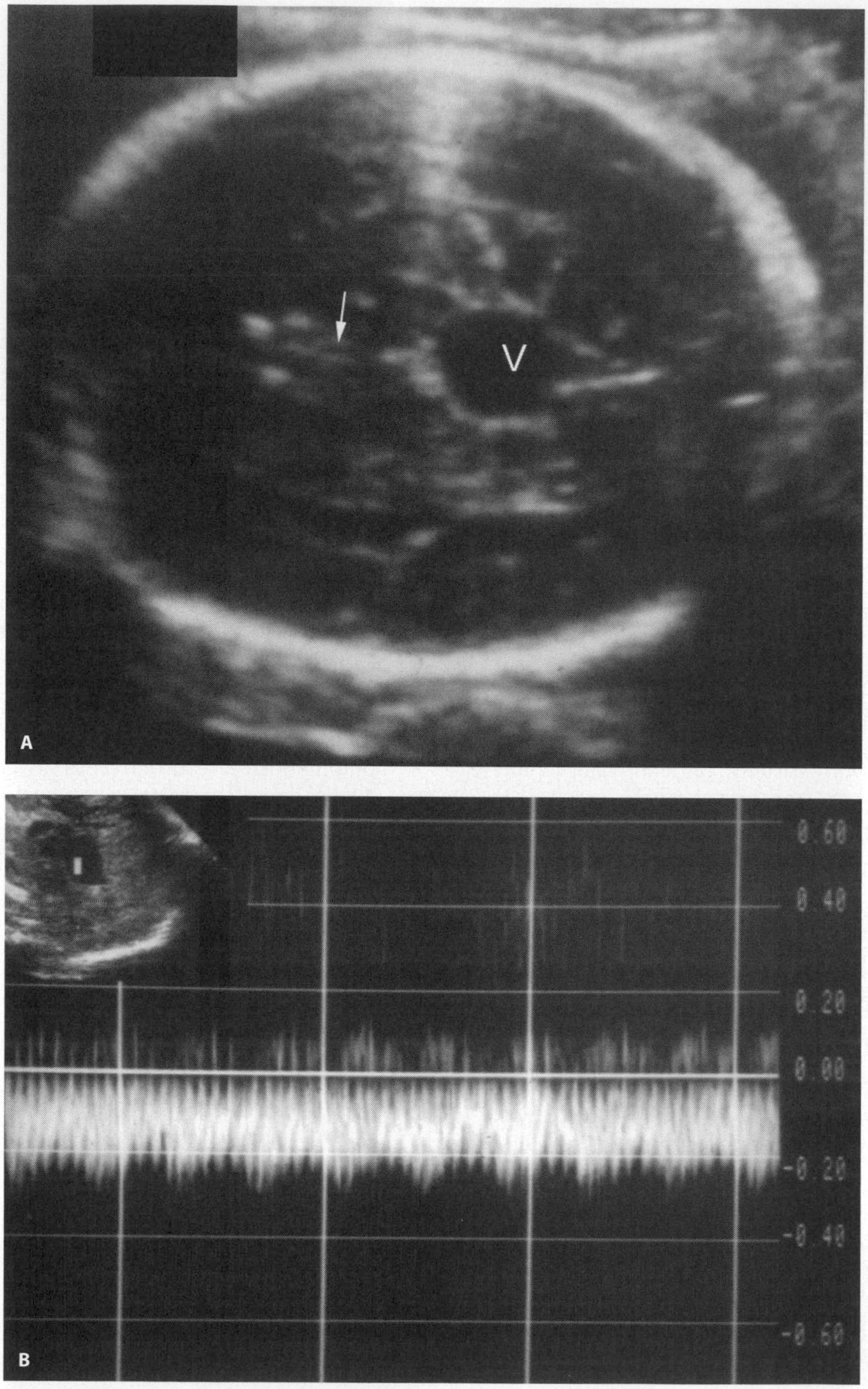

Figure 45-46. ■ *A. Vein of Galen aneurysm. The large cyst* (V) *posterior to the third ventricle* (arrow) *is the clue to the presence of this syndrome. B. Use of Doppler with vein of Galen aneurysm. Either color Doppler or pulsed Doppler will show flow within a vein of Galen aneurysm differentiating the cyst from a normal variant quadrigeminal cyst or arachnoid cyst, which can lie close to where the vein of Galen aneurysm normally forms.*

3. Bleeding into the brain causes an echogenic mass (Fig. 45-47).
4. If any intraventricular bleeding occurs, the ventricles dilate and echogenic clot can be seen within the lateral and third ventricles. Blood can rarely pass through the narrow aqueduct of Sylvius and often results in obstruction at this level.

Arachnoid Cyst. An arachnoid cyst is a fluid-filled space within the brain substance not communicating with the ventricles. This cystic area can be of any shape. Arachnoid cysts arise from the meninges, so a common location is alongside the tentorium (Fig. 45-48). Secondary hydrocephalus can occur. Infratentorial arachnoid cysts can mimic Dandy-Walker syndrome if they are in the midline and low, but the vermis and cerebellum will be present.

Agenesis of the Corpus Callosum. Agenesis of the corpus callosum with associated cyst may look awful, but when isolated, it does not cause symptoms

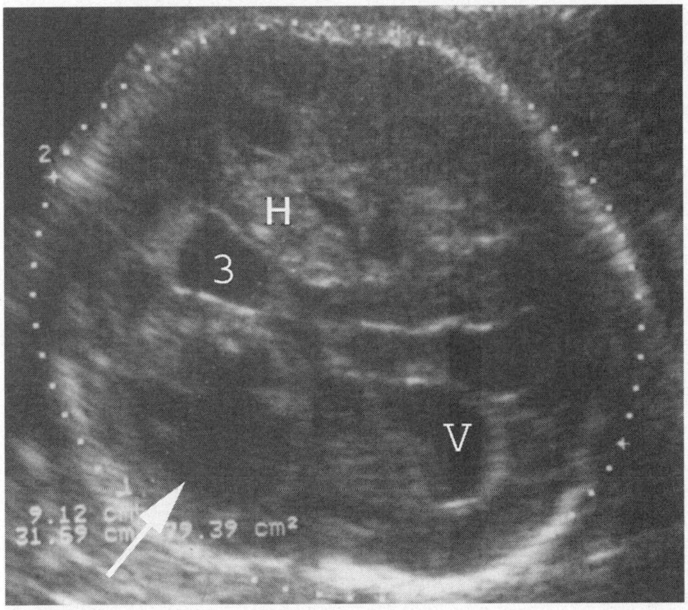

Figure 45-47. ■ *Intracranial hemorrhage. The hemorrhage* (H) *has resulted in ventricular dilation* (V) (arrow). *The third ventricle* (3) *is enlarged. Note the echogenic border to the ventricles—a consequence of the hemorrhage. (Reprinted with permission form Sanders RC, ed.* Structural Fetal Abnormalities: The Total Picture, *2nd ed. New York: Mosby-Year Book Publishers, 2002.)*

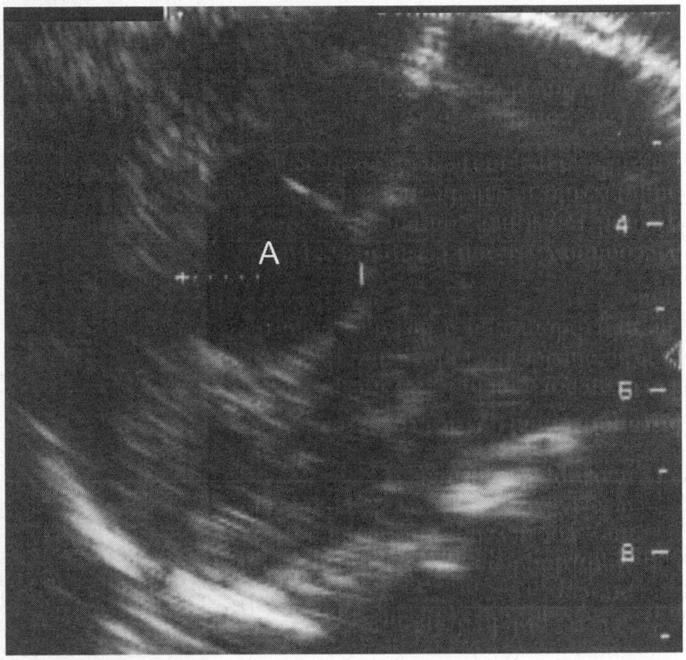

Figure 45-48. ■ *Arachnoid cyst. The cyst* (A) *relates to the meninges. In this case, it lies alongside the tentorium on this sagittal view. Although an arachnoid cyst may cause secondary hydrocephalus, none was present in this case.*

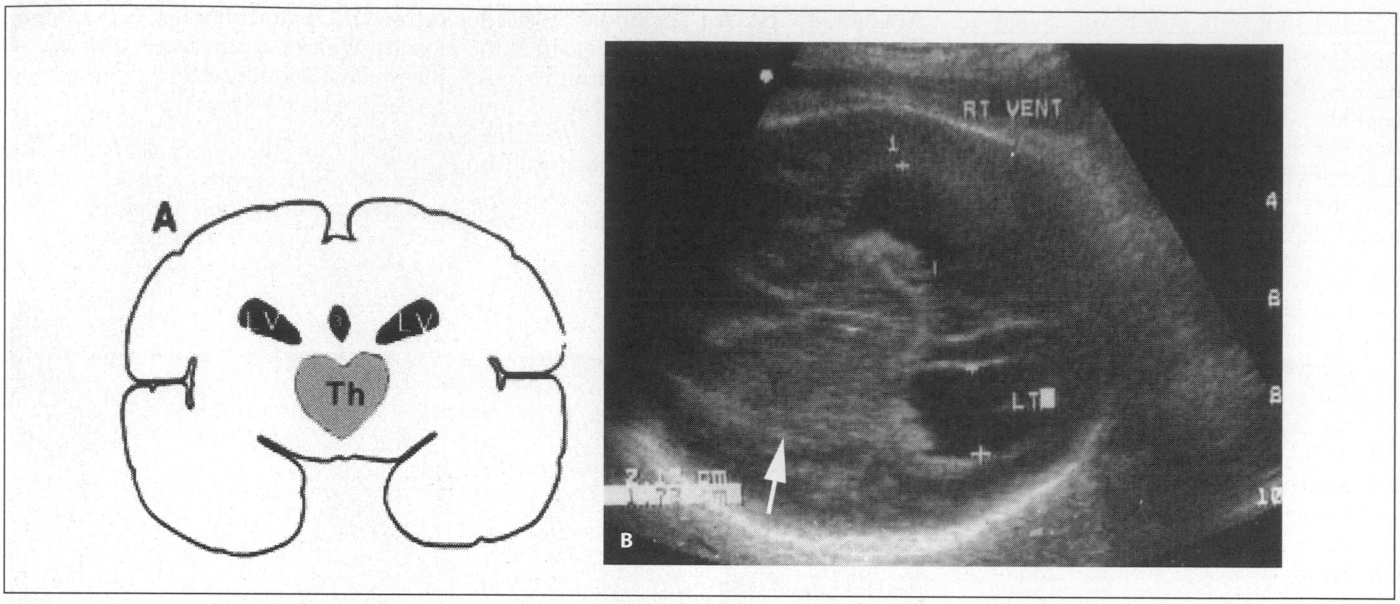

Figure 45-49. ■ *Agenesis of the corpus callosum.* ***A.*** *Coronal view. Standard form of agenesis of the corpus callosum. Note the high position of the third ventricle* (3) *located between the lateral ventricles* (LV) *and lying above the thalamus* (Th). ***B.*** *Colpocephaly. The occipital horns are dilated (see measurement markers), but the anterior horns are normal* (arrow).

apart from occasional epilepsy (Fig. 45-49A,B). Agenesis of the corpus callosum is associated with trisomy syndromes, cardiac anomalies, and a number of cranial conditions. If agenesis is present, it usually worsens the prognosis. The sonographic findings are as follows:

1. Increased separation of the lateral ventricles.
2. Enlargement of the occipital horns and atria (colpocephaly) (Fig. 45-49). Confusion with hydrocephalus is possible.
3. Upward displacement of the third ventricle.
4. Abnormal gyral pattern. The gyri radiate superiorly from the lateral ventricles rather than lie parallel to the lateral ventricles (Fig. 45-50).
5. Possible superior cystic enlargement of the third ventricle (Fig. 45-49A).

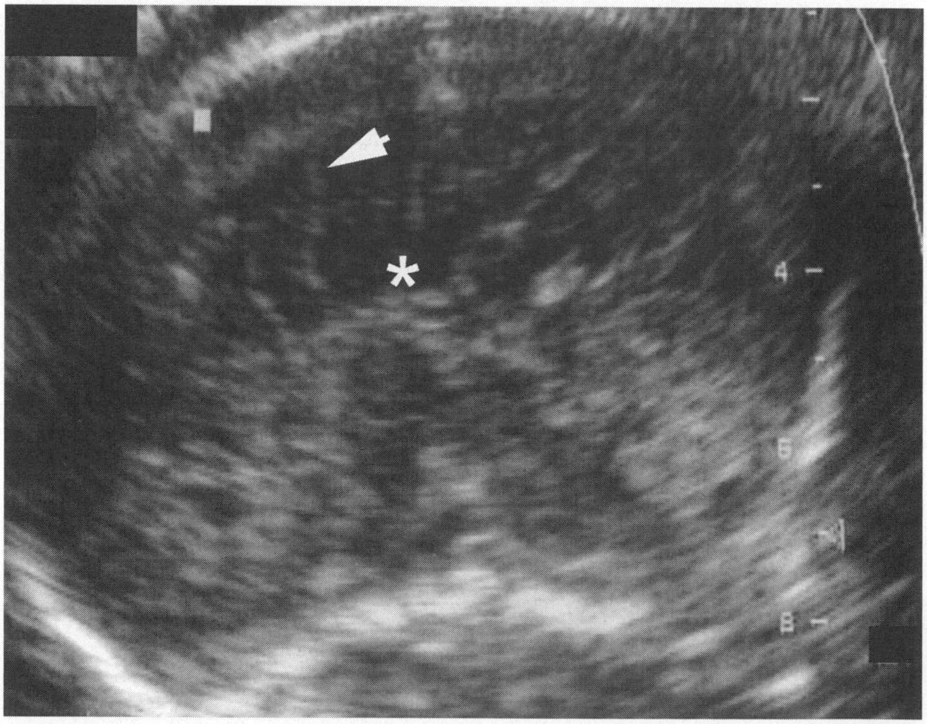

Figure 45-50. ■ *Agenesis of the corpus callosum. The gyri are vertically rather than horizontally aligned* (arrow). *The corpus callosum is not seen on this sagittal view. The asterisk marks the site where the corpus callosum would normally be seen.*

HEAD AND BRAIN MALFORMATIONS

Anencephaly. Only the structures at the base of the brain are present in anencephaly. This brain malformation is thought to be a consequence of the absence of skull formation. The malformation has a different appearance and name, depending on when it is detected.

1. At 11 to 13 weeks, acrania is seen (see Fig. 45-52). No skull is formed. Although a normal amount of brain is present, it has an irregular lobular outline because it is unconfined by the skull.
2. At 14 to 16 weeks, exencephaly is present (see Fig. 45-52). The brain remnant is smaller, and it is now obvious that the skull is absent.
3. From 17 weeks on, anencephaly is present (Figs. 45-51 and 45-52). A "nubbin" of tissue is visible at the cranial end of the trunk. The cerebral hemispheres and cranial vault (skull) are absent. The cranial blood vessels persist and form a vascular mound at the superior aspect of the remaining fetal cranial tissue. When the fetus is

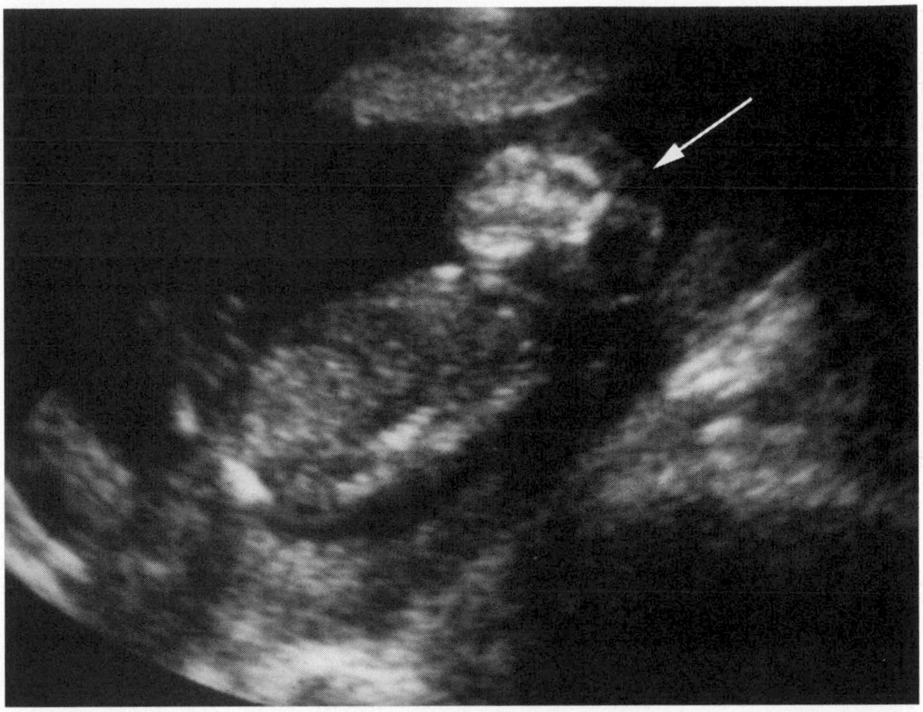

Figure 45-51. ■ *Anencephaly. The skull bones are absent* (arrow), *and the amount of cranial tissue is decreased. (Reprinted with permission form Sanders RC, ed.* Structural Fetal Abnormalities: The Total Picture, *2nd ed. New York: Mosby-Year Book Publishers, 2002.)*

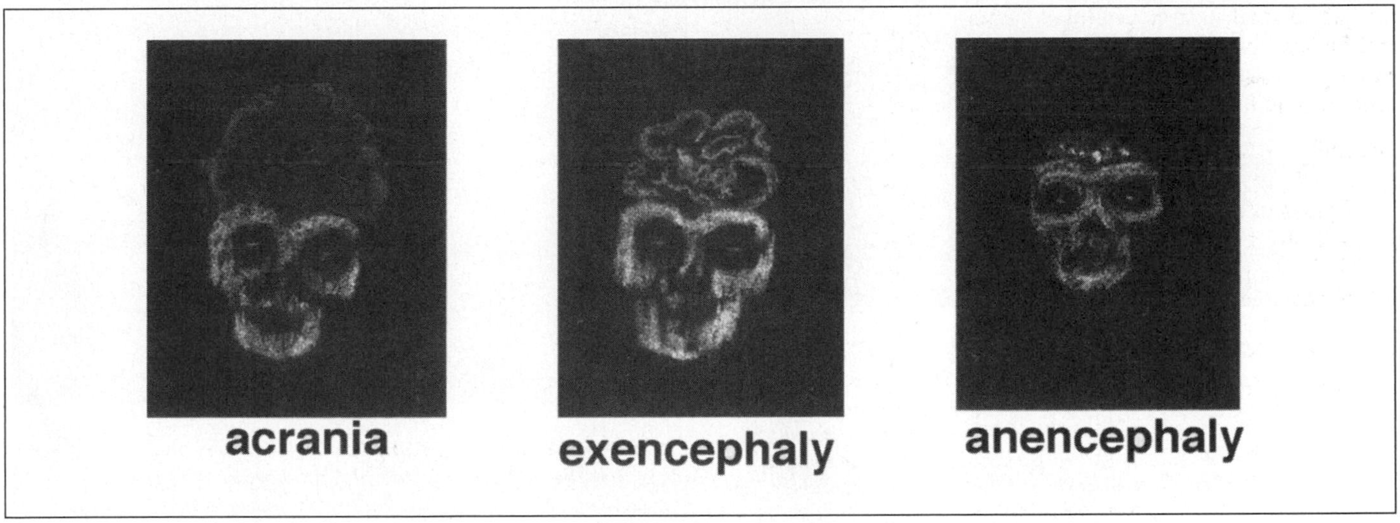

Figure 45-52. ■ *Diagram of anencephaly variants as seen face on. In acrania, the skull is absent. All of the brain is present, but it tends to protrude to the left or right because nothing confines it. In exencephaly, some of the brain is absent. Some has been removed, presumably by trauma. In anencephaly, only a small central bulge occurs above the level of the orbits, representing the blood vessels in the brain, which withstand damage from other structures.*

supine, the facial structures end superiorly with the orbits. When the fetus is prone, the fetal head appears to end with the superior aspect of the spine. Polyhydramnios with much fetal movement is present if fetal swallowing is impaired by brain destruction. Anencephaly is associated with spina bifida and iniencephaly.

Iniencephaly. This rare condition is often associated with anencephaly. The fetal head is retroflexed because there are too few cervical vertebra. The cervical vertebra are unfused with a meningocele present (rachischisis) (Fig. 45-53).

Microcephaly. The head and brain are too small in microcephaly, resulting in mental retardation. The sonographic findings are not straightforward:

1. The cranium is small. Deciding whether the head is small enough to be of concern is not easy. The head may be quite small (greater than two standard deviations below the mean) as a normal variant. An abnormally low head-to-trunk ratio (three standard deviations or less) strongly suggests that the fetus is microcephalic. Serial sonograms show a progressively small head in comparison to the trunk and limbs (Fig. 45-54). The diagnosis can usually not be made before 24 weeks.
2. Ventriculomegaly with a small head is diagnostic of microcephaly. The ventricles dilate because the brain is becoming atrophic. A normal-sized cranium with enlarged ventricles may well be due to atrophy rather than obstruction.
3. Calcification may be seen alongside the ventricle if the cause of microcephaly is cytomegalic inclusion disease. In microcephaly due to toxoplasmosis, there is patchy calcification within the brain.

Intracranial Tumors. Fetal intracranial tumors are rare. Intracranial teratomas are seen as cystic and echogenic areas distributed randomly throughout a greatly enlarged head. Choroid plexus papilloma appears as a bright echogenic mass adjacent to the choroid within the lateral ventricle, with secondary hydrocephalus.

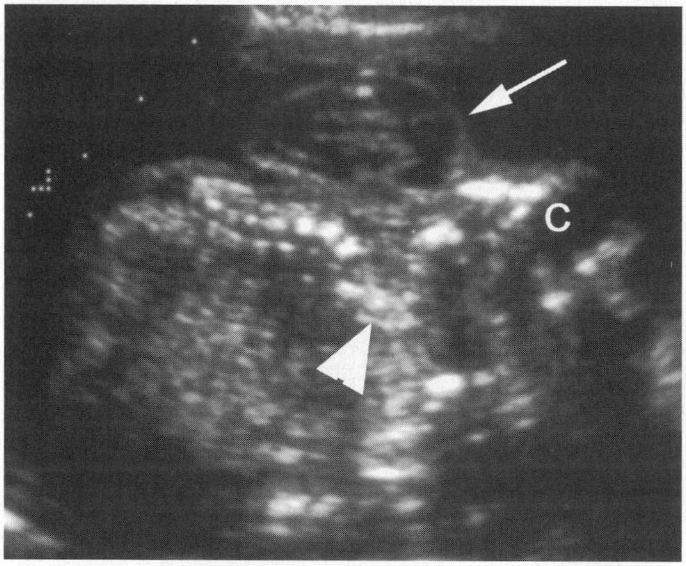

Figure 45-53. ■ *Iniencephaly. There is a severe gibbus deformity* (thick arrow). *Few cervical vertebra are present. An encephalocele* (arrow) *arises from the posterior aspect of the cervical spine and the occipital area of the head* (C). *There was also anencephaly. (Reprinted with permission form Sanders RC, ed.* Structural Fetal Abnormalities: The Total Picture, *2nd ed. New York: Mosby-Year Book Publishers, 2002.)*

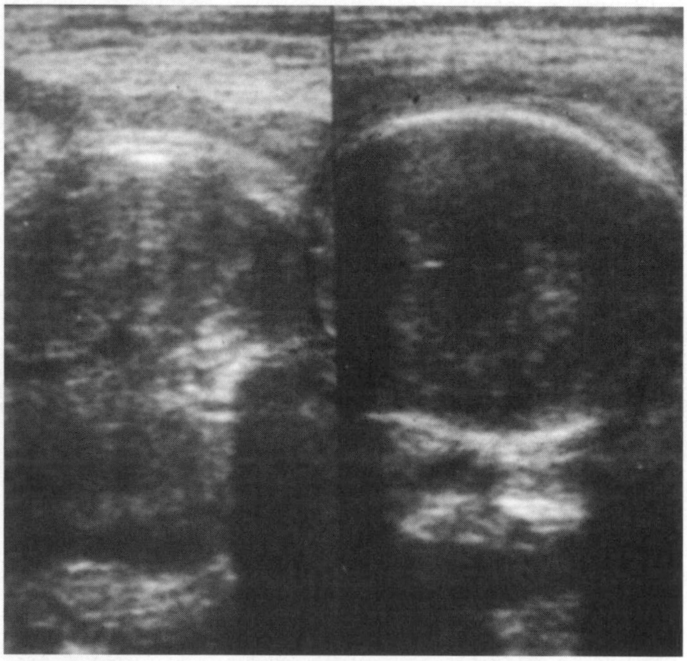

Figure 45-54. ■ *Microcephaly. The fetal abdomen (to the left) is much larger than the fetal head (to the right). In this case of microcephaly, there was no ventriculomegaly, but there was severe mental retardation.*

MASS ARISING FROM THE HEAD OR NECK

Encephalocele

1. With encephalocele, a defect is present, usually in the posterior aspect of the skull, through which portions of the brain substance and perhaps the ventricle prolapse (Fig. 45-55). Encephaloceles usually contain cerebrospinal fluid, but they may contain brain tissue, in which case the prognosis is much worse.
2. The head is often small (microcephaly).
3. Secondary hydrocephalus is a common associated finding.
4. Look for multiple fingers or toes (polydactyly) and enlarged kidneys containing cysts, the main components of the lethal Meckel-Gruber syndrome.
5. A few encephaloceles are on the lateral aspect of the head. Look for an amniotic band if this is the case. Additional features of the amniotic bands such as truncated or swollen limbs, club feet, and cleft palate may be seen.
6. A rare form of encephalocele protrudes between the eyes in an anterior location.

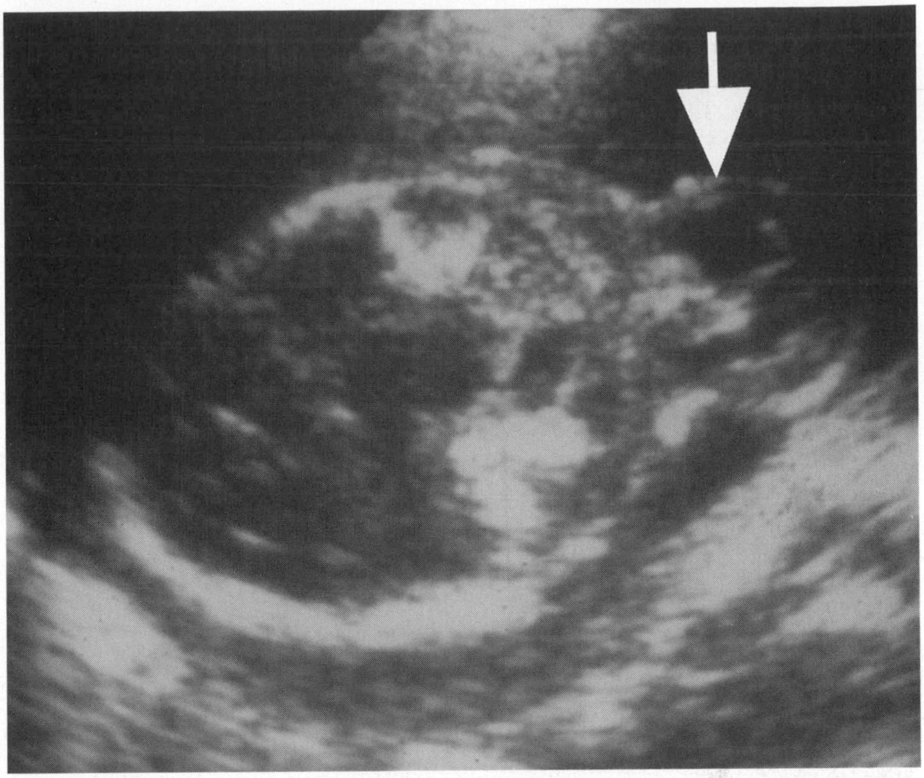

Figure 45-55. ■ *Encephalocele. The occipital encephalocele* (arrow) *protrudes from the cranium posterior to the cerebellum. It contains fluid and some brain tissue, worsening the prognosis.*

Cystic Hygroma. Defective formation of the lymphatic system leads to a buildup of lymph in the neck. Bilateral cysts develop in the neck (Fig. 45-56A,B).

1. In a mild form of cystic hygroma, there is a small cystic area in the posterolateral or posterior aspect of the neck.

   Chromosomal analysis often shows Turner's or Down syndrome when this is an isolated finding. Such cystic hygromas often regress over the course of the pregnancy and disappear.
2. In the more severe form, large cysts on the posterior aspect of both sides of the neck may be in contact with each other (Fig. 45-56A). The find-

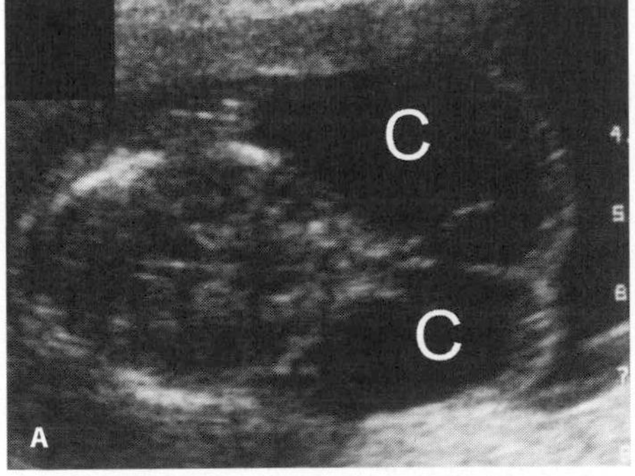

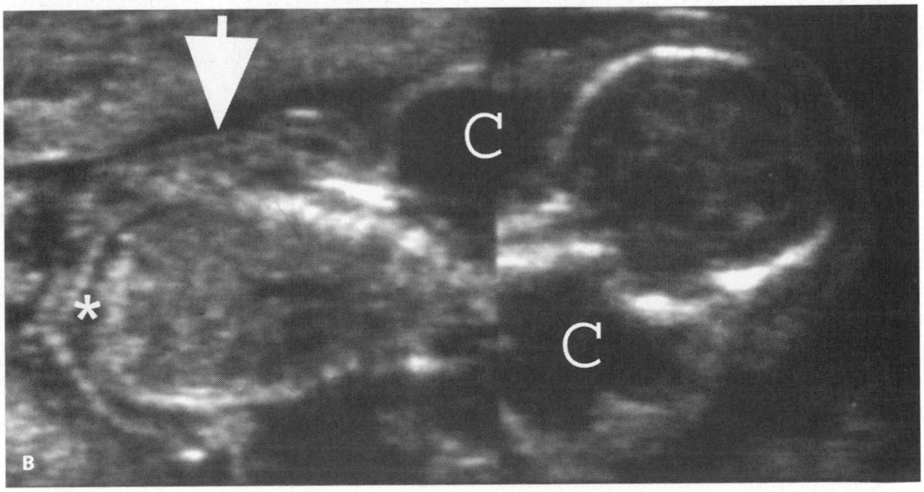

Figure 45-56. ■ *A. Cystic hygroma. The two large cystic structures posterior to the skull* (C) *are large lymphoceles.* ***B.*** *Small cystic hygromas. Combined linear array views. There are two cystic hygromas on either side of the neck* (C)*. When they enlarge, they meet in the midline as in part A. There is marked skin thickening* (arrow) *and a small amount of ascites* (*)*. (A and B are reprinted with permission form Sanders RC, ed.* Structural Fetal Abnormalities: The Total Picture, *2nd ed. New York: Mosby-Year Book Publishers, 2002.)*

ings of hydrops are present (i.e., pleural effusion, ascites, skin thickening, and pericardial effusion).
3. Severe skin thickening is seen. Multiple septa are seen within the thickened skin, sometimes with small cystic areas where lymph has pooled.
4. When hydrops is present as well as cystic hygroma, the condition is always fatal within a few weeks of diagnosis.

Goiter

1. Enlargement of the thyroid leads to a solid mass on the anterior aspect of the neck, often causing head extension.
2. There is severe polyhydramnios, because the neck mass impedes swallowing.
3. A goiter is smooth-bordered and evenly textured. The thyroid gland lies on either side of the fetal trachea. There are normal standards for thyroid size (see Appendix 27).

Teratoma of the Neck. A solid mass of varied echo texture is seen in the anterior neck region when a teratoma of the neck is present. This rare mass usually extends from the jaw to the clavicle.

LIMB SHORTENING

Micromelia is the term used when all limbs and portions of limbs are short. *Mesomelia* is the term used when the distal limbs are most short, and *rhizomelia* is used when the proximal long bones are most affected (Fig. 45-57). These different patterns are associated with different types of dwarfism.

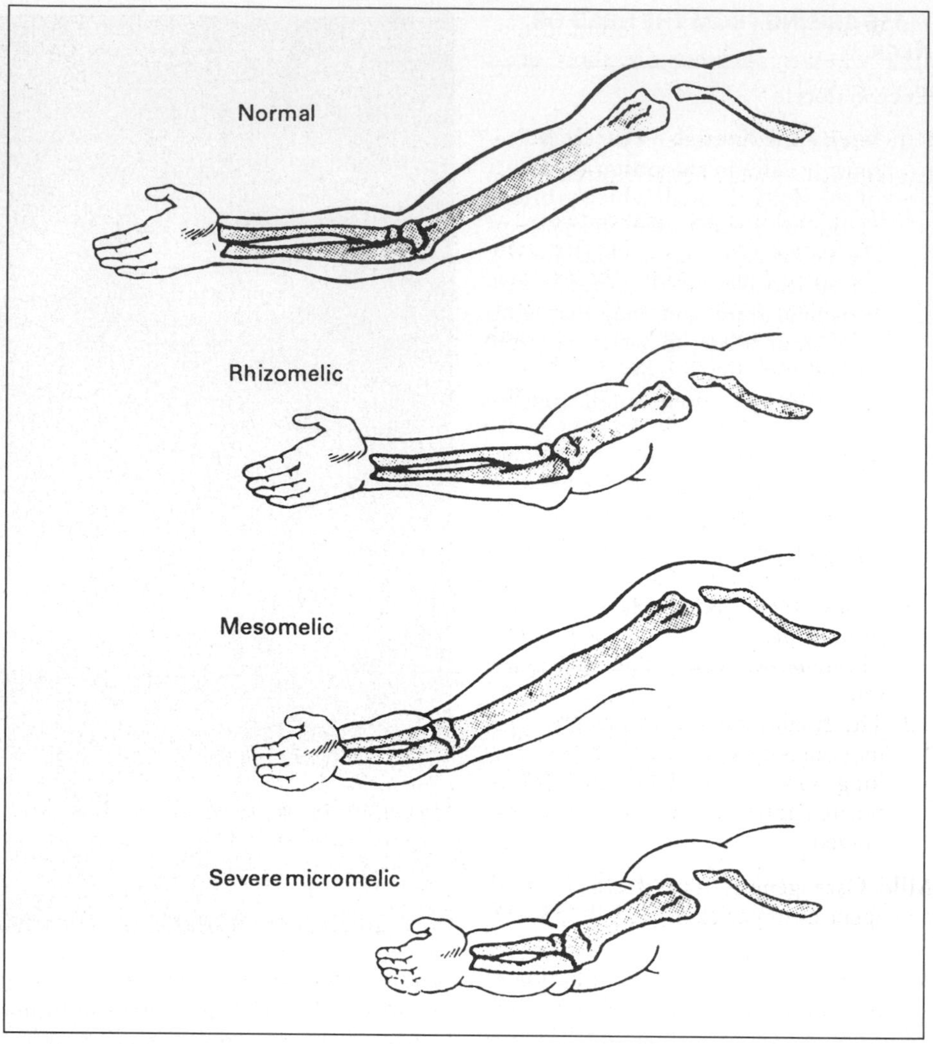

Figure 45-57. ■ *Diagram showing the different types of limb shortening that can occur. The shortening may be only in the proximal limbs (rhizomelia), only in the distal long bones (mesomelia), or throughout the limbs (micromelia). (Reprinted with permission from R. Romero.)*

When a short limb is found, determine whether all limbs are short or if there are only one or two.

Shortening Confined to a Few Limbs

Familial Rhizomelic Limb Shortening

1. If the humerus and femur are mildly shortened (between the 5th and 10th percentile), look at the parents. It is likely that they will also have short proximal limbs. This is a common normal variant.
2. This finding is associated with Down syndrome. Look for other findings of Down syndrome. If this is the only finding, amniocentesis is not usually recommended.

Focal Femoral Deficiency

1. One of the femurs is very short and usually angulated at the midportion. The femoral head is sometimes absent.
2. The fibula and sometimes the tibia may also be short or absent. Other long bones such as the arms or opposite femur may occasionally be involved.

Mild Osteogenesis Imperfecta. In mild osteogenesis imperfecta (Figs. 45-58 and

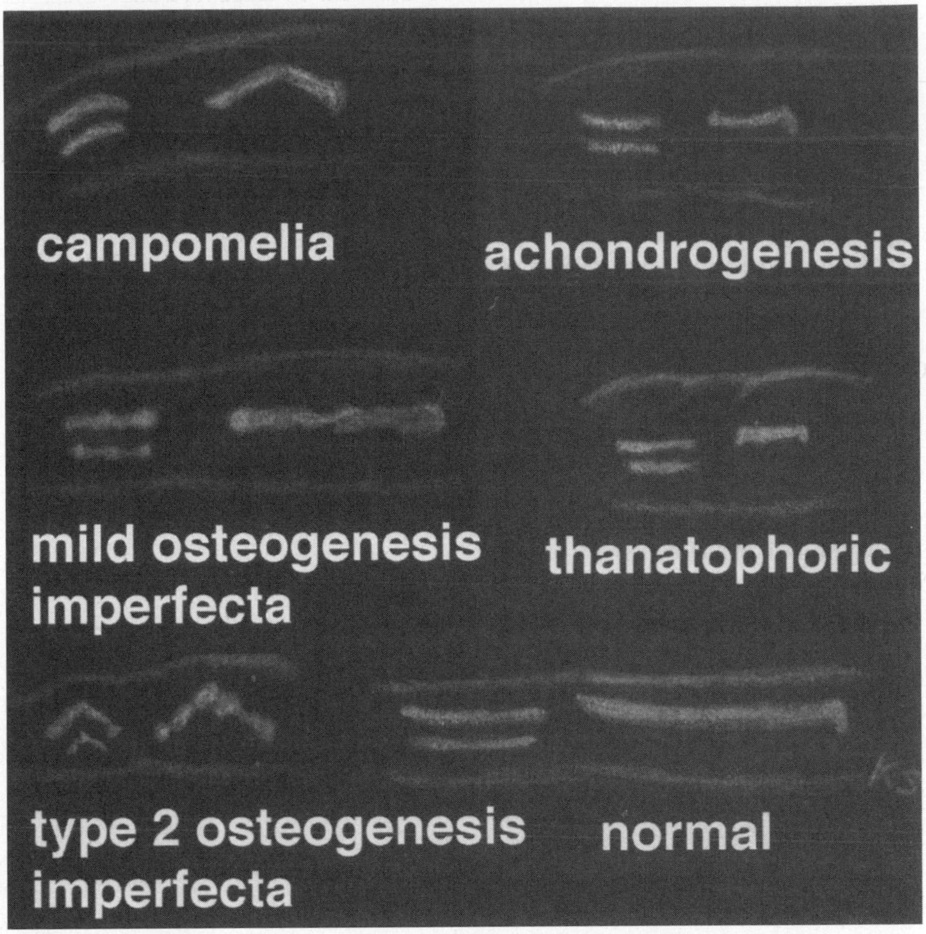

Figure 45-58. ■ *Long bones in various types of dwarfism. In camptomelic dwarfism, the femur is acutely bowed, and the tibia is evenly bowed. Both proximal and distal limbs are mildly shortened. In achondrogenesis, all limbs are extremely short with excessive soft tissues. In mild osteogenesis imperfecta, there is some long bone irregularity and thanatophoric dwarfism; the limbs are extremely short with a telephone receiver appearance to the femur. In type 2 osteogenesis imperfecta, the limbs are very short. Multiple irregularities and fractures are visible. A normal femur, tibia, and fibula are shown for comparison.*

45-59), the following conditions are present:

1. One or more limbs are shortened to a variable extent.
2. The disease tends to affect the lower limbs, notably the femur.
3. The limb is deformed by one or more of the following: bowing, a fracture, a locally thickened midshaft bulge due to callus formation, and overall bony irregularity related to previous fractures.

Generalized Limb Shortening

The severity of the limb shortening may be such that the dwarfism is lethal. Lethal dwarfism is present when the limbs are exceedingly short and, more importantly, when there is severe polyhydramnios and the chest is very small (chest circumference less than 0.081 of abdominal circumference).

Lethal Dwarfisms

There are numerous rare forms of lethal dwarfism. Only the most common and easily recognizable forms will be described.

Thanatophoric Dwarfism. Thanatophoric dwarfism is the most common lethal dwarfism, with the following features (Figs. 45-58 and 45-60):

1. Grossly shortened, bowed limbs. The femur, which is more shortened than the tibia and fibula, usually has a "telephone receiver" shape.
2. Tiny chest with normal-sized abdomen, giving a bell shape to the trunk.
3. Severe polyhydramnios thought to be due to compression of the esophagus by the small chest.
4. Flattened vertebrae. These are difficult to recognize with ultrasound, but they can be seen on a fetal x-ray. On ultrasound, the vertebrae appear unduly close together.
5. Redundant soft tissues. It would appear that the normal quantity of soft tissue surrounds a very short limb.
6. In a rarer form (type 2 thanatophoric dwarfism), the limbs are not as severely shortened and are not bowed. A bulge off the top of the head occurs, a deformity known as a *cloverleaf skull* or *Kleeblattschädel deformity*. This malformation is due to the fusion of some of the skull structures. Cloverleaf changes are seen

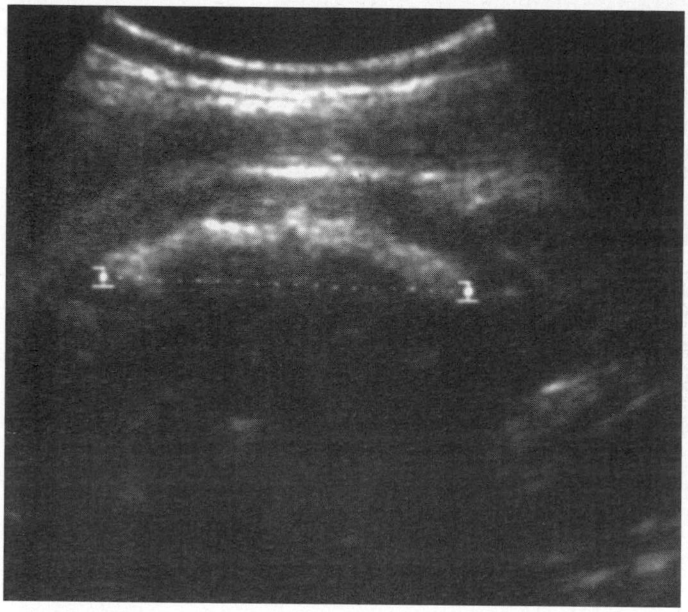

Figure 45-59. ■ *Osteogenesis imperfecta. The femur (between markers) is bowed and has an irregular contour. Several old fractures have left callus and a deformed outline. The femur is shortened for gestational age. (Reprinted with permission form Sanders RC, ed.* Structural Fetal Abnormalities: The Total Picture, *2nd ed. New York: Mosby-Year Book Publishers, 2002.)*

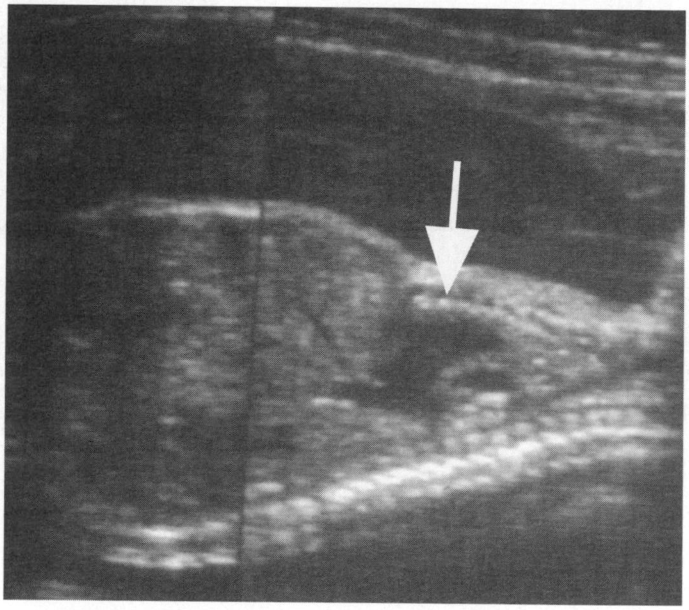

Figure 45-60. ■ *Thanatophoric dwarf. Sagittal view of the chest and abdomen. The heart* (arrow) *is much compressed by the small chest, whereas the abdomen is normal sized (bell-shaped trunk).*

only in this infrequent form, but the head is always large in thanatophoric dwarfism.
7. Short and stubby fingers (triradiate) and feet.

Achondrogenesis

1. Findings in achondrogenesis are similar to those in thanatophoric dwarfism (Fig. 45-58).
2. In the most common variety, the spine is very poorly ossified.
3. Thickening of the skin at the back of the neck occurs with even the formation of a cyst. Hydrops may be present.
4. This condition is always lethal.

Osteogenesis Imperfecta (Lethal Recessive Form)

1. The limbs and ribs are very short with multiple fractures, bowing, and irregular contours (Fig. 45-5).
2. The skull is poorly ossified, so the brain is seen too well. Brain structure close to the transducer and the near skull border can be easily seen. Light transducer pressure over the fetal head will deform the skull.
3. The chest is small, and there are numerous rib fractures.
4. The spine is poorly ossified.
5. Polyhydramnios may be present if the chest is very small.

Nonlethal Dwarfisms

Achondroplasia

1. In the usual heterozygous form of achondroplasia, the limbs do not become short until after 24 weeks. The proximal limbs are more shortened than the distal limbs (rhizomelic shortening). The head is large, and the ventricles may be mildly dilated, as in hydrocephalus.
2. In the homozygous form, in which both parents are achondroplastic dwarfs, the limbs are very short, and the disease is fatal. This condition is indistinguishable (except by family history) from thanatophoric dwarfism.

Phocomelia. The long bones are missing in phocomelia, and the hands and feet arise from the shoulder or hips.

Limb/Body Wall Defect Syndrome (Cyllosoma). The limb/body wall defect syndrome, a lethal multisystem disease, is thought to be due to amnion disruption occurring in the first 2 months of pregnancy. The components are as follows.

1. A variant of gastroschisis in which the liver as well as the small bowel and possibly the heart are outside the abdominal wall.
2. Myelomeningocele, sometimes with hydrocephalus.
3. Absence of one or more limbs.
4. Gross twisting of the spine (kyphoscoliosis), sometimes with loss of the sacrum (caudal regression).
5. Sometimes, amniotic bands are visible.

There is usually oligohydramnios, which, combined with the twisted short spine, makes an examination very difficult.

BLOOD TESTS OR MATERNAL AGE SUSPICIOUS FOR DOWN SYNDROME

The triple screen is a combination of the AFP, estriol, and HCG levels. If estriol and HCG levels are increased and the AFP is depressed, the risk of Down syndrome is increased. A maternal age of over 35 (some would say 32) also increases the risk of Down syndrome (see Table 17-1).

There are several ultrasonic signs that make the diagnosis of Down syndrome more likely. Absence of these signs diminishes the risk for Down syndrome.

Down Syndrome Signs (Trisomy 21)

1. Short femur and humerus length. If the femur and humerus length are less than 0.91 of the expected femur or humerus length for the gesta-

tional age, the risk of Down syndrome is increased.
2. Thickening of the skin on the back of the neck seen on the cerebellar view. A distance of greater than 6 mm is a strong sign of Down syndrome. Skin thickening in this area is most pronounced at 11 to 13 weeks; a long, thin echogenic line along the back of the fetus (called *nuchal translucency*) is measured. Thickening of over 3 mm is strongly associated with Down syndrome (Fig. 45-61A,B). Absence of the nose bone is also associated with Down syndrome (Fig. 45-61B).

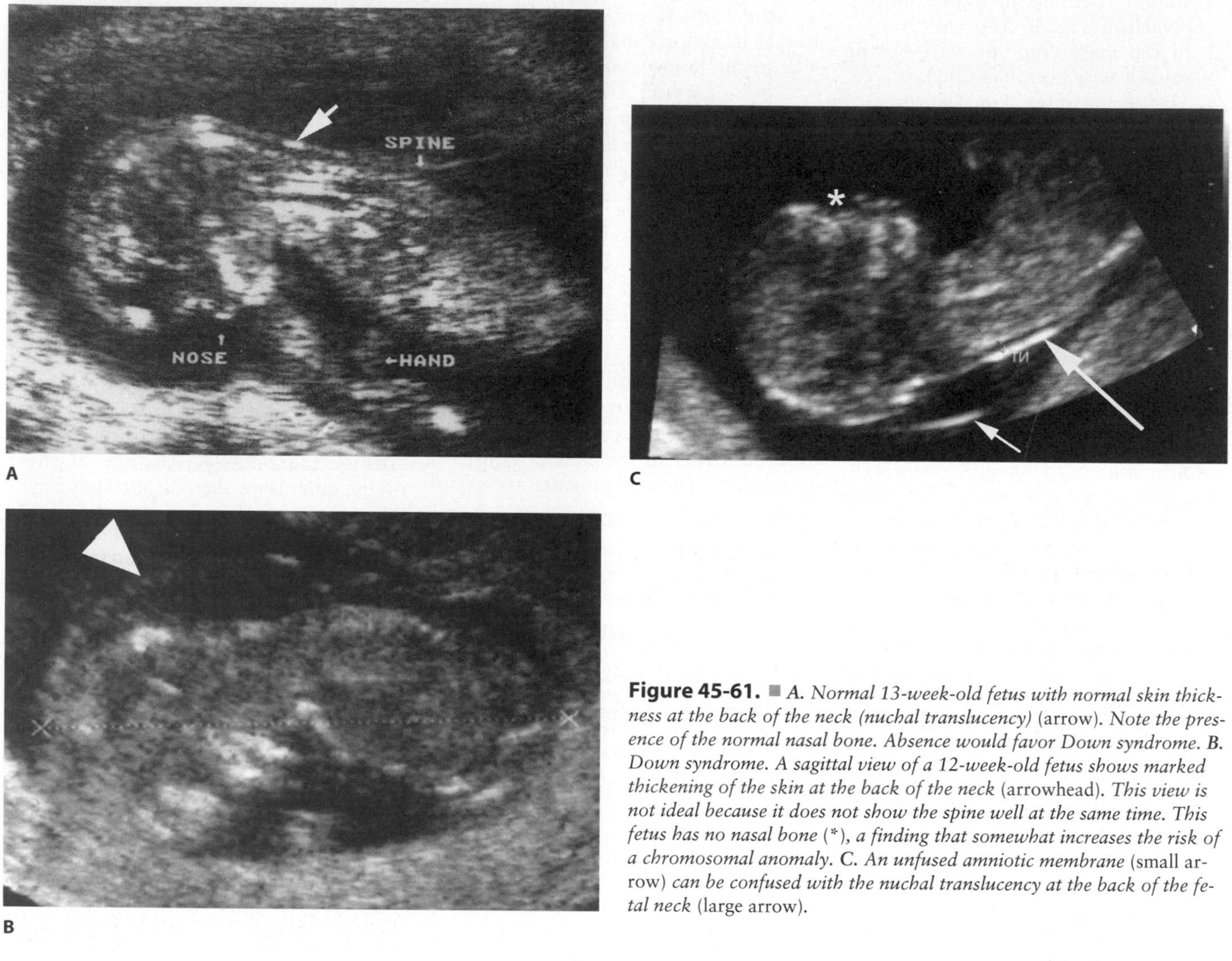

Figure 45-61. ■ *A. Normal 13-week-old fetus with normal skin thickness at the back of the neck (nuchal translucency)* (arrow). *Note the presence of the normal nasal bone. Absence would favor Down syndrome.* **B.** *Down syndrome. A sagittal view of a 12-week-old fetus shows marked thickening of the skin at the back of the neck* (arrowhead). *This view is not ideal because it does not show the spine well at the same time. This fetus has no nasal bone (*), a finding that somewhat increases the risk of a chromosomal anomaly.* **C.** *An unfused amniotic membrane* (small arrow) *can be confused with the nuchal translucency at the back of the fetal neck* (large arrow).

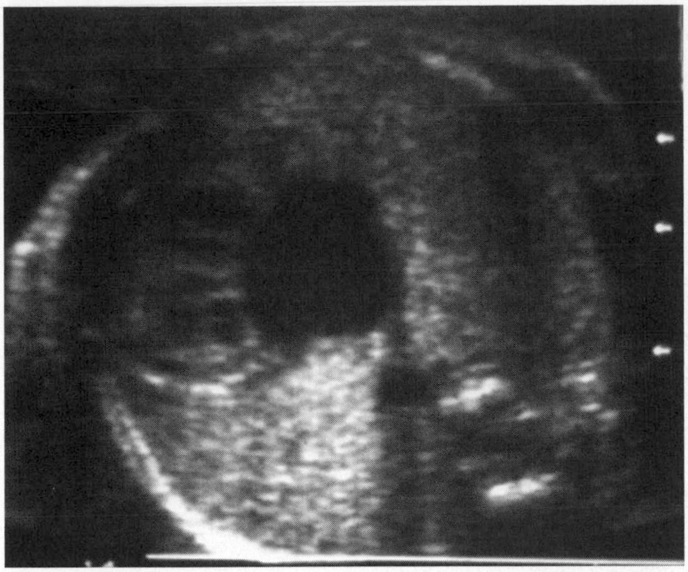

Figure 45-62. ■ *Endocardial cushion defect (A-V canal defect) associated with Down syndrome. There is absence of the ostium primum with a common mitral and tricuspid valve. The axis of the heart is deviated to the left.*

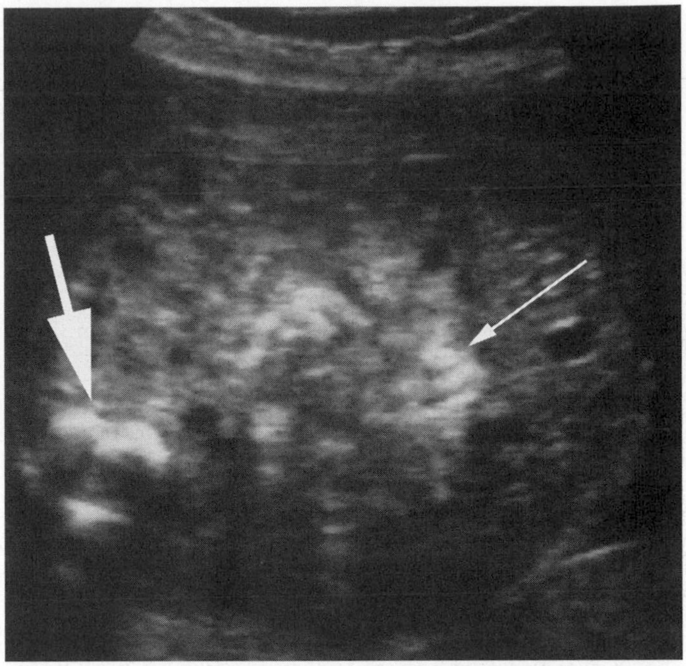

Figure 45-63. ■ *Echogenic bowel. The small bowel is very echogenic* (small arrow). *Bowel echogenicity is machine dependent. The echogenicity has to be as great as the spine* (large arrow) *for the bowel echogenicity to be called abnormal. This was a case of cystic fibrosis.*

3. Endocardial cushion defect. This form of cardiac anomaly (Fig. 45-62)—and, to a lesser extent, other congenital heart defects—is associated with Down syndrome (see Chapter 47).
4. Duodenal atresia (Fig. 45-30). This type of gastrointestinal obstruction and, to a lesser extent, other types of intestinal obstruction have a strong association with Down syndrome.
5. Echogenic bowel. A localized clump of small bowel, which is as echogenic as neighboring bone, suggests Down syndrome, cytomegalic inclusion disease, ingested blood, or meconium peritonitis, or it may be normal (Fig. 45-63) (a weak sign).
6. Sandal toe. The big toe is widely separated from the remaining toes (a weak sign).
7. Small, curved middle phalanx of the little finger (a weak sign).
8. Mild renal pelvic dilation to 4 mm or greater (Fig. 45-18) (a weak sign).
9. Mild cranial lateral ventricular dilation (a strong sign).
10. Echogenic foci in the chordi tendinae or in the moderator band of the right ventricle (Fig. 45-64) (a weak sign).

If the triple screen levels are lowered, then trisomy 18, a lethal chromosomal anomaly, becomes more likely.

Trisomy 18

The features of trisomy 18 are as follows:

1. Clenched fists with overlapping of the ring finger.
2. Early growth retardation (i.e., in the second trimester).

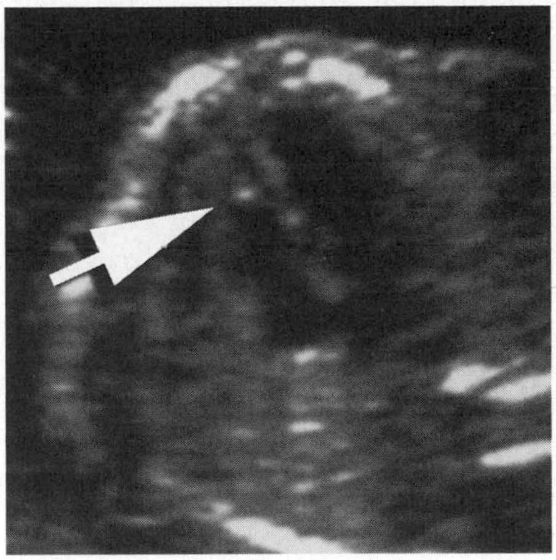

Figure 45-64. ■ *Echogenic focus in the right ventricle* (arrow). *This finding trivially increases the risk of Down syndrome.*

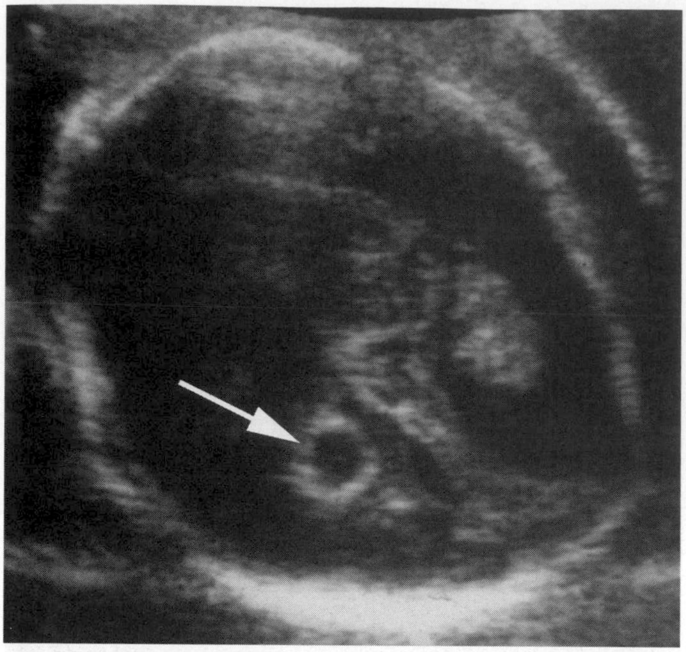

Figure 45-65. ■ *Choroid plexus cyst. A small choroid plexus cyst is present in the left choroid plexus* (arrow).

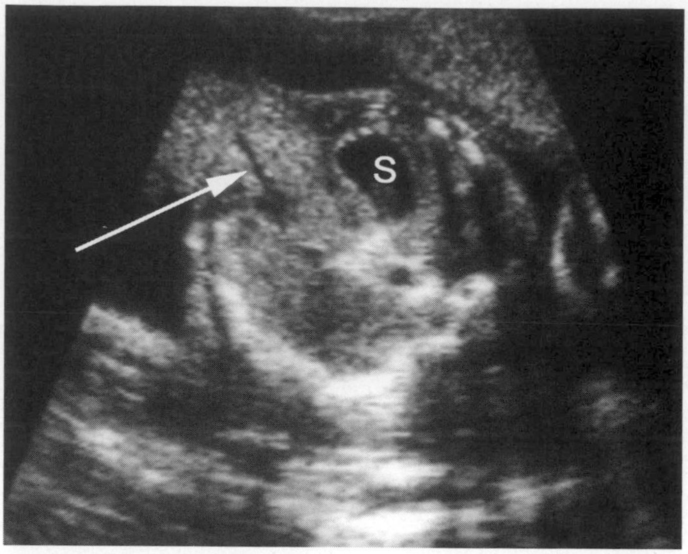

Figure 45-66. ■ *Omphalocele containing liver. A portion of liver surrounding the umbilical vein* (arrow) *protrudes into the omphalocele.* S, *stomach.*

3. Spina bifida and associated neural crest malformations (see Fig. 45-71).
4. Gut containing omphalocele (see Fig. 45-67).
5. Choroid plexus cysts (Fig. 45-65). If the only finding is a cyst in the choroid plexus, most authorities consider this insufficient to perform an amniocentesis. (Our policy is no amniocentesis if the triple screen is normal.).
6. Abnormal fetal heart.

MASS ARISING FROM THE TRUNK

Omphalocele

1. Abdominal contents prolapse through the cord insertion site. Liver (Fig. 45-66) and/or gut (Fig. 45-67) comprise the omphalocele. The cord enters the center of the omphalocele.

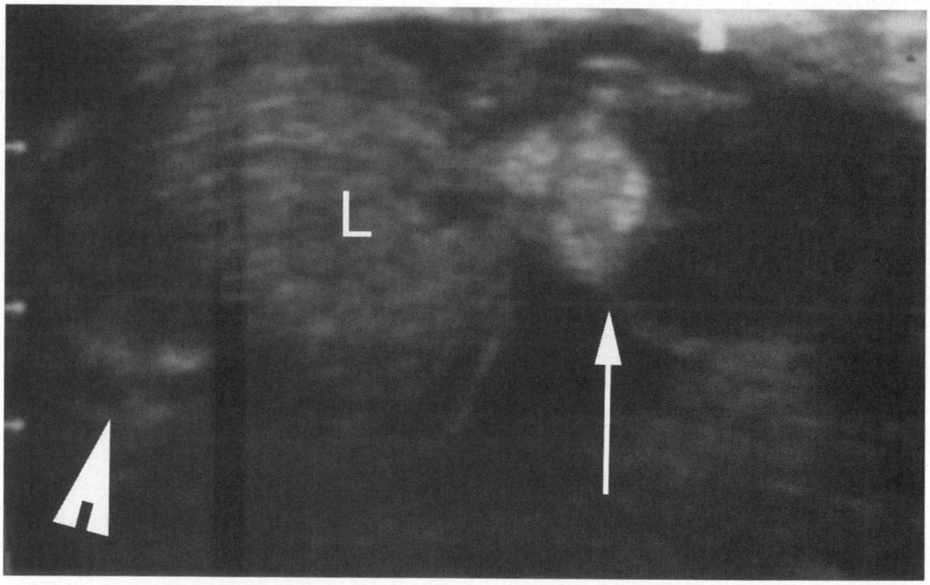

Figure 45-67. ■ *Gut containing omphalocele. The gut* (arrow) *is surrounded by ascites and is enclosed in a membrane.* Arrowhead, *spine;* L, *liver.*

2. Omphalocele may be a component of the pentalogy of Cantrell. Ectopia cordis, the heart outside the chest, and interrupted diaphragm are other principal components.
3. Other anomalies are present with omphalocele about half the time, particularly cardiac problems.
4. If the omphalocele contents are entirely bowel, there is a strong chance of a chromosomal anomaly (Fig. 45-67).
5. A membrane is seen surrounding the herniated contents.
6. Between 8 and 11 weeks, gut normally rotates outside the fetal trunk to give a transitory appearance similar to a gut containing omphalocele.

Gastroschisis

1. Some or all of the gut escapes through a hole in the right lower abdomen into the amniotic fluid (Fig. 45-68). The liver remains in the abdomen. The cord enters at its normal site. In severe cases, the stomach and/or the bladder can lie outside the abdomen.
2. If the abdominal wall opening is small, the gut within the gastroschisis or in the fetal abdomen may be distended. Gut and stomach dilation are now thought to have little relationship to long-term prognosis.
3. This is usually an isolated anomaly.
4. No membrane surrounds the gut; it floats freely in the amniotic fluid.

Sacrococcygeal Teratoma

1. Teratomas occur most often in utero adjacent to the sacrum, where they are known as *sacrococcygeal teratomas* (Fig. 45-69). Arising from the coccyx, they usually extend inferiorly between the legs. They may also infiltrate superiorly, posterior to the bladder.
2. Although they usually contain cysts, many teratomas contain solid areas and calcification.
3. Obstruction of the bladder and kidneys may occur if the tumor has an intrapelvic component (Fig. 45-69).
4. Hydrops may develop, thought to be due to vascular shunting through the mass.

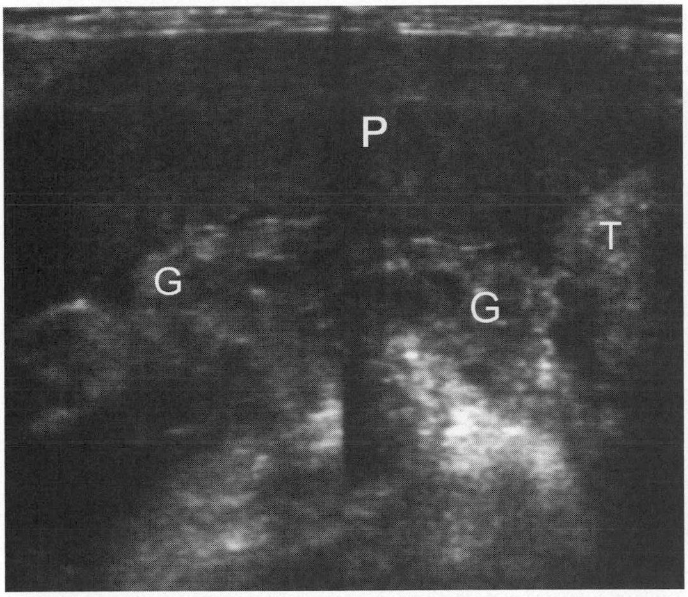

Figure 45-68. ■ *Gastroschisis. Considerable gut* (G) *lies outside the abdomen in the amniotic fluid.* P, *placenta;* T, *trunk.*

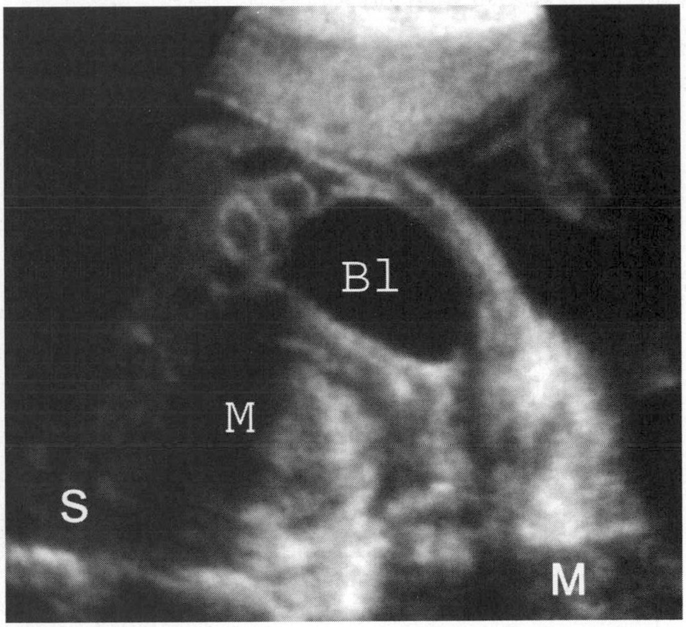

Figure 45-69. ■ *Sacrococcygeal teratoma. On this sagittal view, a mass* (M) *lies posterior to the bladder* (Bl). *In this case, much of the mass was within the fetus, although some extends inferiorly (second M).* S, *spine.*

5. Some teratomas grow to a huge size, so they are as large or larger than the fetus.

Spina Bifida/Myelomeningocele and Related Abnormalities

1. Spina bifida most often occurs in the lumbosacral area, but it may be found in the cervical or thoracic area as well (Figs. 45-70 and 45-71). Almost all types are posterior to the spine, but they may rarely be anterior.
2. The number and level of involved vertebrae influences prognosis. With higher lumbar vertebra and thoracic vertebra involvement, difficulty walking and inability to sit up are probable.
3. If there is no leg movement, and if the feet are clubbed, the prognosis is very poor. On some occasions, leg movement is seen in utero, but once surgery has been performed, movement ceases.
4. After birth, spina bifida causes urological problems, but hydronephrosis and bladder dilation are practically never seen in the fetus.
5. There are various types of spina bifida; some are more severe than others:
   a. Myeloschisis—low termination of the cord with absent spinal processes and widened interpedicular distance. The skin is open over the defect, but no pouch is present.

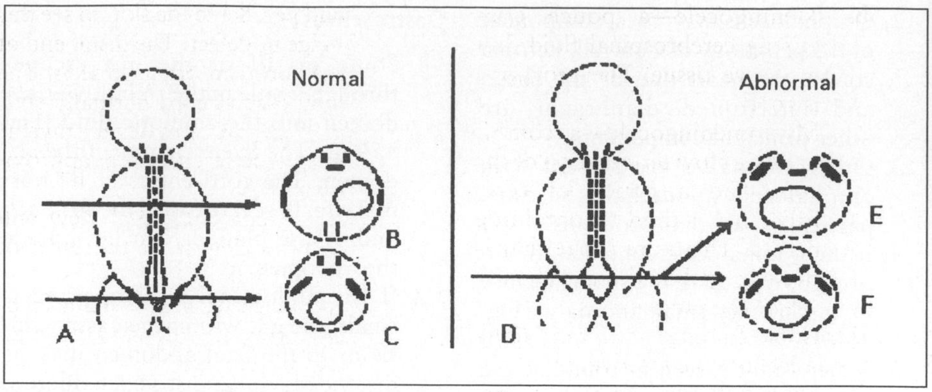

Figure 45-70. ■ *Spina bifida. A. A longitudinal sonographic section of a normal spine has three components. The vertebral arches form two parallel series of echogenic dots. The width of the space between them widens slightly in the cervical and lumbar areas. In the center is another series of echogenic dots that represents the posterior ossification center of the vertebral bodies.* ***B.*** *On transverse section, a circle of echoes is formed.* ***C.*** *Level of the bladder.* ***D.*** *Longitudinal section. In spina bifida, the circle is incomplete, with separation of the posterior element echoes. The space between the arches is widened at the involved level.* ***E.*** *The spina bifida creates a U-shaped gap.* ***F.*** *A fluid-filled sac (a meningomyelocele) may be present.*

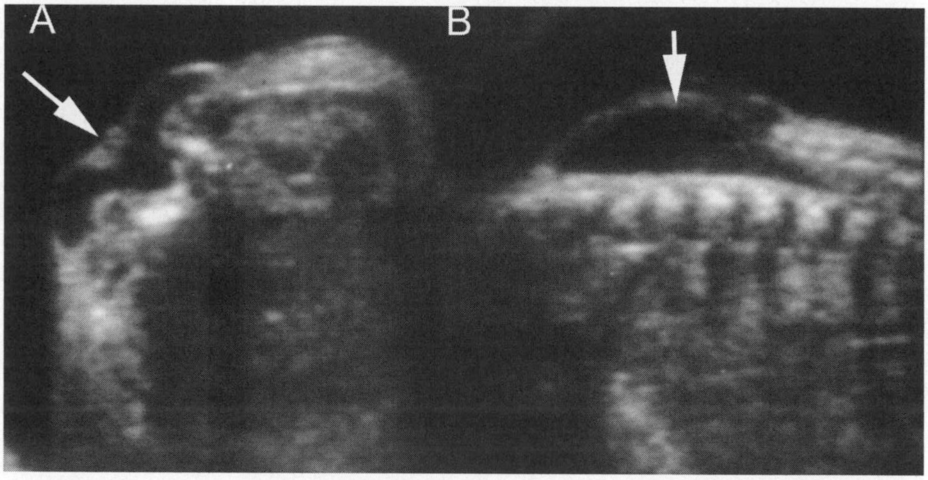

Figure 45-71. ■ *Spina bifida at lumbar level. A. Transverse view shows the widening of the posterior elements of the vertebra and the enclosing membrane (meningocele).* ***B.*** *Sagittal view showing the myelomeningocele* (arrow) *widening the lumbar spine and enclosed by a membrane.*

b. Meningocele—a pouch containing cerebrospinal fluid, but no nerve tissue. The prognosis is good.
c. Myelomeningocele—a combination of low termination of the cord and a pouch of cerebrospinal fluid containing nerves. The more tissue that is present within the pouch, the worse the prognosis is.

6. Ultrasonic findings seen with spina bifida include the following:
   a. Spine. In the normal spine, three echogenic foci are seen on transverse view—an echo from the posterior vertebral body and the two posterior element ossification centers. These three echoes normally form a triangle on transverse views that widens slightly in the cervical and lumbar areas. In spina bifida, the two posterior element echoes are separated, and a U shape is formed (Figs. 45-70 and 45-71).

      In a sagittal view of the normal spine, two parallel lines of echoes representing the posterior elements and the vertebral body are seen. The posterior elements are absent at the level of the defect. A skin defect or a pouch may be seen posterior to the spine at the defect level (Fig. 45-71). Try to place the transducer posterior and parallel to the skin to see this bulge or defect. The distal end of the cord can often be seen. The lumbosacral cord normally ends at L2. In low-level myelomeningoceles, it ends at approximately L5.

      A coronal spinal view will show widening at the level of spina bifida.

      Curved echogenic lines representing nerves may be seen within the pouch.

      The spine may be flexed and angulated at the level of the defect (a gibbous deformity) (Fig. 45-53).
   b. Skull. The cerebellum normally forms two round circles. In spina bifida, the cerebellum forms a banana shape. This shape change indicates the Arnold-Chiari malformation, which is almost always present with spina bifida and may occasionally occur as an isolated process (Fig. 45-41). The cisterna magna will be absent.
   c. Cerebellum. The skull shape often resembles a lemon, with a flattened anterior portion, which is also a consequence of the Arnold-Chiari malformation (Fig. 45-41). This finding may occasionally be seen in the absence of a spinal anomaly.
   d. Lateral ventricles. The lateral ventricles and third ventricle may be dilated.

Diastematomyelia. In a rare variant of spina bifida called *diastematomyelia*, there is widening of the lumbar spine. The cord splits in two around a central bony spur. There is cord tethering. Very disorganized vertebra are seen below the level of the bony spur.

Lipoma. If the cord is tethered and no spinal anomaly is seen, look for an echogenic mass in the spinal canal. Such a mass of fatty tissue is termed a *lipoma*. It is rarely seen in utero.

Vertebral Deformities. Spinal deformities are often found with diabetes mellitus.

1. In hemivertebrae, the spine is angulated slightly at the level of the deformity, and one of the posterior element echoes will be missing.
2. With block vertebra, one of the posterior element echoes will be larger than expected, and the spine will be slightly angulated.

Caudal Regression. In this condition, the spine is too short, and some of the vertebra are missing.

1. Find the iliac crests. The upper aspect of the iliac crest corresponds to L5.

2. Sacral vertebra normally extend down from this level. Sometimes, in addition to the sacrum, some or all of the lumbar vertebra are missing.
3. Club feet with absent leg movement are often found.

STOMACH NOT SEEN

Inability to see the stomach is an important clue that serious pathology exists. Occasionally, it is difficult to see the stomach in obese women with normal fetuses. Coincident polyhydramnios makes a normal variant unlikely. When the stomach is absent, look in the chest, face, and neck for cleft palate, tracheoesophageal atresia, and diaphragmatic hernia.

Cleft Lip and Palate. There are three forms: unilateral, bilateral, and central (Fig. 45-72). Isolated cleft palate without cleft lip is almost impossible to detect with ultrasound in utero. The stomach is

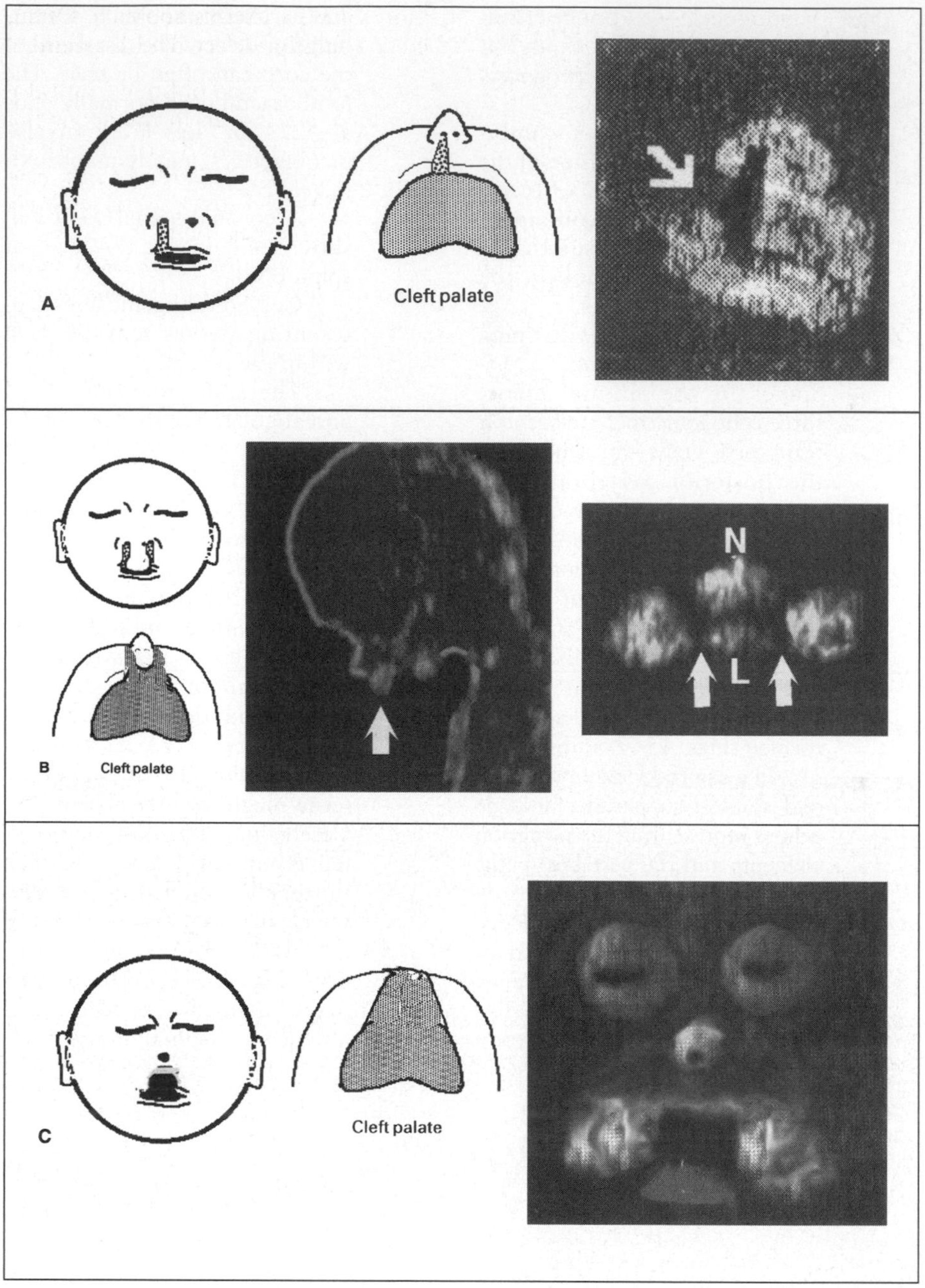

Figure 45-72. ■ *Cleft palate. A. Diagram showing the location of a unilateral cleft lip and palate and a sonogram showing a unilateral cleft* (arrow). *B. Bilateral cleft lip and palate. The central component swings anteriorly and forms a mass* (arrow) *that can be mistaken for a tumor or encephalocele on the lower image.* N, *nose.* L, *lip. The two arrows show the bilateral cleft. C. Central cleft palates of the type that occur with holoprosencephaly and trisomy 18. Note the hypotelorism (close-set eyes) and a single nostril.*

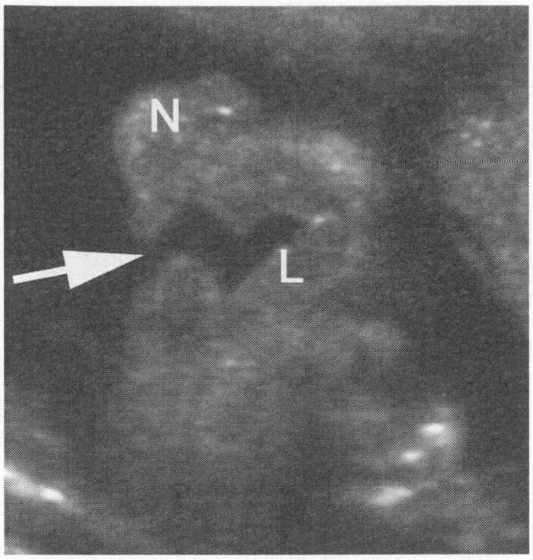

Figure 45-73. ■ *Unilateral cleft. The cleft* (arrow) *extends from the lip* (L) *to the nose* (N). *In this case, it is a right unilateral cleft. (Reprinted with permission form Sanders RC, ed.* Structural Fetal Abnormalities: The Total Picture, *2nd ed. New York: Mosby-Year Book Publishers, 2002.)*

usually visible with this anomaly. Often, there is a family history of cleft palate.

1. Unilateral. An oblique laterally placed gap is seen in the upper lip, which may also affect the maxilla (Fig. 45-73). It extends into the nose. An abnormal hooked nostril is seen on a profile view.
2. Bilateral. A centrally placed mass protrudes immediately below the nose (Fig. 45-74). The upper lip and maxilla are interrupted by the mass. Profile views will show the mass protruding beyond the nose. Additional abnormalities should be sought if either of these cleft types are seen. It is especially important to look for amniotic band deformities.
3. Central. A gap is seen below the nose in the upper lip and maxilla (Fig. 45-75). As a rule, the nose is abnormal and is either absent or there is a single nostril. This type of cleft palate is frequently associated with holoprosencephaly, hypotelorism, and trisomy 13.

Tracheoesophageal Atresia. With tracheoesophageal anomalies, the esophagus is partially absent (atresia), but often it connects (by a fistula) to the trachea, which in turn connects with the stomach. This type of anomaly is often not detectable before birth because amniotic fluid can pass into the gut through the fistula.

1. When the connection to the stomach is narrow, a small stomach is seen.
2. If no connection to the stomach exists (10% of cases), it is not seen on

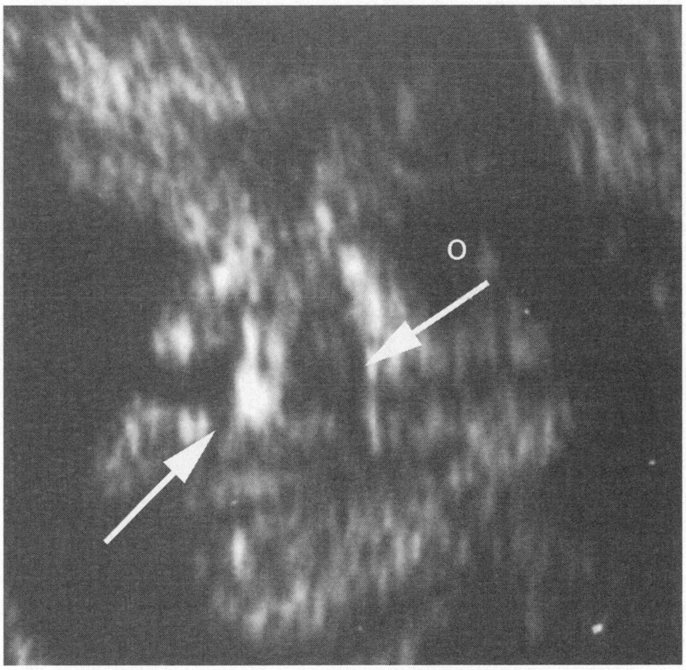

Figure 45-74. ■ *Bilateral cleft. Bilateral cleft lips and palate* (arrows) *extend to the nose. O, orbit. (Reprinted with permission form Sanders RC, ed.* Structural Fetal Abnormalities: The Total Picture, *2nd ed. New York: Mosby-Year Book Publishers, 2002.)*

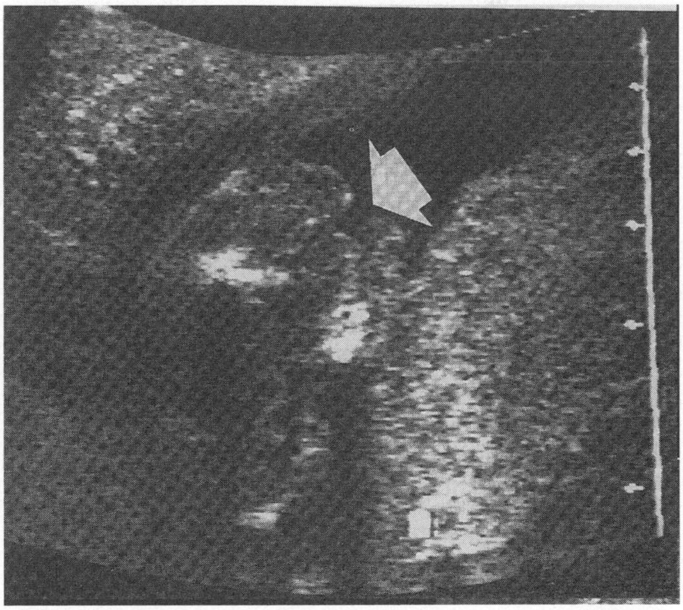

Figure 45-75. ■ *Central cleft. Central cleft lip* (arrow) *seen in a fetus with holoprosencephaly. (Reprinted with permission form Sanders RC, ed.* Structural Fetal Abnormalities: The Total Picture, *2nd ed. New York: Mosby-Year Book Publishers, 2002.)*

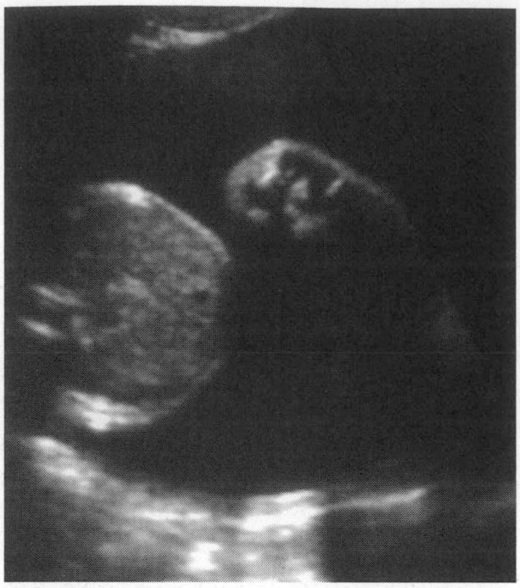

Figure 45-76. ■ *Esophageal atresia. Massive polyhydramnios. A transverse section through the fetal trunk fails to show the stomach.*

ultrasound, and there is very severe polyhydramnios (Fig. 45-76).

3. Cardiac, chromosomal, gastrointestinal, genitourinary, and vertebral malformations may also occur.

Diaphragmatic Hernia. Failure to visualize the stomach in its normal location is often due to diaphragmatic hernia. In left-side diaphragmatic hernia, the stomach is in the chest. (See also Cyst in the Chest section and Fig. 45-37.)

Hydrops. The features of hydrops fetalis are as follows:

1. Ascites
2. Pleural effusions
3. Pericardial effusion if hydrops is severe
4. Polyhydramnios
5. Thick echogenic placenta
6. Skin thickening

The presence of any two of these features allows the diagnosis of hydrops. Isolated ascites or isolated pleural effusion does not represent ascites. There are two main types: immune hydrops and nonimmune hydrops (see Chapter 44).

Immune Hydrops (Rh Incompatibility). If the fetus in a first pregnancy has a different blood group from the mother, antibodies develop at delivery when the two circulations mix. In a second pregnancy, these antibodies pass through the placenta, destroy fetal blood cells, and the fetus becomes anemic. With the anemia come heart failure, pleural effusions, ascites, and other problems.

Immune hydrops can be prevented if RhoGAM is given with the first pregnancy, so it is rare today. Treatment of immune hydrops is by fetal blood transfusion. The blood is usually introduced into the umbilical cord by percutaneous umbilical blood sampling. Transfusion into the peritoneal cavity is a less desirable alternative.

Nonimmune Hydrops. The sonographic findings with nonimmune hydrops are the same as those with immune hydrops, but are usually much more severe, with gross skin thickening. There are many different causes of nonimmune hydrops:

1. Heart diseases, both congenital anomalies such as endocardial cushion defect and irregular rhythms (arrhythmias or dysrhythmias)
2. Lung problems such as cystadenomatoid malformation or pleural effusion that prevent venous return to the heart
3. Infections such as toxoplasmosis and cytomegalic inclusion disease
4. Large placental tumors fed by the blood intended for the fetus
5. Anemic problems such as twin-to-twin transfusion syndrome and alpha thalassemia
6. Gastrointestinal problems such as diaphragmatic hernia and meconium peritonitis
7. Chromosomal problems such as Down syndrome and triploidy
8. Masses with arteriovenous shunting such as sacrococcygeal teratoma and vein of Galen malformations

The basic mechanism of hydrops appears to be anemia or inadequate venous return.

SKIN THICKENING

Skin thickening is seen with the following conditions:

1. Macrosomia. If the fetus is very large (at term over 4,000 g, over 90th percentile for weight at other times), the skin usually becomes thickened and echogenic. There is usually polyhydramnios. Such macrosomia occurs in women with diabetes, particularly the form occurring only with pregnancy (gestational diabetes) and in the fetuses of large women (see Chapter 44).
2. Hydrops. Skin thickening is one of the features of hydrops. In addition, look for pleural effusions, ascites, pericardial effusion, polyhydramnios, and placentomegaly (see Chapter 44).
3. Fetal death. A late sign of fetal death is thickening of the skin. Death should have been recognized by absence of fetal heart movement long before this sign is seen (see Chapter 46).

BILATERAL LARGE ECHOGENIC KIDNEYS

Infantile Polycystic Kidney. Refer to Figure 45-77.

1. The kidneys are much enlarged (see Appendices 15 and 16) and more echogenic than usual. Usually, no cysts are visible.
2. There is normally severe oligohydramnios or no amniotic fluid if the diagnosis is made after 18 weeks.
3. Infantile polycystic kidney is a recessive genetic condition.
4. If infantile polycystic kidney disease is seen in utero, it almost always results in stillbirth.

Adult Polycystic Kidney. Adult polycystic kidney is a dominant condition that can very rarely be detected in utero. Appearances vary from enlarged echogenic kidneys with no obvious cysts to kidneys containing large cysts. Because of the variability in appearance, the parents of any fetus with bilateral enlarged kidneys with possible cystic disease should have their kidneys examined.

Bilateral Multicystic Dysplastic Kidney

1. Variable-size visible cysts that are interspersed with echogenic areas are seen in the bilateral multicystic dysplastic kidney (Figs. 45-25 and 45-26). The cysts are larger and more numerous than those occasionally seen with infantile polycystic kidney.
2. Both kidneys may be large.
3. There can be urine in the bladder (persisting from when the kidneys were functioning), but no amniotic fluid will be seen after 18 weeks.
4. The cysts increase in size as the pregnancy progresses, and may later start to decrease in size while the fetus is still in utero.

ABSENT OR SMALL KIDNEYS

Bilateral Renal Agenesis

1. When there are no kidneys, there is no amniotic fluid after 15 to 18 weeks, and no bladder or kidneys can be seen. Anatomy is difficult to see due to the absence of amniotic fluid.
2. The adrenals assume a flattened discoid shape and tend to be located lower and more lateral than normal (Fig. 45-78). Because they have an

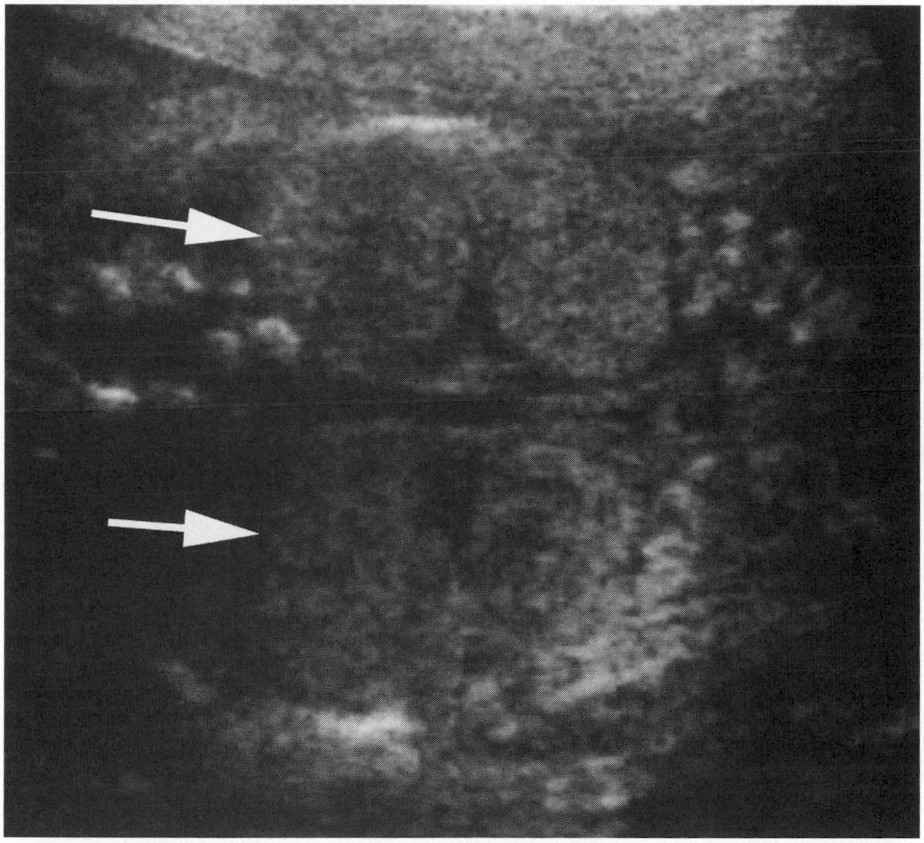

Figure 45-77. ■ *Infantile polycystic kidney disease (autosomal recessive polycystic kidney disease). Very large echogenic kidneys* (arrows) *are present.*

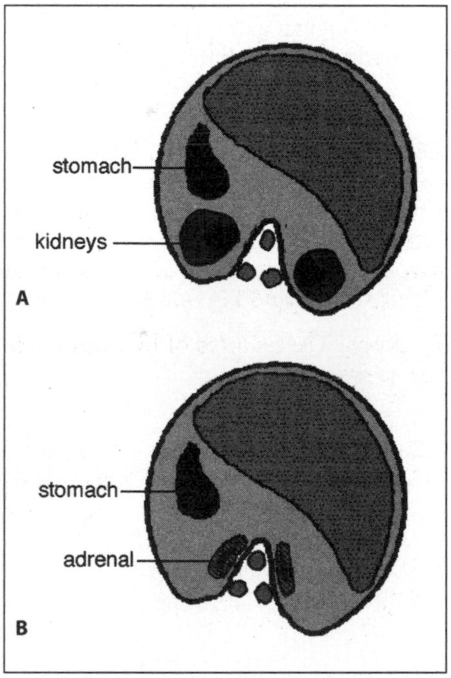

Figure 45-78. ■ *Renal agenesis.* ***A.*** *The normal positions of the kidneys are shown.* ***B.*** *The position of the adrenal glands in renal agenesis is shown.*

echogenic center in utero, they can easily be mistaken for small kidneys (Fig. 45-79).

3. If no fluid is present, it can be hard to decide whether the cause of absent fluid is renal agenesis. Amnioinfusion is a technique that is sometimes performed under these circumstances. A small needle is placed into the amniotic cavity, which may be difficult because there is little or no fluid present. A combination of a dye (indigo carmine) and a sugar-containing fluid is injected into the amniotic space. About 150 mL is usually administered. If the kidneys are present, the fetus will start to swallow, and the stomach and bladder will enlarge. The renal areas will become much easier to see because of the surrounding fluid. In the presence of premature membrane rupture, which is often confused with renal agenesis, fluid leakage through the vagina will occur, and sanitary pads will stain blue.

MASSES IN THE REGION OF THE KIDNEYS

Adrenal Hemorrhage. Hemorrhage in the third trimester may occur spontaneously or as a result of maternal loss of blood pressure. A mass in both adrenals is seen, which is evenly echogenic or partly or completely cystic. The mass will be superior to the kidney and posterior to the liver. A rapid change in acoustic texture over a period of days will be seen as the hemorrhage evolves.

Neuroblastoma. This tumor is common at birth, but is usually so small it cannot be seen. It generally regresses spontaneously. It is frequently densely echogenic, but because it is often associated with adrenal hemorrhage, it may be evenly echogenic or fluid filled. This type of tumor is usually seen in the third trimester but has been reported at 20 weeks. Metastases to the liver may be seen.

Renal Tumor. Renal masses are rare and only occur in the third trimester. They are usually mesoblastic nephroma. Typically, these tumors are large and evenly echogenic, but there may be cystic components. They are almost always associated with severe polyhydramnios.

Fetal Liver Tumors. Several rare liver tumors may occasionally be seen in the third trimester in the fetus. All are extremely vascular. Hemangioendothelioma, the most common tumor, is characterized by large vascular cystic spaces that show up on color flow. Hepatoblastomas are also highly vascular but appear solid.

Second Collecting System. If there is a duplication of the upper half of the kidney and it is obstructed, an echogenic mass containing cysts will be seen due to the development of multicystic dysplastic changes in the kidney. Alternatively, a cystic lesion may be seen representing all that remains of the duplicated kidney.

Extralobar Sequestration. When a portion of the lung forms just above the left adrenal gland, the resulting mass is echogenic with a large supplying artery seen on color flow (Fig. 45-80). Similar appearances to neuroblastoma are seen, but CT scan shows fluid rather than solid tissue.

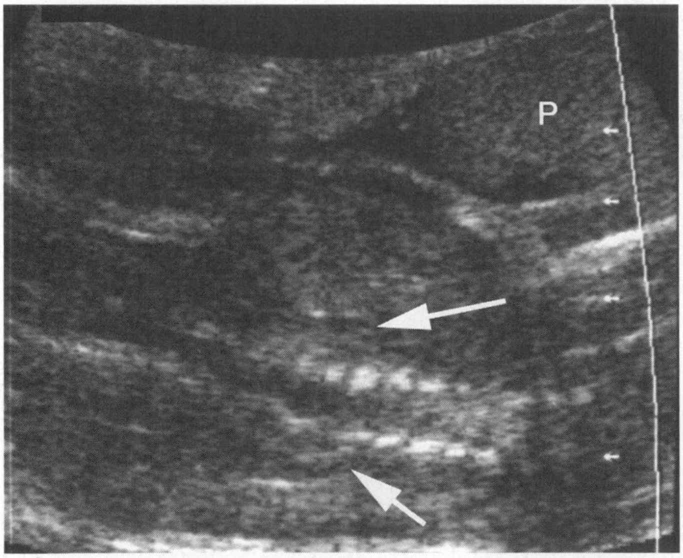

Figure 45-79. ■ *Renal agenesis. The adrenals have assumed a flattened discoid shape and lie alongside the spine* (arrows). *There is no amniotic fluid, so the quality of the image is not good.* P, *placenta.*

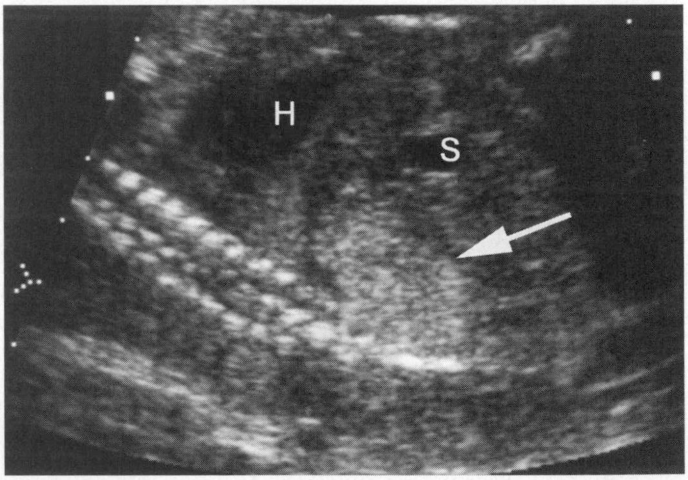

Figure 45-80. ■ *Extralobar sequestration. There is an echogenic mass* (arrow) *located just below the left hemidiaphragm in the region of the adrenal gland. Neuroblastoma may have a similar appearance.* S, *stomach;* H, *heart.*

Pitfalls

1. Sacral spina bifida. Sacral spina bifida is easily missed because the spine ossifies late and curves at this site. Only transverse views may show the abnormality. Apparent spina bifida may be created by angling obliquely and transversely when examining the lower lumbar spine (Fig. 45-81).
2. Femoral length. Limbs may be mistaken to be short if the sonographer is not meticulous about ensuring that the longest bone length views are obtained.
3. Adrenal glands versus kidney. The fetal adrenal glands have been mistaken for kidneys in cases of renal agenesis. The adrenals are smaller and more medial and superior than the normal kidney (Fig. 45-78). There will be no amniotic fluid after 15 to 18 weeks with renal agenesis.
4. Gut versus kidney. Do not mistake gut dilation for a renal cystic anomaly. Renal problems lie in contact with the spine, whereas gut problems lie at a more anterior level.
5. Gut distention. Do not mistake normal loops of bowel for pathologically dilated bowel. On some occasions, the fetal bowel can reach a width of approximately 28 mm and yet not be pathologically enlarged. An examination on another day will probably show that the fluid-filled loops have disappeared. Peristalsis may be seen in normal gut.
6. Gut versus cord. Gastroschisis may be mistaken for a long redundant umbilical cord. In the normal cord, three vessels should be seen, whereas in gastroschisis, only a single tube of bowel is seen, and the umbilical cord enters the trunk at another site. Color flow makes recognition of the cord easy.
7. Pseudohydronephrosis due to distended bladder. If the bladder is large, secondary dilation of the pelvicaliceal system in the kidneys can occur transiently. This dilation disappears when the fetus voids.

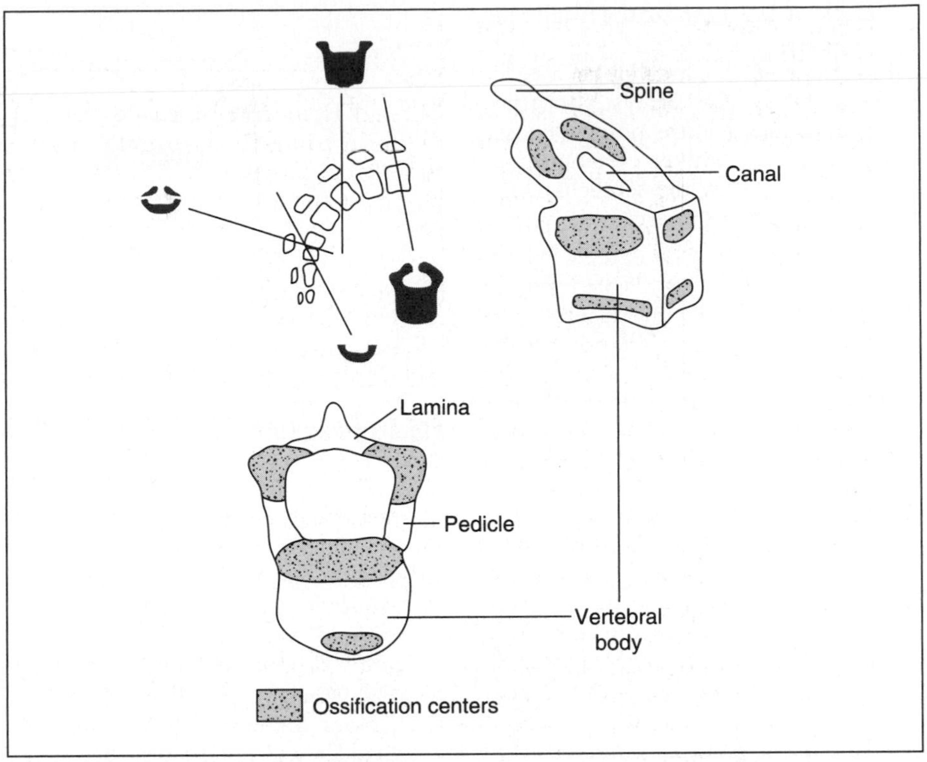

Figure 45-81. ■ *Diagram showing the fashion in which an oblique view through the lower sacrum and lumbar vertebrae can create an apparent spina bifida.*

8. Fetal ear versus mass. To the inexperienced sonographer, the normal ear (Fig. 45-11) with its half-circle shape and two ridges can resemble a mass arising from the side of the head.
9. Physiological gut herniation. Until 11 weeks, fetal gut herniating into the base of the umbilicus is embryologically normal. If liver is seen as well as gut, suspect omphalocele.
10. Colon problems in the third trimester. Colon filled with meconium in the third trimester can be mistaken for cysts (Fig. 45-28). Low-level echoes are seen within the bowel, which can be traced from cecum to rectum. In dehydrated patients, the meconium becomes very concentrated and develops an echogenic appearance.
11. Pseudo-omphalocele. Undue pressure with the linear array on the fetal trunk may distort the trunk's shape so that the abdomen protrudes in a fashion that raises the question of omphalocele. When the fetus turns prone or when the pressure on the transducer is released, the apparent omphalocele will disappear.
12. Pseudohydrocephalus. If the lateral ventricles are examined at an oblique axis, they may appear enlarged. The lateral ventricles and choroid plexus do not change size during the second and third trimester. At any stage, the lateral ventricular width at the posterior aspect of the ventricles (atria) should be no more than 10 to 11 mm, and the choroid plexus should be seen.
13. Pharynx mistaken for a cystic mass in the neck. The pharynx is sometimes visible as a cystic mass in the

neck at the base of the skull (Fig. 45-82).

14. Retrocerebellar arachnoid cyst versus Dandy-Walker cyst. Both present as a cyst in the posterior fossa. The Dandy-Walker cyst will compress and splay the cerebellar lobes as it replaces or inserts in the vermis. An extra-axial cyst will compress, but it will not alter the cerebellum.
15. Dacryocystocele. A cyst develops adjacent to the eye. This cystic structure is found medial to the orbit and represents a dilated lacrimal duct. This is a rare finding. The abnormality will disappear once the baby is born.
16. Pseudoascites. A small amount of fluid may appear to be present in the fetal abdomen located laterally; this is actually abdominal musculature, and it will not be visible around the cord insertion. In true ascites, the liver is seen indenting into the gut.
17. Pseudopericardial effusion. A small amount of fluid may appear to be present around the heart. This fluid represents fat. It is difficult to tell a true pericardial effusion from a pseudopericardial effusion, but a finding of an apparent focal thickening of the fluid at any site favors a diagnosis of true pericardial effusion.
18. Mildly shortened limbs. In patients with a strong family history of short femur or short humerus, a fetus may have a femur or humerus that is at the fifth percentile. This characteristic raises the question of Down syndrome, but more likely it is a familial trait. Look at the parents to see whether they also have a similar configuration.
19. Mildly small/large head. It is not uncommon to find a biparietal diameter and head circumference that is below the 10th percentile or above the 90th percentile as a normal variant. A large head with normal intracranial structure is usually familial, and a parent will be found to also have a large head. Distinction between a small normal head and microcephaly is difficult and is covered in detail in the segment on microcephaly in this chapter. Familial small head is usually the case.
20. Absent stomach. Sometimes, the stomach appears to be absent as a normal variant. At a follow-up study or after a delay, the stomach will be seen.
21. Absent bladder. On occasion, the bladder will not be seen because it has been completely emptied, although as a rule, the fetus does keep some urine within the bladder. Reexamination at the end of the study or at a later date will show the bladder to have some urine within it.
22. Pseudo clubfeet. Especially when there is too little fluid, the foot may be very flexed or extended. When the foot is examined at a later time, it will assume a normal configuration. In a true clubfoot, the foot is bent to one side as well as flexed or extended.
23. Mistaken intracardiac echogenic focus. Spurious echogenic foci from the endocardial cushion, the moderator band, and the tricuspid valve annulus can be mistaken for an "echogenic intracardiac focus" in the left or right ventricle associated with trisomy 18 and 21. These echogenicities have no significance in the diagnosis of chromosomal abnormalities.
24. Choroid plexus cysts. Do not make a diagnosis of a choroid plexus cyst unless the apparent cyst is at least 2.5 mm in diameter.

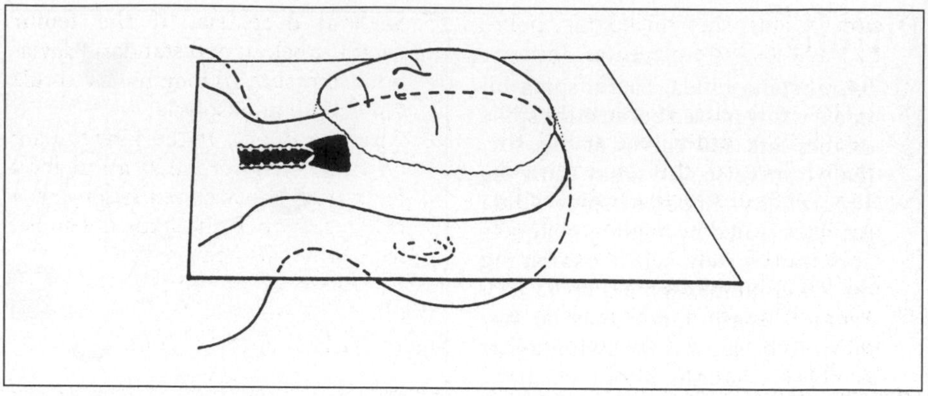

Figure 45-82. ■ *Diagram showing the fluid in the pharynx that can mimic a cystic mass in the neck.*

Where Else to Look

1. Duodenal atresia. There is a strong association with Down syndrome, so look at the heart for atrioventricular canal problems (endocardial cushion defect) (see Chapter 47). Chromosomal analysis for trisomy 21 (Down syndrome) is desirable.
2. Hydrocephalus. If the obstruction level is below the third ventricle, look at the cerebellum for the banana sign of the Arnold-Chiari malformation, and examine the spine for spina bifida.
3. Gastroschisis with liver outside abdomen. Look for the features of the limb/body wall complex: caudal regression, spina bifida, kyphoscoliosis, hydrocephalus, and absent limbs.
4. Infantile polycystic kidney. Consider the possibility of the Meckel-Gruber syndrome. In this syndrome, there are multiple small dysplastic cysts in the kidney, which may be too small to be visible as cysts. Look for polydactyly and encephalocele.
5. Unilateral hydronephrosis. Check for a dilated ureter. Look in the bladder for a ureterocele.
6. Omphalocele. Chromosomal analysis is important. Many other anomalies may be present. Look particularly for heart problems and cystic hygroma.
7. Pleural effusion. Check for the other features of hydrops: pericardial effu-

sion, ascites, skin thickening, polyhydramnios, and placental thickening.

8. Ascites. If ascites is not accompanied by the other features of hydrops, look at the genitourinary tract for an obstructive lesion and at the heart for a cardiac anomaly. Look in the bowel for evidence of meconium peritonitis.
9. Absent stomach. Look for diaphragmatic hernia, cleft palate, and a small jaw (micrognathia).
10. Absent bladder. Look for the kidneys; there could be renal agenesis.
11. Facial anomalies. If hypotelorism and cleft palate are present, look in the skull for holoprosencephaly.
12. Horseshoe-shaped single ventricle in brain. Look for facial anomalies.
13. Severe UPJ. On a coronal view, displacement of the stomach may be seen if the UPJ is left sided. Impingement on the stomach or bowel may cause polyhydramnios.
14. Cleft lip. If cleft lip is found, look for an amniotic band and problems associated with amniotic bands, such as encephalocele and club feet.
15. Skeletal dysplasia. If the femur length is below two standard deviations, measure all long bones to rule out a skeletal dysplasia.
16. Absent kidneys. If the kidneys are absent in their normal location, look for a horseshoe-shaped kidney or a pelvic kidney. If the fetus is female, look for cloacal anomalies.

SELECTED READING

Callen P. *Ultrasonography in Obstetrics and Gynecology*. Philadelphia: W.B. Saunders; 2000.

Fong KW, Toi A, Salem S, et al. Detection of fetal structural abnormalities with US during early pregnancy. *Radiographics* 2004;24:157–174.

Guzman ER, Ranzini A, Day-Salvatore D, et al. The prenatal ultrasonographic visualization of imperforate anus in monoamniotic twins. *J Ultrasound Med* 1995;14:547–551.

Nicholaides KH. Nuchal translucency and other first trimester sonographic markers of chromosomal anomalies. *Am J Obstet Gyn* 2004;191:45–67.

Nyberg D, McGahan JP, Pretorius DH, et al. *Diagnostic imaging of fetal anomalies*. Philadelphia: Lippincott Williams & Wilkins; 2003.

Nyberg DA, Sickler GK, Hegge FN, et al. Fetal cleft lip with and without cleft palate: US classification and correlation with outcome. *Radiology* 1995;195:677–684.

Pilu G, Sandri F, Perolo A, et al. Prenatal diagnosis of lobar holoprosencephaly. *Ultrasound Obstet Gynecol* 1992;2:88–94.

Rotten D, Levaillant JM. Two- and three-dimensional sonographic assessment of the fetal face. 2. Analysis of cleft lip, alveolus and palate. *Ultrasound Obstet Gynecol* 2004;24:402–411.

Rypens FF, Avni EF, Abehsera MM, et al. Areas of increased echogenicity in the fetal abdomen: diagnosis and significance. *Radiographics* 1995;15:1329–1344.

Sanders RC, ed. *Structural Fetal Abnormalities: The Total Picture*, 2nd ed. New York: Mosby-Year Book Publishers; 2002.

Turner SR, Samei E, Hertzburg B, et al. Sonography of fetal choroid plexus cysts. Detection depends on cyst size and gestational age. *J Ultrasound Med* 2003;22:1219–1227.

Winn VD, Sonson J, Filly RA. Echogenic intracardiac focus: potential for misdiagnosis. *J Ultrasound Med* 2003;22:1207–1214.

Fetal Well-Being and Fetal Death

46

MARY MCGRATH-LING

SONOGRAM ABBREVIATIONS

AF	Amniotic fluid
AFI	Amniotic fluid index
BPP	Biophysical profile
BPS	Biophysical profile score
FHM	Fetal heart motion
FHR	Fetal heart rate
LL	Left lower quadrant
LU	Left upper quadrant
NST	Nonstress test
RL	Right lower quadrant
RU	Right upper quadrant
VCR	Videocassette recorder

KEY WORDS

Acoustical Stimulator. Noise-emitting device placed on the maternal abdomen to buzz or wake up the fetus.

Amniotic Fluid Index (AFI). Assessment of the amount of amniotic fluid by measuring and adding the largest vertical pocket in each of the four uterine quadrants.

Biophysical Profile (BPP). An objective test for more accurately diagnosing and subsequently managing fetal oxygen deficiency (hypoxia/asphyxia) consisting of assessment of fluid, breathing, and movements.

Biophysical Profile Score (BPS). All parameters are scored and totalled.

Bradycardia. Slow fetal pulse (less than 110 bpm).

Contraction Stress Test (CST). Fetal heart rate is monitored for accelerations (normal) versus late decelerations (abnormal) in response to uterine contractions.

Doptone. Detection of fetal heartbeat by Doppler. The fetal heart can usually be heard by 12 weeks.

Eclampsia. Severe pregnancy-induced hypertension with protein loss in the urine. It may be associated with convulsions.

Fetal Breathing Movement (FBM). When a diaphragm excursion is observed.

Fetal Hypoxia/Asphyxia. Lack of adequate oxygen supply to the fetus.

Fundal Height (FH). Relative height of uterine fundus at various stages of pregnancy.

Intrauterine Growth Restriction (IUGR). Alternative preferable term for intrauterine growth retardation. Term used to describe compromised fetal growth.

Kick Count. Maternal assessment of fetal movement by counting kicks felt over a 1-hour period.

Lecithin-Sphingomyelin Ratio (L/S Ratio). A ratio of two of the substances (protein and lipids) that are released into the amniotic fluid by the fetus. Measurement at amniocentesis is used in the assessment of fetal lung maturity.

Maceration. Disintegration of the fetus following death. Debris from a dead fetus can be identified in the amniotic fluid.

Modified Biophysical Profile. Sonographic evaluation of fluid volume only, either by amniotic fluid index (AFI) or by largest single pocket done in conjunction with fetal heart rate monitoring (NST).

Nonstress Test (NST). Fetal heart rate is monitored in response to fetal movement.

Placental Insufficiency. Poorly performing placenta, usually due to focal infarcts.

Pre-eclampsia. Pregnancy-induced hypertension with urinary loss of protein.

Presyncopal. Prior to fainting.

Respiratory Distress Syndrome (RDS). Infant breathing problem associated with prematurity.

Robert's Sign. Gas in the fetal abdomen following fetal demise.

Spaulding's Sign. Overlapping of the fetal skull bones as the result of fetal death in utero (FDIU).

Tachycardia. A pulse rate that is too fast (over 180 bpm).

Umbilical Artery Doppler. Doppler evaluation of umbilical arteries to detect abnormal (high-resistance) diastolic flow.

Vanishing Twin. Phenomenon where fetal death of one twin occurs and on subsequent sonograms, the dead twin can no longer be seen. This is due to maceration and eventual disintegration and resorption of the dead twin.

The Clinical Problem

RISKS TO FETAL WELL-BEING

Many pregnancies are at risk for fetal distress or fetal death. Maternal risks include chronic hypertension, pre-eclampsia, eclampsia, diabetes mellitus (including gestational diabetes), alcohol or narcotics abuse, and systemic diseases such as lupus. Placental problems such as placental insufficiency or abruption may result in fetal distress. Multiple pregnancy, intrauterine growth restriction (IUGR), preterm labor, premature rupture of membranes, and fetal anomalies all result in an increased risk of fetal distress. Pregnancies extending beyond 40 weeks' gestation or a previous history of a stillbirth or fetal distress are also risk factors. High-risk patients are monitored more closely for early detection and appropriate management of fetal distress. In the absence of risk factors, the maternal assessment of decreased fetal movement warrants an ultrasonic look for fetal distress.

FETAL ACTIVITY

Fetal activity is easily assessed sonographically. The fetus is most active up to approximately 26 to 28 weeks' gestation. Fetal activity decreases somewhat in the third trimester owing to less available space. It is helpful to ask the mother how much the fetus is moving and whether she has noticed a decrease in activity. Fetal limb and body movements, along with flexion and extension, can be monitored during real-time scanning. The sonographer should always observe fetal movement during any examination and not overlook an inactive fetus. Some unsuspected compromised fetuses may be detected if all third trimester fetal sonograms include assessment of fetal movement. In addition to observing fetal activity, the placenta and amniotic fluid (AF) volume should be evaluated and documented.

THE PULSE RATE

The normal fetal heart rate (FHR) is approximately 140 beats per minute (bpm); the normal range is 110 to 180 bpm after the first trimester (Appendix 25). Brief periods of bradycardia are usually normal if followed by a return to a normal heart rate. Prolonged (greater than 30 seconds) or continuous bradycardia is reason for concern, however, and fetal distress should be considered along with other causes of bradycardia such as cord compression due to decreased AF, arrhythmias, congenital heart lesions, or complete atrioventricular block (see Chapter 47). Fetal tachycardia (greater than 180 bpm) is caused by a number of fetal and maternal conditions including smoking, certain drugs, anxiety, fetal distress, and arrhythmias (see Chapter 47).

When evidence of fetal ill health is discovered, the obstetrician has the advantage of timing the delivery to optimize the likelihood of a favorable outcome. Ultrasound can greatly impact this management decision with the biophysical profile (BPP), which is a useful tool for assessing fetal condition. Good biophysical scores (8 to 10 out of a possible 10) are associated with a favorable perinatal outcome. A fetus at risk for a poor fetal outcome is monitored at appropriate intervals throughout the remainder of the pregnancy.

Because the BPP results impact the timing of delivery, tests are only performed once viability outside the uterus is possible (i.e., 24 to 26 weeks). The nonstress test (NST) is used in conjunction with the ultrasonic BPP. The NST is often nonreactive prior to 28 weeks' gestation and, therefore, is of limited use before that time. Real-time sonography is used to assess AF volume, fetal tone, and fetal breathing.

Although premature delivery may result in respiratory distress syndrome and other complications, the fetus may have a better chance of survival with preterm delivery as opposed to remaining in a hostile intrauterine environment.

FETAL DEATH

Fetal demise is most common in the first trimester (i.e., spontaneous abortion; see Chapter 39). This chapter concentrates on the sonographic appearance and diagnosis of fetal death in the second and third trimesters. Fetal death usually occurs in association with the same risk factors that cause fetal distress (mentioned previously). Fetal demise may also result from structural or chromosomal anomalies in the fetus. Cord problems such as cord compression, if the cord comes first, cord knots, or the cord twisted around the fetal neck are also responsible for some unexpected fetal deaths.

Fetal death is suspected on the basis of absent maternal perception of fetal movement. Failure to detect fetal heart tones by Doppler or failure of the fundal height to grow may also raise suspicion of fetal death. Frequently, fetal heart pulsations go undetected by Doppler because of maternal obesity, retroverted uterus, excessive fetal movement, or fetal position. Real-time ultrasound is essential for confirming or excluding fetal demise.

Technique

BIOPHYSICAL PROFILE

The fetus should be observed for up to 30 minutes to meet the scoring criteria. Most often, a healthy fetus will satisfy all criteria in only a few minutes. Once all the parameters have been observed, the exam can be ended.

The mother should be placed in a semiupright position and made as comfortable as possible. A recumbent left or right lateral position is also acceptable. Having the patient supine may cause compression of the inferior vena cava and a feeling of dizziness; if the patient feels faint, get her to turn on her side as soon as possible. The optimal time for observing an active fetus is after the mother has eaten. If the baby appears to be in a resting state, there are several things the observer can do to enhance fetal activity.

1. Gentle shaking may awaken or stimulate a resting fetus.
2. Give the mother cold water or a sweetened drink.
3. Have the mother breathe in and out deeply several times.
4. Vary the mother's position. Often, she can tell you which positions the baby does not seem to like. Those positions will usually result in the most fetal movement.
5. Use an acoustical stimulator to wake up the baby. Sometimes, the father's voice will work just as well!

The technique for the BPP described in the information to follow is based on work by Manning et al. (see the section entitled Selected Reading at the end of this chapter) and is currently the most widely used by obstetricians.

SCORING PARAMETERS

Each parameter is accorded a score of 0 or 2, as discussed later. There is no score of 1 (Table 46-1).

NST

The NST is an aid in evaluating fetal health; the FHR is monitored over a 20-minute period. A normal fetus responds to fetal movement by an increase in FHR. A reactive (normal) result is when at least two or more accelerations (15 bpm above a baseline) occur in a 20-minute period (Fig. 46-1A). A nonreactive (or positive) NST indicates there have been fewer than two accelerations of FHR over a 40-minute period (Fig. 46-1B). If the result for the first 20 minutes is nonreactive, the NST is continued for an additional 20 minutes using artificial (acoustical) stimulation. If fetal movement is followed after a delay by a lowered fetal pulse rate, this ominous sign of fetal sickness is called a *late deceleration* (Fig. 46-1C). If the results of the NST are negative (reactive), the biophysical profile score (BPS) is 2. If there are fewer than two accelerations of at least 15 bpm above the baseline during the NST, the score is 0. The NST is often nonreactive in the normal pregnancy prior to 28 weeks' gestation.

TABLE 46-1 Biophysical Profile Scoring According to Manning et al.

Parameter	Score of 2	Score of 0
Breathing	Thirty seconds or more of breathing noted in a 30-minute period	Less than 30-second period or no breathing in 30 minutes
Movement	Three or more gross body/limb movements in a 30-minute period	Fewer than three gross body/limb movements in a 30-minute period
Tone	At least two episodes of flexion or extension with return to normal position in a 30-minute period	Failure to observe any flexion or extension in a 30-minute period
Fluid	One pocket of AF measuring 2 cm in both vertical and horizontal planes	Failure to identify fluid pocket measuring 2 cm in any plane
Nonstress test	Negative or reactive test	Fewer than two accelerations of at least 15 bpm

Total possible score = 10.
Amniotic fluid, AF.

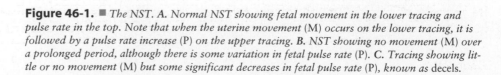

Figure 46-1. ■ *The NST. A. Normal NST showing fetal movement in the lower tracing and pulse rate in the top. Note that when the uterine movement* (M) *occurs on the lower tracing, it is followed by a pulse rate increase* (P) *on the upper tracing. B. NST showing no movement* (M) *over a prolonged period, although there is some variation in fetal pulse rate* (P)*. C. Tracing showing little or no movement* (M) *but some significant decreases in fetal pulse rate* (P)*, known as* decels.

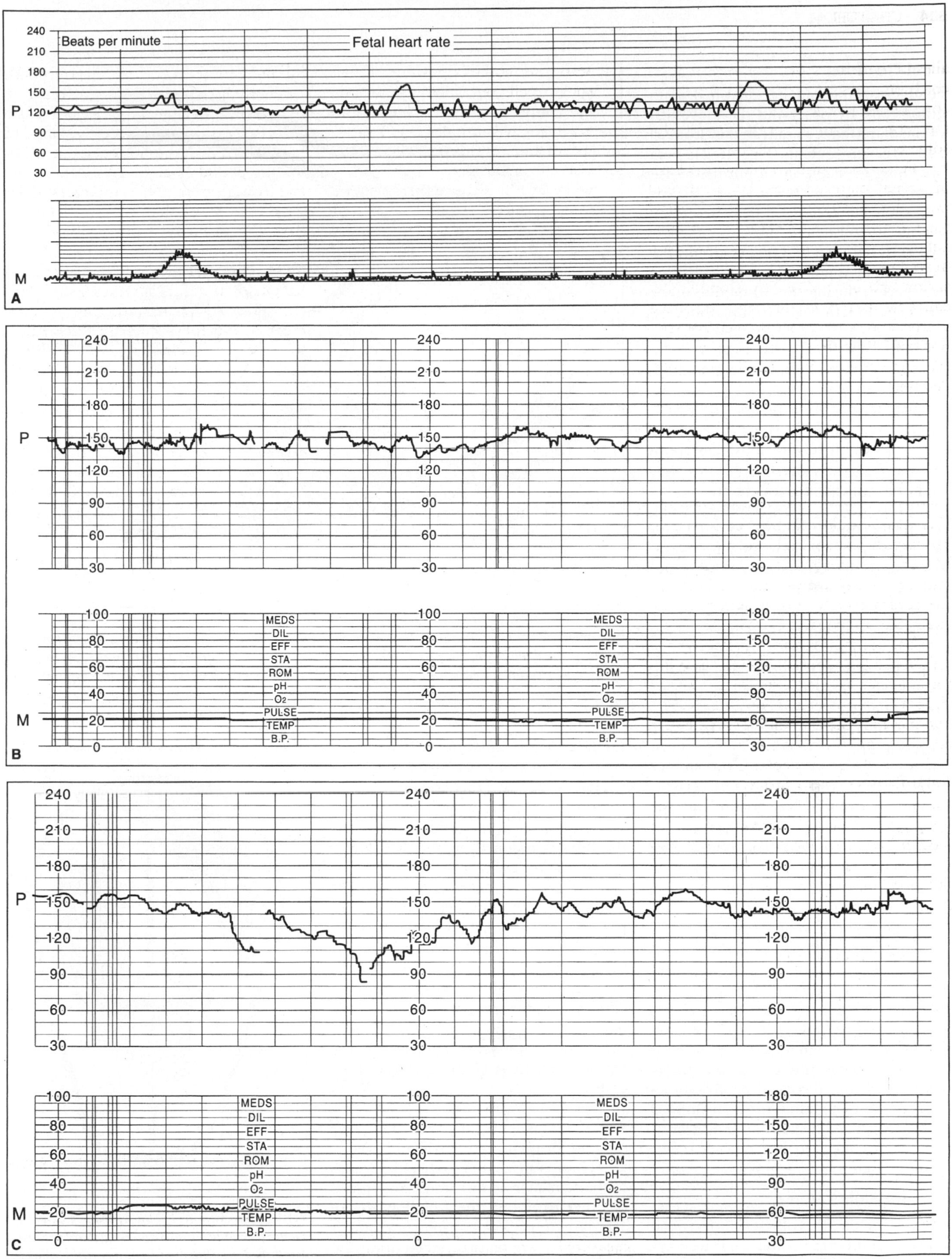
Beats per minute
Fetal heart rate
240
210
180
150
120
90
60
30
P
M
A
B
C
100
80
60
40
20
0
MEDS
DIL
EFF
STA
ROM
pH
O2
PULSE
TEMP
B.P.

Figure 46-1.

Fetal Breathing

Fetal breathing can be identified sonographically by observing the movement of the diaphragm as reflected in stomach and liver movement (Fig. 46-2). Fetal breathing is visible in all normal fetuses from 26 weeks on, but it is intermittent. A prolonged period of fetal breathing, lasting 30 seconds or more, needs to be observed before a BPS of 2 is given. If fetal breathing is not observed for a 30-second period during the 30-minute observation period, the score for breathing is 0.

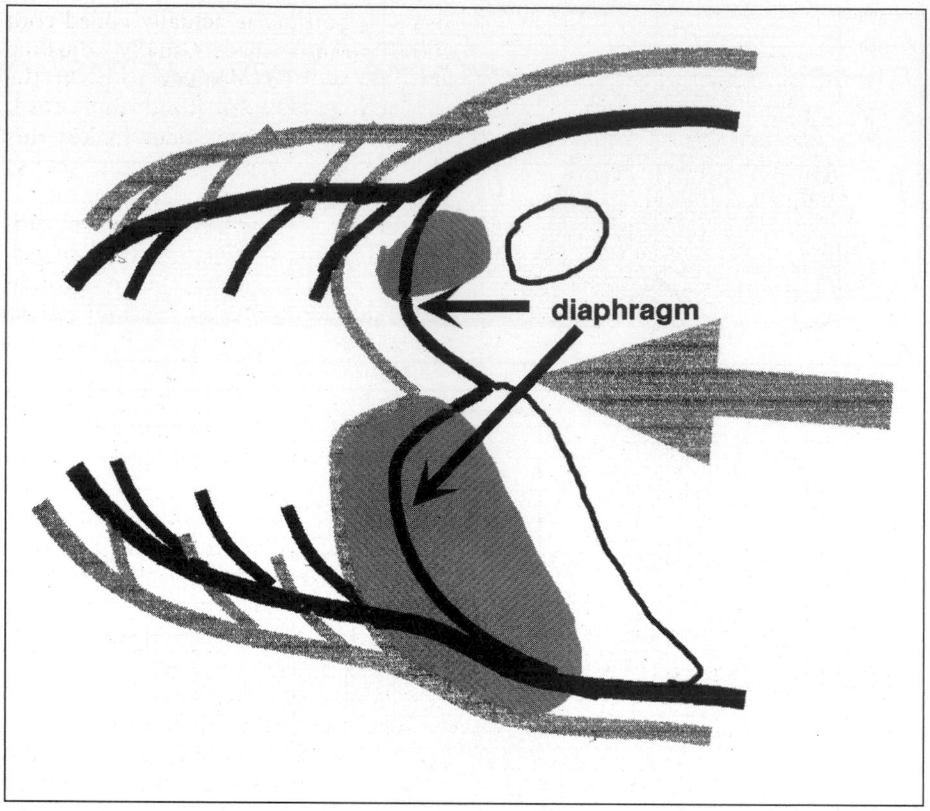

Figure 46-2. ■ *Fetal breathing. The normal position is shown in the black lines. As the fetus breathes, the diaphragm, liver, and stomach move up (shown in gray). Changes in the ribs are minimal. Fetal breathing is easiest to see in the coronal position but can also be seen on a sagittal view.*

Fetal Movement

There should be at least three gross body or limb movements during the 30-minute period for a normal BPS of 2. Fewer than three body or limb movements scores 0. Only significant body movements are scored. Subtle or very slight movements do not count.

Movement is not always easy to assess in the third trimester because only one segment of the fetus can be observed at a time. A healthy fetus will, nevertheless, demonstrate twisting or kicking movements if it is observed over an adequate period of time. Sometimes, a fetus will respond to gentle shaking. If adequate movement is not noted, the fetus can be stimulated by using a noise-producing device. A normal resting fetus will usually respond, whereas a truly sick fetus will not.

Fetal Tone

Flexion and extension movements are monitored. There should be at least one episode of good flexion and extension of fetal limbs or spine followed by return to normal position. Flexion and extension of the arms or legs, arching of the spine, or opening and closing of hands are all good indicators of normal tone for a BPS of 2. Failure to observe any of these movements in the 30-minute period results in a score of 0. This parameter is very closely related to fetal movement; the difference is that specific attention is paid to flexion and extension movements. Caution: if a fetal hand is in an open or limp position for a prolonged period, it is usually a strong indicator of poor fetal tone. Do not overlook this ominous sign.

Amniotic Fluid Volume

Assessment of AF volume is of crucial importance in establishing fetal well-being or sickness. There should be at least one pocket of AF measuring 2 cm in both the horizontal and vertical planes for a BPS of 2. Failure to identify a fluid pocket of at least this size results in a score of 0. Do not include a section of umbilical cord in the fluid pocket when the fluid is minimal, as this will give a false-positive result.

If there is a fluid pocket of less than 2 cm, oligohydramnios is considered present and severe. Less severe changes in AF volume should be noted because the volume rarely decreases enough to meet the zero BPP criteria until fetal demise is imminent. The AF can be evaluated by using the amniotic fluid index (AFI), the largest vertical pocket, or subjective assessment by an experienced operator.

AFI. This is currently the preferred method for quantitating AF volume.

Fluid is measured vertically in each of the four uterine quadrants and added together to obtain the AFI (Fig. 46-3). The largest pocket in each quadrant is measured. Care must be taken not to include segments of the umbilical cord in the measurement. Sometimes, what ap-

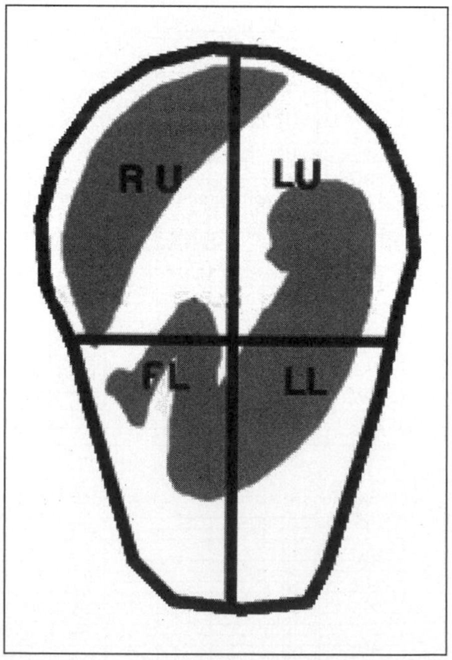

Figure 46-3. ■ *AFI. The AFI is measured by dividing the uterus into quadrants and measuring the longest depth of fluid in each quadrant. The transducer should be positioned longitudinally when the measurement is made.*

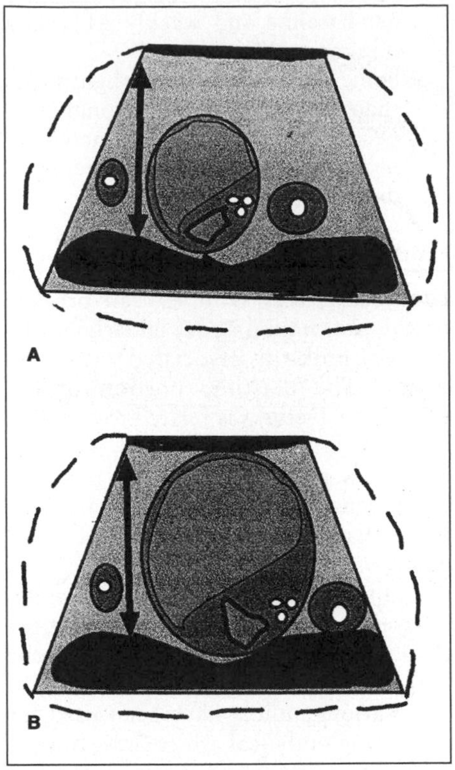

Figure 46-4. ■ *The AFI can be deceptive if the vertical measurement is long but the fluid-filled area is narrow. The same measurement is obtained with a thin, narrow fluid pocket in (B) as in the wide pocket seen in (A).*

pears to be fluid is actually coiled cord filling the entire space. Usually, adjusting the gain will be adequate to make the distinction between fluid and cord. Patient habitus sometimes makes this distinction extremely difficult, so use color Doppler to define the cord.

A sum of 5 or less indicates significant oligohydramnios, regardless of gestational age. A sum of 20 or more indicates polyhydramnios. Normal values are shown in Appendix 24. If there is a fluid pocket that meets the 2 cm criterion in both the vertical and horizontal planes, a BPS of 2 is assigned even in the presence of oligohydramnios by AFI calculation.

The AFI can be falsely reassuring where there are narrow vertical pockets. Conversely, when wide shallow pockets are present, subjective assessment of fluid volume may prove more useful (Fig. 46-4).

Subjective assessment, although quite accurate when done by an experienced observer, has limitations because it cannot provide quantitative information about trends in fluid volume, particularly if a different examiner monitors the patient in subsequent exams.

Largest Vertical Pocket. A single pocket of fluid is measured in the vertical plane, not including segments of the umbilical cord. A measurement of less than 2 cm indicates oligohydramnios, whereas a pocket of 8 cm or more is representative of polyhydramnios. This technique is most helpful when trying to quantitate fluid volume in the multiple-gestation pregnancy or in the assessment of polyhydramnios.

Interpretation of Scores

Assuming a normal AF volume, a BPS of 8 to 10 is normal; 6 is suspicious for chronic asphyxia; and 0 to 4 is highly suggestive of asphyxia (Table 46-2). The clinical significance of the various components of the BPP varies with both the parameter and gestational age. Some components of the BPP are acute markers of fetal asphyxia, and others are chronic. The acute markers are FHR, fetal movement, tone, and breathing, whereas fluid volume is a chronic marker. Interestingly, the biophysical parameters that appear the earliest in pregnancy are the last to disappear with fetal asphyxia. Fetal tone first appears at 7 1/2 to 8 1/2 weeks' gestation. Movement begins at 9 weeks, and

TABLE 46-2 Management Based on Biophysical Profile

Score	Interpretation	Management
10	Normal infant; low risk of chronic asphyxia	Repeat testing at weekly intervals; repeat twice in diabetic patients and patients at ≥42 weeks' gestation
8	Normal infant; low risk of chronic asphyxia	Repeat testing at weekly intervals; repeat testing twice weekly in diabetics and patients at ≥42 weeks' gestation; oligohydramnios is an indication for delivery
6	Suspect chronic asphyxia	If ≥36 weeks' gestation and conditions are favorable, deliver; if at <36 weeks and lecithin-sphingomyelin ratio <2.0, repeat test in 4 to 6 hours; deliver if oligohydramnios is present
4	Suspect chronic asphyxia	If ≥32 weeks' gestation, deliver; if <32 weeks, repeat score
0 to 2	Strongly suspect chronic asphyxia	Extend testing time to 120 minutes; if persistent score ≤4, deliver, regardless of gestation age

Reprinted with permission from Manning FA, Harman CR, Morrison I, et al. Fetal assessment based on fetal biophysical profile scoring. Am J Obstet Gynecol, *1990;162(3):703–709.*

breathing starts at 20 to 21 weeks; FHR control is the last to appear in the late second or early third trimester.

Modified BPP

In some instances, the obstetrician may feel that only a modified version of the BPP is necessary (Fig. 46-5). The modified BPP is the sonographic evaluation of fluid volume only, preferably by AFI and FHR monitoring (NST). Instances when this method is indicated include the following:

1. Postterm pregnancies in which decreased fluid would warrant labor induction due to increased risk of cord compression with resultant fetal compromise or demise
2. Patients who are receiving indomethacin (which can cause decreased fluid production) for preterm labor; these patients often get baseline and weekly AFIs as a minimum
3. Some patients with size slightly less than dates who are not strongly suspected of having IUGR but where more prudent observation seems indicated

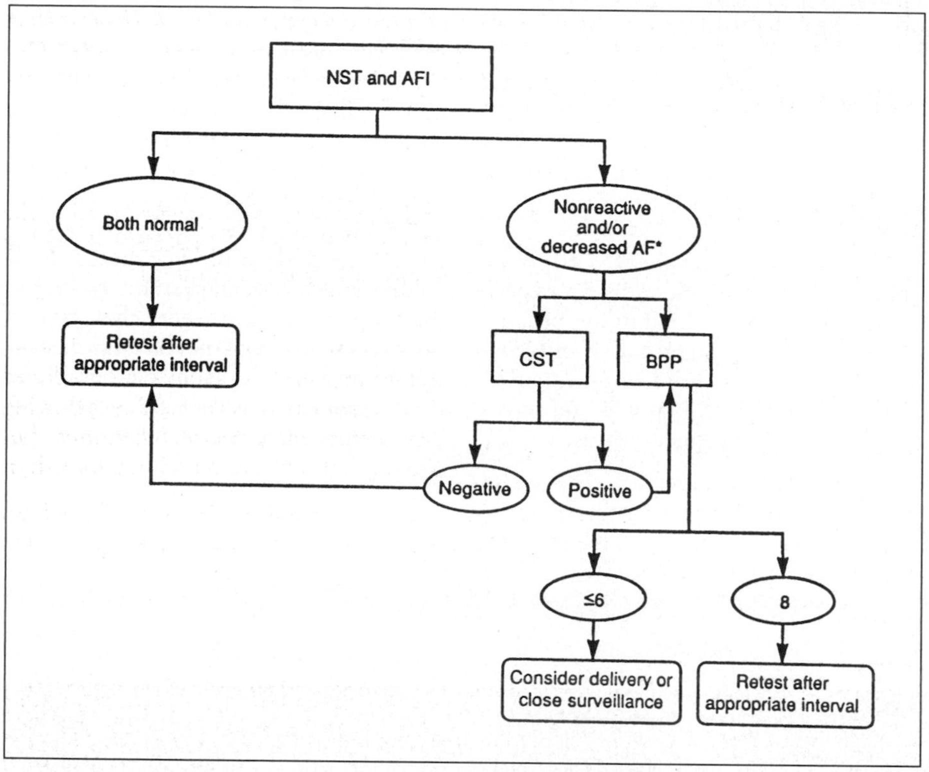

Figure 46-5. ■ *Flowchart for antepartum fetal surveillance in which the NST and AFI are used as the primary methods for fetal evaluation. A nonreactive NST and/or decreased AF are further evaluated using either the contraction stress test or the BPP. If the fetus is mature and if AF volume is reduced, delivery should be considered before further testing is undertaken. (Modified and reprinted with permission from Finberg et al.)*

UMBILICAL ARTERY DOPPLER

Umbilical artery Doppler can provide useful information about underlying circulatory problems associated with pregnancy. The diastolic portion of the Doppler waveform is related to vascular resistance in the placental bed. The normally low resistance decreases throughout pregnancy with a resultant increase in the diastolic velocity. In cases of fetal compromise, there may be an increase in placental resistance resulting in a decreased, absent, or reversed flow through the diastolic portion of the Doppler waveform.

Various indices have been used for measuring umbilical artery flow, but the simplest and most widely used is the A/B ratio:

$$AB = \frac{\text{peak systole}}{\text{end diastole}}$$

The resistive index is also widely used:

$$RI = \frac{\text{systolic flow} - \text{diastolic flow}}{\text{systolic flow}}$$

An abnormal umbilical artery waveform is associated with a poor outcome of the pregnancy.

Technique

If color flow is available, the cord is located as close as possible to the fetal abdomen. The gate is placed over one of the arteries, and the pulsed Doppler is activated. No attempts are made to ob-

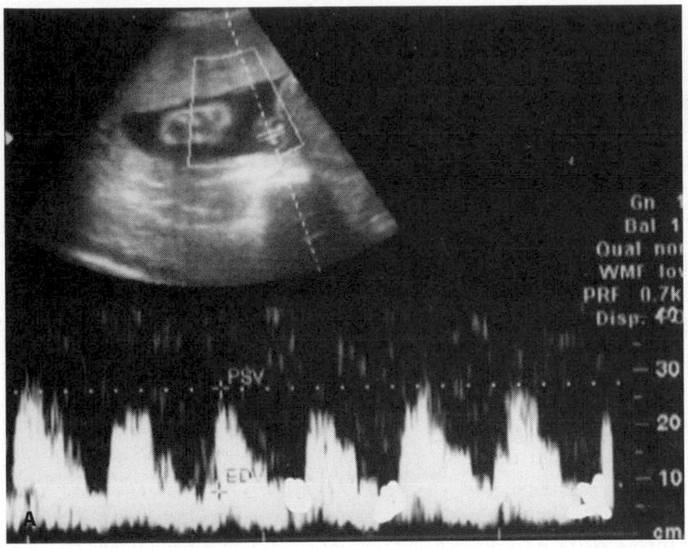

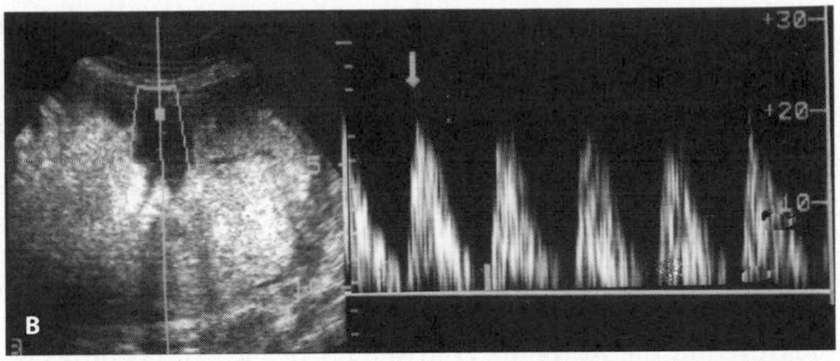

Figure 46-6. ■ *A. Normal umbilical artery pulsed Doppler with the gate placed on the umbilical artery close to the fetal trunk. Note the large amount of diastolic flow. B. Umbilical artery Doppler in a compromised fetus with IUGR; there was no diastolic flow, and the fetus also had an abnormal BPP. Delivery occurred within 1 hour.*

tain a 60-degree angle to the artery because its angle is unknown. If the systole/diastole ratio is lower than 3, or if the resistive index is less than 0.7, results are considered normal (Fig. 46-6A). Levels above these are considered suspicious but of questionable significance if diastolic flow is seen. If no diastolic flow is seen, or if there is a reversal of flow in diastole (Fig. 46-6B), these are worrying findings of clinical significance. The cranial structures are then analyzed using color flow. The middle cerebral vessels (Fig. 46-7) are identified, and Doppler analysis of the middle cerebral artery is performed. If significant cranial diastolic flow is seen with absent diastolic flow in the umbilical artery, this is an ominous sign that many feel would indicate that early delivery should be performed.

Uterine artery Doppler is also performed in some centers in the 16- to 22-week stage of pregnancy, as there is evidence that an abnormal uterine artery Doppler flow at this stage correlates with the development of IUGR later on. This technique is not widely performed in the United States as yet, because there are many false-positive findings.

FETAL LUNG MATURITY

Fetal lung maturity cannot be predicted by ultrasound appearance. The following parameters increase the likelihood but are not indicative of fetal lung maturity:

1. A placental grade of 3 (Fig. 46-8). (When considerable placental calci-

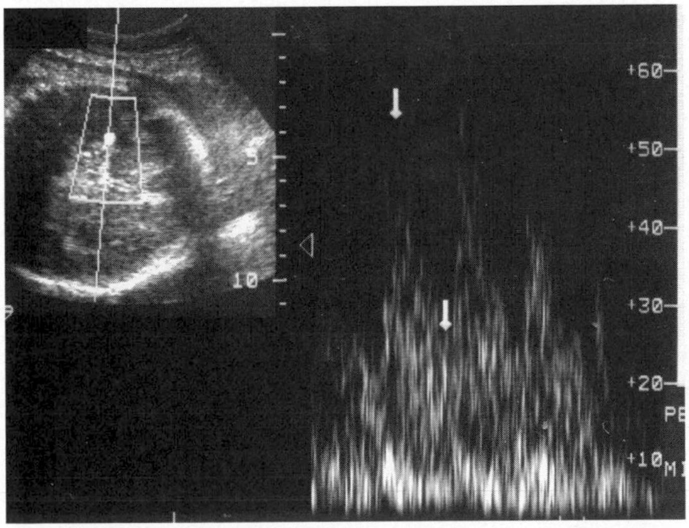

Figure 46-7. ■ *Middle cerebral artery flow. Much diastolic flow is seen in the middle cerebral artery vessels in a compromised fetus. Normally, there should be little diastolic flow.*

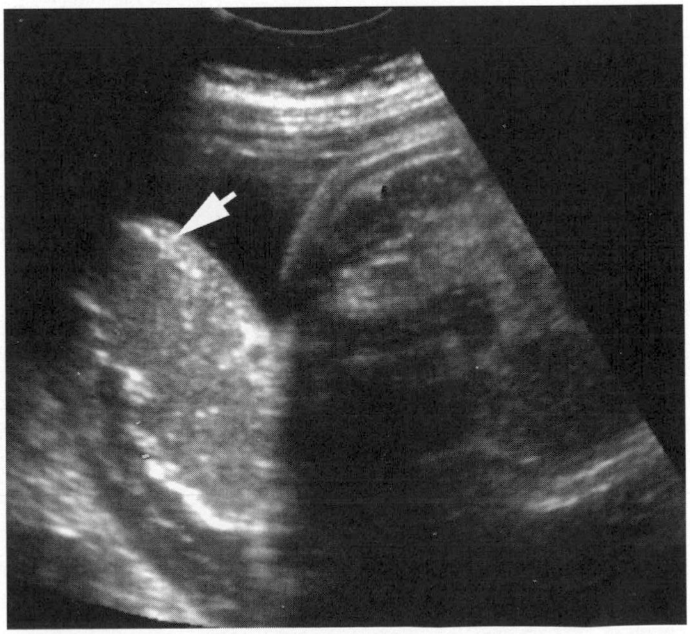

Figure 46-8. ■ *Placental calcification. Considerable placental calcification* (arrow) *in a 32-week compromised fetus with IUGR.*

fication is seen prior to 36 weeks, suspect IUGR).
2. Echopenic meconium in the large bowel.
3. IUGR (the lungs mature earlier in fetuses with IUGR).
4. Proximal humeral epiphyses seen on ultrasound.

The lecithin-sphingomyelin ratio measured in the AF is the gold standard for predicting fetal lung maturity.

Fetal Death

A real-time sonogram is the technique of choice for excluding or confirming fetal demise. Fetal heart motion (FHM) can be detected by real-time ultrasound 5 to 7 weeks after the last menstrual period and as early as 4 1/2 weeks by transvaginal sonography (see Chapter 39).

FHM can be difficult to appreciate early in pregnancy because the fetal chest cavity is so small. Monitor flickering can resemble heart motion but will not be limited to the fetal trunk. Document FHM whenever possible by M-mode, videotape, or Doppler. If an M-mode or VCR is not available, or if there is the slightest doubt concerning heart motion, it is best for two observers to witness FHM and agree upon its presence or absence. If there is no FHM after 2 to 3 minutes of observation, the diagnosis of fetal death in utero can be made.

SONOGRAPHIC APPEARANCES OF FETAL DEATH

Immediately following death, absent FHM is often the only sonographic sign of fetal demise. Within a couple of days, other findings develop (Fig. 46-9).

1. Subcutaneous edema. Appears as a double outline with a sonolucent center surrounding the fetus. Skin thickening may also be seen with fetal hydrops or maternal diabetes.
2. Unnatural fetal position. Usually, the fetus is curled into a tight ball or is in a position of extreme flexion or extension.
3. Spaulding's sign. Overlapping of skull bones is seen in labor as a normal phenomenon, but at other times, it indicates fetal death. Often, the shape of the fetal head becomes grossly distorted after fetal death.
4. Loss of definition of structures in the fetal trunk. Anatomic structures cannot be made out, and abnormal echoes start to appear in the fetal brain.

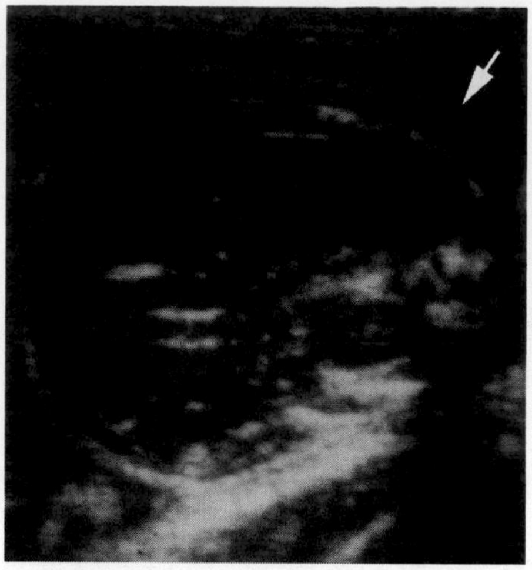

Figure 46-9. ■ *Long-standing fetal death. Transverse view of the fetal trunk shows marked skin edema* (arrow). *There are echogenic areas within the fetal trunk related to maceration and intrafetal gas.*

5. Robert's sign. Gas develops in the fetal abdomen and may obscure fetal anatomy. Shadowing is seen from a strong echo.
6. Maceration causes echoes to develop in the AF.

Pitfalls

BPP

1. Hiccups. Prolonged fetal hiccups will make detection of fetal breathing difficult (Fig. 46-10).
2. Resting fetus. A false-positive BPS result occurs if a normal fetus is observed during a sleep or rest cycle.
3. Oligohydramnios. Fetal movement and tone can be difficult to assess owing to cramped space when fluid is decreased. The postterm pregnancy or pregnancies complicated by premature rupture of membranes are often more difficult to evaluate.
4. Subjective calculation. The assessment of subtle decreases in AF may not be appreciated by an inexperienced observer. Calculating the AFI makes it less likely that oligohydramnios will be overlooked.
5. Cord inclusion. Fluid volume assessment or AFI calculation can be inaccurate when segments of umbilical cord are difficult to see and thus are included in the calculation.

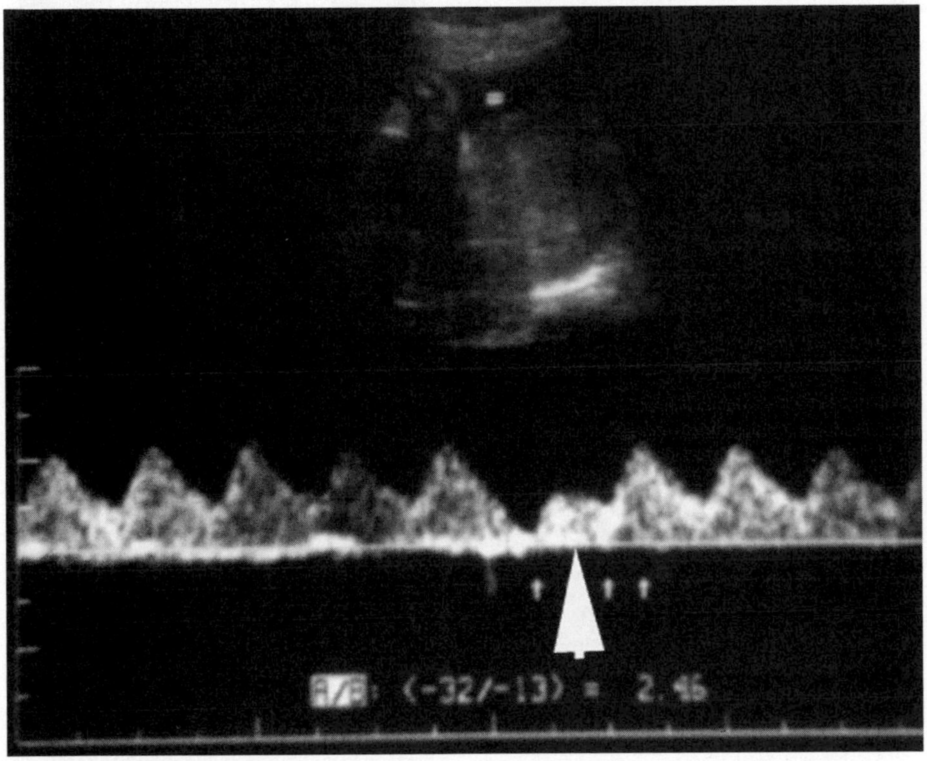

Figure 46-10. ■ *Umbilical artery pulsed Doppler during fetal hiccup* (arrow). *Hiccups have no pathological significance.*

FETAL DEATH

1. Transmitted maternal pulse. Some fetal motion is derived from the maternal aorta. Help clarify that apparent fetal pulsation is maternal by taking the maternal pulse.
2. Maternal habitus. Obesity or excessive scarring may make real-time sonography technically suboptimal. Endovaginal sonography may be helpful, especially in first and second trimester pregnancies, but it is somewhat limited in the third trimester.
3. Frame rate. The use of multiple focal zones decreases pulse repetition frequency, resulting in a significantly lower frame rate. One may fail to demonstrate FHM in a viable fetus if multiple focal zones are used.
4. Persistence. Some ultrasound systems have a variable persistence option. FHM may be present but undetectable with the persistence on.

SELECTED READING

Gabbe SG, Niebyl JR, Simpson JL. *Obstetrics: Normal and Problem Pregnancies*, 4th ed. New York: Churchill Livingstone; 2001.

Manning FA, Basket T, Morrison I, et al. Fetal biophysical profile scoring: a prospective study in 1184 high-risk patients. *Am J Obstet Gynecol* 1981;140:289.

Manning FA, Harman CR, Morrison I, et al. Fetal assessment based on fetal biophysical profile scoring. *Am J Obstet Gynecol* 1990;162:703.

Abnormal Fetal Heart

JOYCE CORDIER

47

KEY WORDS

Angiomas. Echogenic masses that can be situated anywhere in the fetal heart. These tumors are thought to spontaneously resolve.

Annulus. A fibrous ring of tissue where cardiac valve inserts.

Aortic Stenosis. Abnormal aortic valve causing obstruction.

Apex. Inferior portion of heart formed by left ventricle.

Arrhythmia. An irregular heart rate.

Asplenia. Absence of a spleen.

Atresia. Congenital absence or pathologic closure of a normal anatomic opening.

Atrial Isomerism. Both atrial chambers have the anatomic characteristics of a right atrium or left atrium.

Atrial Septal Aneurysm. A thin membrane that bows right to left, sometimes seen at the foramen ovale level.

Atrial Septal Defect (ASD). Defect within the septal wall between the right and the left atrium.

Atrioventricular Valves. Mitral and tricuspid valves. Valves between atria and ventricles.

Autosomal. Not sex related.

Bicuspid Aortic Valve. Aortic valve has two leaflets instead of normal three. May or may not cause aortic stenosis.

Bradycardia. Fetal heart rate less than 100 beats per minute (bpm).

Cardiomyopathy

- **Dilated.** Abnormal dilatation of the heart causing poor function. Seen with critical aortic valve stenosis and heart failure.
- **Hypertrophic.** An abnormal thickening of the septum and ventricular walls. Can be seen in fetus of mother with poorly controlled diabetes.

Chordae Tendineae. Small cord that connects the papillary muscles to the atrioventricular valves.

Coarctation of the Aorta. A localized malformation characterized by deformity of the aortic media, causing narrowing of the lumen of the vessel. Coarctation usually occurs at or near the junction of the patent ductus arteriosus.

Cone (Conus Arteriosus). Part of the embryonic heart that becomes the outflow tracts of the ventricles for the great arteries.

Coronary Sinus. Linear venous structure posterior to left atrium.

Contractility. The property of the cardiac tissue to shorten in response to the appropriate stimulation.

Dextro. Right.

Dextrocardia. The heart is located in the right hemithorax with the apex pointed toward the right. May be associated with cardiac defect.

Double Outlet Ventricle. Both semilunar valves arise from the same ventricle.

Ebstein's Anomaly. One or more leaflets of the tricuspid valve have been displaced apically into the right ventricle, atrializing a portion of the right ventricle.

Ectopia Cordis

- **Abdominal Type.** A gap in the diaphragm through which the heart protrudes into the abdominal cavity.
- **Thoracic Type.** Displacement of the heart outside the thoracic cavity.

Endocardial Fibroelastosis. Hypertrophy of the wall of the left ventricle and conversion of the endocardium into thick fibroelastic coat. The cavity of the ventricle is sometimes reduced, but often increased. Often the walls appear echogenic.

Endocardium. The endothelial lining membrane of the heart.

Eustachian Valve. The valve of the inferior vena cava as it enters the right atrium.

Extrasystoles (Premature Beats). Abnormal atrial or ventricular beats.

Foramen Ovale. An opening in the fetal atrial septum allowing shunting from the right atrium to the left atrium.

Holt-Oram Syndrome. Absence or partial absence of the radius, thumb, and first metacarpal may be present. Atrial septal defect is the most common cardiac defect, but other cardiac defects may be seen.

Hypoplastic. Incomplete development of tissue.

Hypoplastic Left Heart. Incomplete development of the left side of the heart.

Ivemark's Syndrome. Agenesis of the spleen. Commonly associated with cyanotic heart disease and malposition of the abdominal viscera.

Leaflet. A cusp of a heart valve.

Levo. Left.

Lithium. Women who are treated with lithium are at an increased risk of having a child with Ebstein's anomaly.

Lupus (Systemic Lupus Erythematous). A disease in which the body's own immune defenses will damage the connective tissue of an organ. It is associated with congenital heart block in the fetus.

Moderator Band. A band of normal tissue in the right ventricle.

Myocardium. The middle and thickest layer of heart wall.

Papillary Muscle. Striated muscle located in the ventricles of the heart.

Pentalogy of Cantrell. Ectopia cordis, omphalocele, and diaphragmatic defect are present. Can be associated with congenital heart disease.

Pericardial Effusion. Accumulation of fluid around the heart within the pericardial sac. This may result from any type of cardiac failure.

Perimembranous. Thin area of the ventricular septum is inferior to the aortic root.

Phenylketonuria (PKU) (Maternal). In utero fetal damage by elevated phenylketonuria levels (amino acids) in the mother. Possible structure defects include growth deficiency and skeletal and cardiac anomalies (Tetralogy of Fallot, hypoplastic left heart).

Polysplenia. Two or more spleens are sometimes associated with complex congenital heart disease, malformation of the abdominal organs, and absence of the inferior vena cava.

Premature Closure of the Foramen Ovale. May result from underdevelopment of the left side of the heart depending on time of occurrence in utero.

Pulmonary Stenosis. Abnormal pulmonary valve causing obstruction.

Regurgitation. Flow reversal from the ventricles back through the valves into the atria.

Rhabdomyoma. Associated with tuberous sclerosis. A tumor with homogenous bright echo texture. It may occupy any part of the ventricular or atrial walls and chambers. Often associated with rhythm disturbances.

Root. Term used to refer to aorta and pulmonary origin.

Semilunar Valves. Aortic and pulmonic valves.

Skeletal Anomalies. Any type of skeletal anomaly is highly associated with a wide range of congenital heart disease.

Tachycardia. Fetal heart rate greater than 180 bpm.

Tetralogy of Fallot (TOF). Four findings associated are a large perimembranous ventricular septal defect, overriding of the aortic root, pulmonary stenosis (varying from mild valve narrowing to atresia of the valve and artery), and right ventricular hypertrophy (not always seen in the fetus).

Thrombocytopenia. Too few platelets are present.

Thrombocytopenia with Absent Radius (TAR). An inherited, autosomal disease with bilateral absence of the radii and other limb abnormalities. Atrial septal defects and Tetralogy of Fallot are common.

Total Anomalous Pulmonary Venous Return (TAPVR). The pulmonary veins, which normally empty into the left atrium, join to form a confluence that drains into the right atrium, coronary sinus, or superior vena cava. They may form below the diaphragm and drain into a systemic vein in the abdomen.

Transposition of the Great Arteries

D-Transposition of the Great Arteries. The main pulmonary artery arises from the left ventricle and the aorta arises from the right ventricle. Ventricular septal defects are common.

L-Transposition of the Great Arteries (Corrected Transposition). The ventricles are transposed but are correctly connected to the great arteries. Associated with pulmonary stenosis and congenital heart block.

Truncus Arteriosus. A large ventricular septal defect with one overriding great artery.

Tuberous Sclerosis. A familial disease affecting the brain, skin, and kidneys; other organs may be involved. Skin lesions, seizures, and mental retardation are the classic clinical findings. There are varying degrees of severity. Associated with rhabdomyomas.

Turner's Syndrome. A chromosomal abnormality with numerous physical defects, including cystic hygroma, growth retardation, and cardiac defects. Most commonly coarctation of the aorta or other left-sided defects.

Ventricular Outflow Tracts. Term used for views of the aorta and pulmonary arteries as they leave the left and right ventricles.

Ventricular Septal Defect (VSD). A persistent area of dropout within the ventricular septum (see Pitfalls). VSD may be the only finding or may be associated with other cardiac defects.

The Clinical Problem

Congenital heart disease is found in slightly less than 1% of infants. With immediate family history or a prior sibling with congenital heart disease there is an increased risk of congenital heart disease. Entities associated with congenital heart disease are as follows:

1. Fetal cardiac arrhythmia
2. Chromosomal abnormalities
   a. Turner's syndrome
   b. Down syndrome (Trisomy 21)
   c. Trisomy 13
   d. Trisomy 18
3. Familial disease
   a. Ivemark's syndrome
   b. Holt-Oram syndrome
   c. Thrombocytopenia with absent radius
   d. Family history of congenital heart disease
4. Fetal anomalies
   a. Cystic hygromas
   b. Omphalocele
   c. Nonimmune hydrops
      Pleural or pericardial effusion
      Ascites
      Skin thickening
      Polyhydramnios
      Placentomegaly
   d. Intrauterine growth retardation
   e. Duodenal atresia
5. Maternal disease
   a. Diabetes
   b. Lupus
   c. Alcoholism
   d. Medication
   e. Drug abuse

In the presence of complex congenital heart disease a number of management issues arise. The family may elect termination of the pregnancy, depending on the severity of the prognosis. Repeat echocardiograms can follow the progression of the disease. Fetuses with complex congenital heart disease are best delivered at a center with a team of pediatric cardiologists, neonatologists, and pediatric cardiac surgeons.

Anatomy and Physiology

When evaluating the structure of the fetal heart, the sonographer should be familiar with the fetal circulation (Fig. 47-1). The left and right ventricles function in parallel rather than in series, as in the postnatal circulation.

Fetal blood flow patterns depend on the patency of the ductus arteriosus and the foramen ovale. The foramen ovale allows passage of the blood from the right to the left system. The right and left cardiac chambers are approximately the same size in the fetus. Disproportion between the right and left chamber sizes may be the result of obstruction of blood flow through the ductus arteriosus and foramen ovale or the aorta. Maldevelopment of either the right or left ventricle may not cause any hemodynamic problem in utero because of the ductus arteriosus and foramen ovale.

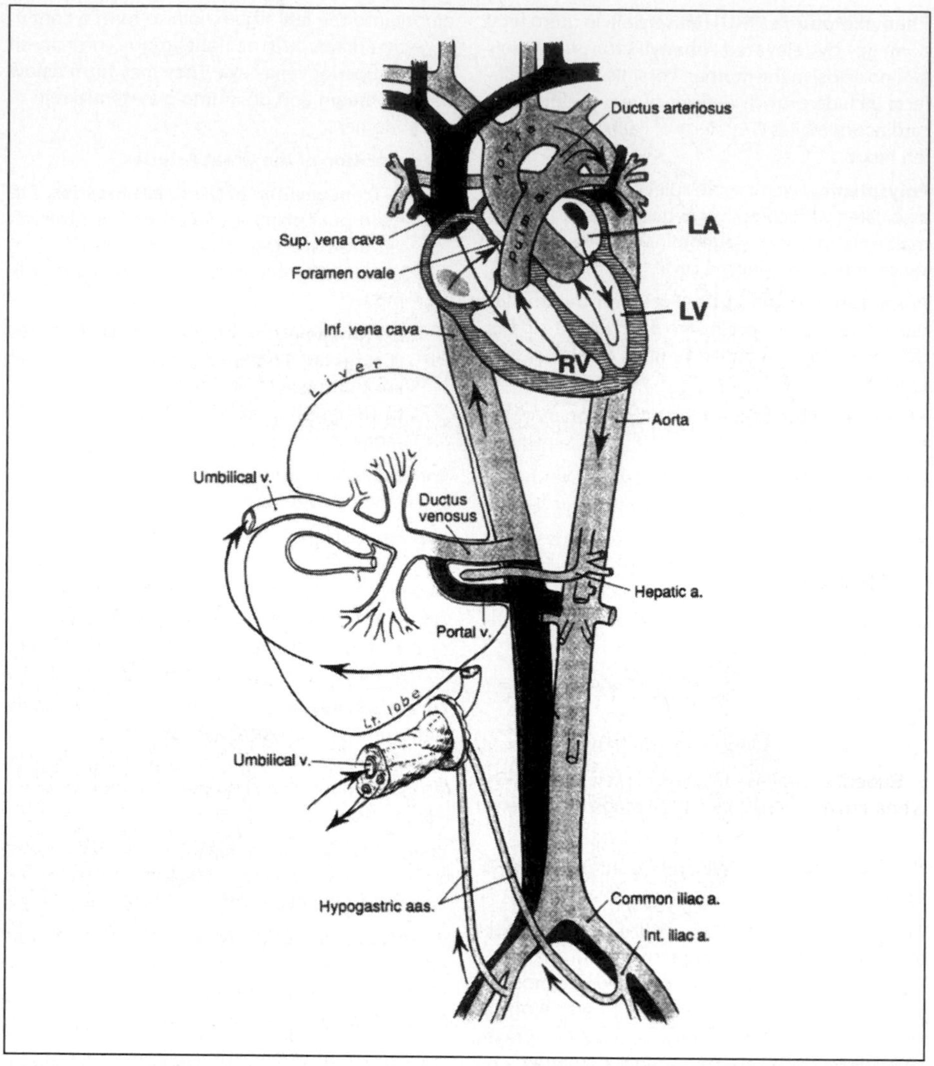

Figure 47-1. ■ *Fetal circulation.*

Technique

First define the fetal position. Correct identification of the right and left sides of the fetus is critical. The stomach is an ideal landmark once abdominal situs is established. The ideal situation is when the fetal spine is down. The following views resemble this position. These views will be oriented differently when the fetus is in different positions, such as spine up.

FOUR-CHAMBER VIEW

The fetal heart lies transversely in the chest. Identify the long axis of the spine and rotate 90 degrees at the level of the thorax, or angle toward the head from the abdominal circumference. The fetal heart should occupy approximately one-third of the thorax and is situated to the left in the chest (Fig. 47-2). Angle perpendicular to the ventricular septum (see Pitfalls) to view the thickness and continuity of the septum (Fig. 47-3A).

1. The right ventricle is situated beneath the anterior chest wall. The moderator band is in the right ventricle, and the walls are trabeculated. The left ventricular walls are much smoother. The left ventricle forms the apex.
2. The left atrium is nearest the spine.

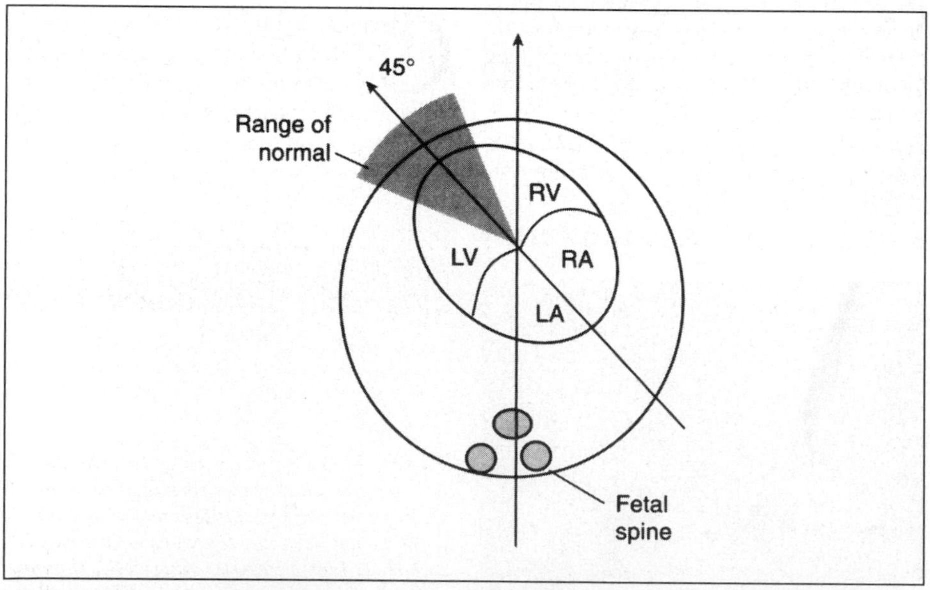

Figure 47-2. ■ *Cardiac axis related to the spine. The normal axis is 45 degrees. A 20-degree variation in either direction is considered within normal limits.*

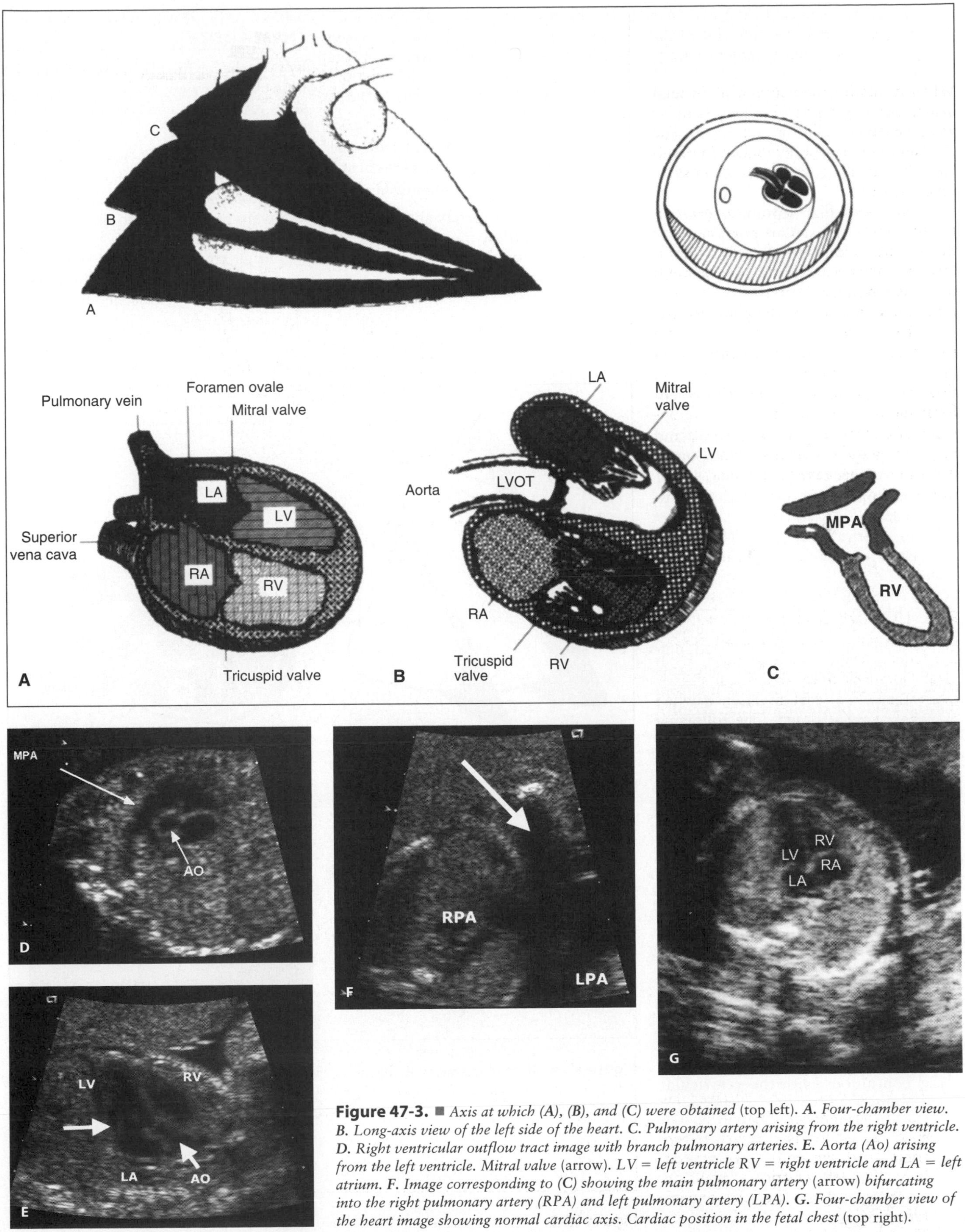

Figure 47-3. ■ *Axis at which (A), (B), and (C) were obtained* (top left). *A. Four-chamber view. B. Long-axis view of the left side of the heart. C. Pulmonary artery arising from the right ventricle. D. Right ventricular outflow tract image with branch pulmonary arteries. E. Aorta (Ao) arising from the left ventricle. Mitral valve* (arrow). *LV = left ventricle RV = right ventricle and LA = left atrium. F. Image corresponding to (C) showing the main pulmonary artery* (arrow) *bifurcating into the right pulmonary artery (RPA) and left pulmonary artery (LPA). G. Four-chamber view of the heart image showing normal cardiac axis. Cardiac position in the fetal chest* (top right).

3. The ventricular cavities are similar in size. At term, the right side of the heart may be slightly larger than the left side.
4. The atrioventricular valves open during diastole.
5. Tricuspid valve insertion into the ventricular septum is slightly more toward the apex than the mitral valve.
6. The ventricular septum is continuous. The muscular portion is of equal thickness to the left ventricular wall. The membranous portion is much thinner.
7. The foramen ovale bows into the left atrium.
8. The atrial chambers are similar in size.
9. The pulmonary veins can be seen entering the left atrium.
10. The cardiac axis is between 30 and 60 degrees to a line from the spine to the midpart of the chest (Fig. 47-2).
11. The thoracic aorta is anterior and to the left of the fetal spine.
12. The inferior vena cava (IVC) should not be seen behind the heart.

LONG-AXIS VIEW OF THE LEFT HEART

At the four-chamber view tilt the scan plane slightly toward the fetal head, pivoting at the apex. The best long-axis view will be obtained when angling from the right side of the heart (Fig. 47-3B). As you angle up toward the aorta, the ventricular septum at this level should be evaluated because many defects occur in this area (see Ventricular Septal Defects). Rotate almost parallel to the fetal spine to demonstrate the left ventricular outflow, interventricular septum, mitral, and aortic valves (see Fig. 47-10A).

1. The aortic valve and root, mitral valve, left ventricle, and left ventricular outflow tract should be seen.
2. Part of the right ventricle is present anterior to the aortic root and ventricular septum.
3. The left atrium sits along the posterior wall of the aortic root.
4. The anterior wall of the aortic root is continuous with the ventricular septum.
5. The posterior wall of the aortic root is continuous with the anterior leaflet of the mitral valve.

PULMONARY ARTERY ARISING FROM THE RIGHT VENTRICLE

Angle slightly more cephalad from the long-axis view of the left side of the heart, pivoting at the apex (Fig. 47-3C,D).

1. The pulmonary artery and right ventricular outflow tract can be seen.
2. Branches of the pulmonary artery can be seen.

SHORT-AXIS VIEW FOR EVALUATING CHAMBER SIZE

Rotate the beam 90 degrees from the four-chamber view. Start at the apex and slide toward the atrioventricular valves (Fig. 47-4B,C).

1. Obtain a view just below the valves to demonstrate the ventricular chamber size and thickness of the walls compared with the ventricular septum.
2. Angle toward the great vessels. The aortic root should be positioned in the center (Mercedes-Benz sign) (Fig. 47-4A).

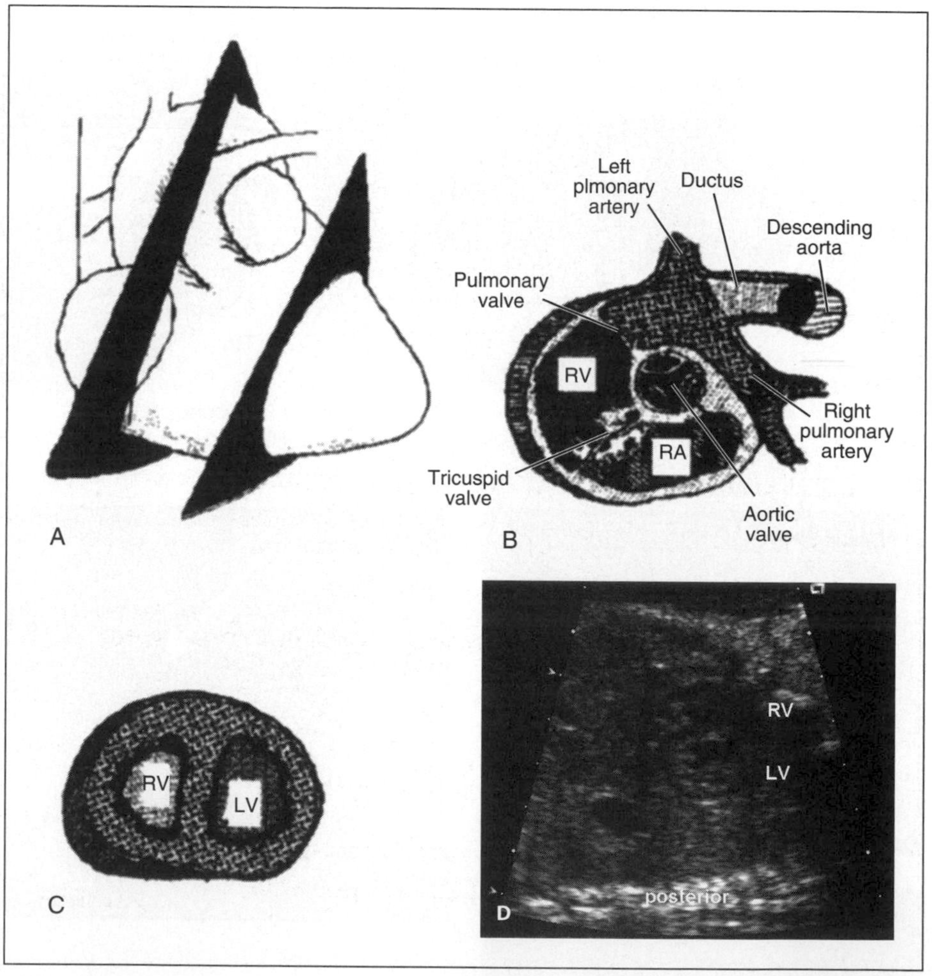

Figure 47-4. ■ *Short-axis views. A. Short-axis view demonstrating great vessels. B. Short-axis view at ventricular level. C. Short-axis view for evaluating ventricular chamber size. D. Real-time image of ventricles.*

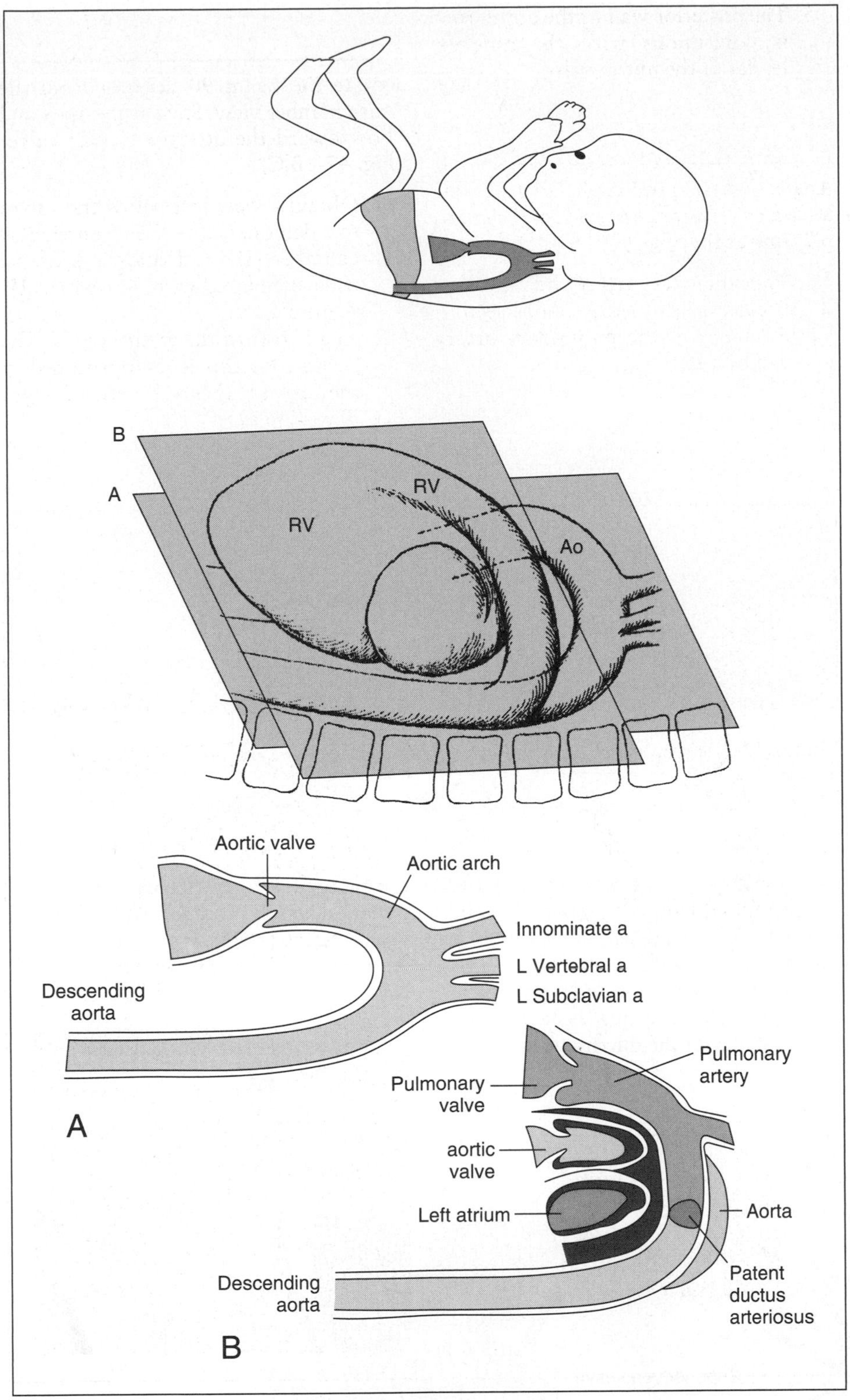

Figure 47-5. ■ *Views required to show the aortic arch and pulmonary artery into the descending aorta. A. Aortic arch into descending aorta. B. Patent ductus arteriosus and pulmonary artery.*

3. The pulmonary artery, right atrium, right ventricle, and left atrium wrap around the aortic valve.
4. Branches of the pulmonary artery may be seen.
5. The size of the aortic root compared with the pulmonic root can be evaluated from this view.

AORTIC ARCH INTO DESCENDING AORTA

Obtain a long-axis of the fetus and direct the beam through the ventral wall of the fetus angling toward the spine (descending aorta) (Fig. 47-5A). When the spine is up (Fig. 47-6), scan laterally (from the left side of the fetus) on the maternal abdomen and angle under the spine. When the spine is down, also scan laterally on the maternal abdomen to visualize the aortic arch.

1. The aorta exits from the center of the heart.
2. The aortic arch gives rise to the head and neck vessels, which include the innominate, left carotid, and left subclavian arteries.
3. The arch curves toward the spine and continues into the descending aorta.

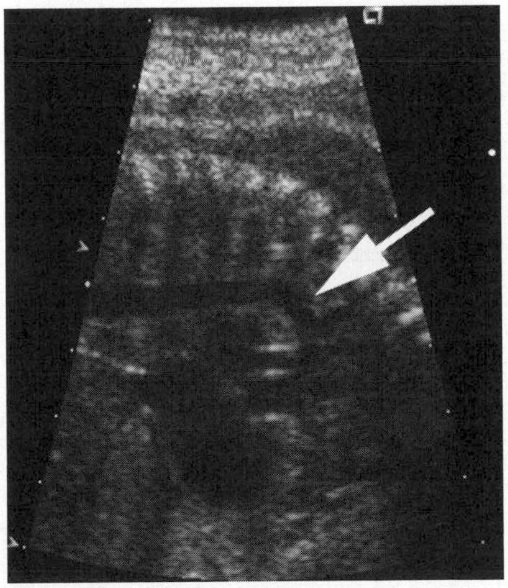

Figure 47-6. ■ *Aortic arch* (arrow) *with fetal spine up.*

PATENT DUCTUS ARTERIOSUS

Stay in the long-axis plane. At the aortic arch view, slide slightly toward the descending aorta (Fig. 47-5B).

1. The pulmonary artery arises from the anterior aspect of the heart (right ventricle) and takes a sharp course straight back toward the descending aorta.
2. The course of the pulmonary artery to the descending aorta (patent ductus arteriosus) resembles the shape of a hockey stick (Fig. 47-7).

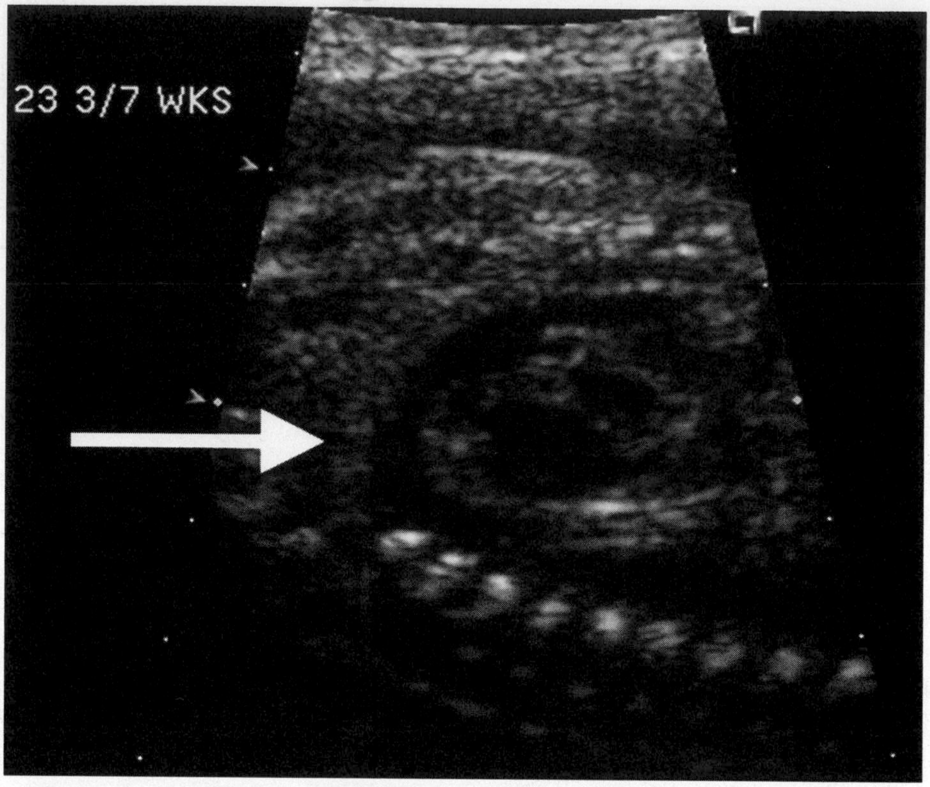

Figure 47-7. ■ *Ductal arch* (arrow). *Note the different shape and entrance point into the cardiac outline.*

INFERIOR VENA CAVA ENTERING THE RIGHT ATRIUM

On the long-axis view of the fetus, direct the beam through the ventral wall of the fetus angling toward the right of the spine (Fig. 47-8). If the spine is up, scan from the right side of the fetus.

1. The IVC enters the right atrium inferiorly.
2. The superior vena cava (SVC) enters the right atrium superiorly.
3. The ductus venosus and hepatic veins can be seen entering the IVC before the IVC enters the right atrium.

PULSED DOPPLER: AN ADDITIONAL TOOL

When performing the fetal echocardiogram, pulsed Doppler can add information or reinforce the suspected diagnosis. The same technique limitations that hold true when performing the two-dimensional examination apply when recording the pulsed Doppler examination. For optimal flow patterns, stay parallel to the blood flow.

In utero, the aortic and pulmonic arterial pressures are equal because of the wide patency of the ductus arteriosus. In the presence of ventricular outflow obstruction and the absence of a ventricular septal defect (VSD), a pressure gradient may cause turbulent flow. Atrioventricular valve regurgitation (e.g., Ebstein's anomaly or atrioventricular canal defect) can be documented with pulsed Doppler.

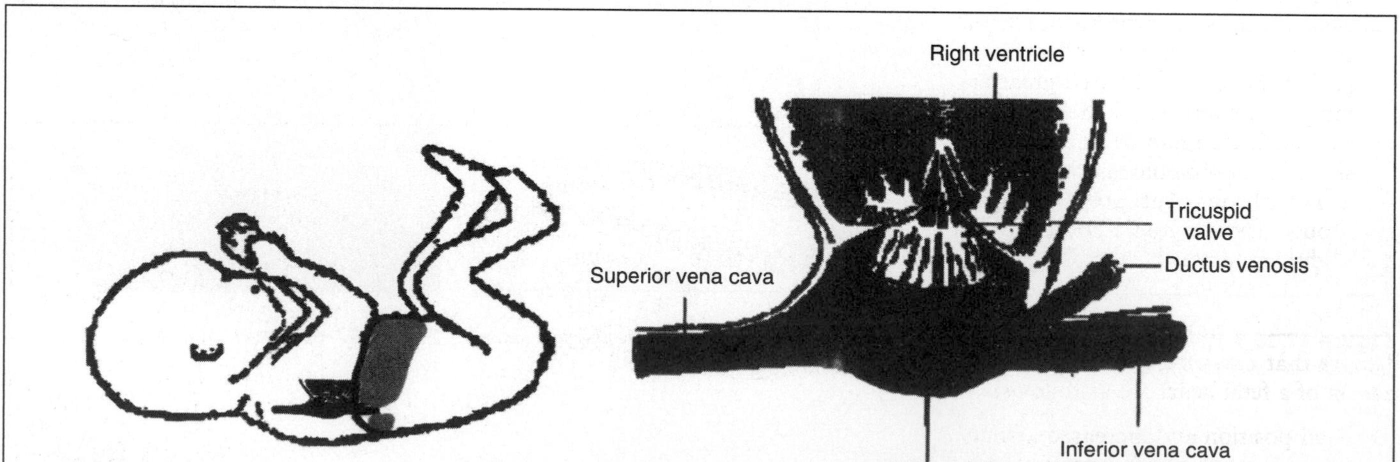

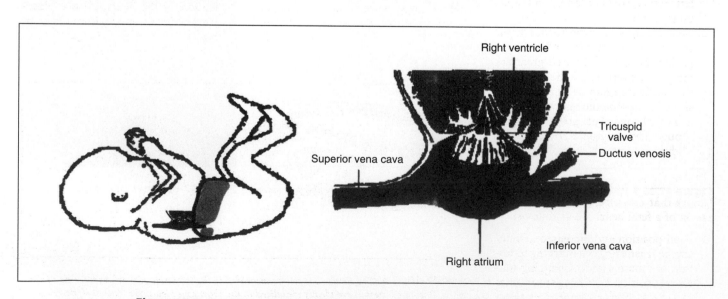

Figure 47-8. ■ *Inferior vena cava and superior vena cava entering the right atrium.*

COLOR DOPPLER

Color Doppler is a very useful tool in fetal echocardiography. Some areas in which color Doppler is useful are as follows:

1. Confirming normal anatomy in the obese or difficult-to-scan patient.
2. Confirming a VSD or proving that the suspected area is not a defect.
3. Visualizing pulmonary vein flow with the Doppler scale low for the low-velocity venous flow.
4. Looking for valve regurgitation in a fetus with atrioventricular canal defect or with signs of hydrops or heart failure.
5. Visualizing sufficient shunt flow across the patent ductus arteriosus and patent foramen ovale.
6. Confirming flow or absence of flow through valves, vessels, or chambers.

Measurements

1. Place an m-mode cursor perpendicular to the ventricular septum to measure ventricular chamber size and ventricular wall thickness just below the level of the atrioventricular valves in the four-chamber or short-axis view (Fig. 47-9). Function of the ventricular chambers can be quantitated by m-mode measurements if there is a concern of poor function. The right and left ventricular chamber sizes and wall thickness should be the same until late in the third trimester, when the right ventricular chamber size may be slightly increased compared with the left. Fetal heart rate can be measured on m-mode.
2. Measure the size of the aortic root in the long or short axis. When comparing the size of the two great arteries, the short axis is helpful (Fig. 47-10). Once again, symmetry in the size of the pulmonic and aortic root is key throughout pregnancy, although the pulmonic root may be slightly larger than the aortic root.

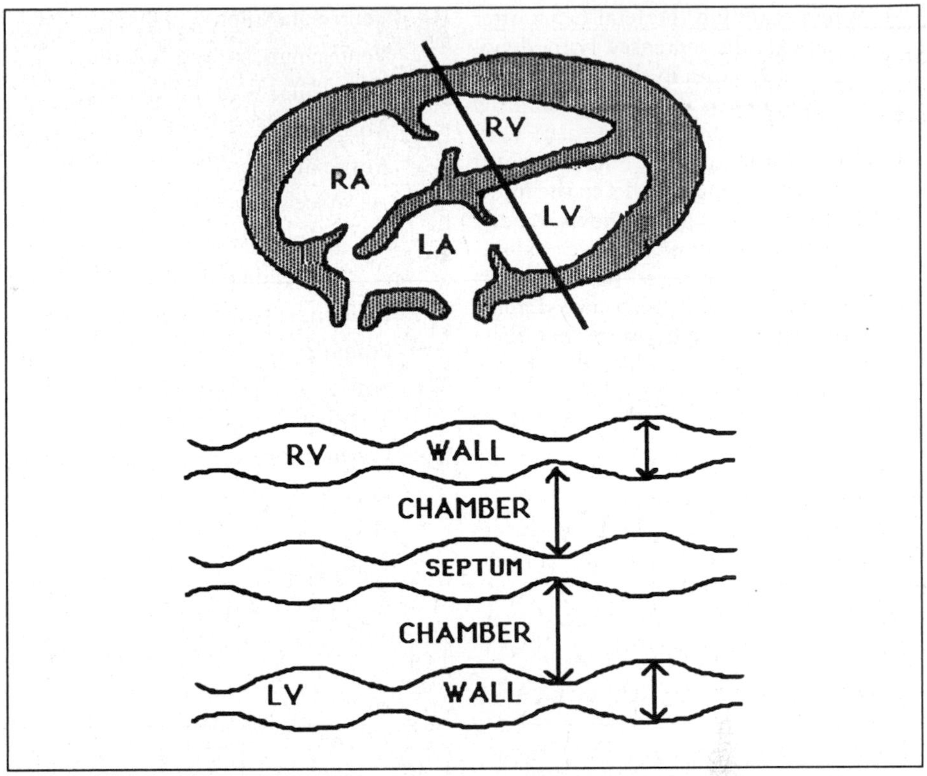

Figure 47-9. ■ *M-mode cursor across the ventricular chambers displays m-mode tracing to evaluate ventricular size and wall thickness. Ventricular heart rate can be measured here.*

TECHNICAL PROBLEMS

Factors that can affect accurate visualization of a fetal heart are as follows:

1. Fetal position and increased activity can be frustrating when trying to obtain optimum views. Changing maternal position by having the mother roll to one side can sometimes affect the fetal position. Having the mother walk around or fill or empty her bladder may also help.
2. Because of a thick body wall, maternal obesity can place anterior reverberations into the chest area. Obesity also increases the distance between the fetus and the probe, making it more difficult to optimize visualization of the heart. Don't rule out using a lower frequency. Tissue harmonics on the newer machines can be very helpful in these circumstances.
3. Decreased or increased amniotic fluid volume can be a problem. Too little fluid prevents ideal visualization of any organ. Too much amniotic fluid can increase the distance between the probe and the fetus, consequently affecting good visualization of the heart. Proper placement of focal zones can be very helpful.

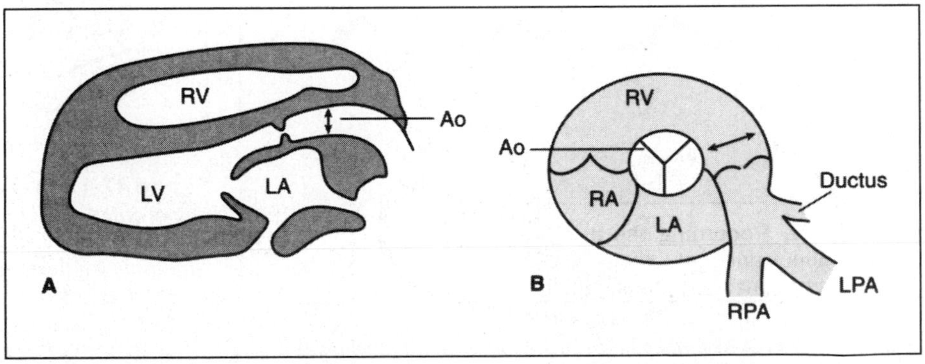

Figure 47-10. ■ *A. The aortic root can be measured in the long-axis view of the left side of the heart. B. Both great vessels are ideally visualized in the short-axis views. Simultaneous measurements can be taken.*

4. When scanning the fetal heart after 32 weeks, the increased bony deposition of calcium in the ribs and vertebral column can cast a shadow through the heart. The ideal window is through the anterior chest wall. By staying parallel to the intercostal spaces, good views of the heart can be obtained.
5. In the postdate heart, the right ventricular chamber can be slightly larger than the left.

CHECKLIST

- Fetal heart rate
- Fetal heart rhythm
- Situs and cardiac position
- Left ventricle
- Right ventricle
- Ventricular septum
- Ventricular size and function
- Ventricular wall thickness
- Aortic valve
- Aortic arch
  - Ascending aorta
  - Transverse aorta (head vessels)
  - Descending aorta
- Pulmonary artery with branching
- Pulmonary valve
- Size of the main pulmonary artery and aorta
- Patent ductus arteriosus
- IVC
- SVC
- Right atrium
- Atrial septum (patent foramen ovale)
- Left atrium
- Pulmonary veins
- Tricuspid valve
- Mitral valve

Pathology

ARRHYTHMIA/DYSRHYTHMIA

If there is a sustained irregular heart rhythm or rate, a more extensive look at the heart is warranted. The normal fetal heart rate varies between 120 and 160 bpm.

1. Record atrial and ventricular contractions simultaneously by directing the m-mode cursor through both the atrial and ventricular walls (Figs. 47-11 and 47-12). Due to the small

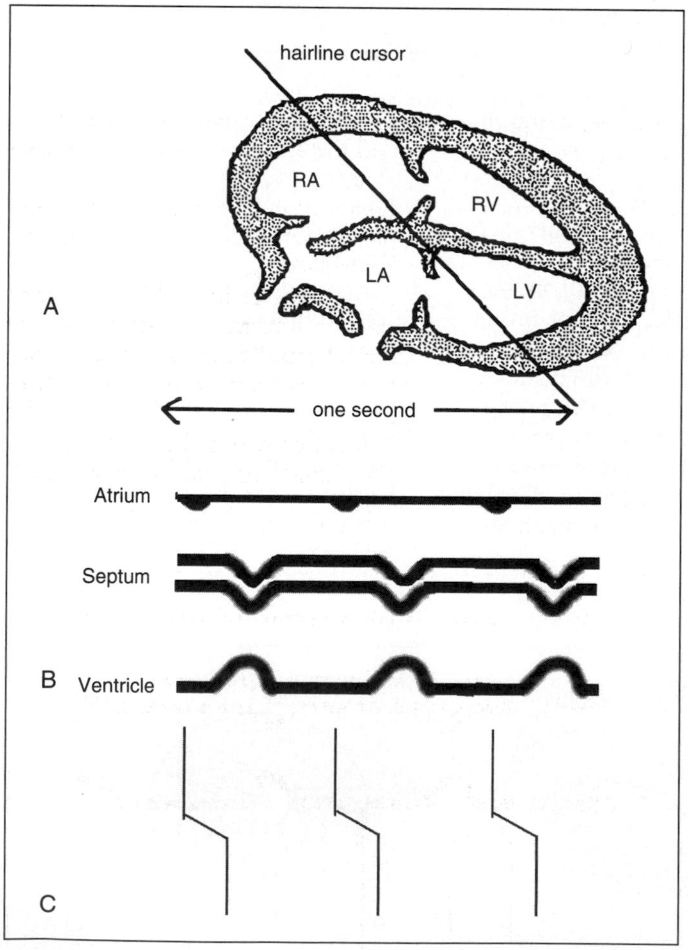

Figure 47-11. ■ *Recording of the atrioventricular contraction sequence. A. Cursor is directed simultaneously through the atrial and ventricular walls. B. M-mode tracing reveals normal ventricular wall contraction after atrial wall contraction. C. Ladder diagram is helpful in evaluating the contraction sequence.*

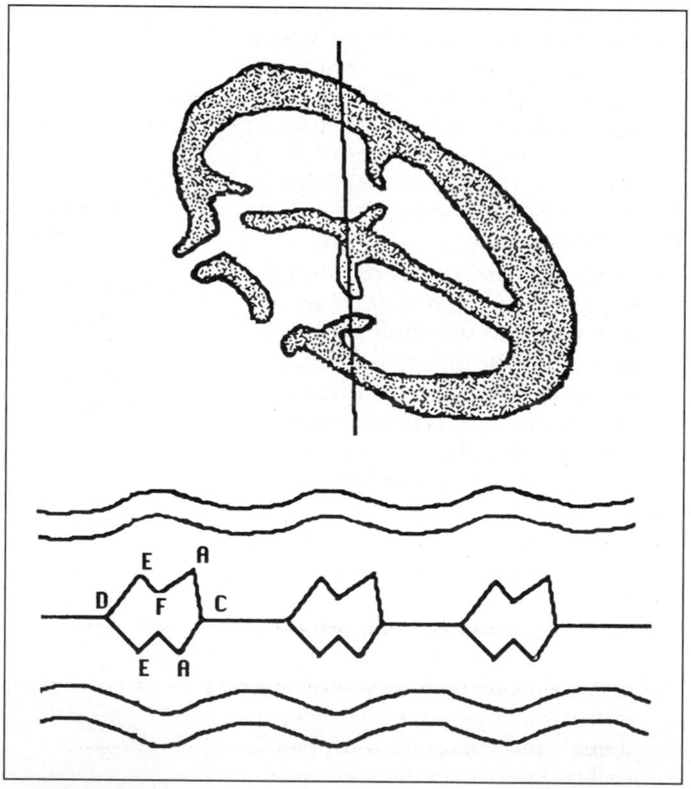

Figure 47-12. ■ *Onset of the A wave can also be observed when evaluating atrial contractions. D = end of ventricular systole, E = peak opening of the valve, F = diastolic closing, A = the peak atrial systole as the atrium contracts, and C = complete valve closure after the onset of ventricular contractions.*

amplitude of the atrial wall during contraction, this can be difficult to record. Atrial contractions can also be recorded by the arrival (onset) of the A-wave of the tricuspid or mitral valve (Fig. 47-13). The atrial contraction will be followed closely by the ventricular contraction (Fig. 47-11B). Do not mistake the foramen ovale tissue motion for the atrial wall contraction.

2. Measure heart rate on the m-mode at the same point on two consecutive beats (Fig. 47-11). Most equipment has this capability built in. Heart rate can be measured as well by pulsed Doppler on most machines.
3. Check for any signs of hydrops. This is associated with fetal cardiac failure and is likely to be present if the dysrhythmia is sustained.
4. Sustained dysrhythmias (especially those with any sign of hydrops) should be followed closely.
5. Dysrhythmias can be associated with structural disease. When the two are both present, the outcome is often poor.

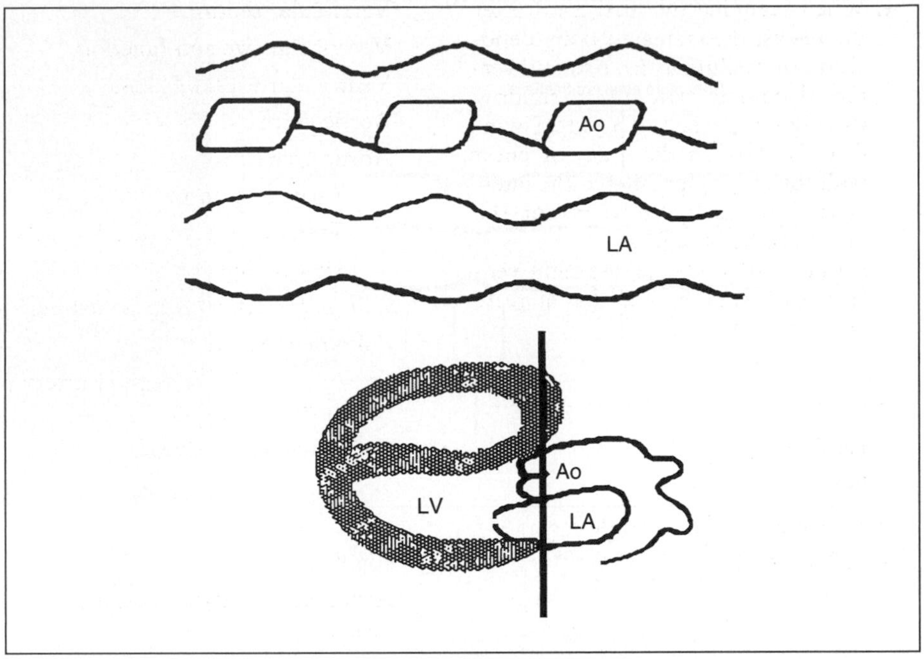

Figure 47-13. ■ *Atrioventricular contraction sequence can be evaluated by angling through a semilunar valve opening and an atrial wall.*

SLOW HEART RATE

Bradycardia

1. Sinus bradycardia is when the heart rate is less than 100 bpm. The atria and ventricles are beating at a 1:1 ratio (Fig. 47-14).
2. Normal to see for brief periods early in pregnancy if it is not sustained.
3. If not sustained, it can be the result of excessive transducer pressure on the maternal abdomen.
4. If sustained, it can be due to cord compression or fetal distress.

Complete Heart Block

The ventricle and atria are not beating at the same rate.

1. Ventricular heart rate is less than 100 bpm, usually 50 to 60 bpm (Fig. 47-15).
2. The ventricle will beat regularly, and the atrial rate will be disassociated.
3. Fifty percent of fetuses with complete heart block will have structural heart disease.
4. Second-degree heart block is when there is intermittent conduction of atrial beats. The atria will beat twice to the ventricle once (2:1) or three times (3:1).
5. Associated with maternal lupus.
6. If sustained maternal drug therapy is used.

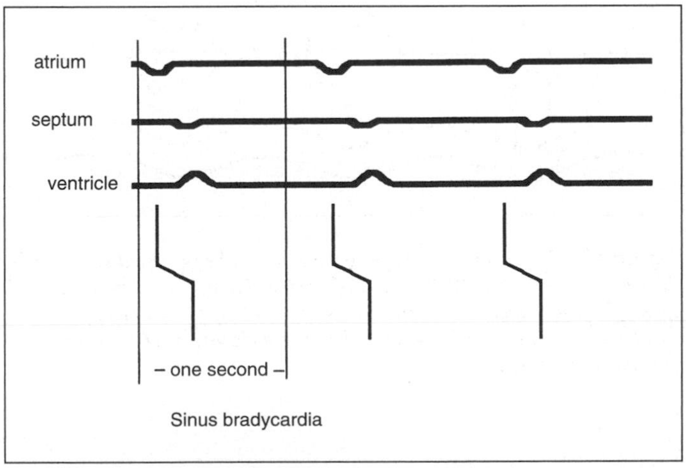

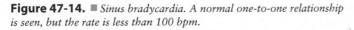

Figure 47-14. ■ *Sinus bradycardia. A normal one-to-one relationship is seen, but the rate is less than 100 bpm.*

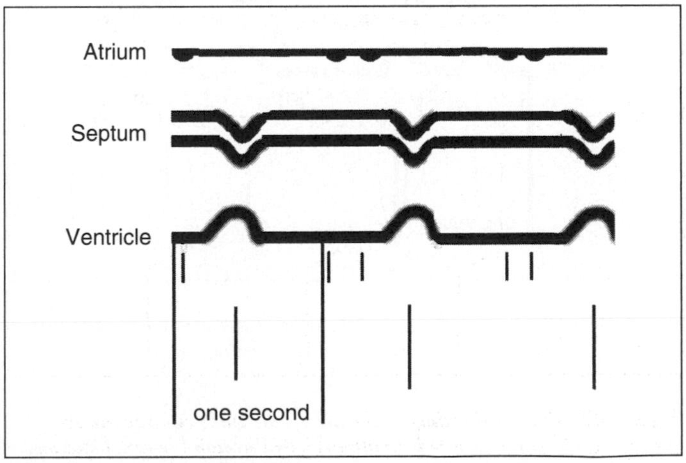

Figure 47-15. ■ *Complete heart block. Rhythm is totally out of synchronization. Ventricular rate is less than 100 bpm.*

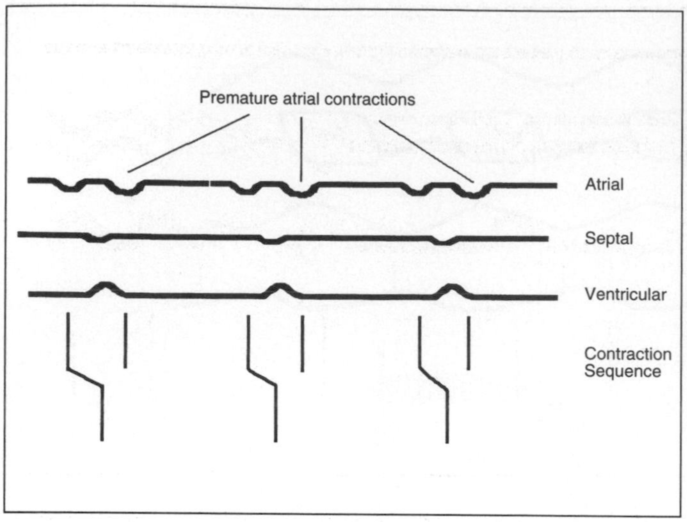

Figure 47-16. ■ *Premature atrial contractions. Early atrial beat is seen without conduction to the ventricle.*

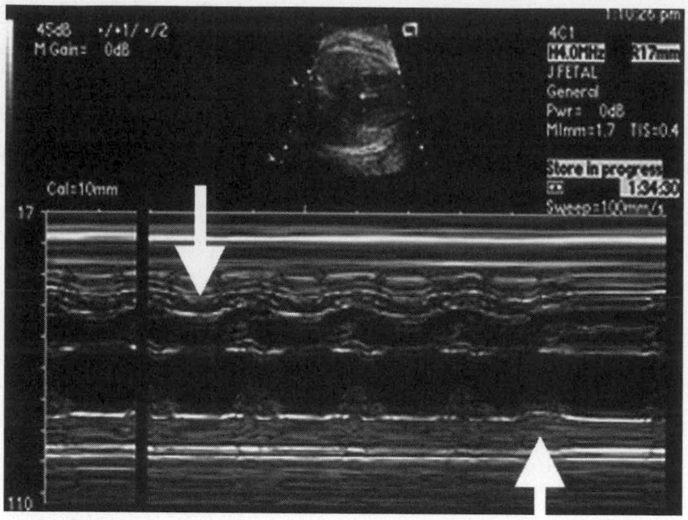

Figure 47-17. ■ *M-mode of conducted premature atrial contraction. Ventricular contraction* (top arrow). *Premature atrial contraction* (bottom arrow).

IRREGULAR HEART RATE

Premature Atrial Contractions

There will be an early atrial contraction that is either conducted or blocked. When conducted, a ventricular beat will follow. When blocked, a ventricular contraction will not follow (Figs. 47-16 and 47-17).

1. Often the foramen ovale is bowed far enough into the left atrium that it is hitting against the atrial wall. This may be the cause of premature contraction of the atrial wall.
2. Can be isolated and may occur only occasionally.
3. Bigeminy is when there are two beats and then a skipped beat or pause. The atria and ventricles will be in a 1:1 relationship (Fig. 47-18).
4. Trigeminy refers to three beats and a skipped beat or pause.
5. If sustained, close fetal monitoring may be considered.

Premature Ventricular Contractions

Premature ventricular contractions are ventricular contractions that are not preceded by an atrial contraction. When isolated, this is usually not of much significance (Fig. 47-19).

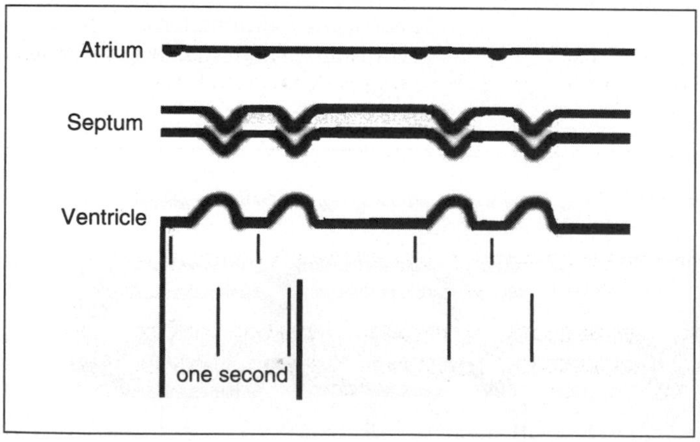

Figure 47-18. ■ *Atrial bigeminy. Two beats are seen in a one-to-one relationship, and there is a pause. Atrial contractions are at the top of the m-mode image.*

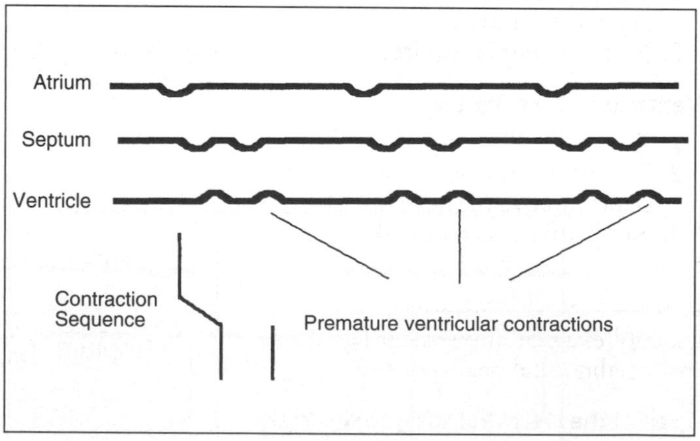

Figure 47-19. ■ *Premature ventricular contractions. Ventricular contraction precedes an early contraction.*

FAST HEART RATE (TACHYCARDIA)

Supraventricular Tachycardia

1. The heart rate will be more than 200 bpm.
2. The ventricle and atria are beating in a 1:1 ratio (Fig. 47-20).
3. If the supraventricular tachycardia is sustained for prolonged periods it will not be well tolerated and the fetus is likely to develop signs of hydrops. Serial echocardiograms are warranted to follow the heart rate and check for signs of heart failure.
4. If sustained maternal drug therapy is used.

Atrial Flutter

1. The atria will beat at a rate of 400 to 600 bpm.
2. The ventricular rate is blocked (not conducted) and will beat at a ratio two to three times slower than the atria (Fig. 47-21).
3. Ventricular rate is usually 200 to 300 bpm.
4. If sustained, it is not tolerated well and the fetus is likely to develop signs of hydrops. Serial echocardiograms are warranted to follow the heart rate and check for signs of heart failure.
5. If sustained maternal drug therapy is used.

Sinus Tachycardia

1. The heart rate will be 180 to 190 bpm (Fig. 47-22).
2. The ventricle and the atria are beating in a 1:1 ratio.
3. No treatment is required.

Ventricular Tachycardia

1. The atria will beat at a normal rate.
2. The ventricles will beat at a rate slightly above the normal heart rate.
3. No treatment is required.

ABNORMAL HEART LOCATION

Initially exclude any noncardiac causes for the abnormal heart position.

Apex of the Heart Pointing to the Right (Dextrocardia, Dextroversion)

The fetal heart is situated on the right side of the body with the apex pointing toward the right.

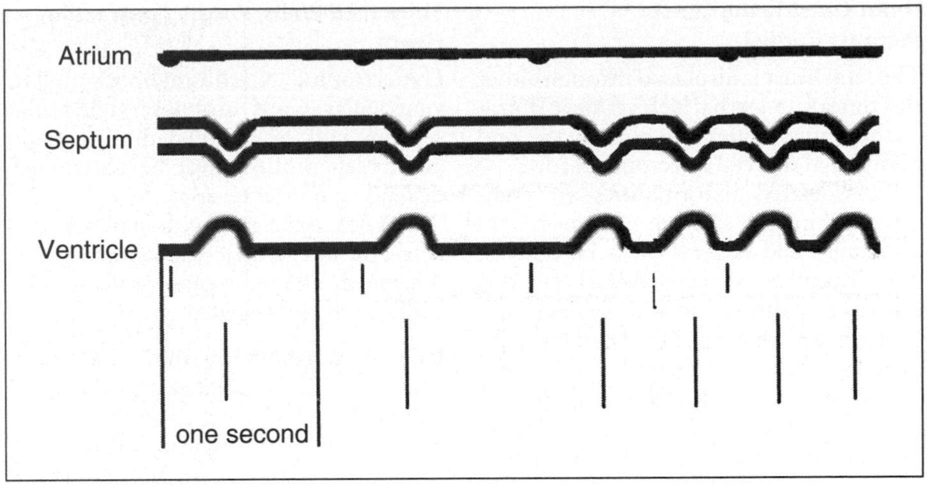

Figure 47-20. ■ *Supraventricular tachycardia. Normal sinus rhythm increased abruptly from 140 to 200 bpm.*

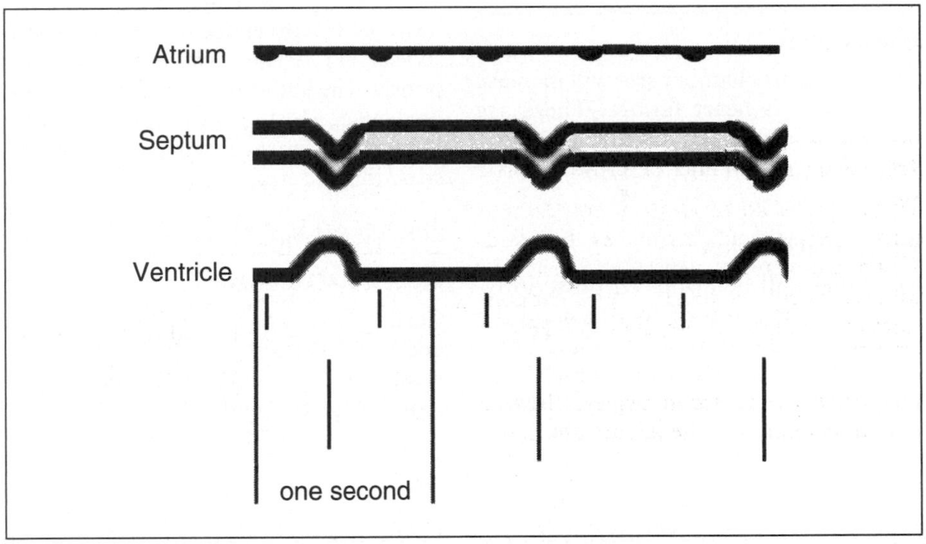

Figure 47-21. ■ *Atrial flutter-2:1 block. Only every other atrial contraction is conducted to the ventricle. Ventricular wall motion is at the top of the m-mode and atria at the bottom.*

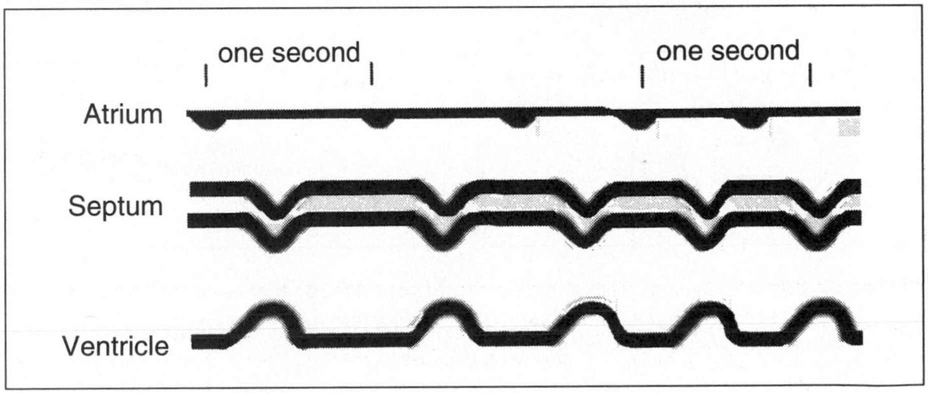

Figure 47-22. ■ *Sinus tachycardia. Gradual increase in the rate is seen.*

Heart Outside the Chest (Ectopia Cordis)

The fetal heart is displaced through either the thorax (a sternal defect) or a thoracoabdominal defect (diaphragmatic and abdominal defects) in ectopia cordis.

Associated abnormalities are common and include central nervous system anomalies and skeletal or facial defects, as well as other cardiac defects. However, due to the malrotation and displacement of the heart, be careful in making the diagnosis of cardiac defects.

When there is a diaphragmatic defect, omphalocele, and abnormal cardiac position, the condition is known as pentalogy of Cantrell. The prognosis is poor. Most die in the neonatal period, but a few have undergone successful surgery.

ENLARGED HEART

Heart Failure

The fetal heart chamber size will increase when there is heart failure. There are many causes of heart failure, including sustained arrhythmias or critical aortic stenosis.

Pericardial Effusion

The lungs will be displaced posteriorly. There will be a rim of fluid around the ventricles of the heart. This should be visualized in more than one view. With pleural effusions, the lungs are floating within the fluid.

Thickened Walls, Poorly Contractile Heart

Hypertrophic Cardiomyopathy. The ventricular walls and interventricular septum will be thickened. The right and/or left outflow may be obstructed, depending on the severity.

When associated with maternal diabetes, the interventricular septum will be thickened. The right anterior ventricular wall can be thickened.

Dilated Cardiomyopathy. The heart chambers will be dilated and the walls will be thin. The heart contracts poorly. This may be due to myocarditis resulting from a bacteria or virus. Mitral and tricuspid valve regurgitation may be present.

Endocardial Fibroelastosis. Echogenic areas may be evident anywhere in the heart walls with endocardial fibroelastosis (see Fig. 47-26). The heart contracts poorly. The left ventricle may or may not be dilated. Most of the time, this is associated with left ventricular outflow obstruction and heart failure.

ECHOGENIC MASS WITHIN THE HEART

Myocardial Tumors

Certain myocardial tumors have been detected in utero. Cardiac tumors are rare; such tumors need to be followed to monitor their growth.

Rhabdomyoma. Rhabdomyoma is an echogenic mass most commonly involving the ventricular walls and/or ventricular septum impinging on the ventricular chambers. They can also be found in the atrial septum and/or atrial walls impinging on the atrial chambers. They are slightly more echogenic than the myocardium (Fig. 47-23). They can vary in size, and some can become quite large. Dysrhythmias can occur with rhabdomyomas.

Teratoma. Teratomas are rare and have the same appearance as rhabdomyoma.

Angiomyomas. Angiomyomas are small echogenic tumors that can be seen anywhere in the heart. They usually resolve on their own.

Endocardial Fibroelastosis. Echogenic areas are seen in different areas of the myocardium.

Normal Structures That Can Appear Echogenic (Fig. 47-24)

1. Moderator band within the right ventricle.
2. Chordae tendineae and papillary muscle within the ventricles.
3. Eustachian valve in the right atrium at the entrance of the IVC.
4. Flap of the foramen ovale within the atrial septum.

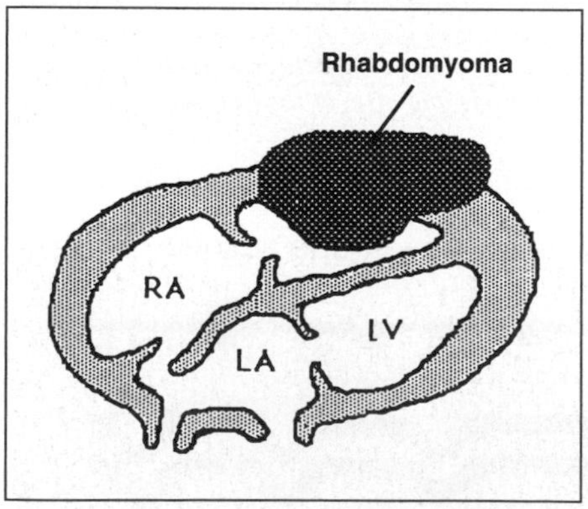

Figure 47-23. ■ *A rhabdomyoma could be missed if texture changes in the myocardium and symmetry in the chamber size are not evaluated.*

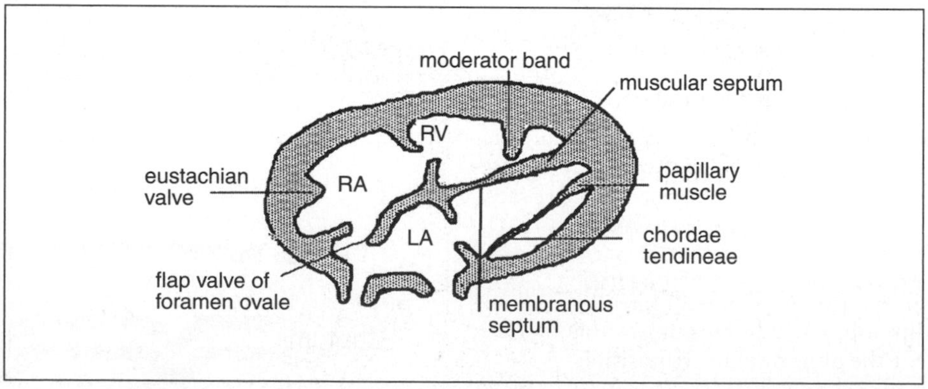

Figure 47-24. ■ *Normal structures within the fetal heart sometimes present as bright echoes, being mistaken for small tumors.*

ABNORMAL FOUR-CHAMBER HEART

Small Left Heart

Hypoplastic Left Heart Syndrome. A wide spectrum of abnormalities affecting the left side of the heart (Fig. 47-25).

1. The left ventricle, aorta, and left ventricular outflow tract are small. The left ventricle does not form the apex of the heart.
2. Most of the time, both the mitral and aortic valves are severely hypoplastic or atretic. Although both valves are usually affected, either one can be normal with the other affected. Mitral valve and aortic valve annulus will be small when compared with the right side of the heart. If atretic, no valve opening will be seen.
3. The left ventricular walls will be thickened. The left ventricle and left atrial chambers will be quite small.
4. The atrial septum is usually intact or has a small patent foramen ovale.
5. The right ventricle will form the apex and be enlarged, but structurally normal. Tricuspid valve regurgitation is often present due to the annulus being stretched.
6. The pulmonary valve annulus and artery will be enlarged.
7. When the aortic valve is atretic the ascending and transverse aortic arch are quite small.
8. There may be a left ventricle chamber present that does not function (Fig. 47-26). The walls of the ventricle are echogenic suggestive of endocardial fibroelastosis.

On real-time imaging, the left side of the heart will be difficult to see in the four-chamber view. If the mitral and aortic valves are both affected, their annulus will be small. No valve opening will be seen. The cross section of the ventricles will show a tiny left ventricle that is not contracting. The left ventricle may be so small it will be difficult to image. The aortic arch will be very difficult to image. The ascending aorta and transverse arch (up to the takeoff of the first head vessel) will be very small. The patent ductus arteriosus will be quite large and easy to confuse for the aortic arch. The origination of the head vessels will be the aortic arch.

There will be no flow by color or pulsed Doppler through the left ventricle when the mitral and aortic valves are atretic. Some flow can be detected across the foramen ovale if it is patent. In the transverse aortic arch, color Doppler will demonstrate retrograde flow from the patent ductus arteriosus into the transverse aortic arch and head vessels.

Small Right Heart

When the right side of the heart is small, there is either inlet or outlet obstruction or both.

Tricuspid Atresia (Inlet Atresia). There is a thin membrane in place of the tricuspid valve when it is atretic. Or there may be a small, hypoplastic valve present that does not allow adequate blood flow through. Hemodynamically, the two function the same. The right ventricle will be small, and the walls will be hypertrophied.

On the four-chamber view, the tricuspid valve annulus will be significantly smaller than the mitral valve annulus. There will be no or little flow through the tricuspid valve by color Doppler.

Pulmonary Atresia (Outlet Atresia). Outlet atresia will result in pulmonary atresia or severe pulmonary stenosis. This usually results in a small right ventricle and small tricuspid valve annulus with minimal flow. If there is atresia of the entire outflow, the pulmonic root may be difficult to visualize. There may be tricuspid regurgitation. VSDs are common. If this is present, the right ventricle will be more developed.

On the four-chamber view the right ventricle will appear small. There may be a small tricuspid valve annulus and/or pulmonic root with little or no flow. Color Doppler will confirm flow or the absence of flow. If the entire outflow tract is atretic and difficult to visualize on real-time imaging, color Doppler will

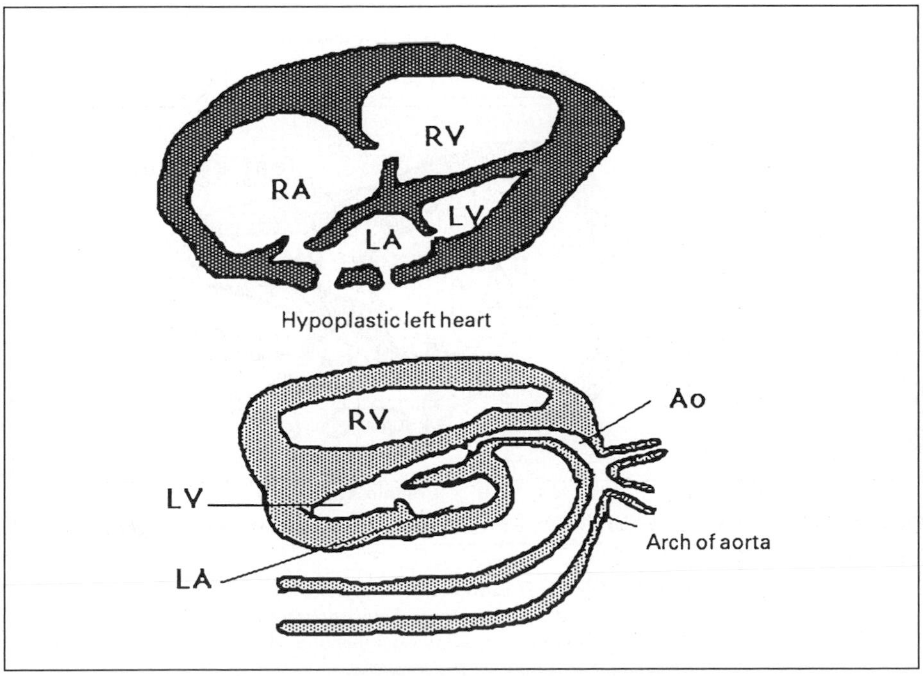

Figure 47-25. ■ *Hypoplastic left heart syndrome. The obvious asymmetry in the four-chamber view can help make the diagnosis* (top). *Ascending and transverse aortic arch will be small and difficult to image* (bottom).

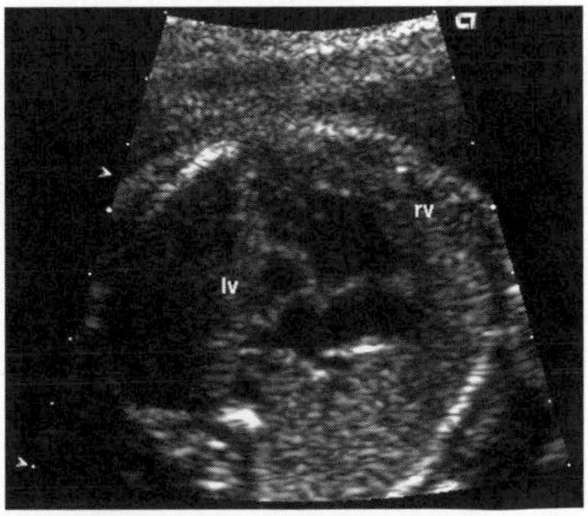

Figure 47-26. ■ *Hypoplastic left ventricle* (lv) *with evidence of endocardial fibroelastosis. Mitral and aortic valve atresia.*

be helpful in outlining the pulmonary artery anatomy. Use color Doppler to look for tricuspid valve regurgitation.

Enlarged Left Heart

Establish whether the entire left side of the heart is enlarged or just the atrium or ventricle is enlarged.

Enlarged Left Ventricle. *Aortic stenosis.* Left ventricular outflow obstruction may be present at one or multiple levels, including a subvalvular membrane, aortic valve stenosis, and supravalvular stenosis. If the valve is stenotic, the valve leaflets will be thickened and echogenic. If the obstruction is mild, fetal echocardiogram may appear normal. However, if the obstruction is severe, the left ventricle may be dilated and function poorly.

There may be secondary endocardial thickening (Fig. 47-27). The four-chamber view may appear normal or the left ventricular wall may be hypertrophied. Color, pulsed and continuous wave Doppler will be helpful in estimating the severity of the stenosis. The color Doppler flow pattern will become turbulent at the point of obstruction.

Enlarged Left Atrium. *Mitral stenosis.* Mitral stenosis is extremely rare as a congenital disease. The valve will appear thickened and echogenic on real-time. Compare the mitral valve annulus with the tricuspid valve annulus. Flow velocity by pulsed/continuous Doppler will be increased.

Mitral regurgitation. If severe, mitral regurgitation will cause left atrial enlargement. Mitral regurgitation is common in a fetus with an atrioventricular canal (see Septal Break and Atrioventricular Canal sections). Another cause of mitral regurgitation is heart failure.

Color Doppler will demonstrate a jet of flow into the left atrium when the mitral valve is closed (systole).

Enlarged Right Heart

Establish whether the entire right side of the heart is enlarged or just the atrium or ventricle is enlarged.

Enlarged Right Atrium. *Ebstein's anomaly of the tricuspid valve.* One or more of the tricuspid valve leaflets are displaced into the right ventricle (Fig. 47-28). The valve annulus remains at the normal level. The septal leaflet is hypoplastic and adherent to the interventricular septum, whereas the anterior leaflet is larger. There are varying degrees of this anomaly, from mild displacement to displacement into the right ventricular apex.

The portion of the right ventricle above the valve becomes atrialized in that it has to function as an atrium, causing enlargement of the right atrium. The amount of tricuspid regurgitation will depend on the severity of the anomaly. Arrhythmias can be associated.

On real-time imaging, the four-chamber view will appear abnormal. The tricuspid valve insertion and opening of the valve will be closer to the apex than normal. There will be enlargement of the right atrium. Color Doppler can help identify the opening of the tricuspid valve and demonstrate the severity of tricuspid valve regurgitation.

Dysplastic pulmonary valve or membranous pulmonary valve atresia. An atretic pulmonary valve will not allow flow through to the main pulmonary artery. The valve will appear as a thin membrane. The rest of the right side of the heart is usually formed normally. The tricuspid valve will appear thickened and echogenic. There will be a massive amount of tricuspid valve regurgitation causing enlargement of the right atrium.

The atrial septum will bow into the left atrium, making the left atrium quite small and difficult to see.

The four-chamber view will show significant enlargement of the right atrium. A membrane will be seen at the level of the pulmonary valve. There will be no opening in the membrane. Color Doppler can be used to confirm the lack of flow across the pulmonary valve and the severity of the tricuspid valve regurgitation.

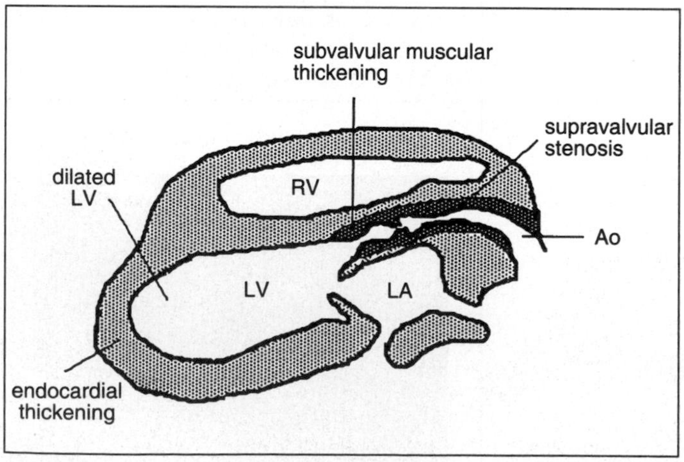

Figure 47-27. ■ *Aortic stenosis. Long axis of the left side of the heart best demonstrates stenosis along the aortic root. One or more areas may be affected; left ventricular hypertrophy is secondary.*

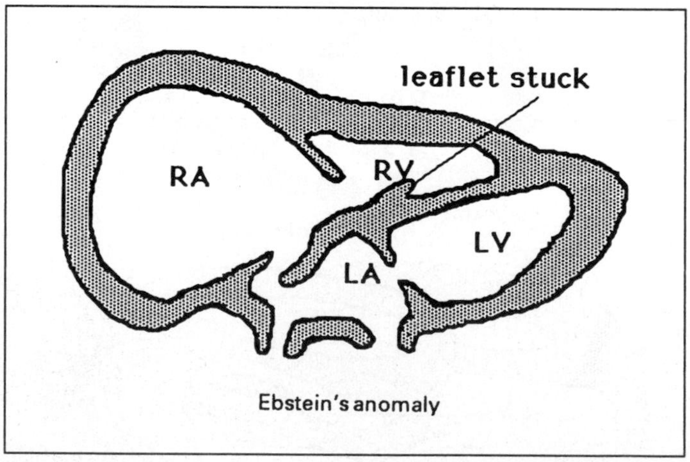

Figure 47-28. ■ *Ebstein's anomaly. Septal leaflet of the tricuspid valve is positioned lower than normal and adherent to the ventricular septum. The four-chamber view allows comparison of the mitral position on the ventricular septum with the tricuspid.*

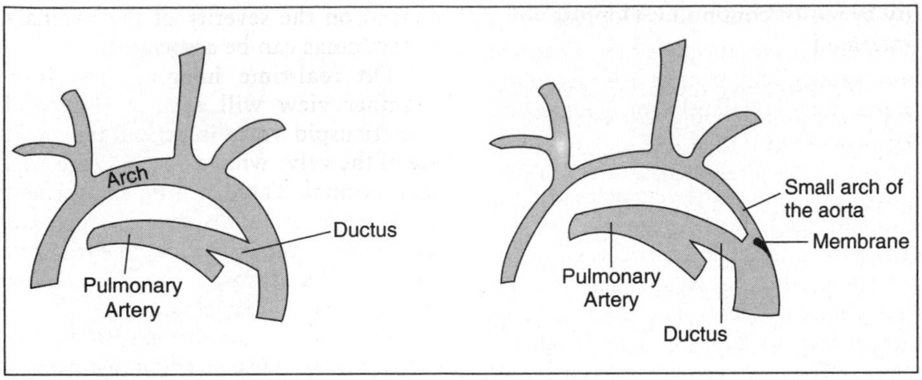

Figure 47-29. ■ *Coarctation of the aorta. Normal aortic arch* (left). *Coarctation of the aorta with a posterior shelf* (right).

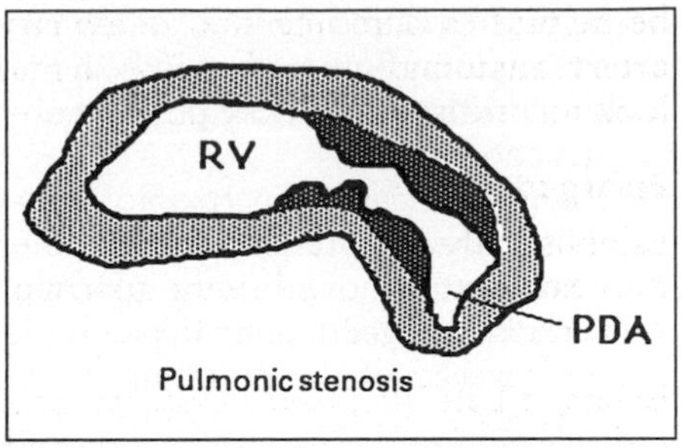

Figure 47-30. ■ *Pulmonary stenosis. Thickening and/or narrowing of the right ventricular outflow tract, thickening of the pulmonary valve, and narrowing of the pulmonary artery may be present.*

Enlarged Right Ventricle. *Coarctation of the aorta.* Coarctation of the aorta is difficult to detect in utero. A posterior shelf above, below, or at the level of the ductus arteriosus may be imaged (Fig. 47-29).

On the four-chamber view the right ventricle may be enlarged. This may be the only finding, and it may be subtle. Other findings include VSD, abnormal mitral valve, and bicuspid aortic valve (difficult to detect on fetal echocardiogram). Color Doppler of the aortic arch may help identify a coarctation if there is severe obstruction.

Although coarctation of the aorta is difficult to identify, hypoplasia of the isthmus (interrupted aortic arch) is more easily identified (Fig. 47-29). The aortic arch will be quite narrow and difficult to identify even with the help of color Doppler. The ductal arch will be enlarged.

Pulmonary stenosis. Pulmonary stenosis can occur at the right outflow in the infundibular portion (before the valve), the level of the valve, or the supravalvular portion (after the valve) (Fig. 47-30). Pulmonary valve stenosis is the most common obstructive lesion involving the right ventricular outflow. The ventricular septum is intact. If obstruction is mild, the valve may appear normal. The right ventricle will function normally.

If the right ventricle is hypertrophied or the right atrium is dilated, severe obstruction is present.

The four-chamber view may appear normal if there is mild obstruction. If the obstruction is severe, the right side of the heart may be enlarged. Measure diameter in the cross section of the aortic and pulmonic valve annulus (Fig. 47-10B). They should be equal in size.

Color Doppler will identify the point of the obstruction and any evidence of tricuspid valve regurgitation. The severity of the obstruction can be estimated with continuous wave Doppler.

Tetralogy of Fallot. Four findings are always present with Tetralogy of Fallot (Fig. 47-31):

1. A large perimembranous VSD that is anterior and to the right of the tricuspid valve.
2. An enlarged aortic root overriding the VSD. The aorta is more rightward than normal.
3. Some type of pulmonary stenosis. There is a wide spectrum of pulmonary disease that ranges from mild pulmonary valve stenosis to pulmonary atresia. The valve may

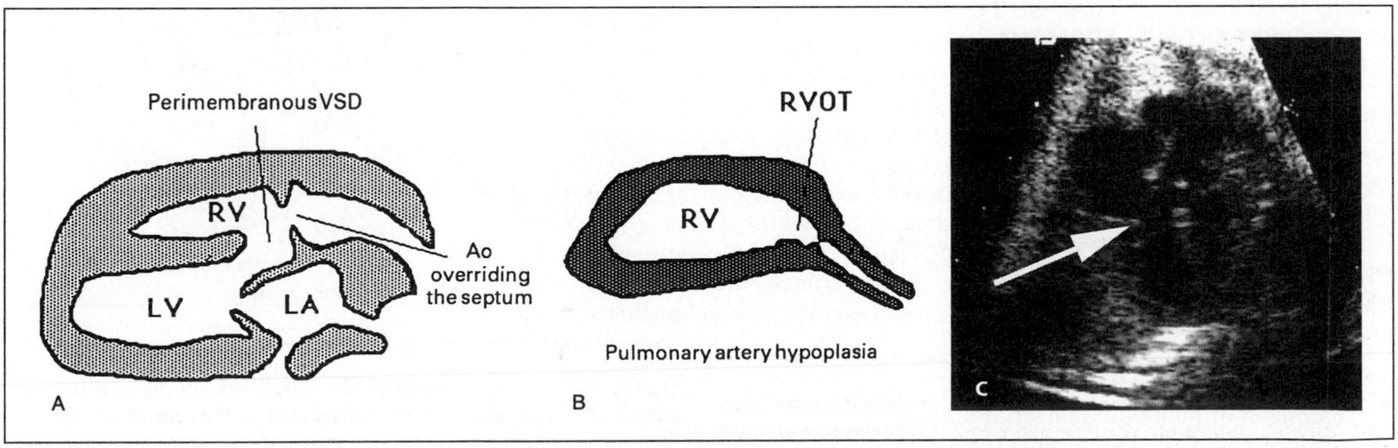

Figure 47-31. ■ *Tetralogy of Fallot. A. Overriding aorta (AO) will be associated with a perimembranous ventricular septal defect (VSD). B. Angling toward the right outflow tract will demonstrate a hypoplastic pulmonary artery in the worst case. C. Short axis demonstrating VSD and aorta overriding both left and right ventricles* (arrow).

be thickened and stenotic, or the entire right outflow tract may be quite small without a discrete point of obstruction.

4. Right ventricular hypertrophy. This is not always present in fetal life. The presence or absence of right ventricular hypertrophy depends on the severity of the pulmonary obstruction.

The four-chamber view may appear normal. The right ventricle may be enlarged. Use real-time imaging to measure the pulmonary and aortic valve annulus. Color Doppler will identify flow across the ventricular septum. Color Doppler will identify the pulmonary anatomy especially if it is small and difficult to see with real-time imaging.

SINGLE VENTRICLE (UNIVENTRICULAR HEART)

A single ventricle heart defect is due to maldevelopment of the interventricular septum.

The atrioventricular junction is connected to one chamber in the ventricular area of the heart. There may be one or two atrioventricular valves. On four-chamber view, there will be one ventricle with one or two atrioventricular valves. No interventricular septum will be seen. Both the aorta and pulmonary arteries will originate from the ventricle. The great arteries may or may not be normally related, or one may be atretic.

There may be a small nonfunctioning ventricle, giving rise to one of the great arteries. In this situation, a VSD will be present.

INABILITY TO VISUALIZE CONTINUITY OF THE GREAT ARTERIES FROM THE VENTRICULAR OUTFLOW TRACTS

Small Aortic Root

For discussion of hypoplastic left heart, see the pertinent information under Small Left Heart earlier in this chapter.

For discussion of aortic stenosis, see the pertinent information under Enlarged Left Heart earlier in this chapter.

Small Pulmonic Root

For discussion of pulmonic stenosis and Tetralogy of Fallot see the pertinent information under Enlarged Right Heart earlier in this chapter.

Double Outlet Right or Left Ventricle

With double outlet right or left ventricle, both of the great arteries arise from one ventricle with bilateral coni. A large VSD will be present (Fig. 47-32).

The four-chamber view may appear normal, or one of the ventricles will appear enlarged. Both great arteries will arise from one of the ventricles when angling toward the great arteries from the four-chamber view. The great arteries may or may not be normally related. The great arteries may or may not be equal in size. Color Doppler will help identify the blood flow pattern from the ventricles to the great arteries.

Truncus Arteriosus

Truncus arteriosus consists of the following findings (Fig. 47-33):

1. Outlet VSD
2. Single semilunar valve
3. Common arterial root that overrides the ventricular septum

The arterial root usually originates from the two ventricles equally. It can originate more from one ventricle than the other. The truncal valve (semilunar valve) may have one to six leaflets. It can have normal flow, regurgitation, or stenosis. There are four types of truncus arteriosus. In all four types, if present, the pulmonary arteries come off the aorta. It can be the main pulmonary artery or one or both of the branches of the pulmonary artery. The position of the pulmonary origin determines the type.

Four-chamber view at the level of the atrioventricular valves can appear normal. A large VSD will be present when angling toward the great arteries from the four-chamber view. One great artery will override the VSD. The artery will be larger than normal. A pulmonary artery must be imaged originating from the aorta to make this diagnosis. The short axis at the base of the heart will be abnormal with only one great artery visualized. This is the only way to differentiate truncus arteriosus from Tetralogy of Fallot with pulmonary atresia.

Color Doppler will show flow from both ventricles into one great artery. It will also show flow from the aorta into the pulmonary artery and help identify this anatomy.

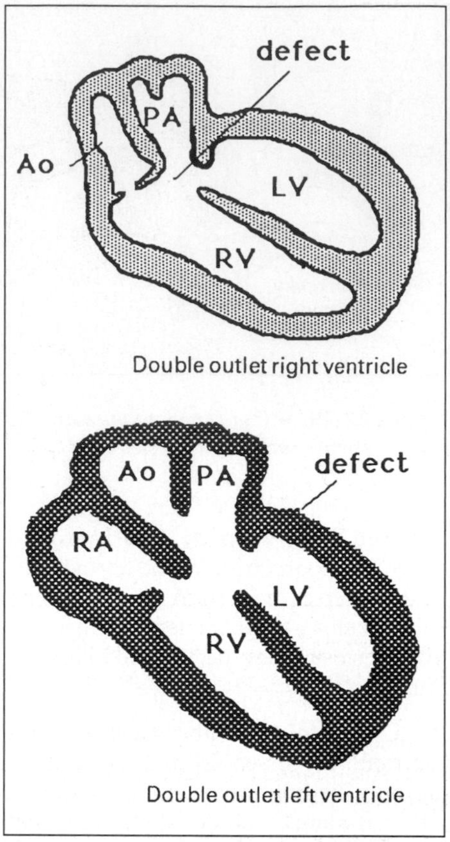

Figure 47-32. ■ *Double outlet ventricle. Simultaneous visualization of both semilunar valves seen originating from the same ventricle.*

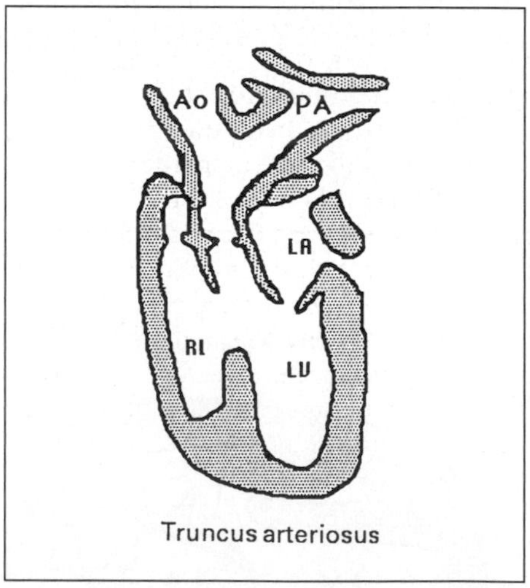

Figure 47-33. ■ *Truncus arteriosus. Large VSD with overriding single great artery.*

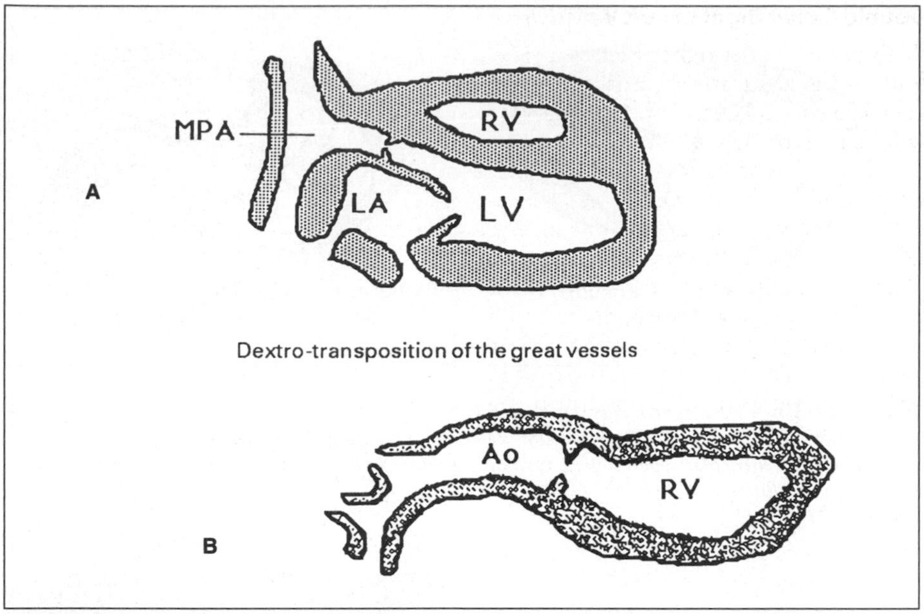

Figure 47-34. ■ *D-transposition of the great arteries. Aorta arises from the anterior right ventricle. Pulmonary arises posterior from the left ventricle and bifurcates.*

Total Anomalous Pulmonary Venous Return

The pulmonary veins join to form a "pulmonary venous confluence" and drain into the right atrium rather than the left.

The confluence can vary in position and be (1) posterior and separate from the left atrium; (2) superior to the left atrium and drain into the right atrium, coronary sinus, or SVC; or (3) inferior to the left atrium or inferior to the diaphragm and drain into the IVC.

On four-chamber view, the left side of the heart will appear smaller than the right. There will be a cystic, vascular structure where the pulmonary vein confluence is located. Pulmonary veins can be difficult to visualize. Color Doppler will help confirm the diagnosis. The color Doppler scale should be set to a low velocity to detect the low venous velocity.

There can be partial anomalous pulmonary venous return. This is associated with a sinus venosus atrial septal defect. One or two of the right pulmonary veins drain into the right atrium. Again, this is a difficult diagnosis to make in utero.

D-Transposition (Dextro-Transposition) of the Great Arteries

The anterior right ventricle will give rise to the aorta. The posterior left ventricle will give rise to the main pulmonary artery (Figs. 47-34 and 47-35). VSDs and pulmonary stenosis can be associated.

The four-chamber view at the level of the atrioventricular valves will appear normal. In the long-axis of the heart, the two great arteries will be parallel when leaving the heart. The short axis will not demonstrate the crossing of the great vessels. To make the diagnosis, the anterior aorta must give rise to the head vessels and the posterior pulmonary artery must bifurcate. Color Doppler will help track the great arteries.

L-Transposition (Levo-Transposition; L-Loop; Corrected Transposition) of the Great Arteries

The ventricles are transposed but are correctly connected to the great arteries. The right atrium is connected to the morphologic left ventricle and the pulmonary artery. The left atrium is connected to the morphologic right ventricle and the aorta. The aorta is to the left of the pulmonary artery most of the time. The aorta and pulmonary arteries will be parallel exiting the heart. Circulation is hemodynamically correct. This can be associated with other defects. The most common defects are pulmonary stenosis, congenital heart block, abnormalities of the tricuspid valve, and VSDs. To make the diagnosis, one must identify the morphology of the atria, ventricles, and great arteries. The ventricle on the left of the fetus has the characteristics of a right ventricle (tricuspid valve closer to the apex and a moderator band).

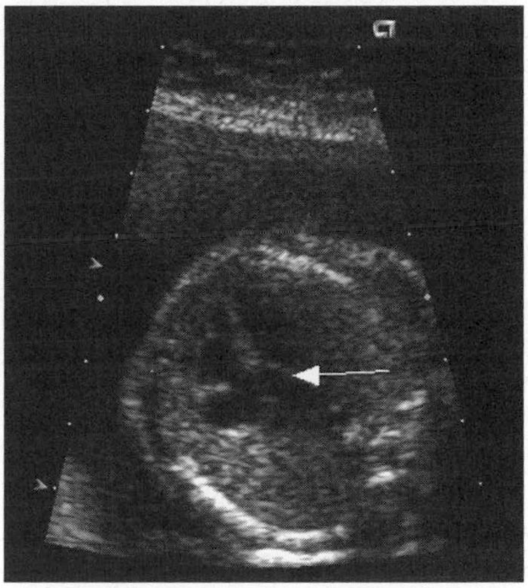

Figure 47-35. ■ *D-transposition. Parallel great vessels* (arrow). *Posterior vessel is pulmonary artery, which bifurcates.*

SEPTAL BREAK

Atrioventricular Septal Defect; Atrioventricular Canal; Endocardial Cushion Defect

There is a wide spectrum of atrioventricular septal defects. A common atrioventricular valve will have superior and inferior bridging leaflets with one or two valve orifices. In a partial form, the common valve leaflet will be displaced downward and connect to the crest of the muscular septum, allowing shunting only across a primum atrial septal defect (Fig. 47-36B). When the valve is free-floating in a complete form (not attached to the atrial or ventricular septum), shunting occurs above and below the valve level (Fig. 47-36A). When the defect is large, the ventricles will have equal pressure and no shunting will be detected.

On four-chamber view, the mitral and tricuspid valves will appear to be one leaflet crossing and/or attaching to the ventricular septum at the same level (Fig. 47-37). The ventricles may be of equal size or one may be larger than the other. The short axis at the level of the atrioventricular valves will demonstrate the anatomy of the valves.

Color Doppler will demonstrate the flow across the atrial and/or ventricular septum. With a large defect, there will not be much flow across the septum because the pressure of the two sides of the heart will be equal. Regurgitation of the mitral and tricuspid valves are common. Color Doppler will help quantitate the amount.

Atrial Isomerism. An atrioventricular canal defect can be a feature of either left or right atrial isomerism. Both atrial chambers assume the same anatomic characteristics. For example, both atria are structured as a right atrium or left atrium. The IVC is often not seen with left atrial isomerism.

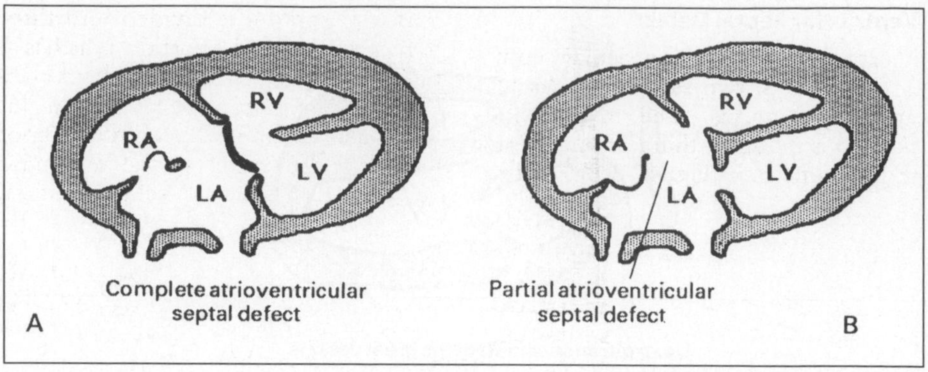

Figure 47-36. ■ *Atrioventricular septal defect.* ***A.*** *Complete atrioventricular septal defect. There is an inlet VSD, ostium primum atrial septal defect, and common atrioventricular valve leaflet.* ***B.*** *Partial atrioventricular septal defect. Ostium primum atrial septal defect with common atrioventricular valve leaflet.*

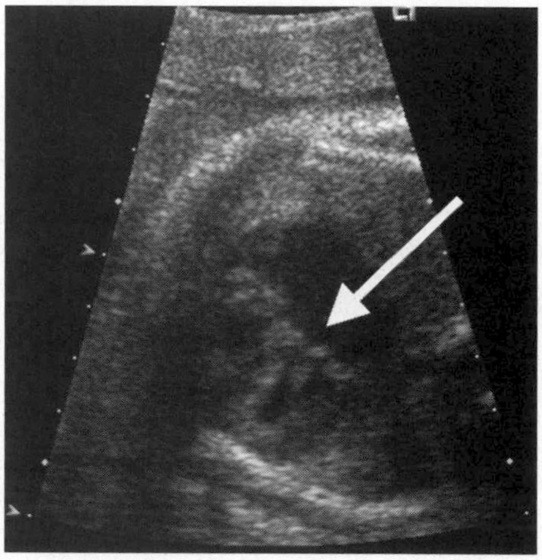

Figure 47-37. ■ *Atrioventricular septal defect. Mitral and tricuspid valves are at the same level* (arrow).

Ventricular Septal Defect

Morphologically the ventricular septum is divided into two segments: muscular and membranous. The membranous portion is the small thin portion inferior to the aortic root (Fig. 47-38B), and the muscular septum is divided into three portions: (1) the inlet portion, which is at the level of the atrioventricular valves (Fig. 47-38A); (2) the outlet or infundibular portion, which is the anterior portion at the level of the semilunar valves; and (3) the muscular septum, which extends from the membranous portion to the apex (Fig. 47-38D). VSDs are common. There can be more than one VSD in the same or different portions of the septum. They are often associated with other types of congenital heart disease.

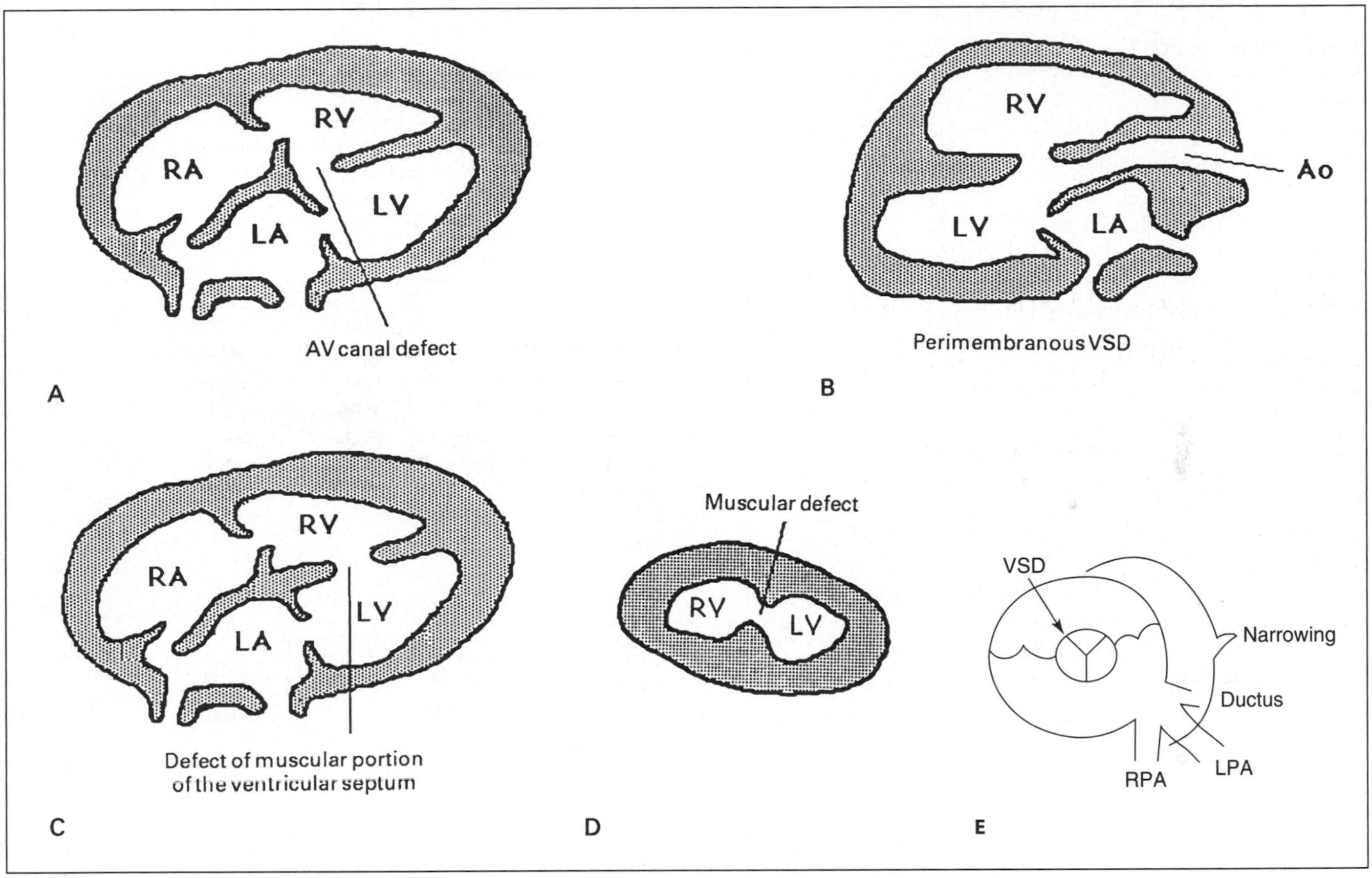

Figure 47-38. ■ *VSD. A. Atrioventricular septal defect. Defect of the inlet ventricular septum. B. Perimembranous VSD. Best demonstrated in the long-axis view. Thin portion of ventricular septum missing. Edge of the muscular septum may appear bright. C. Muscular VSD. Can occur anywhere in the muscular portion of the ventricular septum. Best imaged when perpendicular to the septum. D. Muscular VSD can be imaged from the short axis of the ventricles. Small defects may be difficult to image without color Doppler. E. View through the aortic valve showing VSD at that level.*

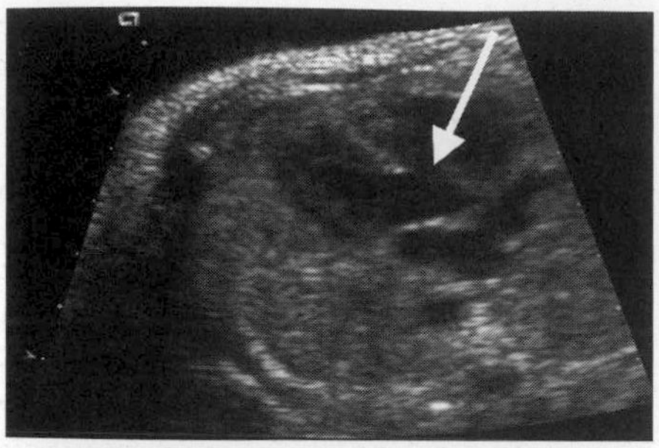

Figure 47-39. ■ *VSD in real-time image* (arrow).

On real-time imaging (Fig. 47-39), there will be persistent dropout in the septum and there should be echogenic borders to the VSD. To best identify number, size, and location of the VSD, multiple views are necessary. The four-chamber view is valuable if one is careful to angle anterior to posterior in the heart. It is helpful to be perpendicular to the septum for best visualization of the VSD and avoid false-positive results (see Fig. 47-42B).

Color and pulsed Doppler are helpful in confirming the presence or absence of a VSD. Being perpendicular to the septum will enhance the Doppler signal. Color Doppler is especially helpful in demonstrating multiple small defects ("Swiss cheese" defects) of the muscular septum.

Atrial Septal Defect

The atrial septum is divided into three portions:

1. The most superior portion is the sinus venosus portion of the septum. Defects in this portion are associated with partial anomalous pulmonary venous return.
2. The midportion (area of the fossa ovalis) of the septum is the secundum portion (Fig. 47-40A). This is the most common area for defects to occur. Because the foramen ovale is

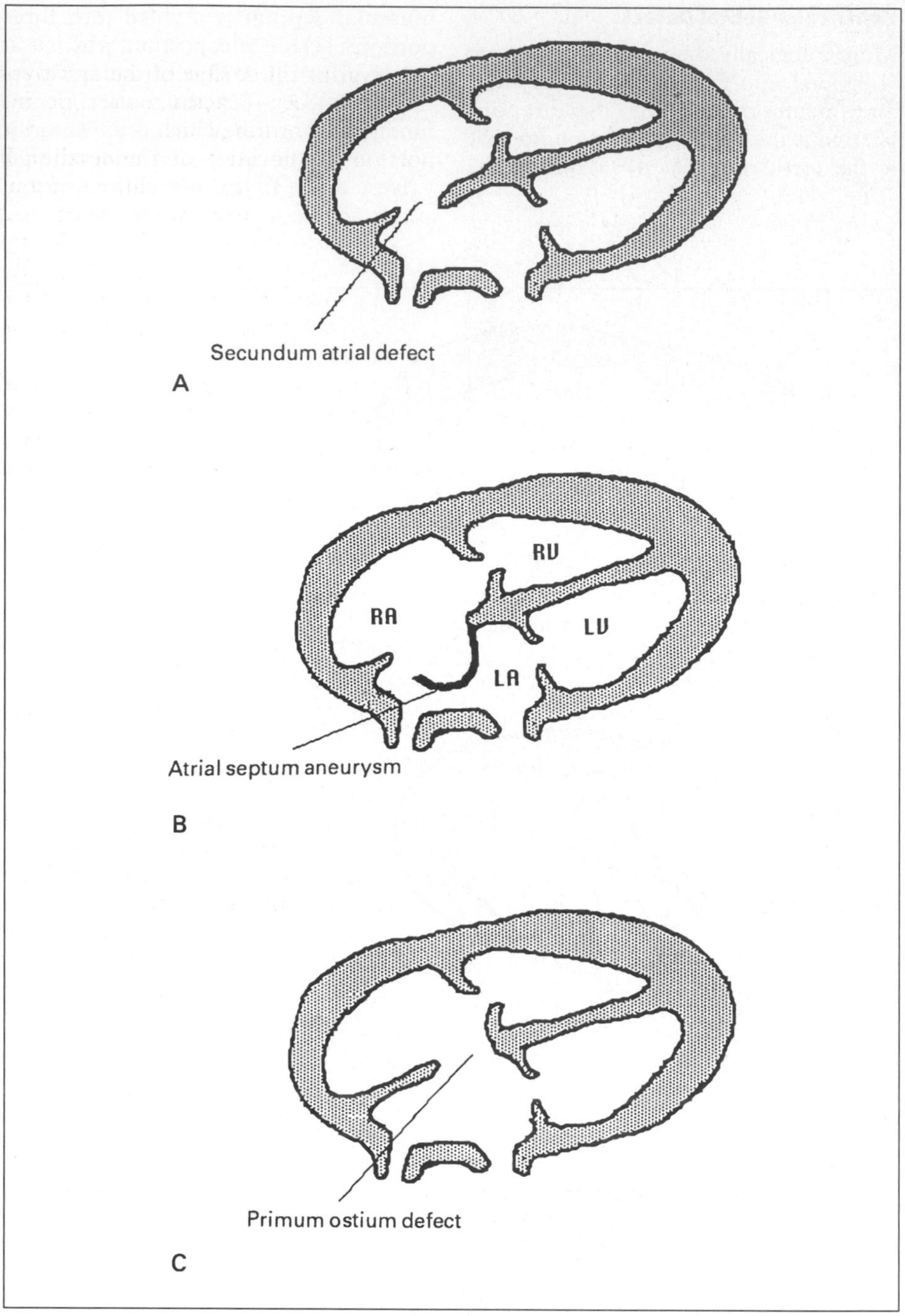

Figure 47-40. ■ *Atrial septal defects.* ***A.*** *Secundum atrial septal defect. Central part of the atrial septum is missing.* ***B.*** *Atrial septal aneurysm. Bowing membrane can be visualized.* ***C.*** *Primum ostium atrial septal defect. Lower portion of the atrial septum is missing.*

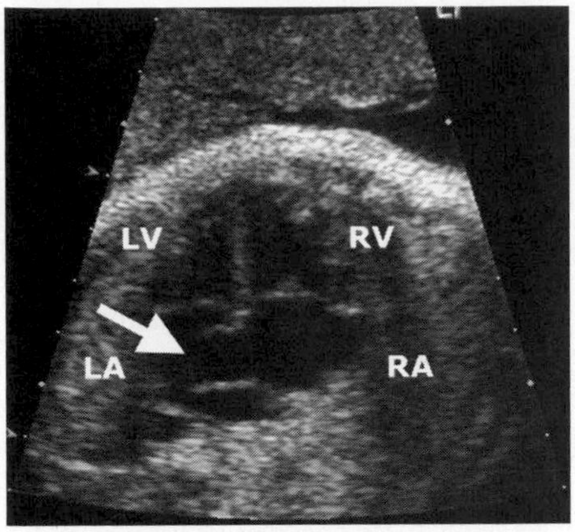

Figure 47-41. ■ *Atrial septal aneurysm* (arrow) *bows into the left atrium.*

patent in fetal life, it is difficult to diagnose a defect in this portion. An aneurysm of this area can occur (Figs. 47-40B and 47-41).

3. The most inferior portion is the ostium primum portion (Fig. 47-40C). A defect in this portion is associated with atrioventricular septal defects.

A four-chamber view that is perpendicular to the atrial septum will demonstrate dropout of the atrial septum. Color Doppler, with the scale turned down, will demonstrate flow across defect. If an atrial septal defect is demonstrated, other associated defects must be ruled out.

Pitfalls

1. Cardiac situs. One of the first steps should be to determine the right and left sides of the fetus.
2. Cardiac location and anomalies. If the cardiac apex is shifted, determine the reason for the shift (i.e., pleural/pericardial effusion, omphalocele, ectopia cordis, or diaphragmatic hernia). Careful attention to the cardiac anatomy is also important.
3. Pericardial versus pleural effusion. A pericardial effusion will push the lungs posteriorly, whereas with a pleural effusion the lungs float within the fluid.
4. Pseudo-pericardial effusion. False-positive pericardial effusion can sometimes be diagnosed. A thin sonolucent rim around the heart is a normal finding. Serial echocardiograms will show it unchanged. A pericardial effusion must be seen in more than one view.
5. There may be a bright/echogenic spot in the left or right ventricle. It is a normal variant when part of the chordae tendinea/papillary muscle. Use multiple views to confirm this is the position of the bright spot.
6. The eustachian valve and flap of the foramen ovale may appear as an echogenic line within the atrium.
7. If there is a question of a cardiac tumor in one of the cardiac walls or chambers, change to a different position. To make a positive diagnosis, demonstrate the tumor in more than one view.
8. Ventricular wall thickness. Differentiating between heart wall thickness and heart wall pathology may be difficult. Different views of the heart walls and m-mode measurements may be helpful.
9. Excessive transducer pressure. Excessive pressure on the maternal abdomen may cause episodes of bradycardia. Release the pressure and the heart rate should return to normal.
10. Patent ductus arteriosus versus aortic arch. The patent ductus arteriosus and the aortic arch can be mistaken for each other on the long axis of the fetus. The aortic arch has the appearance of a candy cane with a tight curve, and the three head vessels originate superiorly. The patent ductus arteriosus resembles a hockey stick with a wider curve (Figs. 47-5B and 47-7).
11. Pseudo-VSD due to transducer angle. In the four-chamber view, angle through the lateral aspect of the heart instead of the apex to avoid dropout and fabrication of an appearance resembling a VSD (Fig. 47-42). Also use color Doppler to confirm diagnosis.

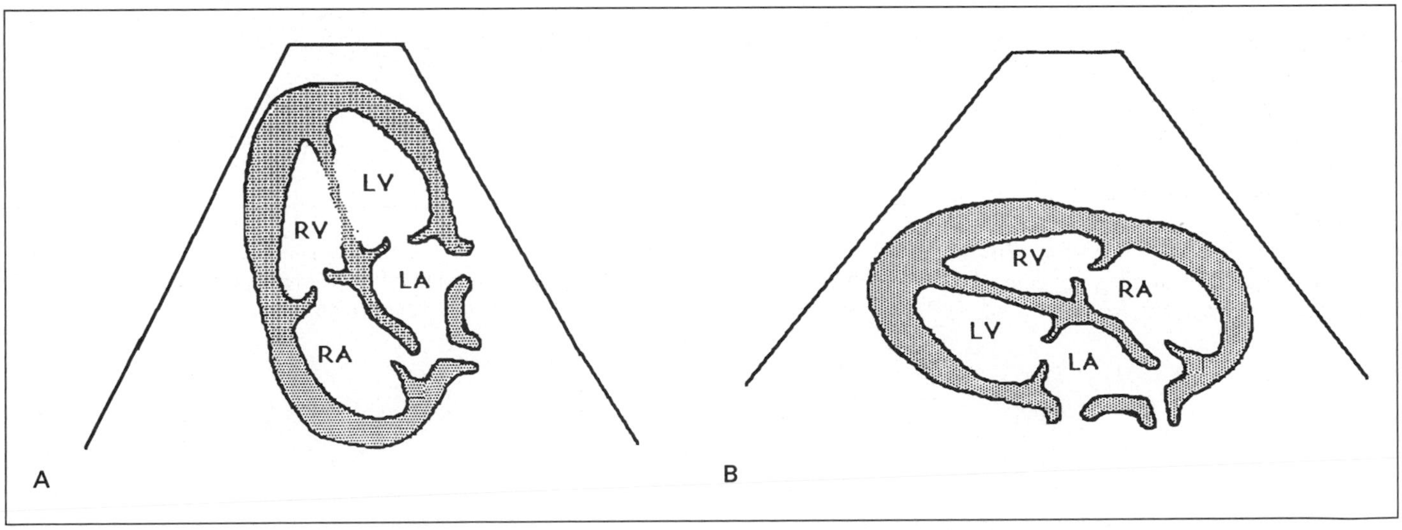

Figure 47-42. ■ *A. Angling through the apex of the heart in the four-chamber view can create dropout of the ventricular septum. B. To avoid this artifact, try to obtain the four-chamber view by angling through the lateral aspect.*

12. Right side of the heart mildly enlarged. Close to term, this is okay. However, it is important to image the aortic arch for a possible coarctation and image the pulmonary vein flow into the left atrium.
13. Use of color Doppler requires attention to the scale settings.
14. Most important to a good fetal echocardiogram is to take your time. False-positives can occur when the fetus is in a difficult to image position. Have the mother walk around, empty or fill her bladder, and then try again.
15. Pseudo-overriding aorta. If possible, obtain the long axis of the left ventricular outflow tract by scanning through the right side of the heart. Remember that the ventricular septum thins out at the aortic root.

SELECTED READING

Abuhamad A. *A practical guide to fetal echocardiography*. Baltimore: Lippincott Williams and Wilkins; 1997.

Drose JA, ed. *Fetal echocardiography*. Philadelphia: Saunders, 1998.

Yagel S, Silverman N, Gembruch U, eds. *Fetal cardiology: Embryology, genetics, physiology, echocardiographic evaluation, diagnosis and perinatal management of cardiac disease*. Baltimore: Lippincott Williams and Wilkins; 1997.

Carotid Artery Disease

REBECCA SCHILLING

48

SONOGRAM ABBREVIATIONS

BIF	Bifurcation
CCA	Common carotid artery
ECA	External carotid artery
EDV	End-diastolic velocity
ICA	Internal carotid artery
PRF	Pulse repetition frequency
PSV	Peak systolic velocity
SUBCL	Subclavian artery
VERT	Vertebral artery

KEY WORDS

Aliasing. A Doppler signal is transmitted before the prior returning signal has been received.

Amaurosis Fugax. Transient blindness.

Bruit. Rumbling sound heard over an artery with a stethoscope.

Plaque. Deposit of fibrinous material on the edge of a vessel due to atheroma that may narrow the vessel significantly.

Pulse Repetition Frequency (PRF). The frequency with which an echo signal is sent into and received from the tissue. A limiting factor in the development of Doppler signals.

Sample Volume. The size of the space from which Doppler signals are being obtained.

Spectral Imaging. A display that shows the various waveforms that make up the pulsed Doppler profile.

Broadening. With flow disturbance, the Doppler signal becomes more varied in pitch, displaying numerous frequencies.

Stroke. Loss of use of a portion of the body due to a brain infarction, hematoma, or embolus.

Subclavian Steal Syndrome. When the subclavian artery is blocked, blood is supplied to the left arm through the left vertebral artery. Flow through the left vertebral artery is thus reversed.

Transient Ischemic Attack (TIA). Transient paralysis of a portion of the body due to temporary interference with blood supply to the brain.

Turbulence. Unusual flow patterns created when an obstructing lesion such as plaque is present within a vessel. The term is incorrect from a physicist's viewpoint—a better term is flow disturbance.

The Clinical Problem

Carotid sonography is the first imaging modality used in the investigation of the extracranial vascular system because it is inexpensive, quick, and noninvasive. Follow-up when positive findings are discovered is generally by magnetic resonance arteriography. The following neurologic symptoms are the typical indications for the ultrasonic examination of the extracranial cerebrovascular system.

1. *Amaurosis fugax*. Transient complete or partial loss of vision. Described as a window shade coming down either partially or completely over the eye. Most often occurs unilaterally and usually indicates the presence of disease in the ipsilateral internal carotid artery (ICA).
2. *Transient ischemic attack*. The patient presents with stroke symptoms that resolve within 24 hours without intervention. Generally caused by an embolus most typically from the carotid or heart. Carotid duplex examination of the carotid arteries can document the extent of disease or rule out carotid disease. A negative duplex test is valuable in suggesting another source of embolus.
3. *Cerebrovascular accident—stroke*. A loss of blood supply to a portion

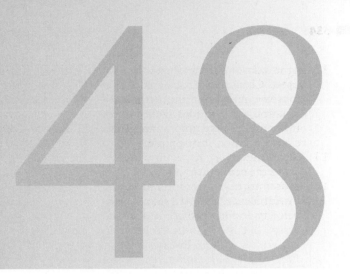

of the brain that causes loss of speech, consciousness, or unilateral motor control for more than 24 hours. If the carotid is the source of the emboli, the symptoms are generally located on the opposite side to the blockage.
4. *Carotid bruit.* An auditory sign caused by tissue vibration produced by turbulence. Can be a sign of high-velocity blood through a diseased vessel, but it is also heard in tortuous vessels without disease.
5. *Elderly surgical candidates.* Stroke risk increases in patients with significant carotid stenosis; it is therefore appropriate to perform a carotid duplex examination in the elderly asymptomatic patient preoperatively to detect any evidence of significant stenosis.
6. *Follow-up of asymptomatic patient with known atheromatous plaque.* Duplex imaging is used to monitor the asymptomatic patient with minimal stenosis to determine when the stenosis becomes significant and requires surgical intervention. When the degree of stenosis is greater than 70%, the patient is considered a candidate for surgery.
7. *Follow-up of patients who have undergone endarterectomy.* Carotid sonography is also the follow-up modality of choice for patients who have had previous carotid surgical intervention. Because many patients develop carotid artery restenosis, duplex imaging is a noninvasive way to monitor postoperative changes before significant stenosis recurs.

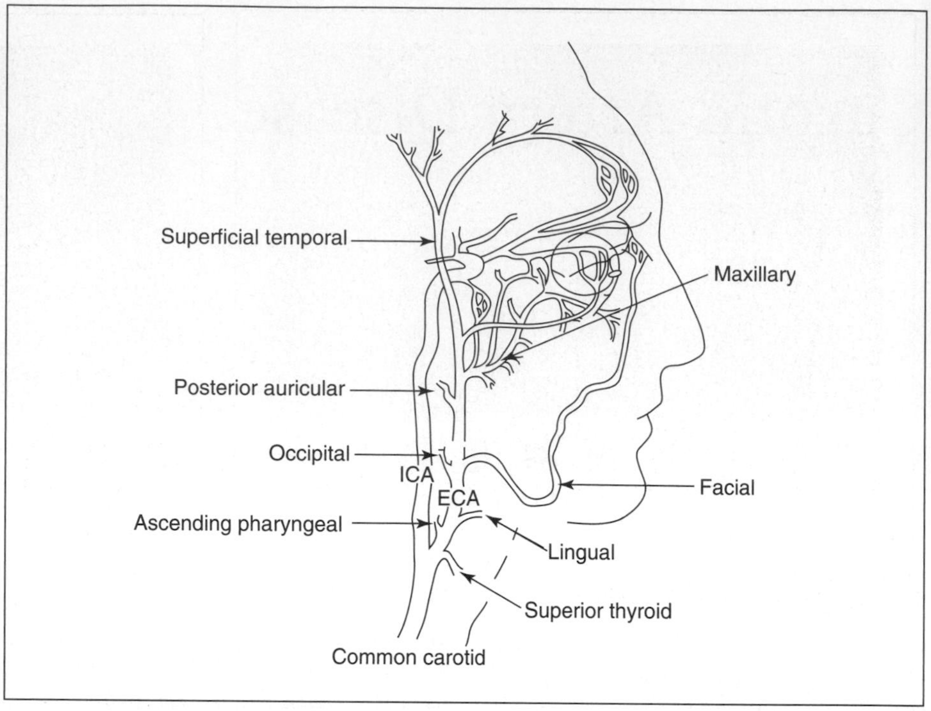

Figure 48-1. ■ *Carotid anatomy.*

Anatomy

The carotid artery supplies blood to the facial structures and brain (Fig. 48-1).

COMMON CAROTID ARTERIES

The left common carotid artery (CCA) is generally shorter than the right because the left carotid branches directly from the aortic arch, whereas the right branches from the subclavian artery. The CCA travels cephalad to just below the mandible and terminates in the carotid bifurcation where the ICAs and external carotid arteries (ECAs) originate.

EXTERNAL CAROTID ARTERIES

The ECAs pursue a posterolateral course from the bifurcation supplying the muscles and structures of the face and scalp. The ECA has eight named branches, and although few are visible with duplex imaging, the branches play an important part in the collateral circulation. In the presence of a severe ICA stenosis or occlusion, the body reroutes the blood supply to avoid a deficiency in blood flow to the brain, which can result in a stroke or transient ischemic attack.

INTERNAL CAROTID ARTERIES

The other branch of the carotid bifurcation is the ICA, which provides most of the blood supply to the brain. It has no branches in the neck and can be very tortuous.

VERTEBRAL ARTERIES

Both vertebral arteries originate from the subclavian arteries and run without branches alongside the spine. The circle of Willis within the cranium normally connects both ICAs and the basilar artery (the latter is formed by the junction of the vertebral arteries); the circle provides a communication between these vessels that may allow adequate blood flow to the brain even when a severe stenosis or total occlusion exists in one of the extracranial carotid arteries (see Chapter 49, Intercranial Vascular Problems).

Technique

- A thorough patient history should be obtained and any suggestive symptoms should be noted, as well as any significant risk factors such as hypertension, high cholesterol, or heart disease.
- The patient is placed on a stretcher with the head turned away from the side being imaged. This allows easy transducer access and makes it more likely that the ICAs and ECAs can be imaged at the same time. A 20- to 30-degree lateral-to-medial transducer angle helps one use the sternocleidomastoid muscle as an acoustic "stand-off." The clinician may need to adjust the position of the patient's head from medial to lateral to "open up" the bifurcation of the ICAs and ECAs. A pillow should not be used unless the patient cannot lie flat due to back or neck problems.

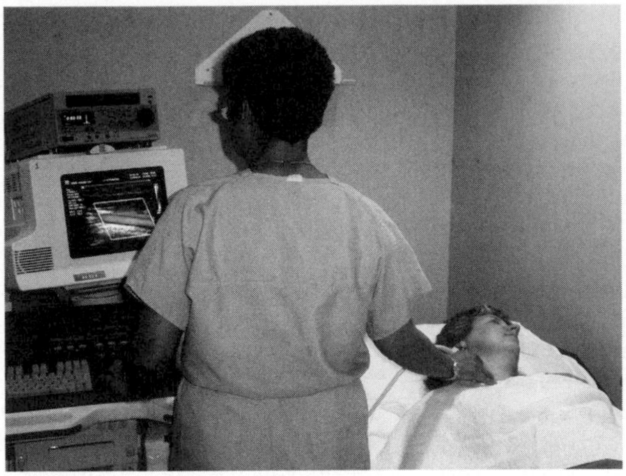

Figure 48-2. ■ *Optimal sonographer position for examining the carotid artery.*

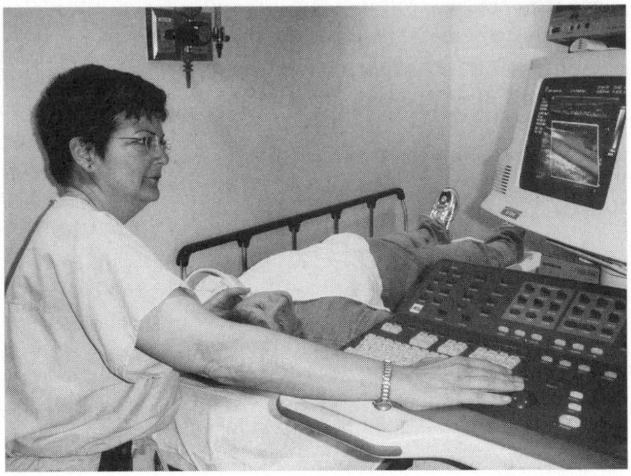

Figure 48-3. ■ *Side view of optional sonographer position.*

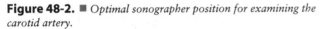

- The sonographer sits at the head of the patient or on the right side with the imaging equipment conveniently located so that she/he can easily reach the controls. Rest the forearm on the stretcher so that tiny changes in the transducer position can be made with simple finger and wrist movements. Position the equipment so that there is sufficient space to change position and sonographic approach (Figs. 48-2 and 48-3).
- Try to make the examination relatively speedy. A quick examination limits the ultrasound exposure to the patient, because the power output levels for pulsed Doppler are higher than those for imaging alone. Second, most patients are elderly and become uncomfortable or unable to cooperate if they are restricted to lying flat for a long time. Finally, technologist fatigue may compromise concentration and examination quality. Initially allow 60 to 90 minutes to complete the bilateral carotid artery interrogation, but try to refine the examination time to 30 minutes.
- Ultrasound coupling gel is applied along the sternocleidomastoid muscle, and a high-frequency (5–10 MHz) linear transducer is placed on the neck at the level of the clavicle. The CCA will be imaged at this level; document in a longitudinal plane any plaque that may be present within the vessel (Fig. 48-4). Transverse imaging is helpful in determining the ideal long axis and obliquity by showing the ICAs and ECAs as they bifurcate from the bulb (area of the bifurcation).
- While keeping the distal portion of the CCA in the image in a longitudinal plane, sweep from medial to lateral with very small movements to image the origin of the ICA. By angling the transducer anteriorly and medially, the ECA can then be imaged. The vessels should be imaged to locate any areas of plaque and to measure any reduction of the lumen at the plaque site (Fig. 48-4).

COLOR DOPPLER

- Color Doppler is a useful tool during the initial examination process and is especially helpful in identifying the extracranial vessels. Color Doppler is based on pulsed ultrasound technology, so the rules of pulsed Doppler apply. As described in Chapter 4, there is no frequency shift at a 90-degree angle when the

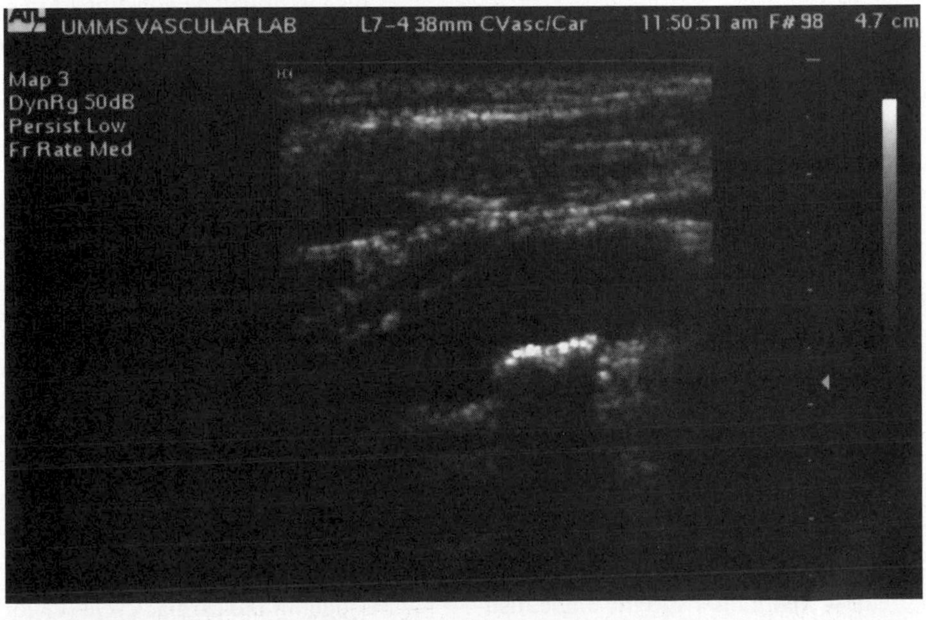

Figure 48-4. ■ *Carotid with plaque.*

ultrasound beam is perpendicular to the flow so there is an absence of color when this occurs. The frequency shift information obtained by color Doppler is displayed as colors on the screen, usually red and blue depending on the direction of blood flow.

- Color Doppler should be used in addition to pulsed Doppler to determine areas of stenosis or turbulent flow. The normal change in direction of the blood flow caused by the tortuosity of the vessel and the division of the internal and external branches can be quickly appreciated within the larger sampling of the color box. At sites of vessel narrowing, the blood flow increases in velocity and color flow shows an aliased color signal, usually converting from red or blue to white.

Color flow has several advantages:

1. With color, it is possible to visualize small amounts of flow in unexpected areas because Doppler signals are strong at angles (0–60 degrees to flow) where imaging (60–90 degrees) is very weak.
2. Vessel identification is rapid.
3. Flow can be visualized on transverse views.
4. The site of critical stenosis can be visualized, and the Doppler sample gate can be placed at the appropriate angle to correspond with the flow.
5. Visualization of good color fill from wall to wall within the vessel eliminates the need to perform a spectral analysis at many locations while moving the sample volume throughout the length of the vessel.

PULSED DOPPLER SPECTRAL ANALYSIS

Common Carotid Artery

- The spectral Doppler examination begins by locating the CCA in the longitudinal plane. Begin low down in the neck and image the most proximal segment of the vessel.
- The Doppler sample volume is placed in the middle of the artery, maintaining an angle of 60 degrees. The Doppler angle must be kept between 45 and 60 degrees for an interpretable signal; many institutions now maintain a specific angle, usually 60 degrees, so a follow-up examination gives comparable results.
- A small gate of 1.5 to 2 mm increases the likelihood of obtaining good central vessel laminar flow information without including the slower-flowing signals from blood near the vessel wall that produce spurious spectral broadening.
- The proximal CCA normally has a very turbulent flow because of a change in flow direction as blood enters the carotid from the subclavian artery. If the velocity is high, there is a stenosis at the origin of the CCA.
- The flow in the mid-CCA is taken at an area where a 60-degree angle can easily be obtained. Accuracy is most important because this velocity is used to calculate the ICA/CCA ratio. The ratio is particularly helpful when there are very high velocities in the ICA or there are diminished velocities throughout the carotid system due to poor cardiac output.

Carotid Bulb

- The CCA is followed cephalad until the bifurcation is imaged. Doppler signals are also obtained in the proximal ECA as well as the proximal, mid, and distal ICA. The information obtained in the spectral analysis is displayed as a velocity, with the units being given in centimeters per second. Depending on the vessel being examined, as well as the signal within the vessel, the spectral analysis will demonstrate different flow characteristics.
- Turbulent flow is normally present in the bulb as the CCA bifurcates into the ECA and ICA.
- The shape or pulsatility of the waveform can provide information about the resistance of the vessel being studied. The ICA provides much of the blood flow to the brain, which has a very low-resistance vascular bed. A low distal resistance causes the entire waveform to show flow above the baseline (low resistance). This monophasic and less pulsatile waveform prevents large changes in flow volume to the brain. A slow acceleration to systole results in a broad, rounded systolic waveform peak and continuous forward flow throughout the cardiac cycle (Color Plate 48-1). The second site for the ICA/CCA ratio is taken at the site of greatest stenosis.
- The CCA provides flow to both the ICA and ECA, but because a significant amount of blood goes to the ICA, the CCA waveform tends to take on the characteristics of the low-resistance flow found in the ICA. The flow in the CCA is changed when there is significant ICA stenosis or occlusion.

External Carotid Arteries

- The ECAs supply the blood flow to the muscles and skin of the face and scalp, which is a high-resistance vascular bed. The typical high-resistance waveform in the ECAs is more pulsatile, displaying a faster acceleration, a high peak systolic velocity (PSV), and an end-diastolic velocity (EDV) that returns to zero, or there may be a reversal of flow below the baseline in late systole or early diastole caused by the high distal resistance (Color Plate 48-2).
- Because the ECAs feed the superficial structures of the face and head, the velocities are not considered as important as those in the ICA. A velocity measurement should be obtained in the proximal ECA to prove the vessel is patent and to demonstrate the quality and direction of flow in the vessel. The normal ECA maintains a high-resistance signal but may develop a low-resistance pattern if the ICA on the same side (ipsilateral) becomes severely narrowed or occluded.

INTERPRETATION

The most common location for an ICA stenosis is in the first 3 cm of its course, and this is fortunate because as the ICA courses more cephalad it becomes deeper, smaller in diameter, and more difficult to image with potential false-positive results. The interpretation criteria described next were calculated on the basis of the diameter reductions measured at arteriography compared with the acquired Doppler velocities at the same site. The combination of the information derived from grayscale images, color flow, and pulsed Doppler at the same site provides an accurate estimation of the severity of the stenosis.

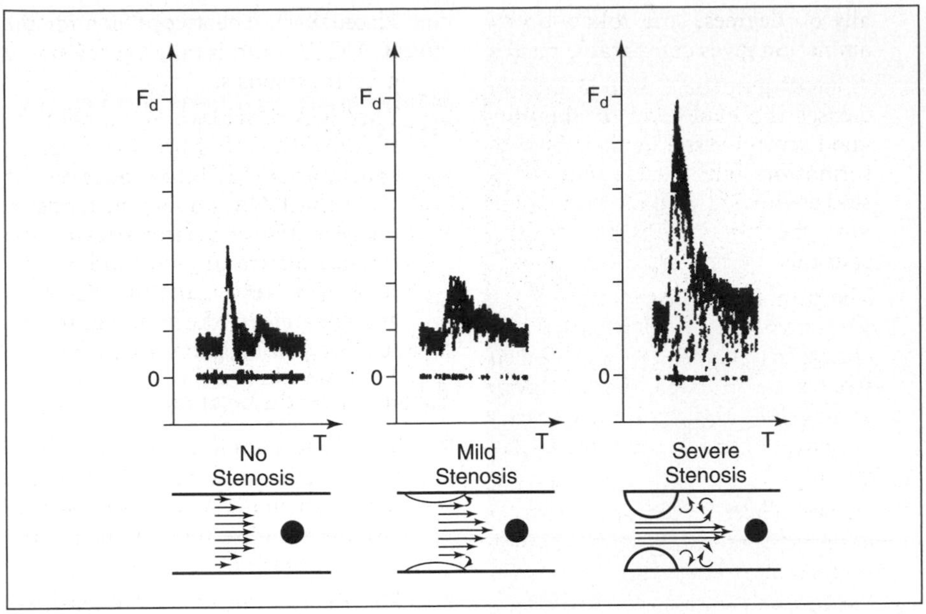

Figure 48-5. ■ *Stenosis profile.*

Stenosis Profile

- Blood flow normally follows certain well-defined patterns. Normal laminar flow is blood flow that flows faster in the center of the stream and slower at the sides. The flow stays in parallel lines with most of the flow at the same speed. On spectral imaging, there is normally a clear spectral window.
- In disturbed or turbulent flow, there is less organized and parallel flow. The waveform spectral window displays significant spectral broadening generally proportional to the disease severity.
- Although spectral broadening is usually abnormal, there can be turbulent flow with spectral broadening when a vessel turns abruptly, kinks back on itself, or branches. One must look carefully for the presence or absence of plaque in a tortuous vessel with turbulent flow.

Doppler Findings with Stenotic Vessels

Because the length of the vessel and the thickness of blood change very little, a decrease in the diameter of a vessel causes a significant change in the velocities within the vessel. A stenosis is considered hemodynamically significant when the diameter reduction reaches 50%, corresponding to an area reduction of 75%. Little change in the hemodynamics occurs when the artery has minimal disease, but as the narrowing becomes more significant, flow effects occur at a rapidly progressive rate. A longer, more involved lesion has a much more profound effect on the overall flow than a small focal lesion (Fig. 48-5).

A hemodynamically significant stenosis causes the following Doppler effects:

1. Proximal to the stenosis, the velocities in the vessel are usually dampened. Flow disturbances may be present.
2. Within the stenosis itself, the Doppler frequencies increase and are displayed as spectral broadening as flow disorganization occurs in the area of the lesion.
3. Poststenotic turbulence takes place at the exit from the stenosis creating flow reversals and currents that appear as disturbed Doppler flow patterns both above and below the baseline.

CLASSIFICATION OF DISEASE (TABLE 48-1)

Normal

A vessel is considered normal when a PSV less than 125 cm/sec is present in the ICA and the vessel walls are smooth with

Table 48-1 Diagnostic Interpretation Criteria

Diameter Reduction (%)	Peak Systolic Velocity (cm/sec)	End-Diastolic Velocity (cm/sec)	
Normal	<125	NA	No spectral broadening; clear spectral window
<50	<125	NA	Minimal spectral broadening present
50–70	125–230	<90	Spectral broadening present throughout systole
>70	>230	90–110	Spectral broadening present; ICA/CCA ratio >4.0
80–99	>230	>110	Spectral broadening present
Occluded ICA	0	0	CCA diastolic flow at zero; ECA signal develops characteristics of ICA

NA, not available; ICA, internal carotid artery; CCA, common carotid artery; ECA, external carotid artery.

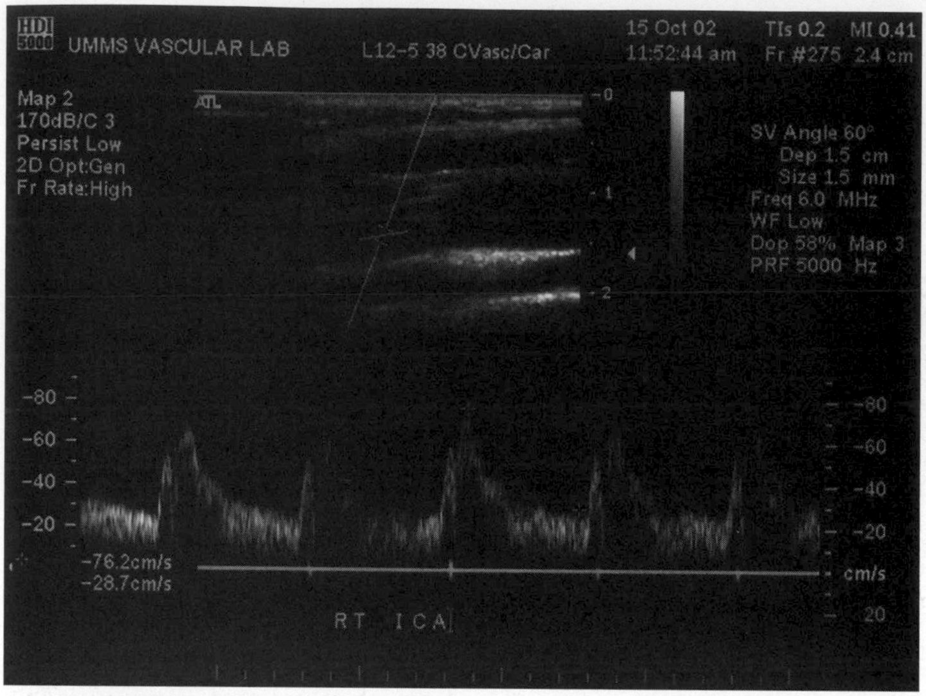

Figure 48-6. ■ *Normal internal carotid artery* (ICA).

no visible plaque in the lumen (Fig. 48-6). Normal flow disturbances and separations will be seen at bifurcations or turns.

Less Than Fifty Percent Stenosis

- This category covers a wide range of stenosis severity. The degree of stenosis is determined by using information obtained from both grayscale imaging and Doppler velocities.
- When the diameter reduction ranges from 1% to 15%, the ICA velocities will still show a PSV of less than 125 cm/sec; there will be a small amount of spectral broadening but no measurable vessel width reduction.
- When the suspected reduction is between 16% and 49%, the amount of spectral broadening will be increased and spectral window may no longer be present. Because the PSV in this category is less than 125 cm/sec, the approximated percentage of stenosis is calculated by considering the amount of spectral broadening and size of any plaque within the vessel lumen.

Fifty Percent to Seventy Percent Stenosis

Until the stenosis severity reaches approximately 70%, diastolic flow is not significantly affected; abnormally high systolic velocities are seen, whereas the EDV remains normal or registers a slight increase. The PSV velocity ranges from 126 to 230 cm/sec, whereas the EDV remains at less than 90 cm/sec (Color Plate 48-3).

Greater than Seventy Percent Stenosis

When the degree of stenosis is greater than 70%, velocity measurement is the primary method of determining disease severity; as the plaque in the vessel becomes more complicated, often partially obscured by calcification, the grayscale image becomes difficult to interpret and therefore less useful. At this stenosis severity, the EDV increases in velocity; the diagnosis of a greater than 70% stenosis requires a PSV greater than 230 cm/sec and an EDV between 90 and 110 cm/sec.

Eighty Percent to Ninety-Nine Percent Stenosis

- Again, Doppler velocities are the best way of determining the location and severity of the lesion because the plaque formation is so complex. The defining criteria for this degree of stenosis hinges on the EDV, which must exceed 110 cm/sec and demonstrate poststenotic turbulence. The PSV will be greater than 230 cm/sec.
- Because it is common for the PSV to exceed the limits set by the PRF, aliasing usually occurs, in which case an accurate measurement cannot be obtained.
- The EDV is more easily obtained and is often the most accurate measurement obtained with this severity of stenosis (Color Plate 48-4).

Occlusion

- Although direct examination of the ICA with color flow will show flow stopping and reversing color at the site of occlusion (Color Plate 48-5), secondary effects on other vessels that relate to the ICA is the key to diagnosing ICA occlusion. With chronic ICA occlusion, the waveforms in the ipsilateral CCA show minimal or no diastolic flow taking on the high-resistance characteristics of the ECA instead of the typical low-resistance waveforms of the CCA and ICA. However, if zero diastolic flow is seen in both CCAs, poor cardiac output is more likely than an occluded ICA.
- After the CCA is imaged, the vessel is followed to the bifurcation and the ECA is imaged. With chronic occlusion of the ICA the ECA takes on the characteristics of the lower-resistance ICA as collateral pathways to the brain develop. With acute ICA occlusion, the ECA will usually maintain the typical high-resistance waveform until collateral routes are established.

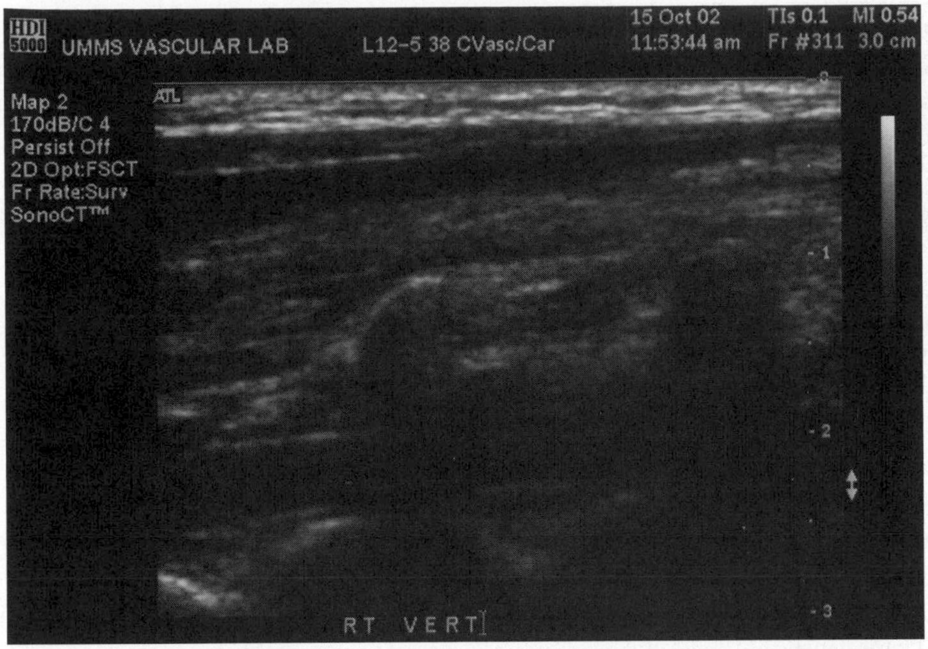

Figure 48-7. ■ *Vertebral artery.*

- In the days after occlusion of the ICA, the contralateral carotid system usually develops compensatory greater flow to accommodate the needs of the brain. There are increased flow velocities throughout the contralateral carotid system with no evidence of plaque disease or vessel tortuosity.

Vertebral Artery

The examination of the vertebral arteries is usually limited to a determination of flow direction. The flow should be in the same direction as that in the CCA, and this is easily seen with color flow Doppler imaging. If flow is in the opposite direction (usually on the left), think of the "subclavian steal syndrome." In this syndrome, the subclavian artery is blocked proximal to the origin of the vertebral artery, and flow in the vertebral artery then reverses so that sufficient blood supplies the left arm, particularly during exercise. This is clinically suspected when there are asymmetric brachial blood pressures and arm pain with exertion.

Vertebral Artery Examination Technique. To image the vertebral artery, follow the CCA to the bifurcation. At this area, angle the transducer posteriorly until the spinous processes are visible. Between these landmarks, the vertebral artery and vein should be clearly visible (Fig. 48-7).

Pitfalls

ALIASING

This artifact appears on the image as a disorganized mosaic of color. Aliasing occurs when very high-flow states are present, or a low pulse repetition frequency is used. Increasing the pulse repetition frequency or decreasing the baseline on the spectral display will allow the higher velocity waveform to be displayed without aliasing.

CONFUSING EXTERNAL AND INTERNAL CAROTID ARTERIES

At times, the ECA and ICA waveforms appear very similar when plaque or stenosis narrows the vessel. The superior thyroid artery branches from the ECA aiding in vessel identification. Also, a slight tap in the temporal area will cause oscillations in the normal ECA waveform but not in the ICA waveform (Fig. 48-8).

NO INTERNAL CAROTID ARTERY WAVEFORM PRESENT

When the ICA is occluded, an ECA branch may be mistaken for the ICA; however, this branch will be smaller than the ICA on duplex imaging and will still have a high-resistance waveform. The signs of an occluded ICA include a lack of diastolic flow in the ipsilateral CCA and blunted reversed flow on the side of the obstruction.

TORTUOUS INTERNAL CAROTID ARTERY

The ICA and ECA can be very difficult to image when they follow a tortuous course through the neck. When the vessels intertwine and acutely bend around

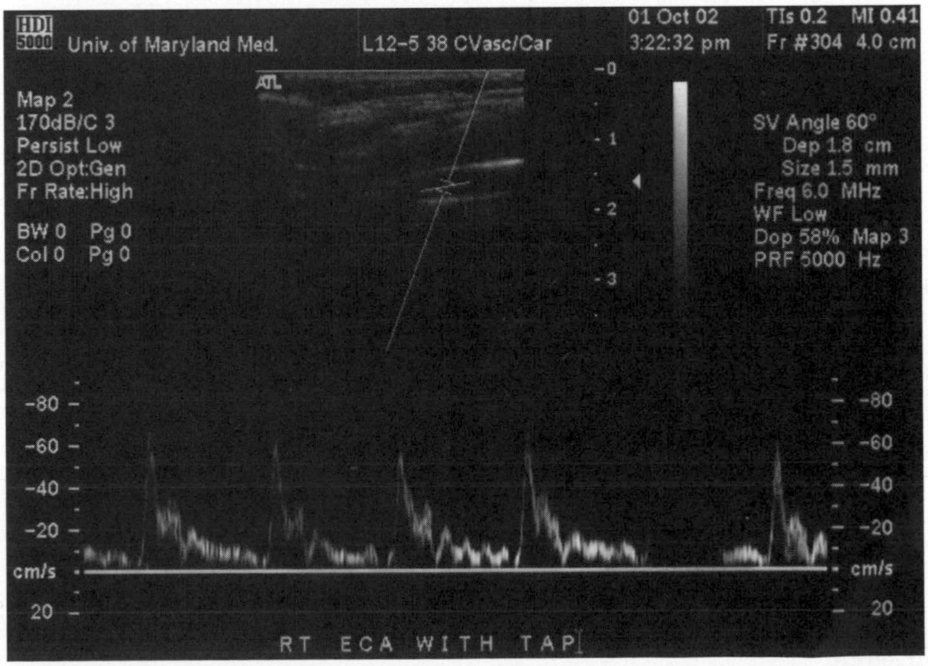

Figure 48-8. ■ *External carotid artery* (ECA) *with temporal tap.*

each other, velocity measurements are compromised and it is almost impossible to obtain an accurate 60-degree angle. A suboptimal angle will result in a poor spectral display, bidirectional flow, and spectral broadening even when no disease is present. An inferior color flow display will also be present because a quality color flow display is also dependant on an adequate angle. Appropriate angling of the color box and small movements of the transducer to follow the course of the vessels are the most helpful techniques until the vessel course is evident.

CALCIFICATION

Pulsed Doppler signals, including color flow, cannot penetrate calcifications. Calcified arterial plaques reflect bright echoes back to the transducer; a highly echogenic area in the vessel wall is seen with shadowing distal to the calcification. One cannot conclude that the vessel is occluded but only that color or Doppler flow cannot be demonstrated due to calcified plaque. The cursor and beam should be angled between calcifications to examine any vessel lumen that is not obscured by shadowing.

LOW-FLOW VELOCITIES

Consistent low-velocity signals on one side of the extracranial system without significant visible disease indicate a more distal lesion. Stenosis or occlusion above the angle of the jaw is impossible to detect with duplex imaging because the lesions are beyond the imaging range. Calculate the ICA/CCA ratio; if only one side is affected, disease superior to the imaged area is considered the likely diagnosis. If a low-flow state is seen on both sides poor cardiac output is assumed to be the cause.

SELECTED READING

Allen P. *Clinical Doppler Ultrasound.* London: Harcourt Publishers; 2000.

Hagen-Ansert S. *Textbook of Diagnostic Ultrasonography.* St. Louis: Mosby; 2001.

Moneta GL, Edwards JM, Chitwood RW, et al. Correlation of North American Symptomatic Carotid Endarterectomy Trial (NASCET). Angiographic definition of 70-99% internal carotid artery stenosis with duplex scanning. *J Vasc Surg* 1992;17:152–160.

Moneta GI, Edwards JM, Papanicolaou G, et al. Screening for asymptomatic internal carotid artery stenosis. Duplex criteria for documenting 60-90% stenosis. *J Vasc Surg* 1995;21:989–994.

North American Symptomatic Carotid Endarterectomy Trial Collaborators. Beneficial effect of carotid endarterectomy in symptomatic patients with high grade carotid stenosis. *N Engl J Med* 1991;325: 445–453.

Strandness DE. *Duplex Scanning in Vascular Disorders.* 3rd ed. Philadelphia: Lippincott Williams & Wilkins; 2002.

Zweibel WJ. *Introduction to Vascular Sonography.* New York: Grune & Stratton; 1992.

Intracranial Vascular Problems

49

GAIL SANDAGER-HADLEY

SONOGRAM ABBREVIATIONS

A Arch	Aortic arch
Aca	Anterior cerebral artery
Acoa	Anterior communicating artery
AW	Anterior window
Ba	Basilar artery
COW	Circle of Willis
ICa	Internal carotid artery
INNa	Innominate artery
LACa	Left anterior cerebral artery
LCCa	Left common carotid artery
LICa	Left internal carotid artery
LMCa	Left middle cerebral artery
MCa	Middle carotid artery
MES	Microemboli signals
MW	Middle window
Oa	Ophthalmic artery
PCa	Posterior cerebral artery
PW	Posterior window
RACa	Right anterior cerebral artery
RCCa	Right common carotid artery
RECa	Right external carotid artery
RICa	Right internal carotid artery
Rva	Right vertebral artery
Sa	Subclavian artery
Va	Vertebral artery

KEY WORDS

Arteriovenous Malformation (AVM). An abnormal communication between arteries and veins.

Basal Intracranial Arteries. Large vessels at the base of the brain.

Butterfly Pattern. The characteristic Doppler velocity spectra seen at the normal middle cerebral artery/anterior cerebral artery bifurcation, displaying the middle cerebral artery flow above the baseline directed toward the probe and the anterior cerebral artery flow below the baseline moving away from the probe. This is a major reference point used for vessel identification.

Collateral Circulation. An alternate circulatory route that is evoked when the normal circulatory pathways are obstructed.

Critical Stenosis (Hemodynamically Significant). A narrowing of the vessel lumen that results in a decrease in pressure and flow.

Endarterectomy. Surgical technique in which a diseased portion of the carotid artery is removed and replaced with a vein.

Foramen. Natural passage or opening.

Genu. Acute bend of the carotid in the brain.

Hyperdynamic Flow. Increased volume of flow gives rise to increased velocities.

Hyperostosis. Bone hypertrophy (overgrowth).

Parasellar. Close to the sella turcica in the region of the pituitary gland.

Range Ambiguity. If a large Doppler sample site is used, a variety of signals will be received giving a wide range of results.

Sickle Cell Anemia. A type of anemia in which the red blood cells are crescent-shaped (sickle).

Supraclinoid. Above the clinoid process, close to the pituitary.

Vasospasm. Constriction or narrowing of the arteries usually occurring after a subarachnoid hemorrhage; velocities become markedly elevated in the presence of vasospasm.

The Clinical Problem

Ultrasonic evaluation of the basal intracranial arteries was, in the past, limited by inability to penetrate the skull with ultrasound. Angiography was, until recently, the only method available for evaluation of intracranial arteries. However, angiography only provides anatomic information with limited functional information. It is too risky and invasive to use as a screening examination. Transcranial Doppler (TCD) is a noninvasive method of examining the intracranial arteries that provides both anatomic and hemodynamic flow information. It is repeatable and can be performed at the bedside, making it the optimum examination for evaluation of the intracranial vessels.

Assessment of the major basal intracranial arteries is important in a variety of clinical conditions. The presenting symptoms or clinical indications will vary depending on the problem.

Clinical indications for TCD include the following:

1. Evaluation of cerebral artery vasospasm: onset, location, severity, and course over time. This usually occurs after a subarachnoid hemorrhage from a ruptured cerebral artery aneurysm.
2. Detection of arteriovenous malformation (AVM).
3. Evaluation of children with sickle cell anemia to identify those at high risk for stroke.
4. Detection of major basal intracranial artery critical stenoses.

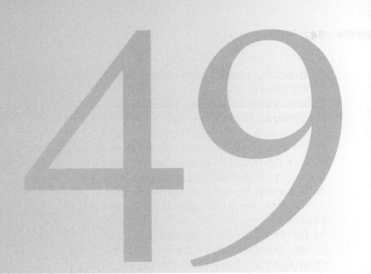

5. Detection of vertebrobasilar insufficiency.
6. Assessment of patterns and extent of collateral circulation.
7. Extension of carotid examination to determine intracranial blood flow velocity in the presence of severe extracranial carotid artery disease.
8. Determining the state of circulation in patients with suspected brain death.
9. Intraoperative monitoring of cerebral hemodynamics during cerebrovascular or cardiovascular surgery.
10. Evaluation of patients posttreatment—success of embolization of AVMs.
11. Determining the effect of subclavian steal on intracranial hemodynamics.
12. Monitor for emboli.

Anatomy

The major basal intracranial arteries form the circle of Willis (COW). The COW is composed of an anterior segment and a posterior segment with right and left sides. The anterior portion of the COW circulation arises from the right and left internal carotid arteries (ICa), whereas the posterior circulation arises from the vertebrobasilar arteries (Fig. 49-1).

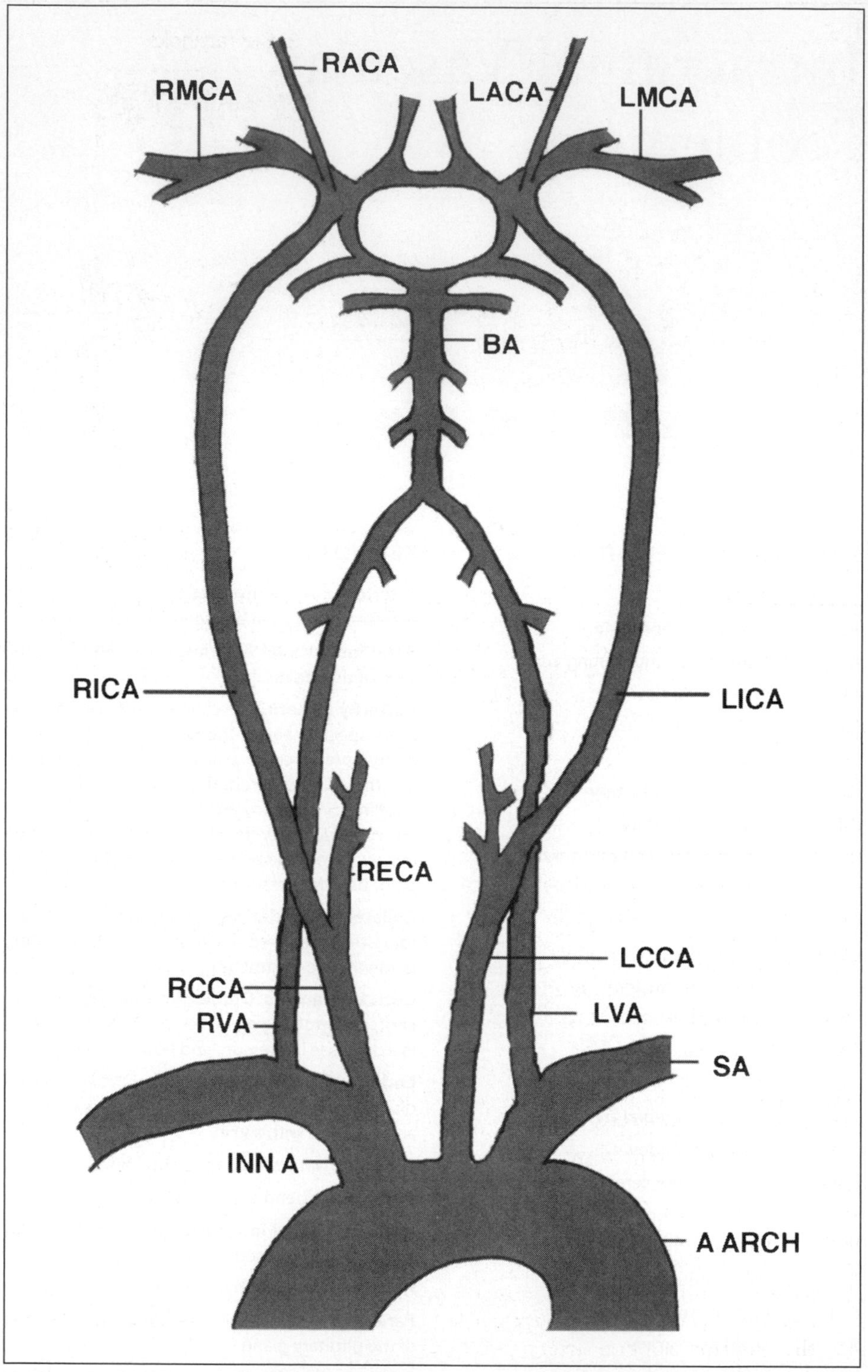

Figure 49-1. ■ *Normal intracranial anatomy.* A Arch, *aortic arch;* INNa, *innominate artery;* Sa, *subclavian artery;* LVa, *left vertebral artery;* LCCa, *left common carotid artery;* LICa, *left internal carotid artery;* LMCa, *left middle cerebral artery;* LACa, *left anterior cerebral artery;* RACa, *right anterior cerebral artery;* RMCa, *right middle cerebral artery;* Ba, *basilar artery;* RICa, *right internal carotid artery;* RECa, *right external carotid artery;* RCCa, *right common carotid artery;* RVa, *right vertebral artery.*

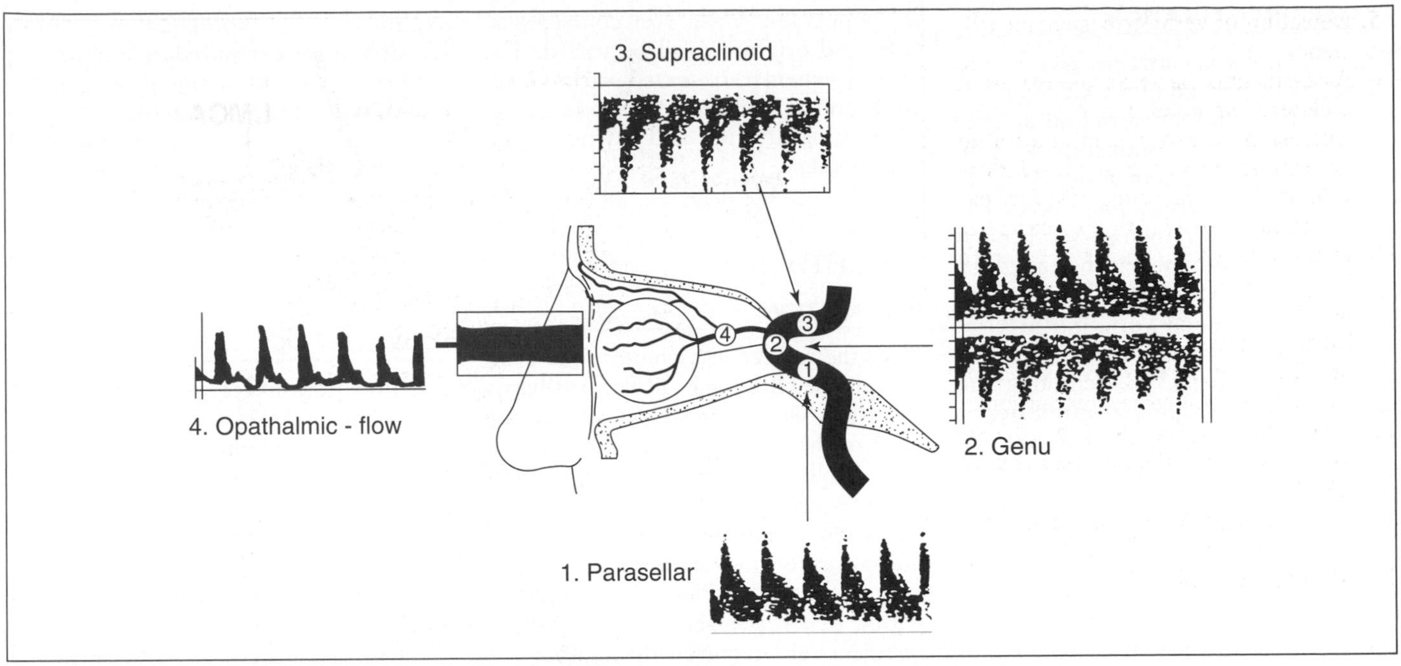

Figure 49-2. ■ *Flow patterns in the carotid siphon. Carotid siphon—lateral view;* 1, *Parasellar—flow toward the probe;* 2,. *Genu—bidirectional flow;* 3, *Supraclinoid—flow away;* 4, *Ophthalmic—flow toward.*

ANTERIOR CIRCULATION OF THE CIRCLE OF WILLIS

The extracranial (neck) segment of the ICa begins at the common carotid bifurcation and ends where the ICa enters the skull. At this point it becomes the intracranial ICa. The intracranial ICa then courses cephalad to the carotid siphon region. At the carotid siphon, the ICa forms an S-like configuration as it first runs anterior, then medial, and then posterior. This segment of the ICa will normally display different flow directions depending on which segment is insonated (Fig. 49-2). This tortuous segment of ICa gives rise to the ophthalmic artery (Oa), which provides blood supply to the eye and surrounding muscles. Just beyond the Oa, the ICa branches into the anterior cerebral artery (ACa) and the middle cerebral artery (MCa). These vessels form the anterior circulation of the COW. The right and left sides of the anterior circulation are connected by the anterior communicating artery. This completes the right and left sides of the anterior portion of the COW (Fig. 49-3).

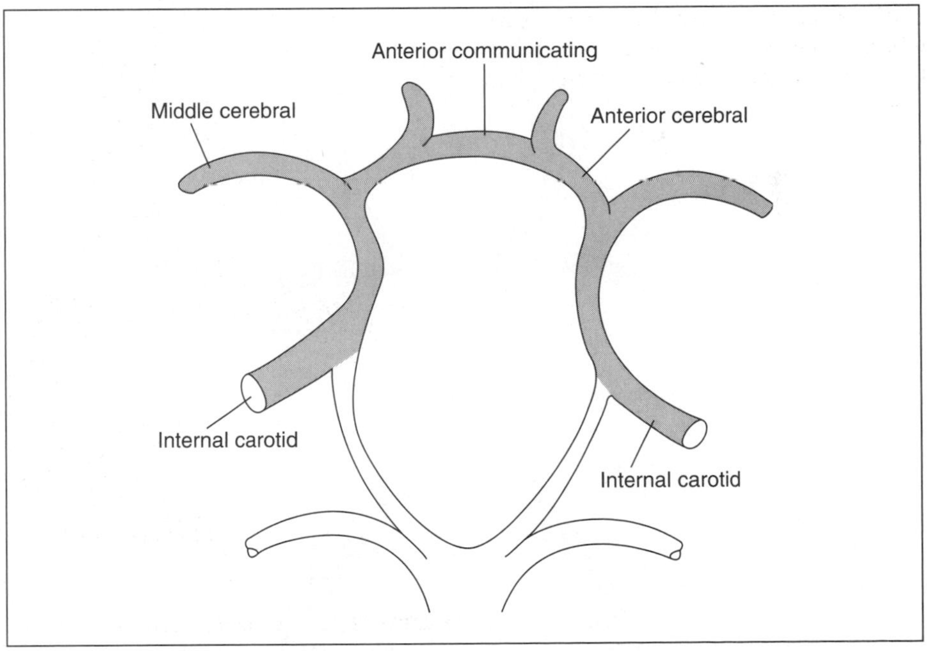

Figure 49-3. ■ *Anterior portion of the circle of Willis (COW).*

POSTERIOR CIRCULATION

The vertebrobasilar arteries give rise to the posterior portion of the COW.

The right and left vertebral arteries originate as the first branch of the subclavian arteries and course superoposterior through the cervical vertebrae. The vertebral artery (Va) then passes through the foramen magnum and becomes the intracranial portion of the Va. The right and left intracranial vertebral arteries join to form the basilar artery (Ba). The Ba is approximately 3 to 4 cm long and branches into the right and left posterior cerebral arteries (PCa). The anterior and posterior segments of the COW are then joined by the posterior communicating arteries. These vessels make up the posterior portion of the COW (Fig. 49-4).

Anatomic variants of the intracranial cerebral circulation are common and reported to occur in up to 50% of the population. Vessel size, course, location, and origin can all be varied. The most frequently observed variants include an incomplete COW, absent communicating arteries, and asymmetry of the Va size.

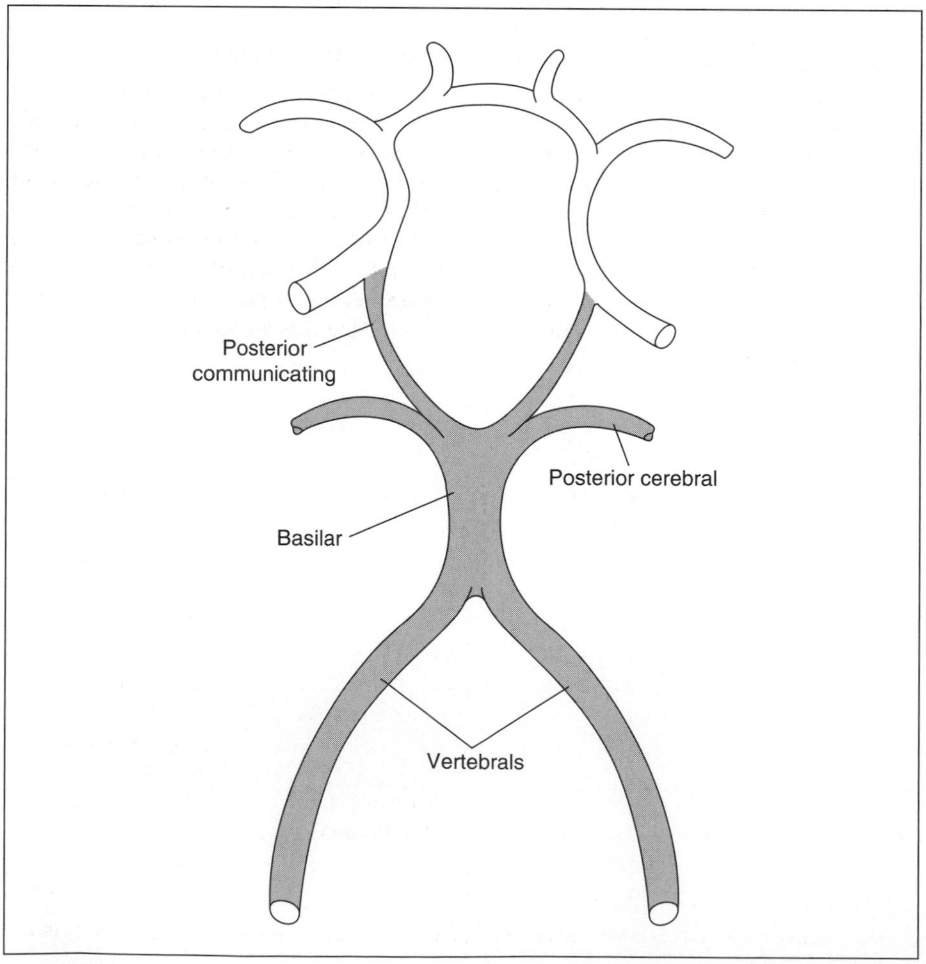

Figure 49-4. ■ *Posterior portion of the COW.*

Technique

PREPARATION

Place the patient in a comfortable position supine with the head flat or slightly elevated. The technologist sits at the head of the patient positioned to maintain stability of the hand with the transducer. A steady hand is essential because slight movement or variation in transducer position may compromise the examination results. Place the equipment within easy reach because frequent adjustments are required throughout the examination; a foot pedal is helpful. Headphones are required to optimize the quality of the audio signal, which is a crucial part of the examination.

The status of the extracranial carotid circulation must be known because obstructive lesions of the extracranial carotid vessels may affect the intracerebral circulation and impact on the TCD findings.

EQUIPMENT

Instrumentation requirements include (1) a 2- to 3-MHz range-gated pulsed Doppler with enhanced power levels to penetrate areas of the skull that are naturally thin; and (2) online spectral analysis that provides time-averaged velocity measurements including peak systole, end diastole, mean velocity, and pulsatility index.

Currently there are two ways for performing TCD. These include a nonimaging system that provides online spectral analysis and color duplex imaging that includes a real-time B-mode image, color Doppler, and pulsed Doppler spectral analysis.

Although several different techniques are used, the only currently available diagnostic criteria are based on Doppler velocity calculations from a 2-MHz nonimaging range-gated pulsed Doppler system. Color duplex imaging provides a road map of the intracranial vessels so anatomic and physiologic information can be accurately obtained from specific sites of interest.

VESSEL IDENTIFICATION CRITERIA

Vessel identification is based on several parameters that should agree to ensure accuracy:

1. Direction of blood flow relative to the transducer
2. Relationship to the acoustic window used—probe orientation
3. Depth of vessel
4. Traceability—distance that the course of the vessel can be followed
5. Spatial relationships to other vessels
6. Hierarchy of blood flow (MCa highest mean velocity, then ACa, and then PCa)
7. Response to common carotid artery (CCa) compression
8. Bony landmarks (used only for imaging studies)

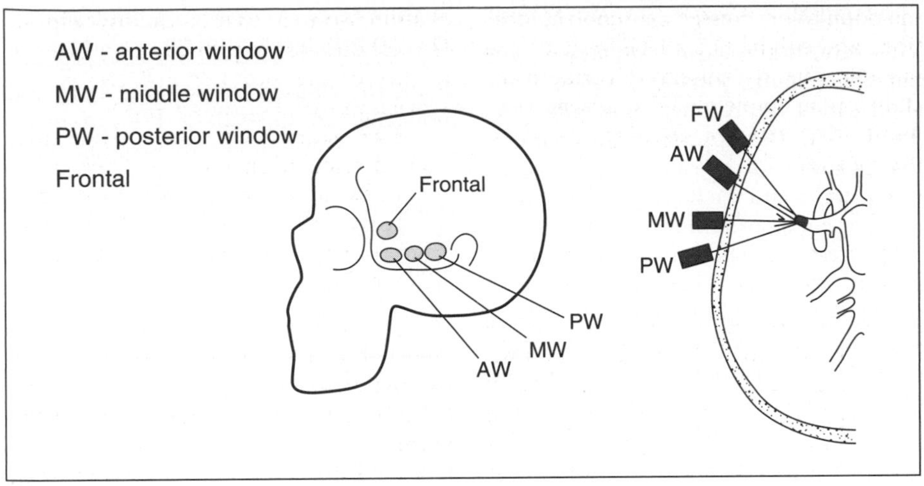

Figure 49-5. ■ *Ultrasonic windows from the transtemporal approach.*

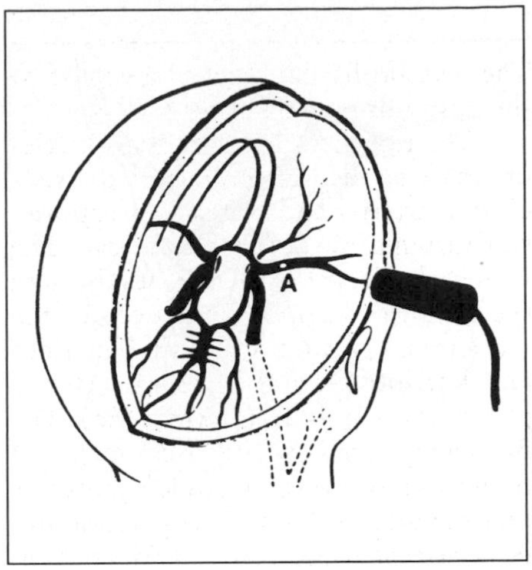

Figure 49-6. ■ *Transtemporal approach.*

ACOUSTIC WINDOWS

There are four ultrasonic windows used to obtain a complete TCD examination: the transtemporal, transorbital, transoccipital, and submandibular approaches. Each window provides information regarding specific vessels of the COW (Figs. 49-5 and 49-6).

Transtemporal Window

A routine examination begins with the transtemporal window on either the right or left side. This window is over the temporal bone immediately superior to the zygomatic arch. The window has four parts: the anterior, middle, posterior, and frontal (Fig. 49-5). The best window will vary from patient to patient; you may find and only use one or you may use a combination of windows. It is important to find the window that provides the highest quality signal. The vessels evaluated routinely from this approach include the MCa, ACa, PCa, and terminal portion of the intracranial ICa. The anterior and posterior communicating arteries are examined using this approach but are not routinely identified owing to size and low flow states under normal conditions. The anterior communicating artery and posterior communicating artery act as collateral pathways that can be identified when flow volume is increased through the vessel. Normal values in each location are shown in Table 49-1.

Transorbital Window

This window is located directly through the eyelid (as opposed to supraorbital) and provides access to the Oa and the intracranial portion of the ICa/carotid siphon. Decrease power levels to 5% to 10% of the maximum power output to minimize ultrasound exposure to the retina because signal attenuation is low when using this window.

Table 49-1 Normal Intracranial Arterial Velocity Values

Artery	Acoustic Window	Depth of Sample Volume (mm)	Normal Mean Velocity (cm/sec)	Color Coding Flow Direction	Normal Direction of Flow
MCa	Transtemporal	35–60	55 ± 12	Red	Toward the probe
ACa	Transtemporal	60–80	50 ± 11	Blue	Away from the probe
PCa(P1)	Transtemporal	60–70	39 ± 10	Red	Toward the probe
PCa(P2)	Transtemporal	60–70	39 ± 10	Blue	Away from the probe
t-ICa	Transtemporal	55–65	39 ± 9	Red	Toward the probe
Oa	Transorbital	40–60	21 ± 5	Not used for the Oa	Toward the probe
Supraclinoid,	Transorbital	60–75	40 ± 11		Away from the probe
Genu,			NA		Bidirectional
Parasellar			47 ± 14	Not used for the carotid siphon	Toward the probe
Va	Transforaminal	65–90	40 ± 10	Blue	Away from the probe
Ba	Transforaminal	80–120	40 ± 10	Blue	Away from the probe

MCa, middle carotid artery; ACa, anterior cerebral artery; PCa, posterior cerebral artery; t-ICa, intracranial internal carotid artery; Oa, ophthalmic artery; Va, vertebral artery; Ba, basilar artery; NA, not available.

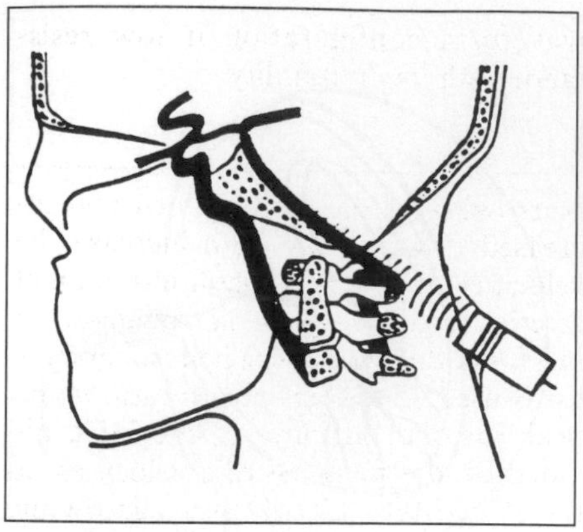

Figure 49-7. ■ *Transoccipital approach for evaluation of the vertebrobasilar arteries.*

Suboccipital Window—Transforaminal

This acoustic window is created by the natural opening found at the base of the skull called the foramen magnum (Fig. 49-7). With this approach, the intracranial portions of the right and left vertebral arteries and the Ba can be insonated. The patient's position is changed to provide access to the posterior portion of the base of the skull. The patient can turn onto either the right or left side with the head flexed forward to create a larger opening between the atlas and the base of the skull. If this position is not comfortable for the patient, almost any position is acceptable that allows forward flexion of the head and adequate space for the transducer.

NONIMAGING TECHNIQUE: RANGE-GATED PULSED DOPPLER

Place the transducer over the temporal bone slightly superior to the zygomatic arch. Start with the sample volume set at 55 mm. Slide the probe across the four windows until an arterial signal is detected. After optimization of the arterial signal, locate the MCa and trace it throughout its course. The MCa runs from depths of 30 to 60 mm with flow directed toward the transducer. The characteristic waveform patterns are low resistance and low pulsatility, with forward flow throughout diastole. Normal mean velocities are 55 ± 12 cm/sec (Fig. 49-8).

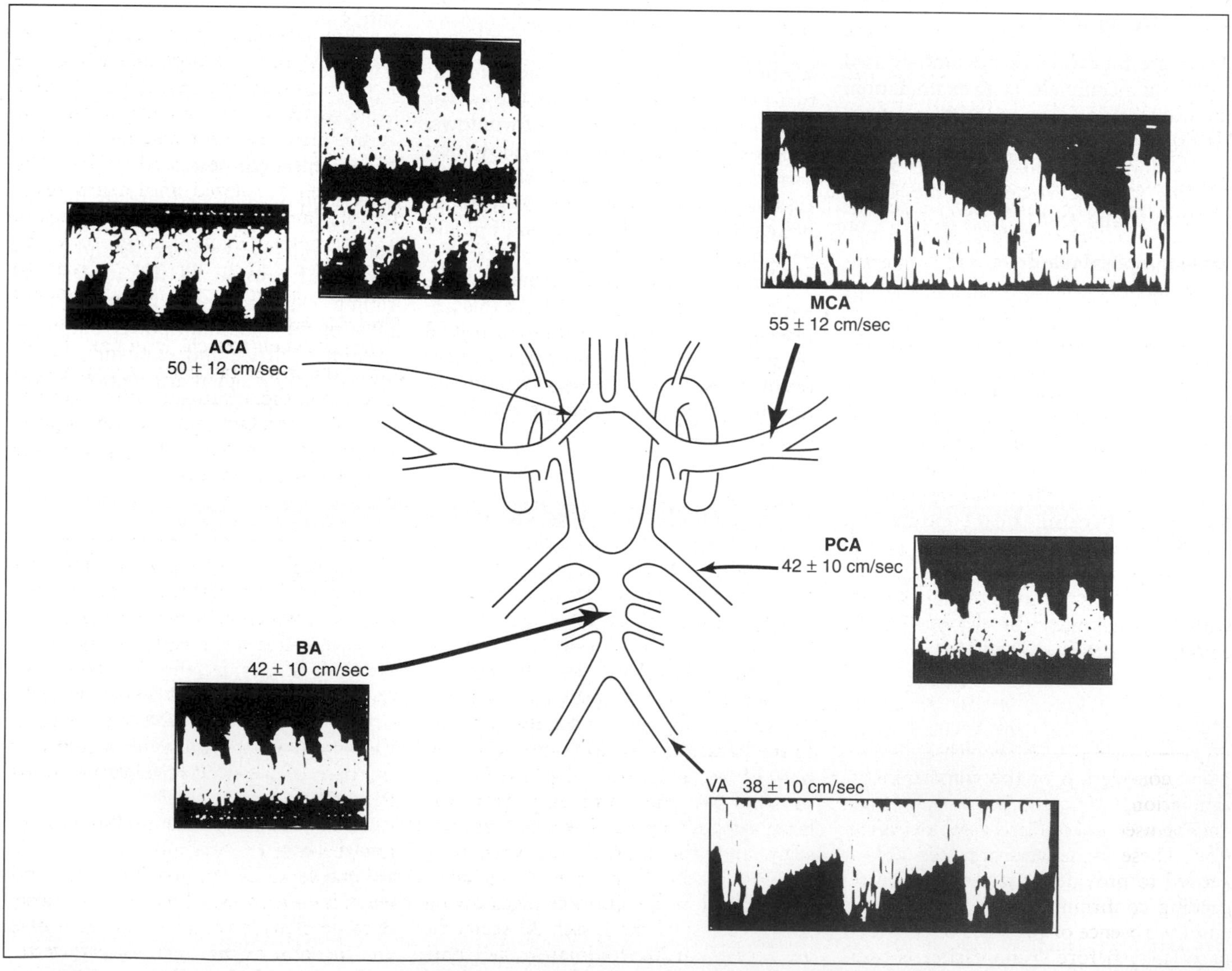

Figure 49-8. ■ *Normal mean velocities and Doppler signals from the COW.*

Complete the evaluation of the MCa, and then locate the MCa/ACa bifurcation. This is identified by moving the sample volume to a depth of 55 to 65 mm and by angling superior and anterior until bidirectional flow is displayed. The large sample volume size (5 mm) causes insonation of both the MCa and ACa at their bifurcation. This pattern is referred to as the "butterfly" pattern and is an important reference point for spatial relationships of other intracranial arteries.

The ACa can be traced from depths of 60 to 80 mm by aiming the ultrasound beam slightly superior and anterior. Flow direction of the normal ACa is away from the transducer with normal mean velocities of 50 ± 11 cm/sec. Once the sample volume depth is moved beyond the MCa/ACa bifurcation, the MCa signal will disappear. After complete investigation of the entire ACa, trace the Doppler signal back to the MCa/ACa bifurcation; this is always the reference point one returns to for tracking the other vessels.

Evaluate the terminal portion of the intracranial ICa by angling the ultrasound beam inferior from the MCa/ACa bifurcation. The sample volume depth remains unchanged. Flow direction is toward the transducer with a normal mean velocity of 39 ± 9 cm/sec. This is generally the only segment of the distal ICa identified.

The PCa is located by directing the ultrasound beam posterior and inferior from the MCa/ACa bifurcation. If the near (P1) PCa precommunicating segment is insonated, the flow is toward the transducer, whereas the contralateral (P2) PCa postcommunicating signal is away from the transducer. The sample volume depth is between 60 and 80 mm with a normal mean velocity of 39 ± 10 cm/sec (Fig. 49-8).

COMMON CAROTID ARTERY COMPRESSION MANEUVERS

After completion of the transtemporal evaluation, CCa compression maneuvers may be used to confirm vessel identification. These maneuvers are used only if needed to provide more information regarding confirming vessel identification and the absence or presence of collateral pathways. Before compression is initiated, the status of the extracranial carotid arteries must be known. Carotid compression maneuvers are contraindicated in the presence of severe carotid artery disease, low carotid bifurcation, or unstable carotid plaque. The decision is made by the appropriate medical personnel; medical supervision should be available during this part of the examination because there is some risk.

CCa compression is performed by palpating the carotid artery in the neck and slowly applying pressure until the pulse disappears. This is done while insonating the intracranial vessel in question. Pressure is applied for only a few seconds, or two to three cardiac cycles; in the presence of an intact COW, compression of the right CCa will cause the right MCa to shrink and flow will be obliterated. The right ACa exhibits either reversal of flow or diminished or obliterated flow. Compression of the left CCa should not affect the contralateral intracerebral vessels unless collateral pathways (cross-filling) has occurred.

TRANSORBITAL APPROACH

The transducer is placed over the closed eyelid with coupling gel. The transducer beam is angled medial with the sample volume depth between 40 and 60 mm. The probe is moved slightly until an arterial signal is located; this is the Oa. The flow direction is toward the probe with normal mean velocities of 21 ± 5 cm/sec. The normal waveform pattern is higher resistance than the other intracerebral vessels. Trace the Oa distal to approximately 65 mm to locate the carotid siphon.

The course of the carotid siphon–intracranial ICa forms an S-like configuration (Fig. 49-2). There are three components to the carotid siphon that form the "S": the parasellar, the genu, and the supraclinoid. All three segments are evaluated by tilting the probe from inferior to superior at depths of 60 to 70 mm.

The proximal parasellar segment is inferior with flow directed toward the transducer. The genu is slightly superior to the parasellar portion with flow seen both above and below the baseline because of the range ambiguity from the large sample volume. The most superior segment is the supraclinoid with flow moving away from the transducer. Although flow direction changes owing to the course of the vessel, all segments are located at approximately the same depth of 60 to 75 mm. The mean velocities detected are the supraclinoid segment at 40 ± 11 cm/sec and the parasellar segment at 47 ± 14 cm/sec. The waveform configuration is low resistance with low pulsatility.

SUBMANDIBULAR APPROACH

Narrowing of the vessel lumen and increased flow volume both increase the velocities of the major basal intracranial arteries. To differentiate narrowing from increased flow volume, a hemispheric ratio is used. The hemispheric ratio is the peak systolic velocities of the MCa divided by the peak systolic velocities of the ICa (MCa/ICa). Vessel narrowing causes increased velocities at the site of narrowing where an increased volume of flow (hyperdynamic flow) causes increased velocities in both vessels. A hemispheric ratio of less than 3 is consistent with hyperdynamic flow, whereas a ratio of more than 3 is compatible with vasospasm.

Velocity measurements of the extracranial ICa are obtained using the submandibular approach. The 2-MHz probe is placed at the angle of the jaw and angled posterior and medial. The power levels are decreased to 5%. The transducer is rotated until a low-resistance ICa signal is located. To ensure proper vessel identification, rock the transducer slightly anterior to listen to the external carotid artery and compare the Doppler signals. By rocking back and forth between vessels, you can distinguish the lower pulsatility signal of the ICa from the more pulsatile external carotid artery. Optimize the ICa Doppler signal and then obtain the appropriate Doppler measurements.

SUBOCCIPITAL WINDOW

The right and left vertebral arteries enter the base of the skull through the foramen magnum, which provides a natural window to evaluate the vertebrobasilar arteries. Change the patient's position so that he or she is lying on either the right or left side with the head flexed forward. This position opens up the window at the base of the skull to facilitate transducer placement.

The probe is placed midline just below the base of the skull with a sample volume depth of 75 mm. The ultrasound beam is aimed toward the patient's nose. Because of wide variations in the course and location of the right and left vertebral arteries, the transducer may need to be moved right and left of midline with the same beam direction until an arterial signal is identified.

Two distinct vessels should be located by rocking the transducer back and forth from right to left and locating two separate arterial signals. Each Va is tracked from depths of 60 to 90 mm with flow moving away from the transducer (Fig. 49-8). The normal mean velocities are 40 ± 10 cm/sec with a low-resistance, low-pulsatility waveform. A second arterial signal may be encountered at depths of 60 to 70 cm, displaying flow in the opposite direction. This is a main branch of the Va, called the posterior inferior cerebellar artery. Because of its course, the signal will disappear when the sample volume depth is moved either in front of or behind the vessel's origin.

Continuing along the course of the Va is the Ba, where the right and left vertebral arteries converge at a depth of 80 to 90 mm with flow continuing away from the probe. The Ba is approximately 3 to 4 cm long. The normal mean velocities are 42 ± 10 cm/sec, approaching the Va (Fig. 49-8).

COLOR DOPPLER IMAGING TECHNIQUE

Color Doppler imaging adds the following: (1) more accurate and confident vessel identification; (2) quicker recognition of anatomic variants; (3) easier location of flow abnormalities; and (4) rapid identification of collateral pathways.

With any commercially available scanner, select the dedicated TCD setup. The two-dimensional B-mode image depth of field is set to 8 cm. Place the transducer over the temporal bone in a transverse oblique orientation, so that anterior is located on the left side of the screen and posterior is on the right side, with lateral along the top of the image and medial at the bottom.

With only the grayscale image, move the probe until an adequate window is found. Optimize the window by aligning the bony and soft tissue landmarks. The temporal window landmarks are the sphenoid wing and petrous portion of the temporal bone, the anterior clinoid process, the foramen lacerum, and the mesencephalic brain stem (Fig. 49-9). Align the sphenoid wing, petrous ridge, and foramen lacerum, and then turn on the color.

Vessels examined from this approach are the MCa, ACa, and PCa. By aiming the beam inferiorly, the intracranial ICa is seen just superior to the foramen lacerum; the foramen lacerum will appear as a small anechoic circle with flow toward the transducer coded in red. With this landmark, angle superior to locate the intracranial basal arteries. The MCa is seen running parallel to the sphenoid wing; flow is toward the transducer and coded in red. Occasionally branches of the MCa are visualized at a depth of 35 mm; this is a normal finding.

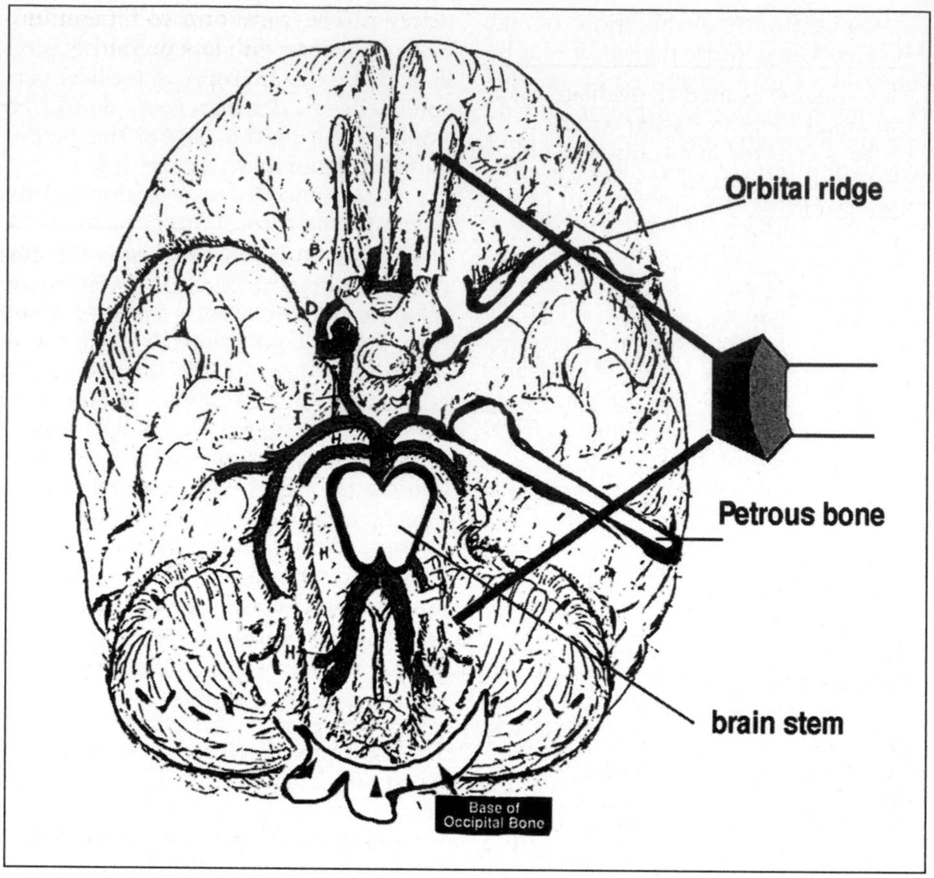

Figure 49-9. ■ *Bony window to the intracranial arteries. Heart-shaped structure is the mesencephalon in the brain stem, which is an obvious landmark. Intracranial vascular problems.*

Because direction of flow is vital to vessel identification, color coding is not changed during the examination. The standard setup displays red toward and blue away from the transducer. The pulsed Doppler information is obtained by tracking the course of the MCa while recording the standard information. Angle correction with color imaging is controversial at this time. Whatever Doppler angle protocol is used, angle-correction measurements or an assumed angle of zero, it must be consistently applied to standardize the procedure and minimize velocity calculation errors.

Trace the course of the MCa with the Doppler until the MCa/ACa bifurcation (butterfly pattern) is located. The ACa will be coded in blue with flow moving away from the transducer. Follow the ACa with the Doppler recording the necessary calculations, always monitoring all the variables for vessel identification. At depths of 70 mm or more, the contralateral ACa is sometimes visualized and will be displayed in red with flow toward the transducer. To investigate the vessels of the opposite hemisphere, the contralateral temporal window is used.

To locate the PCa, optimize the image at the MCa/ACa bifurcation and then angle posterior and inferior. The PCa has the lowest velocities normally, and gain settings or velocity controls may need to be reset to aid color filling. The mesencephalon portion of the brain stem is the major landmark for the PCa. The mesencephalon is a posterior hypoechoic structure (Fig. 49-9). The PCa courses around the mesencephalon. The P1 segment is coded in red, and the P2 segment is coded in blue. Doppler recordings are taken throughout the entire course of the vessel.

TRANSFORAMINAL APPROACH: TRANSOCCIPITAL

This window is used to evaluate the intracranial vertebrobasilar arteries. The probe is oriented in a transverse oblique plane and positioned in the back of the head just below the base of the skull. The probe is angled superiorly toward the patient's nose. Color settings may need to be adjusted for the lower velocities normally seen in the vertebrobasilar arteries. The depth of field is set at approximately 8 cm. By using the B-mode image, locate the foramen magnum, which is circular in appearance with low-level echoes in the center. The right and left vertebral arteries appear to course around the foramen magnum, with flow directed away from the transducer and coded in blue. If the right and left vertebral arteries are not seen in the same plane, move the transducer to the right and left of midline until a vessel is detected.

The vertebral arteries join together to form the Ba at approximately 8.5 cm. To follow the course of the Ba, the transducer may need to be rotated and angled slightly superior. The ultrasound beam should be directed from the base of the neck to the patient's nose. In many cases, only the proximal portion of the Ba can be identified.

TRANSORBITAL WINDOW

The transorbital window is used to evaluate the Oa flow direction and the carotid siphon portion of the intracranial ICa. To minimize acoustic exposure, use the power setting as recommended by the manufacturer. Position the transducer with coupling gel directly over the closed eyelid. The probe is angled slightly medial and superior with the field of view depth set at 7 mm. The Oa is seen at a depth of 40 to 60 mm with flow directed toward the transducer, color-coded red. The carotid siphon is deeper (60–75 mm) with variable flow direction. Flow direction is not meaningful because it is not always possible using color to locate all three segments: parasellar, genu, and supraclinoid of the carotid siphon (Fig. 49-2). Trace the Oa distal to approximately 65 mm to locate the carotid siphon. Although flow direction changes owing to the course of the vessel, all segments are located at approximately the same depth of 60 to 75 mm. The mean velocities detected range from 40 to 47 cm/sec. The waveform configuration is low resistance with low pulsatility.

Pathology

VASOSPASM

The diagnosis of vasospasm is the most widely accepted use of TCD today. Vasospasm is usually seen after a subarachnoid hemorrhage, with a predictable course between days 4 and 14 after the subarachnoid hemorrhage. TCD provides information regarding the location, onset, duration, and severity of the vasospasm. Vasospasm causes narrowing of the arterial lumen, which will increase the mean velocities. The increase in velocity is related to the narrowing; the more severe the narrowing, the higher increase in mean velocities. There are three categories of vasospasm:

Mild: 120 to 140 cm/sec

Moderate: 140 to 200 cm/sec

Severe: >200 cm/sec

There is also a strong correlation between the patient's clinical status and the daily changes in TCD findings. Mean velocities of greater than 250 cm/sec daily are associated with a poor outcome.

ARTERIOVENOUS MALFORMATION

1. Diagnostic criteria for large and medium-size AVMs include changes that occur from the feeding artery to the AVM and within the AVM. The amount of change is dependent on the size and number of vessels involved and communicating with the AVM.
2. In the feeding artery, both systolic and diastolic flow velocity increases are seen with decreased pulsatility. Peak systolic velocity is usually greater than 180 cm/sec with an end-diastolic volume of greater than 140 cm/sec. The pulsatility index can be as low as 0.26.
3. The flow within the AVM is turbulent and chaotic.
4. The velocities between the right and left hemispheres are asymmetric.
5. AVM treatment is to embolize the malformation. TCD is performed pretreatment to obtain baseline values, and then again postembolization to determine the success of therapy. The goal is to embolize and obliterate the AVM.

SICKLE CELL ANEMIA

It is known that children with sickle cell anemia are at high risk for stroke. TCD can be used to identify those children at risk. The examination is performed using the transtemporal and transoccipital windows only. The conduct of the examination is the same as for adults; the only difference is the anatomic location of the COW. The midline of a child aged 8 years is approximately 60 mm (Fig. 49-10). The MCa, ACa, and PCa are routinely evaluated. A mean velocity of 170

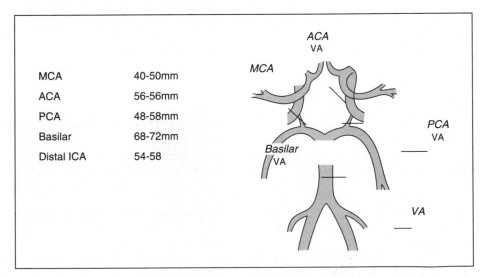

MCA	40-50mm
ACA	56-56mm
PCA	48-58mm
Basilar	68-72mm
Distal ICA	54-58

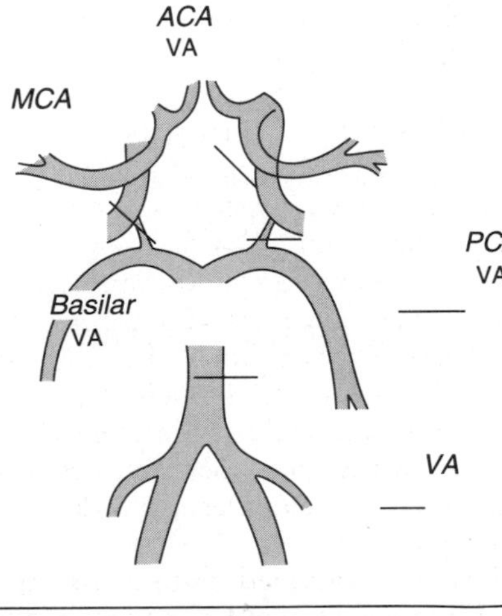

Figure 49-10. ■ *Vessel location for children (8 years of age).*

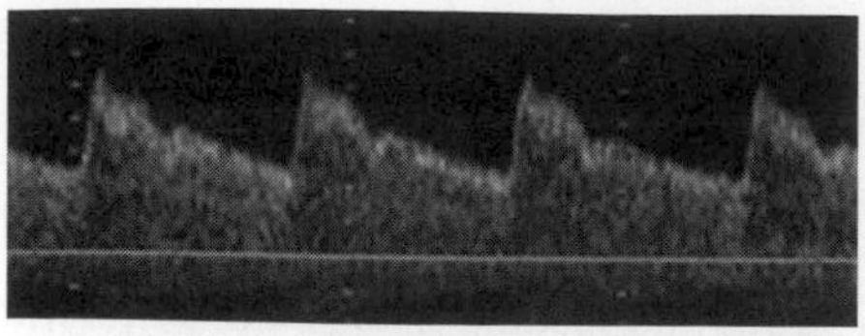

Figure 49-11. ■ *Interpretation criteria for children: for middle carotid artery (MCa), distal internal carotid artery (dICa), MCa/anterior cerebral artery (ACa) bifurcation. Normal, <170 cm/sec; borderline conditional, 170–200 cm/sec; abnormal, >200 cm/sec. This figure shows an MCa: mean velocity of 156 cm/sec.*

cm/sec is normal (Fig. 49-11). Children with a mean velocity of greater than 200 cm/sec are considered to be at risk for stroke. Due to the numerous physiologic variables that affect the velocity, it is important that children with a documented mean velocity of greater than 200 cm/sec be repeated within 7 days to confirm the presence of sustained elevated velocities.

BRAIN DEATH

TCD is a useful tool for documentation of cerebral circulatory arrest and brain death. However, it is not a definitive examination and is only used as a screening tool. Because it is noninvasive and portable, it can help select those patients who may need more invasive studies for which transport is required. Brain death is associated with the absence of cerebral perfusion. This cessation of intracranial flow causes a characteristic Doppler signal that exhibits "to-and-fro flow," forward flow in cardiac systole, and equal net retrograde flow during cardiac diastole. This is associated with an increase in intracranial pressure that causes increased vascular resistance. The Doppler signal varies at different stages of cerebral circulatory arrest (Fig. 49-12); therefore, repeat examinations are performed at various intervals to confirm the findings and the diagnosis.

INTRACRANIAL CEREBRAL ARTERY STENOSES

A stenosis is defined as focal increase (doubling) in the PSV (focal step-up of PSV) that does not extended beyond two sample volume lengths. A PSV that is elevated for an extended length is associated with vasospasm and not a stenosis. Other associated findings may include decreased velocities proximal or distal to the area, delayed systolic upstroke, poststenotic turbulence, and abnormal pulsatility index.

EXTRACRANIAL CAROTID ARTERY STENOSES OR OCCLUSIONS

TCD is an extension of the extracranial carotid duplex examination. It provides information regarding blood flow velocity of the intracranial vessels in the presence of extracranial occlusive disease. Associated findings in the presence of extracranial carotid disease will depend on the amount and extent of disease and the ability of the intracranial vessels to collateralize. Changes observed include decreased blood flow velocity, change in direction of flow, delayed systolic upstroke, decreased pulsatility, and turbulence.

SUBCLAVIAN STEAL

Subclavian steal is caused by a stenosis or occlusion that occurs in the subclavian arteries, or right innominate artery, proximal to the origins of the Va. These lesions can cause a pressure gradient between the Va circulation and the distal subclavian artery. This pressure gradient causes the subclavian artery beyond the origin of the Va to steal flow from the vertebral circulation; flow direction then reverses in the Va. If flow reversal occurs up through the Ba, it can cause brain stem ischemia (Fig. 49-13).

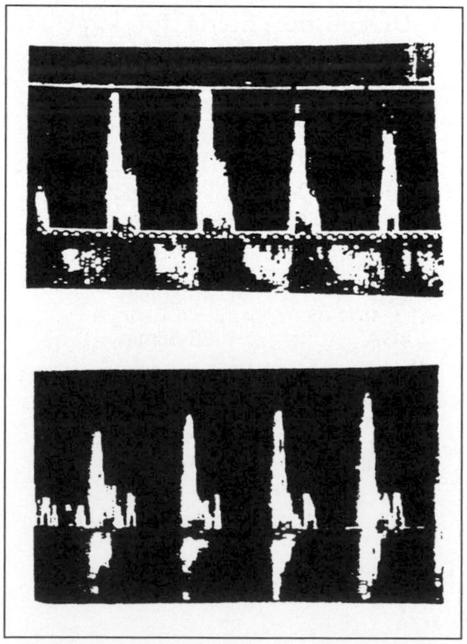

Figure 49-12. ■ *Doppler velocity spectra from the MCa consistent with cerebral circulatory arrest, demonstrating increased vascular resistance and a "to-and-fro flow" pattern.*

Examining the patient for subclavian steal includes extracranial duplex examination of the Va (see Chapter 48) with TCD evaluation of the Va, Ba, and PCa. Diagnostic criteria are based on blood-flow velocity calculations, direction of flow, and waveform configuration.

INTRAOPERATIVE TRANSCRANIAL DOPPLER MONITORING

Intraoperative TCD is used to monitor cerebral blood flow during carotid endarterectomy and cardiac surgery while on cardiopulmonary bypass. This procedure is done through the transtemporal window with the standard nonimaging probe secured onto a headset. This allows for continuous monitoring throughout the surgical procedure. The MCa is the vessel used for monitoring because it is an end vessel that can be reliably insonated.

During carotid endarterectomy when the carotid artery is clamped, TCD is performed to assess the patient's response to carotid clamping. A decrease

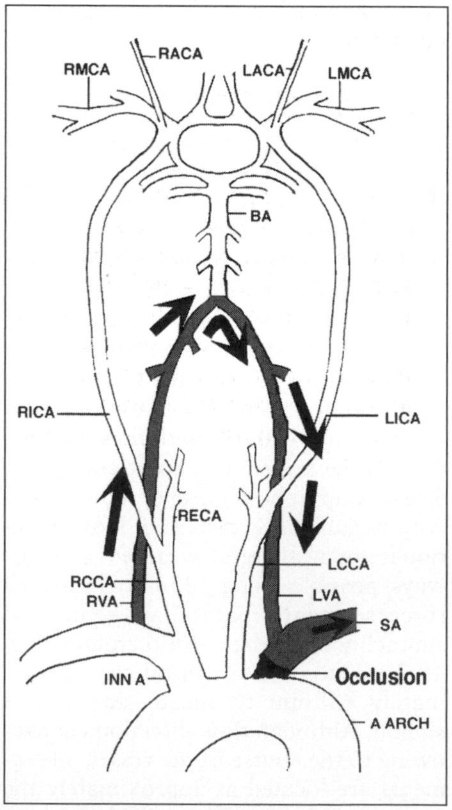

Figure 49-13. ■ *Subclavian steal—proximal left subclavian artery occlusion with reversed flow in the left vertebral artery.*

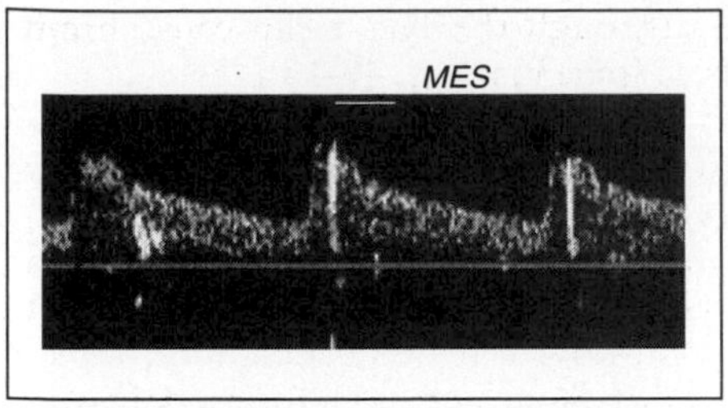

Figure 49-14. ■ *Microemboli.*

in mean blood flow velocity in the ipsilateral MCa of more than 65% from the preclamp value or a decrease to zero is consistent with inadequate collateral flow. These findings help to identify those patients who need a carotid shunt during the endarterectomy.

During reconstructive surgery, coronary or carotid intraoperative monitoring can be used to identify microemboli; both air and particulate matter can be identified. Microemboli signals (MES) have a characteristic signal that is easily displayed in the Doppler spectrum. MES consists of a high-intensity signal reflected back because of the higher density and size of both air and particulate matter (Fig. 49-14). If MES is detected during monitoring, both the frequency and duration are documented.

Pitfalls

1. Temporal window abnormality. Absence of a temporal window occurs in up to 15% of the population, with age, race, and sex being major factors. The most difficult patients to access include older women and African-American patients. Lack of a temporal window may only be unilateral; therefore, always examine both sides.
2. Occlusion versus technical difficulty. If a vessel is not identified, a total occlusion cannot be ruled out, although the cause may be technical difficulty.
3. Operator dependence. The examination is extremely operator-dependent, with a significant learning curve. A number of examinations need to be performed in conjunction with an experienced sonographer to correlate findings before working independently.
4. Lack of patient cooperation. If the patient is uncooperative or cannot hold still, the examination may be incomplete and nondiagnostic. If possible, the examination should be repeated when optimum positioning can be obtained.
5. Aliasing. Aliasing may be a factor when extremely high velocities are encountered with severe vasospasm or critical stenoses (see Chapter 48).
6. Other factors. Variables that may affect examination findings include age, hematocrit, hyperventilation or hypoventilation, cardiac output, and presence of extracranial carotid disease.
7. Anatomic variants. Anatomic variants occur frequently, in up to 50% of the population, with the most common variations including vessel course, size, and origin.
8. Eye surgery. If the patient has undergone recent eye surgery, the orbital portion of the examination may be contraindicated. Approval for the procedure should be given by the ophthalmologist.
9. Color allocation. Confusion can arise if color allocations are changed in the course of the study, so that red is substituted for blue.
10. It is not recommended that the transorbital window be used in children. This does not limit the examination because children universally have good transtemporal windows.

SELECTED READING

Aaslid R, Huber P, Nornes H. A transcranial Doppler method in the evaluation of cerebrovascular spasm. *Neuroradiology* 1986; 28:11–16.

Aaslid R, Markwalder TM, Nornes H. Noninvasive transcranial Doppler ultrasound recording of flow velocity in basal cerebral arteries. *J Neurosurg* 1982;57: 769–774.

Adams RJ, McKie VC, Hsu L, et al. Prevention of a first stroke by transfusions in children with sickle cell anemia and abnormal results on transcranial Doppler ultrasonography. *N Engl J Med* 1998;339:5–11.

Bogdahn U, Becker G, Winkler J, et al. Transcranial color-coded real-time sonography in adults. *Stroke* 1990;21(12):1680–1688.

Diethrich EB. Normal cerebrovascular anatomy and collateral pathways. In: Zwiebel WF, ed. *Introduction to vascular ultrasonography*. Philadelphia: Saunders, 1986.

Fujioka KA, Douville CM. Anatomy and freehand techniques. In: Newell DW, Aaslid R, eds. *Transcranial Doppler*. New York: Raven Press, 1992.

Fujioka KA, Gates DT, Spencer MP. A comparison of transcranial color Doppler imaging and standard static pulsed wave Doppler in the assessment of intracranial hemodynamics. *J Vasc Technol* 1994;18(1):29–35.

Hashimoto BE, Hattrick CW. New method of adult transcranial Doppler. *J Ultrasound Med* 1991;10:349–353.

Jansen C, Ramos LM, van-Heesewijk JP, et al. Impact of microembolism and hemodynamic changes in the brain during carotid endarterectomy. *Stroke* 1994;25:992.

Lindegaard KF, Grolimund P, Aaslid R, et al. Evaluation of cerebral AVMs using transcranial Doppler ultrasound. *J Neurosurg* 1986;65:335–344.

Newell DW, Gradys MS, Sirotta P, et al. Evaluation of brain death using transcranial Doppler. *Neurosurgery* 1989;24:509–513.

Shoning M, Walter J. Evaluation of the vertebrobasilar-posterior system by transcranial color duplex sonography in adults. *Stroke* 1992;23(9):1280–1286.

Pain and Swelling in the Limbs

50

GAIL SANDAGER-HADLEY
ROGER C. SANDERS

KEY WORDS

Baker's Cyst (Popliteal Cyst). Synovial fluid collection adjacent and posterior to the knee joint caused by trauma or rheumatoid arthritis.

Bursa. Inflammatory fluid collection, limited by a capsule, forming adjacent to a joint.

Cellulitis. Inflammation of the soft tissues of the limbs characterized by swelling, hyperemia, and increased echogenicity.

Deep Vein Thrombosis (DVT). Clot in the deep leg veins that may produce symptoms of leg swelling and pain.

Gout. Chronic arthritis affecting feet and hands particularly.

Homans' Sign. Pain in the calves on flexing the toes backward.

Metaphysis. Portion of the long bone adjacent to the epiphysis where no growth takes place.

Popliteum. Area posterior to the knee joints.

Rheumatoid Arthritis. Chronic arthritis affecting many joints, particularly the hands and knees, in which there is an exuberant overgrowth of the synovium of the joint. This is known as pannus.

Synovium. The lining of the joint. It produces the fluid that occupies the joint space and a Baker's cyst.

Tenosynovitis. Inflammation of the synovial membrane that surrounds a tendon. Fluid develops around the tendon, causing a target appearance on ultrasound.

The Clinical Problem

There are multiple causes for leg pain and swelling. Two common causes of pain and swelling in the legs are blood clot (thrombus) in a deep vein (deep vein thrombosis [DVT]) and a burst knee joint space with extravasation of synovial fluid into the surrounding soft tissue (Baker's cyst).

DVTs are common in patients who have recently undergone an operation, who are immobilized in bed, or who have a history of a malignancy. Accurate rapid diagnosis and treatment are important because venous thromboses commonly give rise to emboli that break off from the clot and end up in the lungs. Compression ultrasonography is 95% accurate for the detection of DVTs in the thigh but is less successful in the calf (70% success rate); consequently, many units do not seek calf vein thromboses. Such pulmonary emboli can be lethal. DVTs in the upper extremity occasionally occur but are more often related to indwelling catheters, radiation, or trauma to the upper arm.

The superficial veins of the leg are generally not a source of pulmonary emboli and are not always scanned when evaluating a patient for DVT. Superficial veins are most often evaluated to determine adequacy as a coronary or peripheral arterial bypass graft. This evaluation would include identifying the course, size, location and/or absence of anatomic anomalies, and absence of disease. The superficial veins may develop swelling and redness, apparent to the eye, that are related to thrombus or inflammation of the vein. The danger of emboli to the lungs is minimal unless the thrombus appears at the junction of a superficial vein and a deep vein.

Patients receiving long-term dialysis are at risk for complications related to their arteriovenous shunts. In these patients, a communication between the main artery and the vein is created, usually in the arm, through which dialysis is performed. Either the vein shuts down because of clots or arterial plaque develops.

Masses or collections in limbs are easy to demonstrate with ultrasound. Those located near the knee joint are especially confusing clinically, but are well seen with ultrasound. Baker's cysts are synovial fluid collections that develop posterior to the knee joint and can extend down into the calf. They are common in people with rheumatoid arthritis, and when they rupture they can mimic the clinical features of DVT. Popliteal artery aneurysms occur in the same location. Clinically, other confusing masses such as abscesses, hematomas, and tumors, recognizable by ultrasound, may occur around the knee joint or at any other site in the limbs.

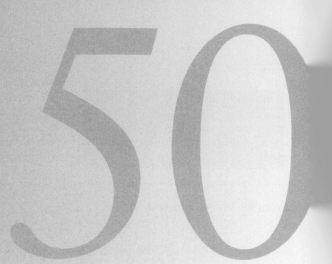

Limb pain, related to infection, can be difficult to analyze. Ultrasound can distinguish between an abscess that needs to be drained, cellulitis (a soft tissue infection without abscess formation), and acute osteomyelitis (bone infection). The latter requires early antibiotic treatment or long-term refractory infection may develop.

Traumatic limb injuries can be examined with ultrasound. Tendon problems are particularly well seen. Distinguishing between a tendon break and a tendon bruise is clinically important. Foreign bodies in the hands or feet can be detected with ultrasound. Muscle tears and muscle injuries are well seen.

Anatomy

VASCULAR SYSTEM

The femoral artery and vein can be found in the inguinal region in the groin lateral to the pubic symphysis. The vein lies medial to the artery (Fig. 50-1) in the

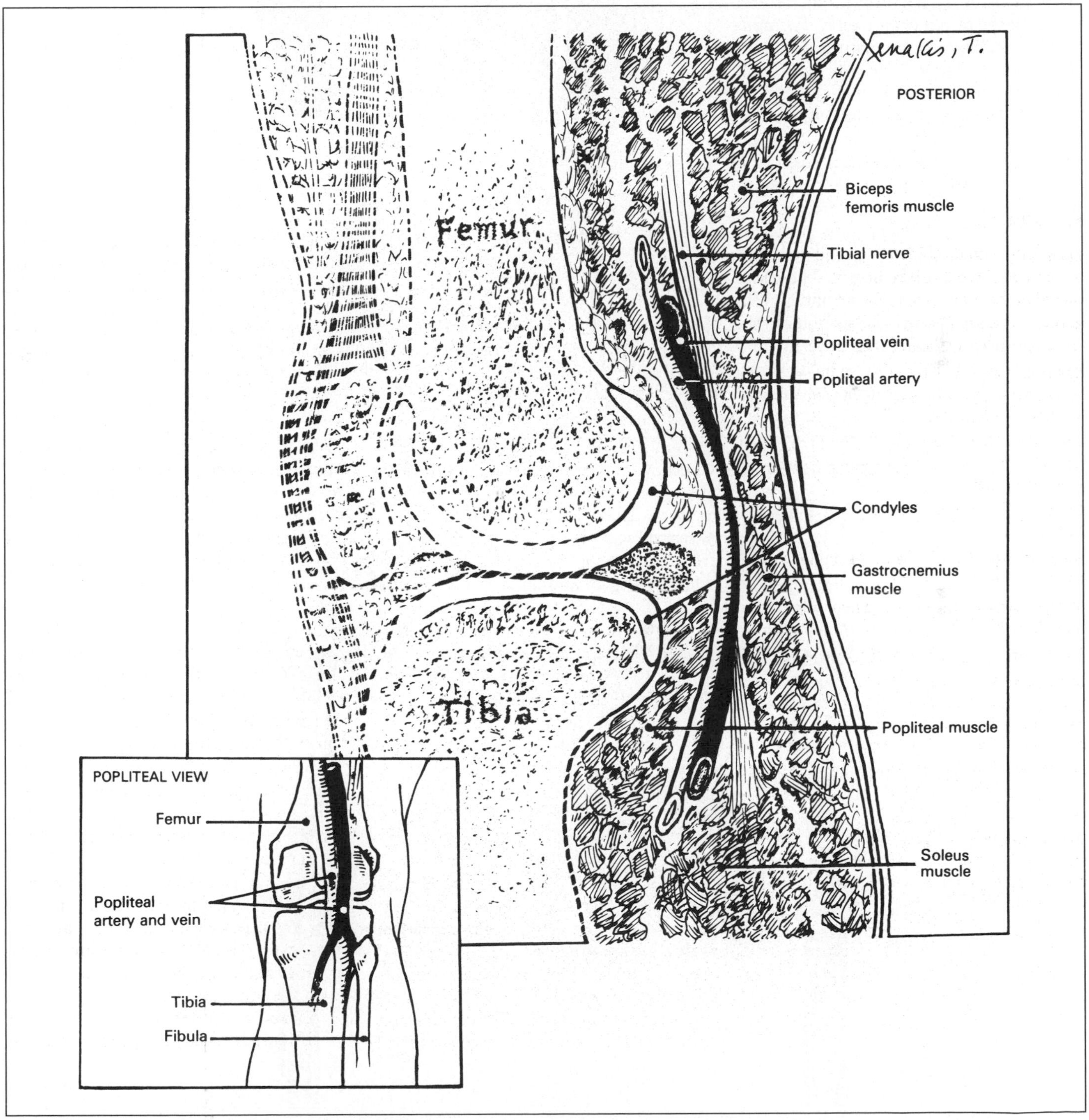

Figure 50-1. ■ *Normal structures visible in the popliteal fossa and the course of the popliteal artery and vein in relation to the knee joint.*

groin. Major branches, the greater saphenous vein (GSV) and the deep femoral vein, join just below the groin (Fig. 50-2). The superficial femoral vein will course into the thigh accompanied by its major landmark, the superficial femoral artery. In the thigh, the superficial femoral vein lies posterior to the superficial femoral artery. The superficial femoral vein is a deep vein. The name is derived from its corresponding artery, the superficial femoral artery. To minimize confusion, some institutions have adopted the name "femoral vein" and dropped the term "superficial." The femoral vein can be traced along the medial aspect of the upper leg as it gradually approaches the popliteal fossa and becomes the popliteal vein. At this point, the vein lies posterior to the artery.

The popliteal artery runs posterior to the knee joint (Fig. 50-1); the popliteal vein runs lateral to the artery. The lesser saphenous vein joins the popliteal vein behind the knee joint. The popliteal vein splits into three veins, the anterior and posterior tibial and the perineal veins, which supply the calf (Figs. 50-3 and

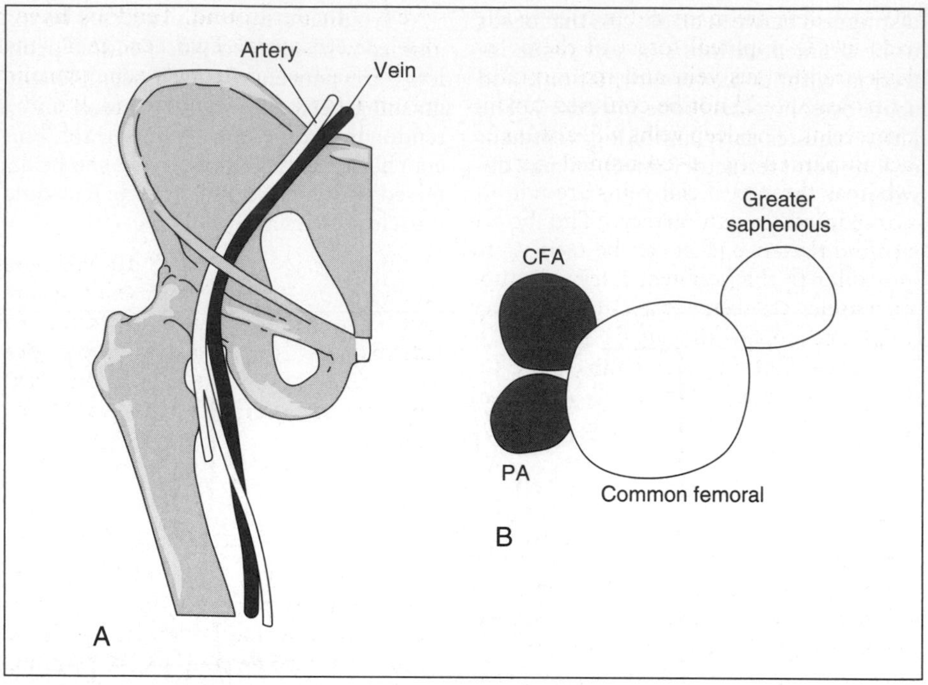

Figure 50-2. ■ *A. The femoral vein is medial to the artery in the groin but is lateral to the artery in the popliteal region. B. Transverse view of the origin of the greater saphenous vein, showing the normal distribution of the arteries and veins on the right. Common femoral artery* (CFA) *is at 10 o'clock, and pulmonary artery* (PA) *(profundal femoris or deep femoral artery) is at 8 o'clock.*

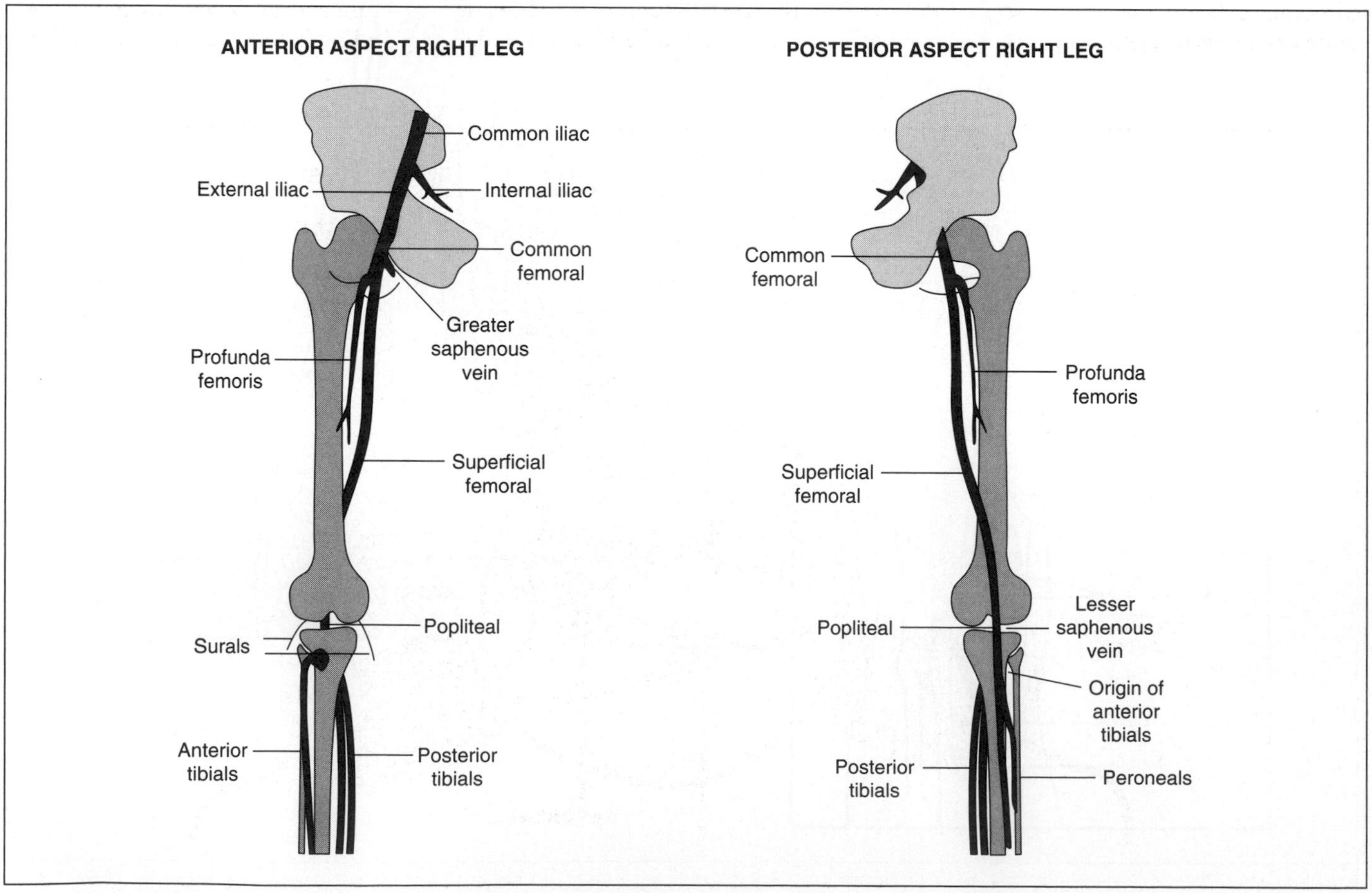

Figure 50-3. ■ *Anterior and posterior views of the legs showing the deep veins that drain the leg.*

50-4). There are many tributaries visualized in the popliteal fossa; of these, the lesser saphenous vein and the muscular branches should not be confused for the deep veins. The deep veins will always be accompanied by a co-named artery, whereas the superficial veins are not accompanied by an artery. The bones around the knee joint can be recognized posterior to the popliteal artery. Groups of muscles are seen in the adjacent lower thigh and upper calf (Fig. 50-4).

The GSV follows a similar course but is much more superficial. Duplication of the common femoral vein and the popliteal vein is common.

MUSCLES

The muscles of the thigh and calf can be individually visualized by the alignment of muscle fibers. Muscles are separated by an echogenic line resulting from connective tissue. As the limb is moved, the muscles move and the individual muscle groups can be distinguished.

BONE

Because bone reflects almost the entire ultrasound beam, only the surface of bone can be seen. Tendons are well analyzed with ultrasound. Tendons have a distinct structure: Two echogenic lines outline a series of strongly echogenic linear structures (see Chapters 52 and 53).

Technique

A linear array with 7- to 10-MHz frequency is preferred. Deeper veins may require a lower-frequency transducer for adequate visualization. Whenever there is concern about a questionable appearance, the contralateral side should be examined.

DEEP VEIN THROMBOSIS VERSUS BAKER'S CYST

The usual study is performed in a warm room with the patient in the supine position, the upper body elevated approximately 45 degrees, and the affected limb mildly flexed and turned laterally. In the supine position, the normal veins may not be easily visualized. To improve visualization, elevate the patient's upper body to approximately 45 degrees. This will promote venous filling. To assist venous filling for evaluation of the calf veins, the limb should be placed in a dependent position. If a Baker's cyst is suspected, place the patient prone and examine the calf.

VEIN RECOGNITION

Place the transducer in the groin to obtain a transverse view. Identify the common femoral artery; immediately medial to the artery is the common femoral vein. Move the transducer inferiorly to identify the termination of the GSV (Fig. 50-3). Identify the termination of the saphenous vein and the deep femoral vein (see Fig. 50-6). The GSV, although superficial, can be mistaken for the deep femoral vein. This can be avoided by following the course of the vessel. The femoral vein is joined by an accompanying artery as it courses into the thigh, whereas the GSV is superficial and has no corresponding artery in the thigh.

EVALUATING DEEP VEIN THROMBOSIS

1. Find the femoral vein by locating the femoral artery with palpation and looking along the medial aspect. Do not confuse the greater saphenous (which is superficial) and the profunda femoris vein (which is deep) with the femoral vein. The GSV will

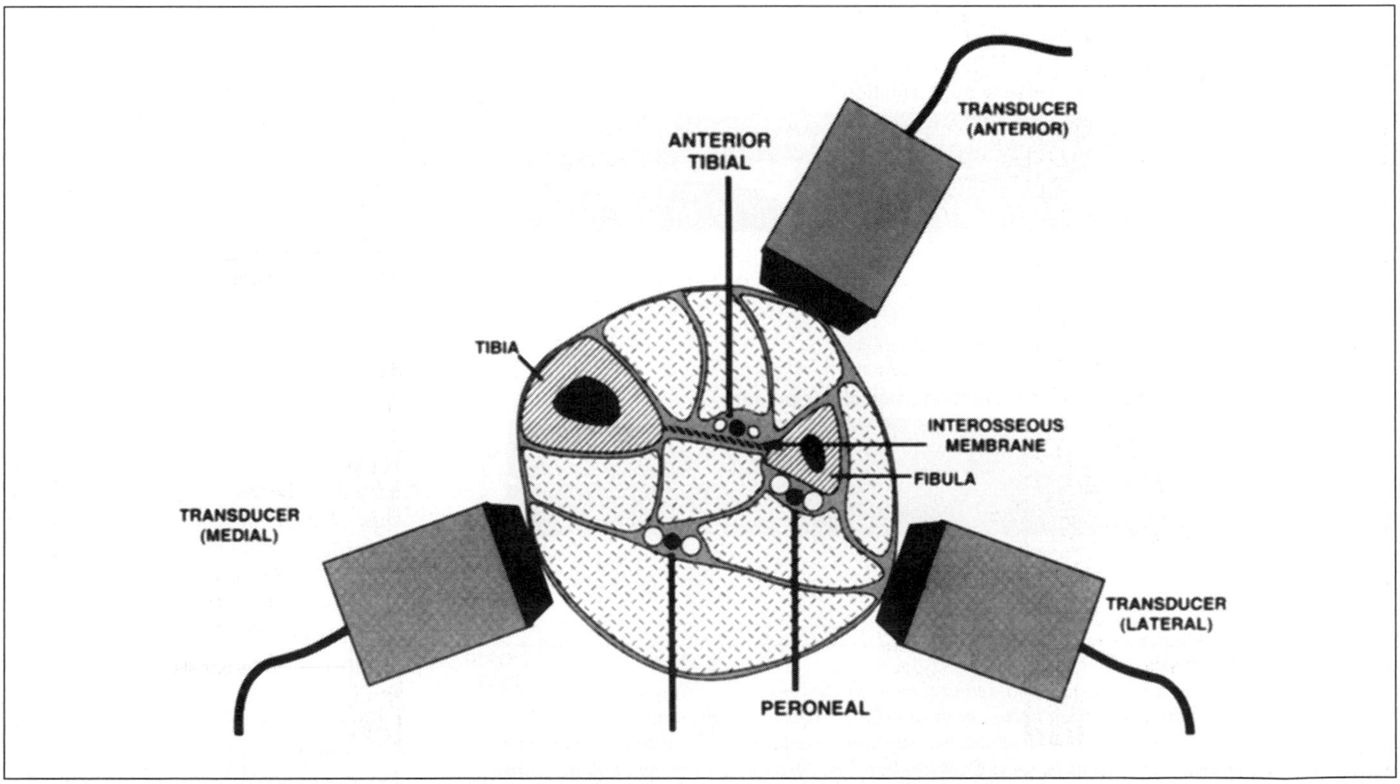

Figure 50-4. ■ *Approach required to demonstrate the calf veins.*

course in the opposite direction of the deep femoral vein. The GSV courses medial, whereas the deep femoral vein courses laterally and will dive deep into the thigh.

2. At each vein intersection with the popliteal vein, take images of the vein at right angles both at rest and with compression so that propagation of any clot can be followed. Typical sites are at the junction with the GSV, the deep femoral vein, the lesser saphenous vein, and the trifurcation. Take sagittal views in between.
3. Compress the vein with the transducer in a transverse position and see whether it changes; this is called "extrinsic compression maneuvers." During compression, the normal vein walls will touch; this is called "coaptation" of the vessel walls (Fig. 50-5A). A vein is normal when both the anterior and posterior walls touch; this should be observed during the compression and during the release of the compression (Fig. 50-5). If there is clot within the vein, the vein will not compress when pressure is applied. If the vein walls completely compress, this rules out the presence of a clot at that site. Compression is most readily demonstrated on the transverse view; if the compression is performed solely in a sagittal fashion, the transducer may slip off the vein. It may appear compressed while the vein is actually not in the field of view. If the vein does not compress, the sagittal views are used to confirm the shape and location of the proximal and distal edges of the clot. Comparison with the other leg's femoral vein (as long as it is normal) may be helpful.
4. Place the Doppler cursor within the femoral vein and listen for the typical low-pitched phasic signal of a vein. Because there is not much flow in veins, it may be normal for no signal to occur. To augment the signal and to determine the presence of phasic venous flow, have the patient take several deep breaths. The increased abdominal pressure during inspiration will cause cessation of venous flow returning from the legs. During expiration, venous flow will return. The waveform will be phasic in response to deep inspiration and expiration. If the patient cannot take a deep breath, venous flow may be augmented by compressing the leg below the level of the transducer (Fig. 50-5B). This will push venous flow up toward the probe.
5. Ask the patient to perform the Valsalva maneuver. The patient takes in a full inspiration, holds it, and contracts his or her abdominal muscles. As the patient lets his or her breath go, there should normally be a venous signal.
6. With the transducer on the vein, squeeze the thigh, below the transducer, over its medial aspect. Flow should occur in the vein when this "augmentation procedure" is performed. Perform the comparison test at several sites.
7. Attempt to follow the vein along the medial aspect of the leg to the popliteal fossa to look for clot.

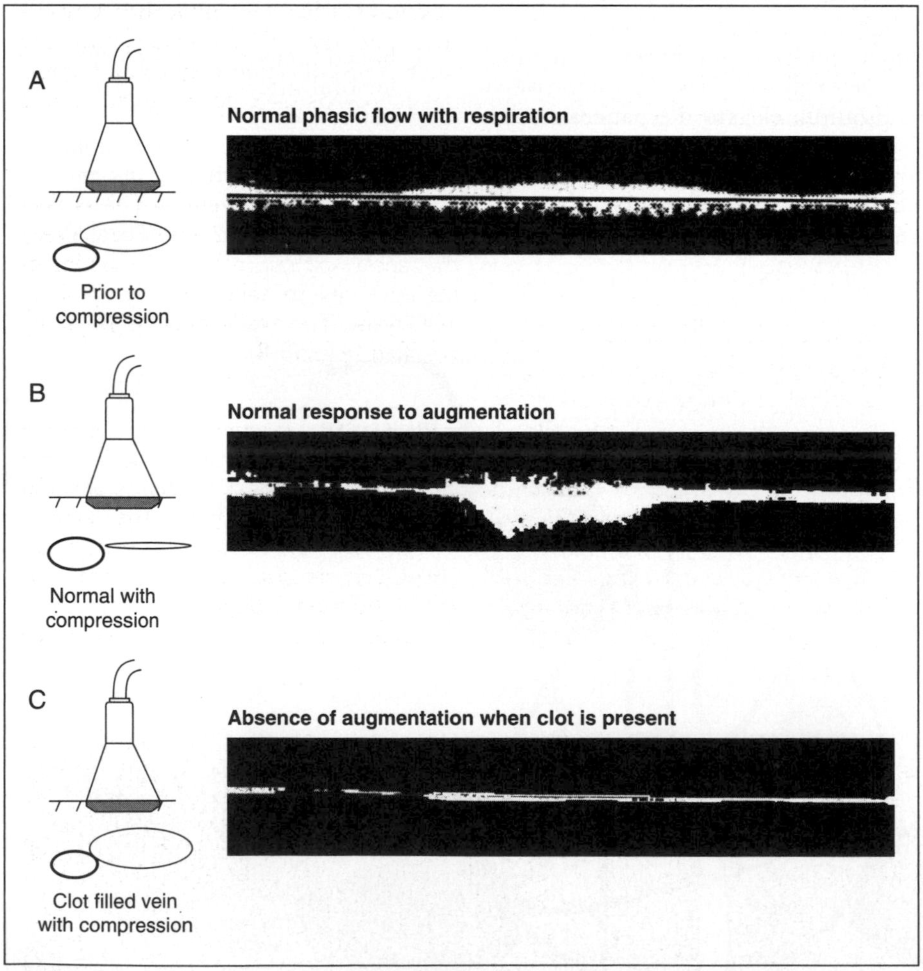

Figure 50-5. ■ *Femoral vein. A. Normal femoral vein shows a normal appearance without compression. Phasic flow with respiration occurs in most normal veins. B. With compression, normal femoral vein collapses. If no flow is seen spontaneously compress the vein distal to the examination point and augmented flow will be seen. C. With deep vein thrombosis, the vein will not compress. Low-level echoes can be seen within the clotted vein. No flow will be seen if the vein is occluded by clot.*

EVALUATING THE POPLITEAL VEIN

1. The popliteal vein is found behind the medial aspect of the knee joint. Look for clot within the vein; compress it with the transducer to confirm vessel wall coaptation. Evaluate this vessel segment with pulsed Doppler to determine the absence or presence of flow.
2. Compress the thigh with the transducer over the popliteal vein. As compression is released, a large venous signal normally occurs.
3. Compress the calf. As compression (augmentation) is performed, a Doppler signal is normally evoked.

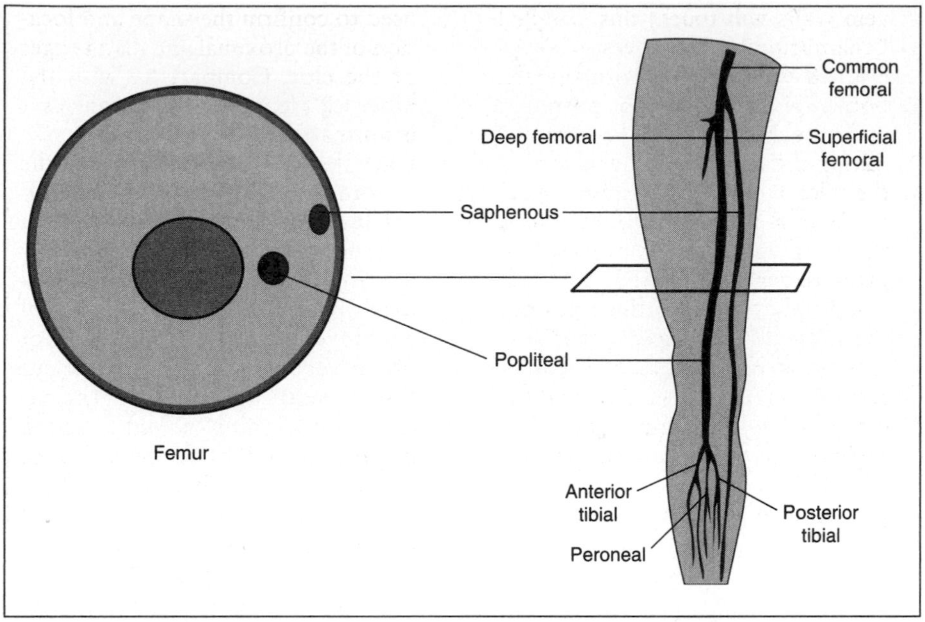

Figure 50-6. ■ *Normal course of the saphenous vein. The saphenous vein is superficial, whereas the popliteal vein is deep.*

Track the popliteal vein into the calf. In the usual examination position, the posterior tibial vein is the easiest of the three veins to follow. Take multiple images and videotape the examination if clot is found. Resolution or worsening of a clot on serial ultrasound studies determines therapy, so consistent, repeatable views should be taken to determine the location and extent of the clot.

SAPHENOUS VEIN MAPPING FOR VEIN GRAFT PROCEDURES

Track the superficial saphenous vein from the popliteal fossa along the medial anterior aspect of the leg (Fig. 50-6). Mark the skin with a grease pencil where the vein is seen. A 10-MHz linear array transducer with color flow is needed for this difficult study. This vein is removed and placed in other body locations if a vein graft is needed or may be kept in its native location and used as a peripheral arterial bypass.

EVALUATING DIALYSIS GRAFTS

1. Use a high-frequency transducer, preferably a linear array. A sector scanner with a stand-off pad is a less desirable alternative.
2. Use Doppler to see whether there is flow (Color Plates 50-1 and 50-3).
3. Examine the wall to make sure there are no small, narrowing plaques. The walls of dialysis grafts are made of Teflon, so they are normally thick and smooth.

INFLAMMATION

Inflammation most commonly affects joints. Lateral or anterior views of the hip joint may reveal fluid that would not otherwise be seen. Views from a lateral or posterior axis of the knee joint are also helpful in showing unexpected bursa or joint fluid. Color flow is helpful in delineating inflammatory problems because vascularity increases if inflammation is present. Both arthritis and infection give rise to increased vascularity.

Pathology

BAKER'S CYST

A Baker's cyst is a fluid-filled collection posterior to the knee joint that may extend into the calf or, rarely, into the thigh. The collection may contain internal echoes or have an irregular outline (Fig. 50-7).

POPLITEAL ANEURYSM

A focal expansion of the popliteal artery that shows pulsation on real-time imaging and may contain clot is a popliteal aneurysm. The walls may be partially calcified (Fig. 50-8).

PSEUDOANEURYSM

After trauma, particularly femoral vein catheterization, an echogenic collection may be seen alongside the artery. Sometimes, these hematomas contain an irregularly shaped echo-free area that shows flow on Doppler, representing a pseudoaneurysm (false aneurysm; see

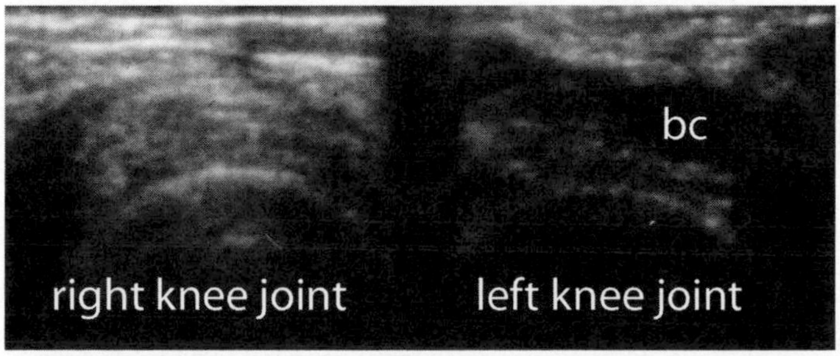

Figure 50-7. ■ *Baker's cyst* (bc) *is a fluid-filled structure extending into the calf that usually communicates with the knee joint. A comparison between the two knee joints shows that a cyst is only present on the left.*

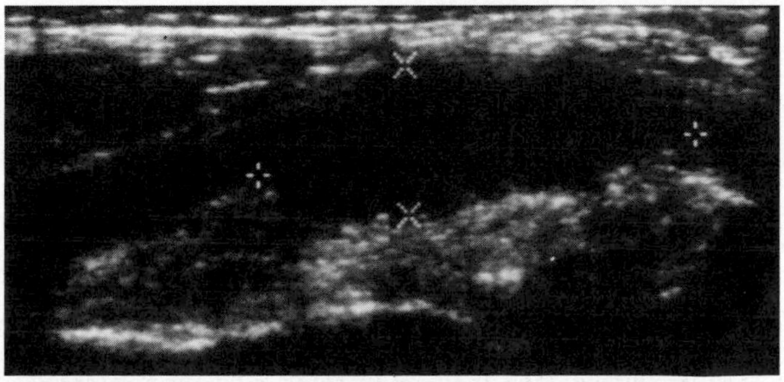

Figure 50-8. ■ *Popliteal artery aneurysm (between markers) expands the popliteal artery posterior to the knee joint.*

Chapter 14). A clot forms the wall of the aneurysm. Flow may be detected in such false aneurysms, even though no echo-free area can be seen. These lesions, which require prompt surgical attention, are elegantly demonstrated by color flow Doppler; a mushroom-like appearance is seen (Color Plate 50-3). Pulsed Doppler shows a to-and-fro motion. After a pseudoaneurysm has been localized with ultrasound, persistent compression (for at least 10 minutes) may cause the aneurysm to clot. A newer, generally more desirable technique, which is gradually replacing compression, is ultrasound-guided injection of thrombin into the pseudoaneurysm.

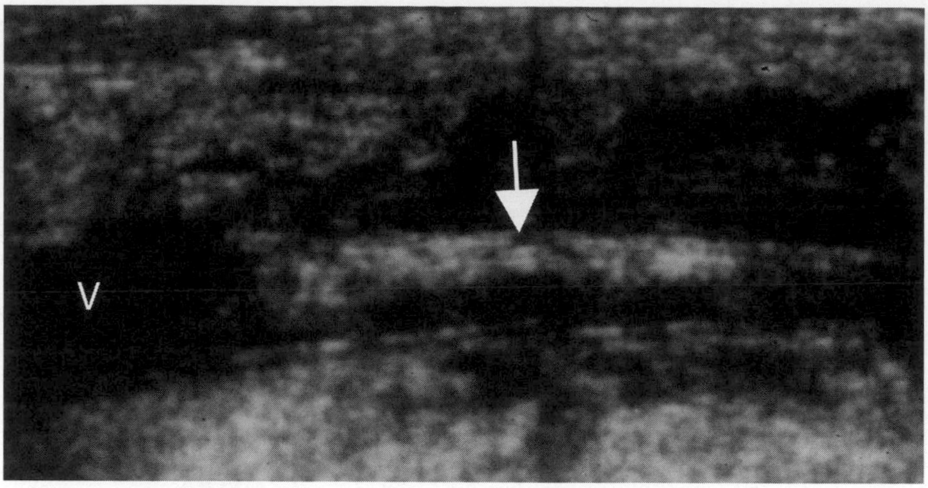

Figure 50-9. ■ *Common femoral vein* (V) *containing old clot* (arrow).

MUSCLES

Hematomas in muscles can either be the result of tearing of the muscles or blunt damage to the limb. If there is a complete muscle tear, the two segments of the muscle are separated by a hematoma, which forms an echopenic area. Older hematomas may be echogenic (see Chapter 19). Localized bruising can produce a fluid collection within the muscle or it can diffusely enlarge the muscle without altering the underlying muscle organization. The muscle should be compared with the contralateral muscle.

Rhabdomyolysis is a rare condition occurring typically in drug addicts who have stayed in the same position with the muscle contracted for hours. An echopenic mass area will be seen within the muscles at the point of tenderness. Normal muscle fibers run through the affected area. The muscles have been partially dissolved by enzymes during the period when they were contracted. Eventually, healing with calcification may take place.

DEEP VEIN THROMBOSIS

Acute Deep Vein Thrombosis

1. A DVT is suspected when there is a low-grade fever of undetermined origin, leg swelling, or pain. The extent of symptoms are related to the amount of thrombus present. The vein may be completely occluded with clot, causing the most dramatic symptoms, or partially obstructed with clot and causing no symptoms (Fig. 50-9). If a patient has a dual venous system, one may be normal, whereas the other has thrombus. The patient may not exhibit symptoms as venous flow is sustained through the second patent system. Thrombus can occur anywhere along the course of the lower extremity deep veins. However, pulmonary emboli that arise from the larger veins in the thigh are more apt to cause fatal pulmonary emboli than those arising from the smaller calf veins.
2. A typical acute clot may cause the vein walls to expand slightly. The vein walls will not be compressible at the site of the thrombus (Fig. 50-5C). Other conditions that limit vein compressibility include severe right-sided heart failure, anatomic location, or other conditions that limit the examiner's ability to apply direct pressure to the vein. Acute thrombus exhibits regular-shaped walls and appears gelatinous in consistency when pressure is applied. A free-floating tip may be seen at the central edge of the thrombus.
3. Venous flow may be completely normal or completely obstructed. This is determined by the volume and extent of thrombus and the absence or presence of collateral vessels.
4. Small, isolated calf vein clots may not be readily visualized.
5. If clot is found in the femoral veins, look at the iliac veins and inferior vena cava; the clot may propagate into these veins. Clot extending into the pelvis may cause a diminished Doppler signal from the common femoral vein. Assessment of the contralateral femoral vein Doppler signal will be more prominent. The iliac veins can be seen on either side of the pelvis with the full bladder lying adjacent to the corresponding iliac arteries.
6. Normally a phasic variation in flow is seen. If the Doppler signal is asymmetric or abnormal, the cause must be determined. A diminished signal may be due to thrombosis or compression of the vein by a mass.

Chronic Venous Disease

Chronic venous disease may be the result of a previous DVT. A chronically diseased vein appears small compared with contralateral normal leg. The walls appear thickened, and flow by Doppler may be diminished or absent and without respiratory variation. The vessel walls may not completely compress due to the scarring on the inside of the vein. Components of the old thrombus may be visualized within the vein segment. The shape of the walls will be irregular. During compression, the irregularity is firm and will not disfigure with compression, whereas an acute DVT will change with pressure. Collateral veins may appear around chronically occluded venous segments.

CELLULITIS

This infection follows soft tissue cuts or trauma. Diffuse thickening of soft tissues occurs with increased vascularity. Tissue borders become more echogenic. No fluid collection is seen.

ABSCESS

Well-defined fluid collections occur with irregular echopenic borders in the center of an inflamed area. A sinus track may be demonstrable. Appearances can be confused with a tumor. If an abscess is demonstrated, drainage under ultrasound control is often initiated.

Pitfalls

1. Leg extension with Baker's cyst. Undue extension of the leg obliterates a Baker's cyst that communicates with the knee joint because the fluid returns into the knee joint proper.
2. Anechoic thrombus. Venous thrombus may not contain echoes and may be recognized only with compression or color flow Doppler.
3. False aneurysm. False aneurysms may be echo-filled as if they were a solid mass. Doppler will show flow.
4. Saphenous versus femoral vein. The GSV may be confused with the femoral vein. It is small and superficial.
5. Problems with compression. If compression views are not obtained in a transverse fashion, the clot may be missed because the transducer slips off the clot (Fig. 50-10).
6. Acute versus chronic DVT. Acute appearances can persist in a vein for a number of weeks. Problems have arisen when a report suggests that a clot is acute when acute appearances are actually longstanding.

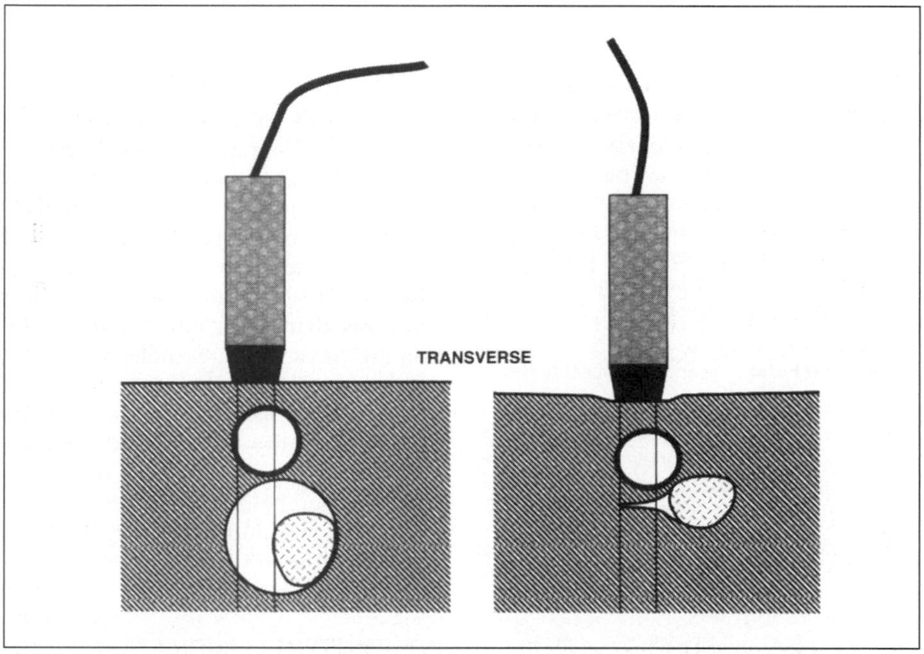

Figure 50-10. ■ *If the clot is asymmetrically placed within the vein, compression of the site that is free of clot may give an erroneous impression that there is no clot within the vein. It is better to use a transverse position, rather than a longitudinal compression, to compress the veins.*

Where Else to Look

1. If a popliteal aneurysm is found, the aorta and the opposite popliteal artery should be examined; abdominal aortic aneurysms are often present in association with popliteal artery aneurysms.
2. If a deep vein thrombus is found in the leg, look in the iliac veins and inferior vena cava.
3. Multiple venous thromboses are said to be associated with carcinoma of the pancreas. Look in the pancreas if there has been more than one episode.

SELECTED READING

Gottlieb RH, Widjaja J, Mehra S, et al. Cynically important pulmonary emboli: does calf vein US alter outcomes? *Radiology* 1999; 211:25–29.

Polak JF. *Peripheral Vascular Sonography,* 2nd ed. Philadelphia: Lippincott Williams and Wilkins; 2004.

Rumswell C, McPharlin M. *Vascular Technology: an illustrated Review.* Pasadena: Davies Publishing; 2003.

Zweibel W, Pellerito J. *Introduction to Vascular Sonography,* 5th ed. Philadelphia: Saunders; 2004.

Arterial Problems in the Limbs

51

GAIL SANDAGER-HADLEY

SONOGRAM ABBREVIATIONS

ABI	Ankle-brachial index
ATa	Anterior tibial artery
Bif	Bifurcation
CFa	Common femoral artery
CFv	Common femoral vein
Cla	Common iliac artery
DPa	Dorsalis pedis artery
Ela	External iliac artery
GSV	Greater saphenous vein
Ila	Internal iliac artery
PERa	Peroneal artery
PFa	Profunda femoris artery
POPa	Popliteal artery
POPv	Popliteal vein
PSV	Peak systolic velocity
PTa	Posterior tibial artery
PVD	Peripheral vascular disease
SFa	Superficial femoral artery
SFv	Superficial femoral vein
TB	Tibioperoneal trunk

KEY WORDS

Abduct. To move a leg away from the other leg.

Ankle-Brachial Index. A ratio of Doppler-derived ankle systolic pressure to Doppler-derived brachial artery systolic pressure (ABI, ankle pressure/highest brachial pressure). The index is an indicator of arterial insufficiency. The normal ABI is greater than 1.0. As the severity of peripheral vascular disease (PVD) increases, the ABI will decrease.

Antecubital Fossa. The anterior aspect of the elbow joint.

Gangrene. Tissue death that can result from inadequate blood supply. Gangrene from peripheral vascular disease (PVD) is identified by its typical distal location on the toes or forefoot.

Geniculate Artery. Small tributary to the popliteal artery in the popliteal fossa.

Fusiform. Spindle shape.

Hunter's Canal. Arterial pathway on the medial aspect of the thigh, just above the knee. The artery is deep within the muscle at this point and difficult to see.

Intermittent Claudication. Means "to limp"; symptoms of leg pain experienced during exercise and relieved with rest. The symptoms are produced by arterial insufficiency.

Laminar. Normal pattern of blood flow in a vessel; the flow in the center of the vessel is faster than at the walls.

Rest Pain. Insufficient arterial supply causing ischemia to the tissues that results in pain at rest in the toes and forefoot.

Saccular. Pouch-like.

Spectral Broadening. Echo fill-in of the spectral window proportional to the severity of the vessel stenosis (see Fig. 4-8). It may also result from poor technique, with too much gain or too large a sample volume.

Sural Arteries. Small branches of the popliteal artery in the popliteal fossa.

The Clinical Problem

Lower-extremity arterial color duplex sonography is useful to identify, localize, and grade the severity of arterial lumen narrowing from peripheral vascular occlusive disease. The most common cause of peripheral vascular disease (PVD) is atherosclerosis. Other problems that affect peripheral circulation are thrombosis, embolism, trauma, and aneurysms. Clinical indications for performing peripheral arterial color duplex imaging are intermittent claudication, limb rest pain, abnormal peripheral pulses, gangrene or tissue necrosis, blue toe syndrome, and arterial trauma, as well as follow-up therapeutic intervention.

INTERMITTENT CLAUDICATION

Claudication is manifested by pain in the various muscle groups of the legs brought on by exercise. The muscle groups that elicit pain are related to the location of the arterial obstruction. Muscle cramping or a tired, aching feeling is experienced during exercise; these symptoms are due to the inability of the arterial blood supply to meet the increased oxygen and nutritive demands of exercise. Because this is a fixed lesion that does not change, without treatment the symptoms always recur. A predictable pattern occurs with respect to the onset of pain, location of pain, and resolution of pain with a brief rest or cessation of exercise. This is the classic presentation of vascular claudication—exercise-pain-rest-relief—and the cycle repeats.

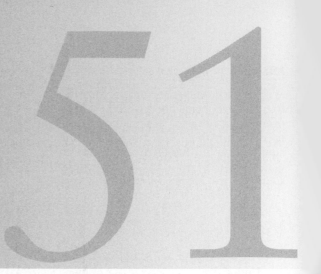

Patients with neurospinal compression present with a similar description of pain that can mimic true vascular claudication. Neurogenic claudication can be differentiated by a thorough history. Neurogenic claudication is not repeatable; symptoms are brought on by a variety of circumstances not related to a specific situation or exercise. Patients' symptoms vary, with good and bad days, and no relief with cessation of exercise.

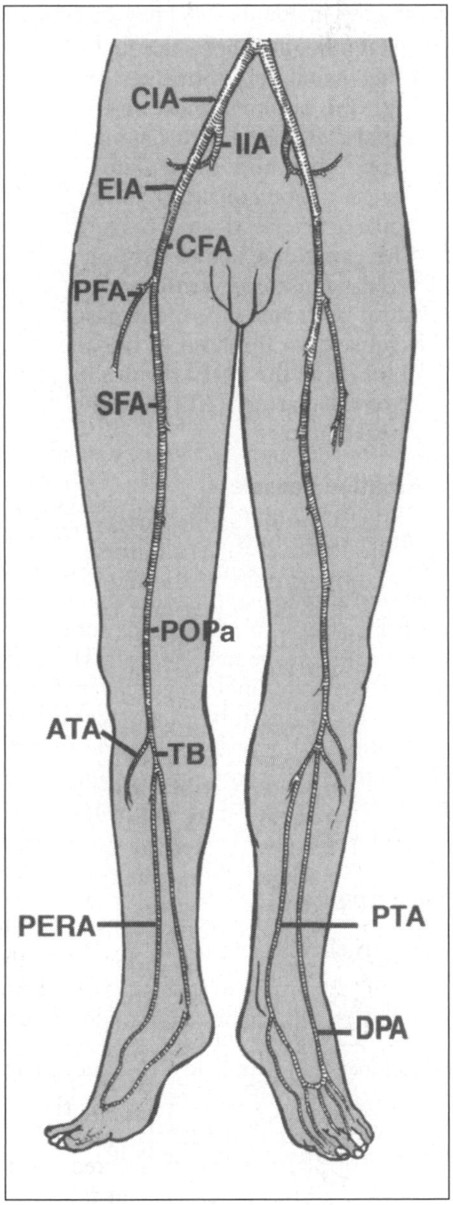

Figure 51-1. ■ *Normal arterial anatomy of the leg.* CIa, *common iliac artery;* IIa, *internal iliac artery;* EIa, *external iliac artery;* PFa, *proximal femoral artery;* CFa, *common femoral artery;* SFa, *superficial femoral artery;* POPa, *popliteal artery;* ATa, *anterior tibial artery;* TB, *tibioperoneal trunk;* PERa, *peroneal artery;* PTa, *posterior tibial artery;* DPa, *dorsalis pedis artery.*

REST PAIN

The patient complains of pain or numbness of the toes or forefoot. This most often occurs at night, causing the patient to awaken from sleep. Rest pain results from the inability of the circulation to meet the demands at rest. Symptoms are pronounced with elevation and will improve with the limb dependent. Patients will often say they have to hang their leg over the bedside to relieve the symptoms.

TISSUE NECROSIS/GANGRENE

These lesions are seen distally on the toes and forefoot and represent tissue loss associated with loss of vascular nutritive supply.

Anatomy

The lower-extremity arteries are the common femoral, profunda femoris, superficial femoral, popliteal, anterior tibial, tibioperoneal trunk, posterior tibial, and peroneal (Fig. 51-1).

FEMORAL ARTERIES

The common femoral artery (CFa) starts at the level of the inguinal ligament and courses lateral to the common femoral vein (CFv) (see Fig. 51-3). The CFa is approximately 3 to 5 cm long and bifurcates into the superficial femoral artery (SFa) and profunda femoris artery (PFa). This arterial bifurcation is just proximal to the confluence of the superficial femoral and profunda femoris veins.

The SFa is anterior to the PFa and medial to the femur; the SFa is the most common site for atherosclerosis. The SFa and superficial femoral vein (SFv) run parallel to each other in the thigh, coursing distally to the adductor canal (Hunter's canal). The SFa terminates at the adductor canal, becoming the popliteal artery (POPa). The PFa courses lateral from its origin going deep into the thigh; only the first few centimeters can be visualized by ultrasound.

POPLITEAL ARTERY

The POPa begins above the knee at the adductor canal and continues inferiorly through the popliteal fossa and into the proximal calf. The POPa has numerous sural branches and geniculate arteries that are a major collateral route in the presence of arterial obstructions (Fig. 51-2). The geniculate arteries supply blood flow to the muscles around the knee, and the sural branches supply the gastrocnemius muscle. At the level of the anterior tibial tubercle, the POPa divides into the anterior tibial artery (ATa) and the tibioperoneal trunk.

TRIFURCATION VESSELS

The ATa is the first tibial artery arising from the POPa. The ATa enters the anterior compartment of the leg between the tibia and the fibula and runs inferior along the lateral aspect of the calf down into the foot, where it becomes the dorsalis pedis artery (DPa).

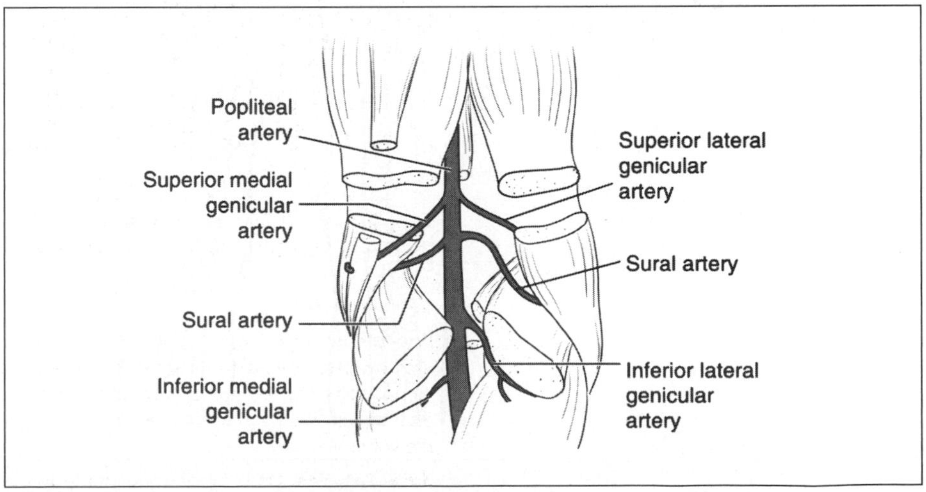

Figure 51-2. ■ *Popliteal artery anatomy.*

The tibioperoneal trunk has a variable length of a few centimeters before dividing into the posterior tibial artery (PTa) and the peroneal artery (PERa). These tibial arteries are located in the posterior compartment of the calf.

The PTa courses along the medial aspect of the lower leg to the medial malleolus. At the level of the ankle, the PTa branches into the plantar arteries.

The PERa runs posterolateral through the posterior compartment to a few centimeters above the ankle. At the ankle, the PERa terminates into branches communicating with the anterior tibial and dorsalis pedis arteries.

Technique

The patient is positioned supine with the head slightly elevated for comfort. The leg being examined is abducted and externally rotated with the knee flexed. Acoustic coupling gel is applied from the groin to the knee medial to the femur. A 5-MHz (or similar frequency) linear array transducer is used with corresponding Doppler frequency. The examination is performed using both transverse and longitudinal views.

UPPER LEG

The transducer is placed in the groin using a transverse orientation. The vessels visualized are the CFa and CFv (Fig. 51-3). The CFa is lateral to the vein with obvious pulsations seen. Compression of the CFv can be performed to distinguish it accurately from the CFa. After correct identification of the CFa, the probe is angled superiorly to visualize the origin or most proximal segment of the vessel at the inguinal ligament.

Move the transducer inferior until the CFa bifurcates into the SFa and the PFa just below the level of the groin. The SFa is the more anterior vessel, whereas the PFa courses lateral and posterior. Generally only the first few centimeters of the PFa will be visualized before moving out of the field of view.

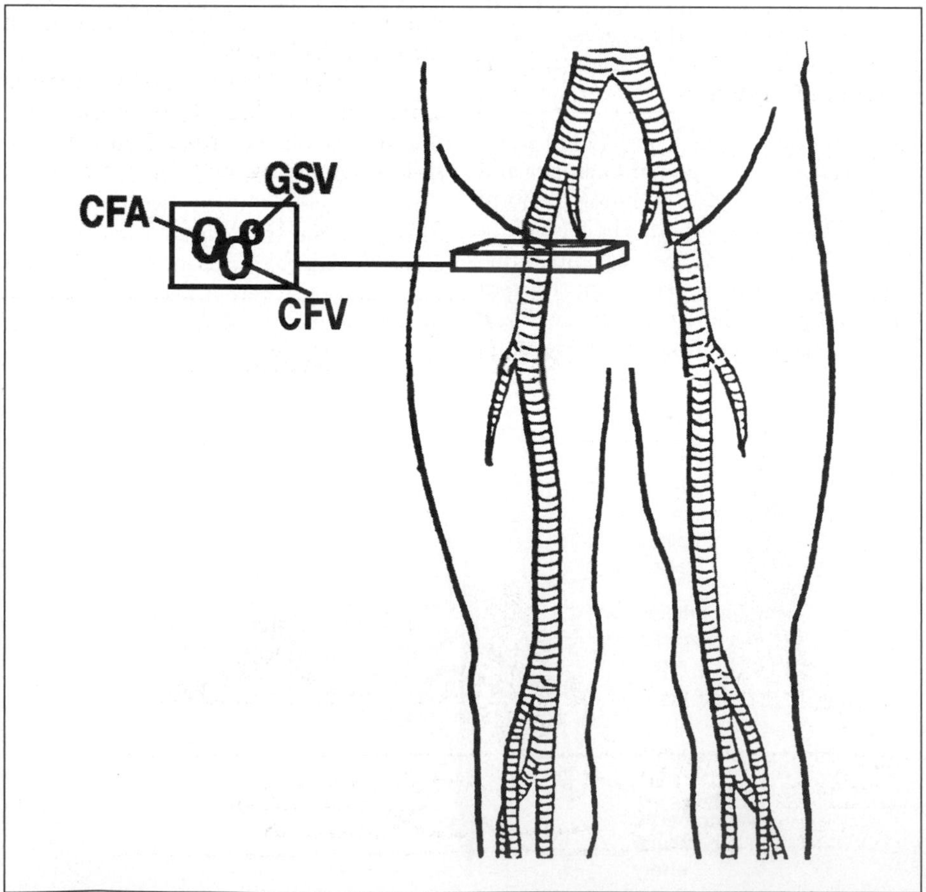

Figure 51-3. ■ *In the groin, the common femoral vein* (CFv) *lies medial to the common femoral artery* (CFa). *The greater saphenous vein* (GSv) *arises from the femoral vein in the groin.*

Just below the arterial bifurcation is the confluence of the SFv and the profunda femoris vein. The SFv is used as a landmark to identify the SFa, as they run parallel to each other throughout the thigh. By using this landmark, follow the SFa/SFv distal. The SFa appears anterior to the vein in the B-mode image. These vessels run medial to the femur in the thigh and can be followed to the adductor canal. At the level of the adductor canal, the SFa will move deeper. At this point, the image quality may be limited owing to the depth of the vessel and the poor penetration through the fascia.

POPLITEAL FOSSA

Because of the anatomic position of the proximal POPa, it is best imaged from a posterior approach. Maintaining a transverse orientation, place the transducer in the popliteal fossa; both the POPa and the popliteal vein are seen, with the artery positioned deeper than the vein. To assess the above-knee portion of the POPa, move the probe superiorly along the posterior thigh until the entire artery has been evaluated. Trace the entire artery back to the SFa, because short-segment occlusions are common at this site. Tendons frequently encountered from a transverse approach may limit its usefulness because the large footprint linear array probe may slide off the tendons. A longitudinal view may provide better image quality. After complete evaluation of the proximal POPa, follow the artery back to and through the popliteal fossa, until its termination below the knee.

THE LOWER LEG

The branches arising from the POPa are visualized from a posterior approach and should not be mistaken for the ATa. The POPa divides into the ATa and the tibioperoneal trunk below the knee. The ATa is the first tibial artery branch arising from the POPa and will course posterior and lateral from the POPa.

Anterior Tibial Artery

The ATa runs along the lateral aspect of the calf, accompanied by the paired anterior tibial veins. The veins and artery run together throughout their course in the calf. If the ATa is difficult to track from its proximal segment, move to the distal segment just above the ankle and scan back to the proximal ATa.

Tibioperoneal and Posterior Tibial Artery

The tibioperoneal trunk is difficult to visualize because of its anatomic location and is only adequately visualized in approximately 70% of the population. From the posterior approach, it is the more anterior vessel at the ATa/tibioperoneal trunk division. The tibioperoneal trunk is relatively short before dividing into the PTa and the PERa. At this point, only one artery can be examined; it does not matter which vessel is scanned first. The PTa runs medial and anterior from the PERa. The vessel origins are difficult to track and can be scanned from the distal segment at the ankle back to their origins. This provides easier and more rapid vessel identification. The PTa is examined by placing the probe just above the medial malleolus; the PTa is medial to the tibia and courses superior with the paired posterior tibial veins.

Peroneal Artery

The PERa can be imaged from either a medial or lateral approach as it runs down the center of the leg. From either approach, it is approximately 3 to 4 cm deep, surrounded by the two peroneal veins, and is next to the fibula. The PERa is the most difficult tibial artery to visualize completely owing to its deep anatomic location in the posterior compartment of the calf. Successful visualization depends on the size of the patient's calf.

The B-mode imaging technique is performed uniformly throughout the lower-extremity arterial tree. Both transverse and sagittal views are performed. The sagittal view is used in conjunction with the pulsed Doppler evaluation. The B-mode image is used to evaluate the quality of the vessel, intraluminal defects, plaque, size, collateral pathways, and anatomic location.

Disease Distribution

Peripheral arterial occlusive disease is most commonly found at arterial bifurcations and distal segments of vessels. The distal SFa is the most prevalent area of disease. However, the disease distribution is different in diabetic patients, with an increased incidence below the knee in the infrapopliteal arteries. In the nondiabetic patient, disease occurs more often in the iliac and the SFa, whereas the younger patient with claudication will have a higher incidence of iliac artery disease.

Peripheral arterial aneurysms commonly occur in the POPa and the femoral arteries and are often bilateral or multiple. If an aneurysm is detected, all other sites are routinely examined (see Chapter 50).

Pulsed Doppler Technique

The entire length of the vessel is examined with Doppler. At a longitudinal view, the pulsed Doppler sample volume (2 mm) is placed center stream or center to a flow jet using an angle of 60 degrees or less. Angles above 60 degrees give erroneous results. The Doppler waveforms are assessed for direction of flow, peak systolic velocity (PSV), spectral broadening, and waveform configuration. End-diastolic velocities are not routinely measured unless there is greater than 50% stenosis.

Record all Doppler calculations at proximal, middle, and distal artery segments. All changes in Doppler velocity spectra are recorded with calculations displayed at the area of change and immediately proximal and distal to the change (Fig. 51-4). If B-mode image abnormalities are detected without a change in Doppler velocity, this is recorded, showing the image abnormality and the corresponding Doppler waveform. All abnormal Doppler findings are repeated from several views to avoid an error in calculations.

The normal lower-extremity arterial waveform is triphasic (three phases): (1) marked systolic upstroke, (2) early diastolic reverse flow, and (3) late forward

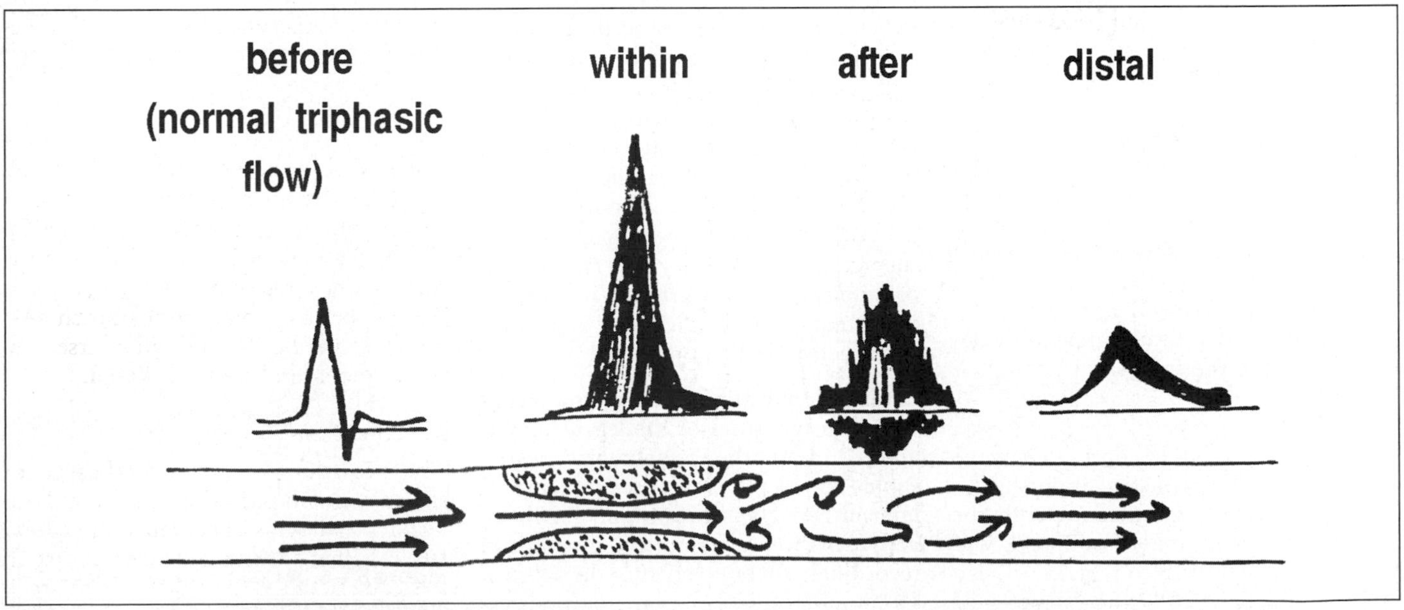

Figure 51-4. ■ *Doppler spectral changes in the presence of a hemodynamically significant stenosis.*

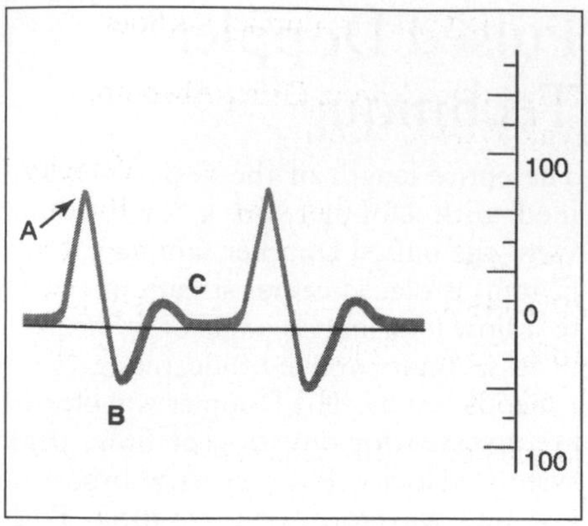

Figure 51-5. ■ *Normal triphasic waveform. A. Systolic upstroke. B. Early diastolic reverse flow. C. Diastolic forward flow.*

flow in end diastole (Fig. 51-5). The third phase of diastolic forward flow exhibits low velocities and may be obliterated if the wall filter is set too high. Wall filters of 50 to 100 Hz are recommended for normal peripheral arterial profiles. PSV in the healthy patient will decrease moving from the aorta to the peripheral tibial arteries.

Examination Protocol

Both anatomic and physiologic testing are used to determine the degree of peripheral vascular occlusive disease. The standard examination for peripheral arterial disease includes ankle-brachial index (ABI) measurement in conjunction with color Doppler sonography.

ANKLE-BRACHIAL INDEX

The ABI is an initial screening assessment to indicate the absence or presence of PVD. Blood pressure levels are taken at multiple sites in the leg and compared with the arm. Arterial narrowing decreases flow with a resultant pressure decrease distal to the stenosis.

Equipment

1. An 8- to 10-MHz continuous wave Doppler and acoustic coupling gel.
2. Appropriate-sized pressure cuffs for the arms and ankles; cuff sizes will vary depending on patient size (should be >20% the diameter of the limb for accurate pressure measurements).
3. A standard sphygmomanometer.

Procedure

The patient is placed supine and at rest for 10 minutes before starting. The pressure cuffs are placed on the upper arms and ankles bilaterally and connected to the sphygmomanometer. With the use of Doppler, obtain the best-quality signal in the antecubital fossa and then inflate the cuff. The pressure in the cuff is inflated to 20 mm Hg above the systolic blood pressure. Deflate the cuff slowly until the first audible arterial signal is detected, and record this as the brachial systolic pressure. Repeat this on the opposite arm. The same procedure is performed at the ankle for the DPa and the PTa. The DPa is located on the top of the foot lateral to the bone, whereas the PTa is just posterior to the medial malleolus (Fig. 51-6).

The ABI is calculated by taking the ankle pressure and dividing it by the highest brachial pressure. This is done for both the DPa and the PTa on both sides. A normal ABI is greater than 1.0.

$$\frac{\text{Highest ankle pressure (mm Hg)}}{\text{Highest brachial pressure (mm Hg)}} = \text{ABI}$$

Example:

$$\frac{\text{Ankle: 124 mm Hg}}{\text{Brachial: 116 mm Hg}} = 1.06$$

COLOR/DUPLEX IMAGING

Patient Selection. The procedure can be used for any patients who have abnormal ABIs and require direct visualization of the arteries. Patients with normal ABIs and no significant clinical history are not routinely examined. A significant clinical history in the presence of normal ABIs includes prominent peripheral pulses suspicious for aneurysm, trauma in proximity to major arteries, symptoms consistent with claudication, or postreconstructive evaluation.

Patient Preparation. The examination begins in the groin of the leg being examined after the patient has rested supine for 10 minutes. If the patient has intermittent claudication and has been active before examination, the initial recordings will be erroneous; therefore, a 10-minute rest before examination is essential. A brief history is taken to define symptoms, previous surgery, and relevant risk factors. The routine examination includes evaluation of the CFa down to the tibioperoneal trunk. Diagnostic parameters and good b-scan information are limited for the tibial arteries, which are therefore not routinely imaged.

B-Scan Imaging. The leg is slightly flexed, abducted, and externally rotated so that all of the major arteries can be examined. The CFa is examined with standard grayscale B-scan imaging in a transverse orientation. The proximal CFa to the bifurcation of the SFa/PFa is imaged first to evaluate the anatomic course and location of the vessels. After correct vessel identification, record the anatomic information, displaying each vessel and its relationship to the vein. All bifurcations are included in the corresponding documentation. This technique is performed throughout the thigh, popliteal fossa, and below the knee to the tibioperoneal trunk.

Doppler Imaging. Repeat the examination using color, pulsed Doppler, and a longitudinal view. Obtain sagittal views of the CFa and place the Doppler sample volume at 60 degrees and in the center of the vessel or center to the flow stream in the presence of disease. Move the sample site throughout the vessel segment being examined. Determine the most accurate representation of the Doppler waveform, and record both the image showing the

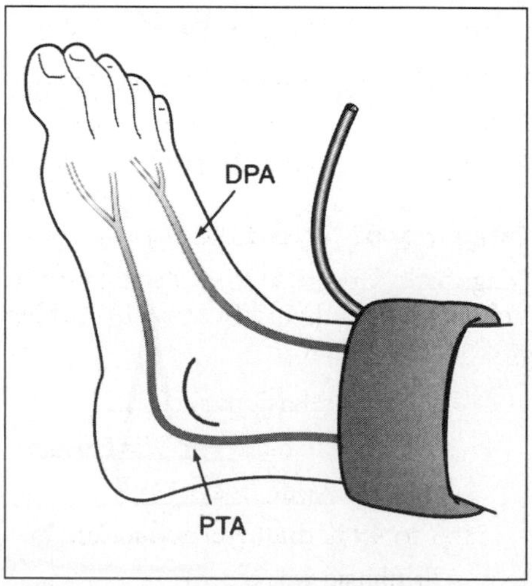

Figure 51-6. ■ *Cuff position for ankle-brachial index (ABI).*

sample site location and the Doppler velocity waveform. Display and record all the necessary Doppler calculations. This technique is repeated and recorded from all segments of the peripheral arterial system.

Documentation. Documentation of abnormal stenotic or occluded areas anywhere in the periphery includes the following:

- Doppler velocity calculations
- Proximal, within, and distal to the area of stenosis (Fig. 51-4)
- Number of lesions
- Location and length of lesions

Vessel diameter measurements are recorded when the examination is performed for aneurysms. The shape of a peripheral artery aneurysm is either saccular or fusiform. The artery is measured from a transverse view with anterior-posterior and medial and lateral external diameter measurements. If an aneurysm is present, an average of three separate measurements is taken from both transverse and sagittal views measuring both the maximum diameter and length. In the presence of an aneurysm the normal vessel diameter immediately proximal to the aneurysm is recorded, along with measurements of the aneurysm in both transverse and sagittal views.

DIAGNOSTIC CRITERIA

Normal PSV Criteria	PSV (cm/sec)	Vessel Diameter (mm)
CFa	114.1 ± 24.9	7–10
Proximal SFa	90.8 ± 13.6	6–9
Distal SFa	93.6 ± 14.1	6–9
POPa	68.8 ± 13.5	5–8

Categories of Percentage of Stenosis

Diagnostic Criteria Using Peak Systolic Velocity Ratios (Modification of Kohler et al. criteria, 1987)

Normal: triphasic waveform
- PSV quasi-steady: no elevation

Normal b-mode image

1% to 49% diameter reduction
- Triphasic waveform
- No appreciable spectral broadening
- ≥30% to 100% focal PSV increase compared with proximal segment of vessel
- Normal PSV and waveform distal to plaque
- B-mode image—visible plaque at site of increase PSV

≥50% to 99% diameter reduction
- Waveform loss of reverse flow component
- Focal PSV increase greater than 100% from normal proximal segment
- Distal waveform monophasic with decreased PSV
- Spectral broadening
- Poststenotic turbulence
- Visible plaque

Occlusion: no detectable Doppler flow from the arterial segment involved
- Proximal signal will vary depending on collateralization
- Monophasic low-velocity waveform distal to occlusion
- Diffuse intraluminal echoes

Diagnostic Criteria Using Absolute Peak Systolic Velocity

	PSV (cm/sec)	Velocity Ratio*
Normal	<150	<1.5:1
30%–49%	150–200	1.5:1–2:1
50%–75%	200–400	2:1–4:1
>75%	>400	>4:1
Occlusion	No detectable color or Doppler flow	

*Velocity ratio PSV at stenosis to PSV proximal artery (Fig. 51-7). (Cossman et al., 1989)

Ankle-Brachial Index Categories

- Greater than 0.945: Normal
- 0.80 to 0.945: Mild disease
- 0.50 to 0.80: Moderate disease (claudication range)
- Less than 0.50: Severe disease
- Less than 0.30: Severe disease associated with ischemia

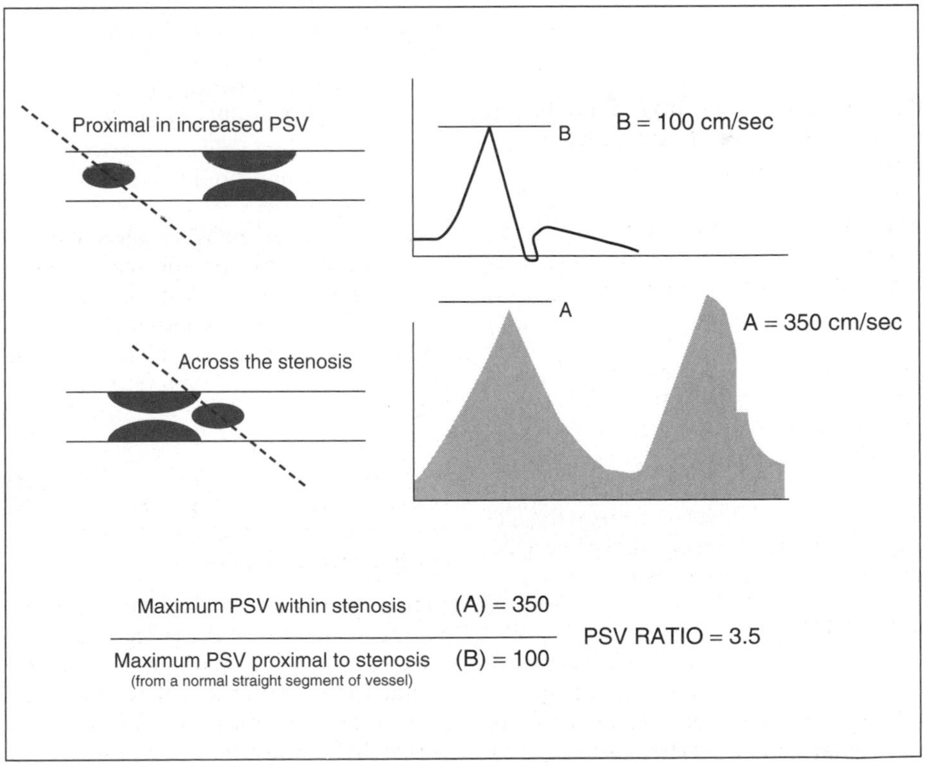

Figure 51-7. ■ *Peak systolic velocity (PSV) ratio calculation.*

Diagnostic Parameters for Peripheral Aneurysm. Measurements of an artery are consistent with an aneurysm when the maximum external diameter of the vessel is 2 cm greater than the diameter of the proximal artery.

DIAGNOSTIC INTERPRETATION

The diagnostic parameters for percentage of stenosis include the PSV ratios (Fig. 51-7), degree of spectral broadening, absence or presence of turbulence, and loss of reverse flow component. The shape of the waveform should be used as an additional tool to support the direct findings. The waveform shape changes immediately distal to a critical stenosis, becoming dampened and monophasic. If a normal, patent CFa is visualized with no evidence of plaque but there is a low-velocity, monophasic waveform with delayed systolic upstroke, one should suspect proximal aortoiliac disease causing compromised flow distal to the stenosis. However, a short focal stenosis greater than 50% can return to normal laminar flow a few centimeters distal to the stenosis. This is why spot-checking with Doppler has a low accuracy.

Pitfalls

1. Proximal aortoiliac artery stenoses or occlusions. A hemodynamically significant lesion in the aortoiliac arteries can alter flow distally by decreasing pulse amplitude and reducing systolic acceleration. These alterations may be very subtle or extremely obvious. With any question of proximal disease, the aorta and iliac arteries should be investigated to avoid this pitfall.
2. Short-segment occlusions. A well-collateralized, short-segment arterial occlusion can be missed, especially in areas of the adductor canal where image resolution is poor. To avoid this problem, always check the relationship of the artery to the vein; any variance should be evaluated. Any distinct change in waveform configuration from level to level calls for reevaluation of the vessel. The only way to detect these changes with a high degree of accuracy is to always be consistent with the Doppler sampling process.
3. Arterial wall calcification. Medial wall calcification is not uncommon in the U.S. patient population. Such calcification can cause acoustic shadowing, causing problems with vessel imaging and obtaining correct Doppler information. This problem has no real solution except to attempt imaging from all possible windows and clearly document the limitation on the record. Arterial calcification also limits the use of the ABI because an accurate blood pressure cannot be determined. In such a case, cuff pressure can exceed 200 mm Hg without causing arterial compression; this is like trying to take a blood pressure on a bathroom pipe. If the ankle artery is calcified and pressure values are inaccurate, a toe pressure should be obtained and documented.
4. Previous vascular surgery. Patients may present with a history of previous vascular reconstruction; information on the nature of the surgery may not be available to the sonographer. Detecting the exact problem is then complicated, because patients do not necessarily return to normal after vascular intervention.
5. Tandem or multiple lesions. A hemodynamically significant proximal lesion causes diminished flow distal to the lesion. The second more distal lesion may not display the true PSV increase; flow is already decreased from the proximal lesion. It is important to document this information in the formal report.
6. Collateral vessels. Distinction between a collateral and an occluded vessel can be difficult. Collateral vessels are generally smaller in diameter than the native feeding artery.

SELECTED READING

Cossman DV, Ellison JE, Wagner WH, et al. Comparison of contrast arteriography to arterial mapping with color-flow duplex imaging in the lower extremities. *J Vasc Surg* 1989;10(5):522–529.

Hatsukami TS, Primozich JF, Zierler RE, et al. Color Doppler imaging of infrainguinal arterial occlusive disease. *J Vasc Surg* 1992; 16(4):527–533.

Kohler TR, Nance DR, Cramer MM, et al. Duplex scanning for diagnosis of aortoiliac and femoropopliteal disease. *Circulation* 1987;76:1074.

Moneta GL, Yeager RA, Lee RW, et al. Noninvasive localization of arterial occlusive disease: a comparison of segmental pressures and arterial duplex imaging. *J Vasc Surg* 1993;17(3):578–582.

52

Shoulder Problems

TOM WINTER

SONOGRAM ABBREVIATIONS

GTR TUB Greater tuberosity

KEY WORDS

Acromion Process. Spinous projection from the scapula that articulates with the clavicle.

Acute Tendonitis. Rapid onset of inflammation of a tendon; symptoms are severe, but the course is short. The term "tendonitis" (also known as tendinitis or tendinosis) is starting to be replaced by the more correct term, "tendinopathy."

Adduction. Movement of a proximal limb toward the body (e.g., moving the arm alongside the chest).

Biceps Tendon. The tendon of the long head of the biceps muscle that arises from the glenoid fossa, arches over the humeral head, and descends through the bicipital groove to insert at the radial tuberosity. The tendon of the short head of the biceps muscle arises from the coracoid process and inserts at the radial tuberosity.

Biceps Tendon Sheath Effusion. Fluid within the dense fibrous sheath covering the biceps tendon.

Biceps Tendonitis. Inflammation of the biceps tendon.

Bicipital or Intertubercular Groove. Deep depression between the greater tuberosity and lesser tuberosity.

Bursa. A small, serous sac between a tendon and a bone.

Calcific Tendonitis. Inflammation and calcification resulting in pain, tenderness, and limited range of motion.

Chronic Tendonitis. Inflammation of a tendon that progresses slowly and has a long duration.

Clavicle. Articulates with the acromion process of the scapula and the upper portion of the sternum to form the anterior portion of the shoulder girdle.

Coracoid Process. Extends from the scapular notch to the upper portion of the neck of the scapula and can be palpated just below and slightly medial to the acromioclavicular junction.

Deltoid Muscle. Originates from the spine and acromion of the scapula and from the lateral one third of the clavicle to insert on the deltoid tuberosity of the humerus.

Deltoid Tuberosity. Ridge on the humerus where the deltoid muscle inserts.

Glenoid Fossa. Oval depression of the scapula that articulates with the head of the humerus.

Greater Tuberosity of the Humerus. Located on the lateral surface of the humerus just below the anatomic neck. Site of insertion for three of the rotator cuff muscles: supraspinatus, infraspinatus, and teres minor.

Infraspinatus. One of the muscles/tendons comprising the rotator cuff that originates from the infraspinatus fossa of the scapula and inserts on the middle posterior portion of the greater tuberosity of the humerus.

Lesser Tuberosity of the Humerus. Located on the anterior surface of the humerus just below the anatomic neck. Site of insertion for the subscapularis, the fourth muscle that comprises the rotator cuff.

Rotator Cuff. Consists of the subscapularis, supraspinatus, infraspinatus, and teres minor muscles and tendons that give support to the glenohumeral joint.

Rotator Cuff Tear. Partial or complete break of one of the four muscles/tendons comprising the rotator cuff. Most rotator cuff tears begin in the supraspinatus.

Scapula. Forms the posterior portion of the shoulder girdle.

Spine of the Scapula. A bony plate projecting from the posterior surface of the scapula.

Subdeltoid Bursa. A bursa located beneath the deltoid muscle that reduces friction in this area.

Subdeltoid Bursitis. Inflammation of the subdeltoid bursa.

Subscapularis. One of the muscles/tendons comprising the rotator cuff that originates from the anterior or costal surface of the scapula to insert at the lesser tuberosity of the humerus.

Supraspinatus. One of the muscles/tendons comprising the rotator cuff that originates from the supraspinatus fossa of the scapula to insert on the highest portion of the greater tuberosity of the humerus.

Synovial Cyst. Accumulation of synovia in a bursa.

Teres Minor. One of the muscles/tendons comprising the rotator cuff that originates from the upper two thirds of the axillary border of the scapula.

The Clinical Problem

Shoulder arthrography, whether using plain films, computed tomography, or magnetic resonance imaging (MRI), requires injection of contrast material into the joint space, which often causes discomfort and limits the examination to one shoulder per visit. MRI without intra-articular contrast is as accurate as ultrasound for evaluation of the rotator cuff but is more expensive; in addition, patients prefer ultrasound to MRI. Ultrasound is noninvasive, painless, less expensive, and allows comparison of both shoulders at one visit.

Often the scan is ordered to diagnose a rotator cuff tear; most of these are chronic conditions and occur late in life, but others are acute injuries from overuse. Rotator cuff tears usually present with one or more of the following symptoms:

1. Shoulder pain
2. Dysfunction, with limited range of motion
3. Weakness and pain with elevation or abduction of the arm
4. Pain at rest from rolling onto the affected shoulder

Other conditions that can be evaluated sonographically include tendonitis, bursitis, cysts, and effusions in the shoulder area.

Anatomy

ROTATOR CUFF

The rotator cuff consists of four muscles and their corresponding tendons whose major function is to hold the humeral head within the glenoid fossa.

Subscapularis Muscle

The subscapularis muscle originates from the anterior or costal surface of the scapula to insert at the lesser tuberosity of the humerus (Figs. 52-1 and 52-2). The lesser tuberosity is located on the anterior surface of the humerus just below the anatomic neck. The subscapularis acts as a medial or internal rotator of the shoulder.

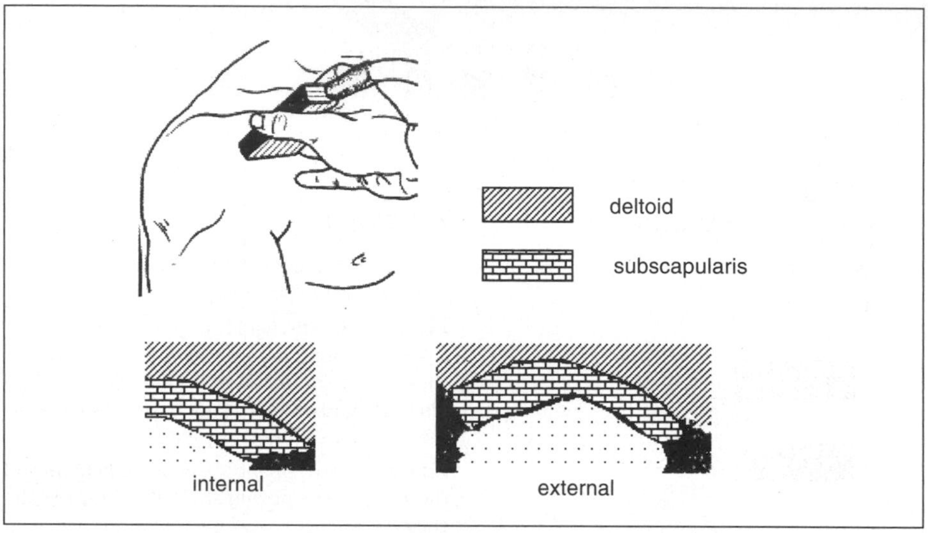

Figure 52-1. ■ *Transducer position and sonographic diagram of the subscapularis tendon. Dynamic imaging with both internal and external rotation should be performed.*

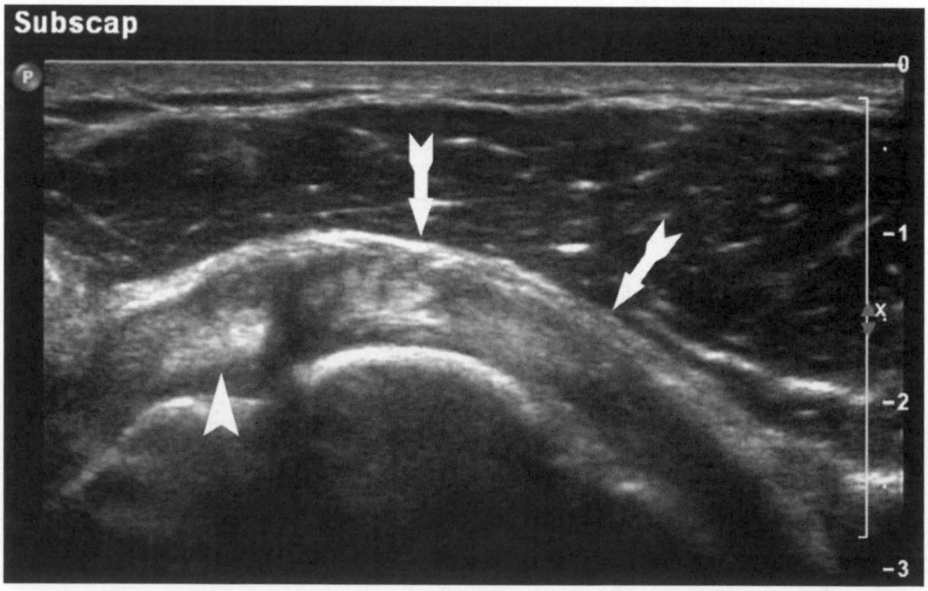

Figure 52-2. ■ *Longitudinal view of the fibers of the right subscapularis tendon* (arrows), *obtained with the transducer position in Figure 52-1. Biceps tendon* (arrowhead).

Supraspinatus Muscle

The supraspinatus muscle originates from the supraspinatus fossa of the scapula, and its tendon passes beneath the acromion to insert on the highest portion or anterior impression of the greater tuberosity (Figs. 52-3 and 52-4). The greater tuberosity is on the lateral surface of the humerus just below the anatomic neck. The supraspinatus works with the deltoid muscle to abduct the shoulder.

Infraspinatus Muscle

The infraspinatus muscle originates from the infraspinatus fossa of the scapula and inserts on the middle posterior portion of the greater tuberosity of the humerus (Figs. 52-5 and 52-6). The infraspinatus

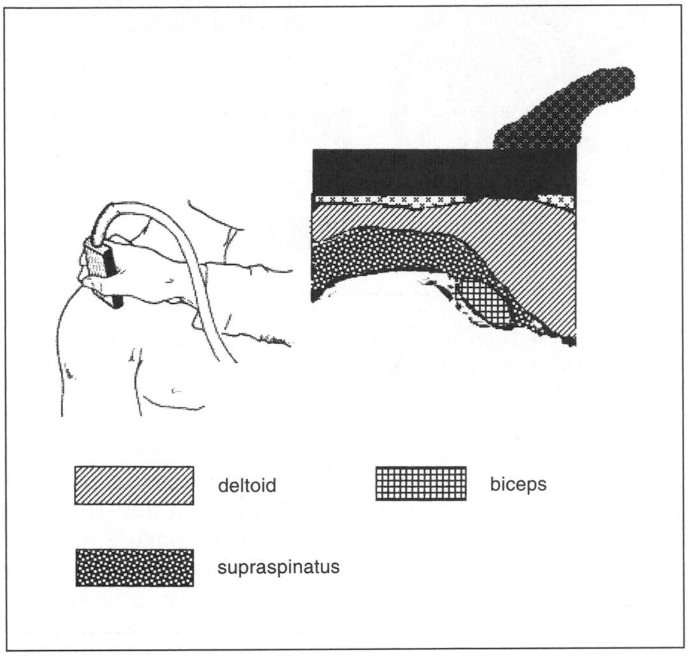

Figure 52-3. ■ *Transducer position and transverse sonographic diagram of the supraspinatus tendon.*

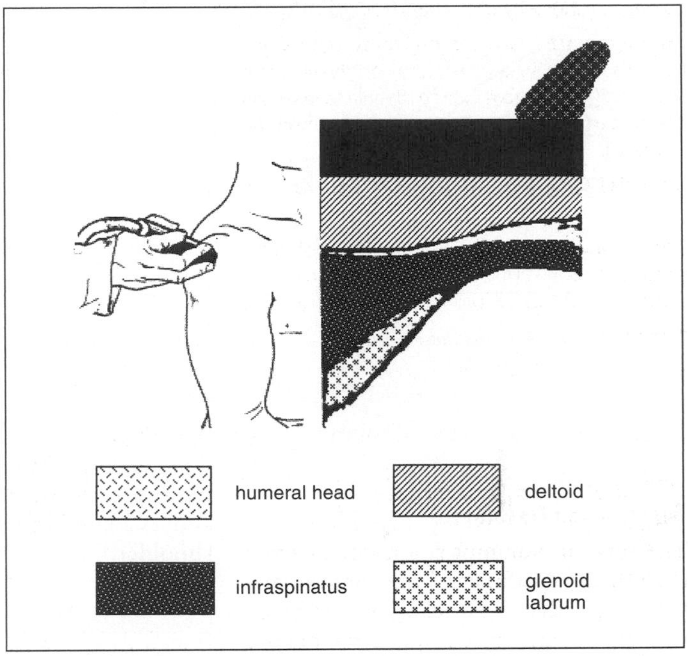

Figure 52-5. ■ *Transducer position and sonographic diagram of the infraspinatus tendon and glenoid labrum.*

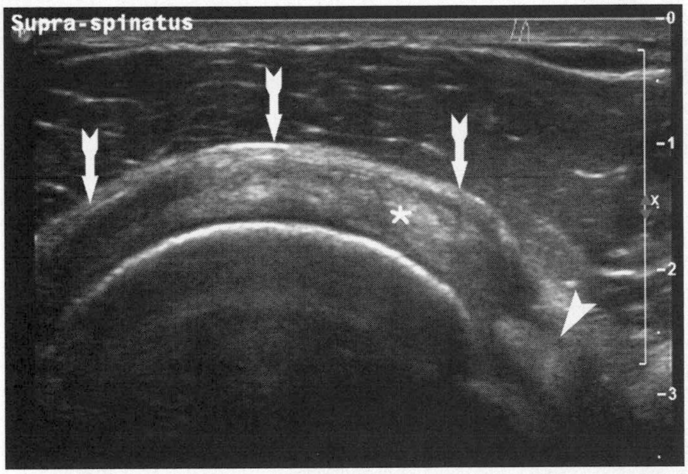

Figure 52-4. ■ *Transverse view of the right supraspinatus tendon* (arrows), *obtained with the transducer position in Figure 52-3. Biceps tendon* (arrowhead); *critical zone* (*), *that portion of the rotator cuff where most tears begin.*

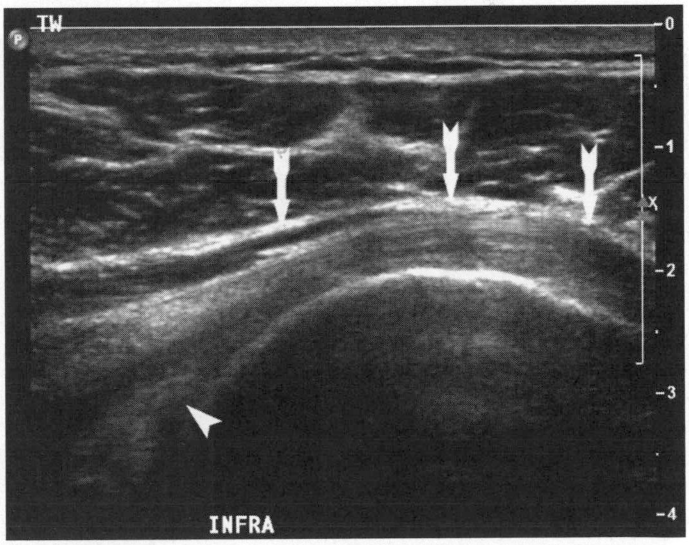

Figure 52-6. ■ *Sonogram of right infraspinatus tendon* (arrows), *obtained with the transducer position in Figure 52-5. Triangular tip of the glenoid labrum* (arrowhead).

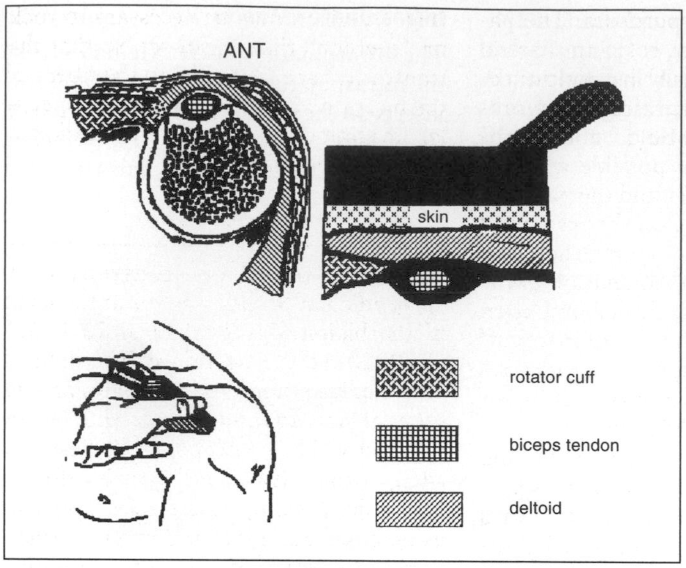

Figure 52-7. ■ *Transducer position and transverse sonographic diagram of the biceps tendon.*

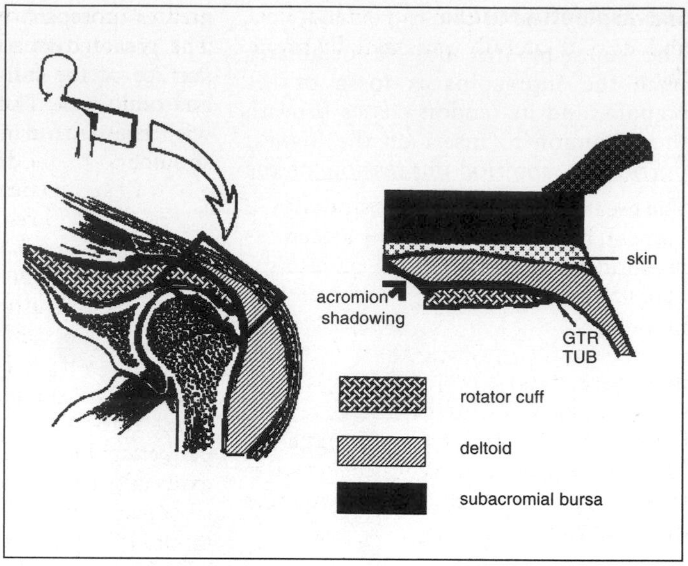

Figure 52-8. ■ *Transducer position and longitudinal sonographic diagram of the rotator cuff and deltoid.*

acts as a lateral or external rotator of the shoulder.

Teres Minor Muscle

The teres minor muscle originates from the upper two thirds of the axillary borders of the dorsal surface of the scapula and inserts at the posterior lower portion of the greater tuberosity. The teres minor acts as a lateral or external rotator of the shoulder.

DELTOID MUSCLE

The deltoid originates from the spine and acromion of the scapula and from the lateral one third of the clavicle to insert on the deltoid tuberosity of the humerus (Figs. 52-1, 52-3, 52-5, 52-7, 52-8, 52-9,

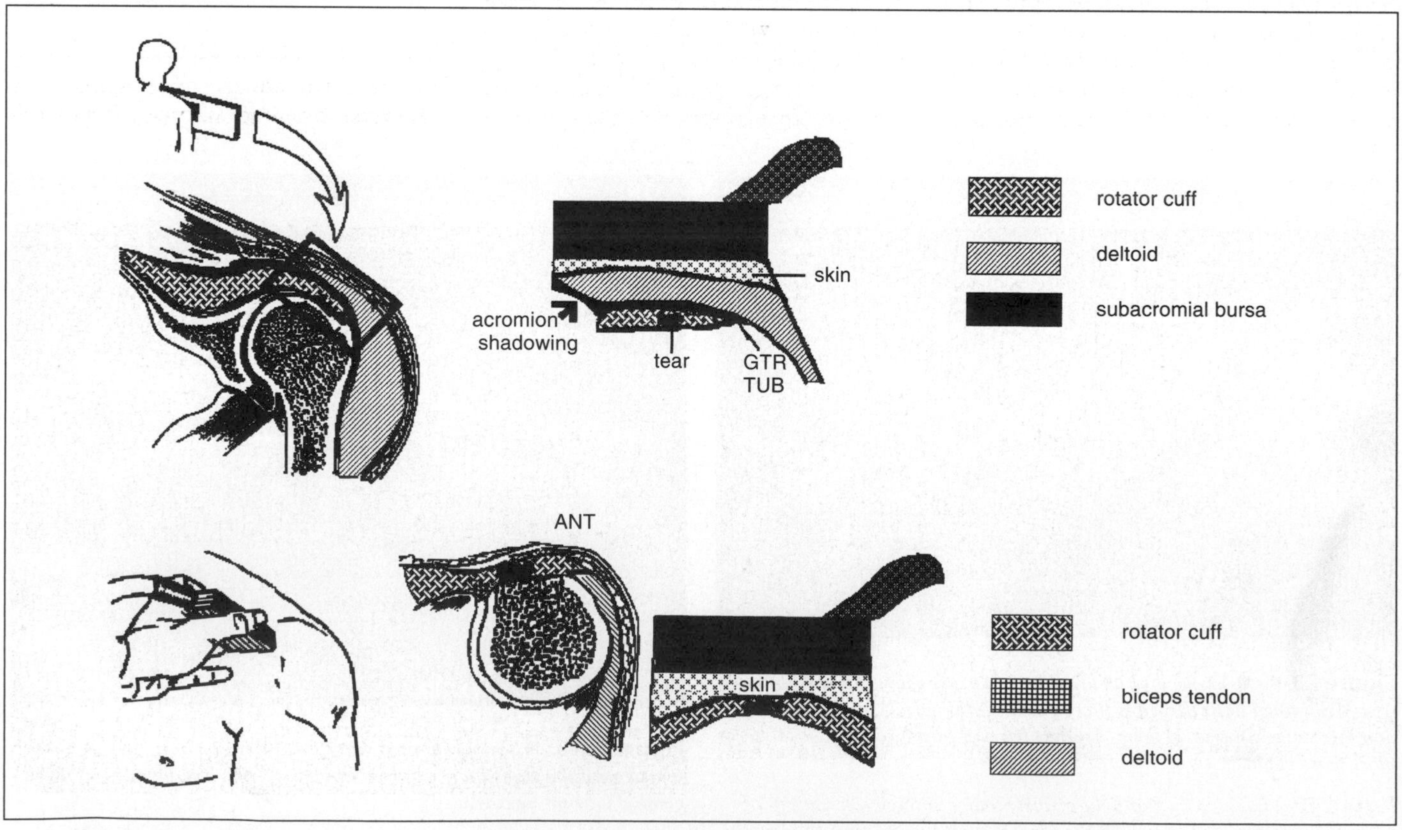

Figure 52-9. ■ *Transducer position and sonographic diagrams of a rotator cuff tear (in both longitudinal and transverse planes).*

and 52-10). The deltoid can extend, flex, abduct, and laterally and medially rotate the shoulder.

BICIPITAL GROOVE AND BICEPS TENDON

The greater and lesser tuberosities of the humeral head are separated by a deep depression called the bicipital or intertubercular groove (Fig. 52-7). The tendon of the long head of the biceps muscle arises from the upper portion of the glenoid fossa, passes through the capsule of the shoulder joint, and arches over the humeral head as it descends through the bicipital groove. The biceps tendon acts to stabilize the shoulder from superior displacement.

SUBDELTOID BURSA

The subdeltoid bursa is located between the deltoid muscle and the rotator cuff, and its purpose is to relieve friction on the tendon of the rotator cuff.

Technique

A small-parts broad bandwidth linear array transducer, covering approximately 12 to 5 MHz, produces the best images. In very large patients, a lower-frequency ("vascular") linear array may be necessary. Both shoulders are examined for comparative purposes. The patient is seated on a low, rotating stool so that he or she can easily be positioned. For examination of the biceps and subscapularis, the arm should be adducted as close to the body as possible with the elbow flexed 90 degrees and the patient's supinated hand resting on the ipsilateral thigh; do not let the patient internally rotate his or her arm or examination of the biceps may be difficult. For examination of the remainder of the rotator cuff (supraspinatus, infraspinatus, and teres minor), have the patient place his or her hand into his or her ipsilateral rear pocket, palm touching the gluteus, and externally rotate the arm as much as possible (e.g., rotate the elbow back toward the middle of his back); this is called the modified Crass position.

BICEPS TENDON/BICIPITAL GROOVE

Begin the examination by placing the transducer transversely over the bicipital groove (Fig. 52-7). The biceps tendon is seen as an echogenic ovoid structure within the bicipital groove. A small amount of hypoechoic fluid may surround the biceps tendon, representing a normal variant.

Rotate the transducer 90 degrees (longitudinally) to visualize the biceps tendon parallel to its long axis. The biceps tendon will appear as an echogenic linear structure anterior to the humerus (Fig. 52-11). It may be necessary to rock or "heel-toe" the transducer, so that the transducer face is parallel to the fibers of the biceps tendon. Otherwise, nonspecular imaging of the tendon may lead to a falsely abnormal image.

SUBSCAPULARIS

Rotate the transducer transversely or perpendicular to the humerus at the level of the bicipital groove (Figs. 52-1 and 52-2). Move the transducer proximally and medially until the subscapularis is seen at its attachment to the lesser tuberosity. The subscapularis is best imaged in this view parallel to its fibers. Dynamic imaging of the subscapularis using passive internal and external rotation is necessary to visualize the entire tendon. When the arm is internally rotated, a portion of the tendon retracts and is obscured behind the coracoid process, but with external rotation, the tendon is drawn out from beneath the coracoid process. Sweep through the entire tendon while passively rotating the arm, and examine it carefully for any irregularities. Repeat this maneuver, imaging the subscapularis longitudinally or perpendicular to its fibers.

SUPRASPINATUS

With the transducer once again in a transverse orientation, move it posteri-

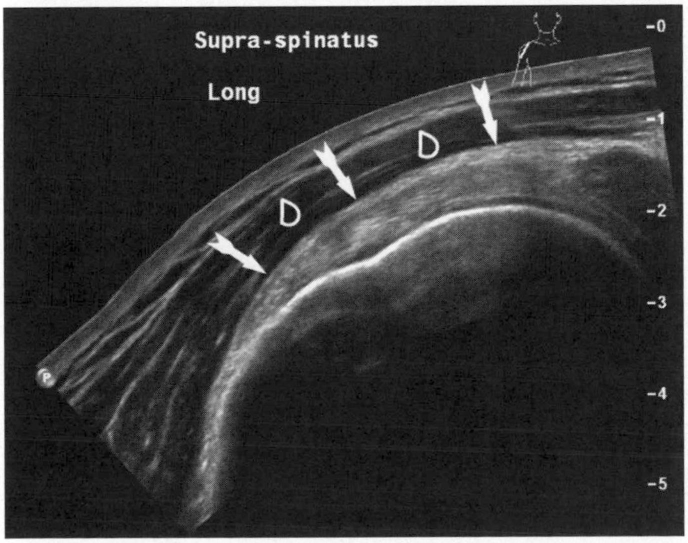

Figure 52-10. ■ *Extended field-of-view image showing the sweep of the supraspinatus tendon (under the* arrows*) as it inserts onto the greater tuberosity. Note the hypoechoic deltoid muscle* (D) *overlying the supraspinatus.*

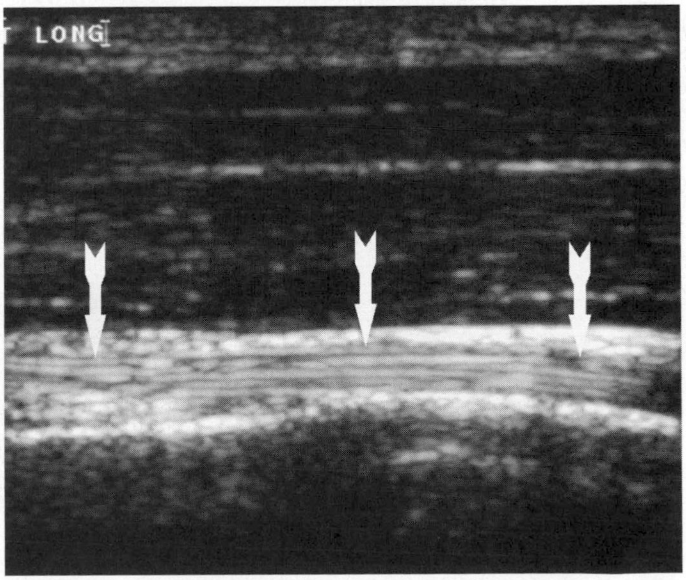

Figure 52-11. ■ *Longitudinal sonogram of the biceps tendon fibers* (arrows). *Note the normal hyperechoic fibrillary pattern obtained when the tendon is perpendicular to the insonating beam.*

orly and laterally from its position over the subscapularis to visualize the supraspinatus, posterior to the biceps tendon (Figs. 52-3 and 52-4). The supraspinatus is seen between the deltoid muscle and the humerus. The echogenicity of the supraspinatus and the rotator cuff tendons is usually greater than the echogenicity of the deltoid muscle, although in older patients the supraspinatus and rotator cuff tendons may be as echogenic or less echogenic than the deltoid. Comparison with the contralateral shoulder shows whether the echogenicity is a normal variant or an indication of a pathologic process. The subdeltoid bursa is visualized between the deltoid and supraspinatus and appears as highly echogenic parallel lines.

Rotating the transducer 90 degrees or longitudinally, the supraspinatus is visualized parallel to its long axis (Figs. 52-8, 52-10, and 52-12). The supraspinatus is seen as a beak-like structure projecting from beneath the acoustic shadowing caused by the acromion. Dynamically visualizing the supraspinatus with passive adduction and abduction of the humerus is important in the detection of pathologic processes within the tendon.

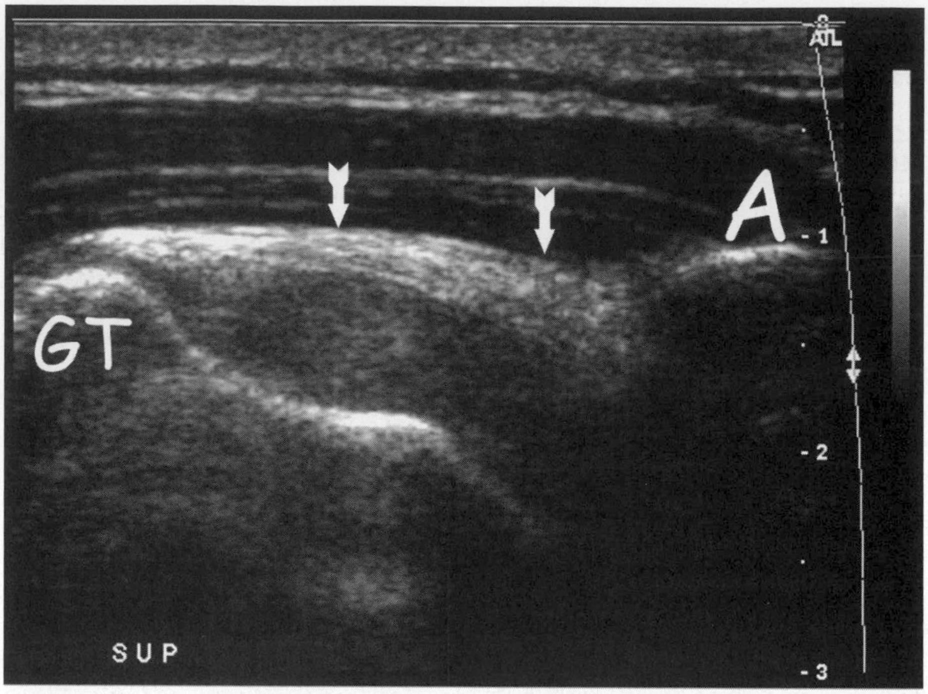

Figure 52-12. ■ *Longitudinal view of the fibers of the right supraspinatus tendon (under the arrows) as they insert onto the greater tuberosity* (GT). *Also note posterior acoustic shadowing beneath the bony acromion* (A), *which obscures visualization of the supraspinatus fibers in this region.*

INFRASPINATUS

With the transducer transversely oriented or perpendicular to the humeral shaft, move posteriorly from the supraspinatus position to visualize the infraspinatus (Figs. 52-5 and 52-6). The infraspinatus muscle appears triangular in shape and tapers to form the infraspinatus tendon, which attaches to the greater tuberosity. The tendon will be visualized parallel to its long axis. Passive internal and external rotation of the arm in adduction enhance visualization of the tendon.

TERES MINOR

Moving the transducer distally (inferiorly) from its position over the infraspinatus reveals the teres minor muscle and tendon. The teres minor appears rhomboid-shaped. Think of the teres minor as the inferior aspect of the infraspinatus; in a certain percentage of patients, these two muscles are actually fused. Passive internal and external rotation of the arm in adduction also enhance visualization of the teres minor tendon. Tears of the teres minor rarely occur in isolation.

Pathology

ROTATOR CUFF TEARS

Rotator cuff tears most frequently involve the supraspinatus tendon anterior and lateral to the acromion process, in an area of decreased vascularity that is just proximal to its insertion into the greater tuberosity (Figs. 52-9 and 52-13). This area, called the "critical zone," is approximately 1 cm posterior and lateral to the biceps tendon, and should be closely scrutinized in every patient. A rotator cuff tear may have one or more of the following features:

1. Focal area or areas of thinning or irregularity of the tendon
2. An entire tendon or a portion of a tendon that cannot be visualized
3. Focal area or areas of echogenicity (not to be confused with calcific tendonitis)
4. Loss of the normal homogeneous echo texture of the tendon
5. A thickened tendon with irregular areas of increased or decreased echogenicity (edema, hemorrhage, or degeneration may be present)

The most reliable signs of a rotator cuff tear are a focal gap or hole in the tendon, or an area of tendon that compresses ("squeezes") when pressure is applied with the transducer; a normal tendon should not compress at all.

BICEPS TENDONITIS

Thickening and irregularity of the biceps tendon are features of biceps tendonitis.

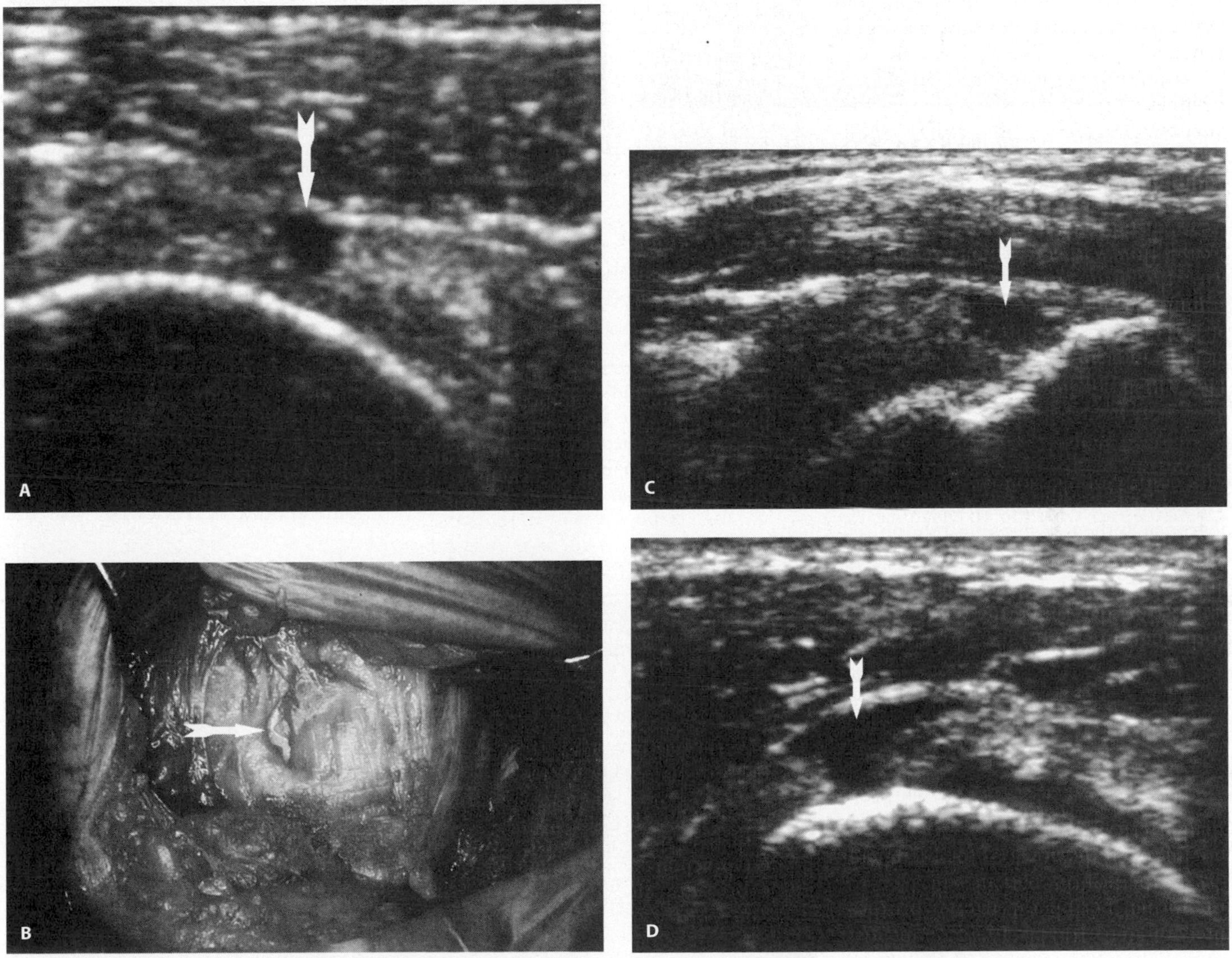

Figure 52-13. ■ *A. Transverse view of a small rotator cuff (supraspinatus tendon) tear* (arrow). *Note the gap or hole in the fibers, as well as the abnormal concave contour to the tendon surface (the tendon surface should be outwardly convex). B. Intraoperative photograph of the tear* (arrow) *in the patient in (A). C. Longitudinal view of a tear* (arrow) *in the supraspinatus tendon in a different patient. D. Transverse view of a tear* (arrow) *in the supraspinatus tendon in yet another patient.*

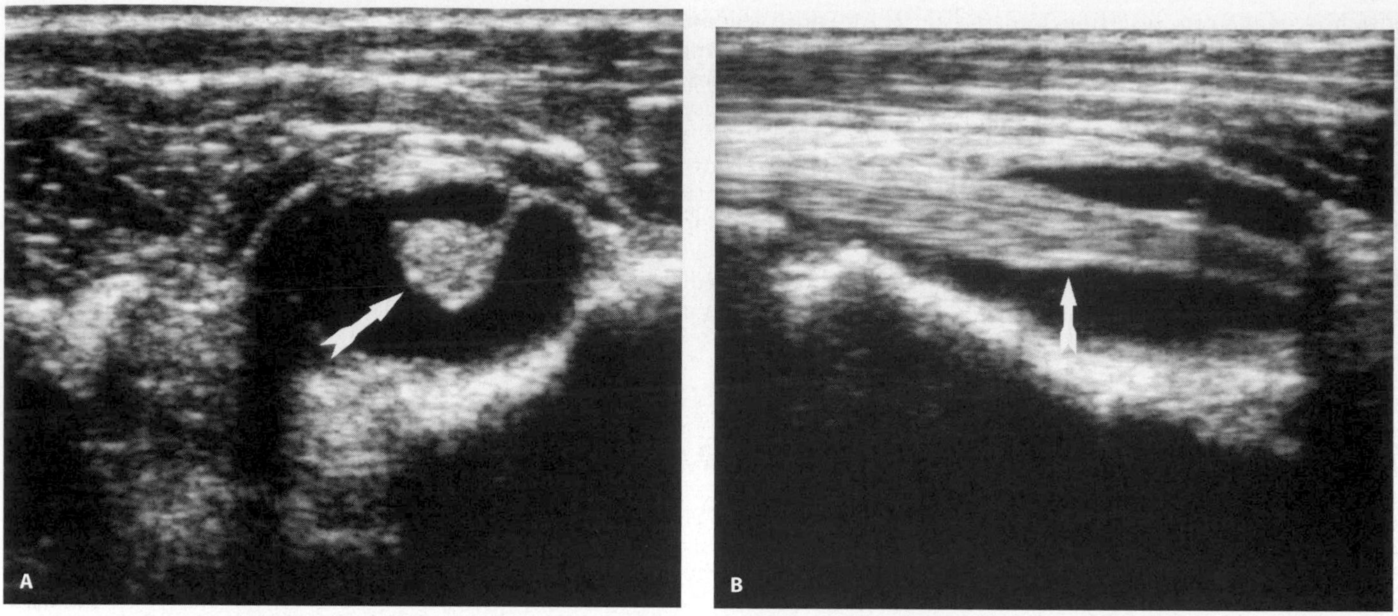

Figure 52-14. ■ *Transverse (A) and longitudinal (B) images of a biceps tendon sheath effusion. Biceps tendon* (arrow).

Many cases of tendinopathy, however, are missed by ultrasound.

Acute Tendonitis

A thickened tendon with decreased echogenicity indicates acute tendonitis.

Chronic Tendonitis

A thickened tendon with decreased echogenicity and a nonhomogeneous appearance indicates chronic tendonitis. Calcifications are frequently present.

SUBDELTOID BURSITIS

In subdeltoid bursitis, an enlarged bursa usually fills with hypoechoic fluid because of inflammatory changes. The bursa will have irregular borders.

BICEPS TENDON SHEATH EFFUSION

A hypoechoic area is visualized surrounding the biceps tendon when there is a sheath effusion (Fig. 52-14).

CALCIFIC TENDONITIS

When tendonitis is calcific, the tendon is usually less echogenic than normal and contains one or more echogenic foci within its substance, with or without acoustic shadowing (Fig. 52-15).

SYNOVIAL CYST

Synovial cysts are most commonly found extending along the biceps tendon and appear as well-defined hypoechoic structures with smooth borders and good through transmission.

Pitfalls

1. Normal anatomy versus pathology. Comparison with the asymptomatic shoulder can help distinguish certain normal variants from pathology.
2. Postoperative rotator cuff. The surgical procedure performed and how it alters the anatomy of the rotator cuff should be reviewed with the

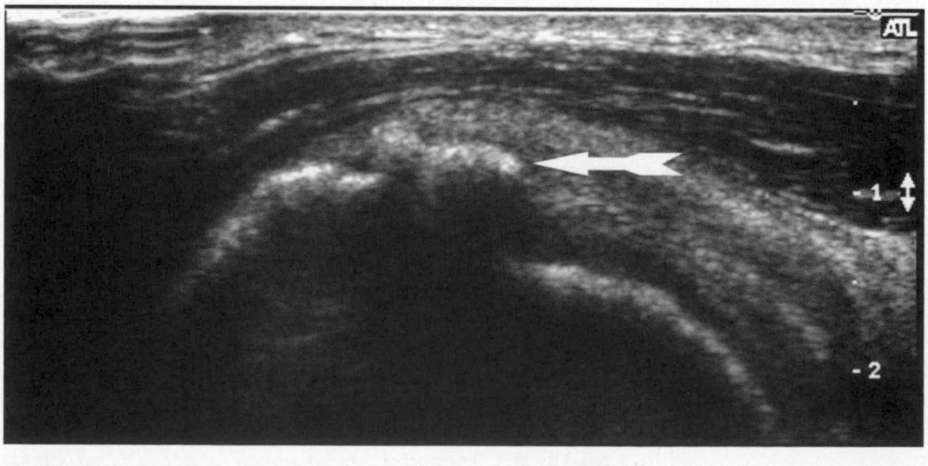

Figure 52-15. ■ *Calcific tendonitis* (arrow) *within the supraspinatus tendon.*

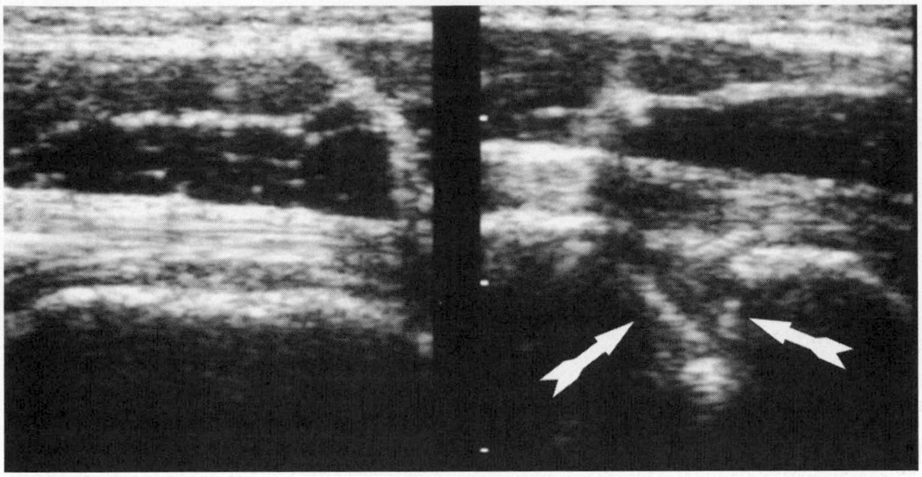

Figure 52-16. ■ *Humeral head fracture noted on ultrasound. Compare the smooth surface of the normal right humeral head* (left), *with the focal divot* (arrows) *in the left humeral head in this orthopaedic nurse who had been thrown directly onto her left shoulder during a martial arts exhibition. The overlying rotator cuff was intact.*

surgeon before sonographic evaluation.

3. Old fractures of the shoulder. Any dislocation of bony anatomy (Fig. 52-16) may alter the appearance of the rotator cuff. Plain radiographs may be helpful in such cases.
4. Shadowing from the acromion process hiding rotator cuff tears. Proper movement and positioning of the arm alleviate this problem.

SELECTED READING

Farin PU, Jaroma H. Sonographic findings of rotator cuff calcifications. *J Ultrasound Med* 1995;14:7–14.

Hollister MS, Mack LA, Patten RM, et al. Association of sonographically detected subacromial/subdeltoid bursal effusion and intraarticular fluid with rotator cuff tear. *AJR Am J Roentgenol* 1995;165:605–608.

Mack LA, Nyberg DA, Matsen FA III. Sonographic evaluation of the rotator cuff. *Radiol Clin North Am* 1988;26:161–177.

Middleton WD, Edelstein G, Reinus WR, et al. Ultrasonography of the rotator cuff: technique and normal anatomy. *J Ultrasound Med* 1984;3:549–551.

Middleton WD, Payne WT, Teefey SA, et al. Sonography and MRI of the shoulder: comparison of patient satisfaction. *AJR Am J Roentgenol* 2004;183:1449–1452.

Middleton WD, Teefey SA, Yamaguchi K. Sonography of the rotator cuff: analysis of interobserver variability. *AJR Am J Roentgenol* 2004;183:1465–1468.

Teefey SA, Hasan SA, Middleton WD, et al. Ultrasonography of the rotator cuff. A comparison of ultrasonographic and arthroscopic findings in one hundred consecutive cases. *J Bone Joint Surg Am* 2000; 82:498–504.

Teefey SA, Rubin DA, Middleton WD, et al. Detection and quantification of rotator cuff tears. Comparison of ultrasonographic, magnetic resonance imaging, and arthroscopic findings in seventy-one consecutive cases. *J Bone Joint Surg Am* 2004;86-A: 708–716.

Van Holsbeeck MT, Kolowich PA, Eyler WR, et al. US depiction of partial-thickness tear of the rotator cuff. *Radiology* 1995;197:443–446.

Wiener SN, Seitz WH Jr. Sonography of the shoulder in patients with tears of the rotator cuff: accuracy and value for selecting surgical options. *AJR Am J Roentgenol* 1993;160:103–107.

Winter TC, Teefey SA, Middleton WD. Musculoskeletal ultrasound: an update. *Radiol Clin North Am* 2001;39(3):465–483.

53 Common Ankle and Foot Problems

JAG DHANJU

SONOGRAM ABBREVIATIONS

ACH	Achilles tendon
ATFL	Anterior talofibular ligament
ATT	Anterior tibialis tendon
EDL	Extensor digitorum longus tendon
EHL	Extensor hallucis longus tendon
FDL	Flexor digitorum longus tendon
FHL	Flexor hallucis longus tendon
PB	Peroneus brevis tendon
PF	Plantar fascia
PL	Peroneus longus tendon
PTT	Posterior tibialis tendon
SOL	Soleus muscle

KEY WORDS

Anisotropy. The echogenicity of a tendon may depend on the orientation of the ultrasound beam relative to the tendon structure. This causes an angle-dependent artifact known as anisotropy. If the tendon is perpendicular to the central axis of the sound beam, then the tendon will appear echogenic, and the fibers of the tendon will be well visualized. However, if the tendon is not perpendicular but is oblique to the central axis of the sound beam, the tendon will appear more hypoechoic, and the fibers will be suboptimally visualized.

Ankle Mortise. Ankle mortise is formed by the lower end of the tibia and its malleolus and the malleolus of the fibula, which together form a mortise for the reception of the upper surface of the talus.

Bursitis. Inflammation of a bursa, a fibrous sac around certain tendons and bones. Bursae have a synovial-lined membrane and secrete synovial fluid.

Plantar. Relating to the sole of the foot.

Perimysium. The sheath of connective tissue enveloping bundles of muscle fibers.

Tenosynovitis. An inflammation of the tendon sheath, sometimes manifested as fluid within the synovial sheath.

Tendonitis. Inflammatory condition of a tendon, often from a strain or repetitive injury.

Tendinopathy. A tendon abnormality resulting from ischemic or degenerative processes rather than inflammation. Most cases of tendonitis would more appropriately be termed "tendinopathy" because pathologically there are no inflammatory cells present, but the word "tendonitis" is still used extensively.

Valgus Test. A clinical maneuver used to apply direct stress to the medial aspect of the joint to test medial instability.

Varus Test. A clinical maneuver used to apply direct stress to the lateral aspect of the joint to test lateral instability.

The Clinical Problem

Ankle and foot injuries affect tens of thousands of people and are often difficult to diagnose and treat. Physicians currently use a variety of imaging technologies to evaluate musculoskeletal disease, from magnetic resonance imaging to arthroscopy to x-ray, with varying degrees of success.

Advances in imaging resolution and improved examination techniques are rapidly making ultrasound the imaging modality of choice in the screening of muscles, tendons, ligaments, and other soft tissue structures around the ankle and foot. Ultrasound is cost-effective and is distinct from other imaging modalities because it allows the imager to apply direct stress to soft tissue structures in a real-time fashion. With ultrasound, we can also simultaneously image the opposite joint for comparison. The examination can be custom-tailored to focus on a specific area (affected area of patient's ankle and foot).

Extra-articular ankle and foot joint pain can be divided into the following regions:

Anterior pain: anterior tibialis tendon (ATT), extensor hallucis longus tendon (EHL), and extensor digitorum longus tendon (EDL)

Medial pain: posterior tibialis tendon (PTT), flexor digitorum longus tendon (FDL), and flexor hallucis longus tendon (FHL)

Lateral pain: peroneus tendons and lateral ligaments

Posterior and plantar pain: Achilles tendon (ACH) and plantar fascia, respectively

Ultrasound can be used also to evaluate soft tissue pathologies around the joint such as ganglion cyst, bursitis, lipoma, joint effusion, and foreign bodies within the foot.

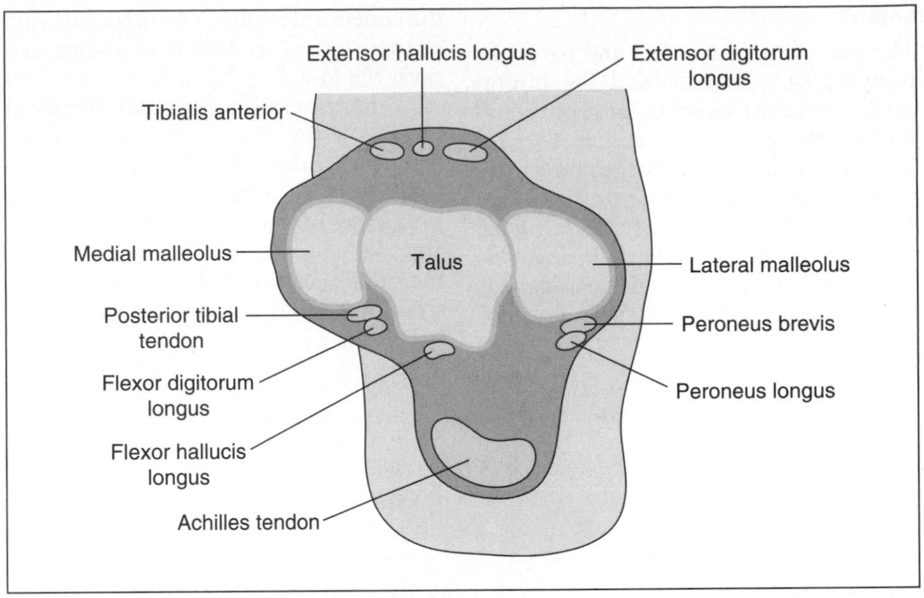

Figure 53-1. ■ *Cross-sectional image of the ankle joint.*

Anatomy

SOFT TISSUE ANATOMY

Ankle Joint

The ankle joint is a synovial articulation acting as a hinge joint, which is formed by mortise (tibia and fibula) and talus. The articulating surfaces of the joint are covered with hyaline cartilage. There is a synovial membrane between the articular margins of the tibia, fibula, and talus. A fibrous capsule surrounds the synovial membrane of the ankle joint. Medially and laterally, there are the collateral ligaments, thickenings of the joint capsule that limit valgus and varus displacement.

Anterior

Passing over the anterior tibiotalar joint space is a group of primary extensor tendons of the ankle that collectively allow dorsiflexion of the joint. From medial to lateral, they consist of the ATT, EHL, and EDL tendons (Fig. 53-1). These extensors are all contained within individual synovial sheaths, which may contain a small amount of normal physiologic fluid. The ATT is the largest in diameter in comparison with the rest of the extensor tendons. The ATT travels medially and then toward the plantar aspect, inserting onto the first medial cuneiform and base of the first metatarsal. Next, located lateral to the ATT, is the EHL tendon; it courses distally over the first toe to insert on the base of the distal phalanx. Lateral to the EHL tendon is the EDL tendon. The EDL branches distally into four separate tendons that insert on the second through fifth toes.

Medial

Posterior to the bony landmark of the medial malleolus and deep to the flexor retinaculum are a group of tendons and a neurovascular bundle. In a medial to lateral direction (see Fig. 53-3), they consist of the PTT, FDL, neurovascular bundle (posterior tibial artery with venae comitantes and tibial nerve), and FHL. A useful mnemonic to help remember this medial arrangement is:

Tom **Di**ck and **A V**ery **N**ervous **H**arry = P**T**T, F**DL** (Posterior Tibial **A**rtery, **V**ein, and **N**erve), and F**H**L

The posterior tibialis muscle originates from the shaft of the tibia and tapers into a long tendon. The PTT hugs the posterior aspect of the medial malleolus and inserts distally onto the tarsal navicular bone. The PTT functions to turn the sole of the foot inward, along with help from the ATT.

The FDL accompanies the PTT and is smaller in diameter. The FDL runs distally along the plantar aspect of the foot to insert on the base of the distal phalanges of the second to fifth toes. The FDL aids in flexing the toes for final push-off in walking.

The FHL originates from the posterior side of the fibula and passes posterior to the talar groove, making it the most lateral of the medial ankle tendons. The FHL inserts onto the plantar aspect of the distal phalanx of the first toe and allows the first toe to flex.

Lateral

The peroneus longus (PL) and peroneus brevis (PB) course behind the lateral malleolus in the retrofibular groove and are held there by a retinaculum (Fig. 53-2). The PB is located more anteriorly than the longus and closer to the fibula. The PB inserts onto the tubercle of the fifth metatarsal base. The PL descends across the lateral aspect of the calcaneus and crosses over plantarly to insert onto the cuneiform region. The main function of these lateral tendons is to abduct and evert the foot.

The anterior talofibular ligament (ATFL) is the most commonly injured ligament of the ankle. The ATFL originates from the anterior-lateral aspect of the distal fibula and passes anteriorly and medially, inserting onto the neck of the talus (Fig. 53-2). It functions to restrain internal rotation of the talus.

Posterior

The ACH connects the calf muscles to the calcaneus (heel bone) and is made of a strong fibrous band. The calf muscles consist of the two heads of the gastrocnemius muscle and the deep soleus muscle. The contraction of the gastrocsoleus muscle group causes plantar flexion of the foot. The ACH does not have a rich blood supply. It is not invested within a true synovial tendon sheath, but a para-

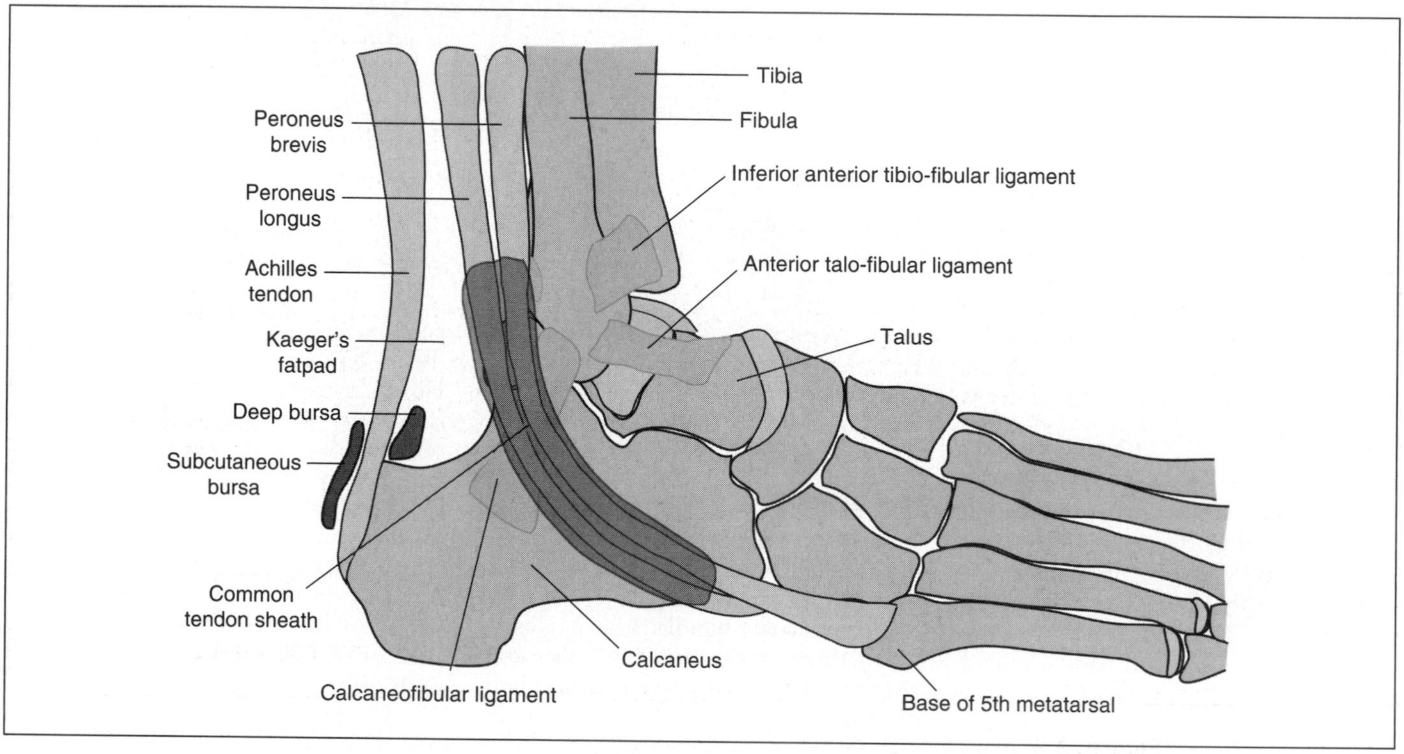

Figure 53-2. *Lateral view of the ankle: peroneal tendons and lateral collateral ligaments.*

tendon composed of fibrous tissue surrounds it. Located deep (anterior) to the distal half of the ACH is Kaegar's triangular fat pad. There is a deep, retrocalcaneal bursa between the distal anterior wall of the ACH and the posterior superior border of the calcaneus bone (Figs. 53-2 and 53-3).

Plantar Foot

The plantar fascia is a dense strip of tissue that runs from the front of the heel bone (calcaneus) to the ball of the foot. There is a large medial band, which originates from the medial tubercle of the calcaneus. A separate, thinner lateral band arises from the lateral tubercle of the calcaneus. The plantar fascia helps to support the longitudinal arch of the foot.

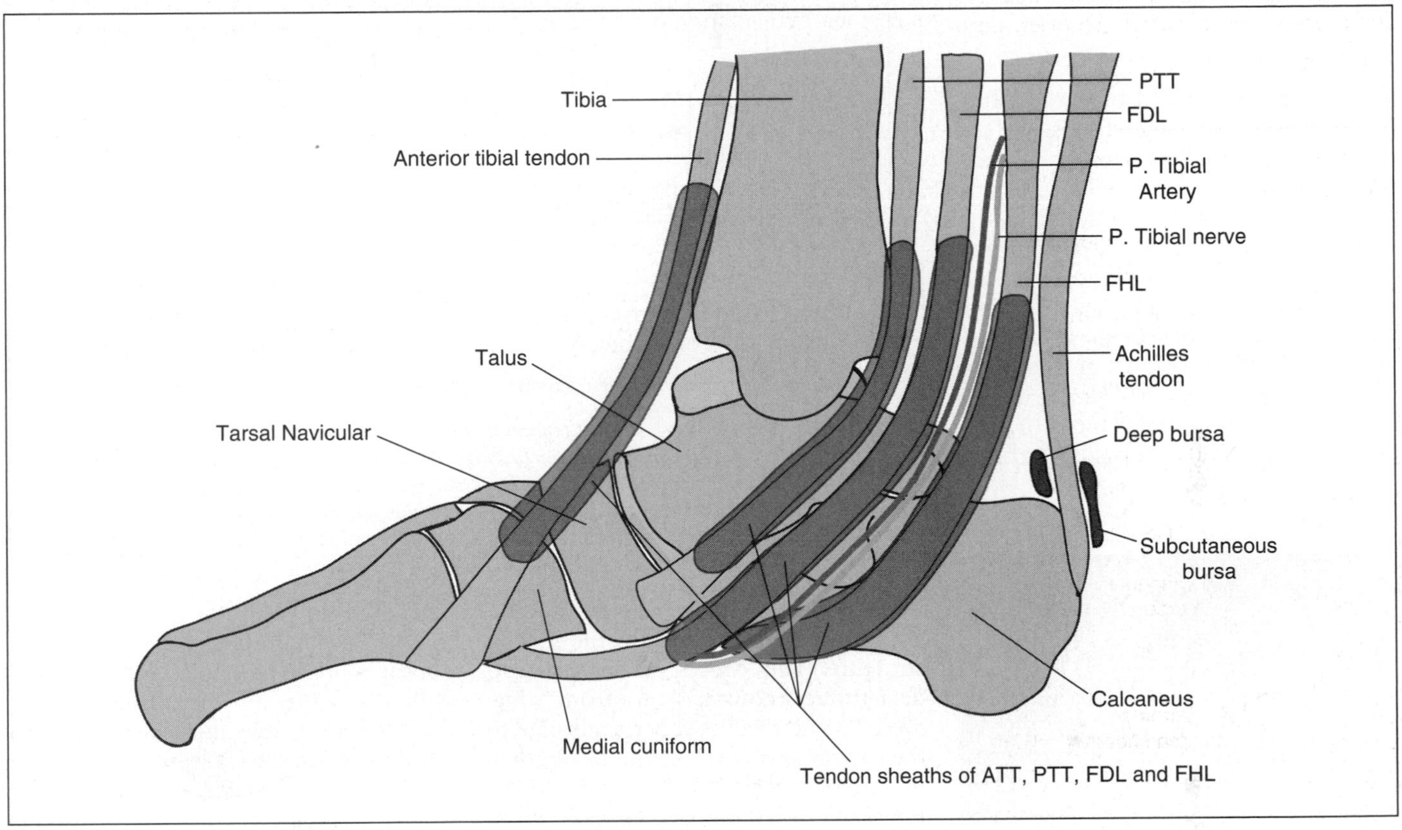

Figure 53-3. ■ *Medial view of the ankle: medial tendons.*

NORMAL ULTRASOUND APPEARANCE OF MUSCLE AND TENDONS

Muscles

Muscle bundles have a hypoechoic appearance. The fibroadipose septa of the perimysium are seen as hyperechoic lines separating the hypoechoic muscle bundles. This appears as a pennate or feather-like arrangement on ultrasound (Fig. 53-4A).

Tendons

Tendons are composed of parallel running fascicles of collagen fibers. We can see these individual fascicles on high-resolution sonography, especially with high-frequency transducers. Tendon fibers appear more echogenic in comparison with their muscle bellies. The fibers of a tendon appear as echogenic parallel lines and give a regular echogenic striated appearance (Fig. 53-4B). There should be no disruptions or tears within the tendon and its borders. The echogenicity of a tendon may depend on the orientation of the ultrasound beam relative to the tendon structure. This causes an angle-dependent artifact known as "anisotropy" (Fig. 53-5). If the tendon is perpendicular to the central axis of the sound beam, then the tendon will appear echogenic, and the fibers of the tendon will be well visualized. However, if the tendon is not perpendicular but is oblique to the central axis of the sound beam, the tendon will appear more hypoechoic, and the fibers will be suboptimally visualized (Fig. 53-6). Therefore, one must remember to continually tilt the transducer depending on the tendon's course. Anisotropy may mimic pathologic conditions such as tendinopathy, tendon tears, and abnormal fluid collections.

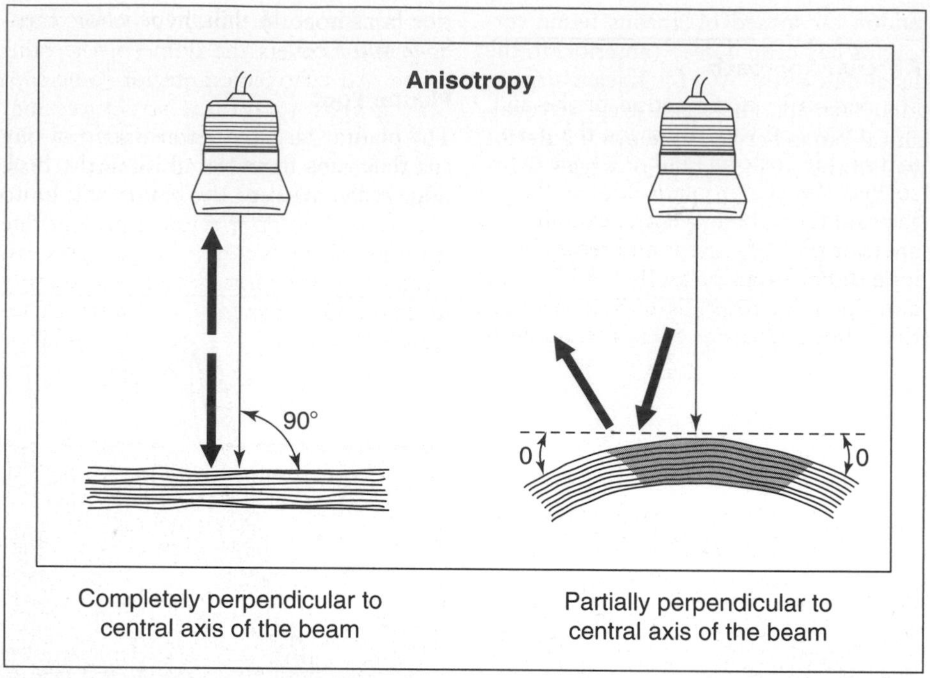

Figure 53-5. ■ *Anisotropy: straight tendon that is perpendicular to the central axis of the sound beam* (left). *In this case, the tendon appears echogenic and the fibers of the tendon are well visualized. Tendon traveling on a curved path* (right). *Portions of this tendon are not perpendicular to the central axis of the sound beam. In this case, the tendon appears hypoechoic along the portions that are not perpendicular. In those areas, the fibers of the tendon will be poorly visualized.*

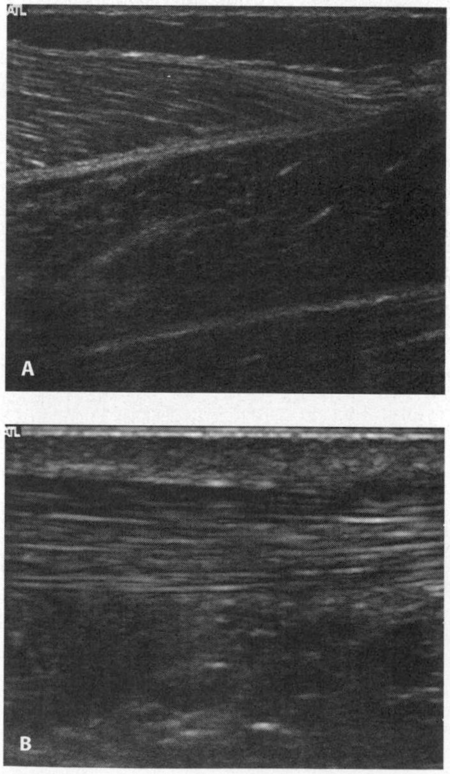

Figure 53-4. ■ *A. Longitudinal image of the medial calf complex shows the feather-like arrangement of a typical muscle bundle. B. Longitudinal image of the Achilles tendon denotes the typical echogenic parallel lines and homogeneous echogenic striated appearance.*

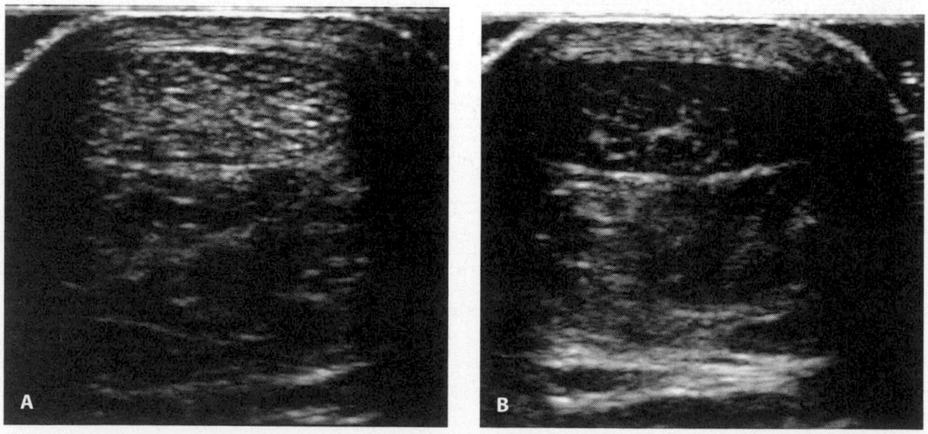

Figure 53-6. ■ *Anisotropy. A. Transverse image of an Achilles tendon that is perpendicular to the central axis of the sound beam. B. Transverse image of Achilles tendon that is not perpendicular but oblique to the central axis of the sound beam. The tendon appears hypoechoic in comparison with images obtained with the ideal angle.*

SCANNING PROTOCOL

Anterior Approach

We begin our examination of the anterior ankle and foot by laying the patient in a supine position, with the knee flexed so that the symptomatic foot is flat on the examining bed. We first examine the anterior tibiotalar joint and recess in the longitudinal scan plane (Fig. 53-7). This anterior joint recess is located between the echogenic distal tibia and dome of the talus bone. A thin, hypoechoic cartilage layer covers the dome of the talus bone. An echogenic anterior joint capsule drapes over these structures and closes off the joint anteriorly, thereby creating the anterior tibiotalar recess. Normally, this recess contains little or no fluid unless joint effusion is present due to an injury or pathologic process. Interrogate the joint medially to laterally to make sure that the entire anterior recess is scanned.

From the longitudinal scanning position of the anterior joint, continue by evaluating each of the extensor tendons. Scan each tendon in both longitudinal and transverse (short axis) planes. The largest and most medial tendon is the ATT. Start examining the ATT from the muscle–tendon junction proximally and then follow the ATT to its insertion onto the medial first cuneiform and base of the first metatarsal (Fig. 53-8). After scanning the ATT, examine the EHL lo-

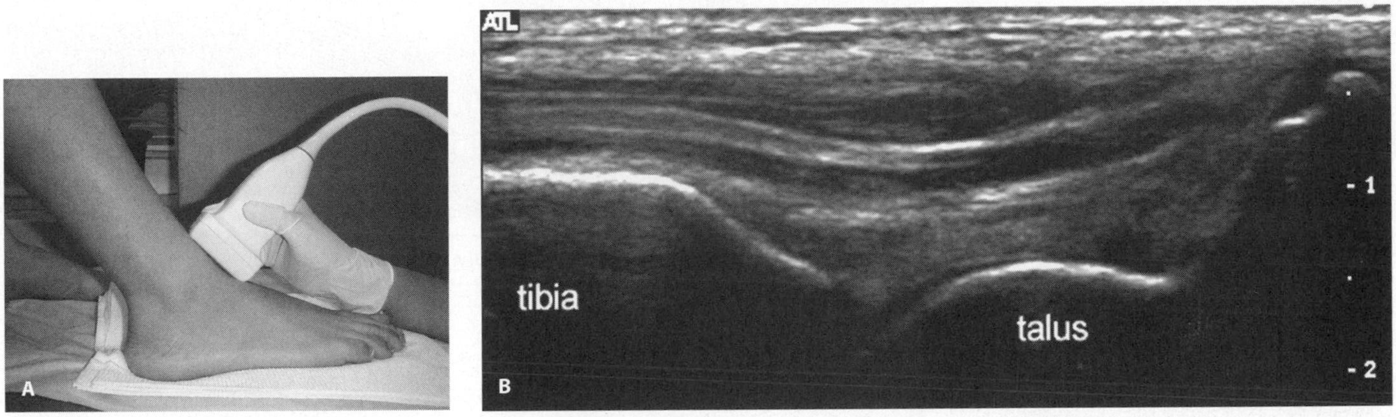

Figure 53-7. ■ *A. Transducer placement for longitudinal view of the anterior tibiotalar recess. B. Longitudinal image of the anterior tibiotalar recess.*

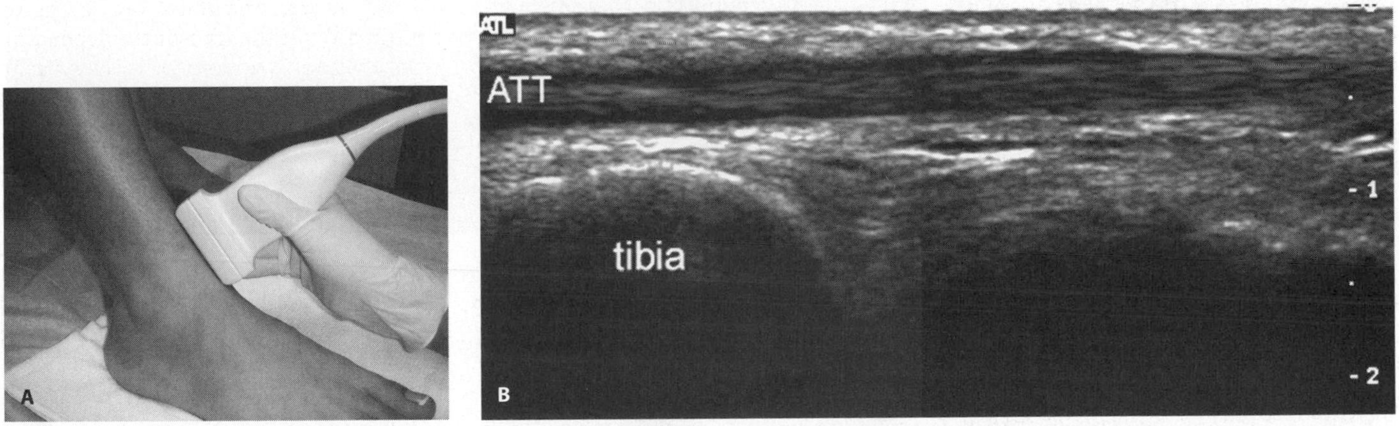

Figure 53-8. ■ *A. Transducer placement for longitudinal view of the anterior tibialis tendon (ATT). B. Longitudinal image of the ATT.*

cated just lateral to it. The EHL is scanned distally to its insertion on the base of the first distal phalanx dorsally (Fig. 53-9). The most lateral of the anterior extensors is the EDL (Fig. 53-10). The EDL branches out distally into four separate tendons that insert on the second through fifth toes.

Lateral Approach

The lateral extra-articular ankle and foot structures are examined by having the patient lie in a semioblique position, with the hip joint slightly internally rotated and the knee flexed so that the lateral aspect of the foot is lifted slightly off of the examining bed. The transducer is positioned over the posterior edge of the

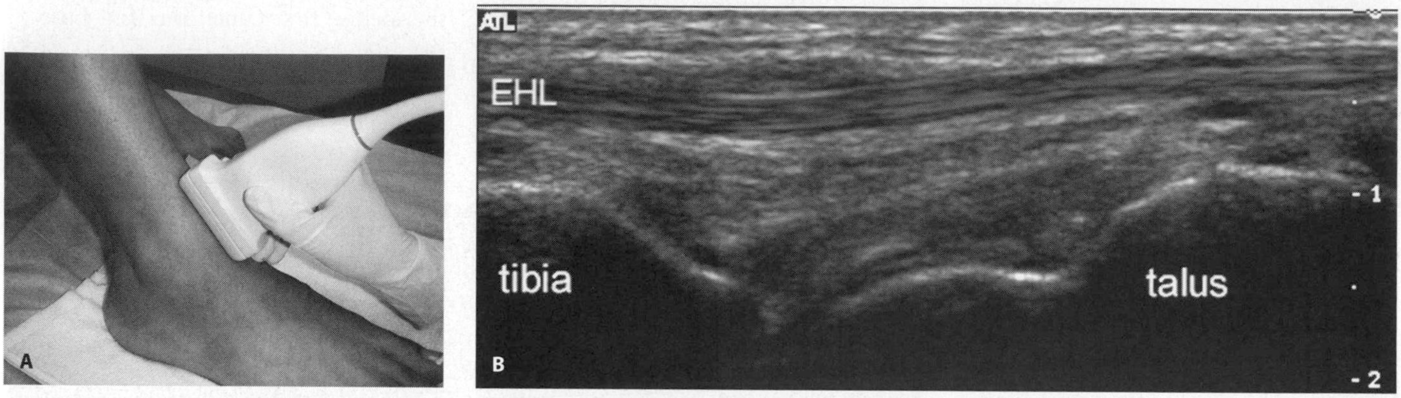

Figure 53-9. ■ *A. Transducer placement for longitudinal view of the extensor hallucis longus tendon* (EHL). *B. Longitudinal image of the EHL.*

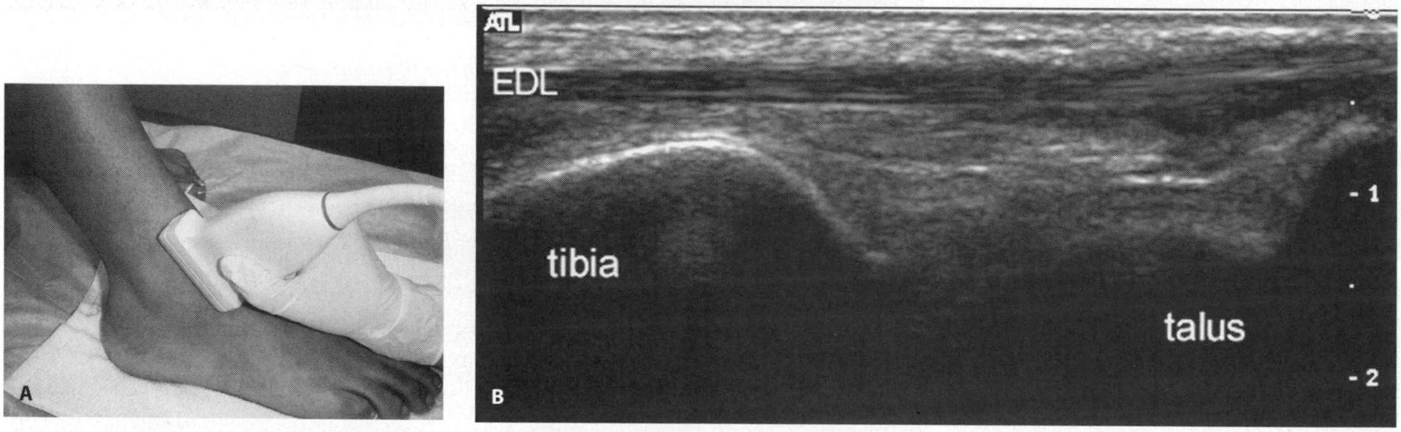

Figure 53-10. ■ *A. Transducer placement for longitudinal view of the extensor digitorum longus tendon* (EDL). *B. Longitudinal image of the EDL tendon.*

lateral malleolus (distal fibula) in a transverse plane. In this plane, we can see the PL and PB course behind the lateral malleolus in the retrofibular groove (Fig. 53-11). The PB is located more anteriorly than the longus and closer to the fibula. After interrogating the peroneal tendons transversely, turn the transducer to the longitudinal axis (Fig. 53-12) and

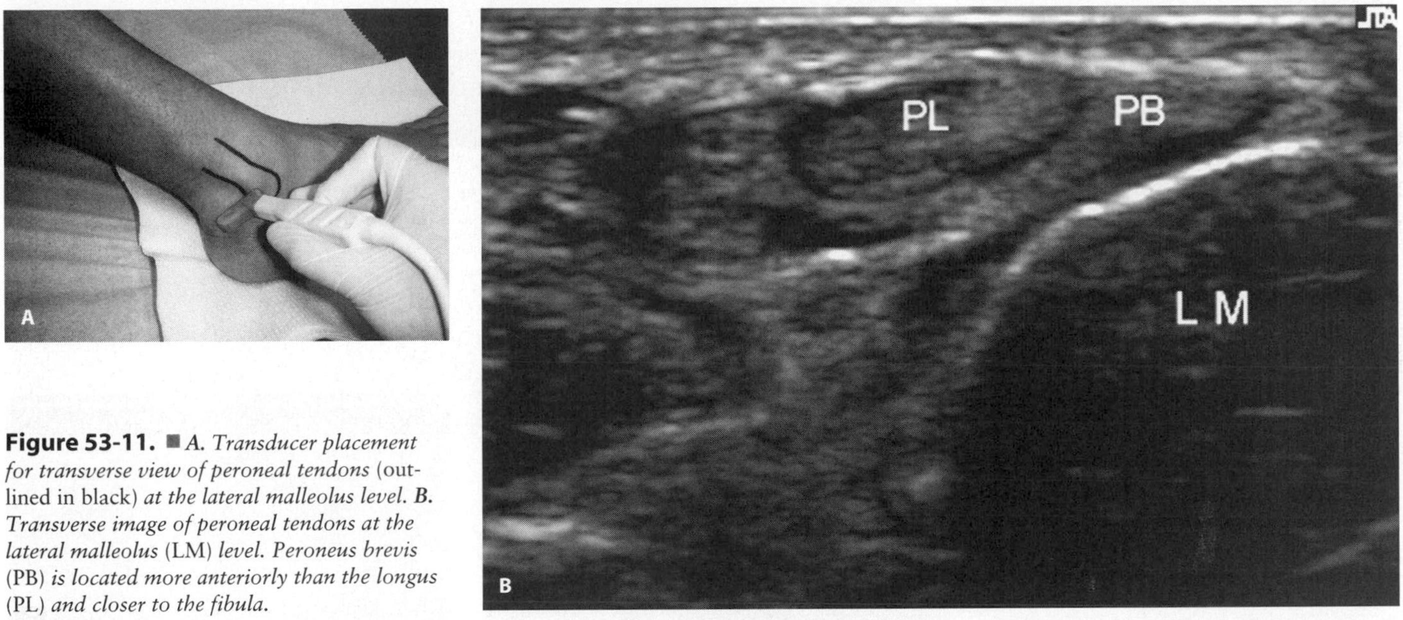

Figure 53-11. ■ *A. Transducer placement for transverse view of peroneal tendons* (outlined in black) *at the lateral malleolus level. B. Transverse image of peroneal tendons at the lateral malleolus* (LM) *level. Peroneus brevis* (PB) *is located more anteriorly than the longus* (PL) *and closer to the fibula.*

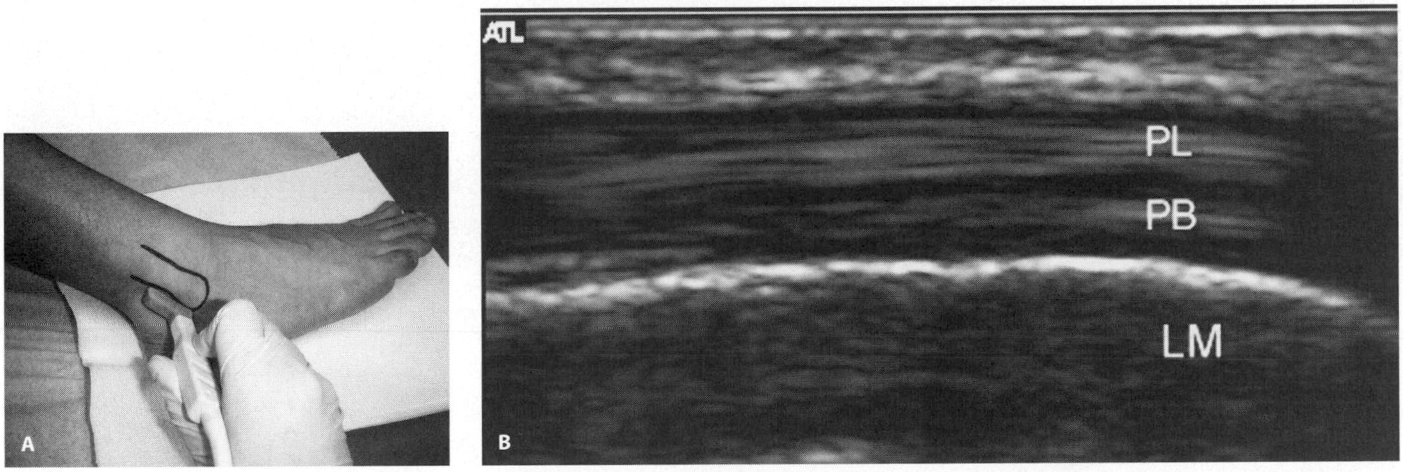

Figure 53-12. ■ *A. Transducer placement for longitudinal view of the peroneal tendons at the lateral malleolus level. B. Longitudinal image of peroneal tendons at the lateral malleolus* (LM) *level.*

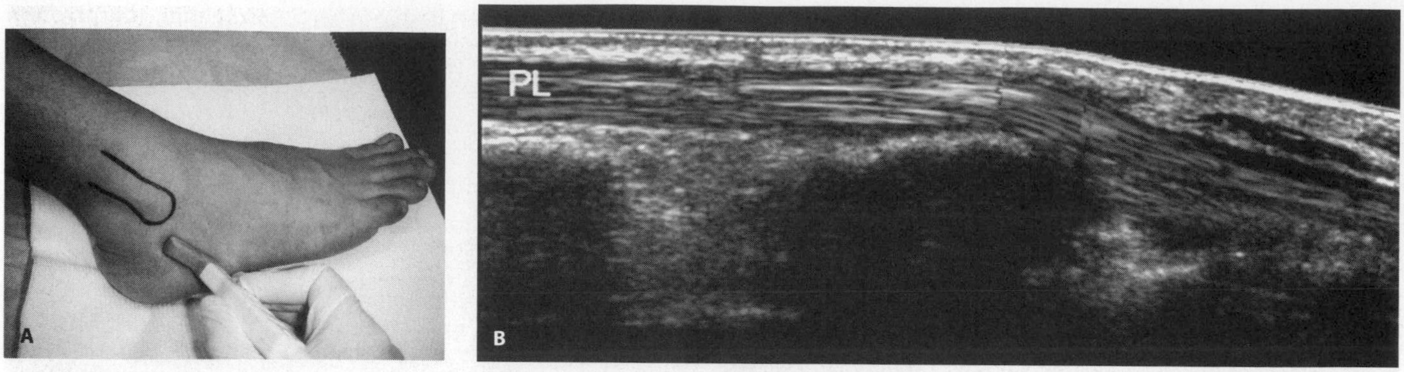

Figure 53-13. ■ *A. Transducer placement for longitudinal view of peroneal longus* (PL) *below the lateral malleolus level. B. Longitudinal image of PL below the lateral malleolus level.*

follow the PB distally onto the tubercle of the fifth metatarsal base (Fig. 53-14). Then the PL is imaged distally to where it dives deep toward the plantar portion (Fig. 53-13). To dynamically test the peroneal tendons for subluxation from their retrofibular groove, position the transducer transversely over the lateral malle-

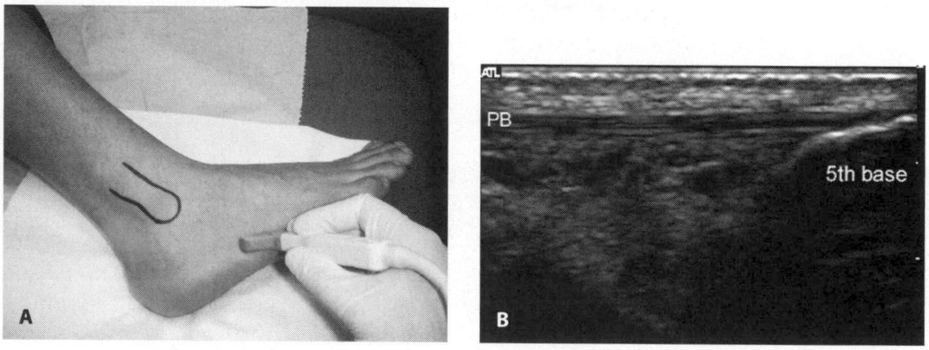

Figure 53-14. ■ *A. Transducer placement for longitudinal view of peroneus brevis even further below the lateral malleolus level. B. Longitudinal image of peroneus brevis* (PB) *below the lateral malleolus level and inserting on the fifth metatarsal base.*

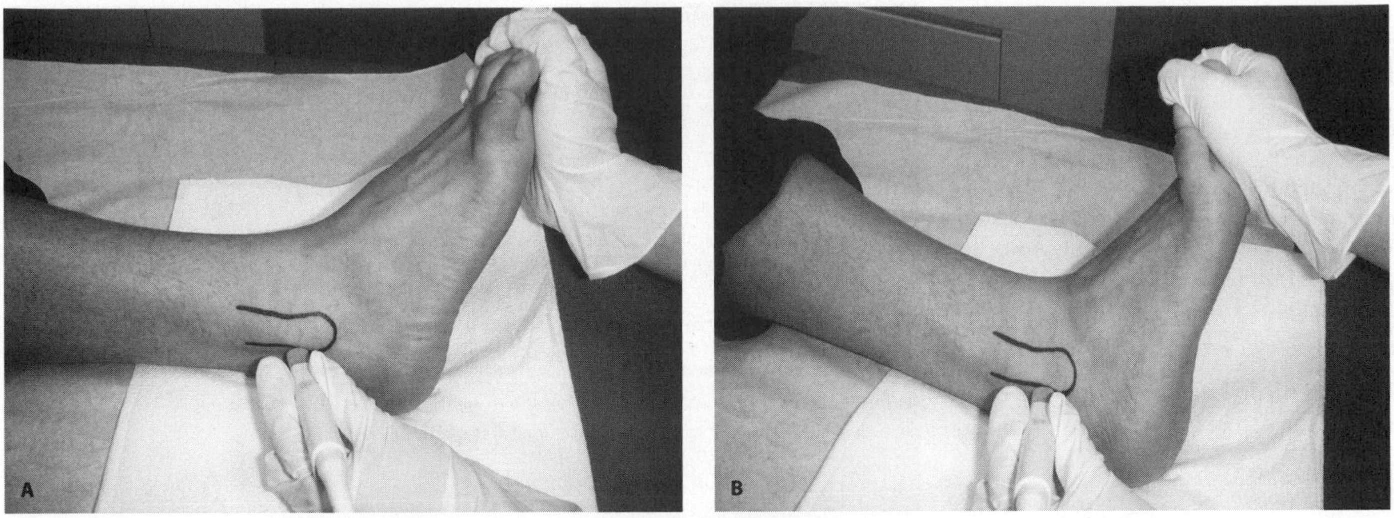

Figure 53-15. ■ *Peroneal subluxation test. A. Neutral rest position: transducer placement for transverse view of peroneal tendons at the lateral malleolus* (outlined in black) *level. B. Stress maneuver: the transducer is held in the same position, and the ankle is dorsiflexed and everted.*

olus with one hand and with the other dorsiflex and evert the ankle (Fig. 53-15). In a positive subluxation test, one or both of the peroneal tendons would pop partially or fully over the lateral malleolus. At the inframalleolar level, it is common to see a small trace of fluid in the tendon sheath.

There are a number of lateral collateral ligaments attached to the distal fibula. The most commonly injured is the ATFL. The ATFL originates from the anterior lateral aspect of the distal fibula and passes anteriorly and medially to insert onto the neck of the talus. The ATFL is seen as a thin, echogenic band (2–3 mm) when the transducer is positioned between the bony distal fibula and the neck of talus (Fig. 53-16).

Medial Approach

In the interest of ergonomics, we have the patient lie supine with the affected leg in a frog position. The hip joint is ex-

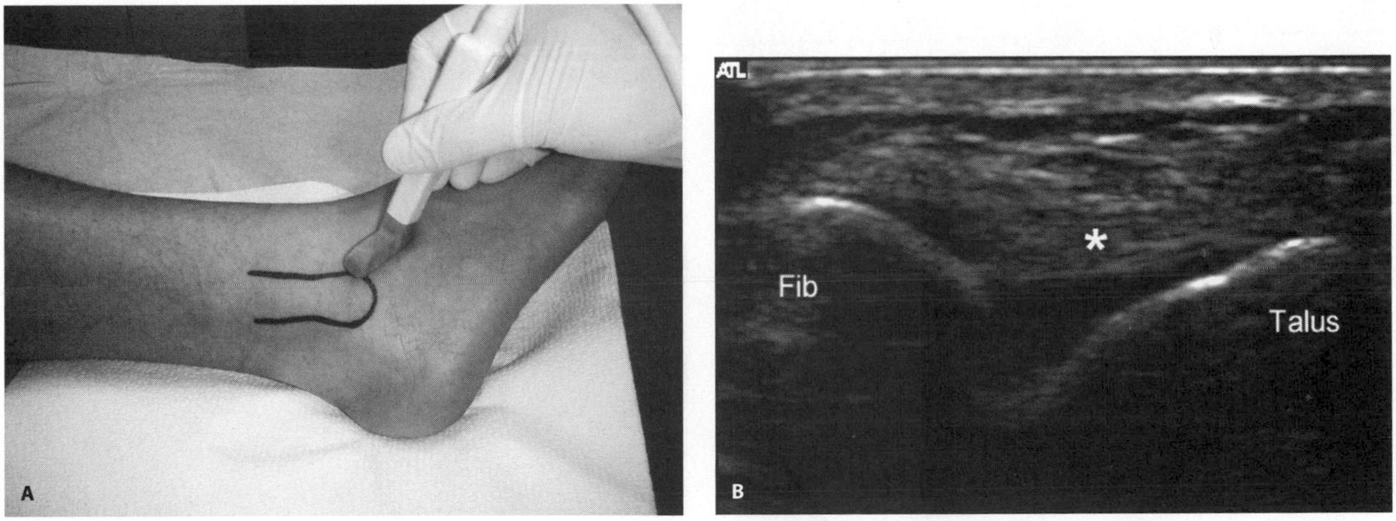

Figure 53-16. ■ *A. Transducer placement for longitudinal view of the anterior talofibular ligament* (ATFL). *Position the transducer between the anterior-lateral aspect of the distal fibula* (Fib), *and then angle anteriorly and medially toward the neck of the talus. B. Longitudinal image of the* ATFL.

ternally rotated, the knee is partially flexed, and the lateral aspect of the foot is in contact with the examination table. This position allows easier access to the soft tissue extra-articular structures between the medial malleolus and ACH. It is important to remember the relationship the medial tendons have to each other and their corresponding bony insertion points. The medial tendon arrangement is better visualized in the transverse (short axis) scanning plane. Positioning the transducer with one end over the medial malleolus and the other end in the direction of the ACH allows us to visualize medial structures in the transverse plane.

The PTT is the most medial of medial ankle tendons and is located next to the medial malleolus. The PTT is scanned in both planes from its muscle tendon junction proximally to the distal insertion onto the tarsal navicular (Figs. 53-17 and 53-18). In longitudinal orientation, the distal PTT fibers can be seen fanning out onto the navicular bone and will appear more hypoechoic. Note that this hypoechoic appearance distally could be mistaken for tendinopathy. Normally at the inframalleolar level, some fluid may be present in the tendon sheath.

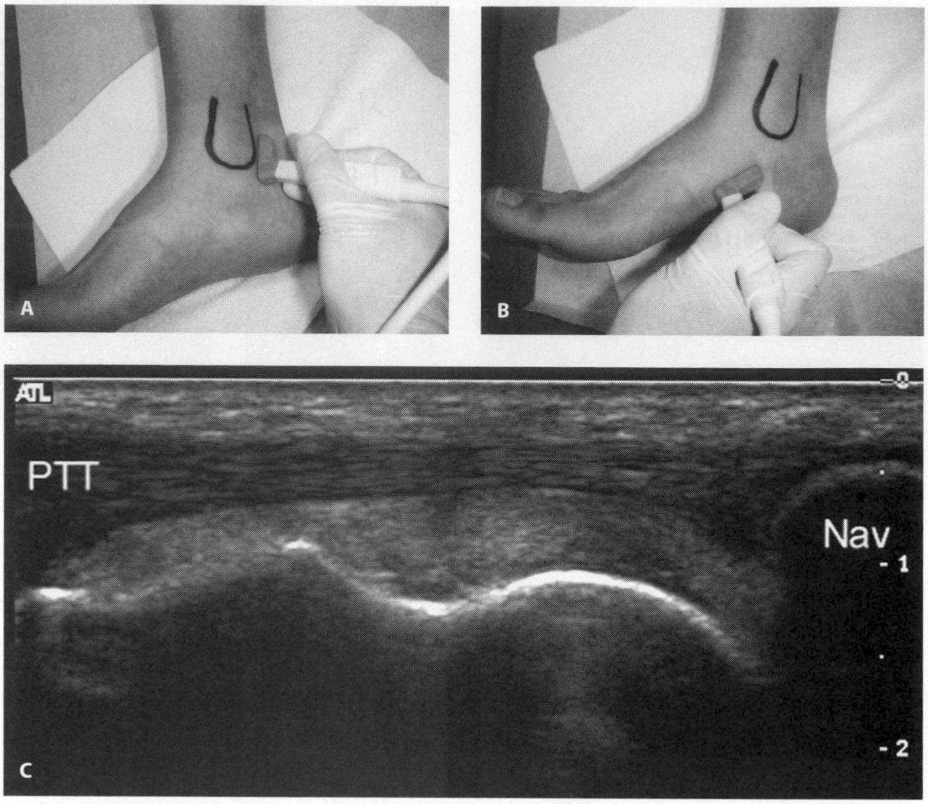

Figure 53-17. ■ *Proximal (A) and distal (B) transducer placement for longitudinal view of posterior tibialis tendon* (PTT) *next to the medial malleolus* (outlined in black). *C. Longitudinal image of the PTT inserting distally on to the tarsal navicular* (Nav).

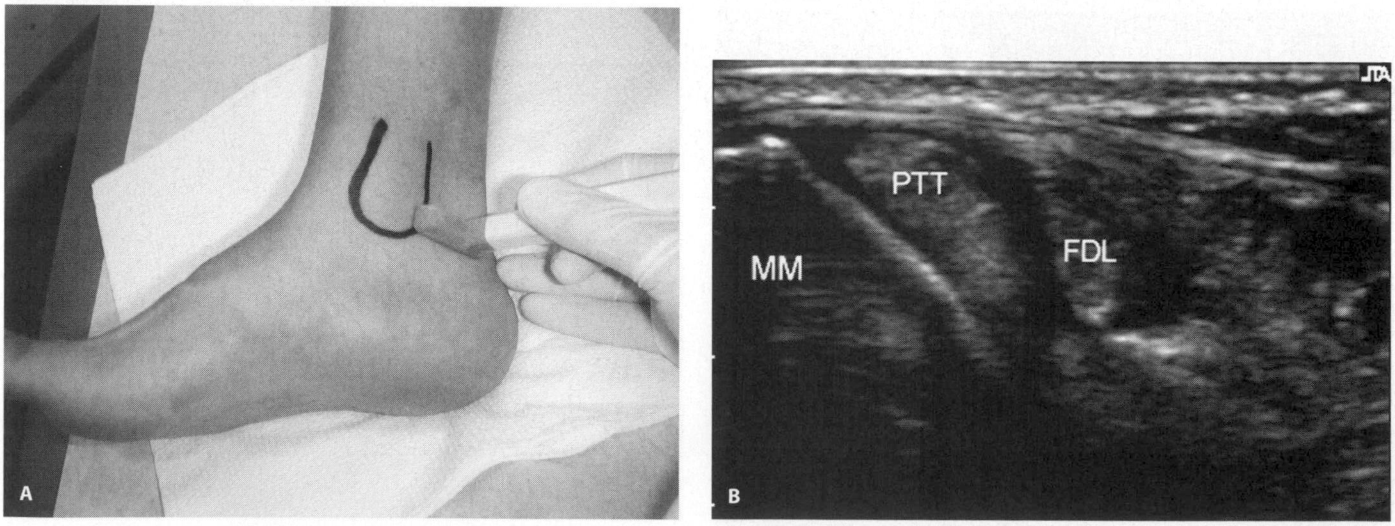

Figure 53-18. ■ *A. Transducer placement for transverse view of posterior tibialis tendon next to the medial malleolus* (MM). *B. Transverse image of the posterior tibialis tendon* (PTT) *and adjacent flexor digitorum longus tendon* (FDL).

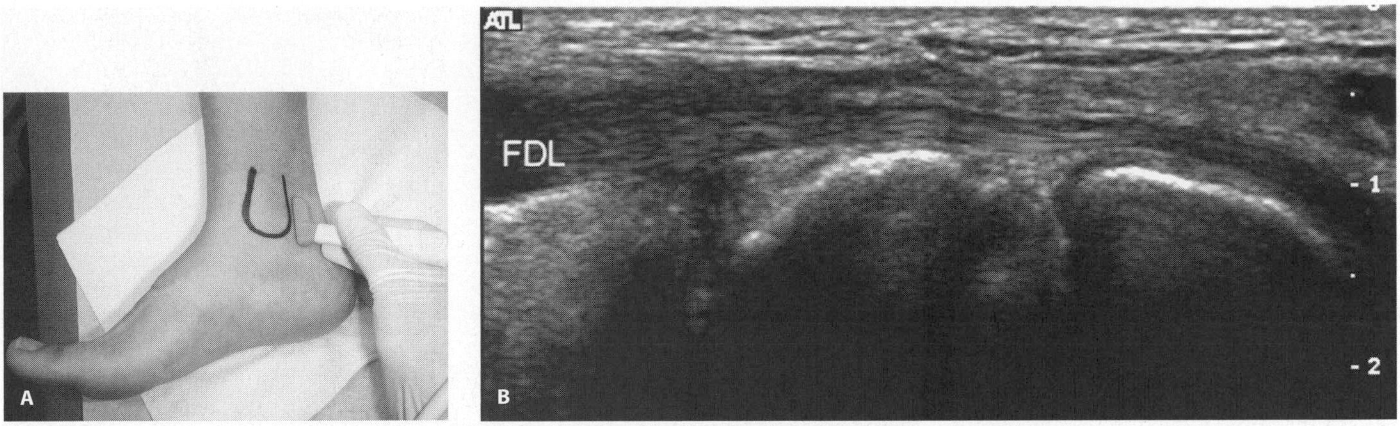

Figure 53-19. ■ *A. Transducer placement for longitudinal view of flexor digitorum longus tendon* (FDL) *laterally from the posterior tibialis tendon. B. Longitudinal image of the FDL.*

Scanning more laterally to the PTT is the adjacent FDL tendon. In the transverse plane, we can appreciate that the FDL has a much smaller tendon diameter compared with the PTT. Routinely, the FDL is imaged distally to where it dives deep toward the plantar portion (Fig. 53-19). It is rare to see pathologic conditions of the FDL distal to this level.

Located between the FDL and the FHL is a neurovascular bundle consisting of the posterior tibial artery, venae comitantes (usually two veins), and tibial nerve. The vascular structures can be more readily identified with the use of color Doppler. The posterior tibial nerve can be visualized around these vascular landmarks with the use of a high-frequency transducer (Fig. 53-20). The posterior tibial nerve will appear more hypoechoic in echogenicity at the ankle joint level in comparison with the surrounding echogenic perineural fat.

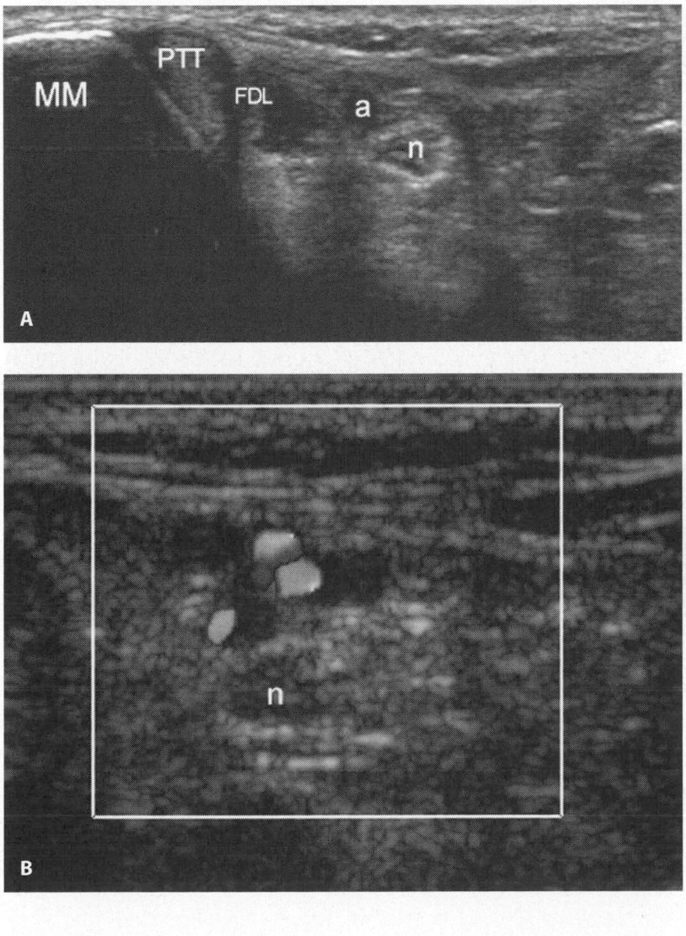

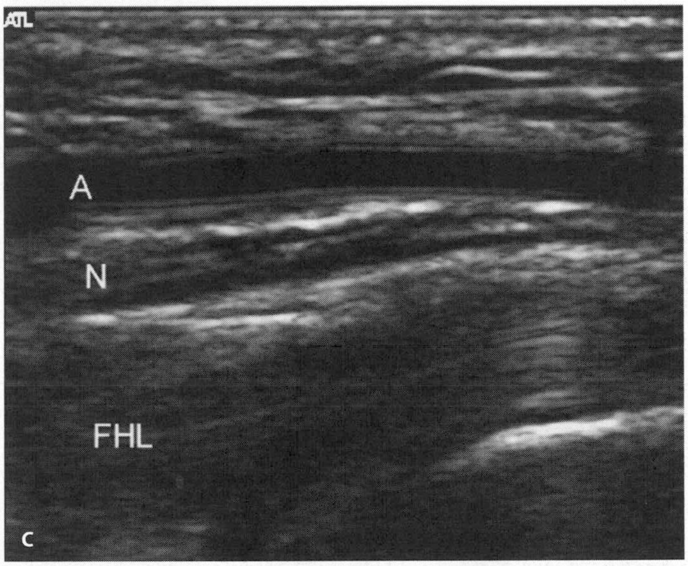

Figure 53-20. ■ *A. Transverse image of the neurovascular bundle. The hypoechoic appearing posterior tibial nerve* (PTN) *is surrounded by echogenic perineural fat. B. Color Doppler imaging easily shows the artery and associated venous structures next to the posterior tibial nerve* (n) *in transverse section. C. Longitudinal image of the posterior tibial artery* (A), *posterior tibial nerve* (N), *and flexor hallucis longus tendon* (FHL).

The FHL is the most deep and lateral tendon of the medial ankle tendons. The FHL tendon is located medial to the ACH. The FHL inserts onto the plantar aspect of the distal phalanx of the first toe (Fig. 53-21).

An easy way to confirm the identity of the FHL in the longitudinal plane is to manually flex and extend the patient's first toe under real-time analysis.

Posterior and Plantar Approach

A common cause of posterior ankle pain is the ACH. Not only is ultrasound exquisite in showing the fine architecture of the ACH, but it is also exquisite in de-

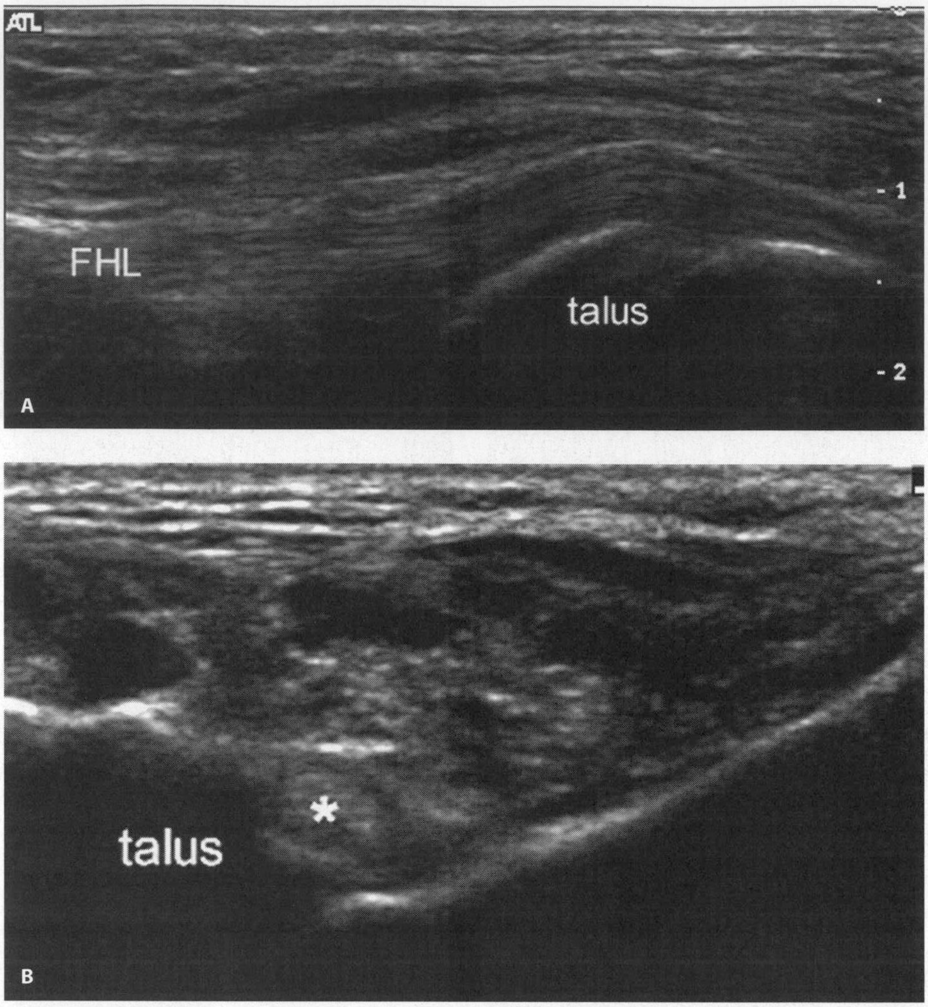

Figure 53-21. ■ *A. Longitudinal image of flexor hallucis longus tendon* (FHL) *posterior to the talus. B. Transverse image of the flexor hallucis longus tendon* (*) *in posterior talar groove.*

picting any surrounding bursal abnormality. The ACH is easy to scan and visualize with ultrasound because of its large diameter and linear course. The patient lies prone with both feet hanging off the end of the examination bed. The patient dorsiflexes the ankle to bring the ACH into a more linear path to reduce any potential anisotropy. Longitudinally, the ACH is interrogated from its origin (gastrocnemius and soleus muscles) to its distal insertion on the calcaneus (Figs. 53-22 and 53-23). When the ACH is scanned transversely, the transducer is positioned slightly more toward the me-

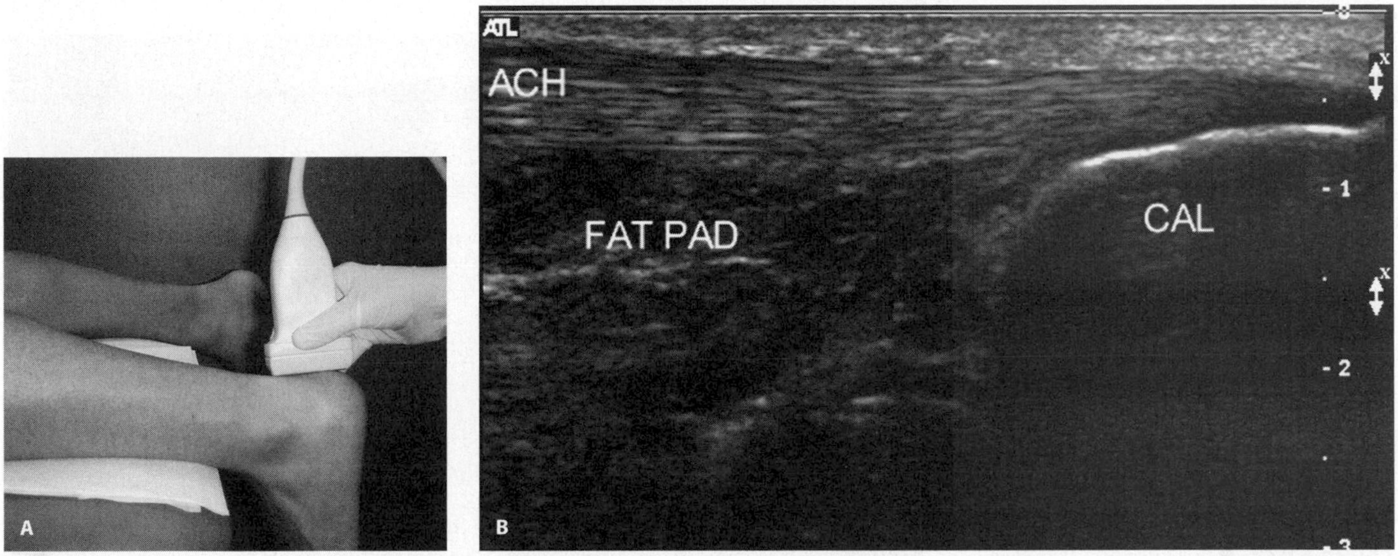

Figure 53-22. ■ *A. Transducer placement for longitudinal view of distal Achilles tendon. B. Longitudinal image of the distal Achilles tendon (ACH).*

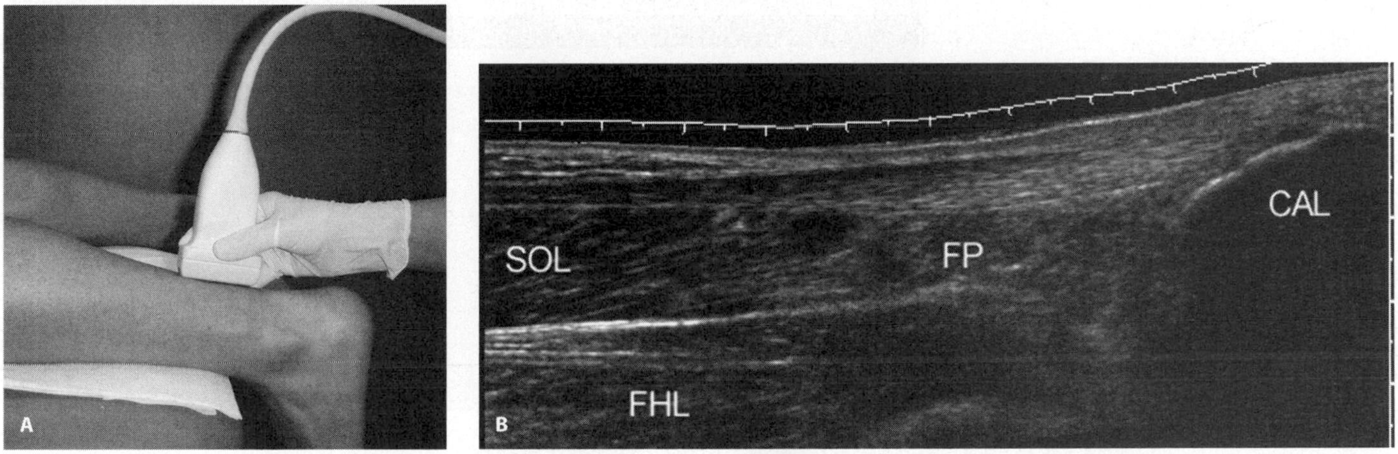

Figure 53-23. ■ *A. Transducer placement for longitudinal view of proximal Achilles tendon. B. Longitudinal extended field-of-view image of the proximal to distal Achilles tendon; fat pad* (FP).

dial aspect of the tendon (Fig. 53-24). This allows us to compensate for the slight medial obliquity of the ACH and achieve a better diagnostic view.

To evaluate the plantar fascia, the patient is scanned in the same position. However, it may help the sonographer to elevate the examining bed to reduce the pressure on the scanning arm. To examine the large medial band of the plantar fascia, the transducer is longitudinally positioned over the medial tubercle of the calcaneus and oriented to follow the medial band to the ball of the foot where it thins out (Fig. 53-25). The lateral band is a small, thinner fibrous band (rarely involved with plantar fasciitis) that can

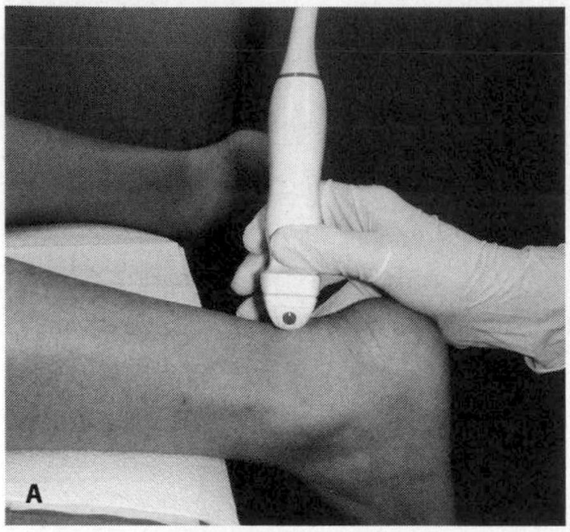

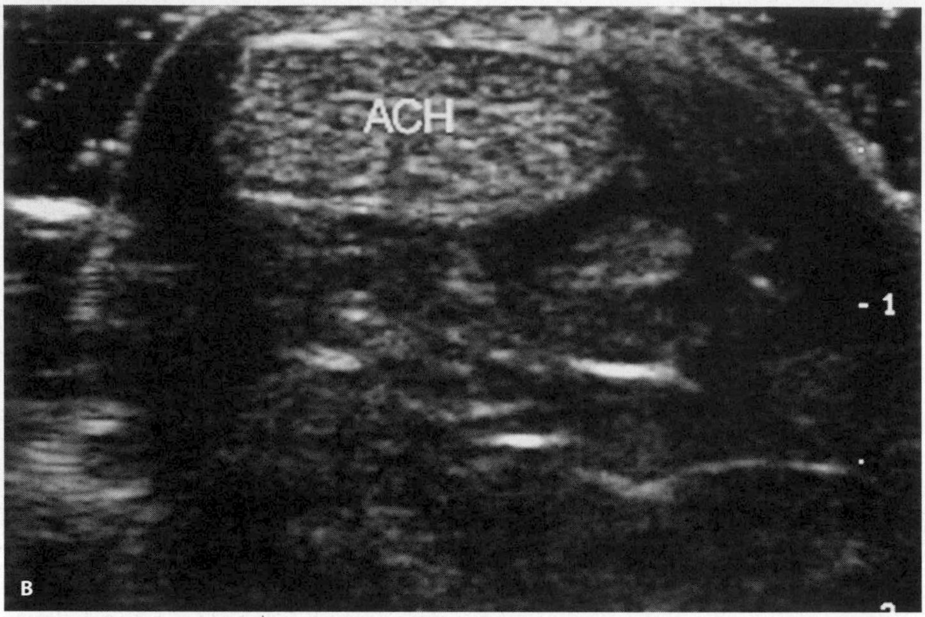

Figure 53-24. ■ *A. Transducer placement for transverse view of mid-Achilles tendon. B. Transverse image of the Achilles tendon (ACH).*

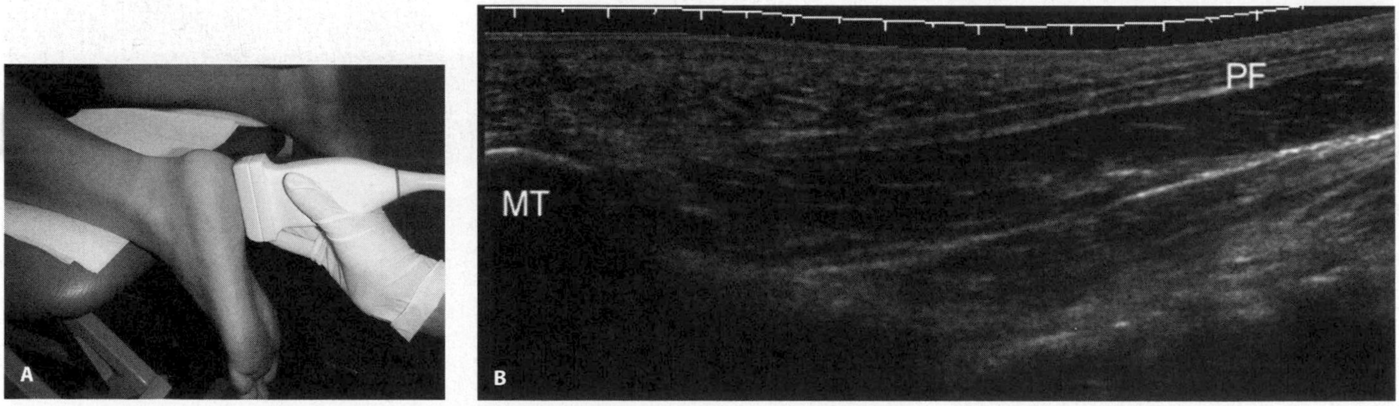

Figure 53-25. ■ *A. Transducer placement for longitudinal view of the medial band of the plantar fascia. B. Longitudinal extended field-of-view image of the medial band plantar fascia (PF) from the medial tubercle* (MT) *of the calcaneus to the ball of the foot.*

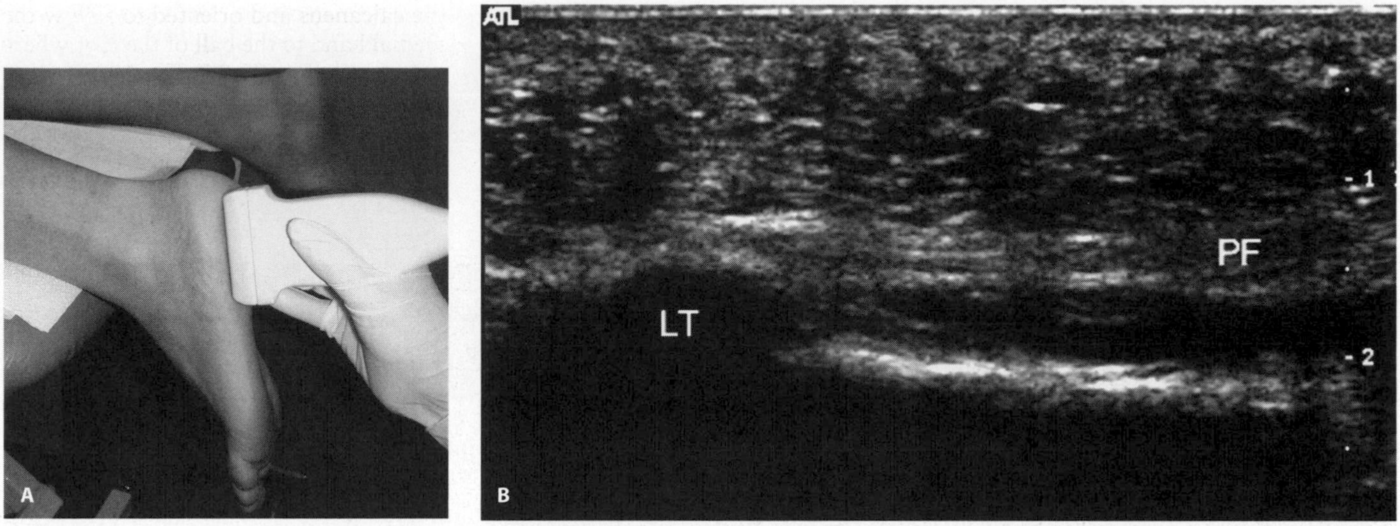

Figure 53-26. ■ *A. Transducer placement for longitudinal view of the lateral band of the plantar fascia. B. Longitudinal image of the thinner lateral band plantar fascia (PF) from the smaller lateral tubercle (LT) of the calcaneus.*

be scanned in a similar fashion (Fig. 53-26).

Common Injuries and Pathologies

ANTERIOR

Ankle Joint Effusion

An acute ankle injury or an intra-articular pathologic process often causes an ankle joint effusion. With ultrasound, fluid in the anterior tibiotalar recess is easily identified as described earlier. The anterior tibiotalar recess will distend with joint fluid (Fig. 53-27). Sometimes loose bodies may be identified within the recess. Clinically, these patients may exhibit difficulty in dorsiflexion of the ankle because of the effusion.

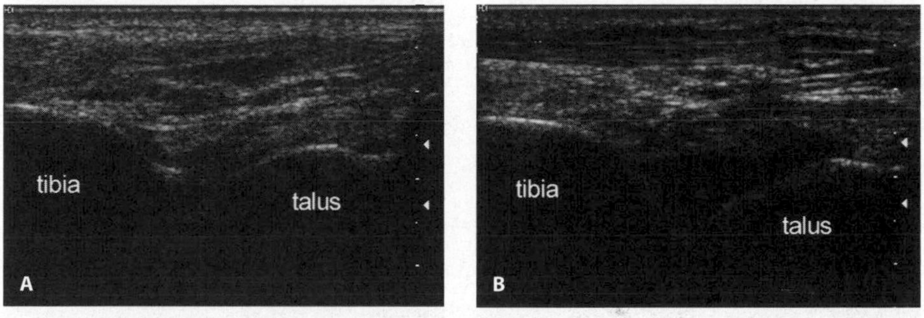

Figure 53-27. ■ *A. Longitudinal image of the asymptomatic anterior tibiotalar recess with no fluid present. B. Longitudinal image of the symptomatic anterior tibiotalar recess with moderate joint effusion seen.*

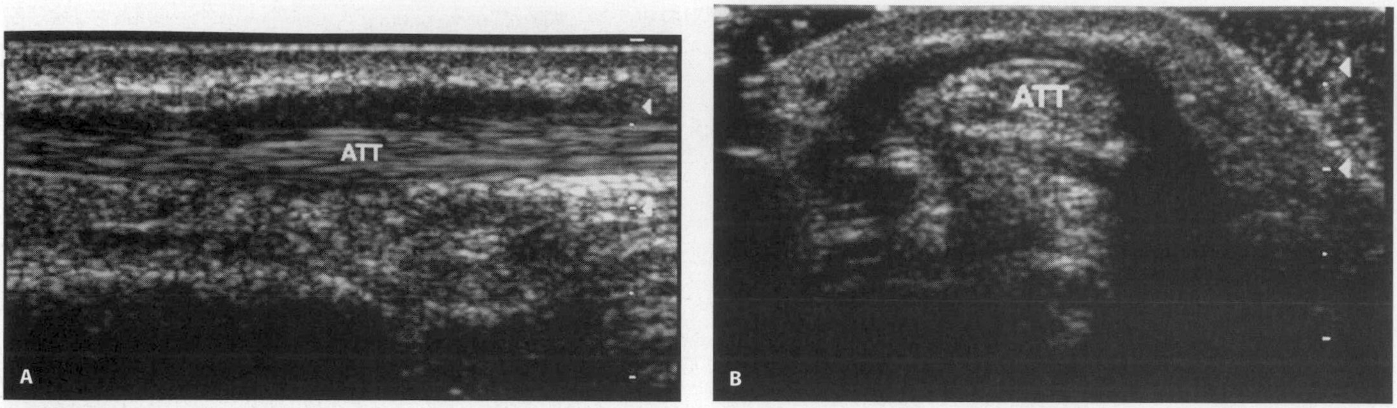

Figure 53-28. ■ *A. Longitudinal image with increased hypoechoic synovial fluid within the tendon sheath of the anterior tibialis tendon (ATT). **B.** Transverse image of the ATT showing the fluid surrounding the tendon.*

Anterior Extensor Tendon Injuries

Soft tissue injuries to the anterior tendon complex of the ankle and foot are less common than those of the medial and lateral compartments. One may sometimes encounter tenosynovitis or a rupture of the ATT. With tenosynovitis of a long tendon such as the ATT, a hypoechoic fluid collection will be seen encompassing the echogenic tendon (Fig. 53-28).

MEDIAL

Posterior Tibial Tendon Tear

As with the anterior tendon complex, the medial complex is also prone to tendinopathy and tendon tears. A patient with PTT tenosynovitis or tear may present with soft tissue swelling posterior to the medial malleolus. The PTT is most susceptible to tendinopathy and tearing at the level where it curves over the distal medial malleolus. When the PTT ruptures, there is complete tendon discontinuity and a tendon gap occurs between the two retracted tendon ends (Fig. 53-29). With acutely ruptured PTT, fluid is frequently seen within the gap, which is maintained by the remaining tendon sheath. With chronic old PTT rupture, echogenic scar tissue may be present instead of fluid.

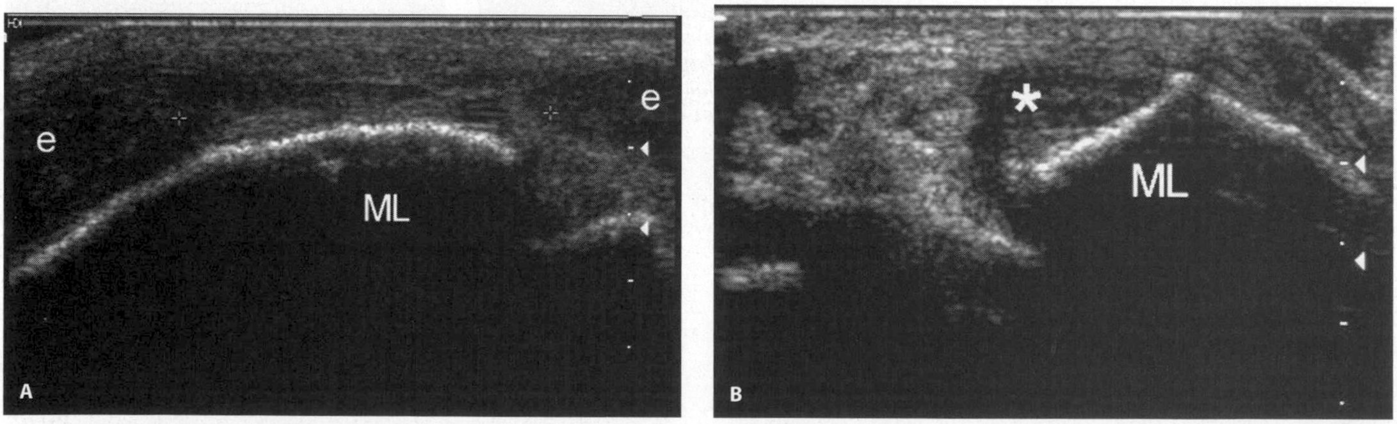

Figure 53-29. ■ *A. Longitudinal image shows complete posterior tibialis tendon rupture at the medial malleolar level* (ML). *Fluid gap is seen between the two retracted tendon ends* (e). ***B.*** *Transverse image at the gap showing tendon discontinuity* (*).

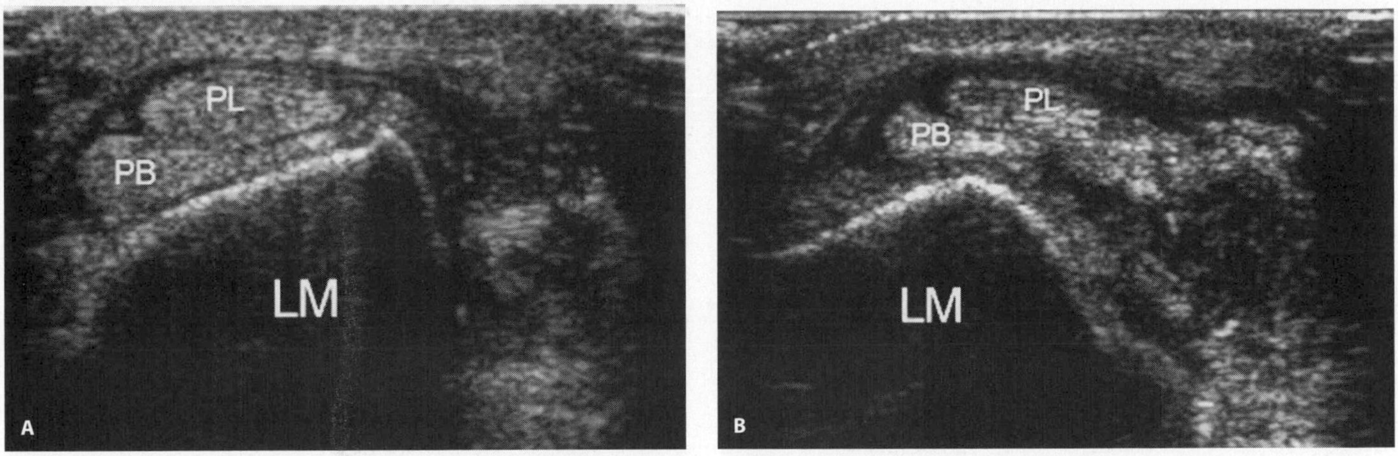

Figure 53-30. ■ *A. Transverse image of the peroneal tendons with the ankle in neutral rest position. The peroneal tendons are seen in the retrofibular groove. B. Transverse image of the peroneal tendons with the ankle dorsiflexed and everted (stress maneuver). The peroneal longus (PL) is seen completely subluxed and the peroneus brevis (PB) partially subluxed from the retrofibular groove.*

LATERAL

Peroneal Tendon Subluxation

Injuries to the peroneal complex are often related to a damaged superior peroneal retinaculum and can lead to subluxation or dislocation of the peroneal tendons. This may result in tenosynovitis, tendinopathy, or tendon split tears. Always dynamically stress the peroneal tendons for subluxation from their retrofibular groove by positioning the transducer transversely over the lateral malleolus with one hand and dorsiflexing and everting the ankle with the other hand. In a positive subluxation test, one or both of the peroneal tendons will pop partially or fully over the lateral malleolus (Fig. 53-30).

POSTERIOR: ACHILLES TENDON

Tendinopathy

The ACH is the most frequently injured ankle tendon. Injuries range from tendinopathy, bursitis, and partial to complete tears of the tendon. In a normal ACH, the fibers are tightly organized and uniform in echogenicity. With moderate tendinopathy, the fibers become more separated, and the tendon appears more hypoechoic in the affected area. The tendon may have an overall fusiform shape. Normal thickness varies in individuals; therefore, bilateral comparison is often done to determine tendon normality. A 2-mm difference in thickness at the same level has been shown to be significant. Normally, the ACH is a relatively avascular structure, but when active tendinopathy exists, hyperemic flow in the swollen tendon can be visualized using power Doppler imaging (Fig. 53-31).

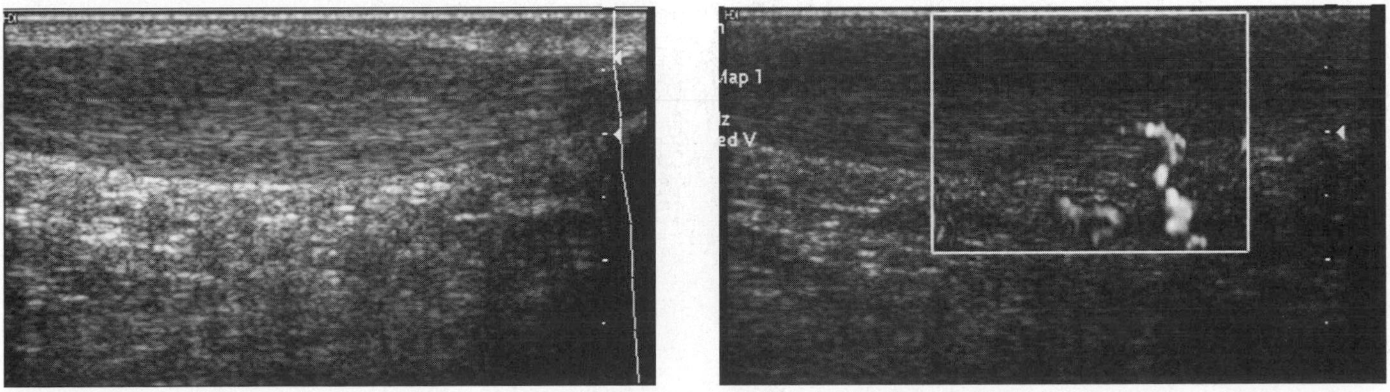

Figure 53-31. ■ *A. Longitudinal image of the Achilles tendon shows moderate fusiform tendinopathy. B. Power Doppler shows hyperemia within the Achilles tendon.*

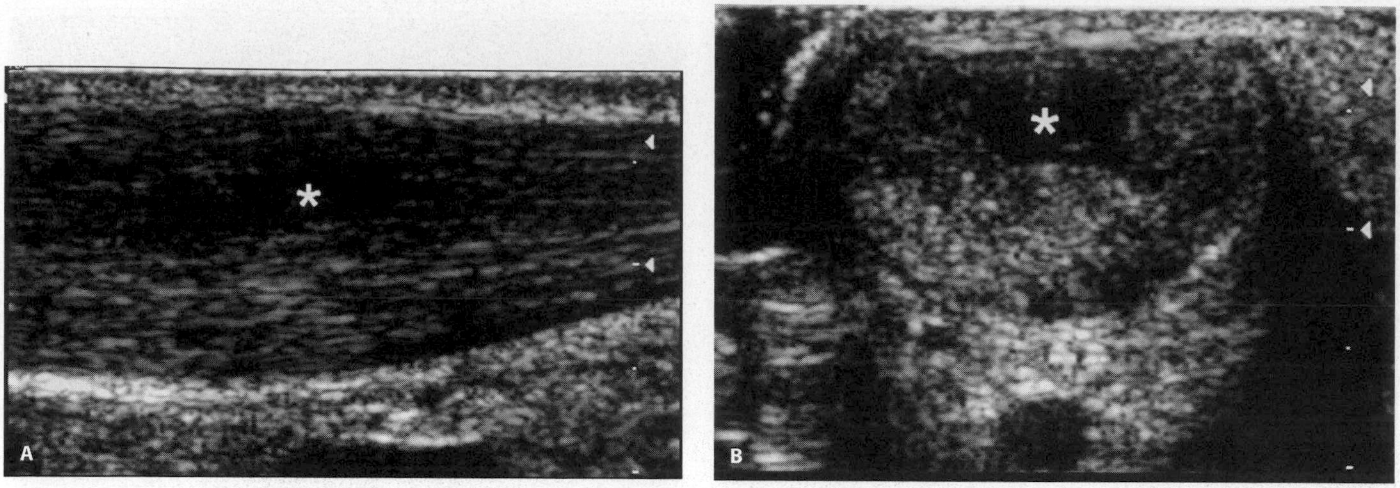

Figure 53-32. ■ *A. Longitudinal image of the Achilles tendon shows midtendinopathy and a partial intrasubstance tear. Hypoechoic defect (*) is visualized within the fibers. B. Transverse image of intratendon hypoechoic defect (*).*

Partial Tears

High-resolution ultrasound is exquisite at detecting small partial intrasubstance tears within a tendon. Partial tears and degeneration within the ACH may predispose individuals to complete ruptures. These partial tears on ultrasound are often seen accompanying tendinopathy. Partial intrasubstance tears display some discontinuity in the fibers of the tendon and often appear as hypoechoic defects within the tendon (Fig. 53-32).

Complete Tears

Ultrasound plays an important role in evaluating complete rupture of the ACH. Clinically it may be difficult to evaluate the tendon for complete tear due to extensive posttraumatic swelling around the area. The following are the ultrasound characteristics of a ruptured ACH (Fig. 53-33):

1. An anechoic or heterogeneous defect due to a recent hematoma
2. Retracted and swollen ends of the tendon, associated with refraction and shadowing
3. Fat filling in the gap

It is important to note that when there is some sparing of some medial fibers of a ruptured ACH, this preserved area may be confused with an intact plantaris tendon. Do not mistake this for a high partial tear of the ACH. Approximately 20% of the population do not have a plantaris tendon. In patients in whom it is difficult to clearly tell the margins of a tear and whether there a complete tear, it is helpful to incorporate a clinical test called the Thompson test (Fig. 53-34). With the patient lying prone, the calf is squeezed. The foot should plantar flex in a patient who does not have a completely torn ACH. Note during this clinical test whether the two ends move separately or as one unit.

Retrocalcaneal Bursitis

A deep retrocalcaneal bursa lies between the distal anterior wall of the ACH and

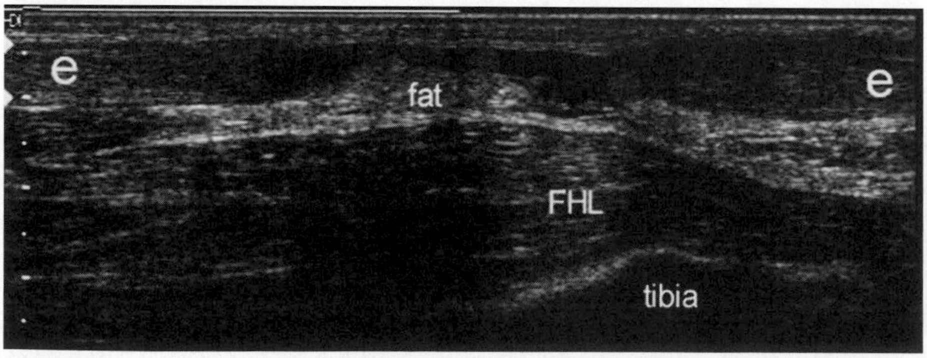

Figure 53-33. ■ *Longitudinal image of the Achilles tendon showing complete rupture. Hypoechoic fluid gap is seen separating the two retracted tendon ends* (e), *and fat is seen herniating into the tear.*

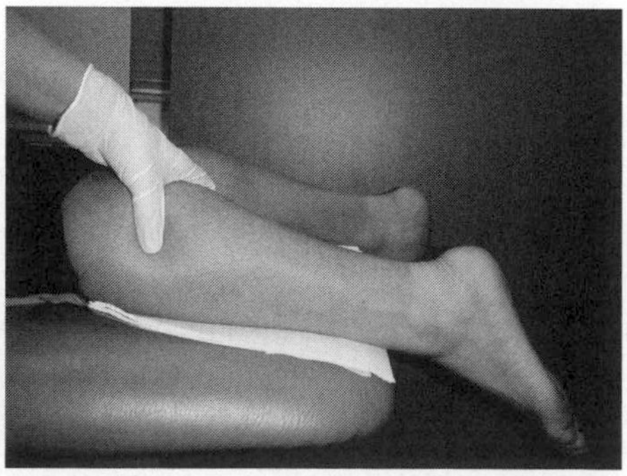

Figure 53-34. ■ *Thompson test. With the patient lying prone, the calf is squeezed. The foot should plantar flex in a patient who does not have a completely torn ACH.*

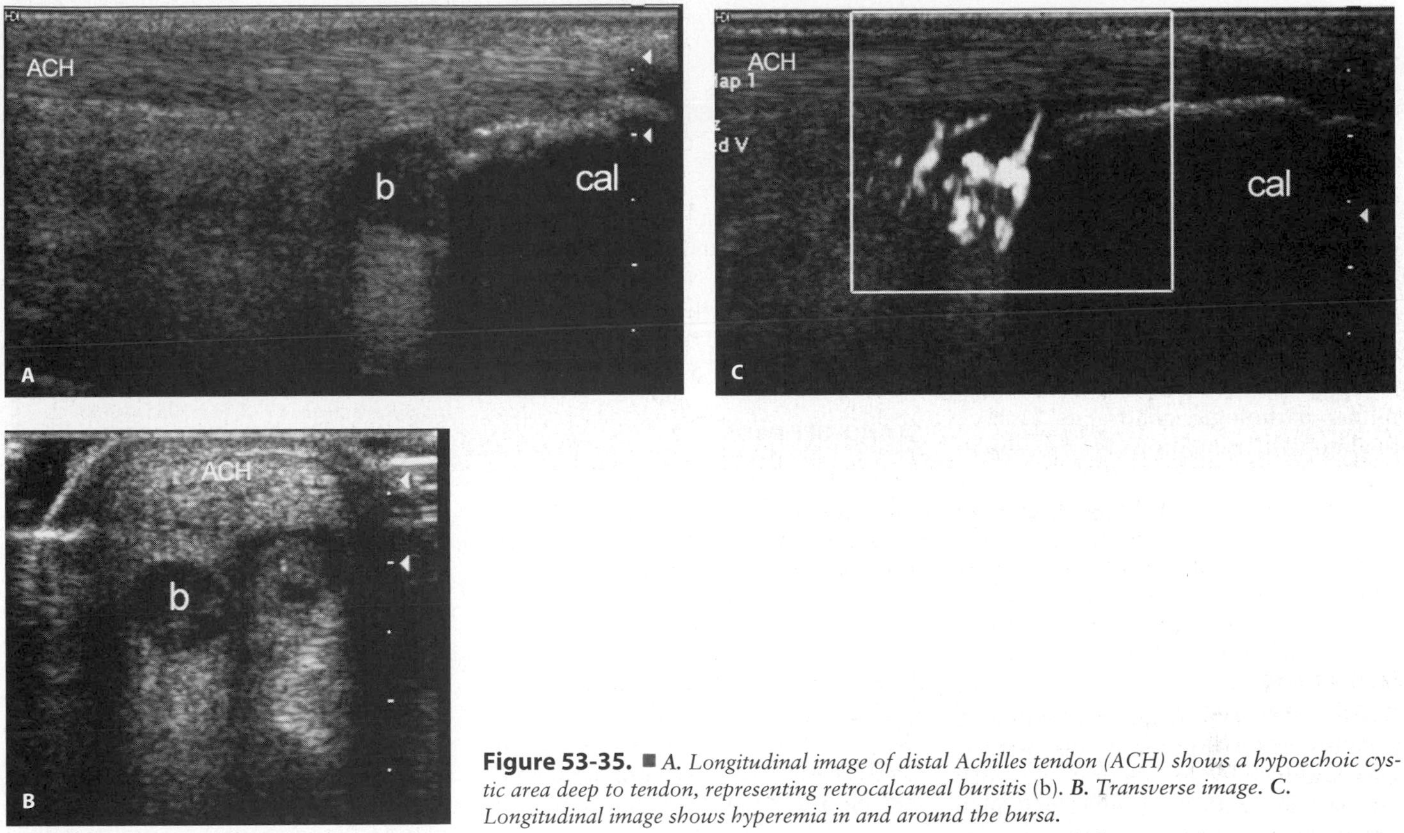

Figure 53-35. ■ *A. Longitudinal image of distal Achilles tendon (ACH) shows a hypoechoic cystic area deep to tendon, representing retrocalcaneal bursitis* (b). ***B.** Transverse image.* ***C.** Longitudinal image shows hyperemia in and around the bursa.*

posterior superior border of the calcaneus. Retrocalcaneal bursitis is usually caused by overuse and can be present with or without an associated Achilles tendinopathy. Often the bursa becomes distended with fluid, and some synovial perforation occurs within the bursa. Power Doppler will show increased hyperemia with an acutely inflamed retrocalcaneal bursa (Fig. 53-35).

Plantar Foot Pain: Plantar Fasciitis

Plantar fasciitis is an inflammation or partial tear of the plantar fascia. Plantar fasciitis can be caused by the stress of repetitive trauma and poor arch support of the foot. Patients usually complain of heel pain. The ultrasound characteristic of plantar fasciitis is a hypoechoic fusiform swelling of the normally hyperechoic plantar fascia, especially at the calcaneal insertion (Fig. 53-36). A calcaneal spur may or may not be present. The calcaneal spur appears sonographically as a strong acoustic shadow near the insertion of the plantar fascia to the tubercle of the calcaneus. In traumatic situations, partial or complete tears may develop in addition to plantar fasciitis. The upper limit of normal posterior anterior thickness for the plantar fascia is 4

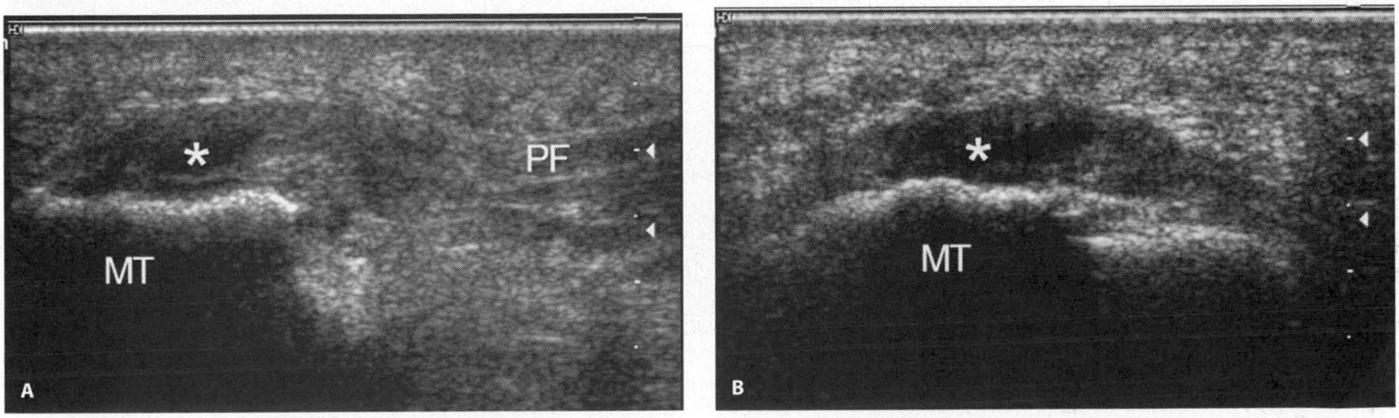

Figure 53-36. ■ *A. Longitudinal image of the medial band of the plantar fascia (PF) at its insertion onto the medial tubercle (MT) of the calcaneus shows a hypoechoic defect (*) within a swollen medial fascia, representing moderate fasciitis with a partial tear.* ***B.** Transverse image showing the partial tear (*) over the medial tubercle of the calcaneus.*

mm, and it is measured near the insertion site but can be measured at any point along the fascia where there is abnormal swelling.

Pitfalls

ANISOTROPY

One must remember to continually tilt the transducer to remain parallel to the tendon as the course of the tendon changes. Otherwise, anisotropy may mimic pathologic conditions such as tendinopathy, tendon tears, and abnormal fluid collections. The echogenicity of a tendon depends on the orientation of the ultrasound beam relative to the tendon structure. This causes an angle-dependent artifact known as anisotropy (Fig. 53-5). If the tendon is perpendicular to the central axis of the sound beam, then the tendon will appear echogenic and the fibers of the tendon will be well visualized. However, if the tendon is not perpendicular but is oblique to the central axis of the sound beam, the tendon will appear more hypoechoic and the fibers will be suboptimally visualized (Fig. 53-6).

PROPER TRANSDUCER SELECTION

Choosing the wrong transducer (or frequency range) can result in poor imaging quality and may result in over- or underpenetration of desired soft tissue structure. Because soft tissue structures of the ankle and foot are superficial, a high-frequency linear array transducer (7.5–15 MHz) would be the ideal selection.

STAND-OFF PADS

Stand-off pads are now obsolete for musculoskeletal ultrasound with the use of today's high-frequency transducers. A generous use of thick ultrasound gel often provides the needed contact around prominent bony structures.

NORMAL ANATOMY VERSUS PATHOLOGY

Comparison of the symptomatic ankle can help distinguish normal anatomy versus pathologic changes.

SELECTED READING

Bianchi S, Zwass A, Abdelwahab IF, et al. Evaluation of tibialis anterior tendon rupture by ultrasonography. *J Clin Ultrasound* 1994;22:564–566.

Cardinal E, Chhem RK, Beauregard CG, et al. Plantar fasciitis: sonographic evaluation. *Radiology* 1996;201:257–259.

Chem RK, Beauregard G, Schmutz GR, et al. Ultrasonography of the ankle and hindfoot. *Can Assoc Radiol J* 1993;44:337–341.

Church CC. Radiographic diagnosis of acute peroneal tendon dislocation. *AJR Am J Roentgenol* 1977;129:1065–1068.

Fessell DP, Vanderschueren GM, Jacobson JA, et al. Ankle ultrasound: technique, anatomy and pathology. *Radiographics* 1998;18: 325–340.

Fessell DP, van Holsbeeck MT. Ultrasound of the foot and ankle. *Semin Musculoskelet Radiol* 1998;2:271–281.

Fornage BD. Achilles tendon: ultrasound examination. *Radiology* 1986;159:769–764.

Gibbon W, Long G. Plantar fasciitis: ultrasound evaluation. *Radiology* 1997;203:290.

van Holsbeeck MT, Introcaso JH. *Musculoskeletal US*, 2nd ed. St. Louis: Mosby Year Book; 2000.

Ultrasound-Guided Interventional Procedures

TOM WINTER

54

KEY WORDS

Activated Partial Thromboplastin Time (APTT). A measure of how well blood clots; APTT measurement is particularly useful in patients taking heparin, a commonly used blood thinner.

Coaxial Catheters. Two or more catheters nested within one another.

Cordocentesis. Puncture of the umbilical cord. See PUBS.

Chorionic Villi Sampling (CVS). Placental tissue is analyzed for the fetal karyotype. A needle is put into the region of the placenta closest to the amniotic fluid, and a portion of the placenta is sucked into a tube. The placenta may be approached through the cervix or through the abdominal wall.

Dermatotomy. Skin incision.

Fentanyl. A drug (narcotic, similar to morphine) used to decrease pain during a procedure.

French. Measure of catheter size.

Hysteroscope. A small, fiberoptic tube inserted through the cervix so the interior of the endometrial cavity can be viewed and samples can be obtained.

Indigo Carmine. A harmless dye that may be inserted into the amniotic fluid when there is a possibility of twins.

International Normalized Ratio (INR). A test designed to better measure the prothrombin time (PT). Most procedures may be safely performed if the INR is less than 1.5.

Laminectomy. Surgical removal of the posterior arch of a vertebra.

Lecithin/Sphingomyelin (L/S) Ratio. Surfactants present in the amniotic fluid that are used as biochemical markers to determine fetal lung maturity. The L/S ratio is gradually being replaced by the fluorescent polarization test, a newer laboratory test on amniotic fluid that can be performed in half the time of the L/S ratio. A third test for assessing fetal lung maturity, the phosphatidylglycerol method, is useful in certain limited situations.

Midazolam. A drug (benzodiazepine, similar to Valium) used for its antianxiety and amnestic (helps the patient forget the procedure) properties during painful procedures.

Myelotomy. Surgical incision of the spinal cord.

Needle Stop. A small clamp that attaches onto any gauge needle; it helps prevent the needle from being inserted past the predetermined depth.

Percutaneous Umbilical Blood Sampling (PUBS, Cordocentesis, Funisocentesis). A small needle is placed in the umbilical cord, and fetal blood is aspirated.

Pigtail Catheter. A catheter with a circular shape at one end. It tends to remain within a cavity. The side holes are placed within the curved region that is known as the pigtail.

Platelet Count. The number of platelets in the blood. Platelets are important for clotting. Most procedures may be safely performed if the platelet count is greater than 50,000.

Prothrombin Time (PT). A measure of how well blood clots; PT measurement is particularly useful in patients taking warfarin, a commonly used blood thinner. See INR.

Syrinx. A fluid collection in the center of the spinal canal.

Tandem. A tube containing radioactive material that is put within the endometrium.

Thermal Ablation. Destroying tumor tissue with either heat (radiofrequency or microwave) or cold (cryoablation).

Trocar. Central insert placed within a tubular needle to give it a point. When it is withdrawn, tissue or fluid can be aspirated.

Vacutainer Tube. Tube that is used for drawing blood. Built-in suction within the tube pulls the blood out at a more rapid rate.

RELEVANT LABORATORY VALUES

Platelet Count: 160–370 K/μL

International Normalized Ratio: 0.9–1.1

Activated Partial Thromboplastin Time: 25.0–35.0 seconds

Lecithin-Sphingomyelin (L/S) Ratio in amniotic fluid: values <1.5–2.0 indicate an increased risk of respiratory distress syndrome at delivery

Reference ranges for individual laboratories may vary slightly.

The Clinical Problem

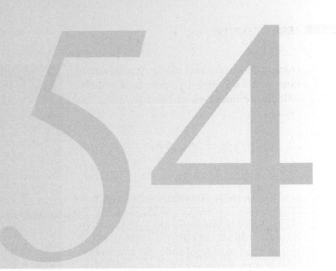

Ultrasound is now used to guide a variety of invasive procedures that previously relied on fluoroscopic or computed tomography (CT) localization or experienced guesswork. Ultrasound is guiding more and more procedures every year that were previously the province of other imaging modalities. If a structure can be seen by ultrasound, it is generally amenable to ultrasound-guided intervention. For abdominal and pelvic pathology, ultrasound is generally cheaper, safer, quicker, and more efficacious than CT. Sonographic guidance allows one to compress the abdominal wall, essentially halving the distance to lesions when compared with CT, making procedures easier in our increasingly obese culture. Ultrasound is also used daily to guide interventions in the operating rooms and in the neck and breast; it is also increasingly used for procedures in the chest wall and mediastinum. Ultrasonic localization should take place immediately before (or during) any potentially difficult fluid aspiration or biopsy.

Approaches to Puncture Procedures

LOCALIZATION WITHOUT GUIDANCE

If the lesion is large and close to the skin, localization is performed with ultrasound but no guidance is necessary. Make sure, however, to use a high-frequency linear or curved linear transducer with color Doppler technology to ensure that there are no prominent blood vessels in the region of the expected puncture site. If these vessels are present, either move the puncture site far away or use direct ultrasound guidance to ensure that these vessels are avoided (Fig. 54-1).

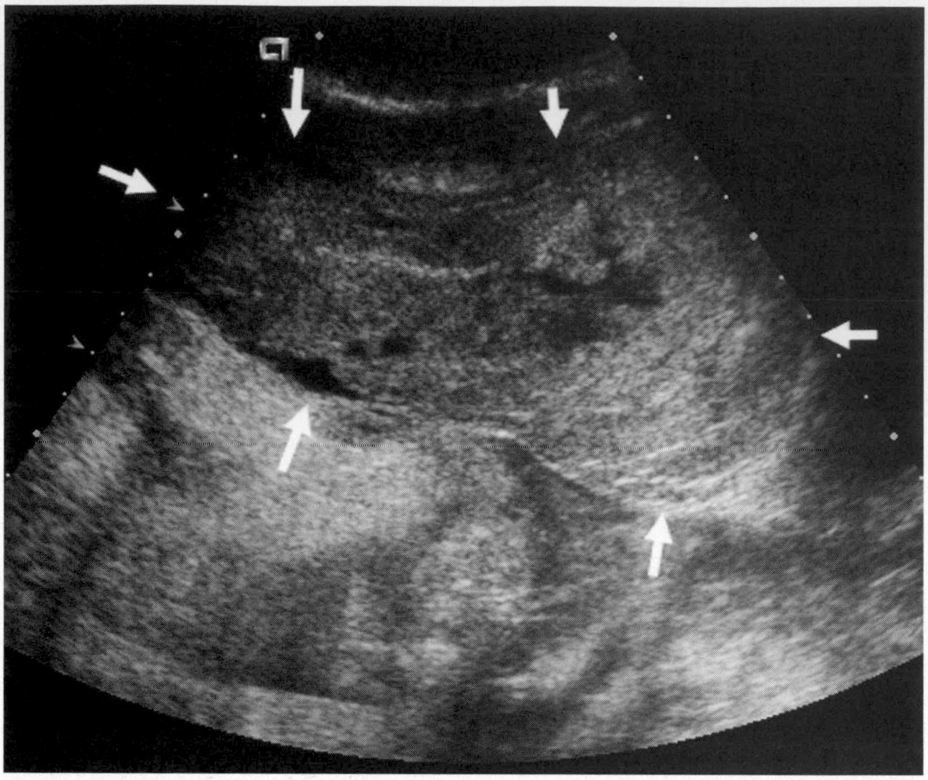

Figure 54-1. ■ *Large (>15 cm) hematoma* (white arrows) *in the anterior abdominal wall after the inferior epigastric artery was inadvertently punctured during a paracentesis.*

RIGHT-ANGLE APPROACH

If the target is located in a space that has an accessible acoustic window at a 60- to 90-degree angle (Figs. 54-2 and 54-3), the following technique is best.

1. Choose a needle insertion site where the lesion can be seen well and where the course of the needle is safe. Avoid a path where you must angle around the bowel or gallbladder.
2. Place the transducer at a nonsterile location where the lesion and needle track can be viewed and that is at approximately right angles to the needle insertion angle. The procedure is usually performed with a curved linear transducer so the angle of the transducer beam to the needle can be readily seen. The transducer should be turned so that the beam is in the same plane as the needle. It is critical to follow subtle angulation changes

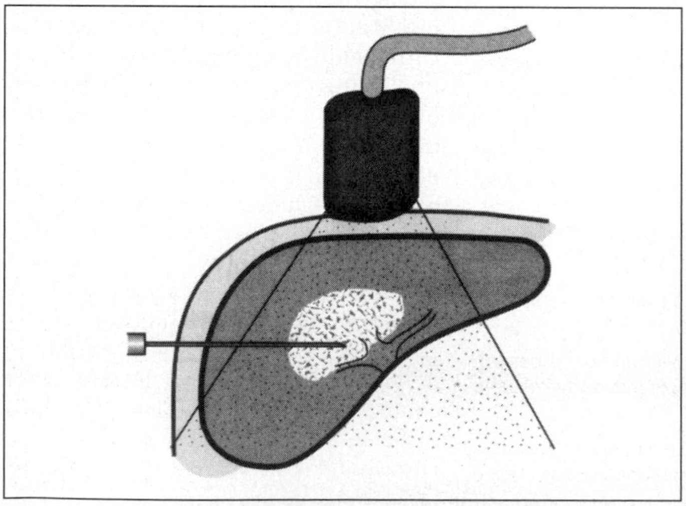

Figure 54-2. ■ *The right-angle technique is used predominantly in obstetrics and for kidney (both native and transplant) biopsies. The transducer is placed over an easily accessible path into the target. The needle insertion site is found by pushing on the skin and watching the image closely. The needle is then placed at approximately right angles to the ultrasonic beam into the mass. Excellent visualization is obtained.*

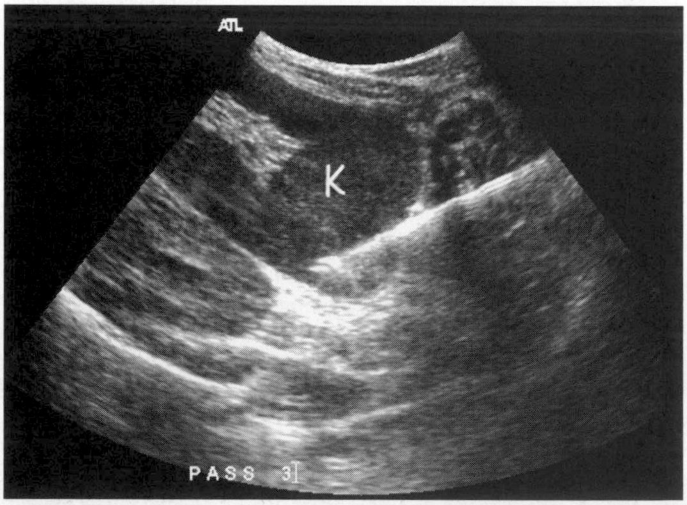

Figure 54-3. ■ *Right-angle approach to biopsy of a transplant kidney* (K) *in the iliac fossa. Note how probe and needle are almost at right angles to each other, allowing for an excellent specular reflection from the needle as it passes into the lower pole of the kidney.*

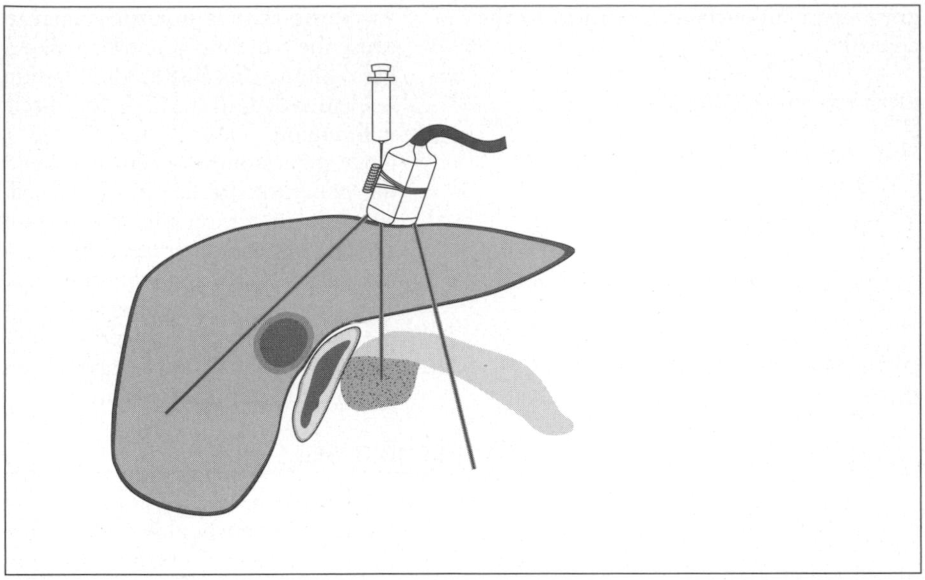

Figure 54-4. ■ *Oblique technique. This pancreatic mass could only be punctured with a needle alongside the transducer because the area around it was obscured by gas. It is difficult to see the needle with this oblique approach, but it can be used if the access is limited. A biopsy guide is helpful with this approach.*

in the needle position with the transducer; aligning the two is essential for successful needle visualization.

3. Before inserting the needle, press with your finger on the skin at the approximate needle insertion site to help show where the needle is about to enter the image. The finger movement can be seen.
4. Localize the lesion in two planes.
5. Provide continuous guidance during the procedure.

Providing the needle location and axis are successfully followed by the sonographer (and this requires skill, experience, and communication between the sonologist and sonographer), even 22-gauge needles can be clearly seen.

It is of particular importance when using a 22-gauge needle to align the bevel and the scan plane to avoid having the needle bend out of the field of view. Needles with centimeter calibrations on them can be very helpful in determining how far the needle has been inserted.

FREEHAND AT AN OBLIQUE AXIS TO THE NEEDLE

The needle can be placed alongside the transducer at an oblique axis to the ultrasound beam (Fig. 54-4). The needle will generally be guided by the physician, who holds both the needle and transducer. The transducer is placed within a sterile plastic cover that has some gel within it. Use a sterile rubber band to tighten the plastic bag neck around the transducer. Sterile tube gauze can be placed around the cable to keep the sterile field intact. Commercially available sheaths cover both the transducer and a good portion of the cable, allowing one to easily maintain a sterile field.

This technique is used when the lesion is large and superficial, access is limited, and some guidance is required. Recognizing the needle path requires skill, because the echoes from the needle may be subtle and only the tip is easily seen. The needle often cannot be seen near the skin. An up-and-down motion with the needle (jiggling), movement of the inner stylet within the needle, rotating the needle to expose the beveled tip, use of modern cross-beam technology, and use of a sonographically reflective coating on the needle tip all help with needle visualization.

USING A BIOPSY ATTACHMENT

Biopsy attachments are occasionally helpful when the ultrasonic access is limited and the target is small (Fig. 54-5).

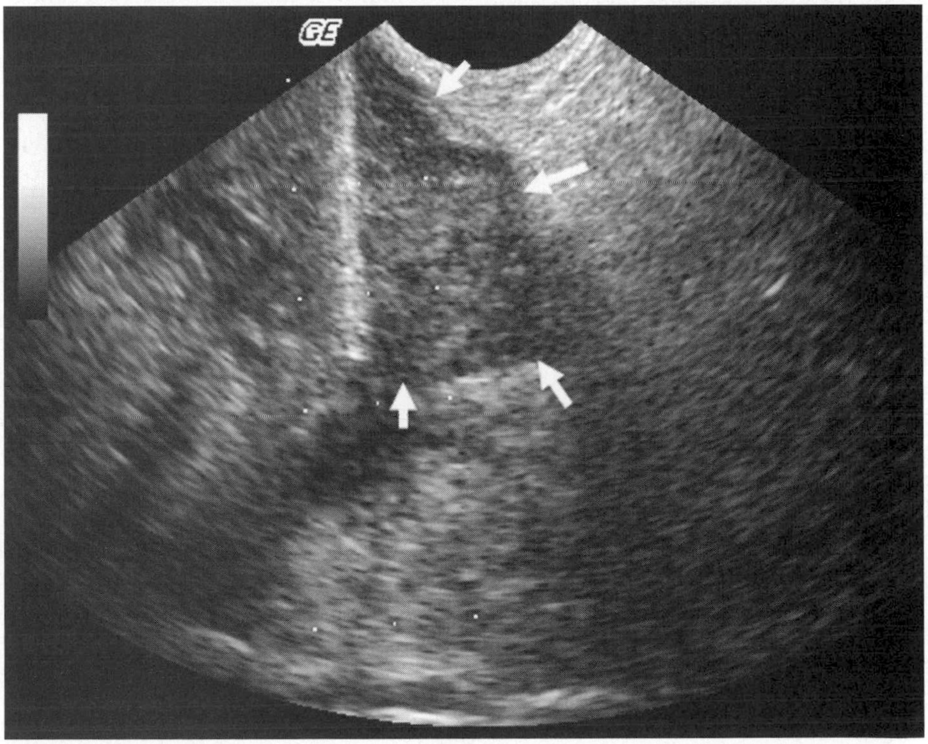

Figure 54-5. ■ *Lung cancer metastasis* (white arrows) *on the pelvic sidewall in an elderly smoker being biopsied with a transvaginal approach using a biopsy guide. Because the tumor deep in the pelvis could not be safely approached percutaneously (from the front or back) because of overlying structures, a biopsy guide and an endovaginal approach were used for a safe and easy successful biopsy. Note dotted lines from the biopsy guide software, which predict the needle trajectory. Needle* (heavy white line) *passing into the mass.*

Biopsy attachments are available for almost all transducers. The needle is inserted through a guide so the needle enters the image and the body at a preset oblique axis, shown on the monitor as a dotted line or template. The transducer axis can be changed so that the target lies in the middle of the dotted line. The needle may not be easy to see unless it is large because the needle is almost on the same axis as the sound beam; however, improvements in ultrasound hardware and software make needle visualization easier and easier. Needle tip visualization is improved by using a needle that has a roughened tip or commercially applied polymer coating to make it more echogenic. The sonographer must be adept at recognizing subtle tissue movement as the needle enters the tissues. The needle will enter the image obliquely and may not follow the expected template route. Thin needles tend to bend out of the plane as they meet tissues of different consistency. Although very experienced sonographers and sonologists may not need to use a biopsy guide for any but the most difficult of procedures, we find that use of a guide generally makes procedures much easier for beginners or those who only practice ultrasound intermittently.

Practical Steps

OBTAIN CONSENT FORMS

Punctures of any kind carry potential risks, and a full explanation of the risks and benefits of the procedure must be given to the patient. The alternative diagnostic and therapeutic maneuvers that are available should be discussed. The patient will then sign a consent form before the puncture. Consent forms are obtained by the physician performing the procedure, but such matters can be overlooked in any busy laboratory; the sonographer should therefore double-check that the form has been signed. The sonographer usually acts as a witness to the consent.

FIND THE PUNCTURE SITE

Demonstrate the following:

1. Where the mass or collection is
2. How deep it is
3. What lies between the patient's skin and the mass, such as bowel or vessels

DETERMINE THE OPTIMUM NEEDLE DEPTH

1. *Make sure that the patient is comfortable.* This is imperative because the patient must lie still for the duration of the procedure. However, the position should give the physician easy access to the target, preferably in a vertical axis without the need to angle the needle. If an oblique position is necessary, stabilize the patient with sponges or pillows.
2. Move the patient so that as few structures as possible lie in the path of the needle. Piercing the liver, small bowel, or stomach is undesirable if it can be avoided by a change in the angulation of the patient or the approach. One should never puncture the large bowel (colon).
3. Watch the patient's respiration. Scanning and locating the site during quiet breathing is best. Respiration should be suspended when the needle is inserted. The needle may move greatly, especially in the kidney, when the patient breathes.
4. The puncture site must be marked in such a way that the mark will not be scrubbed away when the patient's skin is cleaned. A simple but effective method is to imprint the skin by pressing on it with a localizer. Among the many possible "scientific puncture site localizers" that are used are retracted ballpoint pens, plastic needle caps, and pen caps. Anything that is not too sharp to cause the patient discomfort will do. Press on the skin just before the skin is cleansed, and a small red circle will remain.
5. Once the lesion has been found and the puncture site has been marked, leave an image on the screen with the calipers demonstrating the depth of the lesion and angle of approach. This can serve as a reference during the set-up for the procedure, enabling the physician to review the depth and approximate angle.

REMOVE GEL

The gel that has been used in performing the scan must be thoroughly removed before the skin antiseptic cleaning solution is applied, or otherwise adequate sterility cannot be obtained. A dry towel, or rarely alcohol, is usually sufficient to remove the gel. The povidone-iodine (Betadine, Purdue Pharma L.P., Stamford, CT) skin-cleaning solutions of the past are gradually being supplanted by chlorhexidine-isopropyl alcohol mixes (ChloraPrep, Medi-Flex, Inc., Leawood, KS); the latter have the advantage of better antimicrobial activity and do not cause staining of the patient's clothes.

DOCUMENT THE PROCEDURE

Make sure that the ultrasound of the actual puncture site has been recorded on film or the Picture Archiving and Communication System. No matter how carefully a procedure is carried out, tissue or fluid is not always obtained, and documentation of an appropriate approach is therefore important. For example, an apparent collection may in fact be an organized hematoma, and nothing can be aspirated even though the needle is correctly placed. If a procedure using a biopsy guide allows visualization of the needle placement, this also should be documented. CINE clip capability, if available, allows definitive recording of the needle pass into the target.

PUNCTURE EQUIPMENT

The following sterile supplies should either be available as a basic tray or assembled before a procedure (Fig. 54-6). Prepackaged kits for specific examinations are readily available and should include the following:

Sterile drapes (one with a hole for access to the puncture site).

Two containers (for antiseptic solutions).

Glass tubes (for collecting specimens).

5- or 10-mL syringe and 30- and 22-gauge needles (for local anesthetic); 30-gauge needles cause much less pain at the skin surface when injecting lidocaine than do 25-gauge needles.

Cleansing sponges.

To be added:

Needle of choice; should have an echogenic tip for improved visualization. If commercial polymer enhanced-visualization needles are not available, simply roughing the tip with a scalpel blade improves sonographic visualization.

20- and 2-mL syringes for amniocentesis.

Syringe of choice (depends on the size of the collection).

Extension tubing (desirable for targets that move with respiration; e.g., kidney).

Sterile ruler (to measure the correct depth on the needle).

Needle stop (to screw on the needle at the correct depth).

Local anesthetic (usually 1% lidocaine).

Sodium bicarbonate 8.4%. Some physicians believe that buffering the lidocaine (1 mL bicarbonate to 9 or 10 mL lidocaine) decreases the burning sensation felt when lidocaine is injected.

Alcohol wipes (for cleaning off the rubber stopper on any bottles, such as lidocaine, radiographic contrast media, anaerobic culture bottles).

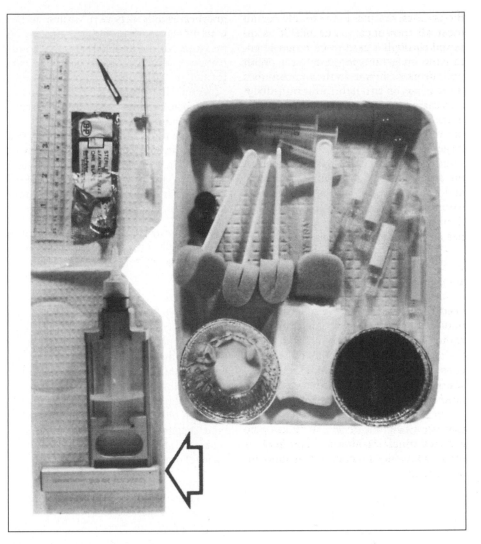

Figure 54-6. ■ *Supplies needed for a basic tray for a sterile procedure include containers for iodine and alcohol; prep sponges; a 5-mL syringe; 18- and 30-gauge needles for drawing up local anesthetic and then producing a skin wheal; glass culture tubes; some 3 × 4 gauze pads; and sterile drapes (at least one fenestrated). A sterile ruler, a scalpel blade, and the appropriate needle and sterile needle stop must be added. Aspiration device* (arrow) *that can be attached to a 20-mL syringe to help apply more negative pressure during biopsies.*

Sterile gloves (latex-free available if patient has a latex allergy).

Biopsy guide attachment for transducer if necessary.

Sterile plastic bag to cover the transducer, with sterile rubber bands or sterile pipe cleaner to secure bag in place. Commercial transducer drape sets include all necessary fasteners.

No. 11 scalpel blade (to perform dermatotomy).

Obstetric Puncture Procedures

PRENATAL CHROMOSOMAL ANALYSIS

Needles are most commonly placed within the uterus during pregnancy to obtain material for chromosomal analysis. The technique used depends on the stage of pregnancy. In the first trimester, chorionic villi material is obtained by chorionic villi sampling (CVS). In the early second trimester, amniocentesis is the usual technique. Later in the second trimester, percutaneous umbilical blood sampling (PUBS) used to be required because it gives the speediest result. With the advent of newer analysis techniques (fluorescent in situ hybridization), PUBS for diagnostic purposes has become much rarer; PUBS is now generally reserved for therapeutic procedures (e.g., transfusions).

Amniocentesis is also performed in the third trimester to evaluate the amniotic fluid for fetal lung maturity; this information is valuable if the obstetrician is thinking of inducing labor or considering a procedure that may precipitate labor.

Chorionic Villi Sampling

Chromosomal material can be obtained in the first trimester (~11–14 weeks) by taking a sample from the placental implantation site. Most commonly, a catheter is inserted through the cervix and guided under ultrasound to the thickest portion of the gestational sac; a portion of the chorion is aspirated. If the gestational sac is at an inaccessible site (e.g., in an acutely anteverted or retroverted uterus), a needle can be placed into the uterus through the abdominal wall. This route is less likely to introduce infection than the vaginal route, but it may be slightly more painful. CVS gives material that allows chromosomal analysis in 2 days to 2 weeks (depending on the technique used) at a very early stage of pregnancy; however, it is statistically slightly more hazardous than amniocentesis, alpha-fetoprotein amniotic fluid analysis cannot be performed, and maternal cells may occasionally be confused with fetal cells. Occasionally, persistent amniotic fluid leakage may occur. CVS is a technique that requires a skilled operator and is best performed at a site where a maternal-fetal medicine specialist (perinatologist) is available. With the advent of more widespread first-trimester nuchal translucency screening programs for aneuploidy, the number of CVS procedures will likely increase.

In addition to the early and quick availability of chromosomal information with CVS, it is also possible to take the tissue and extract DNA to test for certain specific diagnoses, such as cystic fibrosis and sickle cell anemia.

Amniocentesis

Amniocentesis for chromosomal analysis is usually performed between 15 and 18 weeks. It is safe, with a less than 0.5% abortion rate; cell growth occurs within 6 to 17 days. Alpha-fetoprotein can be measured in the amniotic fluid. Second-trimester amniocentesis is generally performed to rule out chromosomal and congenital defects at a stage early enough to give the parents the option of termination if a fetal anomaly is found.

In the third trimester, amniocentesis is performed to obtain fluid to determine whether the fetal lungs are mature. There is relative oligohydramnios in the third trimester, and the procedure can be more difficult to perform.

Percutaneous Umbilical Blood Sampling (PUBS, Cordocentesis, or Funisocentesis)

PUBS is performed later in pregnancy when access to the fetal circulation for diagnostic or therapeutic purposes is desired. A needle is inserted into the cord at either the placental or, less often, the fetal end of the cord. Cordocentesis is done either when the pregnancy is close to the abortion limit or when the fetus may be viable but has an anomaly that raises the question of a chromosomal abnormality. New diagnostic techniques like fluorescent in situ hybridization that can be performed rapidly on amniotic fluid have decreased the necessity for diagnostic PUBS. PUBS is the most dangerous of the three techniques but is still surprisingly safe; we quote a 1% loss rate, but the exact hazard is unknown.

AMNIOCENTESIS TECHNIQUE

When amniocentesis is performed in the second trimester, the site is easily localized. There are several important points to be remembered when choosing a site:

1. Avoid the placenta. This may be impossible if the placenta covers the entire anterior surface of the uterus (Fig. 54-7); then it is still possible to take a needle path through the placenta unless Rh incompatibility has been diagnosed. Penetrating the placenta will aggravate the basic condition in these cases.
2. Avoid the fetus. The chances of striking the fetus are slim; however, do not choose a puncture site with a fetus in the field of view. Monitor continuously during the procedure.
3. Avoid the umbilical cord. The cord can easily be seen floating in the fluid (Fig. 54-7). If the puncture has to be performed through the pla-

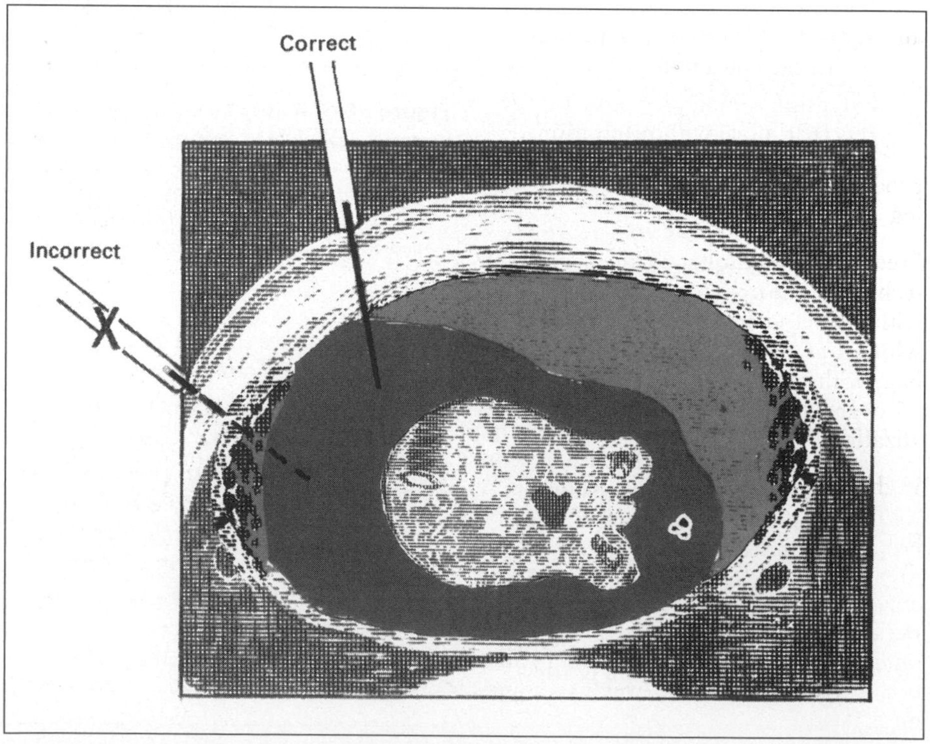

Figure 54-7. ■ *Transverse section through a pregnant uterus. A small area of amniotic fluid is present. The correct angle for obtaining fluid from this site is shown. Avoid the large vascular sinuses that would be punctured if a lateral approach were used.*

centa, be sure to avoid the site of the cord entrance.

4. Avoid a site that is too lateral. The uterine arteries run along the lateral walls of the uterus. Fortunately, these arteries are generally visible on the sonogram as large sonolucent areas (Fig. 54-7). Color Doppler will help identify them if there is confusion.
5. Document the site. The site should be recorded on film or Picture Archiving and Communication System using calipers to show the correct depth.
6. Speed of needle insertion. The needle should be inserted quickly, particularly in second-trimester amniocenteses, to avoid tenting of the amniotic membrane.

Amniocentesis Equipment

A 3-mL syringe is used to take off the first few milliliters of fluid collected so that any maternal blood is cleared from the main sample. Either a 20- or 22-gauge needle is used for amniocentesis; those with a roughened tip or echogenic coating can be seen in fluid with a 3.5- to 5-MHz transducer. Prepackaged amniocentesis sets are available.

Opaque tubes are necessary to keep light from reaching fluid samples and breaking down the bilirubin pigments if an Rh problem is being investigated.

Amniocentesis Guidance

Regardless of your choice of technical approach, it is important to monitor the procedure continuously in real time during amniocentesis.

Freehand Technique. With a freehand technique, the operator guides the needle with one hand and holds the transducer, which has been covered with a sterile bag, with the other hand. Insertion at a 45-degree angle allows good needle visualization.

Right-Angle Technique. The right-angle technique, in which a second individual holds the transducer at a right angle to the needle, is very effective. Needle visualization is optimal with this approach. Because the transducer is used from a site outside the sterile field, a sterile bag does not have to be placed over the transducer.

Use of a Biopsy Guide. The use of a biopsy guide attached to the transducer may be helpful if the amniotic fluid volume is very limited and avoiding the fetus is tricky.

Third-Trimester Problems

If it is difficult to find a big enough fluid pocket in the third trimester, turning the patient to an oblique position allows a small pool to form. If no pocket is available, the physician can push the fetal head out of the pelvis, creating a small pocket of fluid not previously seen.

Twins

When performing an amniocentesis on twins, take care to avoid tapping the same amniotic sac twice (see Fig. 44-1). Find the amniotic sac membrane and choose puncture sites on either side of the membrane. Perform the first amniocentesis and leave the needle in place, injecting a small amount of indigo carmine dye through it to color the fluid in that sac only.

Perform the second amniocentesis at a site localized on the other side of the membrane. The fluid should be a clear, yellow color. If there is any question as to whether the dye has crossed the intra-amniotic membrane, more fluid can be aspirated out of the initial needle site to compare the color of the fluid from the two different sacs.

Check Fetal Heart Motion

Before amniocentesis, check for fetal heart motion. If fetal death is found, it will not be attributed to the amniocentesis and potential legal problems can be avoided. After amniocentesis, check and document the fetal heart motion again. It is reassuring for the parents to see that the fetal heart is beating after the procedure is finished and provides legal confirmation that the fetus was living at the end of the procedure.

CHORIONIC VILLI SAMPLING TECHNIQUE

Two methods of performing CVS are currently used. In the most popular technique, the transducer views the catheter insertion through a transvesical approach (Fig. 54-8). The catheter is followed as it is placed through the vagina and cervix. A sample of the villi is obtained from the thickest portion of the gestational sac. Ultrasound delineates the precise location of the catheter and monitors fetal heart rate. Small bleeds are not uncommon at the time of the CVS.

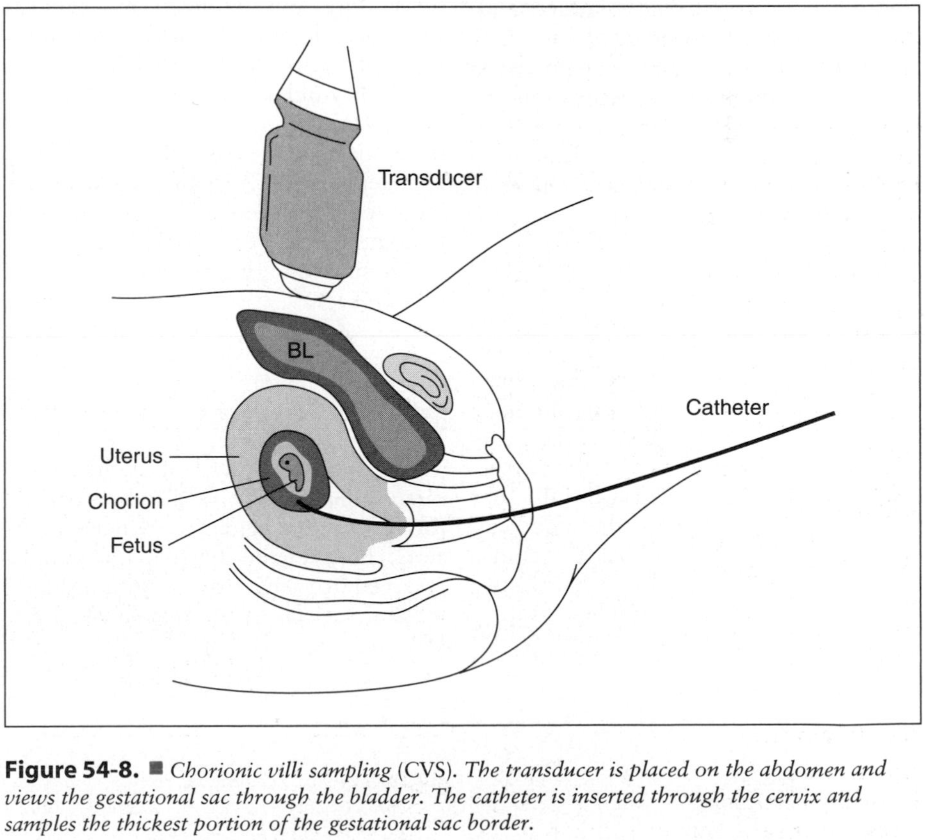

Figure 54-8. ■ *Chorionic villi sampling* (CVS). *The transducer is placed on the abdomen and views the gestational sac through the bladder. The catheter is inserted through the cervix and samples the thickest portion of the gestational sac border.*

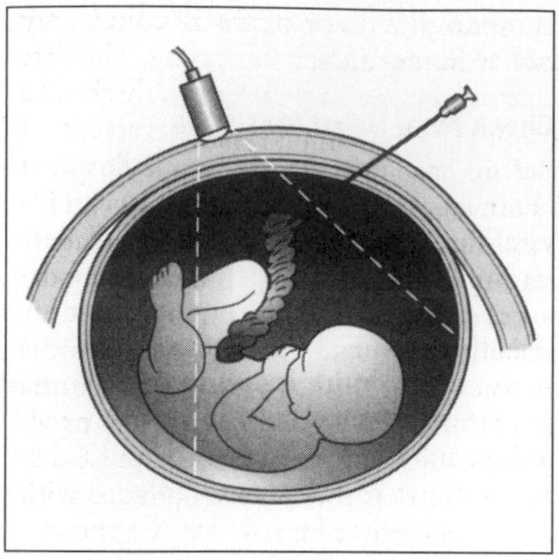

Figure 54-9. ■ *Percutaneous umbilical vein sampling. With the transducer in an oblique axis, the needle is inserted into the cord at the site where it leaves the placenta. The placenta in the image shown is in the optimal position. It is much more difficult to perform this procedure when the placenta is posteriorly located.*

The transabdominal approach is much the same, except that the needle is placed obliquely to the transducer and enters through the abdominal wall. The transabdominal approach is similar to the technique for ovum aspiration (see discussion accompanying Fig. 29-22). A full bladder is required, and the needle is inserted just above the bladder and placed within the gestational sac. The needle can be monitored as it proceeds through the abdominal contents by viewing it through the bladder.

PERCUTANEOUS UMBILICAL BLOOD SAMPLING TECHNIQUE

PUBS requires careful cooperation between sonographer and physician (Fig. 54-9). The cord insertion into the placenta is localized. Ideally the insertion site is anterior, but if it is posterior or lateral, the procedure can still be performed. The sonographer places the transducer at right angles to the needle insertion site. The needle is carefully followed as it moves toward the umbilical artery and vein. The fetal heart is monitored at intervals to ensure that no damage has occurred. An attached biopsy guide may be useful.

POTENTIAL COMPLICATIONS

Possible complications of amniocentesis, CVS, and PUBS include the following:

1. Premature labor
2. Vaginal fluid leakage
3. Onset of infection after a delay
4. Intrauterine bleeding
5. Cord laceration
6. Fetal damage or death

Fluid Collection, Aspiration, and Drainage

Ultrasound can be used to guide cyst puncture, tapping of ascites, and fluid pocket drainage. Mark a site, preferably below the ribs, as close to the fluid pocket as possible. When the fluid collection is obtained from the abdomen it is prudent to locate the inferior epigastric arteries, because inadvertent puncture of these vessels can lead to a large hematoma and complications (Fig. 54-1). Use a high-frequency linear or curved linear transducer with Doppler to find these vessels. Then choose one of the guidance techniques described earlier to aid in obtaining fluid (Figs. 54-2–54-5). Fluid is normally sent for culture and cytology. Biochemical analysis to determine whether the fluid is lymph or urine may be helpful.

If the fluid is being removed for therapeutic as opposed to diagnostic purposes, it may be desirable to leave a catheter in place. A small pigtail catheter mounted on a needle is available and is helpful when there is massive ascites or if it is desirable to drain a cyst to completion.

Mass Biopsy

The techniques described at the beginning of this chapter are also appropriate for ultrasound guidance of mass biopsies. The freehand approach should be reserved for large or very superficial masses, such as in the thyroid (Fig. 54-10).

There are two basic ways of obtaining pathologic material: thin-needle aspiration and core biopsy. Both have similar setups. Aspiration biopsies, used for masses in the pancreas and liver, where leakage or bleeding is a concern, are done with 20- or 22-gauge needles. The length is determined by the depth of the lesion. Only a small specimen is obtained by using a repetitive back-and-forth motion to pack cells into the needle until blood is seen at the needle hub. Suction generally degrades the sample by aspirating too much blood, but may be used for very fibrous lesions. The cells are either flushed through the needle into cytology solution or immediately smeared on a slide for cytologic analysis. Ideally, a cytologist is on hand in the room to provide feedback on whether the sample contains diagnostic material.

For routine renal or liver biopsies that are performed for diffuse organ diseases, or for masses in less vascular areas, core biopsy is performed. Consider obtaining the core from the outer margins of masses where potentially viable cancer cells are located, as opposed to the necrotic center of the mass where decomposing cells may prevent the pathologist from making an accurate diagnosis

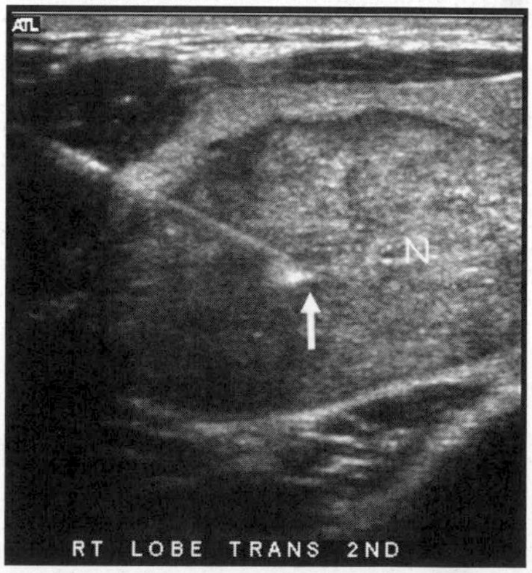

Figure 54-10. ■ *Ultrasound-guided fine-needle aspiration of a benign colloid nodule* (N). *Tip of 25-gauge needle in center of nodule* (white arrow).

(Fig. 54-11). Biopsy is most commonly performed using a single-use core biopsy gun. There are a wide variety of single-use guns available, ranging in size from 14 to 22 gauge; 18 gauge generally suffices for most purposes. These devices consist of a notched needle within an outer sheath that is mounted within the "gun," and a spring-loaded device that allows rapid, controlled passage of a needle into tissue, usually for a 1.8- to 2.3-cm long sample (newer devices allow one to choose lengths from 13 to 33 mm). The rapid spring-driven acquisition minimizes bleeding and discomfort as it obtains a core of tissue. The core is sent to the pathology laboratory in a formalin solution.

As with all invasive procedures, prior informed consent is necessary and premedication ("moderate sedation") is helpful. Prothrombin time, partial thromboplastin time (or international normalized ratio), and platelet count are generally obtained for renal and liver biopsies and when there is a history of bleeding diathesis. Although the actual biopsy takes only a few minutes, the procedure can feel quite lengthy to the patient. Make sure the patient is going to be comfortable, especially if he or she has been obliqued for the procedure. Deciding on a site, even if a small lesion has been defined by a previous CT scan, can take some time. In many cases, the site can only be localized at one particular phase of respiration, so it is a good idea to practice a few times with the patient before cleansing the skin and localizing the site with ultrasound.

Abscess Drainage

Drainage of an abscess involves the insertion of a large catheter, which is required because the infected fluid is often very thick. The procedure can be painful, and premedication or moderate (conscious) sedation is typically given. Because the procedure can be hazardous, vital signs are obtained at appropriate intervals. The main difference from the other puncture techniques described here is that different and larger catheters are required. Abscess drainage is often best performed with an ultrasound system in the fluoroscopy suite so that guide wire and catheter placement can be visualized fluoroscopically.

One of two systems is commonly used to access an abscess cavity. The first is a 21-gauge needle on which are mounted two coaxial catheters: a 4 French that is tapered to the needle and a 6 French mounted on the 4 French. This system can be introduced into the collection in one pass (after a small dermatotomy) or by using an 0.18-inch guide wire through the needle to allow exchange for the two coaxial catheters. Once the 6 French catheter is in the collection, the 4 French catheter and 0.18-inch wire are removed and replaced with a 0.38-inch wire, over which can then be passed a succession of dilators, enlarging the tract to the desired size. (The 0.18-inch wire is too flimsy to allow an exchange of dilators.) The second system is simpler. A thin-walled 18-gauge long needle is passed into the abscess, allowing immediate placement of a large (0.38-inch) exchange guide wire.

Systems commonly used for abscess drainage are (1) a Cope-type self-retaining pigtail catheter set and (2) a straight or curved catheter with many side holes. The first pus aspirated is sent for culture. Platelet count and prothrombin time should be known before the procedure is done.

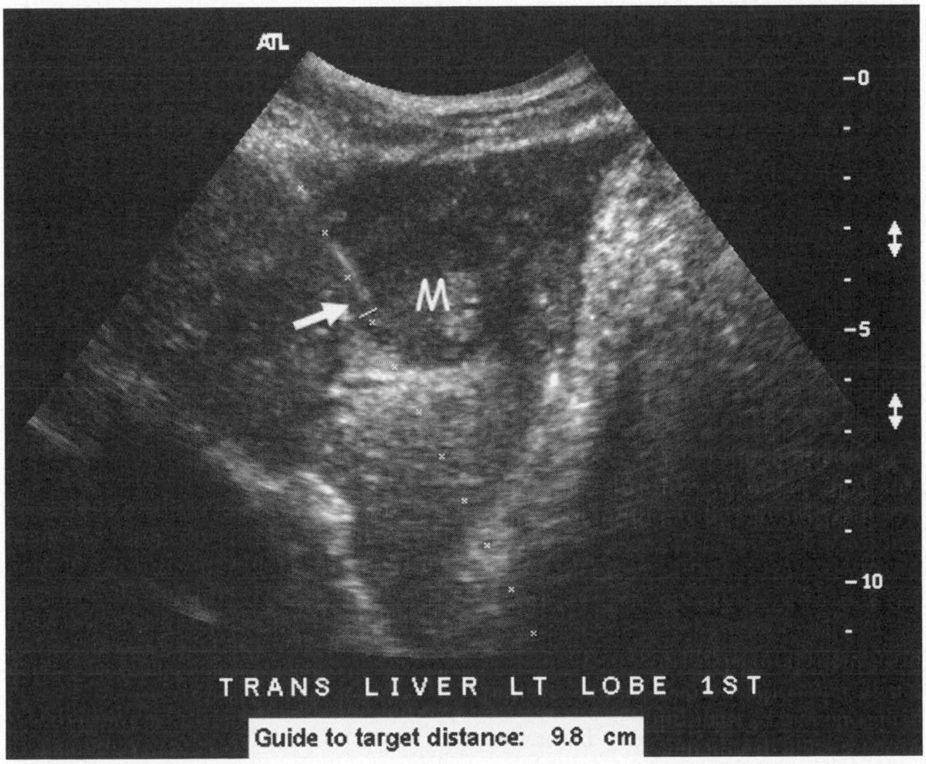

Figure 54-11. ■ *A 76-year-old man with metastatic pancreatic cancer to the liver. Previous core biopsies from the center of the mass were nondiagnostic, consisting of only necrotic cells. This core (needle tip,* white arrow*) at the edge of the tumor* (M) *contained diagnostic cancer cells.*

Biliary Duct Drainage and Percutaneous Nephrostomy

Ultrasound plays a limited role in percutaneous nephrostomy and biliary duct drainage, but is particularly useful to guide left hepatic duct puncture because fluoroscopic guidance often results in a significant dose to the operator's hands. It is mainly used to localize the site and establish the depth for the initial puncture. Because the catheter is often left in for a very long period of time, full sterile precautions including masks, gowns, and caps must be maintained.

These procedures are potentially hazardous and painful, and adequate medication must be given. The procedure should be explained to the patient, and a consent form should be obtained in advance of the medication. Again, one should monitor for evidence of bleeding by watching the patient's pulse and blood pressure.

Breast Intervention

CYSTS

Cyst aspiration is a common procedure performed by sonologists under ultrasound guidance or, if palpable, by the clinician in the office. Small cysts can be difficult to puncture because of the mobility of the breast. Often the operator will hold the transducer in one hand and the needle in the other hand. Assistance from the sonographer may be helpful to immobilize the breast for puncture.

The challenge for the sonographer is to include the needle, the mass, and the predicted needle path in the same longitudinal plane. The choice of skin site for initial needle insertion should be based on the following:

1. The nipple and the retroareolar area should be avoided.
2. The site should be approximately 3 cm from the lesion if it is deep on the chest wall, but if it is superficial, less than 1 cm is fine.

The technique is similar to that used for cyst puncture, described earlier in this chapter.

The use of a Vacutainer tube allows one-handed aspiration. Simple cyst aspiration is often done to alleviate symptoms, and the fluid is discarded. Fluid can be sent for cytology from complex cysts or a bloody aspirate, but a negative cytology should not obviate core biopsy or excision of a suspicious cystic mass. Sterile prep is used.

CORE BIOPSY

Unlike core biopsy of other organs, imaging-guided core biopsy of the breast usually requires at least five passes with a large-bore (14-gauge) biopsy needle mounted in a gun, either as a one-use device or as a reusable one. With improved sonography and increasing interest in distinguishing benign from malignant sonographic characteristics of breast masses, there has also been a significant increase in ultrasound-guided, large-gauge core biopsy. Using large-bore needles does increase the risk of hematoma, but the risk is still small (0.5%). The use of local anesthesia is mandatory, however, and 2% lidocaine with epinephrine can be used to deter bleeding, particularly for very large-gauge vacuum-assisted biopsies.

One helpful device now used is a 13-gauge metallic sheath with cutting stylet. Before sterile prep, the lesion is scanned and a skin site for puncture is picked. A site is chosen approximately 5 cm from the mass so a more shallow approach can be used. This facilitates visualization, is safer, and keeps the sheath stable. The skin is then prepped and infiltrated with 1% lidocaine. A small nick is made using the 13-gauge sheath stylet or a scalpel, and a 20-gauge spinal needle is passed along the anticipated tract to the lesion. Two percent lidocaine with epinephrine is then injected around the lesion (under ultrasound visualization), and the needle is withdrawn as the tract is infiltrated with anesthetic. The sheath is then introduced along the same tract just to the front edge of the lesion. This sheath then serves as a conduit through which passes the 14-gauge needle mounted in the biopsy gun, enabling multiple passes without traversing the entire path of breast tissue each time. Specimens are sent in formalin for analysis.

Yet another refinement in biopsy technology now available is called a mammotomy device. This consists of a 9- or 11-gauge needle with a window cut into the side that uses vacuum assistance to obtain larger samples. Within this needle a rotating blade is advanced, cutting a small specimen off and storing it inside the needle. Multiple samples can thus be obtained rapidly and very accurately by directing the window toward the lesion. This is performed under stereotactic or sonographic guidance. Although this is primarily a sampling device similar to core biopsy, there is some evidence to suggest that it may be able to remove the entire lesion in some cases, thus replacing lumpectomy. Currently the device can be used to remove benign masses; clinical trials are under way evaluating the device's ability to remove breast cancers.

Percutaneous Gastrostomy

Gastrostomy and gastrojejunostomy tubes are often placed percutaneously using fluoroscopic guidance to facilitate guide wire and catheter exchange. However, ultrasound imagery before the procedure is extremely useful to document the edge of the left lobe of the liver and to help choose an appropriate skin site for puncture.

Vascular Access

Ultrasound guidance helps obtain difficult or unusual vascular access by using duplex and color flow visualization of the vessel. The popliteal artery or vein can be accessed using this technique. Access of the popliteal artery can allow angioplasty of femoral artery stenoses that are not accessible by conventional groin puncture. Extensive deep vein thrombosis has been successfully thrombolysed using directed puncture of the popliteal vein. Central venous access (subclavian or internal jugular veins) can be expedited using ultrasound guidance. In these procedures, the sonographer finds the vessel and helps guide access by showing the best needle insertion site, vessel depth, and appropriate angle. The needle is tracked with ultrasound as it is placed in the vessel. The recent advent of relatively inexpensive "handheld" or compact ultrasound units has resulted in the use of sonography for vascular access on a much greater basis.

Intraoperative Ultrasound

Intraoperative ultrasound can help surgeons by showing masses or calculi within organs. By using high-resolution transducers directly on the surface of an organ, ultrasound can provide information not available preoperatively. Several studies have shown that high-frequency intraoperative ultrasound is more sensitive at detecting liver lesions than are CT, magnetic resonance imaging, or positron emission tomography. Small lesions in the liver or brain can be pinpointed. This can change the surgical approach and shorten operating time.

Several dedicated operating room units have been developed, but standard high-resolution equipment and probes are usable. In addition, the relatively new laparoscopic transducers may be placed through small incisions in the patient's skin and used to guide minimally invasive surgical procedures. Scanning with laparoscopic ultrasound probes is best accomplished with guidance from a conventional optical laparoscope placed through another "port" (small skin incision). Some transducers can be gas-sterilized (check with the manufacturer); all can be covered with sterile sheaths.

Sterile gel should be used inside the sheath (for the rare instance when the sheath may develop a leak). The transducer cable should also be covered because it will inevitably lie in the sterile field. The body cavity being scanned is usually filled with saline as a coupling aid. Generally, an initial scan is done as soon as the area of concern is exposed and before much tissue dissection has taken place. Guidance is performed as needed during surgery (often delineating relevant vascular structures that need to be sacrificed or avoided), and then a final scan at the end of the procedure reassures the surgeon that the margin of the resection is tumor-free, that the cysts are completely drained, or that all the stones have been retrieved.

RENAL SURGERY

In patients in whom renal calculi—usually staghorn—cannot be removed by means of lithotripsy or percutaneous stone extraction, intraoperative ultrasound can easily localize remaining stones, regardless of their composition. This is especially useful when the stone is surrounded by soft blood clot; the clot hinders the surgeon's ability to feel the stone but does not interfere with the ultrasound beam. A Keith needle is inserted under ultrasound guidance until it touches the stone.

More often, ultrasound is used during partial nephrectomy to localize and define the extent of renal neoplasms (Fig. 54-12). If there is uncertainty from preoperative tests about whether a nephron-sparing approach is appropriate, intraoperative ultrasound can determine a tumor's relationship to the hilar structures and the capsule, and find accessory lesions. Adjacent structures can be evaluated, such as the vena cava, adrenal gland, or liver, for possible tumor extension. Ultrasound is also used for open renal biopsies and the unroofing and evaluation of renal cysts.

A transducer with multiple frequencies is optimal; 7.5 MHz is generally used, but 10 or 5 MHz may be necessary during the procedure, and it would be time-consuming and expensive to prepare three different transducers. Duplex Doppler helps to assess tumors for vascularity, differentiates renal veins and arteries from dilated collecting systems, and detects tumor spread in venous structures. If regional hypothermia is used, it is especially important to get a thorough scan before clamping the renal vessels to minimize ischemia time.

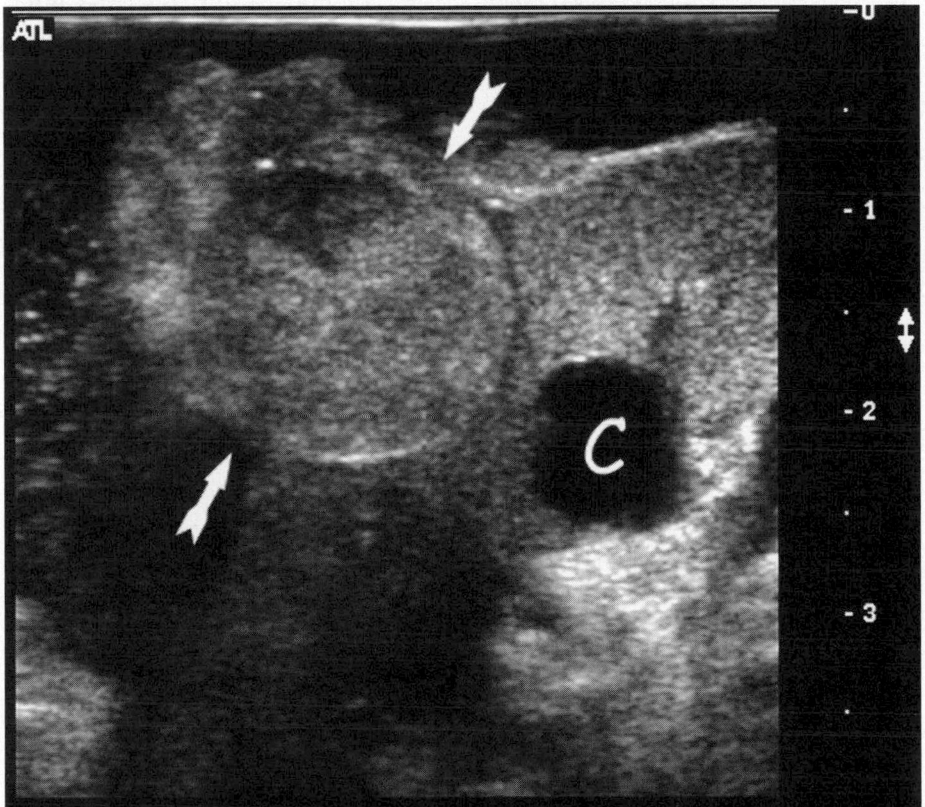

Figure 54-12. ■ *Intraoperative sonogram beautifully defines an exophytic renal cell carcinoma* (arrows) *that partially protrudes from the cortex of the left kidney. C, simple cyst.*

NEUROSURGERY

Initial intraoperative scanning of the brain takes place through a burr hole, while the dura is still intact, or directly on the brain surface after the calvarium has been removed. A multiple-frequency transducer is again preferred because the pathology may be superficial or deep-seated; 7.5 MHz is a reasonable compromise. Modern broad-bandwidth transducers make it even easier to use just one transducer, rather than a variety of low- and high-frequency probes. A dedicated unit is not essential, but the probe should have a small footprint to enable maneuverability in the small surface available. Color Doppler is very helpful when lesions are isoechoic, particularly vascular lesions such as arteriovenous malformations or hemangioblastomas, which may show up only with color flow.

Intraoperative scanning of the spine takes place through a saline-filled cavity, after the initial laminectomy and before the dura is opened (Fig. 54-13). The

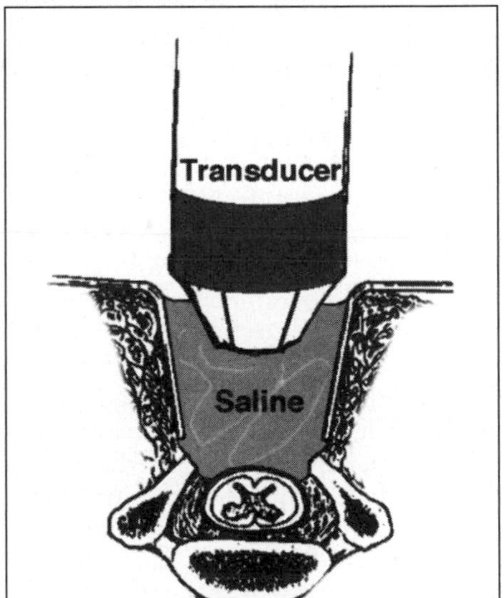

Figure 54-13. ■ *Intraoperative technique for examining the spine. After the spine has been exposed, saline fills the cavity and the probe is placed within the saline to view the spinal cord.*

spinal cord and central canal, the dorsal surface of the dural sac, the posterior portion of the spinal subarachnoid space, and the dentate ligaments are well seen. The water path technique allows some distance between the transducer and the cord, so near-field reverberations do not interfere with the image; in addition, the water path provides a safety margin, because the delicate spinal cord should not be touched with the transducer if possible. Usually, some air bubbles and a layer of blood are present in the saline-filled cavity. A 7.5- or 10-MHz transducer is appropriate for this technique.

Cysts and tumors—both intramedullary and extramedullary, and intradural and extradural—and syringomyelia can be localized for resection, drainage, or biopsy. Because of the precision of the localization, the size of the myelotomy can be limited, and scans during and after the procedures verify the presence of any residual tumor or fluid collections. It is also possible to see developing intramedullary hematomas due to the surgery. Serial scans are especially important when draining fluid cavities in syringomyelia, because the cavities may not be connected with each other and could require multiple drains.

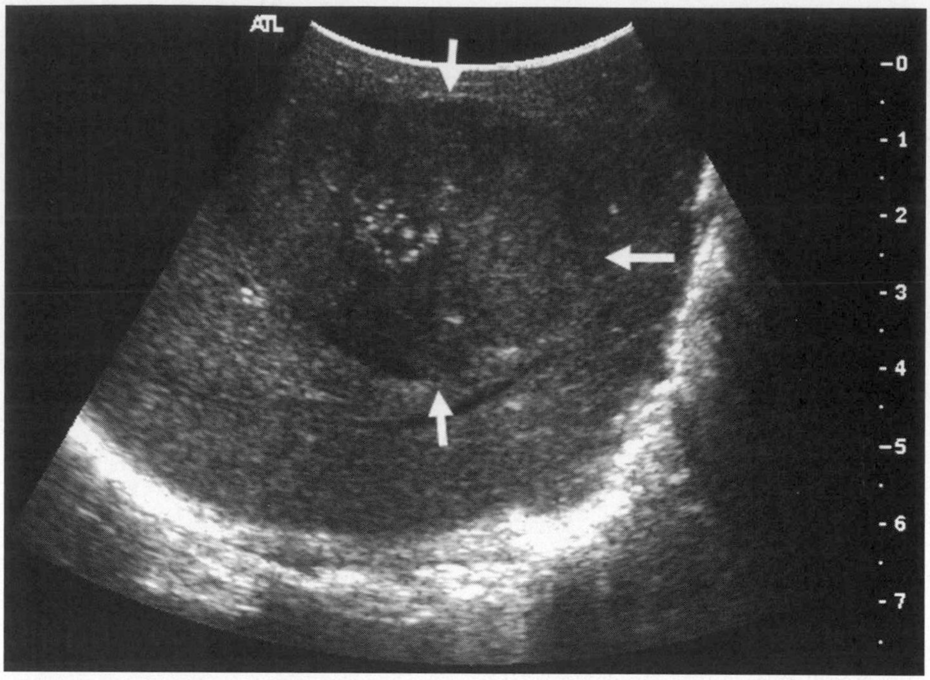

Figure 54-14. ■ *Intraoperative liver ultrasound. Intraoperative ultrasound image of the colon cancer metastasis* (white arrows) *in Color Plate 54-1.*

HEPATOBILIARY AND PANCREATIC SURGERY

In the abdomen, intraoperative ultrasound is used for a wide variety of procedures, from resecting tumors to localizing foreign bodies and stones. Needle and catheter placement is guided for biopsy, fluid aspiration, agent injection (e.g., alcohol into malignant tumors, chemotherapeutic drugs into arteries), tumor thermal ablation (Fig. 54-14 and Color Plate 54-1), and contrast media injection for radiographic studies. The biliary tree can be carefully evaluated for stones, polyps, and tumors, and decompressed under ultrasound guidance. Although it is possible to use a needle-guide attachment, most needle placement is done using the freehand technique discussed earlier in this chapter.

There are flat or curved small footprint linear-array transducers with a side-viewing capability that are optimal for obtaining good contact with the liver surface (Color Plate 54-1). A broad-bandwidth 5- to 8-MHz transducer is generally used, but ultrasound is most helpful here in demonstrating nonpalpable lesions, and a lower-frequency transducer may be rarely needed to see them. One trick to see deep lesions in the liver is to also scan from the back (posterior) surface of the liver, thereby allowing better imaging of this area. Color Doppler is useful both for defining vascular structures and lesions, and for watching needle movement during guidance. A pencil-thin probe is preferred for biliary structures, and sometimes in the pancreas. The so-called hockey-stick probe is very nice for the pancreas and for scanning intraoperatively when there is not a lot of room for a larger probe. The abdominal cavity is filled with saline, allowing the transducer to stand-off from the area of interest. Otherwise, a tiny bile duct may get lost in near-field artifact. Scan the pancreas directly on its exposed surface. If necessary, however, the pancreas can be scanned through the gastrocolic ligament, stomach, or liver.

GYNECOLOGIC SURGERY

Intraoperative ultrasound decreases the risk of uterine perforation with hysteroscopic procedures such as myomectomy or endometrial adhesion resection; it is used in conjunction with the laparoscope to ensure that the resection is complete. Ultrasound has also been useful in fluid aspiration, stone and foreign body removal, and tandem radiotherapy placement (Fig. 54-15). Intraoperative ultrasound may be used during uterine evacuation, both to avoid uterine perforation and to ensure completion of the procedure when uterine anatomy is unusual.

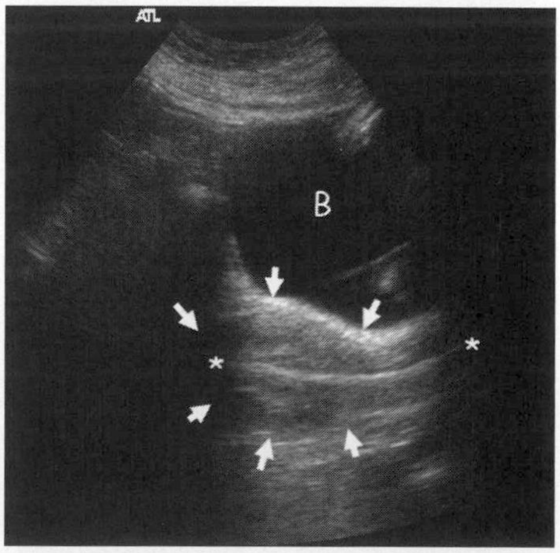

Figure 54-15. ■ *Ultrasound guidance provided in radiation therapy for a 400-lb patient with inoperable endometrial cancer. The hollow tube* (curved echogenic line between the two asterisks) *used to place the radioactive seeds was guided into the center of the uterus* (white arrows). *The urinary bladder* (B) *was filled with saline through a Foley catheter before the procedure to obtain visualization of the uterus.*

Scanning is performed transabdominally through a saline-filled bladder; a 3.5-MHz transducer is probably optimal because of the increased depth to the areas of interest. There is continuous monitoring with real time during the procedure.

ULTRASOUND-GUIDED RADIATION TREATMENT

The outline of periaortic nodes or organs such as the prostate can be marked on the skin, before setting up radiotherapy ports, with ultrasound. This technique has been largely replaced with CT scans that can be directly integrated into the data on the radiotherapy planning computer in a way that cannot be done with ultrasound. Since 1985, transperineal radioactive seed implantation using a template with ultrasound guidance has largely replaced open laparotomy seed placement for the treatment of early stage prostate cancer. Specially designed 18-gauge needles are loaded with radioactive palladium 103 and iodine 125 seeds; these are placed into a custom needle holder at appropriate coordinates according to a template matched to a transrectal scan of the prostate. With the patient in lithotomy position under spinal anesthesia, an ultrasound probe is placed in the rectum and attached to a stepping unit that allows precisely controlled placement of the seeds (up to 100) throughout the entire gland.

SELECTED READING

Dodd GD, Esola CC, Memel DS, et al. Sonography: the undiscovered jewel of interventional radiology. *Radiographics* 1996;16:1271–1988.

Fisher AJ, Paulson EK, Sheafor DM, et al. Small lymph nodes of the abdomen, pelvis, and retroperitoneum: usefulness of sonographically guided biopsy. *Radiology* 1997;205: 185–190.

Kandarpa K, Aruny J. *Handbook of Interventional Radiologic Procedures,* 3rd ed. Philadelphia: Lippincott Williams & Wilkins; 2002.

Kliewer MA, Sheafor DH, Paulson EK, et al. Percutaneous liver biopsy: a cost-benefit analysis comparing sonographic and CT guidance. *AJR Am J Roentgenol* 1999;173: 1199–1202.

Letterie G, Kramer D. Intraoperative ultrasound guidance for intrauterine endoscopic surgery. *Fertil Steril* 1994;62:654–656.

Leroux PD, Winter TC, Berger MS, et al. A comparison between preoperative magnetic resonance scans and intraoperative ultrasound tumor volumes and margins. *J Clin Ultrasound* 1994;22(1):29–36.

Parker SH, Dennis MA, Stavros AT, et al. Ultrasound guided mammotomy: a new breast biopsy technique. *J Diag Med Sonogr* 1996;12:113–118.

Rausch P, Nowels K, Jeffrey RB Jr. Ultrasonographically guided thyroid biopsy: a review with emphasis on technique. *J Ultrasound Med* 2001;20:79–85.

Reading CC. Intraoperative ultrasonography. *Abdom Imaging* 1996;21:21–29.

Sheafor DH, Paulson EK, Simmons CM, et al. Abdominal percutaneous interventional procedures: comparison of CT and US guidance. *Radiology* 1998;207:705–710.

Nursing Procedures

DEROSHIA STANLEY

55

KEY WORDS

Body Mechanics. The use of the human body as a machine. Performed properly, body mechanics aid in the safe movement of people and objects.

CPR Barrier Device. Various devices such as an Ambu bag and a mask with a one-way valve that allows performance of rescue breathing without direct mouth-to-mouth contact.

Effective Communication. The use of spoken words, body language, and the environment to reduce patient anxiety and obtain patient cooperation and satisfaction.

Fowler's Position. A sitting position. This position aids breathing and prevents reflux of gastric contents.

Handwashing. The reduction of microorganisms on the hands through the use of water, soap, and friction. It is the single most important aspect of infection control.

High Filtration Mask. A nose/mouth mask worn when providing care to a patient on airborne precautions such as tuberculosis (TB).

Infiltration. If an intravenous device becomes dislocated from the vein, fluid continues to infuse into the soft tissue. This mishap is termed infiltration.

Intake and Output (I&O). I&O is the recording/reporting of the amount and type of food and fluid that a patient receives as well as the loss of any fluids from the body.

NPO. Abbreviation for *non per os,* meaning nothing by mouth.

Orthostatic (Postural) Hypotension. Low blood pressure occurring as a result of the patient sitting or standing too quickly. It is commonly experienced in the elderly and in patients with significant blood loss. It causes dizziness, which may lead to a fall.

Sim's Position. Patient is placed left side down with the right knee bent toward the chest. This position aids insertion of rectal devices.

Sterile Technique. A procedure that prevents the contamination or introduction of microorganisms and spore into/onto a person, object, or solution. Sterile technique is required when penetrating the skin or mucous membranes and accessing the urinary system.

Standard Precautions. Practices mandated by the Centers for Disease Control and Prevention that reduce the transmission of blood-borne pathogens such as hepatitis B virus and human immunodeficiency virus. Precautions are instituted when handling blood or other body fluid.

Supine Position. Patient is placed flat on his or her back with a pillow under the head. This position aids blood flow to the heart/brain.

Water Seal Chest Catheter. When a catheter is placed into the pleural space, there is the risk that if it becomes detached, air may be introduced and cause a tension pneumothorax. To prevent this, the catheter is connected to a water container.

Restraints. Devices used to immobilize a patient to aid scanning or prevent injury.

Introduction

Nursing care is an important aspect of patient service. To promote patient cooperation and satisfaction, you must be able to attend to the patient's physical, emotional, and cultural needs. Incorporating nursing into your care provides a level of service that ensures the best scans possible.

Effective Communication

The basis of patient cooperation and satisfaction is effective communication. To cultivate a positive relationship, you must demonstrate respect, acceptance, and support for the anxiety and/or limitations that a real or potential health problem can impose on a patient (Table 55-1).

We live in a diverse society. So as not to appear discourteous or rude to patients who have different values and beliefs, become familiar with other cultures and customs. Obtain assistance from your institution's international office or use the Internet as a resource. If unsure of how to approach a patient, take your cue from the patient or family.

Before starting a scan, first make sure you have the correct patient. To identify a hospitalized patient, always check his or her arm bracelet. If the patient does not have an ID bracelet, notify the patient's nurse. To identify an outpatient, call out the last name then have the patient tell you his or her first name.

Address the patient by his or her full name unless the patient directs you otherwise or is a child. Introduce yourself. Do not arbitrarily invite an adolescent or adult patient's family/friend to observe a scan. Avoid distracting or annoying habits, such as chewing gum. Provide privacy and confidentiality; close the examination room door and drape the patient. If necessary, assist the patient with hygienic needs.

Patient Hygiene

DRESSING AND UNDRESSING THE PATIENT

A patient who has limited mobility in an extremity because of disease, intravenous (IV) line, or injury may require your assistance to disrobe. Be sure to remove only the clothing necessary for the scan. To remove clothes easily, start with the patient's unaffected extremity and proceed to the affected one. First, remove cloths above the waist, put a gown on the patient, and then remove the cloths below the waist. Secure belongings in a locker or keep with the patient. Reverse the order to redress.

TOILETING NEEDS

Direct (or assist) a patient who needs to evacuate to the nearest toilet or provide the patient with a bedpan (Fig. 55-1) or urinal. Wear gloves (and gown if necessary) when assisting the patient. When applicable, measure and record/report intake and output.

Bedpan Assistance

To position a regular bedpan (Fig. 55-1A), first make sure the patient is positioned properly on the stretcher or table (see Body Mechanics). Tell the patient to raise his/her buttocks. Slide the bedpan (the broad flat end toward the sacrum) under the buttocks. Tell the patient to lower the buttocks onto the bedpan; the high, narrow end should be visible under the upper thighs. If the patient is unable to raise the buttocks, turn him/her onto his/her side and place the bedpan against the buttocks. Roll the patient back onto the bedpan and adjust if necessary. To simulate the normal position of evacuation, elevate the head of the stretcher unless it is contraindicated.

A fracture bedpan (Fig. 55-1B) is used for the elderly patient, debilitated patient, or patient in traction; it requires minimal patient movement. To position a fracture bedpan, use the same procedure as for a regular bedpan, except place the flat narrow end under the patient's sacrum and the handle end under the patient's upper thighs.

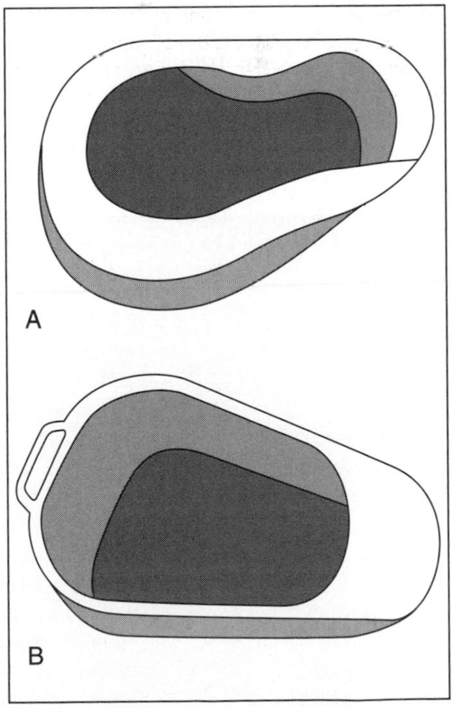

Figure 55-1. ■ *A. Regular bedpan. B. Fracture bedpan.*

Table 55-1 Effective Patient Interaction

Communication	Service
Introduce yourself when you first meet the patient and maintain eye contact.	Be prompt.
Address the patient by full name and what she/he chooses to be called.	Provide physical support for patients as needed when ushering the patient to the examination room.
Explain delays and what to expect. Offer choices when possible.	Provide clear instructions.
Avoid discussions with others that exclude the patient.	Assist with hygiene and positioning as needed.
Humor; use judiciously.	Avoid criticizing staff.
Listen attentively and pay attention to nonverbal messages.	Don't chew gum, smoke, pick your nose, etc.
Assure the patient of privacy and confidentiality.	Maintain a clean/neat appearance and uncluttered examination room.
Speak clearly and respectfully.	
Monitor your nonverbal messages; they may alarm the patient.	

After placing a female patient on a bedpan, tell her to part her thighs slightly to prevent the deflection of urine. Stabilize the bedpan when removing it from under the patient. Once it is removed, cover and dispose of the contents as soon as possible. If necessary, clean the patient's perineal area from the urethral meatus to the anus. Remove gloves (and gown) and wash hands.

Urinal Assistance

When assisting a male patient with a urinal, hold the urinal by the handle and use the rim to lift and place the penis within. Advance the urinal along the shaft of the penis, and then rest it between the patient's thighs. After use, remove the urinal, cover and empty as soon as possible. Remove gloves and wash hands.

Infection Control

Patients with various illnesses are scanned daily on the same system. This exposes you and the patient to the hazard of cross infections. Hospital-acquired (nosocomial) infections are especially dangerous because they can prolong hospitalization and increase morbidity.

HANDWASHING

The primary means of spreading bacteria and other microorganisms is through touch. Hands are frequently used to touch people, animals, and objects; therefore, washing your hands properly is crucial to preventing the spread of potentially harmful organisms. Wearing gloves does not replace effective hand washing.

Hand washing is performed between patients, after toileting or blowing your nose, before setting up for sterile procedures, before preparing drugs or eating, and as directed by your institution's policy. Wet, soap, and lather the hands. Wash your hands including the nails for at least 10 to 15 seconds. After washing your hands, turn off the faucet using a paper towel. Alcohol-based cleaners that do not require water may be used if the hands are not visibly soiled.

TRANSDUCER CARE

The scanning probe, which acts as an extension of your hand, should also be "washed" after each use. To disinfect the probe, use isopropyl alcohol, 70%, or follow the manufacturer's recommendations. Wipe the probe (and cable) several times to thoroughly clean them.

Probes that have been in contact with blood or body fluid require a higher level of disinfection. Before using the probe, cover it with a disposable sheath. After use, discard the sheath. Clean the probe of all gross soil, and then immerse it in an activated glutaraldehyde or orthophthalaldehyde solution. (Do not immerse the cable connection.) Immersion time can vary depending on type of solution. After thoroughly disinfecting the probe, rinse it thoroughly using tap or sterile water. Wipe dry and store (see Appendix 30).

Stand-off pads, if not disposable, are disinfected after each use. Clean thoroughly with soap and water, and then wipe with isopropyl alcohol, 70%.

SANITATION

Routinely clean counters, tables, and technical units. Floors, walls, and ceiling fixtures should be cleaned to prevent dust and dirt accumulation, which can harbor spores and mites. Cover bedpans and urinals until they are emptied, and then rinse and dispose of them properly. To avoid releasing microorganisms into the air, handle soiled linens gently and dust with a damp cloth.

ISOLATION PRECAUTIONS

Because you cannot be certain whether a patient is infected with the human immunodeficiency virus, which is responsible for acquired immune deficiency syndrome (AIDS) or hepatitis B virus, blood and body fluids precautions or "standard precautions" are recommended for use with everyone. Always wear gloves when there is a possibility of coming in contact with any blood or body fluid. When splattering may occur wear a gown, mask, and goggles. Do not re-cap, clip, or bend needles or blades. Place them directly into an impervious container from which they cannot be removed. Precautions instituted for other means of infectious transmission are outlined in Table 55-2.

Table 55-2 Required Elements for Precaution Categories

	Standard	Airborne	Contact	Droplet	Pediatric Droplet
Mask	Fluid splatter	Yes*	No	Close to patient	Close to patient
Goggles	Fluid splatter	No	No	No	No
Gown	Fluid splatter	No	Yes	Yes	Yes
Gloves	Contact with blood/body fluids	??	Yes	Yes	Yes
Probe cover	Contact with blood/body fluids	No	Yes	Yes	Yes
Disposable items:					
Biohazard bag		Sputum/oral secretions	Yes	Yes	Yes
Linen	Place in moisture-resistant bag located in room				
Disinfect equipment/ supplies	Sodium hypochlorite 0.05% (bleach solution)				
Specimens	Place in special transport bags				
Handwashing	Chlorhexidine gluconate preferred				

**Requires a high filtration mask.*

When requested to do a portable scan on a patient in isolation, consult with the patient's nurse before entering the room. Disinfect the ultrasound machine before leaving the unit. If supplies must be sent elsewhere to be disinfected, place them in an isolation bag, label, and secure the bag with tape.

STERILE TECHNIQUES

Sterilization is the chemical process by which items are rendered sterile (free of organisms and spores). Procedures that pierce the skin or mucosa and that invade the urinary tract or vascular system require the use of sterile techniques (Table 55-3).

Skin Prep

The skin is the body's first line of defense against microbes. Before an incision or needle pierces the skin, the skin is cleaned with isopropyl alcohol 70% and/or a povidone-iodine solution. Povidone-iodine is also used to clean mucosal linings such as the vagina; alcohol,

Table 55-3 Principles of Surgical Asepsis

Field	Dry Items	Solutions	Nonsterile Person	Sterile Person
Prepare as close as possible to time of use.	Open wrapped item distal, lateral, lateral, proximal.	Do not discard antiseptics/disinfectants unless expired, contaminated, or left open.	Open wrapped/pouched sterile items and flip them onto the sterile field.	Don sterile gloves: —Peel down pouch. —Remove inner wrap. —Pull back flaps. —Pick up first glove at the fold of cuff (use nondominant hand). —Hold the opposite hand palm up and slide it into glove. —With gloved hand, pick up the second glove by slipping fingers under the edge of cuff. —Palm up, slide hand inside glove. —Adjust for proper fit. —If wearing gown, cuffs must extend over gown cuffs.
Do not leave unattended.	Open pouched items by "peeling down" from the top.	Before pouring into a sterile container, pour off some; pour with label facing you.	Pour solution into sterile container. Avoid splashing.	Keep hands above waist and in front of chest.
Open and place sterile drape over table to create a sterile field (handle edges only).	Consider edges of pouch contaminated; do not allow item to touch edges.	Lay caps/lids/tops down with the insides facing up.	Refrain from reaching over sterile field.	Avoid leaning over a nonsterile area.
Consider edges nonsterile.	Consider a sterile item that comes in contact with a nonsterile item/person contaminated.	Avoid using multiple dose vials with more than one patient.	Do not turn back to sterile field.	Face field when passing.
Any item extending off the field is contaminated and removed.	Keep handling of pouches and wrappers to a minimum (pressure forces sterile air out and replaces it with room air).	Discard vial within 30 days unless an earlier expiration is indicated.	Face field when passing and allow one foot of margin safety.	Avoid coughing/talking over a sterile field.
Cover a contaminated area with a sterile folded drape.	Look for the word "STERILE" on package.	Prep the entry site of vial with an alcohol wipe before inserting needle.	Keep examination room door/curtain closed.	If a gown is required, put it on before donning gloves.
	Do not use if package is wet, torn, or seal is broken.	Discard hydrogen peroxide 7 days after opening.		Don sterile gown: —Open wrap. —Lift gown by neck, gently shake loose. —Slide arms into sleeves. —Have nonsterile person secure ties.
	Check expiration date.	Discard solutions without preservatives, i.e., irrigation solutions, 24 hours after initial use.		

because of its "burning" effect, is not used. If a patient is allergic to povidone-iodine, chlorhexidine gluconate may be used.

After the skin is cleaned, a sterile drape is placed around the site to create a sterile field. Postprocedure, the site is covered with a band-aid or other sterile dressing. If a sterile dressing impedes your ability to scan around an area, remove the dressing only after consulting with the physician or nurse. Discard the dressing. Apply a new dressing afterward.

Scanning within a sterile field will require you to (1) wear sterile gloves, (2) use a sterile couplant, and (3) use a sterile probe.

Probe and Needle Guide Sterilization Techniques

Cold Chemical Soak. After thoroughly cleaning the probe, immerse it for the required amount of time in an activated glutaraldehyde solution (see Appendix 30). (Do not immerse the cable connection.) Put on sterile gloves. With a sterile hand remove the probe from the solution. With the other hand, hold a sterile water container and rinse the probe. Place the probe on a double-folded sterile towel, and wrap and seal with tape. Carry it to the examination room and use it immediately. Follow the same procedure for a needle guide.

Sterile Disposable Covers. Most probes can be rendered sterile by using sterile probe covers. Covers are included in "needle guide kits" and are also available separately. After placing a sterile cover onto a sterile field, don sterile gloves. Hold open the sterile probe cover. An unsterile person squirts couplant inside the cover (or the couplant may be put directly on the probe). The unsterile person then places the probe within the cover. Unfold the sterile cover over the probe and secure it with a rubber band or tie (Fig. 55-2).

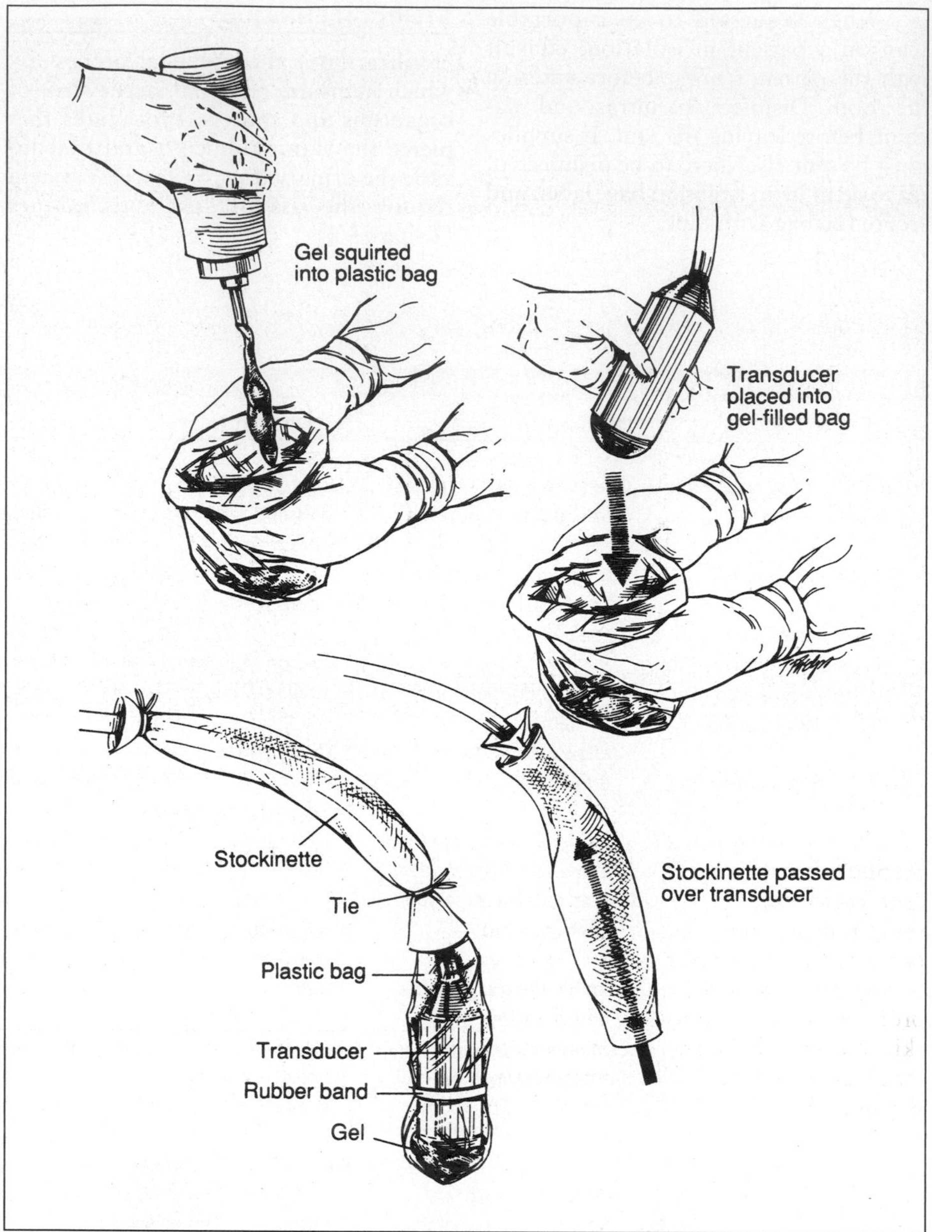

Figure 55-2. ■ *Method of rendering a probe sterile. Sterile covers (which are commercially available in various sizes) can be fabricated from 6- × 3- × 15-inch plastic bags as shown. Application of sterile covers: The sterile bag is folded open; fingers are placed under the fold. Gel (sufficient to cover probe face) is squirted into the bag away from the seam. The probe is placed onto the gel inside the bag. The bag is rolled over the probe and secured. Sterile stockinette, if needed, is slipped over the bag to cable and secured. (Reprinted with permission, The nurse's role in ultrasound.* Ultrasound Q *1989;7(1):73–104.)*

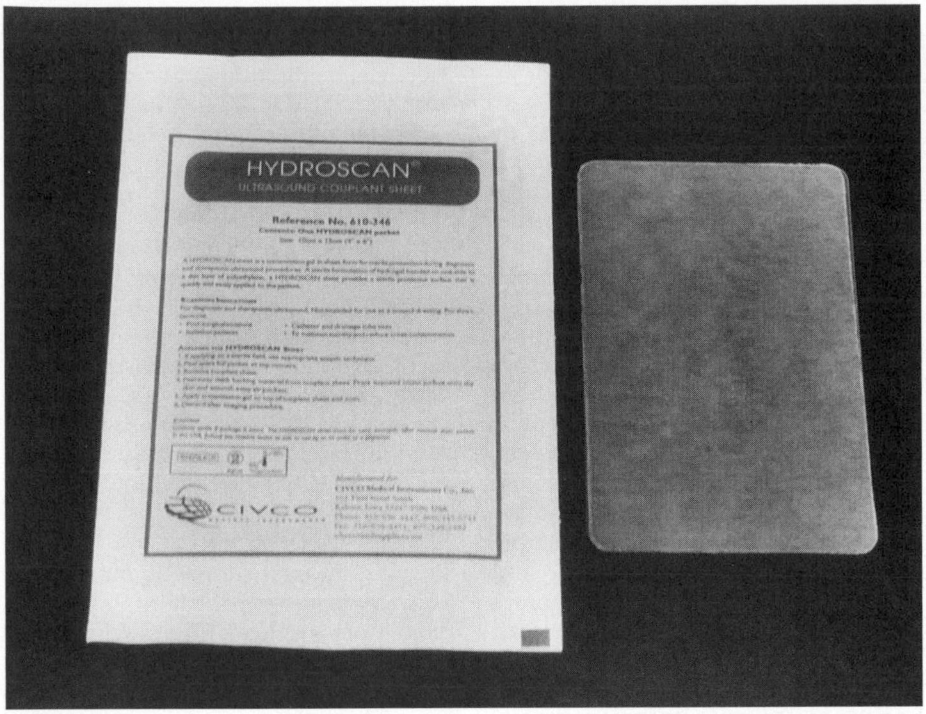

Figure 55-3. ■ *Hydroscan Ultrasound Couplant Sheet (4 × 6 inches) distributed by CIVCO Medical Instruments, Kalona, Iowa.*

Sterile Barrier. To scan over a fresh or recent postoperative site, such as a renal transplant wound, a sterile gel-film skin barrier (Fig. 55-3) may be used. The skin barrier eliminates the need for a sterile probe and sterile couplant. Handle the skin barrier only by the edges and extend it at least 1 inch beyond the periphery of the wound.

Body Mechanics

Proper transport, transfer, and positioning techniques help to ensure patient safety. In addition to decreasing the risk of injury, the use of proper body mechanics can increase comfort and conserve energy for yourself as well as the patient. If your institution has ergonomic devices, use them.

TRANSPORT

When transporting a patient, your goal is to reduce personal back strain and protect the patient's head from possible injury. Stand close behind the wheelchair and push from the handles; push a stretcher from the two adjacent corners nearest to the patient's head. Walk beside an ambulatory patient and, if needed, have him or her hold your arm for support and guidance.

TRANSFER

Before transferring a patient onto the examination table, assess his/her ability to assist with the move, and then decide on the best method of transfer. Guidelines are as follows: (1) transfer across the shortest distance; place a wheelchair as close to the examination table as possible; place a stretcher level with the table and against it; (2) stabilize the transport vehicle and the examination table, lock the brakes, and raise the footrests on a wheelchair; (3) do not permit a patient to climb onto the examination table, rather, place a step stool beside the table, turn the patient's back toward the table, and tell the patient to step onto the step stool from the side; (4) support, if necessary, the patient's head/neck, spine, and/or legs during a transfer and do not permit the patient to support himself by holding the back of your neck; (5) to avoid orthostatic (postural) hypotension, sit a patient up slowly from a supine position and have him/her sit momentarily on the side of the table before standing. If the patient sits or stands too quickly, his/her blood pressure may decrease causing dizziness and loss of balance, which could lead to a fall; (6) use the two-carrier lift (Fig. 55-4) to transfer

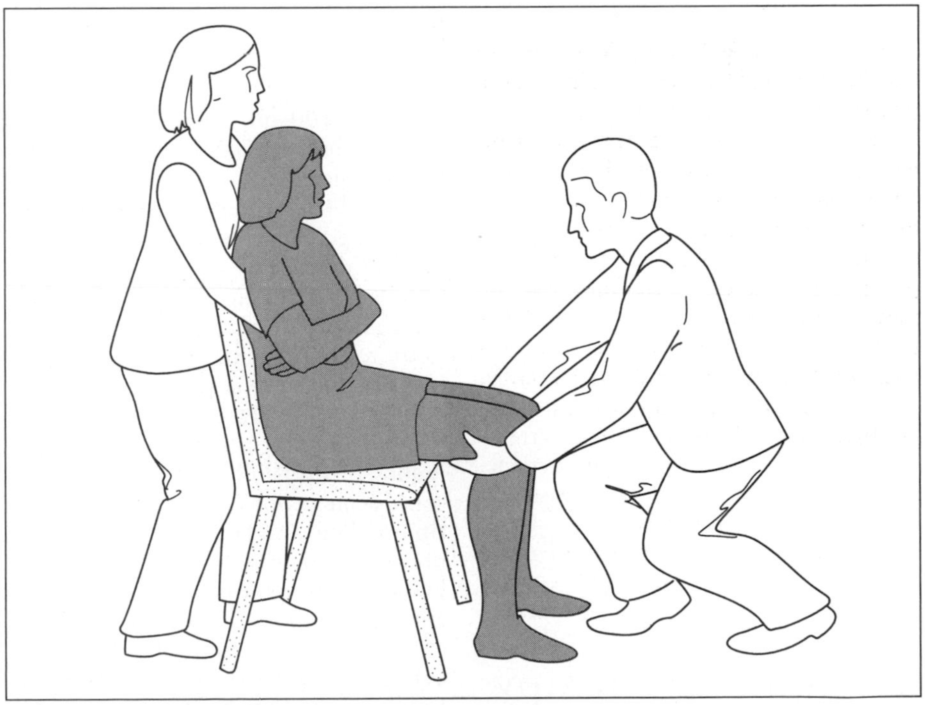

Figure 55-4. ■ *Two-carrier lift. Place patient's arms across his/her chest; bend your knees slightly and place your arms around the patient's chest and knees. On signal, lift the patient and place on stretcher.*

a patient who cannot stand; (7) before leaving a patient alone, secure the safety straps and railings. Place a call bell within reach.

POSITIONING

Move the patient up on a stretcher or ultrasound table.

When the head of a stretcher or table is elevated, the patient may slide toward the foot. This can impede the patient's ability to breath as well as exert pressure on bony prominences. To reposition the patient: (1) Lock the wheels and lower the head of the stretcher; (2) raise the stretcher to comfortable level; (3) you and another person position yourselves on opposite sides of the stretcher and face in the direction of the move; (4) you each place one foot in front of the other and slightly bend your knees; (5) the person on the left of the patient slips his/her right arm under the patient's left shoulder and puts the left arm behind the back to the other shoulder; (6) the person on the right of the patient slips his/her left arm under the right shoulder and puts the right arm behind the back to the patient's left shoulder; (7) if possible, bend the patient's knees to help reduce drag; and (8) on a signal, step forward, carrying the patient with you.

LIMB RESTRAINTS

Restraining or immobilizing a patient is occasionally necessary to aid scanning or to protect the patient and others from harm. Before applying restraints, obtain a doctor's order and explain the need to the patient/family. Pad the skin to protect it from possible abrasions. Secure the restraint to the stretcher, chair, or table frame out of the patient's grasp and in a way that allows for quick release and removal in case of an emergency. Restraints should be loose enough to allow adequate circulation to the extremity. Signs and symptoms of impaired circulation can occur distal to the restraint and include an absent or weak pulse, coldness, numbness, burning, tingling, cyanosis (or pallor), and edema.

Intravenous Therapy

IV therapy is the insertion of a device into a vein for the purpose of providing hydration, blood products, medications, or diagnostic agents. When caring for a patient with an IV line, you are responsible for ensuring that the flow is not impeded and the line and insertion site are not compromised. To detect a potential or real problem, check the patient's IV before bringing him/her into the room, during the scan, and after returning him/her to the waiting area.

General guidelines: (1) keep tubing as close to insertion site as possible; (2) keep tubing off the floor; (3) do not allow tubing to dangle by the wheels where it could become entangled and pull apart; (4) place tubing in front of the patient when transferring or positioning the patient; (5) instruct the patient to push the IV pole with the hand that does not have the IV; (6) hang an IV container at least 18 to 30 inches above the infusion site; (7) plug in IV infusion pumps; and (8) report complications immediately.

TROUBLESHOOTING COMPLICATIONS

No Infusion Rate/Flow

The flow of a fluid is checked by observing the drip rate. Verify a very rapid rate or "wide open" rate with the nurse/doctor. If fluid is not dripping, check the IV line from the container to the insertion site. Eliminate any kinks or sharp bends in the tubing and raise the height of the container. If flow does not resume, notify the nurse.

Check the fluid level in the container. Notify the nurse if the fluid level is below 100 mL. If the container is empty or breaks, close the clamp and notify the nurse.

Fluid that requires close monitoring is regulated by an infusion pump. If there is any impedance to flow, the pump sounds an alarm and may also display a message as to what the problem is and how to correct it. Keep the pump plugged in whenever possible.

Disconnections

Pulling on an IV line is the primary reason disconnections occur. Your responsibility should an IV line disconnect is to prevent fluid loss from the tubing and blood loss from the patient. (1) If the disconnection occurs between tubings, clamp off tubings. Wipe the ends with alcohol 70% or povidone-iodine solution. Reconnect and unclamp tubings. Check for flow. If the tubings touched the floor (or other soiled surface) or air has entered the lumen of tubing connected to the patient, notify the nurse. (2) If tubing disconnects from the hub of the IV device, clamp the tubing and apply pressure over the vein 1/2 to 1 inch above the insertion site or insert a 1-mL syringe into the hub of device. Notify the nurse.

Device Pulled Out

An IV device that is pulled out is immediately checked for breakage. If the tip is missing, tell the patient to decrease movement. Apply a tourniquet high up on the extremity; palpate a distal pulse to verify arterial flow. Apply a sterile dressing over the site, and then promptly notify the physician, who may order an x-ray film to help locate the tip.

Circulatory Overload

Preparation for a transabdominal pelvic scan can cause a patient to experience circulatory overload. The rapid infusion of IV fluids may be more than the patient's vascular system can accommodate. The patient may have one or more of these symptoms: difficulty breathing, headache, and chest pain. The patient's blood pressure would be elevated. Slow the infusion rate and notify the doctor/nurse.

Infiltration

An IV device that slips out of the vein into the surrounding tissue has infiltrated. Signs and symptoms include edema (compare muscle mass with the opposite extremity), pain, and cool skin over the site. The dressing may be wet due to fluid leaking out of the site. Clamp off the infusion and then notify the nurse.

Phlebitis

Inflammation of a vein can be caused by the (1) infusion of irritating drugs (i.e., potassium and antibiotics), (2) overuse of a vein, or (3) rubbing of the IV device against the vein's inner wall. Signs and symptoms of phlebitis include redness, warmth, and pain. An induration along the course of the vein may also be felt. Notify the nurse.

Catheters, Tubes, and Drains

As with an IV line, avoid putting tension on a catheter, drain, or tube that may be attached to the patient. A subsequent disconnection or displacement may require the patient to undergo a painful reinsertion and place the patient at risk for a serious complication. Other guidelines are as follows: (1) prevent drainage from backflowing into the patient by not draping the tubing over the side rail; (2) keep the drainage receptacle upright and below or at the level of the site being drained; (3) obtain a doctor's permission before removing a dressing covering a drain, catheter, or tube; (4) if a catheter, drain, or tube falls out, cover the skin site (if applicable) with a sterile gauze dressing; and (5) notify the physician or nurse of any problem.

NASOGASTRIC/NASOENTERIC TUBES

The primary purpose of a nasogastric (NG) or nasoenteric (NE) tube is for decompression of the gut. In general, patients who have NG/NE tubes are *non per os* (NPO). This means he/she is not permitted any food and/or liquids by mouth. The major risk of having an NG/NE tube is aspiration of gastric secretions into the lungs. An aspiration can cause pneumonia. Always keep the patient's head elevated 30 to 90 degrees, particularly when fluids such as tube feeding are being instilled. Tube feedings should be stopped before scanning the anterior and lateral sides of the neck.

Some tubes are connected to suction or straight drainage. When the suction or drainage is interrupted for any length of time, the patient may vomit around the tube. Position the patient in an upright sitting position (Fowler's). If unable to sit, place the patient on his/her right side and raise his/her head. If the patient must remain flat, turn his/her head to the side. Notify the nurse.

CHEST CATHETERS

A disruption in a chest catheter drainage setup requires immediate correction to prevent the patient from experiencing a tension pneumothorax. A tension pneumothorax is caused by the excessive accumulation of fluid/air in the pleural space *or* by an occlusion in the setup. Signs and symptoms are shortness of breath, increased respirations, increased pulse, decreased blood pressure, dizziness, and tracheal deviation. The receptacle of a water-sealed chest catheter must remain upright at all times to prevent spillage and shifting of fluid. Promptly notify the physician and the nurse when any of the following occur. (1) The chest catheter falls out of the chest wall: Cover the site immediately with an occlusive dressing such as petrolatum gauze, and leave one corner of dressing open to vent. Elevate the patient's head 45 degrees (semi-Fowler's position). (2) The receptacle breaks: Disconnect the tubing from receptacle and place at least 2 inches of tubing into a container of sterile irrigation saline. (3) The tubing disconnects from the catheter: Clean off the exposed ends with alcohol 70% or povidone-iodine solution and reconnect.

URINARY CATHETERS

Three of the most common urinary catheters that you will encounter are (1) a condom catheter that covers the penis, (2) a straight catheter that is inserted through the urethra into the bladder for procedural use only, and (3) a Foley catheter that is inserted like the straight catheter except it has a balloon near the distal tip; when inflated, the balloon helps anchor the catheter in the bladder. A Foley catheter is also referred to as an indwelling or retention catheter.

Guidelines to follow when caring for a patient with a urinary catheter are as follows: (1) Do not pull on the catheter unless attempting to remove it; (2) do not drape catheter tubing over the side rails; (3) keep the drainage bag below the urinary bladder and off the floor; (4) notify the nurse if the drainage bag is full/bulging; and (5) use sterile technique when disconnecting a catheter from its drainage bag.

Oxygen Therapy

When a patient receiving oxygen arrives, check the two gauges on the oxygen tank's regulator. One gauge registers the oxygen pressure per square inch (PSI); the other registers the liter flow per minute (LPM). The LPM gauge may be set from 0.25 to 15. The PSI gauge should be greater than 500. If the PSI is less than 500, a replacement tank may be needed; follow your institution's procedure for obtaining a tank.

To ensure sufficient oxygen in the tank for transport and to eliminate the need to check the tank periodically and possibly replace it, use piped in oxygen when available. The wall oxygen regulator has only an LPM gauge for setting the flow rate. Set the wall regulator to the same setting as on the tank; disconnect the oxygen tubing from the cylinder and connect it to the wall regulator. Turn off the tank.

Aerosol may be added to an oxygen delivery system to prevent excessive drying of the mucous membranes. If a distilled water container is attached, keep it upright to prevent spillage. Condensation buildup in the tubing can block the flow of oxygen, and the patient may say he/she cannot feel the oxygen or you no longer see a fine mist coming from the oxygen mask. Disconnect the tubing from the water container and the patient's mask. Dump the water and reconnect the tubing.

Do not permit anyone to smoke within the vicinity of a patient receiving oxygen; there is the potential danger of an explosion. The use of oil-based lubricants should also be avoided.

Emergencies

A medical emergency can arise with any patient in your care. When one occurs, you need to respond quickly and accurately. Always have a nurse or physician present when scanning a monitored patient or a baby in an isolette/warmer.

GENERAL GUIDELINES

1. Plan ahead.
   a. *Maintain basic cardiac life support training.* Basic cardiac life support or cardiopulmonary resuscitation is performed on a patient who is unresponsive with absent or highly questionable pulse and/or breathing. To eliminate direct mouth-to-mouth contact when giving breaths, use an Ambu bag, a resuscitative airway, a mask with a one-way valve, or a plastic mouth shield with a one-way valve.
   b. *Be familiar with medical emergency equipment.* Equipment should be centrally located and may consist of the following:

      Automated external defibrillator is easier to operate than a standard defibrillator and converts ventricular tachycardia/fibrillation to a rhythm compatible with life.

      Twelve-lead electrocardiogram machine displays and records heart rhythm.

      Pulse oximeter displays oxygen saturation and pulse.

Suction removes fluids from airway.

Dinamap displays and records vital signs.

Code Cart contains items necessary for advanced life support including drugs.

c. *Know how to contact essential personnel.* Post emergency numbers by phones. When speaking with the contact, give the exact location and type of emergency.

2. Never leave the patient alone unless absolutely necessary; call out for help.
3. Keep the area clear of spectators. Maintain the patient's privacy and confidentiality.
4. Clean and replace equipment/supplies soon after the emergency.
5. Document in the medical record and, if required, complete an incident report.

SYNCOPE (FAINTING)

Position the patient supine and loosen tight clothing. Place inhalant ammonia, a respiratory stimulant, under the patient's nose to attempt to arouse him/her.

INSULIN REACTION

A diabetic patient required not to eat (NPO) in preparation for a scan may experience low blood sugar (hypoglycemia). Signs and symptoms occur suddenly and include headache, nervousness, shaking, dizziness, sweating, cold-clammy skin, blurred vision, numbness of lips or tongue, and hunger. If the patient must remain NPO, the physician may request dextrose 50% for IV administration or glucagon, and 1 mg for subcutaneous or intramuscular injection. If the patient can eat, give him/her sugar, such as hard candy, juice, or milk. Provide him/her a well-balanced meal as soon as possible. Diabetic patients should have early morning appointments when required to be NPO.

VASOVAGAL REACTION

Patients undergoing transrectal scans, carotid studies, and invasive procedures such as biopsies may experience a decrease in blood pressure and pulse brought on by stimulation of the vagus nerve. Pain or anxiety usually triggers this reaction. Signs and symptoms include pallor, warmth, nausea/vomiting, dizziness, and cold-clammy skin. Immediately stop the procedure and remove the offending device such as the needle or probe. Place a cool damp cloth to the patient's forehead and position him/her supine; if the patient has an advanced pregnancy, put her in the left lateral position. Elevate the legs. Notify the physician or nurse. If the patient does not improve, IV fluids and atropine 1 mg may need to be administered.

SEIZURE

Protect the patient from injury by placing padding under his/her head and removing sharp or hard objects. Do not restrain the patient. Loosen tight clothing. Observe and time the seizure closely. After the seizure, turn the patient onto the side nearest you and check for breathing. If respirations are absent, open the airway by tilting the head and lifting the chin. If breathing does not resume, initiate cardiopulmonary resuscitation.

CHEST PAIN

Immediately notify the nurse or doctor when a patient experiences chest pain or discomfort. Chest pain can be a symptom of (1) coronary artery disease, (2) pulmonary disease, (3) gastric reflux, or (4) musculoskeletal disease. Until the cause is determined, stop the examination and have the patient rest. Place the patient in Fowler's position. An elderly patient may have atypical pain in the upper abdomen. When performing a deep venous thrombosis scan, avoid manipulating the leg excessively to prevent the possibility of a pulmonary embolus.

Procedures Integral to Scans

FILLING A URINARY BLADDER

The bladder may be filled by four methods. In general, how quick the bladder fills is determined by how well the patient is hydrated; the more hydrated, the more urine is produced. To check for bladder fullness, (1) ask the patient, (2) scan the bladder, or (3) palpate lightly above symphysis pubis. Always attempt to fill the bladder by the least invasive method. After the scan, provide the patient with a means for prompt evacuation. If applicable, record/report intake and output.

DRINK LIQUIDS

Consuming 32 ounces of water usually fills the bladder in 1 to 2 hours. Make sure the patient is not NPO. To prevent nausea and vomiting, caution the patient against gulping down the water. Avoid using this method with the elderly, who in general have delayed gastric emptying.

CLAMP INDWELLING URINARY CATHETER

A Foley catheter may be clamped if the patient does not have any of the following contraindications: urinary tract infection, recent renal transplant, bladder spasms, and spinal cord injury T6 or higher. Providing there are no contraindications, clamp the catheter using

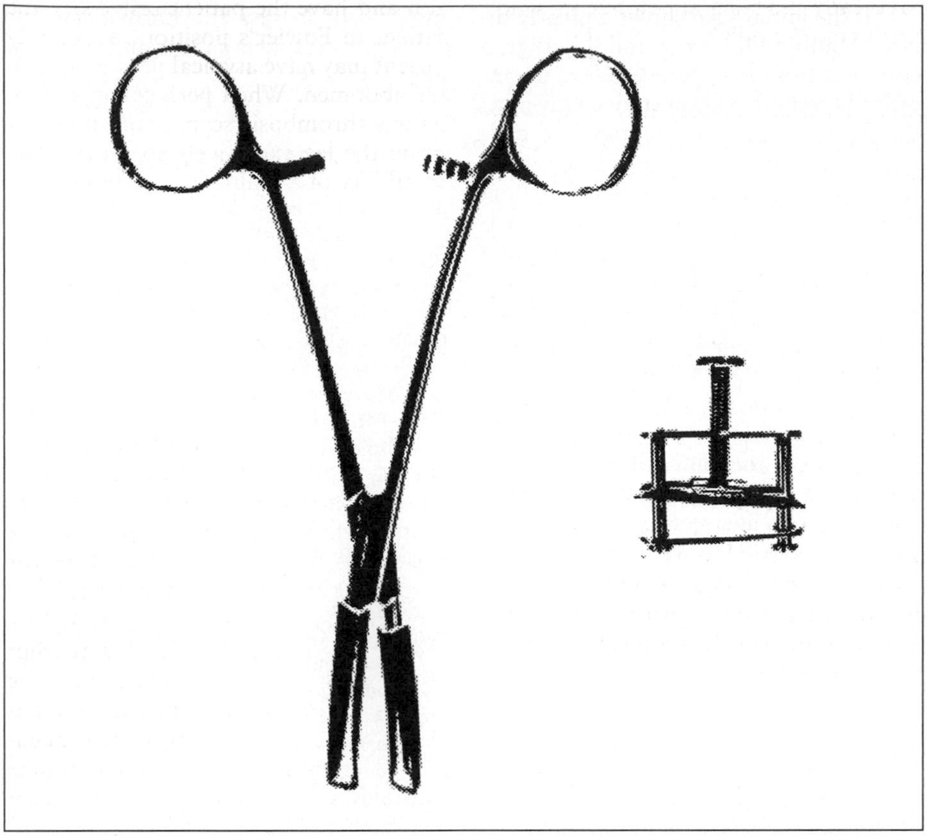

Figure 55-5. ■ *Clamps: Hoffman* (left); *padded Halsted* (right) *(gauze can also be used for padding).*

a Hoffman clamp or a padded straight forceps (Fig. 55-5) (these clamps will not puncture or exert excessive pull on catheter). Check the patient for bladder distention every 20 to 30 minutes. Unclamp the catheter once the scan is completed.

INCREASE INTRAVENOUS FLOW RATE

Before increasing the flow rate of an IV solution, obtain permission from the patient's physician. Diseases affecting fluid and electrolyte balance and solutions containing medications may contraindicate this method. Check for bladder distention every 15 to 20 minutes (once a full bladder is obtained, reduce the rate). Do not allow the fluid bag to run dry; notify the nurse if fluid level is below 100 mL. Observe the patient for fluid overload. If she/he experiences headache, difficulty breathing, and/or lightheadedness, reduce the rate and notify the nurse or physician. Avoid using this method with the very young and elderly.

FILL THROUGH A CATHETER

Interrupting a closed urinary drainage system is discouraged. Retrograde filling of the bladder carries the risk of contamination and possible urinary tract infection. Do not use this method with patients who are immunosuppressed or have a urinary tract infection. Adhere to sterile technique when preparing the setup. (1) Connect irrigation tubing to a bag of irrigation 0.9% sodium chloride (saline). (2) Position the roller clamp under the drip chamber and close it. (3) Suspend the solution bag and squeeze the drip chamber several times to fill it. (4) Open the clamp and purge the tubing of air by allowing some of the saline to flow through; close the clamp. (5) Clamp the catheter (Fig. 55-5) and disconnect the urinary drainage bag. Wrap the exposed end of the drainage bag tubing inside an alcohol wipe or sterile 4 × 3 gauze and lay it aside. (6) Connect the irrigation set to the catheter and unclamp both. Allow the saline to flow into the bladder gradually. (7) Once the bladder is full, close the roller clamp and perform the scan. (8) After scanning, decompress the bladder by lowering the bag below the level of the bladder. Open the roller clamp, thus allowing drainage.

For babies and toddlers, saline may be instilled through a syringe that is connected to the catheter. However, the risk of contamination is increased and it requires at least two people.

If the patient does not have a catheter and there is no other means of filling the bladder, the nurse or doctor can insert a straight catheter.

ENDORECTAL PROCEDURES

Procedures that require the insertion of a device into the rectum can be very uncomfortable to the patient. Proceed with caution in patients with spinal injury above T6 to prevent autonomic dysreflexia. If the patient has hemorrhoids or rectal irritation lidocaine jelly may be used as a lubricant. To insert the device, place the patient in the Sim's position (on left side with right knee bent and left leg straight). Do not have the patient perform the Valsalva maneuver (bear down). This could potentially cause a cardiac event in susceptible people. After scanning, direct (or assist) the patient to a toilet or provide a bedpan (see Toileting Needs).

Water Enema

When the distinction between a pelvic mass and colon is unclear, a water enema may occasionally be needed. (1) Close the clamp on an enema bag, and fill the bag with 500 to 700 mL of warm water. Purge the tubing of air by allowing some of the water to flow through and reclamp. (2) Place the patient in the Sim's position. (3) Liberally lubricate the tip of the enema tubing. (4) Separate the patient's buttocks to see the anus. (5) Angle the enema tip toward the patient's umbilicus and gently insert and advance it 3 to 4 inches into the rectum. To help the patient relax the abdominal muscles, instruct him/her to breathe deeply and slowly in through the nose and out through the mouth. If resistance is felt, reangle the tip or allow a little water to flow through. If resistance is still felt, stop and notify the doctor or nurse. (6) Once the tip is inserted, tape it in place. Tell the patient to tighten the anal sphincter to help retain the water. (7) Position the patient supine and unclamp the tubing. Allow the water to flow in gradually.

Transrectal Scan

Imaging of the prostate gland and other perirectal masses require the insertion of a rectal probe. Fecal material in the lower rectum can make it impossible to obtain a satisfactory scan. Therefore, before arriving the patient may be instructed to eat a light meal the day of procedure and administer a cleansing enema, such as a Fleet sodium phosphate enema. A sodium phosphate enema should not be administered to patients who have inflammatory bowel diseases such as Crohn's disease or ulcerative colitis.

If the patient did not perform the enema, you may need to assist. Follow the same procedure as outlined in steps 2–5 under Water Enema above. Once the tip is inserted, squeeze the container until empty. Tell the patient to retain the solution until he/she feels the urge to defecate (usually in 1 to 2 minutes). To insert the rectal probe, use the same technique but advance the probe 4 to 5 inches into rectum.

DRUG ADMINISTRATION

Very few diagnostic or contrast agents are administered as a part of ultrasonography. Microbubbles for enhancement of masses are on the horizon but are not yet standard. Methylcellulose, used as an acoustic window when evaluating the stomach/pancreas, is difficult for most patients to consume. Follow these guidelines when administering drugs: (1) Obtain a doctor's order; (2) prepare the correct drug by reading the label on the container three times, when taking the container off the shelf, preparing the dose, and discarding or returning the container; (3) prepare correct dose by having a conversion chart or table of equivalents available; (4) identify the patient by checking ID bracelet or asking his/her name (as opposed to saying "Are you Mrs. X?"); (5) check the patient's allergy history; (6) administer the drug at the correct time and by the correct route; and (7) document the administration in the patient's medical record.

FATTY MEAL

To properly examine the gallbladder and common bile duct, the patient should not eat anything 5 to 6 hours before the scan. This helps to ensure that the gallbladder will be distended. Clear liquids such as water and Jell-O are permitted.

If the initial scan shows a greatly dilated gallbladder or a mildly dilated common bile duct, Neo-Cholex, or another liquid fatty agent may be given to the patient by mouth to stimulate gallbladder contraction or bowel excretion. If the patient is not permitted anything by mouth, cholecystokinin may be administered IV. Nausea and vomiting is a common transient adverse effect of Neo-Cholex and cholecystokinin. After administering the agent, re-scan the gallbladder in 15 to 20 minutes.

ENSURE™

Evaluation of the pancreas and superior mesenteric artery may entail the administration of an agent to increase peristalsis and thus blood flow. Ensure™, a balanced nutrient drink, can be given to the patient. It is easy to tolerate and may also be used as a "fatty meal." The patient is re-scanned in 15 minutes.

SEDATION

Attending to comfort needs is essential when planning the care of a patient undergoing a biopsy. With the exception of "blood thinners," patients scheduled for biopsies should continue to take their medicine(s) as prescribed. On arrival, the patient's pain level and anxiety state are assessed. If medication is warranted, the nurse or doctor will administer it.

The patient may receive sedation by mouth, intramuscular injection, or conscious sedation. Anesthesia may be required for a pediatric patient or a patient with uncontrolled pain. Antianxiety medications include lorazepam (Ativan), diazepam (Valium), alprazolam (Xanax), and midazolam (Versed). Pain medications include acetaminophen (Tylenol), oxycodone, Sublimaze (fentanyl), and morphine. Conscious sedation requires the patient to have an IV device. The nurse or doctor must monitor the patient's vital signs, including the use of pulse oximetry, continuously throughout the procedure. Sublimaze and midazolam are the drugs of choice for conscious sedation. Emergency equipment and reversal drugs should be readily available.

Summary

Nursing procedures are not performed solely by a nurse. The sonographer and sonologist, to affect a positive outcome, must also possess the knowledge and skills to assess their patient and intervene appropriately.

SELECTED READING

Ashton K. Following the standard. *Advance for Nurses* 2002;4(5):33–34.

Borton D. Isolation precautions, part I: how to protect your patients and yourself. *Nursing* 2001;31(6):14.

Combating infection. Handwashing: first defense against infection. *Nursing* 2001; 31(6):20.

Craven R, Hirnle C. *Fundamentals of Nursing,* 3rd ed. Philadelphia: Lippincott; 2002.

Deering CG, Cody DJ. Communicating with children and adolescents. *Am J Nurs* 2002; 102(3):32–41.

Fulginiti SP. When your client has a spinal cord injury. *Advance for Nurses* 2002;4(7): 31–34.

Gonzalez R, Gooden MB, Porter C. Eliminating racial and ethnic disparities in health care. *Am J Nurs* 2000;100(3):56–58.

Holmes HN. *Nursing Procedures,* 3rd ed. Springhouse Corporation, PA: Springhouse; 2000.

Incredibly easy. Understanding chest pain. *Nursing* 2001;31(12):28.

Lazzara D. Eliminating the air of mystery from chest tubes. *Nursing* 2002;32(6):36–43.

Lipson JG, Dibble SL, Minarik PA, eds. *Culture and Nursing Care: A Pocket Guide.* San Francisco, CA: UCSF Nursing Press; 1996.

Malozemoff W, Gentleman B. Dizziness in elders: defined and differentiated. *Nurs Spectr* 2003;13(6DC):14–16.

Mercer TA. JCAHO patient safety goals. *Advance for Nurses* 2002;4(17):21–22.

Moureau N. Preventing complications from vascular access devices. *Nursing* 2001;31(7): 48–50.

Nelson A, Owen B, Lloyd JD, et al. Safe patient handling and movement. *Am J Nurs* 2003; 103(3):32–43.

Noble K. Name that tube. *Nursing* 2003;33(3): 56–62.

O'Donnell JM, Bragg K, Sell S. Procedural sedation: safely navigating the twilight zone. *Nursing* 2003;33(4):36–44.

Sammer CE. How should you respond to hypoglycemia? *Nursing* 2001;31(7):48–50.

Web Sites

www.advancefornurses.com
www.engenderhealth.org
www.infodotinc.com
www.nursingcenter.com
www.omhrc.gov
www.patientsafety.com

Work-Related Musculoskeletal Disorders in Sonography

56

CAROLYN COFFIN
SUSAN MURPHY

KEY WORDS

Work-related musculoskeletal disorders (WRMSDs), or musculoskeletal disorders (MSDs). Refers to injuries of muscles, tendons, and joints that result from work activities.

Biomechanical Factors. Body movements, postures, or activities that contribute to injury risk.

Ergonomics. The science of designing a work environment to fit the individual employee.

Engineering Controls. One of three ergonomic principles for reducing or eliminating work-related injury.

Definition

Work-related musculoskeletal disorders (WRMSDs), or musculoskeletal disorders (MSDs), are defined as injuries that are caused by or aggravated by workplace activities. They account for up to 60% of all workplace illnesses, and survey data have shown that more than 80% of sonographers have some form of MSD that can be attributed to their work activities.

Causes and Risk Factors

The causes of MSD can be attributed to three groups of factors:

- Biomechanical factors—awkward scanning postures, excessive force used in performing an exam, workspace design
- Faulty work organization—infrequent breaks, overtime and on-call incentives, poor employee training
- Injury management—delayed injury reporting and diagnosis, improper injury management, returning worker to injury-producing environment

Work activities that contribute to injuries in sonographers are repetitive motions, forceful exertions or strain, awkward or unnatural positions, uncomfortable positioning of the limbs, static postures, overuse, and frequent reaching above shoulder level.

There are a number of individual factors that also increase one's risk for MSD, including sonographer height and weight, age, gender, systemic illnesses, level of physical fitness, and hand dominance. Shorter workers are forced to reach to access their patients, and taller workers may have to use awkward postures to scan their patients or to view the ultrasound monitor. Muscle strength usually peaks between 25 and 35 years of age, which is why older workers are at higher risk for injury. Male workers generally have more muscle mass and muscle strength than female workers. Systemic illnesses that may compromise blood flow to muscles and tendons increase one's risk for musculoskeletal injury.

In addition, there are certain leisure activities that can aggravate injury, such as playing musical instruments, running, sewing, and racket sports. These activities put extra strain on the muscles of the hands and forearm and the intervertebral discs of the back.

The current use of filmless storage in sonography has contributed to the increase in MSDs because this now allows sonographers to move rapidly from patient to patient without sufficient rest periods. The use of narrow transducers for certain examinations requires a tighter, or "pinch," grip that causes excess stress on the fingers and forearm muscles. Chairs or stools and examination tables that are not adjustable result in excessive reaching and twisting to reach to the patient during an examination. Increases in workloads are due to downsizing and shortages of skilled sonographers. Thus, each sonographer is performing more patient examinations during the workday, often necessitating more overtime and fewer work breaks.

Symptoms

Symptoms of musculoskeletal injury are as follows:

- Pain
- Inflammation
- Swelling
- Loss of sensation
- Numbness
- Tingling
- Burning
- Clumsiness
- Muscle spasm

Symptoms of MSD can occur after months or years of overuse and have been staged according to their reversibility and outcome.

Stage 1—aching and fatigue that subside with overnight rest and do not result in a reduction in work performance.

Stage 2—recurrent aching and fatigue that do not subside with overnight rest; symptoms occur earlier in the workday and affect performance at work.

Stage 3—aching, fatigue, and weakness result in reduced performance in work and leisure activities; pain occurs with nonrepetitive movements; symptoms disturb sleep and may last years.

Types of Musculoskeletal Disorders

Specific disorders of MSD are as follows:

- Tenosynovitis/tendonitis—inflammation of the tendon sheath and tendon
- Carpal tunnel syndrome—entrapment of the median nerve due to inflammation and edema of the soft tissues in the carpal tunnel of the wrist
- Cubital tunnel syndrome—entrapment of the ulnar nerve due to inflammation of the soft tissues in the elbow
- Trigger finger—inflammation of the tendon sheath of a finger, entrapping the tendon within and preventing flexion and/or extension of the finger
- de Quervain's disease—tendonitis specific to the thumb
- Lateral/medial epicondylitis—inflammation of the epicondyles of the distal humerus caused by repeated twisting of the forearm and exerting pressure with the arm
- Rotator cuff injury
- Bursitis of the shoulder
- Thoracic outlet syndrome—entrapment of the brachial plexus and/or the subclavian vessels by the muscles of the chest or the first rib
- Spinal degeneration—caused by constrained postures causing increased pressure between the vertebrae of the spine
- Neck/back sprains—caused by standing or sitting in awkward postures during an examination

Muscle Physiology

Muscles and tendons are designed to be used regularly. However, when frequency and duration of loading exceed the ability of the muscles and tendons to adapt, inflammation occurs, followed by degeneration, microtears, and scar formation. Once a tendon is injured, the muscle to which it is attached must compensate by working harder to provide support for the extremity and joint. An increase in the level of muscle support results in fatigue and strain. This type of stress is a function of the transducer time a sonographer maintains daily, particularly when performing the same type of examination. Work pace, recovery time, and level of muscular effort lead to these injuries. Studies have shown that a sonographer may exert up to 40 pounds of pressure during an examination. Muscles require an adequate supply of oxygen to function properly. Oxygen is pumped into muscles, and wastes are removed through the normal contraction of muscles during dynamic movement. Static postures prevent this process from occurring, resulting in decreased oxygen to the muscles and a buildup of lactic acid followed by fatigue and potential injury. Nerve damage results from arm abduction, flexion, and extension of the wrist and/or fingers. These motions cause swelling of the soft tissues that compress and entrap the nerves of the wrist or fingers.

Impact of Musculoskeletal Disorders

The impact of MSDs ranges from minor discomfort to career-ending injury. There are a number of emotional and financial implications for the injured worker, as well as an impact on the employer, coworkers, and Worker's Compensation.

Treatments

Once an accurate diagnosis of musculoskeletal injury has been made, treatment ranges from analgesics and anti-inflammatory medications to surgery. However, treatment of work-related MSDs has a poor outcome because sonographers are often expected to return to the same work environment that caused the injury initially. It is important, therefore, to *prevent* injury by addressing the risk factors in the workplace.

Injury Prevention

The keys to prevention are *education* and *ergonomics*. For example, employers must be aware of work schedules and allow for adequate breaks. They should provide separate monitors so that the patient and the sonographer do not have to share the monitor on the equipment. Examination gloves with textured fingers, which make it easier to grip the transducer, should be available. Equipment manufacturers must develop ergonomic transducer shapes, lighter cables, and adjustable keyboards and monitors. Scanning rooms can be ergonomically designed to fit each individual sonographer, with attention to room layout and proper lighting. Engineering controls, which address the physical hazards present in the workplace, are the most effective means for reducing WRMSDs.

INDIVIDUAL PREVENTION METHODS

Sonographers must learn to change the behaviors that have led to pain in the past. This can be done by using adjustable chairs or stools with backs and height-adjustable examination tables. Taking the time to position the equipment and the patient close to them can significantly reduce reaching and twisting. Attention should be given to arranging a patient's room during bedside examinations so that the sonographer can scan the patient comfortably without ex-

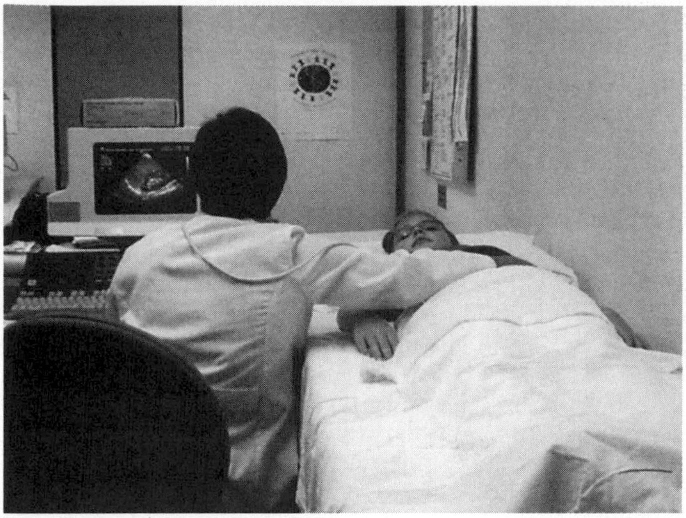

Figure 56-1. ■ *Bad posture can lead to pain and discomfort while scanning.*

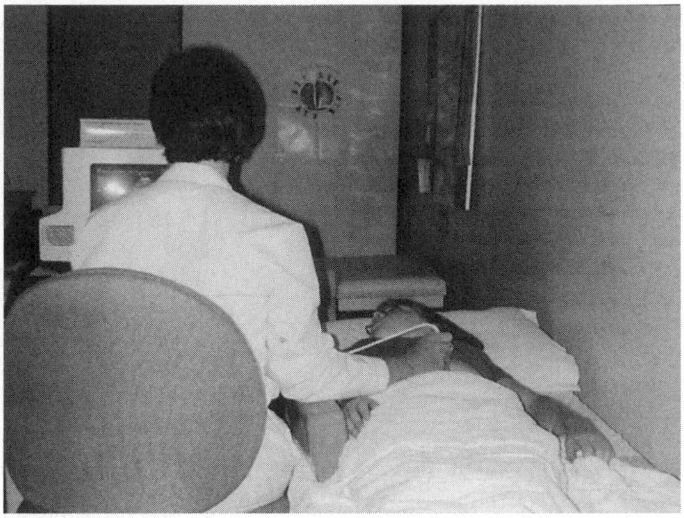

Figure 56-2. ■ *The correct position for a sonographer is to sit close to the patient with properly abducted arm and shoulder (not more than 30 degrees).*

cessive reach or abduction of their upper extremities (Figs. 56-1 and 56-2). The simple practice of taking multiple "mini-breaks," stopping to relax the neck and shoulder muscles, opening and closing hands, and resting the eyes can make a significant difference in the level of muscle strain and fatigue. Using cushions to support the scanning arm drastically reduces the amount of muscle activity in the arm, thus reducing fatigue and risk for injury. Sonographers should also learn to perform stretching and strengthening exercises designed to condition the shoulder, arms, and hands. During an acute injury, it is recommended that any leisure activities that aggravate the pain be limited.

DEPARTMENTAL CHANGES

Department managers should encourage sonographers to take rest breaks during the workday. Examinations should be scheduled so that the same examinations are not scheduled together, thus reducing repetitive motions. Employees should be instructed in the proper use of all examination room equipment. Bedside examinations should be reserved for patients on life support only and should be shared among staff members. Ideally, a hospital transporter should be used for the transport of hospital patients to the ultrasound department.

ERGONOMIC PRINCIPLES

Ergonomics is the "science" of designing a job to fit the individual worker. In ultrasound departments where a number of different sonographers are employed, adjustable examination room equipment and furnishings and the use of adaptive equipment while scanning best achieve this. Ergonomic engineering control measures, which attempt to fit the job to the employee, ultimately lead to improved operator productivity. Current equipment designs, from ultrasound equipment to examination room tables and chairs, are beginning to incorporate more ergonomic principles. As ultrasound departments replace old equipment or purchase additional equipment, they will be able to choose products that have been designed with the sonographer's safety as a priority.

ERGONOMIC EQUIPMENT

The ultrasound machine should have a height-adjustable monitor that swivels and tilts. The keyboard should also be height-adjustable and moveable independently of the monitor. Frequently used keys should be positioned so that minimal reach is needed to access them. Transducers should be easy to exchange and connect. The machine should be easy to move and position and should have brakes.

The examination table should also be height-adjustable and easy to move. The height range should be between 22 and 40 inches. The table width should be between 24 and 27 inches. If there are side rails on the table, they should retract completely below and beneath the table so that there is no additional distance between the sonographer and the patient. Other specifications for examination tables will depend on the specific studies performed in each ultrasound facility.

An ergonomic examination room chair, which is often overlooked when designing ultrasound facilities, is extremely important in contributing to injury prevention.

The chair should have an adjustable seat pan, allowing sonographers of different heights to have good support for their thighs. It should be height-adjustable and capable of rising high enough to allow for a sit–stand position. It should have five or more casters for stability, a footrest, and lumbar support. The back of the chair should also be adjustable to accommodate workers of different heights. A saddle-shaped design for the seat of the chair has been shown to promote the most upright and comfortable posture.

Sonographers should use support cushions during an examination to support the arm and, thus, prevent the upper extremity muscles from supporting the entire weight and activity of the arm. Once the arm is extended more than 30 degrees from the body, muscle strain and fatigue occur because the muscles are "firing" 100% of the time to maintain this position. Supporting the arm allows the muscles to rest and minimizes injury risk.

ERGONOMIC ADAPTATIONS OF CURRENT EQUIPMENT

Newer equipment designs incorporate ergonomic principles that may not be available in existing examination room equipment. Injury prevention is most effectively achieved by the purchase and use of ergonomically designed chairs, examination tables, and ultrasound equipment. However, until current equipment is replaced, there are a number of ways that equipment can be made more ergonomic or used in a more ergonomically correct way. Injuries can be minimized in a number of ways:

For examination room chairs whose height cannot be adjusted, something can be added to the chair, such as a folded towel, a lumbar support cushion, or an air-filled seat cushion. There may be other chairs that are not in use elsewhere in the hospital or ultrasound facility that might be more appropriate for an ultrasound department. Standing up while scanning may allow the sonographer to maintain a more comfortable posture and places less compression force on the spine than sitting in a poorly designed chair. The key is for sonographers to position themselves high enough to reduce the reach and abduction of the scanning arm. Most standard chairs do not achieve the necessary height. A properly designed ergonomic chair should also encourage an upright posture, thus reducing the pressure between the vertebrae of the spine.

Working with current examination tables requires that the patient be positioned close to the sonographer. This prevents unnecessary reaching and arm fatigue. It may be helpful to sit on the bed with the patient, especially in those cases when the patient cannot move. A height-adjustable table is critical in reducing the risk for injury to the upper extremity and neck. Fixed-height tables do not allow the sonographer to make the adjustments necessary to reduce the abduction of his or her scanning arm. For examination tables that are not height-adjustable, mattresses can be added or subtracted in an attempt to obtain an optimal height. Neck and upper extremity structures can be scanned with the patient seated in a wheelchair or a chair with arms, thus allowing the sonographer to get closer to the patient and maintain a more comfortable position.

If the monitor on the ultrasound equipment is stationary, the engineering department of the hospital or ultrasound facility may be able to modify the monitor of the ultrasound equipment to make it height-adjustable. It is wise to check with the ultrasound equipment manufacturer to make sure this modification will not void the warranty on the equipment. Adding an external monitor for the patient so that the monitor is not shared between the sonographer and the patient is an inexpensive solution. This prevents the need to twist the neck and back to view the monitor.

For equipment with fixed-height monitors, a small, second monitor may be added on top of the equipment for viewing examinations while standing.

CHANGES IN SCANNING AND WORKSTATION PRACTICES

Bedside Examinations

Try to share these examinations with other colleagues in the department and do portable examinations only when absolutely necessary, not because it is just more convenient.

Computer Equipment

Many departments now use picture archiving and communications (PAC) systems for image storage. Placement of this equipment can be as important as the equipment in the examination rooms. Place the PAC tower so that there is free leg room under the table. Try to obtain a height-adjustable chair or make the adjustments to the chair to keep arms in a neutral position, close to the body. Place the monitor on something, if necessary, to raise it to eye level. Note the position of the keyboard and raise it to a comfortable position.

It is important that sonographers take responsibility for how they practice their profession.

On Call

Limit call to only one institution, and try not to take call more than one 24-hour period at a time.

Breaks

Take lunch breaks. Don't give this up to accommodate add-on patients just to leave work on time at the end of the day; the muscle recovery time achieved by taking a break is more important.

Scanning Practices

Use mild transducer pressure. Don't be "image-driven." Avoid sacrificing musculoskeletal health for a "pretty picture" that does not affect the diagnosis.

Use a light grip on the transducer and use textured-finger gloves when possible, which improves the grip on the transducer, thus reducing the force required to hold it.

If the transducer is so narrow that it requires a "pinch" grip to hold it, try to use adaptive products that can be slipped over the transducer to widen it. The hand is four times stronger in a palmar or "power" grip than in a "pinch" grip. If available in your department, use lightweight transducers and transducers with lightweight, flexible cables.

Support your scanning arm by placing support cushions or a rolled-up towel under the elbow.

When performing endovaginal examinations, position the equipment at the foot-end of the examination table, and sit between the patient's legs with your scanning arm supported on towels or a cushion resting on your thigh. Position the equipment and the patient close enough to reduce the reach of both upper extremities.

Self Care

Practice strengthening exercises regularly at home to strengthen arm and shoulder muscles. Stretch before starting to scan each day. Exercise putty or a large rubber band can be used for hand-stretching exercises to increase blood supply to the hand and fingers. Take "mini-breaks" during patient examinations. Mini-breaks require only a few seconds and add only approximately 2 minutes to each examination. Put the transducer down and relax your scanning arm and hand. Gently shake the hand and arm, open and close your fist, and close your eyes momentarily. Get plenty of rest and practice good nutrition.

Have your eyes examined to ensure that corrective lenses are appropriately adjusted for an 18- to 22-inch screen distance. This helps reduce eyestrain and headaches and prevents the need to lean closer to the monitor. Room lighting should be easy to reach from the sonographer scanning location and should have dimming capabilities. Make sure the examination room lighting is adjusted to prevent glare on the monitor.

When one has an acute injury, try to limit the time spent on a home computer, especially avoiding a lot of mouse work or graphics all at one time. Limit leisure activities that use the upper extremity, such as gardening, needlework, knitting, playing musical instruments, and racket sports.

Following these suggestions, many of which are readily available within each facility or are very affordable adaptations, can make any ultrasound department more ergonomic and reduce sonographer exposure to MSD risks.

SELECTED READING

Browne CD, Nolan BM, Faithfull DK. Occupational repetition strain injuries. *Med J Aust* 1984:140;329–332.

Carson R. Reducing cumulative trauma disorders. *AAOHN J* 1994;42(6):270–276.

Ergoweb Inc. Available at: http://www.ergoweb.com.

Grieco A, Molteni G, DeVito G, et al. Epidemiology of musculoskeletal disorders due to biomechanical overload. *Ergonomics* 1998;41(9):1253–1260.

Kroemer K, Grandjean E. *Fitting the Task to the Human,* 5th ed. Philadelphia: Taylor & Francis, Inc.; 2000.

Handbook of Human Factors. In: Salvendy G, ed. New York: John Wiley & Sons, 1987. Chapters 5.1–5.4.

Melhorn JM. Cumulative trauma disorders and repetitive strain injuries: the future. *Clin Orthop* 1998;(351):107–126.

Pike I, Russo A, Berkowitz J, et al. The prevalence of musculoskeletal disorders among diagnostic medical sonographers. *JDMS* 1997;13(5):219–227.

57 Artifacts

ROGER GENT

KEY WORDS

Attenuation. Reduction in intensity with increasing depth of penetration.

Aliasing. Misrepresentation of Doppler shifts, caused by inadequate sampling rate (PRF).

Analog and Digital. Analog—Echo signals that have not been computer processed have an infinite number of patterns, more than a computer can manage. This unmodified (unmodulated) signal is termed analog. Digital—To allow a computer to display the image, the picture is broken up into multiple small areas (pixels), and numeric values are given to patterns and echo levels. Glossy photographs represent an analog image, whereas the small dots that compose a newspaper photographic image were composed digitally. Analog signals are continuous and therefore have an infinite number of values, like a ramp. Digital signals have a discrete number of values, like a staircase.

Artifact. Ultrasonic image appearance that does not accurately represent the region being displayed.

Azimuth. Depth axis.

Beamwidth. Dimension of the beam in the scan plane (cf. Slice Thickness).

Beamwidth Artifact. Display of echoes as lines rather than dots, caused by the finite width of ultrasound beams.

Comet Tail. Short-range reverberation.

Dirty Shadow. Acoustic shadow containing reverberation echoes.

Elevation Plane. See Slice Thickness.

Enhancement. Increased brightness of echoes deep to low-attenuating structures.

Frame Rate. Frequency of image formation; usually between 10 and 30 frames per second.

Grating Lobe. Ultrasonic energy radiating at an angle to the main lobe, in array transducers.

Harmonic Imaging. Receiving at twice the transmit frequency to reduce artifact.

Intrinsic Spectral Broadening. Misleading increase in bandwidth of Doppler signals.

Lateral Beam Spread. Widening of the transducer focus as the beam passes through tissues at increasing depths.

Main Bang. High-level echoes at the skin's surface, caused by the transmission signal passing into the receiver.

Mirror Artifact. Duplication of part of the display, caused by reflection of the beam at a specular reflector.

Nyquist Limit. The maximum frequency shift that can be unambiguously detected in Doppler, equal to PRF/2.

Pulse-Repetition Frequency (PRF). The number of pulses transmitted each second, measured in kilohertz.

Range Ambiguity Artifact. Display of echoes more superficially than their true depth of origin.

Refraction. Bending of a beam when it passes into tissue with a different speed of sound.

Resonance. Vibration of a structure at its natural frequency.

Reverberation. Bouncing of sound between two or more interfaces, causing multiple echoes in the display, at increasing depths.

Ringdown. Resonance phenomenon occurring in gas bubbles and resulting in a shaft of bright echoes.

Scan Plane. The plane in which the ultrasound beam sweeps.

Shadow. Region where there is no useful echo information because it has not been interrogated by the beam.

Side Lobe. Lobes of energy surrounding the main lobe and radiating at various angles to it.

Slice Thickness. The dimension of the beam perpendicular to the scan plane.

Specular Reflector. A reflector that acts like a mirror.

Twinkle Artifact. Multicolored artifact in color Doppler, arising from crystalline material and simulating blood flow.

Introduction

Artifacts are appearances in ultrasound images that do not accurately represent the structure or characteristics of the region being displayed. They occur because of physical limitations of ultrasound imaging and when inappropriate control settings are used in the acquisition of images. An understanding of the appearances and causes of artifacts is essential to the proper interpretation of ultrasound images to maximize the available information and to avoid diagnostic errors.

Diagnostic ultrasound systems necessarily operate under several assumptions. The main ones are as follows:

1. Ultrasound beams travel in straight lines.
2. The beams are extremely thin.
3. The speed of sound is constant throughout the tissues being imaged.
4. Attenuation is uniform throughout the tissue displayed in any one image.

The fact that these assumptions are not true, to varying degrees, gives rise to a range of appearances described as artifacts. Although we refer to them as artifacts, they are in fact accurate representations of the interaction of ultrasound beams with patient tissues.

The Clinical Problem

Artifacts are often present in ultrasound images. Some, such as shadowing and enhancement, provide useful diagnostic information. Many artifacts, such as reverberation, refraction, side lobe, and slice thickness effects, are undesirable and cause degradation of the images, resulting in loss of information. Some artifacts cause misleading appearances that, if unrecognized, can lead to incorrect diagnosis and inappropriate management of the patient.

It is important to recognize that some of the undesirable artifacts can be reduced or avoided by manipulation of the transducer (position, angulation, and pressure) and by adjustment of control settings according to the scanning circumstances. Recognizing and then minimizing or avoiding undesirable artifacts is one of the responsibilities of a sonographer, but one that is all too often overlooked.

Techniques for avoiding or minimizing artifacts are described, where relevant, in the following sections.

Types Of Artifact

Artifacts can be divided into four categories.

1. **Acoustic artifacts**—these relate to the way in which the beam interacts with the patient tissues.
2. **Equipment settings artifacts**—these result from inappropriate control settings used at the time of acquisition of the images.
3. **Doppler artifacts**—various appearances relating to the way in which Doppler information is acquired.
4. **Electronic noise and electrical interference effects**—inherent to electrical equipment.

Acoustic artifacts, the largest group, can be divided into four categories.

1. **Attenuation artifacts**, resulting from variations in attenuation in different tissues.
2. **Depth of origin artifacts**, causing echoes to be displayed at incorrect depths from the transducer.
3. **Beam dimension effects**, resulting from the finite dimensions of ultrasonic beams.
4. **Beam path artifacts**, resulting from deviation of the beam from its intended and assumed path.

Some of the acoustic artifacts have parallels in optics, useful for gaining an understanding of their origin and possible avoidance.

ACOUSTIC ARTIFACTS

Attenuation Artifacts

Acoustic Shadowing. Interfaces or structures that highly attenuate ultrasound beams cause acoustic shadows to appear deep to the structure. The shadow represents an area that has not been interrogated by the beam and from which no information is available. Bone, calculi, gas, scar tissue, and foreign bodies are common causes of shadowing. Shadows from calculi and foreign bodies are usually echo-free and are useful in identifying the presence of the abnormality (Fig. 57-1). The focal zone should be set at the

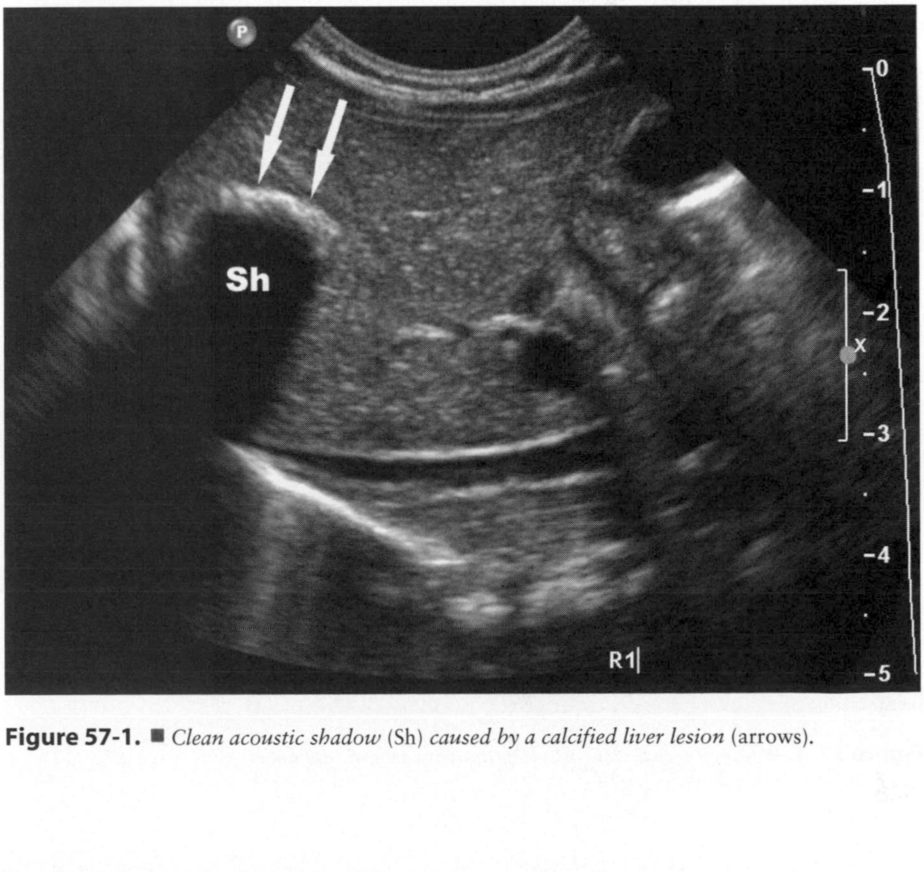

Figure 57-1. ■ *Clean acoustic shadow* (Sh) *caused by a calcified liver lesion* (arrows).

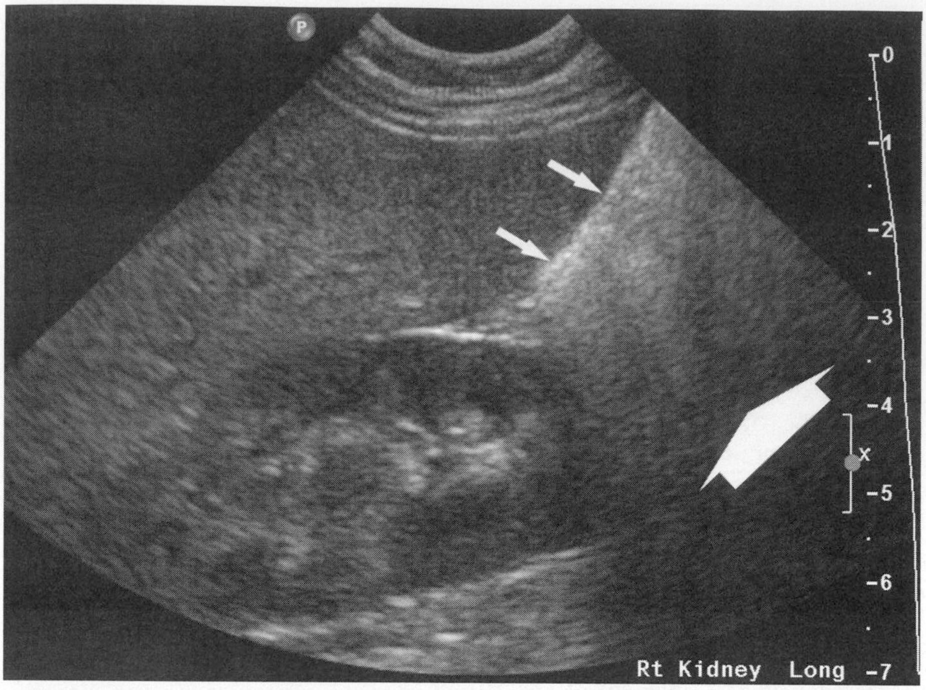

Figure 57-2. ■ *Longitudinal view of right kidney. The lower pole is obscured by dirty shadow* (large arrow) *arising from bowel gas* (small arrows).

depth of any suspected calculus to maximize the possibility of eliciting a shadow. Shadows caused by a gas-filled structure are often filled with reverberation echoes, sometimes referred to as "dirty shadowing" (Fig. 57-2).

Shadows deep to a calculus may not be apparent when scanning with multiple focal zones or with spatial compounding on. When trying to elicit a shadow from a suspected calculus, it is appropriate to use a single focal zone operating without compounding.

Acoustic Enhancement. Acoustic enhancement is essentially the opposite of acoustic shadowing, appearing as an area of increased brightness, usually seen deep to fluid-filled structures (cysts, gallbladder). The increased brightness results from the low level of attenuation within fluid, so the echoes arising from tissue deep to the fluid have greater amplitude than those from adjacent tissue (Fig. 57-3). Acoustic enhancement is helpful in identifying abnormal fluid-filled structures. Note that not all fluid-filled structures are echo-free. Abscesses, hemorrhagic cysts, and fluid structures with a high protein content may contain echoes. Posterior enhancement is therefore useful as an indicator of the fluid nature of the structure. Enhancement may be less apparent when using spatial compounding or automatic time gain compensation (TGC) functions.

Edge Shadowing. Edge shadowing is a reflective/refractive effect seen deep to the margins of rounded structures that have a speed of sound different from the surrounding tissue. These artifacts are frequently seen arising from cystic structures, appearing as very narrow shadows in line with the beam direction, arising immediately deep to the edge of the structure (Fig. 57-4). They may also be seen arising from the edge of the right kidney, which has a different speed of

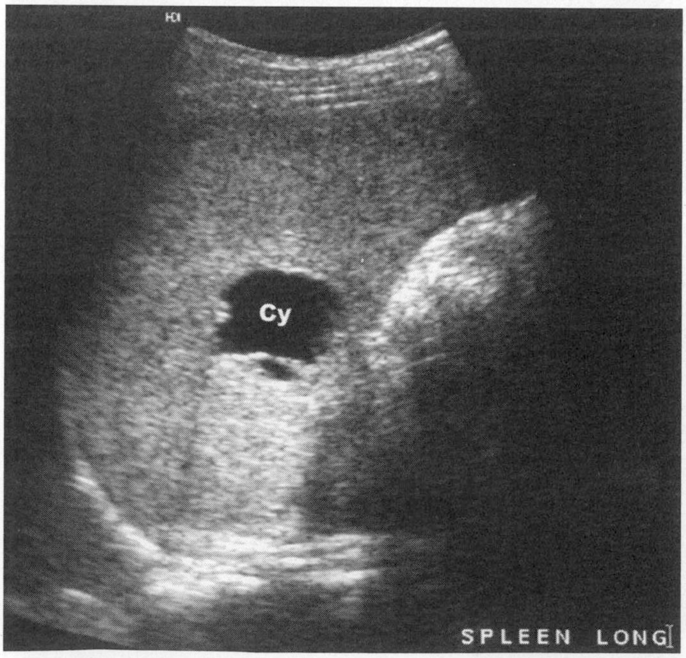

Figure 57-3. ■ *Longitudinal view of spleen showing acoustic enhancement deep to a splenic cyst* (Cy).

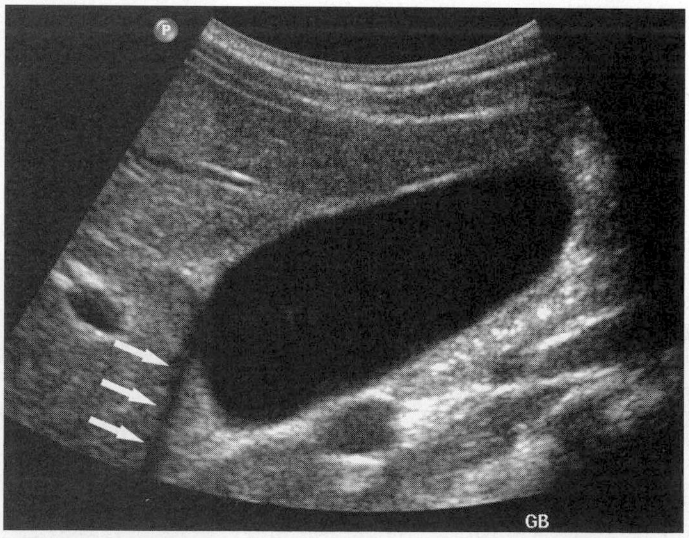

Figure 57-4. ■ *Edge shadow* (arrows) *arising from the edge of the gallbladder.*

sound from the adjacent liver. Edge shadows may not be apparent when using multiple focal zones.

Depth of Origin Artifacts

Reverberation. Reverberation is the process when the beam "bounces" repeatedly between two or more interfaces. Each reverberation cycle, some echoes return to the transducer, causing multiple echoes at increasing depth in the display (Fig. 57-5). Reverberation echoes are always displayed deeper than the interfaces they arise from. The transducer–skin interface is often one of the interfaces involved, but not necessarily so. Reverberation can be discrete, diffuse, or a combination of both. Discrete reverberation occurs between specular reflectors, especially when they are parallel and when the beam approaches them perpendicularly (Fig. 57-6). The distance between the reverberation echoes equals that between the interfaces causing them. This effect is often seen in the anterior part of the urinary bladder, caused by reverberation between the fascial planes of the abdominal wall and the transducer.

Diffuse reverberation often occurs in subcutaneous fat, appearing as a "snowstorm" superimposed on the deeper structures and adversely affecting contrast resolution in this region (Fig. 57-7). Reverberation echoes from the abdominal wall are readily apparent when displayed in structures that are

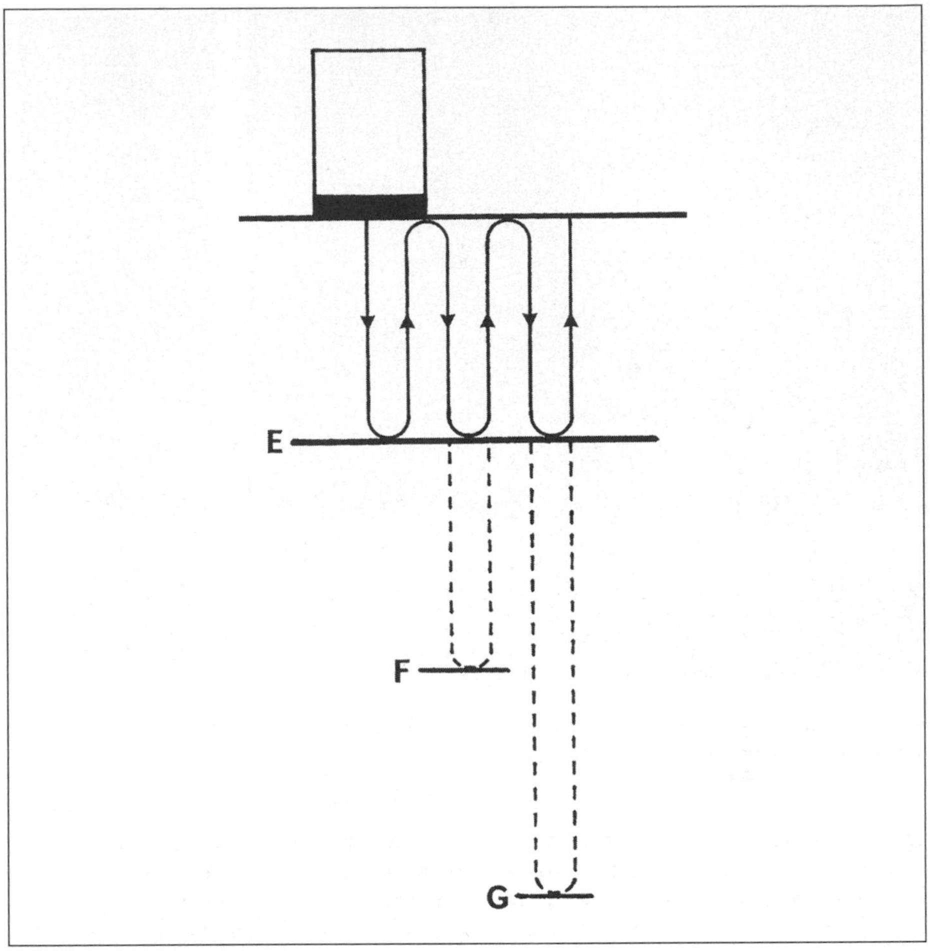

Figure 57-5. ■ *Diagram showing origin of reverberation echoes. Sound bounces between interface E and the transducer, causing echoes at F and G. For the sake of clarity, the reverberation paths in the diagram are shown side by side, but in reality, they occur along the same line.*

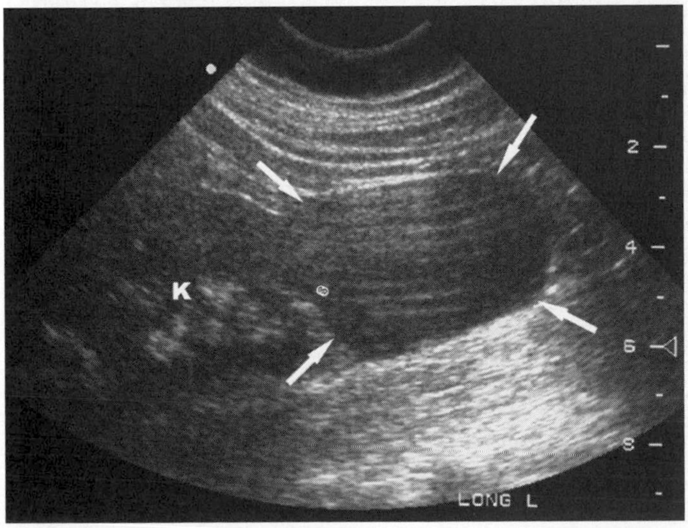

Figure 57-6. ■ *Longitudinal view of cyst* (arrows) *on lower pole of left kidney* (K). *Discrete and diffuse reverberation from overlying tissue planes obscures the cyst.*

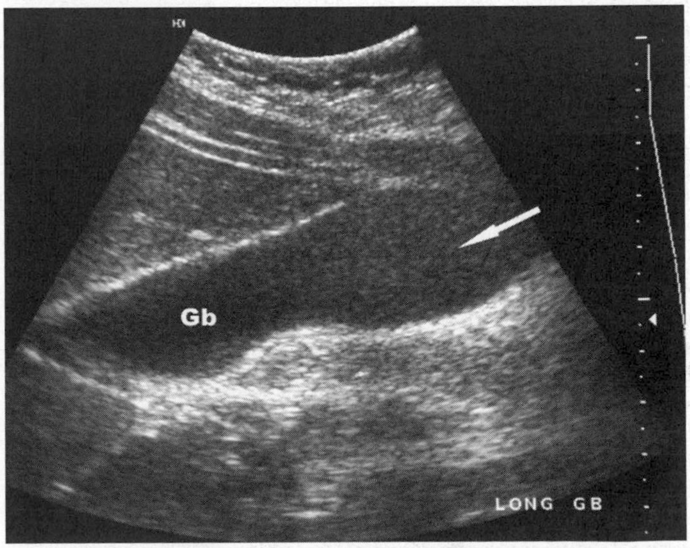

Figure 57-7. ■ *Longitudinal view of gallbladder* (Gb). *Diffuse reverberation* (arrow) *from the abdominal wall fills much of the lumen, simulating sludge.*

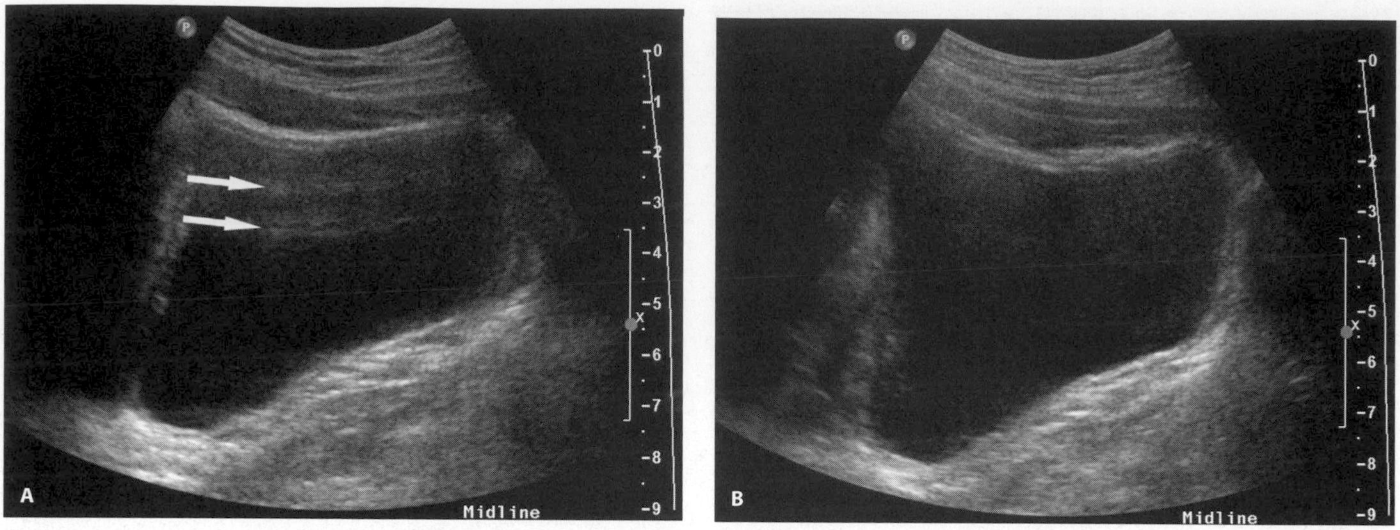

Figure 57-8. ■ *A. Longitudinal view of bladder showing reverberation artifact* (arrows). *The artifact is mostly gone when the transducer is angled, avoiding the perpendicular approach to the bladder wall (B).*

normally echo-free (e.g., the urinary bladder) (Fig. 57-8A) but are less obvious over the liver where they are superimposed on the liver echoes. Diffuse reverberation artifact can easily obscure small structures situated close to the abdominal wall, particularly if they are cystic.

Avoidance/Minimization. Use of harmonic imaging can reduce or eliminate diffuse reverberation artifact, thereby improving contrast resolution.

Reverberation can be avoided or minimized by avoiding a perpendicular approach to any specular interfaces involved, which can often be achieved by angling or tilting the transducer (Fig. 57-8A,B).

In the abdomen, transducer pressure can often reduce the depth of tissue overlying the region of interest and reduce reverberation artifact.

Comet Tail. The comet tail artifact is a localized reverberation artifact, often seen deep to crystalline material such as cholesterol stones (Fig. 57-9), and also arising from metal structures such as surgical staples or needles. This appearance was originally described arising from metal pellets after a shotgun injury. The reverberation effect is typically over a short range, with the brightness of the artifact reducing over a short distance. This artifact is also described as arising from air in the lung surface at the diaphragm.

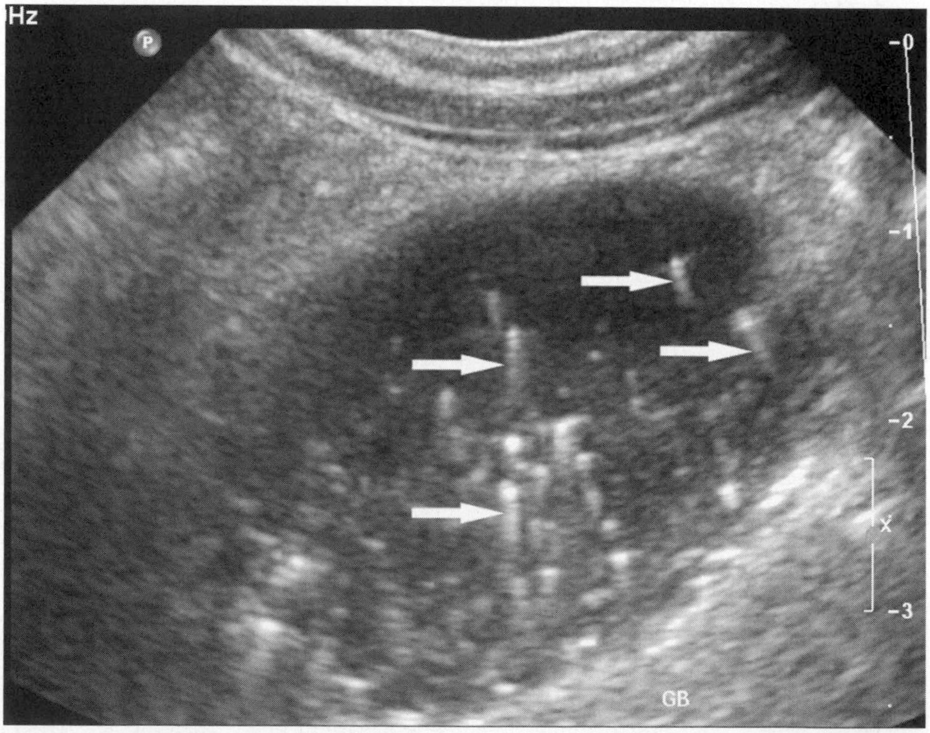

Figure 57-9. ■ *Multiple comet tail artifacts* (arrows) *arising from cholesterol crystals within a gallbladder.*

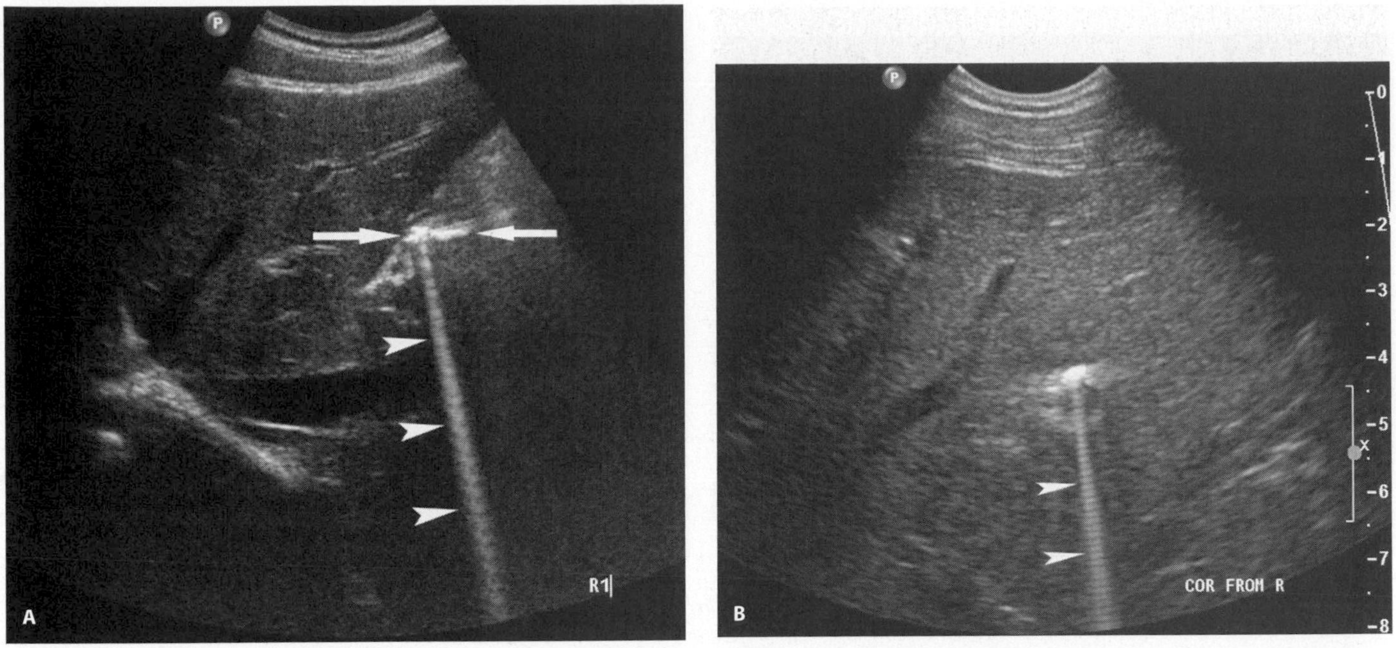

Figure 57-10. ■ *A. Ringdown artifact* (arrowheads) *from gas bubbles in bowel. The artifact does not arise across the full width of the gas margin* (arrows), *but only where there are bubbles. B. Focal ringdown artifact (arrowheads) arising from gas bubbles in an intrahepatic bile duct.*

Ringdown. Ringdown is a resonance phenomenon arising from gas bubbles. It has been shown experimentally that groups of gas bubbles with a bugle configuration may resonate when insonated, causing a stream of strong echoes to return to the transducer. The artifact is frequently seen in abdominal imaging, arising from bubbles of bowel gas (Fig. 57-10A). Ringdown is typically a bright artifact, extending from the gas bubbles through to the bottom of the display, and is a useful indicator of the presence of gas bubbles in abnormal areas such as the biliary tree (Fig. 57-10B).

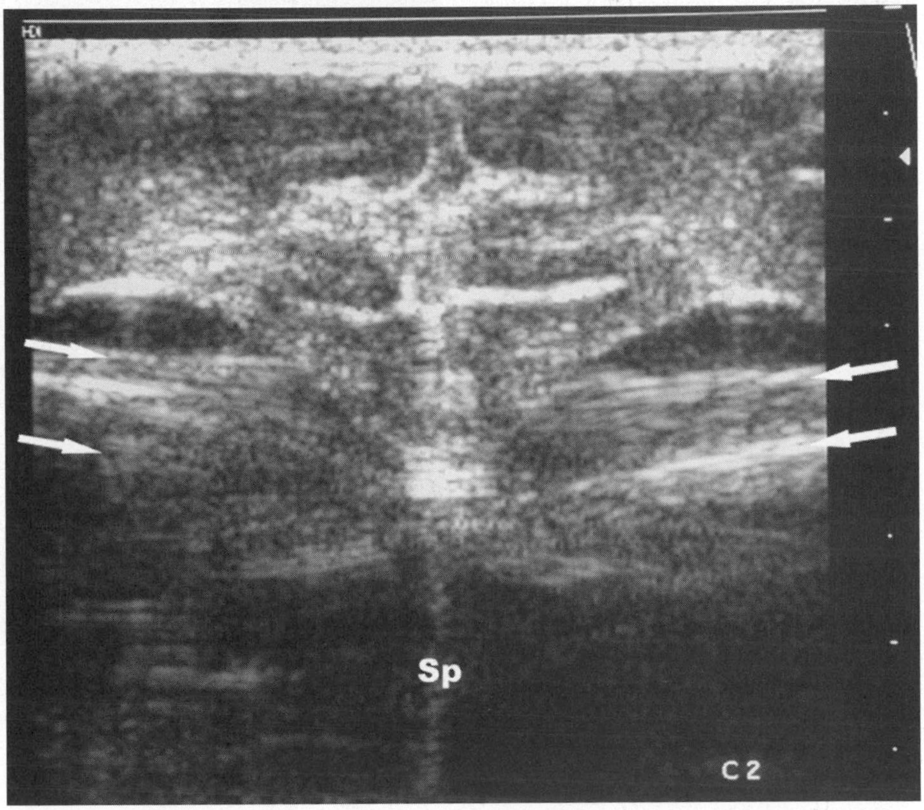

Figure 57-11. ■ *Coronal view of brain surface in patient with markedly dilated cerebral ventricles. Range ambiguity artifact* (arrows) *is apparent within the ventricles.* Sp, *septum pellucidum.*

Range Ambiguity Artifact. Echoes are placed at a depth in the display according to their time of arrival after the last pulse transmission. When large fluid-filled areas are scanned with a small field of view, echoes may return much later than allowed for due to the increased depth of penetration in the low attenuation fluid. Echoes returning after transmission of the next pulse will be attributed to that pulse and therefore placed at the wrong depth, more superficially than their true depth of origin. These are called range ambiguity artifacts (RAAs) and are usually obvious because they appear within the echo-free fluid (Fig. 57-11). RAAs are also seen in ultrasound

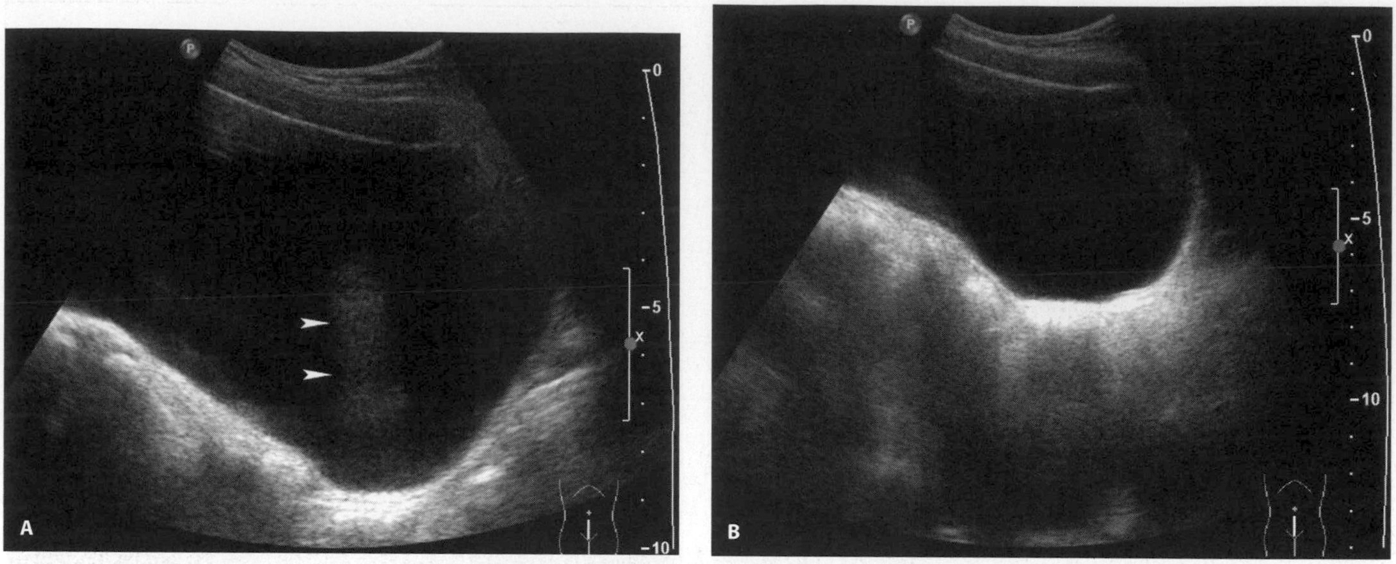

Figure 57-12. ■ *A. Range ambiguity artifact* (arrowheads) *within a bladder, resulting from the operation of concurrent beams. The artifact disappears when the depth of display is increased (**B**).*

systems that scan using multiple concurrent beams (Fig. 57-12) and are commonly encountered when scanning fluid-filled regions while using multiple focal zones (discussed below).

Avoidance/Minimization. RAA occurring with a single focal zone can be avoided by increasing the depth of field of view.

Beam Dimension Effects

Beamwidth Artifact. Ultrasound beams have finite dimensions, but the echoes they produce are assumed to have come from their central axis. The echo from a point reflector appears as a line (perpendicular to the beam axis) in an ultrasound image because it returns an echo for as long as it remains within the beam. This is referred to as beamwidth artifact (Fig. 57-13). The length of the line equals the beamwidth at that depth, and the center of the line is the true position of the reflector. The effect is often apparent deep to the focal zone because of beam divergence in this region, causing echoes to appear smeared. This type of artifact is often seen projecting into the bladder,

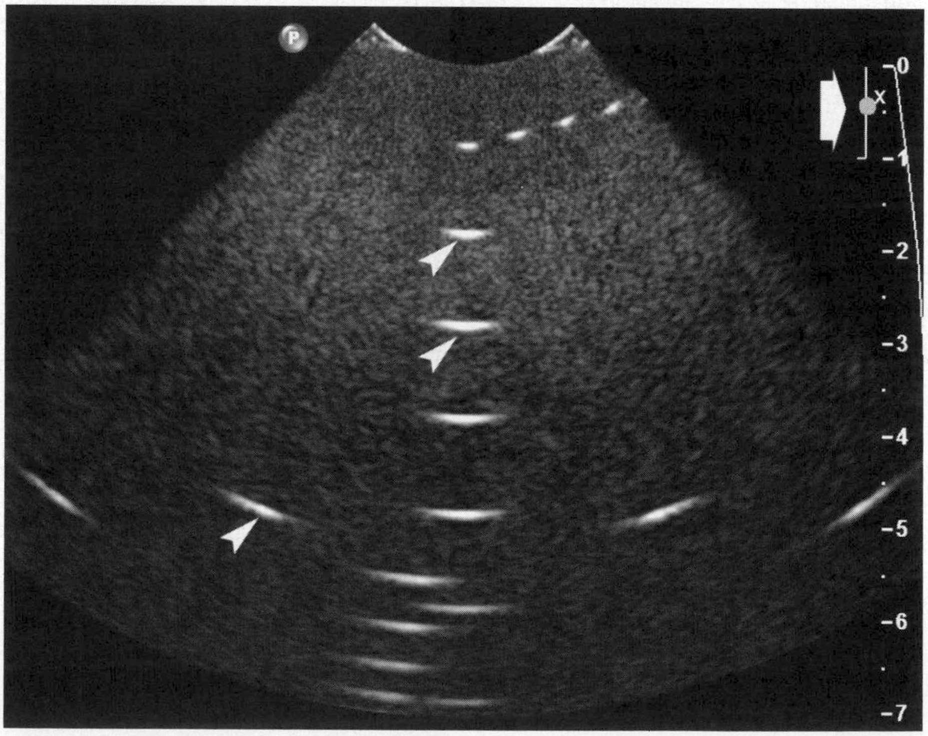

Figure 57-13. ■ *Beamwidth artifact in a phantom. The filaments are less than 1 mm in diameter but appear as lines* (arrowheads) *several millimeters long because of beam divergence deep to the focal zone* (arrow).

arising from highly reflective bowel gas intersected by the beam edge (Fig. 57-14). It is minimal in the focal zone, where beamwidth is smallest. Beamwidth artifact may be particularly obvious when the transmit aperture is compromised due to poor transducer contact with the patient or partial obstruction of the beam by an overlying rib. The resultant beam is very wide, causing smearing of echoes. Beamwidth artifact is also responsible for making thin membranes appear thick when they are intersected obliquely by the beam.

Avoidance/Minimization. Beamwidth artifact can be minimized by the use of multiple focal zones. When a single focal zone is used, it should be set at the depth of main interest to minimize the artifact in this region.

Side Lobe Artifact. All ultrasound beams have side lobes surrounding the main lobe, propagating at various angles to it and capable of producing echoes. Side lobes in modern transducers are of low intensity but nevertheless produce echoes from strongly reflective interfaces, such as gas and bone. All echoes detected by the transducer are assumed to have arisen from the center axis of the main lobe. Echoes received from side lobes are therefore displayed well away from their true position (although at the correct depth). In essence, this is an extension of the beamwidth situation, but with the error in placement of the echoes much greater. Side lobe artifacts are most obvious when they arise from a strong reflector such as gas or bone and when the artifact is displayed in a region expected to be echo-free, such as the urinary bladder or amni-

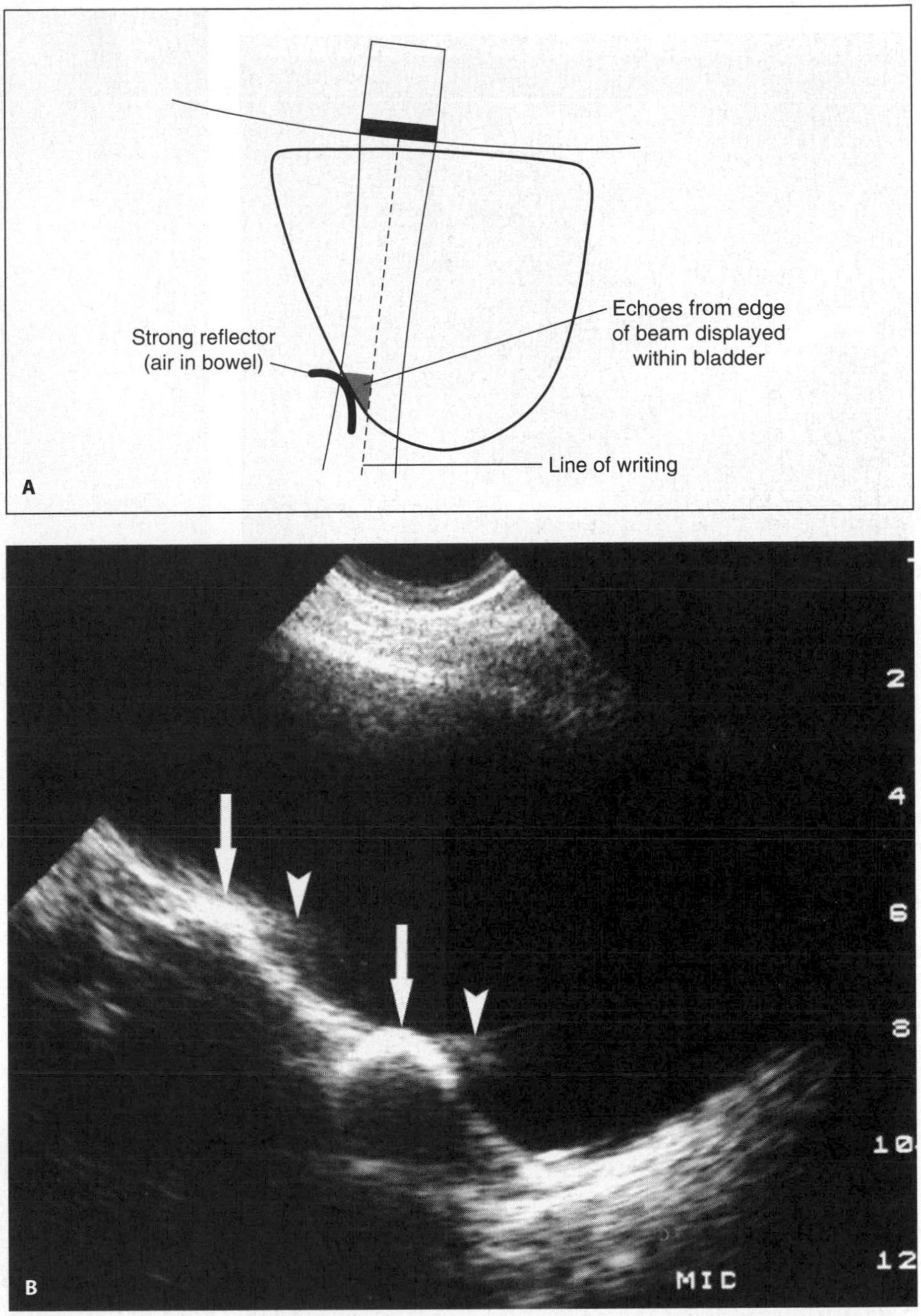

Figure 57-14. ■ *A. Origin of beamwidth artifact in the bladder. Echoes detected by the edge of the beam are displayed as if they have arisen from the center.* ***B.*** *Clinical example of the situation shown in (A), with the artifact* (arrowheads) *clearly arising from bowel gas* (arrows) *adjacent to the bladder.*

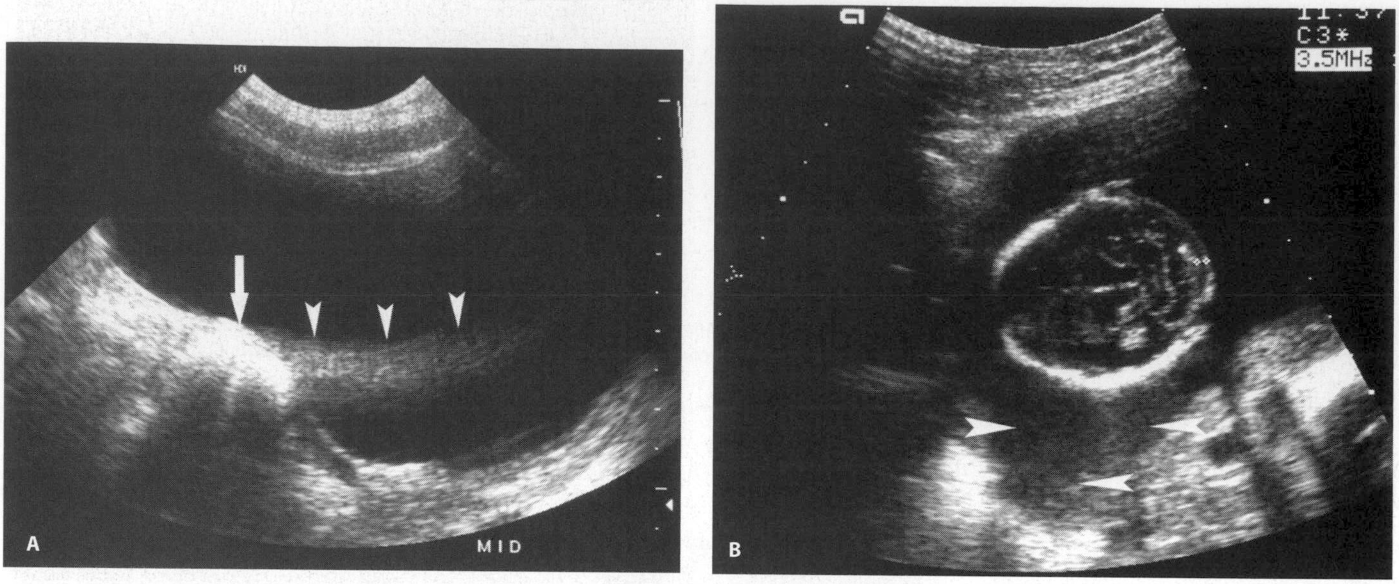

Figure 57-15. ■ *Longitudinal view of urinary bladder (A) showing sidelobe artifact* (arrowheads) *arising from bowel gas* (arrow) *and extending well into the bladder. B. Obstetric scan showing sidelobe artifact* (arrowheads) *deep to the fetal head, simulating placenta. (Image courtesy of Piotr Niznik.)*

otic fluid (Fig. 57-15). With increasing depth from the transducer, side lobe echoes are further from their true position because the side lobes diverge from the main lobe.

Avoidance/Minimization. Side lobe artifacts are more apparent when excessively high gain is used and can be minimized by ensuring the image is not "overwritten." These artifacts can also be reduced or eliminated by using harmonic imaging (Fig. 57-16).

Grating Lobe Artifact. Grating lobes occur in array transducers because of the regular and fine spacing of the crystal elements, which causes the array to act like a diffraction grating. Grating lobe artifacts are similar to those resulting from side lobes, but only occur in the plane of the array (not in the slice thickness dimension). They are most apparent with phased-array transducers because grating lobe production is exacerbated by electronic steering of the beam. They are

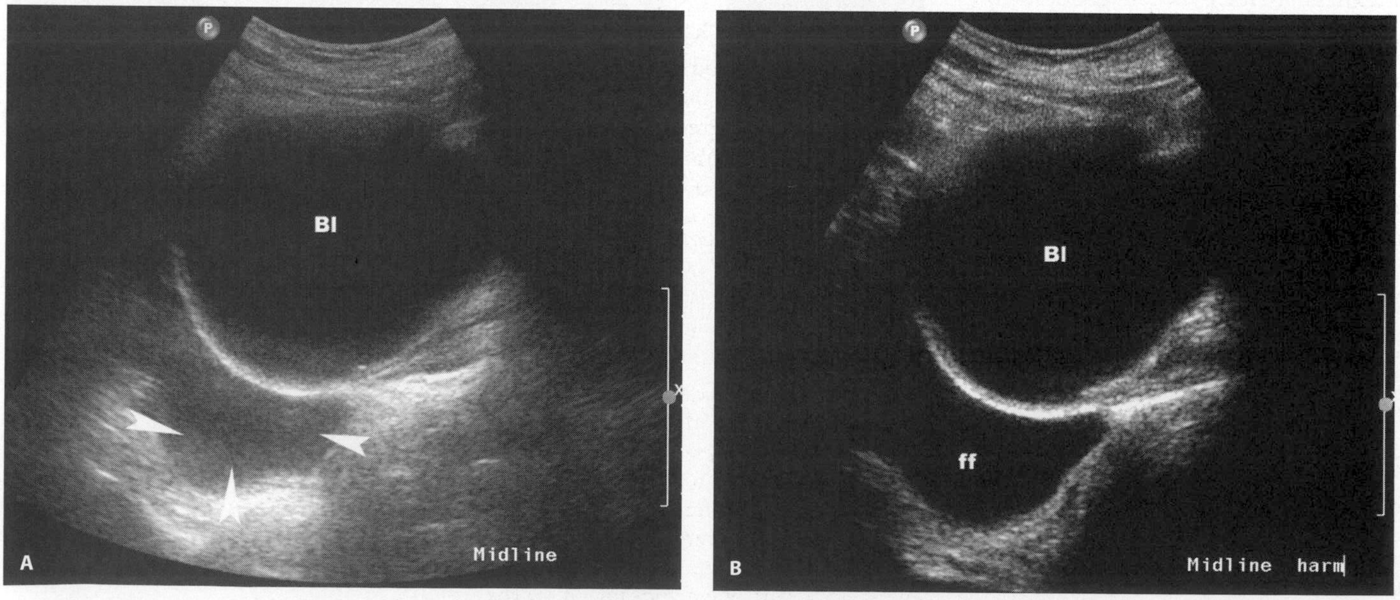

Figure 57-16. ■ *A. Longitudinal view in the pelvis, with sidelobe artifact* (arrowheads) *obscuring visualization of free fluid adjacent to the bladder. The artifact disappears when harmonic mode is used (B).* Bl, *bladder;* ff, *free fluid.*

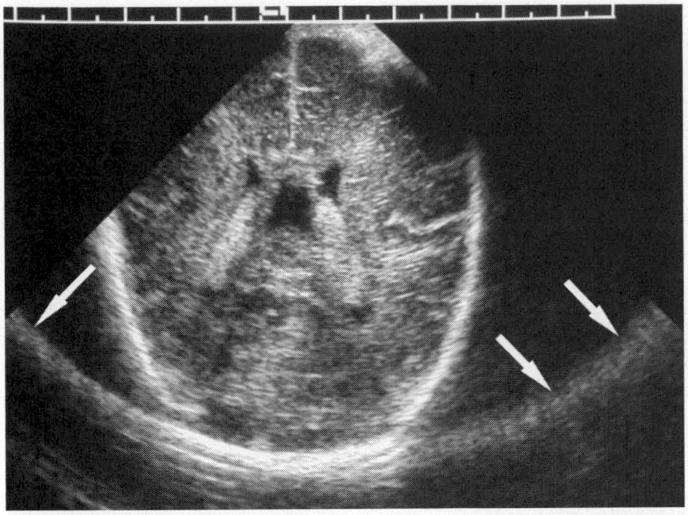

Figure 57-17. ■ *Coronal view of a neonatal brain using a phased array transducer. A grating lobe artifact* (arrows) *is seen arising from the occipital bone and extending laterally to the edge of the display.*

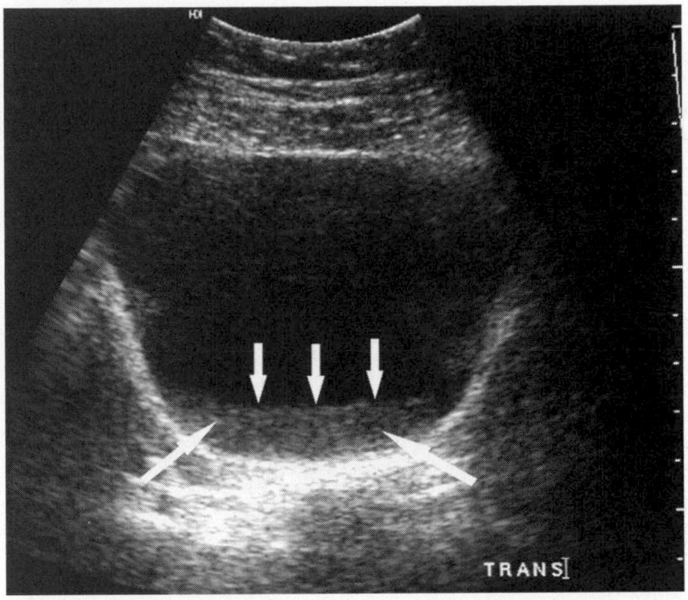

Figure 57-18. ■ *Transverse view of urinary bladder showing slice thickness artifact simulating sludge* (arrows). *The artifact has arisen from bowel gas superior to the bladder.*

commonly seen arising from strong reflectors such as gas and bone, extending a long way from their origin (Fig. 57-17).

Slice Thickness Artifact. Echoes displayed in two-dimensional ultrasound images have arisen from the three-dimensional volume scanned by the beam. Compression from three-dimensional to two-dimensional images results in slice thickness artifact, when echoes from outside the assumed plane of origin appear in the display. It is the equivalent of the partial volume effect seen in computed tomography imaging. Side lobes in the slice thickness plane contribute to slice thickness artifact. This type of artifact is frequently seen within fluid-filled structures (bladder, blood vessels, gall bladder), especially when gas is adjacent in the slice thickness (elevation) plane. In transverse views of the urinary bladder, it often simulates a dependent layer of sludge and may be misinterpreted as such (Fig. 57-18). Artifact can only be reliably differentiated from sludge by rolling the patient to one side to see if the echoes are dependent. Slice thickness artifact causes a loss of contrast resolution; small cystic or tubular structures may be difficult or impossible to see if they are filled with slice thickness artifact.

Avoidance/Minimization. When scanning a very superficial structure, it is advantageous to use a stand-off pad so that the region of interest is within the elevation plane focal zone, where slice thickness artifact is minimal. Use of 1.5D (matrix) transducers reduces this type of artifact because of their ability to reduce the elevation beam dimension.

Beam Path Artifacts

Refraction. Refraction is the bending of an ultrasound beam when it passes through an interface between tissues with different speeds of sound, when the angle of approach to the interface is not perpendicular. The degree and direction of refraction depend on the relative speeds of sound in the two mediums. Echoes arising from the refracted part of the beam pass back to the transducer along the same (refracted) pathway but are assumed to have arisen from along the original beam path (Fig. 57-19). Refraction occurs at many sites where there is "nonuniformity" of tissue, but its effects are commonly seen deep to muscle–fat and muscle–cartilage interfaces and also deep to junctions between muscle bodies. It can result in significant distortion (defocusing) of ultrasound beams, resulting in a loss of resolution. The optics equivalent is apparent when looking at traffic lights through a rain-spattered windscreen, where irregular refraction causes distortion of the light rays.

In transverse views of the abdomen, the double lens-shaped rectus abdominis muscles are a frequent source of refraction, resulting in double or even triple images of structures near the midline ("ghosting"). This effect can be mislead-

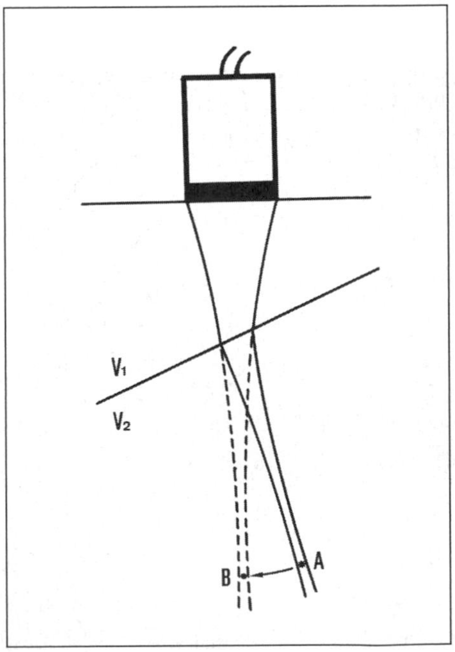

Figure 57-19. ■ *Effect of refraction on placement of echoes. An echo from (**A**) is displayed as if it came from (**B**).*

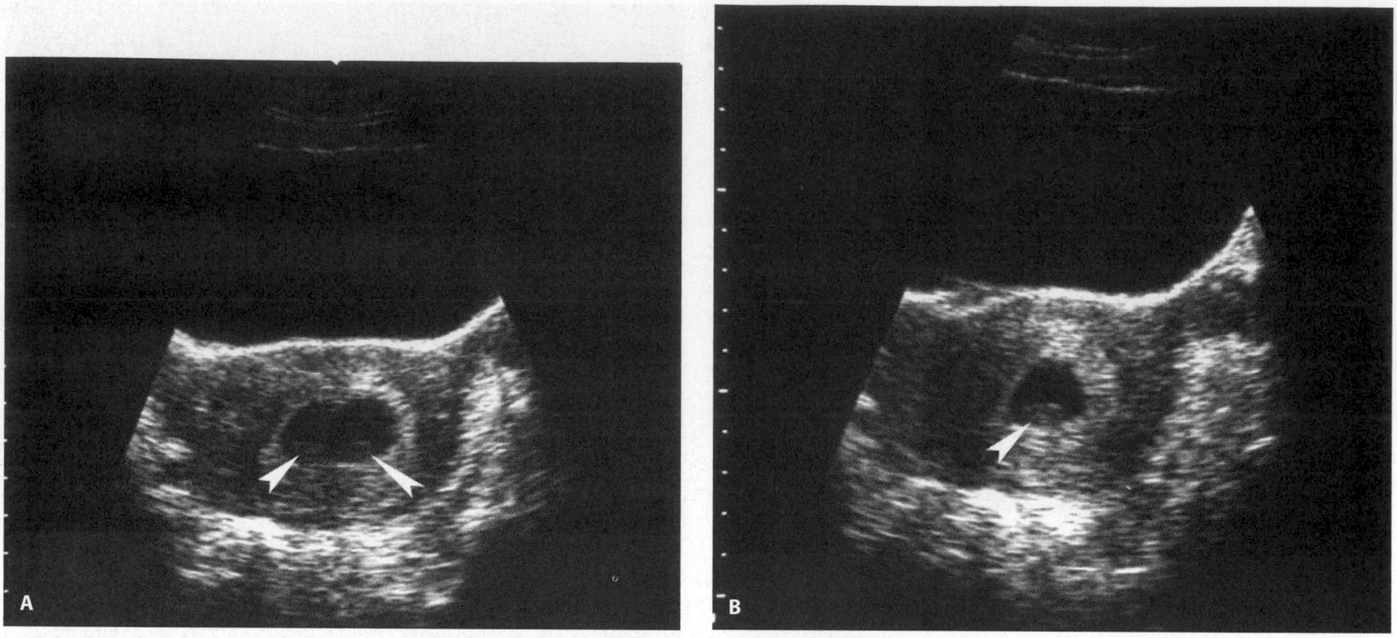

Figure 57-20. ■ *Transverse abdominal view of early pregnancy.* ***A.*** *Refraction in the rectus muscles causes the "ghosting" of the fetal pole* (arrowheads), *suggesting a twin pregnancy. Transverse view with the transducer moved to one side (**B**), avoiding the double refraction effect and showing a single fetal pole* (arrowhead). *(Images courtesy of Jeff Siegmann.)*

ing, causing a single gestational sac to appear as two sacs (Fig. 57-20), suggesting a twin pregnancy, or causing a single bladder calculus to appear as two. The optical equivalent of this effect can be seen when looking at a single structure through two adjacent drinking glasses, causing the structure to be seen twice (Fig. 57-21). Refraction at muscle–cartilage interfaces can cause distortion of the beam, with resultant image degradation, sometimes appearing as disruption of the

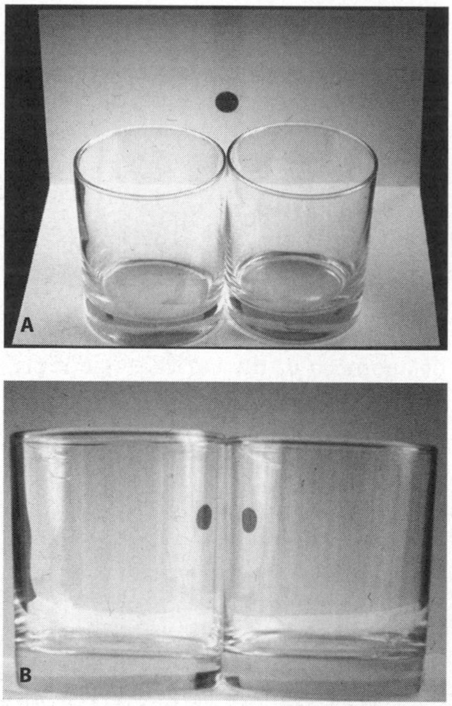

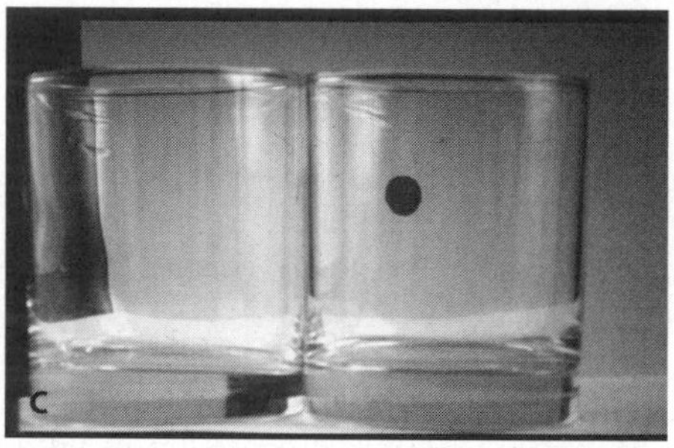

Figure 57-21. ■ *Optics equivalent of "ghosting." A single dot is present on the cardboard behind the drinking glasses (**A**). Two dots are seen when looking through the glasses (**B**). Moving to one side avoids the effect (**C**).*

renal margin or diaphragm margin (Fig. 57-22). This also occurs in coronal views of the neonatal brain taken through the anterior fontanelle, when refraction occurs in the interhemispheric fissure, distorting midline structures (Fig. 57-23). The degradation may be apparent as smearing in the affected part of the image, similar to beamwidth artifact.

Avoidance/Minimization. Image degradation from refraction can often be avoided by adjusting transducer position to avoid the nonuniform tissue. In the rectus abdominis case, movement of the transducer to one side avoids the double refraction effect, allowing the anatomy to be displayed accurately (Fig. 57-21C). Refraction in the interhemispheric fissure in neonatal brain images can also be avoided by shifting the transducer to one side. Use of endocavity transducers avoids the beam distortion caused by propagation through the nonuniform abdominal wall (and has the added advantage of improved resolution from use of a higher frequency). In abdominal scanning, use of transducer pressure will often allow bowel to be compressed, resulting in less distortion of the beam and less artifact interfering with visualization of deeper structures.

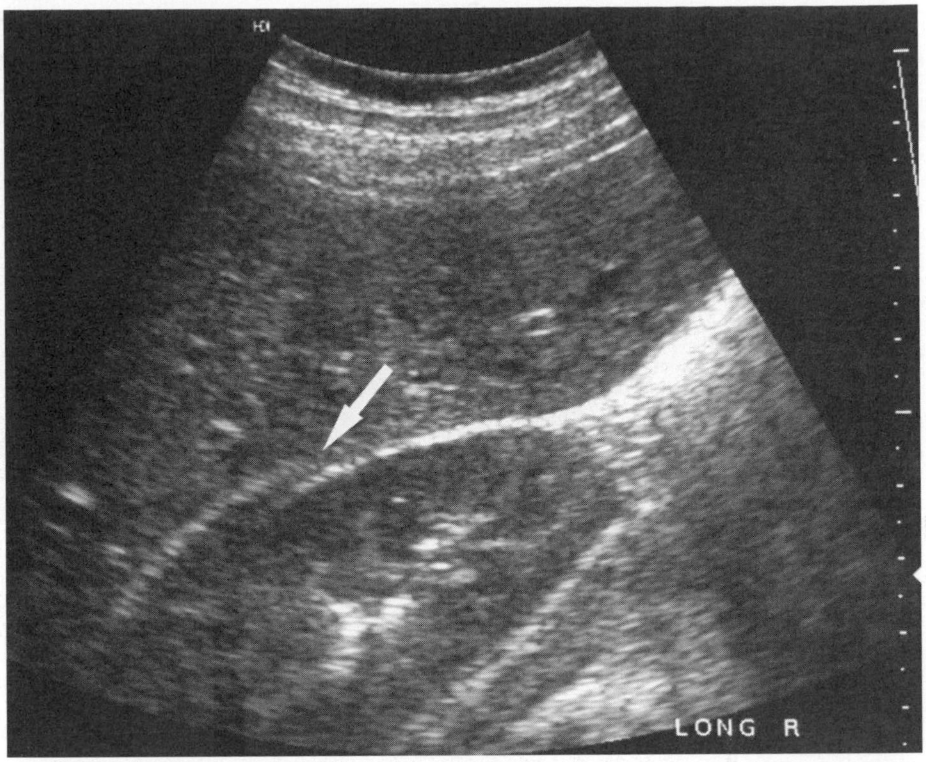

Figure 57-22. ■ *Longitudinal view of right kidney. Refraction at the muscle–cartilage interface in the abdominal wall causes disruption* (arrow) *of the anterior renal margin.*

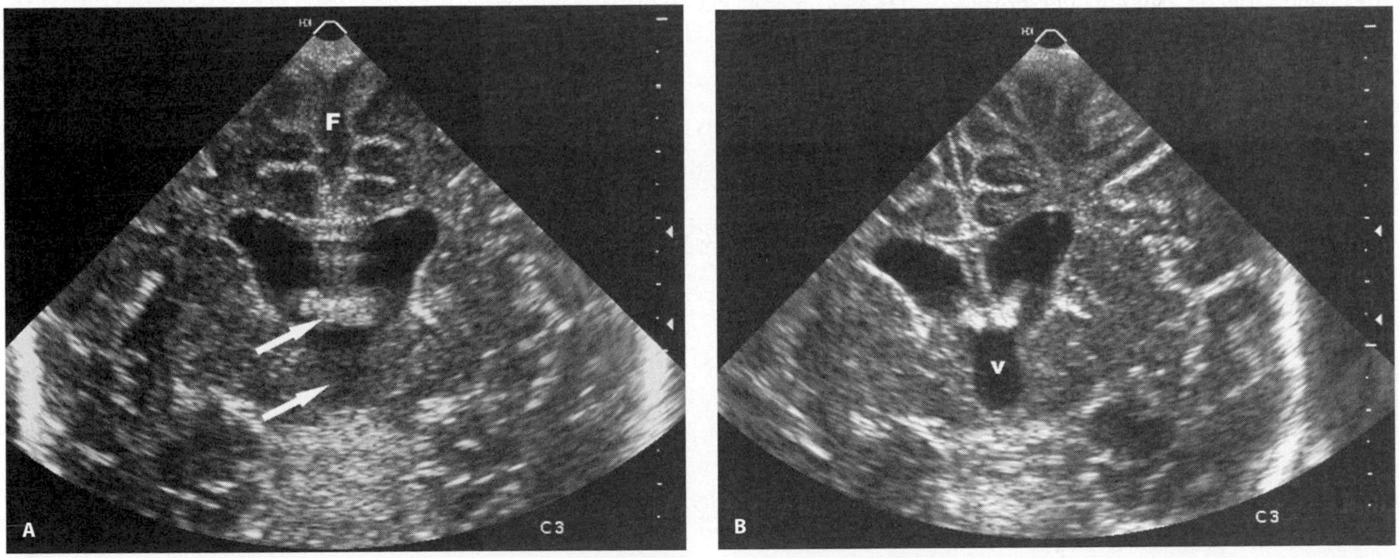

Figure 57-23. ■ *Coronal view of neonatal head. Refraction in the region of the interhemispheric fissure* (F) *causes smearing of midline structures* (arrows) *when the transducer is over the midline* (**A**). *The artifact is avoided by moving the transducer to one side* (**B**), *allowing the third ventricle* (V) *to be seen.*

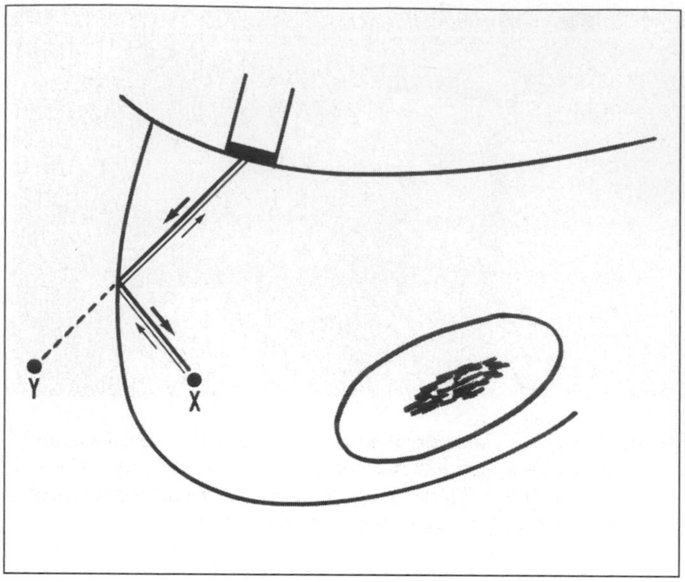

Figure 57-24. ■ *Mechanism for mirror image production. An echo from X is displayed at Y.*

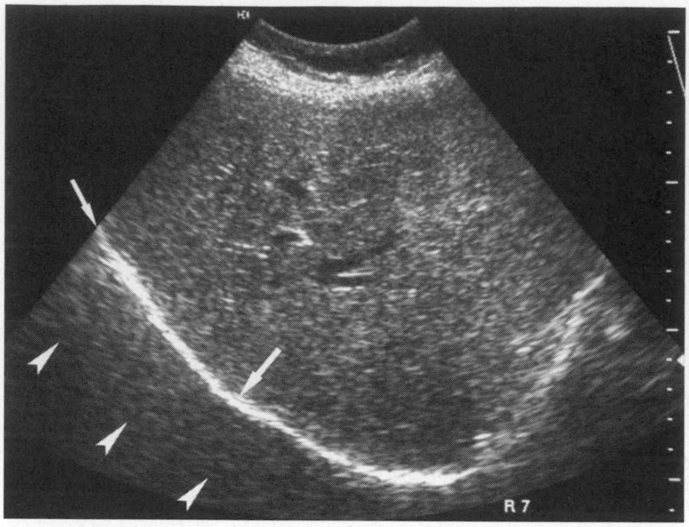

Figure 57-25. ■ *Clinical example of Figure 57-24. A longitudinal view in the right upper quadrant showing mirror artifact* (arrowheads) *of liver tissue mirrored in the diaphragm–lung interface* (arrows) *and appearing in the chest.*

Mirror Artifacts. Strong (high impedance mismatch) specular reflectors can act as mirrors for ultrasound beams, causing tissues adjacent to the mirror to be displayed twice, with the mirror in between. Tissues adjacent to the mirror are interrogated twice, once as the beam propagates toward the mirror and again after it has reflected from the mirror (Fig. 57-24). Echoes from the reflected beam return to the transducer via the mirror but are displayed as if they have arisen from along the original beam path, deep to the mirror. Smooth layers of gas (at the diaphragm or in bowel) and bone surfaces are common sites for mirror artifact, which is regularly seen in the right upper quadrant, where air in the lung acts as a mirror, causing liver echoes to be displayed above the diaphragm (Fig. 57-25). Focal lesions within the liver or spleen may also be visible in the mirror image (Fig. 57-26).

Mirror artifacts can be misleading if not recognized as such. Gas in the rectum may result in a mirror image of the bladder appearing as a cystic mass in the pelvis (Fig. 57-27). A singleton pregnancy can appear as twins if images of

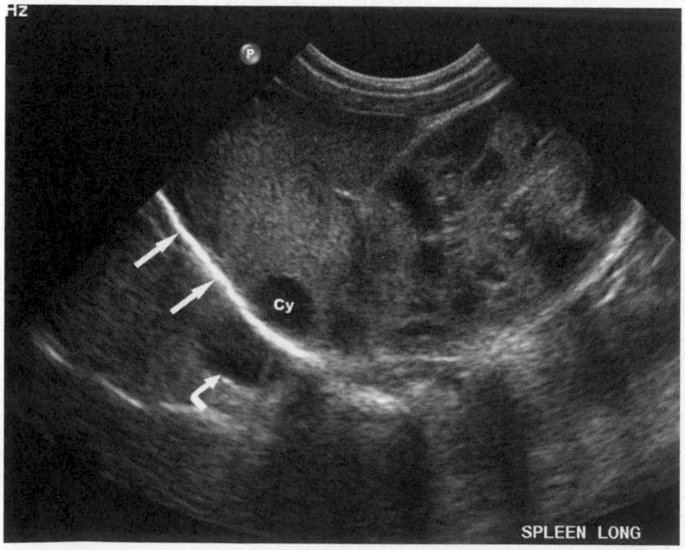

Figure 57-26. ■ *Longitudinal view in left upper quadrant. Mirror image of the spleen is seen above the diaphragm* (arrows), *including a mirror image of the splenic cyst* (curved arrow). Cy, *cyst.*

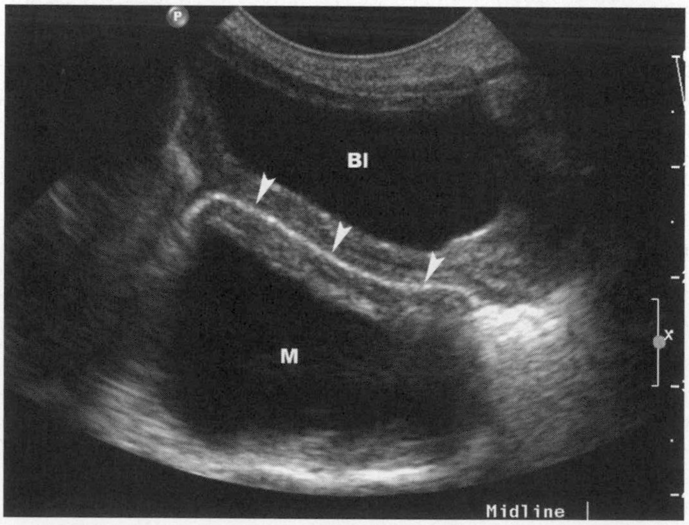

Figure 57-27. ■ *Longitudinal view of urinary bladder* (Bl) *in a baby. A smooth layer of gas in the rectum* (arrowheads) *acts as a mirror, resulting in a mirror image* (M) *of the bladder simulating a cystic mass behind the bladder.*

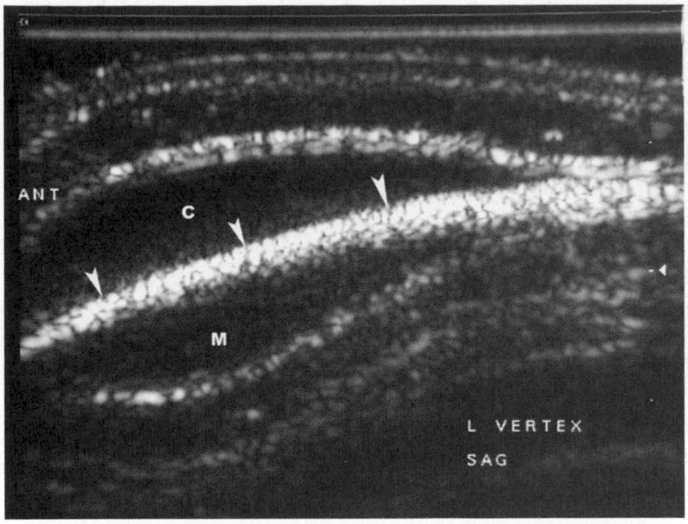

Figure 57-28. ■ *Mirror image* (M) *of a cephalhematoma* (C), *mirrored in bone* (arrowheads) *of the skull and simulating a subdural hematoma.*

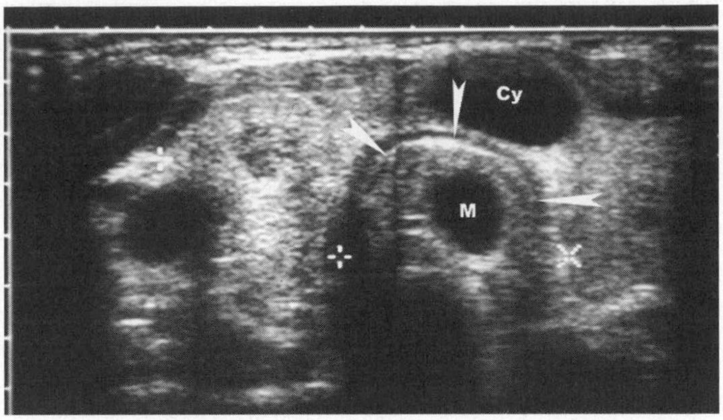

Figure 57-29. ■ *Transverse view of thyroid. The thyroid isthmus and a cyst* (Cy) *within is mirrored in air in the trachea* (arrowheads). *The mirror image* (M) *is a different shape from the cyst because of the curvature of the mirror. (Image courtesy of Peter Murfett.)*

the fetus are mirrored in adjacent bowel gas. The uterus can appear duplicated in adjacent bowel gas when scanned transvaginally. Mirror image of a scalp mass such as a cephalhematoma (Fig. 57-28) can be misinterpreted as a subdural hematoma, leading to unnecessary further investigation with computed tomography.

It should be understood that the appearances on each side of the mirror are not necessarily identical. This is seen when the mirror is curved, causing distortion of the mirror image, and when the mirror is angled relative to the scan plane. The thyroid isthmus is frequently seen mirrored in air in the trachea, but the mirror image is distorted by curvature of the air margin (Fig. 57-29). Angulation of the mirror is encountered in transverse views of the upper abdomen, because of the obliquity of the diaphragm. Reflection of the beam from an angled mirror means that echoes on each side of it are from different planes, so that a focal lesion may be visible in the liver but not in the mirror image, and vice versa.

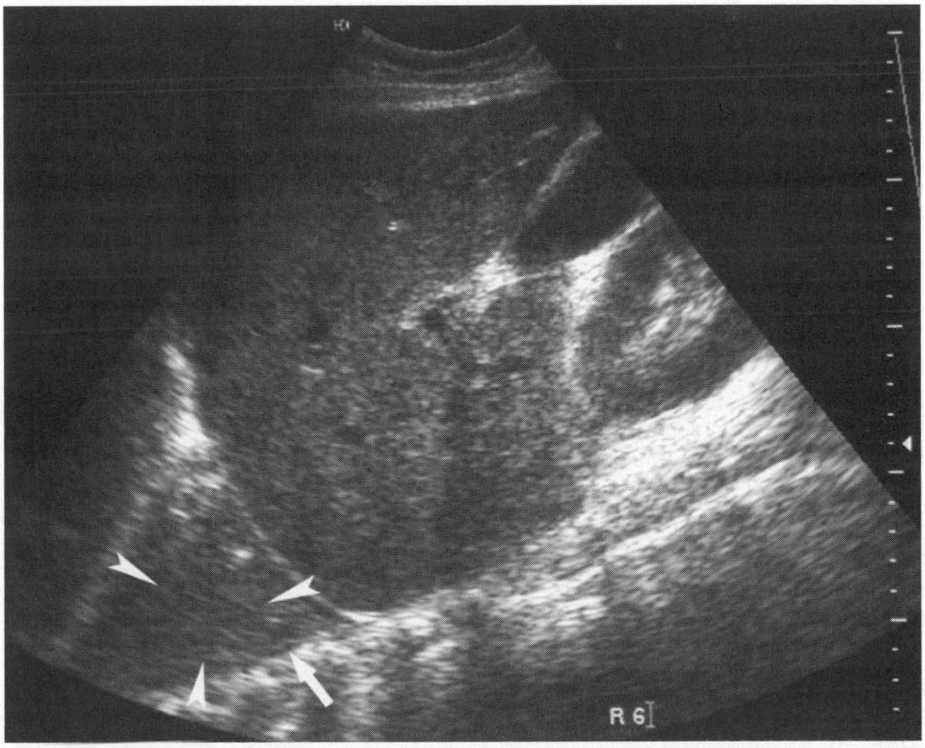

Figure 57-30. ■ *Longitudinal view of liver. Echoes* (arrowheads) *above the diaphragm represent consolidated lung but could easily be interpreted as mirror artifact. The diaphragm echo is reduced in brightness, and the posterior chest wall* (arrow) *is seen through the lung.*

It is important to recognize that not all echoes above the diaphragm represent mirror artifact. Pathology (lung consolidation or collapse, neoplasms) within lung bases adjacent to the diaphragm is often mistaken for mirror artifact, but careful analysis of the images should reveal the correct diagnosis. In cases of pathology (Fig. 57-30), the diaphragm echo is less bright (soft tissue–soft tissue interface instead of soft tissue–gas) and the posterior chest wall is likely to be seen, continuous with the posterior abdominal wall. Echo-free pleural effusions are easily identified in liver images, but echogenic lung pathology is easily mistaken for mirror artifact.

Avoidance/Minimization. In many cases, nothing can be done to avoid mirror artifact. If bowel gas is acting as the mirror, re-scanning the patient after the gas has shifted, or scanning from another angle, may resolve any uncertainty. When scanning near a bone surface, variation of transducer pressure allows differentiation between mirror artifact and "genuine" echoes. Mirror artifact will change inversely with transducer pressure, corresponding to the depth of tissue between the transducer and the bone.

EQUIPMENT SETTING ARTIFACTS

These result from inappropriate settings of such controls as TGC, gain, and frame rate, and may result when using multiple focal zones.

Time Gain Compensation Artifacts. When TGC settings are not correct, a band of increased (TGC too high) or decreased (TGC too low) brightness appears in the image, suggesting a variation in reflectivity that can be misinterpreted as pathology. The band will be equidistant from the transducer face, appearing horizontal in linear array transducers and curved in curved arrays (Fig. 57-31). This can be corrected by adjusting the TGC controls corresponding to the region of the band, until image brightness is uniform.

Avoidance/Minimization. Careful adjustment of TGC controls should be made throughout each examination, according to the type of tissue and transducer frequency. Newer ultrasound systems have adaptive TGC functions that operate automatically.

Gain Settings. Inadequately high or low gain settings can cause misleading appearances. High gain reduces contrast resolution by masking subtle differences in echogenicity between different tissues. Excessively high gain can also cause artifactual echoes (side lobe, slice thickness, reverberation) to be displayed in cystic structures (Fig. 57-32), causing them to appear complex or be missed. Excessively low gain settings can cause echogenic structures to appear echo-free, misrepresenting their true nature.

Avoidance/Minimization. Gain level should always be set high enough to display low-level echoes but not so high that artifacts appear.

Movement Artifact. Movement of the patient during acquisition of an image may result in blurring of the echoes in the display. This is more likely when scanning rapidly moving structures (cardiac) and when using low frame rates (using multiple focal zones or a large depth of field of view) or effectively low frame rates that result when using a high degree of frame averaging (persistence).

Avoidance/Minimization. When movement artifact is present, adjustment of controls causing low frame rates is necessary. This includes use of a single focal zone and selection of a low level of frame averaging. Some equipment allows the operator to choose between high resolution/low frame rate and low resolution/high frame rate modes according to the circumstances.

Multiple Focal Zone Artifacts. Multiple focal zones can cause RAAs to appear, particularly when scanning fluid-filled structures. The low attenuation within the fluid allows much greater depth of penetration of pulses, so that echoes return over a longer period than allowed for. Distant echoes arising from one pulse, returning after transmission of the next pulse, are placed in the focal zone of the latter, more superficially than their true position. In some cases, these artifacts have very sharp upper and/or lower

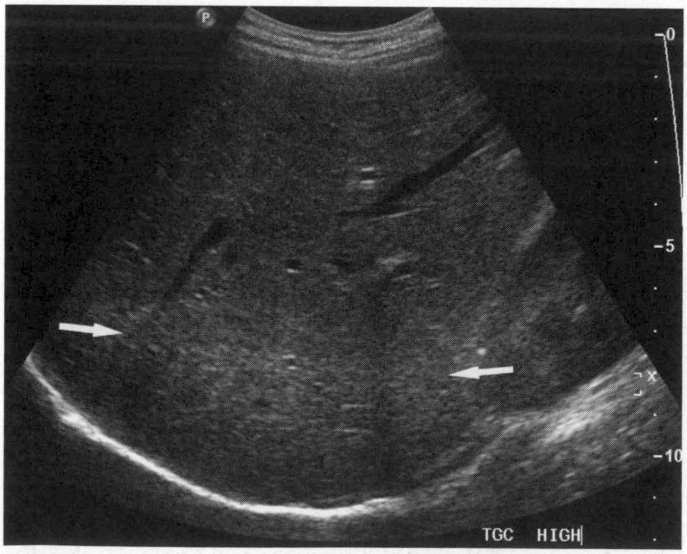

Figure 57-31. ■ *Inappropriate time gain compensation* (TGC) *setting causing a band of increased echogenicity* (arrows) *within the liver.*

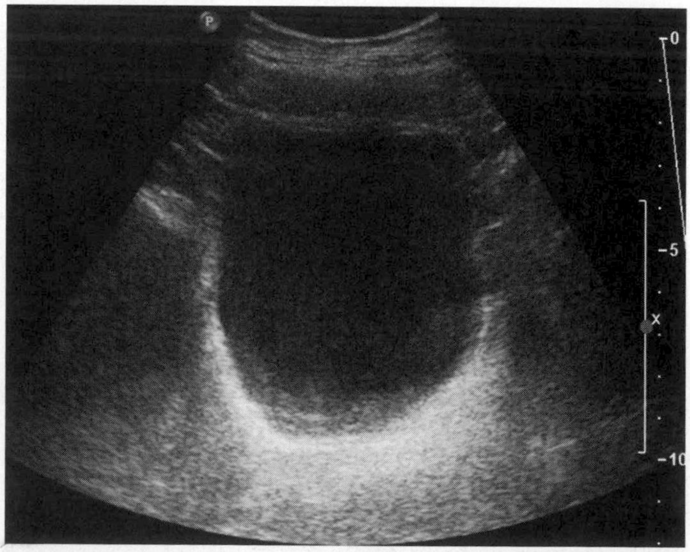

Figure 57-32. ■ *Transverse view of pelvis. Excessive gain has resulted in sidelobe, slice thickness, and reverberation echoes appearing throughout the bladder, which should be echo-free.*

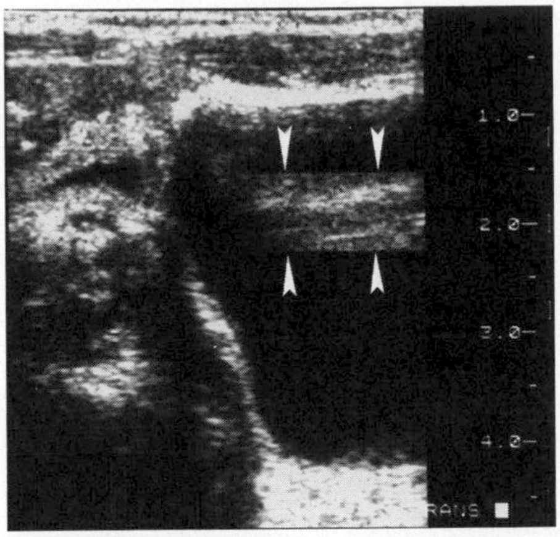

Figure 57-33. ■ *Transverse view of urinary bladder showing range ambiguity artifact* (arrowheads) *resulting from use of three focal zones. Echoes from deep in the pelvis are displayed within the second focal zone, but only within the bladder, where the attenuation is very low. Reverting to a single focal zone removes the artifact.*

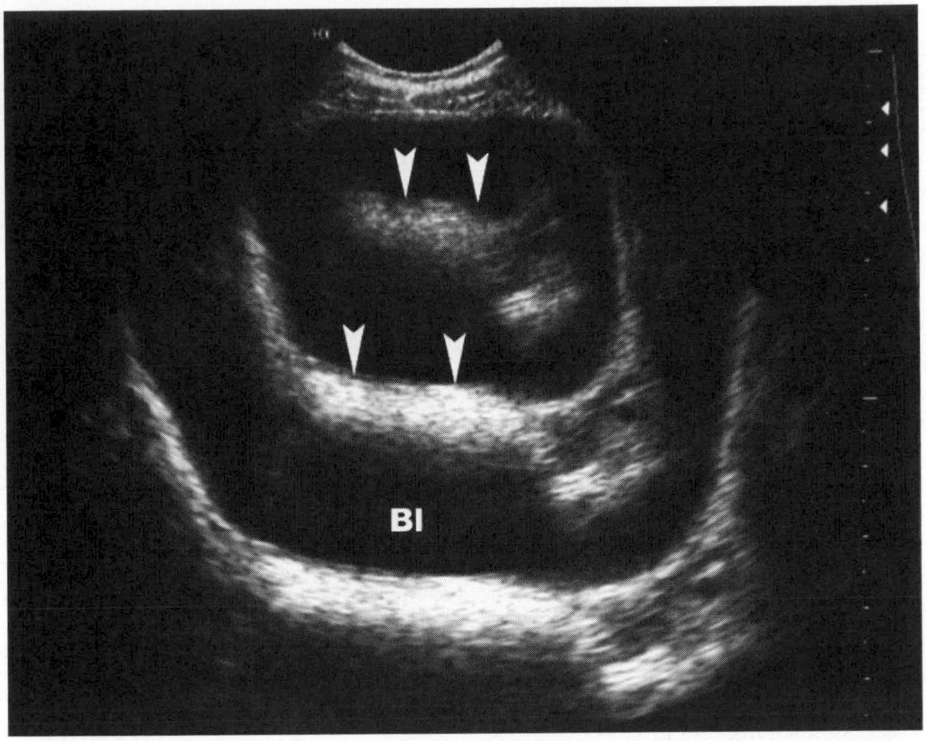

Figure 57-34. ■ *Transverse view of urinary bladder* (Bl) *using three focal zones. Range ambiguity artifact is present, appearing as two miniature versions of the bladder* (arrowheads).

margins (Fig. 57-33), corresponding to the junctions between focal zones. They may also result in one or more miniature images of a structure being displayed within itself, with the appearances varying according to the number and depth of the focal zones. Such an appearance can be seen in the urinary bladder (Fig. 57-34) and in neonatal head scans, especially when there is ventricular dilatation. These artifacts can give the misleading impression of solid tissue within a cystic structure (Fig. 57-35). It is a common misconception that these artifacts result from a different speed of sound in the fluid, but this is not correct. They result from the very low attenuation of sound by the fluid.

Avoidance/Minimization. RAAs resulting from multiple focal zones can invariably be removed by reverting to a single focal zone.

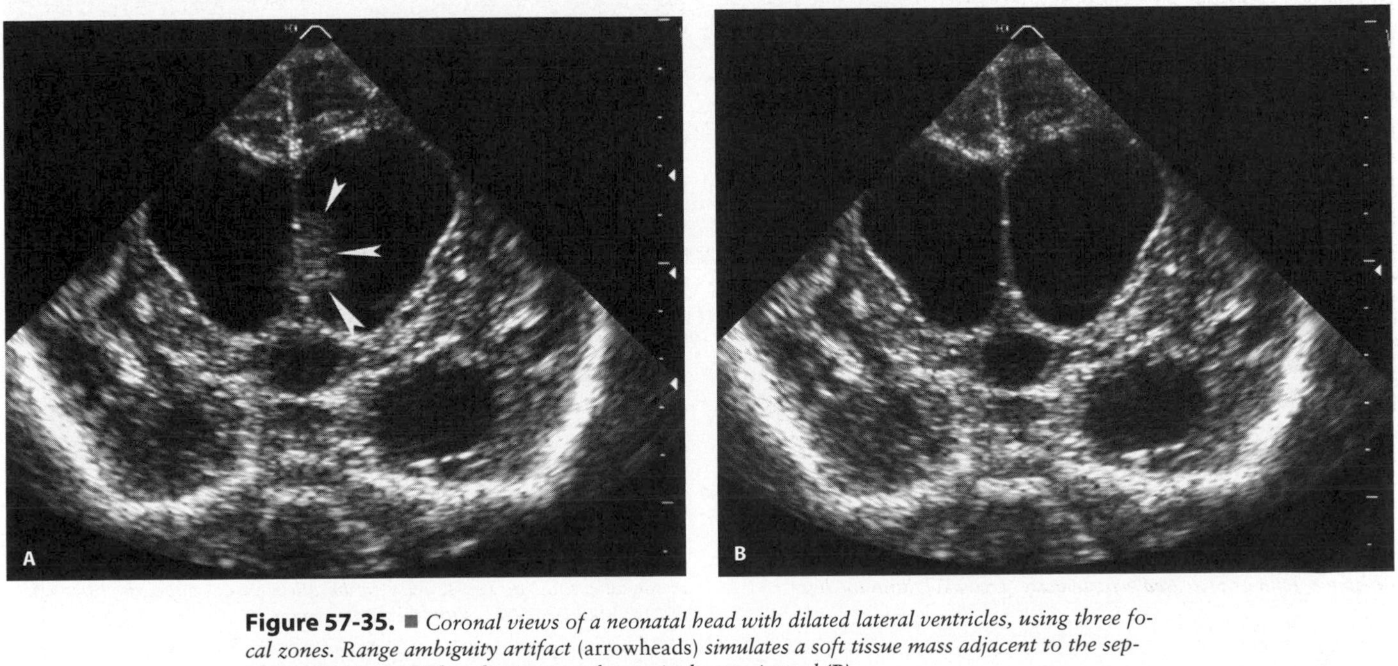

Figure 57-35. ■ *Coronal views of a neonatal head with dilated lateral ventricles, using three focal zones. Range ambiguity artifact* (arrowheads) *simulates a soft tissue mass adjacent to the septum pellucidum (A), but disappears when a single zone is used (B).*

DOPPLER ARTIFACTS

Artifacts also occur in Doppler modes of operation. Some of these are Doppler versions of artifacts described above, whereas others occur because of the way in which Doppler information is acquired.

Spectral and Color Doppler Noise. When operating in spectral Doppler mode with excessively high gain, "noise" appears throughout the display, masking genuine signals from blood. Noise has random frequency and phase and therefore appears as a "snowstorm" in both channels in spectral Doppler (Fig. 57-36) and as a random mixture of forward and reverse colors throughout the color box in color Doppler. Excessively high gain in color Doppler also causes color to "bleed" into tissue around vessels.

Avoidance/Minimization. In each case, reducing the gain level avoids the problem.

Color Doppler Flash Artifact. Sudden movement of the patient (cough, sneeze) or transducer causes Doppler shifts to be detected throughout the color box so that it fills with a "flash" of color.

Avoidance/Minimization. Acquire color images when the patient is able to remain still.

Aliasing. Aliasing is an artifact resulting from inadequate sampling of the Doppler signals, causing some of the detected Doppler shift to be displayed in the wrong channel. Only those frequency components that exceed the Nyquist limit (pulse-repetition frequency [PRF]/2) are aliased. Aliasing is easily identified in spectral Doppler, with the peaks of each systole being displayed in the opposite channel (Fig. 57-37). In color Doppler, an abrupt change in color occurs between the aliased and nonaliased part of the display (Color Plate 57-1), without a black line between the colors. Aliasing should not be confused with color change caused by flow rever-

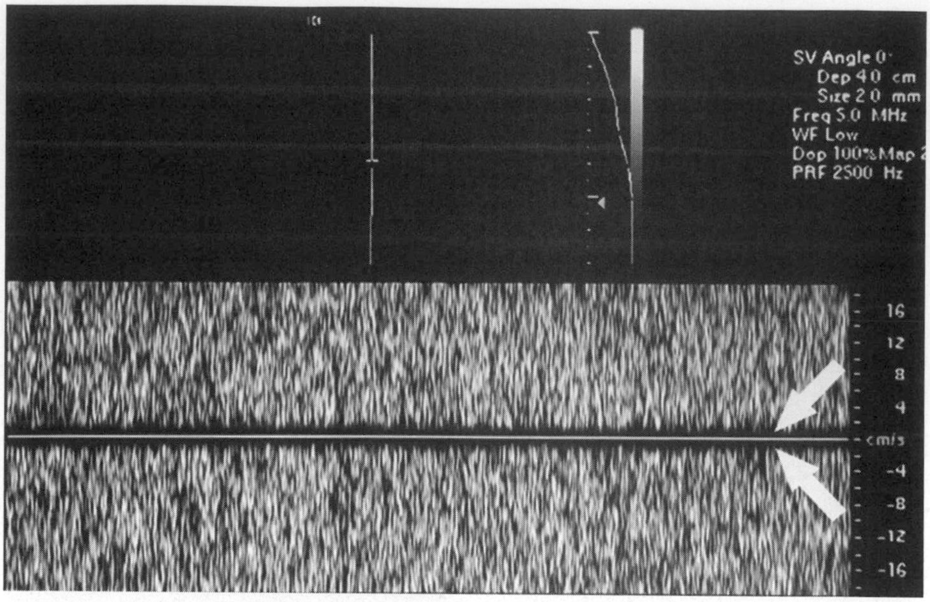

Figure 57-36. ■ *Spectral Doppler display. Excessive gain fills the display with noise except for the region on each side of the baseline* (arrows), *where signals have been removed by the wall filter.*

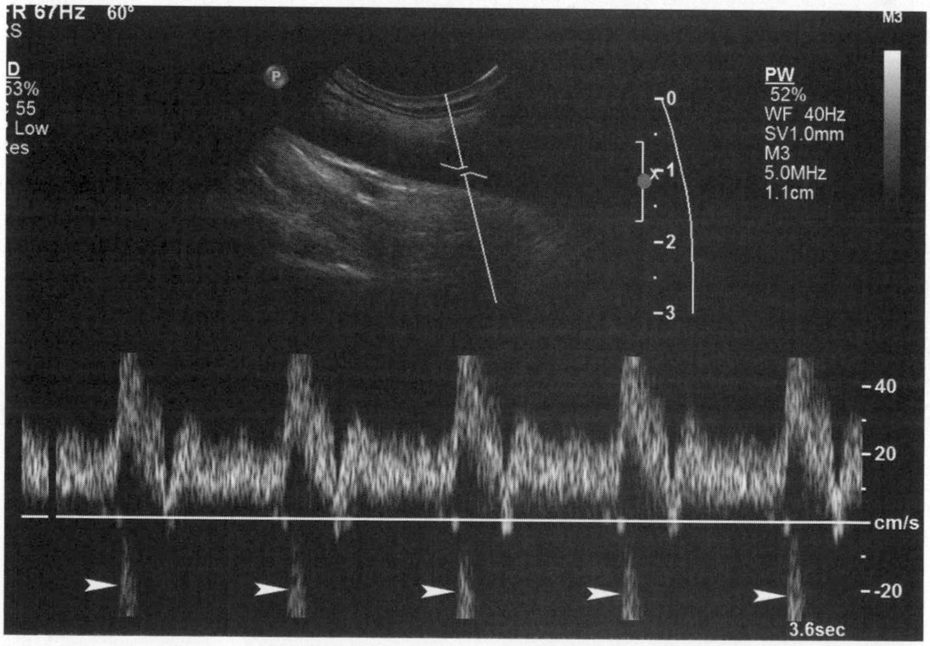

Figure 57-37. ■ *Spectral Doppler display showing aliasing. Peaks from each systole* (arrowheads) *are displayed in the reverse channel. In this case, lowering the baseline would overcome the problem.*

sal, which shows a black line (representing the wall filter) between the colors of the different channels.

Avoidance/Minimization. Various adjustments can be made to eliminate aliasing. For spectral and color modes, these include increasing the PRF (scale, velocity range) and expanding the velocity range in one channel by shifting the baseline. Additional techniques available in spectral Doppler include using high PRF technique (multiple sample gates), increasing the Doppler angle, using a lower transmit frequency, and using Doppler (CW).

Intrinsic Spectral Broadening. Spectral Doppler signals appear in both channels when a Doppler beam is perpendicular to the vessel being interrogated (Fig. 57-38), suggesting bidirectional flow. This seems to contradict the Doppler equation, which indicates that no shift should be detected at 90 degrees. In reality, echoes from the sample volume approach the finite aperture of the transducer over a range of angles, causing upward and downward Doppler shifts to be detected and resulting in signals in both channels. This effect is known as "intrinsic spectral broadening" because it is inherent to the finite aperture used to acquire signals.

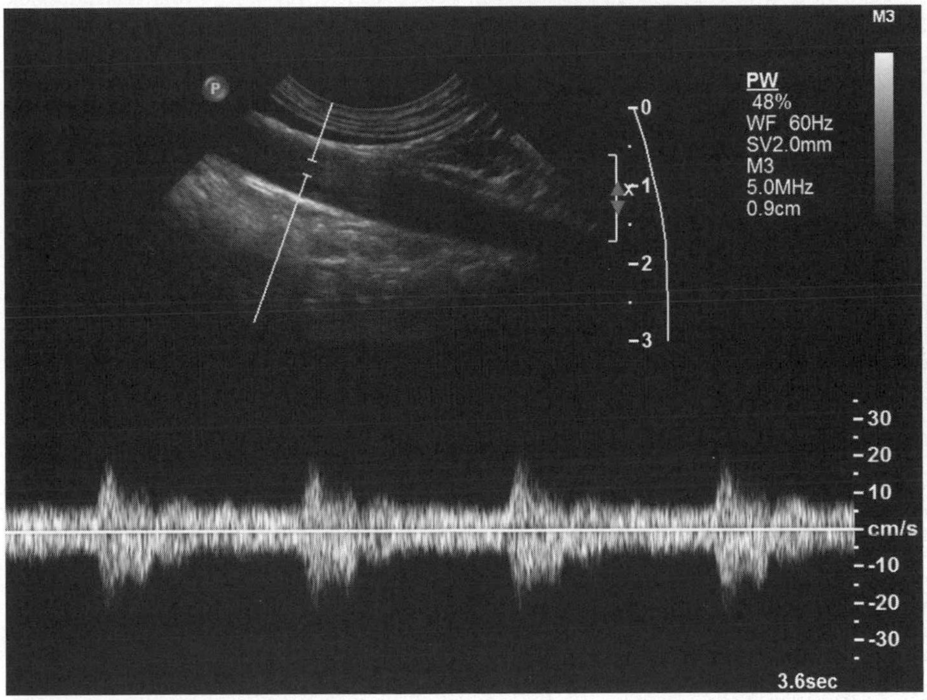

Figure 57-38. ■ *Spectral Doppler display showing intrinsic spectral broadening. The center axis of the Doppler beam is perpendicular to the vessel but shows signals in each channel because of the range of angles over which echoes return to the transducer aperture.*

Avoidance/Minimization. This effect can be minimized by using an appropriate Doppler angle (<70 degrees).

Color Doppler Mirror Artifact. Color Doppler mirror artifacts are the same as their grayscale counterparts, with color signals seen on each side of a mirror. Examples include mirroring of subclavian vessels in the apex of the lung, and of the inferior vena cava in the lung base (Color Plate 57-2), particularly during deep inspiration. Color in the aorta is sometimes seen mirrored in calcified plaque within the wall. The color coding of the mirror artifact may be different from that in the "true" vessel, depending on the scanning format, orientation of the vessel and mirror, and shape of the mirror (Color Plate 57-2).

Avoidance/Minimization. Approaching from a different angle may avoid the surface acting as the mirror.

Twinkle Artifact. In color Doppler mode, multiple reflections occurring in crystalline structures (e.g., calculi and urate crystals) produce phase shifts in the returning signals that are interpreted as Doppler shifts and therefore displayed in color. The multiple reflections produce a range of phase shifts that are displayed as a mixture of colors of the forward and reverse channels (see Color Plate 20-1 and Fig. 9-15). Variation in the detected phase shift over time results in a "twinkling" appearance during real-time scanning, suggestive of blood flow. This appearance is useful in identifying small calculi.

ELECTRONIC NOISE, INTERFERENCE, AND MALFUNCTION

Electrical Interference. Nearby electric fields can occasionally result in an interference pattern on the display, typically as repetitive lines or dots (Color Plate 57-3). These usually do not significantly interfere with interpretation of the images.

Avoidance/Minimization. Identify and, if possible, switch off the offending equipment. Use of a shielded power supply reduces the likelihood of such artifacts.

Electronic Noise. The generation of spurious signals known as electronic noise is inherent to electronic equipment. At high gain levels, the noise may be apparent in the display, as a fine "snowstorm" visible throughout the region of high gain (Fig. 57-39).

Avoidance/Minimization. Reduction of the TGC or gain level is likely to rectify the problem.

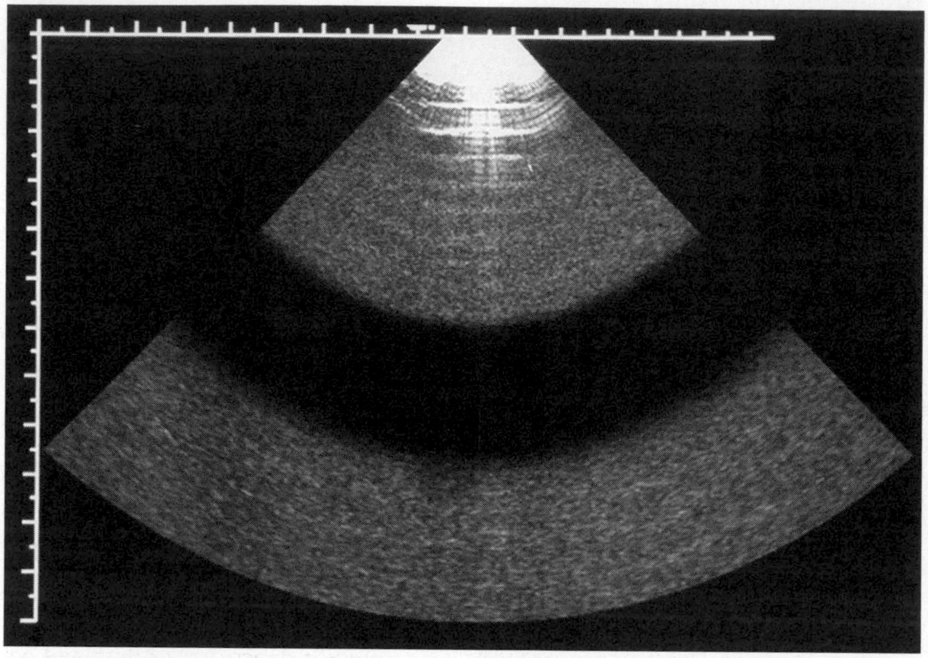

Figure 57-39. ■ *Electronic noise throughout the display, except for a region where the TGC is set low. This noise is caused by operating at maximum gain.*

ACKNOWLEDGMENTS

Thanks to Piotr Niznik for assistance with preparation of the images and diagrams.

SELECTED READING

Hedrick WR, Peterson CL. Image artifacts in real-time ultrasound. *JDMS* 1995;11:300–308.

Hykes D, Hedrick WR, Starchman D, eds. *Ultrasound Physics and Instrumentation*, 4th ed. Philadelphia: Mosby, 2005.

Kamaya A, Tuthill TA, Rubin JM. Twinkling artifact on color Doppler sonography: dependence on machine parameters and underlying cause. *AJR Am J Roentgenol* 2003;180: 215–222.

Kremkau FW, Taylor KJ. Artifacts in ultrasound imaging. *J Ultrasound Med* 1986;5:227–237.

Lim JH, Lee KS, Kim TS, et al. Ring-down artifacts posterior to the right hemidiaphragm on abdominal sonography. *J Ultrasound Med* 1999;18:403–410.

Reading CC, Charboneau JW, Allison JW, et al. Color and spectral Doppler mirror-image artifact of the subclavian artery. *Radiology* 1990;174:41–42.

Sauerbrei EE. The split image artifact in pelvic ultrasonography: the anatomy and physics. *J Ultrasound Med* 1985;4:29–34.

Thickman DI, Ziskin MC, Goldenberg NJ, et al. Clinical manifestations of the comet tail artifact. *J Ultrasound Med* 1983;2:225–230.

Wilson SR, Burns PN, Wilkinson LM, et al. Gas at abdominal US: appearance, relevance, and analysis of artifacts. *Radiology* 1999; 210:113–123.

Equipment Care and Quality Control

58

ROGER GENT

KEY WORDS

Axial. Along the axis of the ultrasound beam.

Axial Resolution. Ability to resolve closely spaced structures at different depths along the axis of the beam, determined mainly by pulse length.

Calibration. The accuracy of measurements made from ultrasound images. See Vertical and Horizontal Calibration.

Horizontal Calibration. Accuracy of measurements taken from side to side in an image (cf. Vertical Calibration).

Lateral Resolution. Ability to resolve closely spaced structures, side by side at the same depth, determined by the beamwidth.

Registration. The correct placement of echoes in a two-dimensional image, determined by the accuracy of tracking of the beam direction in the X-Y plane.

Spatial Resolution. Ability of a system to distinguish closely spaced targets. See Lateral and Axial Resolution.

SUAR. Sensitivity, uniformity, axial resolution phantom (obtainable from Gammex RMI of Middleton, WI).

Tissue-Equivalent Phantom. Phantom used to test real-time ultrasound systems, having properties similar to soft tissue (attenuation, speed of sound, and reflectivity).

Vertical Calibration. Accuracy of measurements taken from top to bottom in an image (cf. Horizontal Calibration).

Clinical Problem

Ultrasound systems are precision instruments that require careful handling and regular maintenance to ensure optimum performance. Put another way, ultrasound systems are like people: They don't respond well to rough treatment or lack of attention. Simple practical equipment checks decrease downtime and maximize image quality.

PREVENTIVE MAINTENANCE

1. Liquids other than contact gel should not be stored on the equipment. Spills may cause equipment malfunction or damage. The hand used to adjust control settings should be kept clean to ensure that contact gel does not affect the trackball or other functions.
2. Cables and transducers should be inspected visually for worn areas or cracks. Damaged cables may be potential safety hazards or the causes of intermittent malfunctions. Gel left on the transducer and cable causes brittle transducer housings.
3. Careless placement of the transducer and cable on the machine can cause cable damage. Cables should be properly stored when moving equipment to avoid damage if they are run over by the system wheels. Transducers should be placed in proper holders to avoid stress on cables.
4. When taking ultrasound equipment to wards, it should be moved carefully to avoid sudden impact, which may dislodge printed circuit boards from their connectors, resulting in failure of operation.
5. Many ultrasound systems have cooling fans with overlying air filters to prevent deposition of dust and particles on circuit boards within the unit. These should be cleaned periodically (weekly), especially if used in carpeted areas. They can usually be removed, cleaned with soap and water, and replaced. Always refer to the manufacturer's instructions to see whether an air filter is in use and for any recommended cleaning regimen. Neglect may cause equipment to overheat owing to decreased airflow.
6. Error messages should be noted and recorded for referral to service personnel.

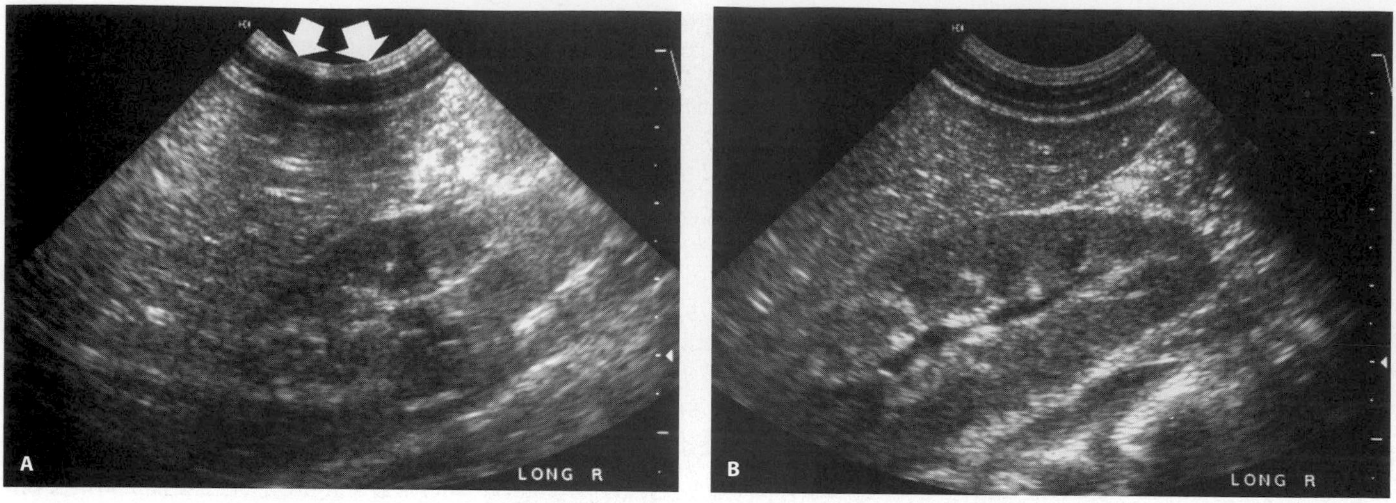

Figure 58-1. ■ *A. Longitudinal view of a kidney in a neonate. Voids* (arrows) *are present in the image, corresponding to nonfunctioning elements. This transducer is not acceptable for clinical use. The extent of the image degradation is apparent when the image in* (**A**) *is compared with one acquired with a nondamaged transducer (same type)* (**B**).

TRANSDUCER CARE

Transducers are delicate instruments and require careful handling. Transducers that have been dropped or treated roughly may have "dead" elements that no longer transmit or receive signals. This results in dark areas extending from the transducer through the full depth of the display (Fig. 58-1) of varying width depending on how many elements are involved. These damaged regions may also be apparent as voids in the reverberation echoes arising within the transducer when it is not in contact with a patient (Fig. 58-2). Running a needle or paper clip along the length of the transducer is a simple means of detecting dead elements. In a normal transducer, reverberation echoes from within the metal are seen but diminish in brightness or disappear when the needle is over nonfunctioning elements.

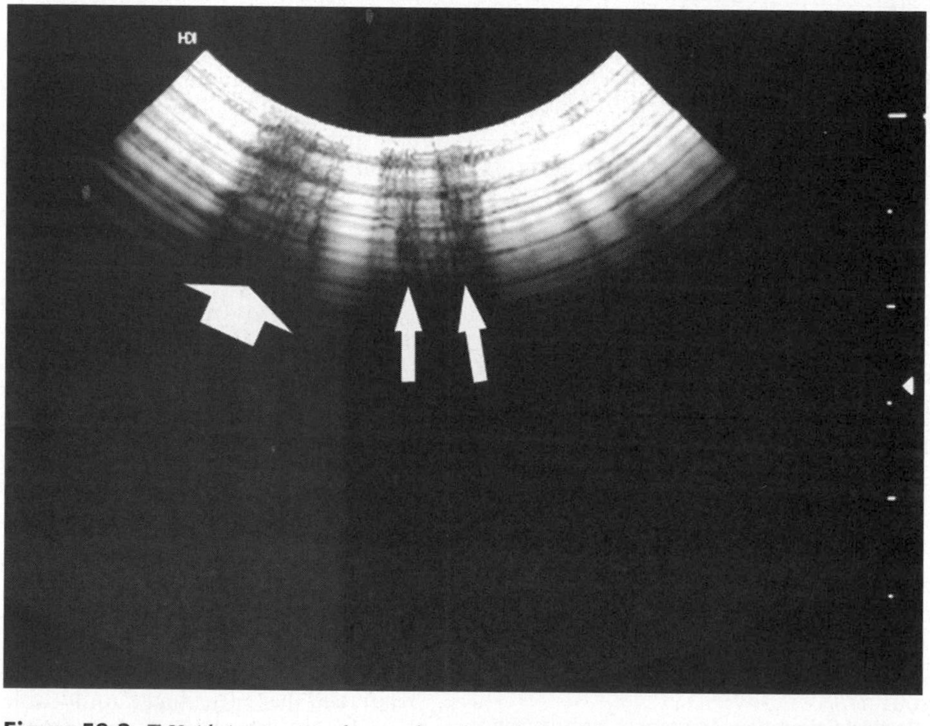

Figure 58-2. ■ *Voids* (arrows) *in the reverberation echoes of the transducer used in Figure 58-1A.*

Transducers should be cleaned after each patient with an alcohol sponge or transducer disinfectant, particularly if the patient has an open wound or a skin problem. Plastic freezer bags are an inexpensive means of covering the transducer to avoid contact with open wounds and avoid contamination. Some transducers can be immersed in Cidex up to the handle for sterilization. Approximately 10 minutes immersion is required for adequate sterilization (see Appendix 30). Users should always refer to the manufacturer's instructions for suitable cleaning agents for transducers to avoid damage to cables or transducer housing.

CONTACT AGENTS

Use a commercial water-soluble coupling gel to ensure good acoustic contact between the transducer and patient. Thick, high-viscosity gels are desirable when scanning the patient in an erect position because they don't slide off easily. Thicker gels are also helpful for obstetric patients with large abdomens.

It is desirable to heat gel in a commercially available heating device. However, make sure that there is enough

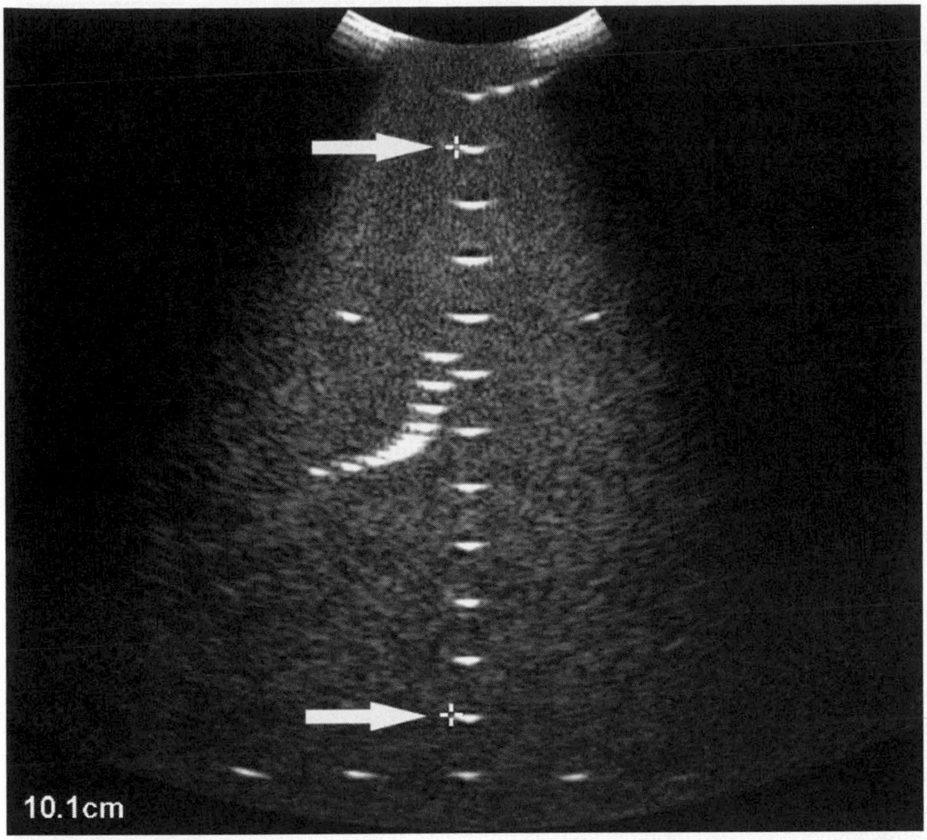

Figure 58-3. ■ *View of a phantom confirming that vertical calibration (top to bottom) is accurate. Measured distance between the selected pins is 10.1 cm, compared with the true value of 10.0 cm (an error of 1%).*

gel in the container because gel can be overheated if only a small amount is present. Gel temperature should be tested before application to the patient, particularly in pediatric cases. Gel warmers that do not have thermostat control should not be left on indefinitely because they pose a potential fire hazard.

Use disposable gloves when scanning a patient to avoid the risk of infection. Spread the gel around the abdomen with the transducer rather than by hand. Do not handle the controls with gel on your hand or glove.

QUALITY ASSURANCE

Quality assurance tests may be tedious to perform but are worthwhile because it may be difficult or even impossible to detect calibration and measurement distortions from examination of the images alone. Clearly, major clinical problems may result if erroneous measurement data are produced. Quality assurance checks should be performed on a quarterly basis with most systems or more often if a problem is suspected (e.g., if a transducer has been dropped or measurements are consistently higher or lower than expected).

Quality Control Tests

The standard tests performed to ensure that the system is working satisfactorily are (1) aspect ratio and calibration tests, (2) resolution tests (both axial and lateral), and (3) a comparative power output test that equates to a depth of penetration measurement. All of these tests are performed on a tissue-equivalent phantom (RMI 413A or equivalent).

Aspect Ratio and Calibration. The aspect ratio and calibration test measures whether distances are accurate in both directions (X [horizontal], Y [vertical]) and whether these measurements are correctly displayed on a hard-copy device (Figs. 58-3 and 58-4). When the phantom is scanned, the vertically (spaced 1 cm apart; see Fig. 58-3) and horizontally (spaced 1 cm apart; see Fig. 58-4) aligned pins should measure the correct distance apart when using electronic calipers. The distance measured by caliper can be compared with the known distance between the pins in the phantom and the error calculated. Errors of 1% to 2% are acceptable. The measurements obtained by electronic caliper should also match those taken from the vertical and horizontal scale markers on the hardcopy images, measured with a handheld caliper. One centimeter measured vertically on an image should be equal to the same distance measured horizontally.

Resolution. Axial and lateral resolution capability can be determined using closely spaced pins in a phantom. The arrangement of pins varies from phantom to phantom. In the example shown

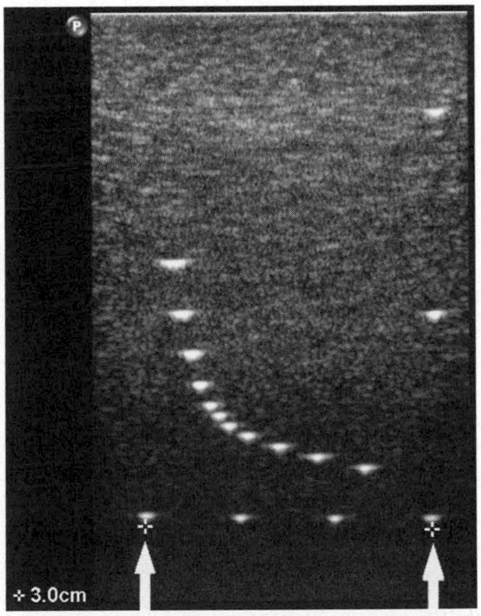

Figure 58-4. ■ *View of a phantom confirming that horizontal calibration (side to side) is accurate. Measured distance between the selected pins* (arrows) *is 3.0 cm, equal to the true distance between them.*

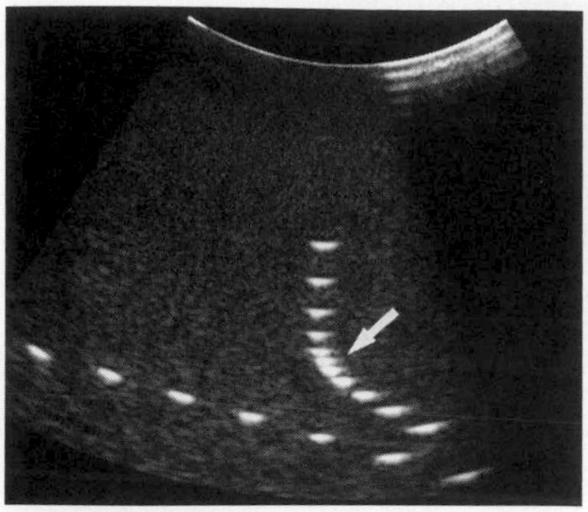

Figure 58-5. ■ *Axial resolution assessment using pins progressively closer together along the axis of the beam. The closest pins* (arrow) *are 0.5 mm apart and are resolved, so that axial resolution for this transducer is better than 0.5 mm.*

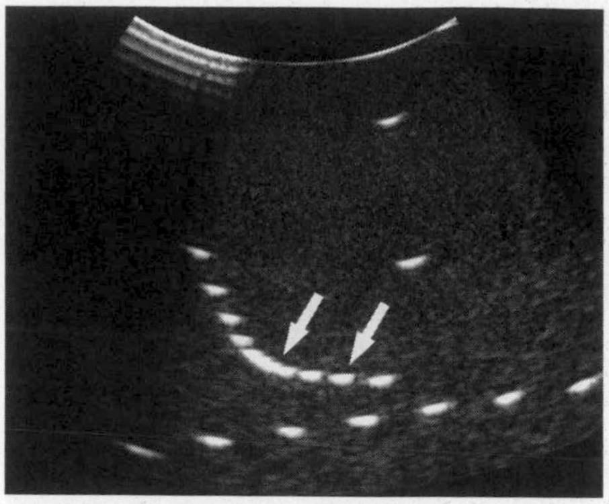

Figure 58-6. ■ *Lateral resolution assessment using pins progressively closer together from right to left* (arrows), *across the axis of the beam. The third and fourth pins (1 mm apart) are resolved, whereas the fourth and fifth pins (0.5 mm apart) are not. Lateral resolution is better than 1 mm for this transducer.*

(Fig. 58-5), a curved array of pins is used, with transducer position adjusted to make use of the vertically (axial resolution) or horizontally (lateral resolution) aligned pins. Some phantoms provide separate pin groups for axial and lateral resolution assessment.

Axial resolution is assessed by seeing whether the pins can be resolved vertically (Fig. 58-5). The spacings between the closest pins in the phantom shown are 3, 2, 1, and 0.5 mm. In Figure 58-5, the spacing can be seen between all the pins; therefore, the axial resolution is better than the smallest distance (0.5 mm). Lateral resolution is assessed in Figure 58-6, with the pins *(arrows)* aligned across the beam. Resolution capability is expressed as the closest pin spacing that can be resolved.

Comparative Power Output. The test for comparative power output determines whether the sound beam emitted by the transducer can reach a depth adequate to see deep structures (Fig. 58-7). The test is performed at full power output (in Fig. 58-7 the highest power output is 0 dB), and the time gain compensation is set at maximum at the area of depth visualization. The measurement is taken from the top to the deepest area at which good information is still obtained. In Figure 58-7, the deepest area satisfactorily imaged is 73.5 mm (7.35 cm) deep. This model of the RMI phantom had an attenuation factor of 0.7 dB/cm/MHz, and the transducer had a frequency of 5 MHz. These numbers are used to determine the output capabilities of the system with this transducer. The comparative power output can be calculated as follows:

$$\text{Attenuation factor } (0.7) \times \text{Depth } (7.35) \times \text{Transducer frequency } (5) = 25.725 \text{ dB}$$

This number is recorded in the quality-control logbook as the output for this transducer using this phantom. Repeat tests should give the same result. For the comparison of results to be valid, all settings must be the same each time the test is undertaken. This is a useful test to see whether transmitter and/or receiver characteristics are changing over time.

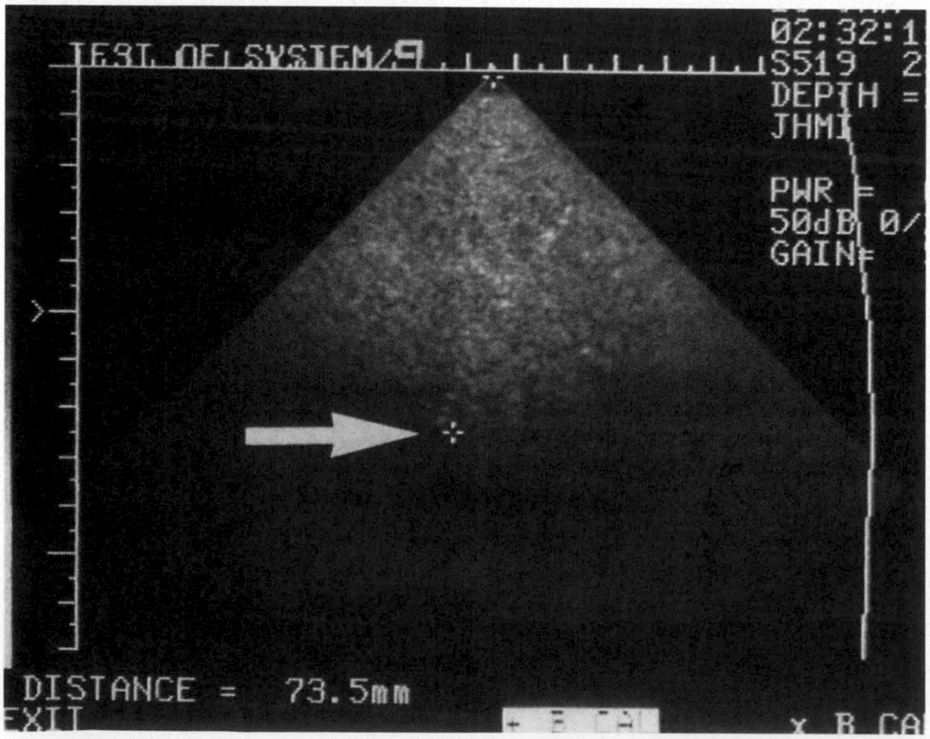

Figure 58-7. ■ *Depth at which structures can be viewed with a sector scan transducer (7.4 cm)* (arrow).

MALFUNCTION

Modern ultrasound systems are very reliable but occasionally can malfunction, resulting in disruption of images. This is rare in modern systems, but when it occurs it is usually obvious with clear disruption of the images. The disruption may relate to circuitry for a specific transducer, so the equipment may still be useable with different transducers until the problem can be rectified.

Software errors occasionally occur and can often be rectified by switching the ultrasound unit off and on again, allowing the system to reboot.

SELECTED READING

Hedrick WR, Hykes DL, Starchman DE. *Ultrasound Physics and Instrumentation,* 4th ed. Philadelphia: Elsevier, 2005.

Hykes DL, Hendrick WR, Milavickas LR, et al. Quality assurance for real-time ultrasound equipment. *JDMS* 1986;2:121–133.

Kremkau F. *Diagnostic Ultrasound: Principles and Instruments,* 6th ed. Philadelphia: WB Saunders, 2002.

59 Photography

ROGER C. SANDERS
TOM WINTER

KEY WORDS

Brightness. Controls the intensity of the CRT background.

Cathode Ray Tube (CRT). The sonographic image is displayed on the screen of a CRT. A second CRT displays the image for the multiformat camera.

Contrast. Controls the amount of gray-level echoes seen; that is, how many medium- and low-level echoes are visible.

DICOM. *D*igital *I*maging and *Co*mmunications in *M*edicine standard permits distributing and viewing any kind of medical image regardless of its origin. DICOM is an agreed on common language so that medical images acquired by any machine, made by any manufacturer, are usable by any other system.

F-Stop. Controls the aperture of the lens; wider apertures (which correspond to lower f-stop numbers) present more light to the film.

PACS. *P*icture *A*rchiving and *C*ommunication *S*ystem. A computer-based method for archiving, displaying, and transmitting image data.

Time (T). Sets the time interval of exposure (e.g., 0.5 second, 1 second, etc.).

Photographic Systems

Several different methods of recording the image are in use; each has virtues and disadvantages.

POLAROID CAMERA

Polaroid has the following advantages: The camera is cheap and easy to use, film development is rapid, and resolution is almost as good as that with the cathode ray tube (CRT) image. However, the film is costly, fades with time, and is difficult to store. Camera settings are not easy to maintain. With approximately three patients per day and an average number of films, one can save the price of a multiformat camera during the course of a year by not using Polaroid film.

THERMAL-SENSITIVE PAPER PRINTER

A cheaper alternative to Polaroids is a paper printer that uses durable thermal paper. The camera operates much like the multiformat cameras with brightness and contrast controls. No processor is required. Image quality is good. Color images can be recorded.

At the time of writing, the cost of an image on a thermal printer was one-tenth the cost of a Polaroid image and a sheet of x-ray film cost approximately twice as much as a Polaroid image. Each sheet of film may contain four to nine images. Images recorded on thermal paper start to decay after approximately 6 months.

MULTIFORMAT CAMERAS

Multiformat cameras have the following advantages: They use relatively cheap film, the film is easy to store and view, and exposures are relatively easy to set. However, the initial purchase of a multiformat camera is expensive, a processor is required, and personnel are needed to handle the film, chemicals, and so on.

Multiformat cameras come with various features, some of which are well worth having. The smaller and more compact versions are as cheap as the larger systems and are preferable because they can be placed on a portable real-time system. One feature that is unimportant is whether the system is "on axis" (i.e., whether the lens lines up with the CRT image directly). A variable-format system is not of much practical importance because the sonographer almost always uses the same settings (usually six on one film). This format displays an image of satisfactory size, but putting nine images on one film provides optimum cost savings. Processing systems are now available that do not require a darkroom or additional chemicals. These "dry" systems are expensive.

There are several important features to consider in your choice of a multiformat camera:

1. Rapid exposure time
2. Compact size
3. A method of preventing double exposure
4. Convenient brightness and contrast controls (not buried inside the camera)

5. A "flat-face" screen (which means that a measurement at the periphery of the image will be reliable)

"Laser" multiformat cameras yield a consistent quality image because they compensate for poor-quality image settings. They are expensive.

35-MM CAMERA

Cameras using 35-mm film are cheaper than multiformat cameras but less convenient. The advantages of these systems are that the film and camera are very inexpensive. More than six exposures can be made without changing the film or cassette. However, the system needs a processor. Film can be wasted when you want to photograph and view the images from a single patient because the roll of film could take many more pictures.

VIDEOTAPE

Some advocate videotaping all examinations. This makes the examination difficult to view at a later date because videotape review is lengthy. Image quality may not be optimal.

Videotapes decay with time unless they are reexamined at biannual intervals.

PICTURE ARCHIVING AND COMMUNICATION SYSTEMS

Image acquisition to a computer is practical because new hard drives can accommodate terabytes of data, computer processing capabilities have improved dramatically over time, and there have been marked decreases in costs of the necessary hardware. Newer ultrasound units transmit the digital data to the Picture Archiving and Communication System (PACS) directly; for older units, an acquisition box connected to the ultrasound system accumulates images that are then downloaded to a central computer. Image quality is excellent when the images are reviewed. Benefits of this type of system are the absence of lost films, long-term cost economies because no film is used, the capability to instantaneously send images electronically to viewing computers throughout the hospital or clinic system (or for that matter, anywhere in the world over the World Wide Web), infinite image archival life, and the ability to process and improve the images on the computer. Digital Imaging and Communications in Medicine capability of the newest units addresses both image standardization and Health Insurance Portability and Accountability Act privacy concerns. PACS allows direct integration of the ultrasound examination with the radiology report and electronic medical record. Digitally stored images may be easily accessed for teaching and research purposes. Precise comparison of ultrasound with all other digital imaging techniques (e.g., computed tomography, magnetic resonance imaging, and positron emission tomography) at the same level facilitates diagnostic problem solving. Previous ultrasound studies are immediately available for comparison with the current examination.

Difficulties with a system of this type in the past have included frequent system failures and difficulty printing images when they are requested by clinicians or when they are needed at another site. Comparing images from a current series with previous studies required several display facilities. Retrieval of earlier images could be tedious unless a "jukebox" was available for the digital media on which the information was stored. Because there was no standardization of computer image acquisition, initial high expense and inability to exchange images had been drawbacks. All of the above problems have essentially been solved with modern technology. Practically speaking, the only disadvantages to a good digital PACS are cost and the necessity for adequate computer support; however, the older analog systems discussed above are more than adequate in many situations and can be more economical.

Setting Up the Camera

Setting the photographic controls on the ultrasound system is one of the most important and difficult parts of obtaining a satisfactory long-term record of the examination. Subtle changes in brightness and contrast greatly alter the image. Although observation of the graybars helps in setting up the image, a clinical scan showing an area such as the liver and kidney, where there are both high- and low-level echoes, is of more value. A tissue-equivalent phantom that has pseudometastatic and pseudocystic lesions within it can also be used. Although use of a PACS system obviates many of these concerns, even an all-digital system requires careful setup and attention to the image transfer and display process, although in a different manner than that with optical analog systems.

MULTIFORMAT CAMERA SETUP

Warm-up time adjustments may be avoided by making sure that the scanner and multiformat camera have been turned on a half hour before they are adjusted or used. Most multiformat cameras will not allow an image to be photographed until the camera is warmed up.

Practical Maneuvers

1. Lower the background and contrast all the way. Select the mode (black or white background) for display.
2. Find the optimal background display by changing the brightness level. Fine-tune settings with no image on the screen until you see an acceptable background for white or black imaging. Note the setting.
3. Put graybars on the screen. Move the contrast to a level at which all graybars can be seen at the same time, keeping the background brightness at an optimal level, perhaps by reducing the brightness slightly.
4. Obtain a good-quality image of the liver and right kidney on a longitudinal view; include a gallbladder with some artifactual echoes and see if you can reproduce those low-level echoes.
5. Now vary the contrast and compensate with the brightness until you achieve an optimal setting. Photograph each setting and record the different levels. Unfortunately, both controls usually need to be varied at the same time.

6. Once the ideal photographic settings have been obtained, lock and record them (Fig. 59-1). It takes time to set up a camera correctly; a casual knob-fiddler can destroy an hour's work.
7. Multiformat cameras are not very sturdy and can easily malfunction if mistreated. An important part of practical maintenance is keeping the air filters clean (check daily for dust accumulation). Do not put the multiformat camera in too confined a space because it tends to overheat. The internal monitor must be adjusted periodically to maintain optimum photographic capability.

POLAROID CAMERA

Technique is different on Polaroid cameras; the f-stop and time (shutter speed) must be adjusted. The f-stop on Polaroid cameras has an opposite effect on exposure from that in a multiformat camera because the Polaroid image is a positive image. A decrease in the f-stop number brightens the picture. Polaroid camera setup includes adjusting the camera CRT to display an acceptable image and then varying the f-stop and time to capture the image properly on film.

Ideally, only one variable should be changed at a time (i.e., the background is adjusted for optimum brightness, and the contrast is then varied for proper echo levels superimposed on this brightness level), but this is not entirely practical. The adjustment of either brightness or contrast could change the background.

Maintenance of Polaroid cameras requires cleaning the rollers with an alcohol swab on a daily basis. The rollers are easily detachable from most Polaroid cameras. Do not unwrap Polaroid film before it is to be used because humidity and heat decrease the sensitivity of the film. Develop the film within a few minutes. If the film is left undeveloped for longer than this, it adheres to the film

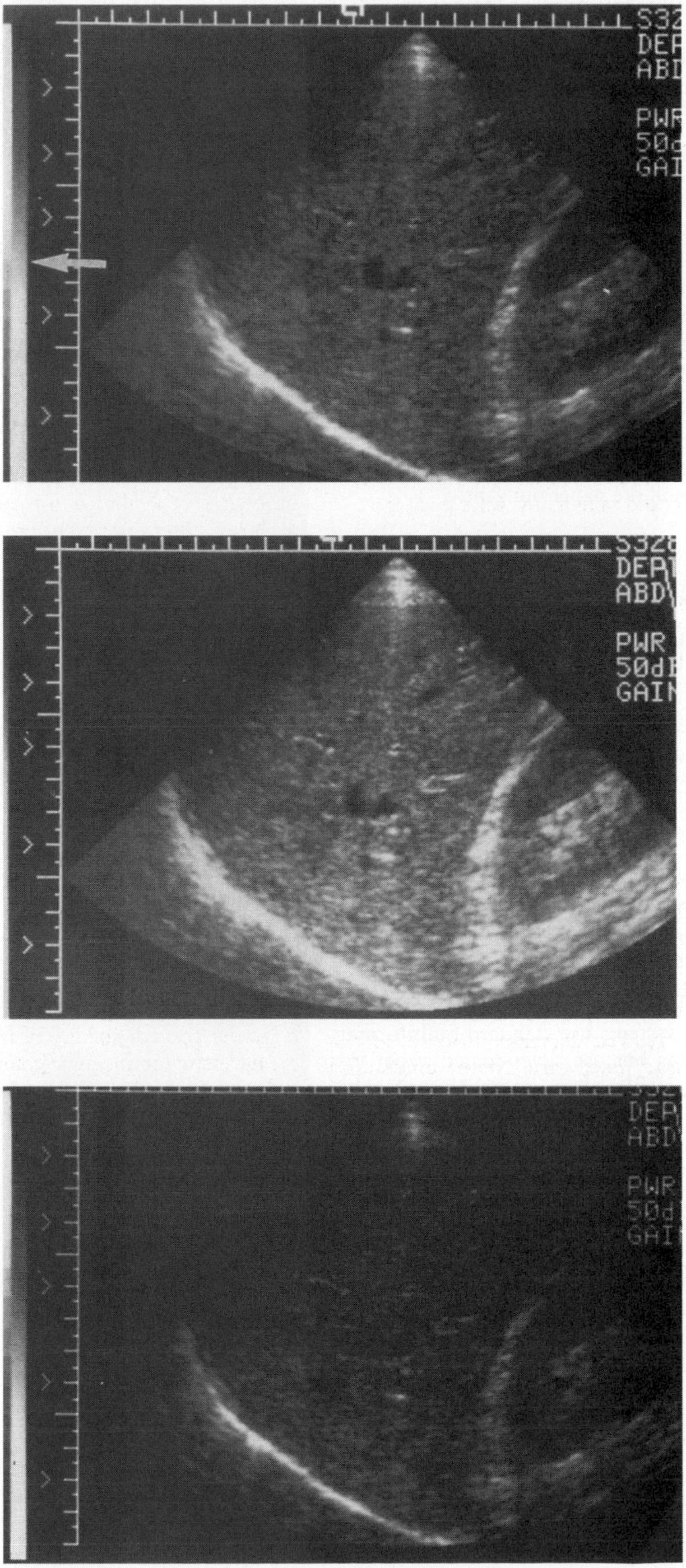
A

B

C

Figure 59-1. ■ *Obtaining correct photographic settings. **A.** Satisfactory photographic image. Note the grayscale bars* (arrow). ***B.** Excessive brightness. Compare the grayscale bars with those in (A). **C.** Incorrect contrast settings with suboptimal grayscale bar display.*

back. Pull the Polaroid tab straight through the rollers or streaks may appear on the image and paper segments may break off in the rollers.

THERMAL-SENSITIVE PAPER

Thermal-sensitive paper printers require special maintenance procedures. Dust and dirt can collect on the thermal printing head. A head-cleaning sheet is usually provided. If the thermal head overheats, prints may come out totally black. Allow the temperature of the printing head to drop by not printing, then continue. When the printer is suddenly exposed to a temperature change, moisture may condense inside the unit and the paper can adhere to the roller, causing a jam. Let the printer dry out for a couple of hours and then pull the paper out gently.

Film Choice and Storage

FILM

There is a choice of film that can be used with multiformat cameras. All manufacturers make both a film with a clear base and a film with a blue-green base. We prefer the clear base because we think there is a chance that low-level echoes may be overlooked against a blue-green background, but many think that the blue-green format is more attractive.

SILVER-COATED PAPER

Some systems use standard multiformat cameras but use silver-coated paper instead of film. Because paper cannot be viewed through a viewbox, this system is cumbersome for teaching large groups. However, this method is acceptable if showing the image to an audience is not part of your practice, because paper is inexpensive and easily stored.

THERMAL-SENSITIVE PAPER

Store paper rolls in a cool, dry area away from heat and sunlight. Printed images are said to last approximately 5 years if kept in a clear plastic case. The print could be damaged if brought into contact with solvent such as alcohol.

Photographic Problems

1. *Fogging* along the edge of the film may occur (Fig. 59-2). Either the cassette has not been pushed completely into the multiformat camera

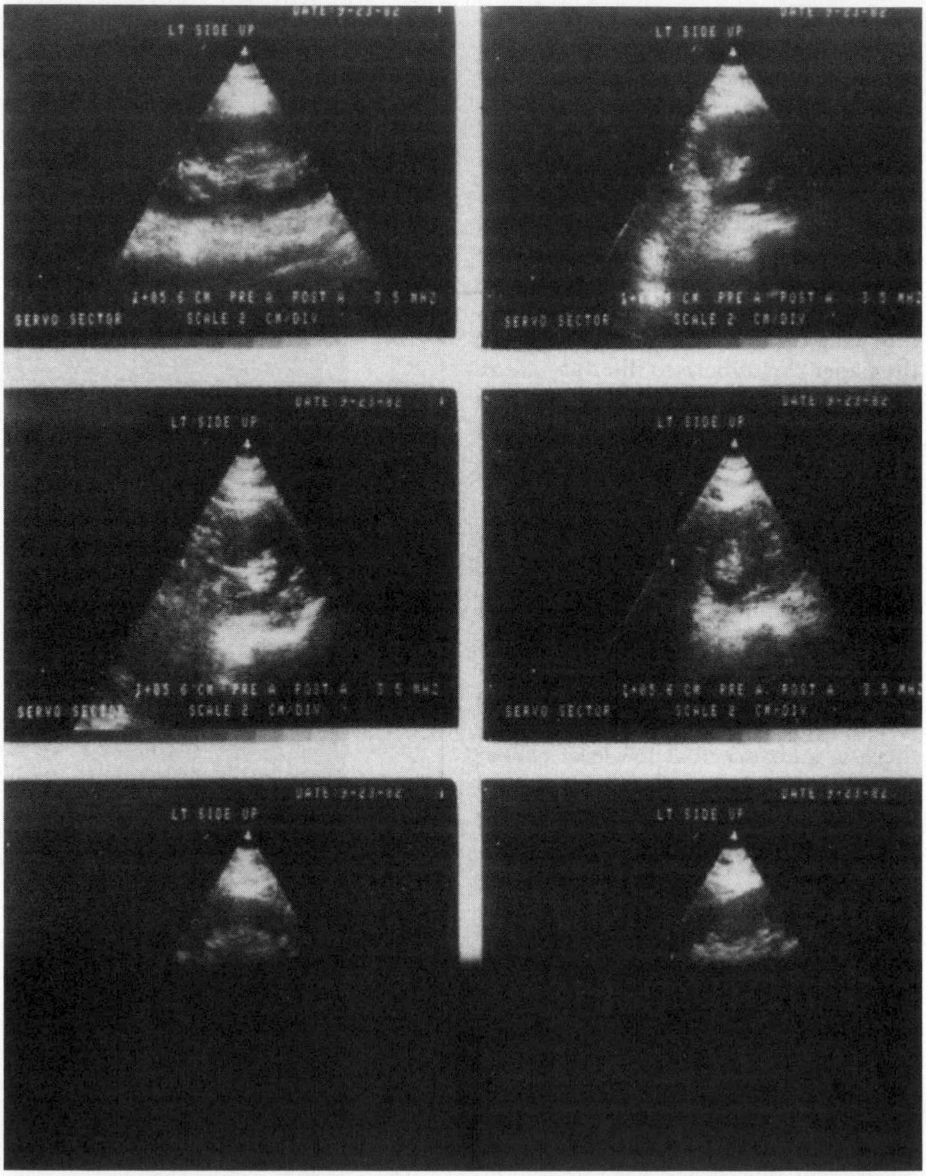

Figure 59-2. ■ *This film has been partially exposed to light at the bottom. Check the cassette for cracks and light leaks.*

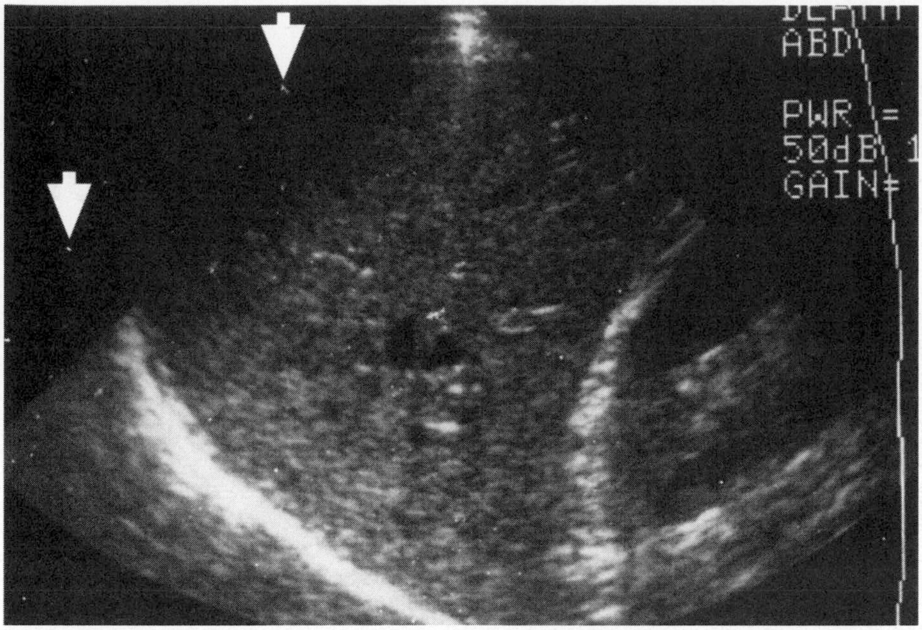

Figure 59-3. ■ *White marks caused by dust on the CRT will appear on sequential films in the same area.*

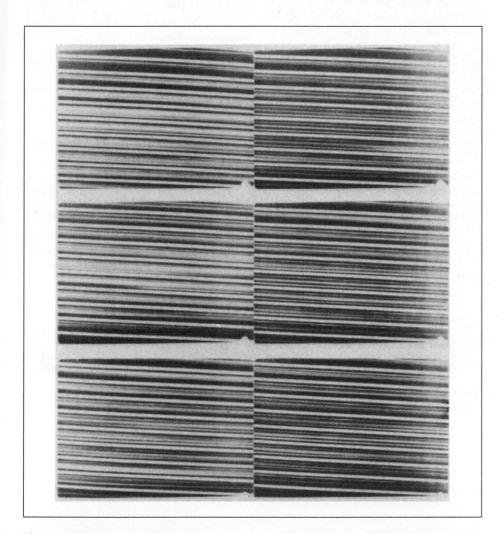

Figure 59-4. ■ *Diagonal linear artifact usually caused by defective horizontal hold on the CRT.*

or there is a light leak along one edge of the cassette. Cassettes are fragile and develop light leaks with rough usage.

2. There may be white marks on the film (when using white-on-black mode) that appear in the same place on sequential films (Fig. 59-3). Dust is present on the camera lens or on the CRT face. Clean the camera.
3. The film won't expose, although it seems to be in a good position. Push the cassette properly into its housing.
4. The film may be unexpectedly dark or light. The possibilities are that (1) the multiformat camera or ultrasound system has not warmed up; (2) the wrong type of film is in the cassette; (3) the processor has not been warmed up (is the film damp?); (4) the developing mixture is wrong; or (5) someone has altered the camera settings.
5. If the processed image is crisscrossed with diagonal lines (Fig. 59-4), the horizontal hold of the CRT is out of adjustment. You won't be aware of this unless you look at the camera monitor.

Preliminary Reports

60

ROGER C. SANDERS

KEY WORDS

Anechoic. Echo free.

Attenuating Lesion. A sound-absorbing lesion.

Contour. The shape and borders of a lesion or organ.

Echogenicity. The number of echoes within a structure.

Echotexture. The arrangement of echoes within tissue.

Posterior Enhancement. Increased echogenicity directly behind a structure.

Preliminary Report. The unofficial report that precedes the final, detailed report.

Preliminary Reports

Preliminary reports should give the key sonographic findings so that the clinician does not have to wait for the official dictation to be typed (which may take several days). Immediate action may be indicated by the sonogram findings. Preliminary reports by the sonographer are required when the sonologist is not present at the examination.

WHO WRITES THEM?

Some ultrasound departments are well staffed with physicians who write preliminary reports; others depend on the sonographer. Sonographers entrusted with this task should confine themselves to describing the sonographic findings without offering a conclusion about pathology unless prior physician approval has been obtained. Preliminary reports should be accurate, clear, complete, concise, and timely.

TYPICAL REPORTS

Normal Study

Liver No lesion seen; normal size.

Common bile duct 4 mm (normal for age).

Gallbladder No evidence of sludge or calculi. Normal wall thickness.

Pancreas No abnormality seen. No evidence of dilated ducts or focal lesions.

Spleen No focal lesions seen; normal size.

Kidneys Right, 10 cm. Left, 10 cm. No evidence of hydronephrosis, calculi, or mass.

No fluid seen in the abdomen.

Abnormal Study

(The pathologic lesion described is noted here in parentheses.)

Liver Echopenic region in the right posterior lobe 4 × 5 × 3 cm. (Primary or metastatic lesion in the liver.)

Gallbladder Gallstones. Gallbladder wall 5 mm thick. Local tenderness over the gallbladder. (Acute cholecystitis.)

Pancreas Highly echogenic pancreas with irregular border and calcification. (Chronic pancreatitis.)

Kidney Cystic structure at the right lower pole with septation and irregular superior border. (Complex cyst suggesting a neoplasm.)

OBSTETRICS

1. The lateral ventricles are 16 mm at the level of the atrium (top normal 10 mm) with an abnormal shape to the cerebellum and skull. The distance between the posterior elements of the spine is increased, and there is an adjacent cystic area at L3–S1. (Spina bifida with hydrocephalus.)
2. There is a fluid pocket of greater than 8 cm noted. (Polyhydramnios.)
3. There is an anterior placenta that completely/partially covers

the internal os. (Placenta previa before or after 20 weeks.)

Pathologic descriptions can be used if there is well-accepted standard terminology and there is not a subjective element involved.

For the clinician, the report gives an indication of relevant sonographic findings without a conclusion about the pathologic diagnosis. (This is considered the physician's privilege/liability/burden.)

The sonologist conveys a clinical opinion in addition to the factual data.

Interpretation and Documentation

MEASUREMENTS

If the examination includes a description of organs that are measurable, it is good practice to include these measurements in the report. Consistent measurement (e.g., inner to outer, inner to inner, or outer to outer) should be used. The same charts and tables should be used all the time, and the measurements described by the author when the chart was developed must be followed (see Appendices 2–22).

Established normal measurements may be mentioned in the report. Organs that need measuring on a routine basis include the following:

1. Kidney
   a. Length (longest possible length, with even cortex surrounding the sinus).
   b. Anteroposterior (A-P) (perpendicular to the length measurement on the same image).
   c. Width (90 degrees from the length view at the level of renal vein) may be helpful.
2. Common bile duct
   In the sagittal plane, measured at the point where the duct crosses anterior to the main portal vein and the hepatic artery. Measure from inner wall to inner wall. Magnify an image before measuring to increase the accuracy.
3. Uterus (measured abdominally)
   a. Length (showing the linear endometrial canal).
   b. A-P (perpendicular to the length measurement on the same image).
   c. Width (obtained at the widest diameter of the uterus, 90 degrees from the length view).
   The uterus can also be measured during an endovaginal examination, in which case the length from the fundus to the uterocervical junction is measured. This point is a little indefinite, although often echogenic glands are seen at this site.
4. Ovary
   a. Length (sagittal plane).
   b. A-P (perpendicular to the length measurement on the same image).
   c. Width (90 degrees to the length view, in the transverse plane).
5. Prostate
   a. Length (obtained in the sagittal plane).
   b. A-P (perpendicular to the length measurement on the same image).
   c. Width (transverse plane, widest diameter of gland).
6. Urinary bladder
   a. Length (greatest length measured postvoid, sagittal plane).
   b. A-P (perpendicular to the length measurement on the same image).
   c. Width (90 degrees to the length view at the widest diameter of the bladder in the transverse plane). Prevoid measurements are given only if your sonologist requests it. Postvoid measurements are required if the patient has prostate problems, urinary tract infections, or neurologic problems.
7. All masses should be measured.

SONOGRAPHIC APPEARANCES

Organs that need to be evaluated for texture and mentioned in the preliminary report are the liver, kidneys, pancreas, and spleen. Statements of relative echogenicity are acceptable in the preliminary report.

Echogenicity

The echogenicity of an organ can indicate the functional state of that organ. The normal range of echogenicity of abdominal viscera from greatest to least is as follows:

renal sinus → pancreas → spleen → liver renal cortex → renal medullary pyramids

A kidney with echogenicity greater than the adjacent liver or spleen suggests renal pathology, except in the neonate. A pancreas that is less echogenic than the adjacent liver makes one suspicious of acute pancreatitis, except in the small child.

Through Transmission

The echogenicity posterior to a structure or lesion should be mentally quantitated because it relates to the internal composition of that structure. Enhanced echogenicity behind an area of interest usually indicates a fluid-filled structure. Decreased echogenicity posterior to a structure indicates a solid, sound-absorbing lesion.

Contour

Demarcation. A structure that is well circumscribed should be described as such; this indicates a confined process with no surrounding tissue invasion. Irregular borders raise the question of tissue intrusion as by inflammation or neoplasm.

Shape Changes. Note whether a structure appears enlarged or smaller than usual. Changes in shape with time may occur on a physiologic basis; for example, the kidney enlarges when fluid is administered and the uterine size changes with puberty, the menstrual cycle, and menopause. Most often, however, shape changes indicate pathology.

When to Telephone

New findings that require urgent management change should be conveyed to the patient's physician immediately. Typical examples of urgent findings are as follows:

1. Strong suspicion of ectopic pregnancy
2. Fetal death
3. Major fetal anomalies
4. Abruptio placentae
5. Markedly abnormal fetal heart rate
6. Leaking aneurysm
7. Unexpected neoplastic mass
8. Unexpected periorgan hematoma
9. Renal artery occlusion in a transplant
10. Obstructed bile ducts
11. Placenta previa if there is vaginal bleeding

12. Unexpected renal obstruction
13. Tendon or muscle tear
14. Undiagnosed deep vein thrombosis
15. Markedly narrowed carotid or limb vessels
16. Incompetent cervix
17. Absent fetal movement and low fluid, especially with marked intrauterine growth restriction
18. Testicular fragmentation by trauma
19. Testicular torsion

Information that is too sensitive for the patient to carry should also prompt a telephone call.

1. Fetal death
2. Fetal anomalies if not discussed with the patient previously
3. Findings indicative of acquired immune deficiency syndrome
4. Neoplastic mass if not discussed with the patient previously

Findings that are subjective in nature may be better conveyed by a phone call.

1. Unexpected absence of fetal movement in the presence of normal measurements
2. Reporting on structures inadequately visualized that are strongly suspicious for pathology, such as the fetal head being deep in the pelvis, but appearing to contain an intracranial abnormality

Malpractice and Ultrasound

ROGER C. SANDERS

61

KEY WORDS

Defendant. The individual or entity, whether physician or hospital, that is the target of the suit.

Plaintiff. In this area, this is the patient or the patient's representative, for example, a mother who is initiating the suit.

Sonographer. The skilled technologist who performs the study, most often under the supervision of the physician.

Sonologist. Physician reporting and sometimes performing the sonogram.

Causes of Malpractice

Malpractice from a legal point of view as it relates to ultrasound comes in two forms:

1. "Battery." The patient is injured during the examination by assault or inadequate care, for example, falls off the table. Failure to obtain informed consent is another type of "battery" injury.
2. Negligence. The examination is performed in a fashion that is "below the standard of care."

Standard of care is defined as the way in which a "reasonable and prudent" physician or sonographer would act under the same circumstances. In our court system, the standard of care is established in several different ways.

1. Expert witnesses testify as to the standard of care.
2. Guidelines such as the "AIUM practice guidelines for the performance of an antepartum obstetric ultrasound examination" or American College of Obstetricians and Gynecologists technical bulletins set national standards.
3. Local hospital, radiology, or obstetric department policy statements also set the standard of care.

The American Institute of Ultrasound in Medicine (AIUM) practice guidelines set the standard for a "basic" ultrasound performed in an obstetrician's office or a clinic; however, it is important to note that although there are no written guidelines, there is an implied higher standard for a referral ultrasound unit or perinatologist's office that specializes in fetal anomaly detection.

RESPONSIBILITIES OF THE PHYSICIAN OR SONOGRAPHER REPORTING THE STUDY

The physician or sonographer reporting the study is required to accurately describe the findings on the examination including pertinent negative findings with a clinical conclusion about the presence or absence of an abnormality. Suggestions about additional procedures or follow-up studies may be required. Problems in the performance of the study such as obesity or suboptimal patient position should be covered in the narrative portion of the report. In the United States, the physician reporting the study is responsible for the accuracy and quality of the report even though she/he may not actually see the patient.

Sonographers are frequently named defendants in a malpractice suit but he/she will not be held liable for a diagnostic error unless he/she reports out the study. The sonographer often has a different employer—such as a hospital, clinic, or mobile group—and this gives the plaintiff a second and perhaps larger target (the doctrine of "deep pockets"). Typically the doctor is an independent contractor with separate insurance from the hospital.

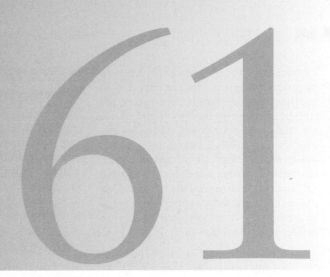

A preliminary report is not considered legally hazardous as long as the sonographer does not attempt to make a diagnosis. If a sonographer is working for a sonologist, the sonographer is not responsible for errors in the study, providing that the study is performed according to standards set by the sonologist, even if the study is of poor quality. The sonographer is not liable if he/she uses a technique that creates an image that looks like pathology but is not. Some examples of misleading findings or wrong technique that are not the sonographer's legal responsibility if uncorrected by the sonologist are the following:

1. Pseudohydronephrosis as the result of a full urinary bladder.
2. Sludge-filled gallbladder due to an overgained image.
3. Not following up on a pathologic finding, such as missing hydronephrosis with a pelvic mass.
4. Missing a pancreatic mass by not trying different scanning techniques such as erect scanning or having the patient drink to fill the stomach to create an acoustic window.
5. Missing stones in the gallbladder or kidneys due to a failure to use a high-frequency transducer.

Although the sonographer is not held legally responsible for these errors, there is the moral and ethical element to consider.

RESPONSIBILITIES OF THE PHYSICIAN OR SONOGRAPHER PERFORMING THE EXAMINATION

The primary responsibility is to perform a comprehensive examination that conforms to the national standards. One should care for the patient and make sure that the patient comes to no harm by rough treatment or carelessness. Confidentiality must be observed.

Some examples of situations in which a sonographer is liable are:

1. Physically molesting the patient. (It may be wise for a sonographer or physician to seek a chaperone when performing an examination with a vaginal or rectal probe on a patient of the opposite sex.)
2. Letting a patient fall, causing injury.
3. Giving the patient or accompanying doctor a wrong diagnosis (e.g., "no abruption" when abruption is present and subsequently correctly reported by the sonologist).
4. Revealing confidential information about the contents of the sonogram or disclosing any information that has adverse effects on the patient.

LEGALLY HAZARDOUS SITUATIONS

Emergency Studies

Emergency ultrasound studies often modify clinical management from conservative to aggressive and, because any management changes hinge on the sonographic findings, the examination may be legally hazardous. Litigation is common when a wrong diagnosis leads to immediate consequences. Some examples of emergency situations often followed by litigation are as follows:

1. Failure to recognize ectopic pregnancy (fortunately the use of the vaginal probe has markedly reduced litigation in this area).
2. Failure to diagnose testicular torsion. There is an approximate 4–8 hour window of opportunity to repair a torsed testicle, so delay is disastrous. Doppler signs of arterial occlusion may be intermittent with partial torsion making the diagnosis difficult.
3. Misdiagnosis of fetal death. Wrongly diagnosing fetal death with the subsequent delivery of a live but damaged infant can occur but is very rare with today's equipment.
4. Failure to diagnose abruptio placenta. This clinical situation is unusual because most severe abruptio placenta are clinically recognized and never undergo an ultrasound examination. The findings with abruptio placenta may be subtle and only recognized by comparison with previous studies and have resulted in litigation on a number of occasions.

Failure to Diagnose a Fetal Anomaly

Fetal abnormalities are a common cause of litigation because the monetary award for a missed anomaly is so large. (Awards are calculated by computing the cost of health care and loss of earnings until the expected age of death for someone of the same gender. This amount from birth to age 70 to 80 years is often many millions of dollars for a chronically disabled infant such as one with spina bifida.) Litigation related to obstetrical ultrasound is many times more frequent than for all other types of ultrasound combined.

Common missed fetal abnormalities resulting in litigation are as follows:

1. Missed spina bifida. Spina bifida may be subtle and difficult to see in the spine. The "lemon" and "banana" signs in the skull are almost always present. The "cerebellar" view, now required by the AIUM obstetric guidelines, which shows the "banana" sign, may be difficult to obtain. The cerebellum may not be seen because it has been pulled by the tethered cord into the upper cervical spine.
2. Hypoplastic left heart syndrome. This cardiac abnormality is very hard to correct surgically and requires lifelong medical treatment or is lethal. This defect is visible on a four-chamber view of the heart (required by the guidelines). (Recent information has shown that this anomaly may not be present at 18 weeks and may develop over the course of pregnancy.)
3. Absent limb or limbs. Until recently, the AIUM guidelines did not require all the limbs to be examined; however, suits related to absent limbs were common because it seems obvious to a layperson that it should be easy to detect the absence of a limb. The latest version of the AIUM guidelines does require visualization of all four limbs.
4. Down syndrome signs. Suits related to failure to diagnose Down syndrome are common. Failure to mention that two (or more) subtle signs of Down syndrome are present, such as a mild renal pelvic dilation, an echogenic focus in the heart, or an echogenic bowel may result in litigation.
5. Hydrocephalus. The upper limit of normal cranial lateral ventricular size is 10 mm on an axial view. Failure to comment on a slight enlargement of the lateral ventricle or a disorganized lateral ventricular appearance, as in holoprosencephaly, commonly results in litigation.

Failure to Diagnose Major Obstetric Findings

Some obstetric ultrasound findings that have been overlooked and that have serious consequences to pregnancy management are as follows:

1. Twins or triplets. Failure to diagnose twins or triplets can lead to severe long-term disability if the presence of twins is first discovered at delivery.
2. Unrecognized placenta previa during a sonographic examination may lead to a major bleed at delivery.

3. Breast cancer that is misdiagnosed as merely a breast cyst. Failure to diagnose breast cancer is the most common cause of imaging litigation. Most suits relate to mammography, but breast cancer ultrasound cases are occurring increasingly.

SUBSTANDARD REPORTING OF THE ULTRASOUND STUDY

Careless language in a report has often resulted in litigation. Typical examples are as follows:

1. Dating an obstetric study in the third trimester. The range of possible dates for a series of obstetric measurements such as the biparietal diameter, head circumference, femur length, and abdominal circumference in the third trimester is ±3 to 4 weeks, so accurate dating if the patient presents in the third trimester is not possible. This error is so well known that the obstetrician and radiologist share responsibility if delivery is performed before fetal viability under these circumstances. Although this error was much more frequent in the past, it still occurs.
2. Dating or weight estimation with unsatisfactory measurement data. It is not always possible to obtain a quality abdominal circumference or fetal head measurements with an unusual fetal position. Problems of this type should be noted in the report. Not reporting these problems may result in wrong clinical decisions about delivery or the presence of intrauterine growth restriction (IUGR).
3. Failure to compare the dates or weight on the current examination with earlier sonographic studies may mean a failure to diagnose IUGR.

TARDY REPORTING

Delayed reporting of an ultrasound study or delayed transmission of an ultrasound report to the referring doctor can lead to litigation. Findings that change management, such as the discovery of an ectopic pregnancy or a low biophysical profile score of 0 to 2, require a telephone call. Some examples of serious consequences of a delayed report are as follows:

1. Failure to telephone a report of a placenta previa resulted in the loss of the pregnancy in a patient with heavy vaginal bleeding.
2. Two-week delay in transmitting a report of IUGR resulted in the loss of the pregnancy.

FAILURE TO PERFORM AN APPROPRIATE ULTRASOUND STUDY WHEN A PATIENT PRESENTS WITH A FAMILY HISTORY OF A MALFORMATION OR A DRUG HISTORY PREDISPOSING TO A MALFORMATION

A common indication for an ultrasound study is a family history of a fetal malformation or when the patient is taking a drug, such as Valproic acid, that causes a fetal malformation. Specific views of potential malformation sites such as the lumbar spine with Valproic acid, or the face with a family history of cleft lip and palate, need to be obtained and reported.

AMNIOCENTESIS PROBLEMS

Amniocentesis for chromosomal abnormality or to establish fetal lung maturity is commonly performed and is standardly performed under ultrasound guidance. Suits related to fetal damage or fetal death due to the procedure are common. Documentation of the amniocentesis site, of fetal viability after the procedure, and a written report of the way in which the procedure was performed are helpful in avoiding litigation and defending complaints. By convention, only two passes are made if aspiration of amniotic fluid is unsuccessful.

Malpractice Insurance: Who Needs It?

Any sonographer performing freelance work (i.e., moonlighting or on a mobile service) should invest in malpractice insurance. Sonographers employed by a hospital or other institution do not generally need to purchase insurance because they are covered by the hospital's or clinic's policy.

SELECTED READING

American Institute of Ultrasound in Medicine Standards and Guidelines. Available at: http://www.aium.org/provider/standards/standards.asp.

Sanders R. Changing patterns of ultrasound-related litigation: a historical survey. *J Ultrasound Med* 2003;22:1009–1015.

62 Accreditation Chapter

CAROL MITCHELL

ABBREVIATIONS

ACR	American College of Radiology
AIUM	American Institute of Ultrasound in Medicine
ARDMS	American Registry of Diagnostic Medical Sonography
ARRT	American Registry of Radiologic Technologists
CCI	Cardiovascular Credentialing International
ICAVL	Intersocietal Commission on Accreditation of Vascular Laboratories
ICAEL	Intersocietal Commission on Accreditation of Echocardiography Laboratories

KEY WORDS

Accreditation. Process that determines that an institution has met a certain standard.

Certification. Award given when an individual or institution has met a certain standard.

Credential. Written evidence of a qualification. May be given to an individual (occupational credentialing) or an institution.

Professionalism. Individuals show "professionalism" when they adhere to professional methods, standards, and character.

The Problem

Evidence from multi-institutional studies such as the RADIUS study and from litigation shows that the quality of diagnostic ultrasound varies greatly. Ultrasound laboratory accreditation offers a means to ensure that a minimum standard of ultrasound is in place at any given institution that performs diagnostic medical sonography. Accreditation is currently voluntary. Currently, accreditation is confined to ultrasound laboratory accreditation. Certification of sonographers by the American Registry of Diagnostic Medical Sonography (ARDMS) and American Registry of Radiologic Technologists (for general, obstetric and gynecologic, and vascular ultrasound) is currently available and is a requirement for employment by many institutions. Certification for cardiac sonographers is available through the ARDMS and Cardiovascular Credentialing International (CCI). No certification for physicians has yet been put in force in the United States, although a certifying examination distributed by the Jefferson Ultrasound Research and Education Trust is widely taken by physicians in other countries.

One of the most recent examples of implementation of standards and improvements in patient outcome can be seen in the discipline of mammography. On October 27, 1992, Congress passed the Mammography Quality Standards Act (MQSA). In North Carolina, the quality of mammography improved the very first year that the MQSA was enforced. In 1987, when the American College of Radiology Mammography Accreditation Program was voluntary, only 31.9% of facilities applying for accreditation passed the first inspection. After federal legislation, phantom scores improved and 78.2% of facilities passed inspection. Pisano and colleagues argue that this improved pass rate is linked to improved quality-control practices and adherence to set standards, and that improved quality will ultimately result in earlier detection and improved breast cancer outcomes for women living in North Carolina. With the precedent of MQSA, there is no reason to think that accreditation for diagnostic medical sonography laboratories will not impact patient care and practice in a similar fashion.

Organizations That Offer Diagnostic Medical Sonography Laboratory Accreditation

ORGANIZATION: AMERICAN COLLEGE OF RADIOLOGY

Contact Information

http://www.acr.org/accreditation/index.html

1891 Preston White Drive, Reston, VA 20191-4379

Disciplines Accredited through the American College of Radiology

- Breast Ultrasound
- Obstetrical Ultrasound
- Gynecological Ultrasound
- General Ultrasound
- Vascular Ultrasound
- Combination of any of the above

ORGANIZATION: AMERICAN INSTITUTE OF ULTRASOUND IN MEDICINE

Contact Information

http://www.aium.org/accreditation/whatis.asp

Disciplines Accredited through American Institute of Ultrasound in Medicine

- Abdominal/General Ultrasound
- Breast Ultrasound (Diagnostic and Interventional)
- Gynecologic Ultrasound
- Obstetrics (Complete) and Trimester Specific

ORGANIZATION: INTERSOCIETAL COMMISSION ON ACCREDITATION OF VASCULAR LABORATORIES

Contact Information

http://www.intersocietal.org/icavl/apply/standards.htm

410-872-0100

8840 Stanford Boulevard, Suite 4900, Columbia, MD 21045

Disciplines Accredited

- Vascular Ultrasound
  - Extracranial Cerebrovascular
  - Intracranial Cerebrovascular
  - Peripheral arterial
  - Peripheral venous
  - Visceral vascular
  - Screening

ORGANIZATION: INTERSOCIETAL COMMISSION ON ACCREDITATION OF ECHOCARDIOGRAPHY LABORATORIES

Contact Information

http://www.intersocietal.org/icael/apply/standards.htm

410-872-0100

8840 Stanford Boulevard, Suite 4900, Columbia, MD 21045

Disciplines Accredited

- Echocardiogram
  - Adult Transthoracic
  - Adult Transesophageal
  - Adult Stress
  - Pediatric Transthoracic
  - Pediatric Transesophageal
  - Fetal

Steps for Accreditation

1. Contact organization.
2. Submit fee to purchase application and self-study materials. Most organizations offer an electronic application.
3. Receive application and self-study information.
4. Assign a physician and sonographer to work as a team and organize the application process.
5. Inform administration about the extra time needed to complete this process.
6. Schedule administrative time for the physician and sonographer to complete the accreditation application.
7. Schedule regular meetings with deadlines for the laboratory to complete the various portions of the application.
8. Mail the completed application and application fee to the accreditation organization.
9. Wait for feedback and accreditation.
10. All of the above organizations list detailed information on how and who to contact to begin the accreditation process. The organizations are happy to consult and help laboratories to become accredited. Accreditation should not be viewed as a pass/fail experience but rather as an opportunity to evaluate one's practice policies and quality assurance (QA) methods.

Sonographer/Physician and Laboratory Facility Requirements for Accreditation

ORGANIZATION: AMERICAN COLLEGE OF RADIOLOGY

Sonographer Requirements

1. At initial accreditation, sonographers must have either American Registry of Diagnostic Medical Sonographers (ARDMS) or American Registry of Radiologic Technologists (ARRT) sonography certification.
2. If a sonographer is not certified at the time of initial application, he or she must be certified within 1 year of the initial accreditation.
3. By the time of accreditation renewal, sonographers must be certified.
4. If vascular accreditation is being sought, at least one sonographer must be certified with the ARDMS Registered Vascular Technologist (RVT) credential, ARRT vascular sonography (VS) credential or CCI Registered Vascular Specialist (RVS) credential.

Physician Requirements

1. Completion of an approved residency program in which physicians are involved in 500 ultrasound examinations and passing the written and oral boards.
2. Fellowship in which physicians were involved in 500 ultrasound examinations.
3. If physicians took their training before 1982, they must have 10 years of experience in interpreting ultrasound examinations.
4. Two years of ultrasound experience with at least 500 examinations and copies of the records of these examinations are required for physicians without a formal fellowship or post graduate training.

Laboratory Facilities

1. Written protocols that follow the American College of Radiology standards for each examination at a minimum.

2. Appropriate examination rooms interpreting areas and storage.
3. Active QA program with reviews.
   - Equipment maintenance on a regular basis

ORGANIZATION: AMERICAN INSTITUTE OF ULTRASOUND IN MEDICINE

Sonographer Requirements

1. Must be certified by the ARDMS or become certified before the next accreditation cycle.
2. Sonographers not ARDMS certified at the time of initial application must submit 30 continuing medical education credits. If the lab is applying for breast accreditation, 10 of the 30 continuing medical education credits must pertain to breast sonography.

Physician Requirements

1. Thirty American Medical Association Physician's Recognition Award category 1 CME credits over 3 years.
2. Meet established guidelines for physicians who evaluate and interpret diagnostic ultrasound examinations and a predetermined number of examinations in each specialty seeking accreditation for or participate in a double-read QA program.

Laboratory Facilities

1. Written policy and procedures that address patient safety, patient confidentiality, management of patient complications, infection control, and protocols for all exams following the AIUM standards at a minimum.
2. Appropriate examination rooms, interpreting areas, and storage.
3. QA program with reviews.
   - Equipment maintenance
   - Correlation of report interpretation and final outcome
   - Correlation of ultrasound findings with surgery, laboratory, radiological and pathology findings
   - Plan for monitoring clinical practice and personnel

ORGANIZATION: INTERSOCIETAL COMMISSION ON ACCREDITATION OF VASCULAR LABORATORIES

Sonographer Requirements

Technical Director

1. Technical Director must be an appropriately credentialed sonographer in vascular testing and must complete a minimum number of exams for each specialty the lab is applying for accreditation in.
2. Fifteen hours of continuing medical education relevant to vascular testing every 3 years.
3. Three years of vascular testing experience with completion of at least 1,800 noninvasive vascular tests with appropriate distribution in testing areas being performed by the vascular laboratory.
4. Fifteen hours of CME relevant to vascular testing per year.

Technical staff must meet one of the following:

1. The technical staff must have appropriate training, technical certification or documented experience. Examples of these criteria would be a credential in vascular testing, formal ultrasound training or postsecondary education plus 12 months of full-time ultrasound experience. Educational training criteria are completion of a formal 2-year allied health program, bachelor's degree, MD, or DO degree. Documented experience is defined as 12 months of vascular testing with performance of 600 vascular testing exams under the supervision of qualified medical or technical staff.
2. The technical staff must obtain 15 hours of continuing medical education related to vascular testing every 3 years.

Physician Requirements

Medical Director

1. Legally qualified physician
2. Demonstration of appropriate training and experience by one of the following criteria:
   i. Formal training that meets established guidelines for evaluation and interpretation of a predetermined number of exams in each specialty area that the lab is applying for accreditation in.
   ii. Informal (or self-study) training program that provides training and experience for proper qualifications to interpret non-invasive vascular laboratory studies. This can be achieved through formal accredited postgraduate education (ICAVL Essentials and Standards, Part I: Vascular Laboratory Operations—Organization, p. 2).
      a. Forty hours of continuing medical education category I acquired in a 3-year time period. Eight hours must be applicable to each of the testing areas.
      b. Eight hours of supervised practical experience observing or participating in testing procedures (preferred to be completed in an accredited lab) and documented number of examination interpreted.
3. Established practice, 3 years of work in a vascular laboratory, and has interpreted a predetermined number of examinations.
4. Fifteen hours of continuing medical education every 3 hours.

Medical Staff Requirements:

1. Legally qualified physician.
2. Documentation of an appropriate level of training by one of the following:
   i. Formal training program that provides experience in interpreting a predetermined number of studies under supervision. (ICAVL Essentials and Standards, Part I: Vascular Laboratory Operations—Organization, p. 8.)
   ii. Informal (or self-study) training performed by accredited postgraduate education.
   iii. Established practice for at least 3 years with a minimum number of interpreted vascular examinations.
3. CME requirements.

Laboratory Facilities

1. Must demonstrate reasonable examination areas, interpretation space, and storage space.
2. Written policies for all procedures and quality assurance programs performed in the laboratory.
3. Standards for reporting and archiving examinations.
4. Adherence to patient confidentiality policies.
5. Quality Assurance.
   - Documentation of exam volume for each specialty area applying for accreditation
   - Documentation of equipment maintenance

- Correlation and confirmation of results
- Documentation of Case Reviews

ORGANIZATION: INTERSOCIETAL COMMISSION ON ACCREDITATION OF ECHOCARDIOGRAPHY LABORATORIES

Sonographer Requirements

Technical Director

1. Qualified sonographer. A qualified sonographer must meet one of the following criteria:
   i. Credentialed in echocardiography.
   ii. Graduate of a Committee of accreditation of allied health programs (CAAHEP) or Canadian Medical Association (CMA) ultrasound or cardiovascular technology program.
   iii. Graduate of a two-year allied health program, bachelor's degree, MD or DO degree, with 12 months of full-time echocardiography experience.
   iv. 3 years of echocardiography experience with a predetermined minimum number of exams completed.
2. Technical Directors must also maintain 30 hours of continuing medical education credits in a 3-year time period.

Technical staff must be recognized as a qualified sonographer by one of the following criteria:

1. Qualified sonographer. A qualified sonographer must meet one of the following criteria:
   i. Credentialed in echocardiography.
   ii. Graduate of a Committee of accreditation of allied health programs (CAAHEP) or Canadian Medical Association (CMA) ultrasound or cardiovascular technology program.
   iii. Graduate of a two-year allied health program, bachelor's degree, MD or DO degree, with 12 months of full-time echocardiography experience.
   iv. One year of echocardiography experience with a predetermined minimum number of exams completed.
2. Technical staff must also obtain 15 hours of continuing medical education credits within a 3-year time period.

Physician Requirements

Medical Director

1. Medical Director must be a legally qualified physician and meet one of the following criteria:
   i. Completion of 12-month formal echocardiography training program.
   ii. Completion of a 6-month formal echocardiography training program and 1 year of experience interpreting a predetermined minimum number of exams.
   iii. Three years of echocardiography experience with interpretation of a predetermined minimum number of exams.
2. Medical Directors must also maintain 30 hours of AMA Category I continuing medical education credits in echocardiography within a 3-year time period.

Medical staff requirements are as follows:

1. Medical staff must be legally qualified physicians and meet one of the following criteria:
   i. Completion of a 6-month formal echocardiography training program and experience interpreting a predetermined minimum number of exams.
   ii. Three years of echocardiography experience with interpretation of a predetermined minimum number of exams.
2. Medical Directors must also maintain 15 hours of AMA Category I continuing medical education credits in echocardiography within a 3-year time period.

Laboratory Facilities

1. Standards for examination interpretation and archiving.
2. Written protocols for all procedures and Quality Assurance programs performed in the laboratory.
3. Laboratory space.
4. Adherence to patient confidentiality policies.
5. Quality Assurance.
   - Documentation of exam volume for each specialty area applying for accreditation
   - Documentation of equipment maintenance
   - Correlation and confirmation of results
   - Documentation of Case Reviews
   - QA conferences with physicians and sonographers

SELECTED READING

American College of Radiology. ACR Ultrasound Accreditation Program Overview. Available at: http://www.acr.org/accreditation/index.html. Accessed March 14, 2006.

American Institute of Ultrasound in Medicine. Practice Accreditation. Available at: http://www.aium.org/accreditation/whatis.asp. Accessed March 14, 2006.

Federal Register, Part VII, Department of Health and Human Services, Food and Drug Administration, 21 CFR Part 900, Mammography Facilities—Requirements, for accrediting Bodies and Quality Standards and Certification requirements; Interim Rules. Pp. 5–18.

Freidson E. *Professional Posers: A Study of the Institutionalization of Formal Knowledge.* Chicago, IL: University of Chicago Press; 1986.

Intersocietal Commission for the Accreditation of Echocardiography Laboratories. Laboratory Accreditation A commitment to quality patient care and diagnostic evaluations. Available at: http://www.intersocietal.org/icael/apply/standards.htm. Accessed March 14, 2006.

Intersocietal Commission for the Accreditation of Vascular Laboratories. ICAVL office directory. Available at: http://www.intersocietal.org/icavl/apply/standards.htm. Accessed March 14, 2006.

Pisano ED, Schell M, Rollins J, et al. Has the Mammography Quality Standards Act affected the mammography quality in North Carolina? *AJR Am J Roentgenol* 2000;174:1089–1091.

Poppiti R. Sociopolitical symposium: accreditation gaining insight. *JDMS* 1997;13:195–197.

Troiano L. Ultrasound lab accreditation. *RT Image* 2001;14(3):3740.

INDEX

Page numbers followed by f indicate a figure
Page numbers followed by t indicate a table

A

C

M

Q

R